PLASTIC and RECONSTRUCTIVE SURGERY of the BREAST

PLASTIC and RECONSTRUCTIVE SURGERY of the BREAST

Edited by

R. BARRETT NOONE, M.D.

Clinical Professor of Surgery
University of Pennsylvania School of Medicine
Philadelphia, Pennsylvania

Chief, Service of Plastic Surgery
Bryn Mawr Hospital, Bryn Mawr, Pennsylvania

Chief, Division of Plastic and Reconstructive Surgery
Lankenau Hospital
Philadelphia, Pennsylvania

Illustrated by

DAVID W. LOW, M.D.

Assistant Professor of Surgery
University of Pennsylvania School of Medicine
Philadelphia, Pennsylvania

B. C. Decker
An Imprint of Mosby–Year Book, Inc.

Publisher

B. C. Decker
320 Walnut Street
Suite 400
Philadelphia, Pennsylvania 19106

Sales and Distribution

United States and Puerto Rico
Mosby-Year Book Inc.
11830 Westline Industrial Drive
Saint Louis, Missouri 63146

Canada
Mosby-Year Book Limited
5240 Finch Ave. E., Unit 1
Scarborough, Ontario M1S 5A2

Australia
McGraw-Hill Book Company Australia Pty. Ltd.
4 Barcoo Street
Roseville East 2069
New South Wales, Australia

Brazil
Editora McGraw-Hill do Brasil, Ltda.
rua Tabapua, 1.105. Itaim-Bibi
Sao Paulo, S.P. Brasil

Colombia
Interamericana/McGraw-Hill de Colombia, S.A.
Carrera 17, No. 33-71
Apartado Postal, A.A., 6131
Bogota, D.E. Colombia

Europe, United Kingdom, Middle East, and Africa
Wolfe Publishing Limited
Brook House
2-16 Torrington Place
London WC1E 7LT England

Hong Kong and China
McGraw-Hill Book Company
Suite 618, Ocean Centre
5 Canton Road
Tsimshatsui, Kowloon
Hong Kong

India
Tata McGraw-Hill Publishing Company, Ltd.
12/4 Asaf Ali Road, 3rd Floor
New Delhi 110002, India

Indonesia
P.O. Box 122/JAT
Jakarta, 1300 Indonesia

Japan
Igaku-Shoin Ltd.
Tokyo International P.O. Box 5063
1-28-36 Hongo, Bunkyo-ku,
Tokyo 113, Japan

Korea
Mr. Don-Gap Choi
C.P.O. Box 10583
Seoul, Korea

Malaysia
Mr. Lim Tao Slong
No. 8 Jalan SS 7/6B
Kelana Jaya
47301 Petaling Jaya
Selangor, Malaysia

Mexico
Interamericana/McGraw-Hill de Mexico, S.A. de C.V.
Cedro 512, Colonia Atlampa
(Apartado Postal 26370)
06450 Mexico, D.F., Mexico

New Zealand
McGraw-Hill Book Co. New Zealand Ltd.
5 Joval Place, Wiri
Manukau City, New Zealand

Portugal
Editora McGraw-Hill de Portugal, Ltda.
Rua Rosa Damasceno 11A-B
1900 Lisboa, Portugal

Singapore and Southeast Asia
McGraw-Hill Book Co.
21 Neythal Road
Jurong, Singapore 2262

South Africa
Libriger Book Distributors
Warehouse Number 8
"Die Ou Looiery"
Tannery Road
Hamilton, Bloemfontein 9300

Spain
McGraw-Hill/Interamericana de Espana, S.A.
Manuel Ferrero, 13
28020 Madrid, Spain

Taiwan
Mr. George Lim
P.O. Box 87-601
Taipei, Taiwan

Thailand
632/5 Phaholyothin Road
Sapan Kwai
Bangkok 10400
Thailand

Venezuela
McGraw-Hill/Interamericana, C.A.
2da. calle Bello Monte
(entre avenida Casanova y Sabana Grande)
Apartado Aereo 50785
Caracas 1050, Venezuela

Notice

The authors and publisher have made every effort to ensure that the patient care recommended herein, including choice of drugs and drug dosages, is in accord with the accepted standards and practice at the time of publication. However, since research and regulation constantly change clinical standards, the reader is urged to check the product information sheet included in the package of each drug, which includes recommended doses, warnings, and contraindications. This is particularly important with new or infrequently used drugs.

Plastic and Reconstructive Surgery of the Breast

ISBN 1-55664-192-3
D-03623

Library of Congress catalog card number: 90-81826

10 9 8 7 6 5 4 3 2 1

Dedication

To my wife, Barbara, and to my children—Bob, Megan, Genevieve, Becky, and Teri. More than family, you are my best friends and greatest sources of support and inspiration. You generously sacrificed the time I needed to prepare this book. Its completion would not have been possible without your unselfish encouragement.

Contributors

CHRISTINA Y. AHN, M.D.
Assistant Professor, Division of Plastic Surgery, University of California, Los Angeles, University of California School of Medicine, Los Angeles, California

GREGORY A. ANTOINE, M.D.
Chief Resident, Division of Plastic Surgery, Georgetown University School of Medicine, Washington, D.C.

LOUIS C. ARGENTA, M.D.
Professor of Surgery and Chairman, Department of Plastic and Reconstructive Surgery, Bowman Gray Medical School of Wake Forest University, Winston-Salem, North Carolina

PHILLIP G. ARNOLD, M.D.
Professor of Plastic Surgery, Mayo Graduate School of Medicine; Chief, Department of Plastic and Reconstructive Surgery, Mayo Clinic, Rochester, Minnesota

FRITZ E. BARTON, JR., M.D.
Professor and Chairman, Division of Plastic Surgery, University of Texas Southwestern Medical Center at Dallas, Southwestern Medical School, Dallas, Texas

JOHN BOSTWICK III, M.D.
Professor of Plastic and Reconstructive Surgery, Emory University School of Medicine; Chief of Plastic Surgery, Emory University Hospital, Atlanta, Georgia

GARRY S. BRODY, M.D.
Clinical Professor of Plastic Surgery, University of Southern California School of Medicine, Los Angeles; Chief of Plastic Surgery Research, Rancho Los Amigos Hospital, and Chief of Surgery, Downey Community Hospital, Downey, California

A. JAY BURNS, M.D.
Assistant Professor, Division of Plastic Surgery, University of Texas Southwestern Medical Center at Dallas, Southwestern School of Medicine, Dallas, Texas

I. KELMAN COHEN, M.D.
Professor and Chairman, Department of Surgery, Division of Plastic and Reconstructive Surgery, Medical College of Virginia, Richmond, Virginia

STEVEN R. COHEN, M.D.
Assistant Professor of Surgery, Division of Plastic and Reconstructive Surgery, University of Michigan Medical School; Chief, Pediatric Plastic Surgery, C.S. Mott Children's Hospital, and Director, Craniofacial Anomalies Program, University of Michigan Medical Center, Ann Arbor, Michigan

EUGENE H. COURTISS, M.D.
Assistant Clinical Professor of Surgery, Harvard Medical School; Consultant, Massachusetts General Hospital, Boston; Chief, Plastic Surgery, Newton-Wellesley Hospital, Newton Lower Falls, Massachusetts

ROBERT W. CRICHLOW, M.D.
William and Bessie Allyn Professor of Surgery, Dartmouth Medical School; Chairman, Department of Surgery, Dartmouth-Hitchcock Medical Center, Hanover, New Hampshire

FRANCIS X. DELONE, JR., M.D.
Clinical Associate Professor in Plastic Surgery, University of Pennsylvania School of Medicine, Philadelphia, Pennsylvania

VINCENT R. DIGREGORIO, M.D.
Clinical Associate Professor of Surgery, State University of New York Health Science Center at Stony Brook School of Medicine, Stony Brook; Chief, Section of Plastic and Reconstructive Surgery, Winthrop University Hospital, Mineola, New York

RICHARD V. DOWDEN, M.D.
Head, Section of Breast Surgery, Cleveland Clinic Foundation, Cleveland, Ohio

G. W. EKLUND, M.D.
Assistant Clinical Professor of Radiology, University of Illinois College of Medicine at Peoria; Medical Director, Susan Komen Breast Center, Peoria, Illinois

L. FRANKLYN ELLIOTT, M.D.
Clinical Instructor, Plastic Surgery, Emory University School of Medicine, Atlanta, Georgia

JACK FISHER, M.D.
Assistant Clinical Professor of Plastic Surgery, Vanderbilt University School of Medicine, Nashville, Tennessee

MARCIA A. FITZPATRICK, M.D.
Clinical Instructor in Surgery, Jefferson Medical College of Thomas Jefferson University, and Clinical Instructor in Surgery, University of Pennsylvania School of Medicine, Philadelphia, Pennsylvania

THOMAS G. FRAZIER, M.D.
Assistant Professor of Surgery, Jefferson Medical College of Thomas Jefferson University, Philadelphia; Senior Attending Surgeon, Bryn Mawr Hospital, Bryn Mawr, Pennsylvania

GARY D. FRIEDMAN, M.D.
Chief, Plastic Surgery, Mount Zion Hospital, San Francisco, California

SPENCER W. GALT, M.D.
Resident in Surgery, Dartmouth-Hitchcock Medical Center, Hanover, New Hampshire

DAVID N. GOLDBERG, D.O.
Assistant Professor of Obstetrics and Gynecology, University of Medicine and Dentistry of New Jersey School of Osteopathic Medicine; Attending Physician, Kennedy Memorial Hospitals University Medical Center, Stratford, New Jersey

ALVIN F. GOLDFARB, M.D.
Professor of Obstetrics and Gynecology, and Director of Education, Department of Obstetrics and Gynecology, Jefferson Medical College of Thomas Jefferson University, Philadelphia, Pennsylvania

GEORGE T. GRACE, M.D.
Clinical Associate Professor, Department of Surgery, Division of Plastic and Reconstructive Surgery, University of Maryland, Baltimore, Maryland

JAMES C. GROTTING, M.D.
Associate Professor of Surgery, Division of Plastic and Reconstructive Surgery, University of Alabama at Birmingham School of Medicine, Birmingham, Alabama

RONALD P. GRUBER, M.D.
Clinical Instructor, Stanford University School of Medicine, Stanford, California

CARL R. HARTRAMPF, JR., M.D.
Clinical Professor, Division of Plastic Surgery, Department of Surgery, Emory University School of Medicine; Atlanta Plastic Surgery, P.A., Atlanta, Georgia

T. RODERICK HESTER, JR., M.D.
Associate Professor of Plastic and Reconstructive Surgery; Staff Attending Physician and Chief of Plastic Surgery, Egleston Hospital for Children, Atlanta, Georgia

SAUL HOFFMAN, M.D.
Clinical Professor of Plastic Surgery, Mount Sinai School of Medicine of the City University of New York; Chief of Plastic Surgery, Doctors Hospital, and Attending Surgeon, Division of Plastic Surgery, Beth Israel Hospital and Mount Sinai Hospital, New York, New York

JOHN R. JARRETT, M.D.
Clinical Instructor in Plastic Surgery, University of Oregon Health Sciences Center, Portland; Attending Surgeon, Sacred Heart Memorial Center, Eugene, Oregon

ROBERT J. JOHNSON, M.D.
Emeritus Professor of Anatomy, University of Pennsylvania School of Medicine, Philadelphia, Pennsylvania

DON LAROSSA, M.D.
Associate Professor of Surgery, University of Pennsylvania School of Medicine, Philadelphia, Pennsylvania

JOHN WILLIAM LITTLE, M.D.
Professor and Director, Division of Plastic Surgery, Georgetown University School of Medicine, Washington, D.C.; Consultant, National Cancer Institute, National Institutes of Health, Bethesda, Maryland

DAVID W. LOW, M.D.
Assistant Professor of Surgery, University of Pennsylvania School of Medicine; Attending Physician, Hospital of the University of Pennsylvania and Children's Hospital of Philadelphia; Chief of Plastic Surgery, Veterans Administration Medical Center, Philadelphia, Pennsylvania

W. EARLE MATORY, JR., M.D.
Assistant Professor, Graduate Biomedical Sciences, University of Massachusetts Medical School; Co-Director, Breast Science, and Director, Hand and Microsurgery, University of Massachusetts Medical Center, Worcester, Massachusetts

G. PATRICK MAXWELL, M.D.
Assistant Clinical Professor of Plastic Surgery, Vanderbilt University School of Medicine; Director, Institute for Aesthetic and Reconstructive Surgery, Baptist Hospital, Nashville, Tennessee

R. MICHAEL McCLELLAN, M.D.
Clinical Associate Professor in Plastic Surgery, University of Pennsylvania School of Medicine; Chief, Division of Plastic Surgery, Crozer-Chester Medical Center, Chester, Pennsylvania

N. BRADLY MELAND, M.D.
Assistant Professor of Plastic Surgery, Mayo Graduate School of Medicine; Staff Surgeon, Department of Plastic and Reconstructive Surgery, Mayo Clinic, Rochester, Minnesota

J. BRIEN MURPHY, M.D.
Clinical Assistant Professor of Surgery, University of Pennsylvania School of Medicine, Philadelphia, Pennsylvania

R. BARRETT NOONE, M.D.
Clinical Professor of Surgery, University of Pennsylvania School of Medicine; Chief, Service of Plastic Surgery, Bryn Mawr Hospital, Bryn Mawr; Chief, Division of Plastic and Reconstructive Surgery, Lankenau Hospital, Philadelphia, Pennsylvania

JEAN-YVES PETIT, M.D.
Chief of Breast Surgery, Faculte Medecine, Kremlin-Bicetre, Villejuif, France

PAULE REGNAULT, M.D.
Former Clinical Professor, University of Montreal College of Medicine; Former Chief of Plastic Surgery, St. Luc Hospital, Montreal, Quebec, Canada

MARIO RIETJENS, M.D.
Chief Resident, Breast Surgery, Faculte Medecine, Kremlin-Bicetre, Villejuif, France

ROSS RUDOLPH, M.D.
Associate Clinical Professor of Surgery, University of California San Diego School of Medicine, San Diego; Head, Division of Plastic and Reconstructive Surgery, Scripps Clinic and Research Foundation, La Jolla, California

JAMES J. RYAN, M.D.
Associate Professor of Plastic Surgery, Johns Hopkins University School of Medicine; Chief of Plastic Surgery, Children's Hospital, Baltimore, Maryland

WENDY S. SCHAIN, Ed.D.
Psychosocial Director, Adult Oncology, Memorial Cancer Institute, Long Beach, California

WILLIAM W. SHAW, M.D.
Professor and Chief, Division of Plastic and Reconstructive Surgery, UCLA Medical Center, Los Angeles, California

ARTHUR G. SHIP, M.D., D.M.D.
Clinical Professor of Plastic and Reconstructive Surgery, Albert Einstein College of Medicine of Yeshiva University; Attending Plastic Surgeon, Montefiore Medical Center, New York, New York

SUMNER A. SLAVIN, M.D.
Assistant Clinical Professor of Surgery, Harvard Medical School; Associate in Plastic Surgery, Beth Israel Hospital, and Consultant in Surgical Oncology, Dana-Farber Cancer Institute, Boston, Massachusetts

SCOTT L. SPEAR, M.D.
Professor of Plastic Surgery, Georgetown University School of Medicine, Washington, D.C.; Deputy Director, Division of Plastic Surgery, Georgetown University Hospital, and Consultant, National Institutes of Health and National Naval Medical Center, Bethesda, Maryland

JAN OLOF STRÖMBECK, M.D.
Professor and Former Head, Department of Plastic Surgery, Sabbatsbergs Sjukhus, Stockholm, Sweden

DANIEL L. WEINER, M.D.
Attending Surgeon, New York Eye and Ear Infirmary, New York, New York

Preface

Advances in science over the past two decades have contributed to the explosion in techniques available to the reconstructive surgeon in general. When these techniques and scientific developments are directed toward improvements in breast surgery, an ideal opportunity exists for restoration and improvement of the quality of life of the patient. Less obvious, but also important, are the benefits experienced by the surgeon. The ability to use this wide range of basic principles and reconstructive techniques to achieve an artistic, gratifying result provides a great source of satisfaction for the present-day plastic and reconstructive surgeon. We achieve our results from the use of alloplastic implants and basic techniques such as skin grafting and from the more complex innovations of musculocutaneous flaps and microvascular surgery.

Because of these substantial developments, surgery of the breast has become a major part of the specialty of plastic and reconstructive surgery over the past two decades, and it occupies an appreciable part of the practice of almost every plastic surgeon. This growth is due in part to an increasing recognition by general surgeons and other colleagues in medicine that aesthetic and reconstructive surgery of the breast is a necessary component in the overall surgical rehabilitation of the patient.

A field such as plastic surgery of the breast can never be considered static. Perhaps for this reason a major, comprehensive reference textbook, with multiple contributors, has not been attempted previously. As the field has developed, there have been numerous scientific publications, smaller texts and monographs, and excellent text-atlases on the subject. Clearly the time had arrived for a complete, detailed, and comprehensive reference text, with contributions by recognized experts in all areas of breast aesthetic and reconstructive surgery. I sensed the appropriate timing when I was asked by the publisher to edit and coordinate such a project; most of the basic techniques that evolved during the 1970s and 1980s were settling into a refinement mode. They are the foundations on which the future is to be built.

The book's essential feature is the participation of 53 authors, all recognized experts in science or surgery related to the breast. The very nature of this book militates against a single authorship. No one person has the experience or the ability to be expert in all the areas covered in this text.

The chapters were grouped in sections progressing in sequence from basics to the more complex reconstructive challenges. The first section, Basic Science, forms the foundation on which the other four sections can be based. It covers basic scientific principles—including anatomy, embryology, physiology, and silicone chemistry—and contains detailed discussions of diagnostic imaging as it relates to reconstructive surgery.

The four remaining sections are organized to allow detailed and comprehensive presentations of the evaluation and treatment of mammary developmental deformities, hypoplasia, hypertrophy, and acquired absence of the breast. The male breast is also subject to developmental abnormality, and gynecomastia is the only male condition covered in the book.

Sections 3, 4, and 5 comprise the greater part of the book. In Section 3, topics dealing with the clinical applications of silicone implants are addressed, including techniques of placement, philosophies of augmentation mammaplasty, issues of regulation, and potential complications. The chapters in Section 4 present the major techniques in reduction mammaplasty.

The largest and final section is devoted to reconstruction of the breast after surgical removal, radiation damage, or trauma. An overview of the surgical treatment of breast cancer is included, in addition to a chapter on the psychological benefits of reconstruction. Because modern treatment of breast cancer also involves lesser excisional procedures combined with radiation therapy, I have included a discussion of innovative techniques of partial mastectomy directed toward better aesthetic results.

I have attempted to include the most complete and up-to-date concepts and techniques for all areas of plastic surgery of the breast. Repetition has been eliminated except when necessary in more than one context. For example, in the reduction mammaplasty section, references to historical development of vascularized pedicle techniques may appear in more than one chapter.

The contributors were encouraged to use illustrations and photographs liberally throughout their chapters. Dr. David Low's artistry contributes a unique feature to the book. A plastic surgeon and medical illustrator, Dr. Low was able to communicate the illustrative desires of each author to the sketch pad. His surgical background and experience with the techniques he was to demonstrate gave us the opportunity to produce a book we feel is unique among surgical textbooks. The publisher has shown great expertise in sizing and placing the 147 drawings by Dr. Low in an artistic and tasteful manner.

It is my belief that this text is sufficiently detailed to provide the well-trained modern plastic surgeon with the knowledge needed to perform any reconstructive surgical procedure on the breast. It is my sincere hope that the many patients who suffer the physical and psychological trauma of breast deformity will benefit from the care provided by the surgeons who read its pages.

R. Barrett Noone, M.D.

Acknowledgments

A comprehensive textbook is not possible to develop without the dedication and cooperation of the numerous contributing authors, all experts in their respective areas. Although heavily committed to clinical duties, research, or academic responsibilities, they have given freely of their time to meet deadlines leading to the completion of this book.

My personal growth in the subspecialty area of plastic surgery of the breast has been stimulated from many sources: my patients, who have greeted their surgical results with appreciation and satisfaction; the residents in the University of Pennsylvania plastic surgery program over the past 18 years, whose enthusiasm was a stimulus for the teacher; and my own mentors and teachers.

Special recognition goes to Dr. Henry P. Royster, founder and first professor of the plastic surgery residency program at the University of Pennsylvania, and his resident at the time, Dr. William P. Graham, III, who guided an inquiring intern toward a specialty that was exciting, dynamic, and one of the most fulfilling in medicine over the past two decades; my surgery chairman, Dr. Jonathan E. Rhoads, whose program in general surgery provided the surgical background needed by every plastic surgeon. My early teachers in plastic surgery also included Dr. Herndon B. Lehr, Dr. Peter Randall, Dr. Ralph Hamilton, and Dr. Robert A. Chase. I thank them all for sharing their experiences with me. Dr. Linton A. Whitaker, currently chief of plastic surgery at the University of Pennsylvania, encouraged me to tackle the task of this textbook and has been a constant source of encouragement through its completion.

Few books in surgery have been illustrated as completely and as clearly as this textbook. Dr. David W. Low, who follows a dual career as a plastic surgeon and medical illustrator, began this project with me when he was a resident and together we saw its completion as his young practice of plastic surgery developed. His knowledge of the specialty, combined with a superb artistic talent, presented a unique opportunity for us to produce a textbook which is uniformly illustrated.

My colleagues in plastic surgery, many of whom are contributing authors, have been generous in sharing their concepts and techniques with me and other plastic surgeons. Only through mutual cooperation and communication can an area as dynamic as plastic surgery of the breast continue to evolve.

I am also indebted to my general surgery colleague, Dr. Thomas G. Frazier, who, recognizing the emotional gratification breast reconstruction provided his patients, stimulated pioneering efforts of reconstruction at the time of mastectomy. My associate, Dr. J. Brien Murphy, deserves special recognition for extra help with clinical duties during the time I spent in preparation of this text.

I am grateful to the staff at B.C. Decker, a cooperative publishing house which has been most gracious and understanding in extending deadlines and providing support needed for publication of this book. Mary E. Mansor, medical editor, and Kimberly A. LoDico, project editor, could not have been more helpful or understanding. Special thanks is also extended to my research assistants, Megan J. Noone and Genevieve C. Noone, who turned part-time college jobs into a pleasure for their dad; and to my tireless, loyal, and good-humored secretaries, Lynne S. DeRita, Suzanne Duell, and Deborah W. Lander, who helped with the typing, coordination and mailing of the manuscripts.

This book is dedicated to my family for good reason. Although I was advised by many friends that editing a multi-contributor textbook was a thankless and difficult task, my wife and children encouraged me to spend the time necessary, and they were very understanding when my thoughts wandered from their worlds to the all-encompassing task at hand. Never once did they complain that my time and attention were diverted from them. They are a unique group of people, and I am fortunate to have their love and support.

R.B.N.

Contents

SECTION 1

BASIC SCIENCE

SECTION 2

DEVELOPMENTAL DEFORMITIES

SECTION 3

AUGMENTATION MAMMAPLASTY

SECTION **4**

REDUCTION MAMMAPLASTY

SECTION 5

BREAST RECONSTRUCTION

SECTION 1

BASIC SCIENCE

CHAPTER 1

Anatomy of the Breast and Related Areas

ROBERT J. JOHNSON, M.D.

MAMMARY GLAND PROPER

The glandular elements of the breast consist of some 15 to 20 *lactiferous ducts*, each of which is prolonged into a branching system of epithelial (epidermal) tubules. The precise histologic anatomy of these tubules of ectodermal origin varies with the age of the woman and during pregnancy and lactation. At puberty, the distal ends of the ducts show an increase in the number of branches, but the extremity of each ending is a small, solid mass of cells (*potential alveolus*) that during pregnancy will become an actual alveolus, each with a central lumen.

During pregnancy and lactation the ductal system further elongates and becomes more complicated in its branching at the distal ends. Thus, each of the 15 to 20 ducts with all of its branches forms a *lobe*, while the more terminal branches and their ending alveoli of secreting cells form *lobules*. The total ductal system of each lobe with its lobules and alveoli is surrounded by fibrous connective tissue that supports and ensheathes the glandular elements within the substance of the breast. Fat cells in clusters are interspersed between the fibrous sheaths of the epithelial lobes, lobules, and alveoli, thus obscuring the glandular tissues and making it difficult to trace the full extent of the glandular structures on gross dissection.

Each lactiferous duct as it approaches the nipple shows a slight, fusiform expansion of its lumen, the *lactiferous sinus*, which lies deep to the areola and extends up into the *mammary papilla* or *nipple* for a short distance. Beyond the sinus the duct narrows again and continues upward in the nipple to expand slightly once again as it approaches the surface, forming a slender, cone-shaped final segment or *ampulla*, whose larger end opens on the surface of the nipple. The ampulla is lined with stratified squamous epithelium, which tolerates the cannulation that may be necessary during mammography.

Microscopic cross sections of the nipple reveal that the lactiferous sinuses are lined with a collapsed and much folded epithelial wall surrounding the lumen. They probably serve as reservoirs for milk during lactation. Surrounding the lactiferous ducts, and within the nipple, is a network of smooth muscle fibers arranged both longitudinally and circumferentially to the axis of the nipple. These muscle fibers are caused to contract reflexly by tactile stimuli to the nipple or by chilling, leading to erection of the nipple.

The fibrous tissue stroma of the breast consists of both collagenous and elastic fibers, which are chiefly arranged in irregular sheets or septa between the lobes and lobules of the glandular parenchyma. Many of these sheetlike connective tissue partitions extend superficially toward the skin of the breast, becoming tapered into points and bands (*retinacular ligaments of Cooper*) that anchor to the corium of the skin. Carcinomatous disease of the mammary gland may lead to such fibrotic shortening of these ligaments of Cooper that pitting or dimpling of the skin occurs overlying the diseased area. These rather gross pits are to be contrasted with the fine pits that occur at each hair follicle as the skin of the breast becomes edematous where it overlies a cancerous growth, and the finely indented hair follicles cause a resemblance to the skin of an orange (peau d'orange) or to pigskin.

The lactiferous ducts radiate away from the nipple and areola in all directions and extend much farther outward than they are usually shown as doing in illustrations in the literature. Of the 15 to 20 ducts that radiate away from the nipple, several never grow to the length of the others and remain perpetually underdeveloped, both in length and in functional ability. Hicken[1] suggested that 95 percent of the function of the mammary gland is performed by only six to eight of the lobes or lactiferous duct systems, the other ducts and their ramifications remaining small and feebly developed. Using cadavers, Hicken showed, after injecting methiodal sodium (Skiodan) into the ducts of 385 breasts whose ductal ramifications were displayed by roentgenography, that many of the ducts extended well beyond the usually portrayed length. In 95 percent of the breasts the visualized ducts ascended around the lateral border of the pectoralis major and extended for varying distances up into the axillary fossa. This extension of breast tissue, when well developed, can be dissected grossly and is seen to perforate the *axillary fascia.* This fascia bridges the interval between the anterior and posterior axillary folds and thus forms the base of the pyramidal-shaped axillary fossa. This extension of the mammary gland proper is known as the *axillary tail of Spence* and sometimes is felt to be enlarged and tender during lactation. In some women it may show palpable tenderness in phase with the menstrual cycle.

In 15 percent of the breasts Hicken studied, the lactiferous ducts extended across the costal margin and into the epigastrium superficial to the rectus abdominis. In 2 percent of the breasts, the visualized ducts extended horizontally around the lateral wall of the chest to cross the anterior border of the latissimus dorsi. In two of the 385 breasts some element of the duct system actually crossed the midsternal or median line of the chest. This extensive ramification of the lactiferous ducts had not been appreciated because gross dissection in the cadaver does not allow one to trace the finer calibered distal ends of the ducts, and because most dissecting room cadavers are elderly, and glandular development in the breast is in a state of involution.

The use of dyes and radiopaque materials to delineate the ductal system of the living patient at surgery, combined with careful study of the removed specimen, has largely confirmed Hicken's data. Such studies have also revealed the close proximity to the skin of elements of the ductal system, thus explaining the great difficulty in performing a complete subcutaneous mastectomy.[2-4]

THE SUPERFICIAL FASCIA

The glandular tissue of the breast lies in the central stratum of the superficial fascia (the subcutaneous fat layer) overlying the anterolateral wall of the chest. Therefore, there is a superficial layer of the superficial fascia that overlies the glandular tissue, and also a deeper layer of the superficial fascia of the pectoral region that lies deep to the mammary gland proper. This deeper layer is often referred to as the *retromammary* or *submammary fascia.* It is more areolar and less fatty than the layer on the superficial side of the mammary gland proper. Because it allows easy cleavage for separating the mammary gland from the *deep* or *muscle fascia* that lies on the surface of the pectoralis major, it is common to refer to this retromammary fascia as the retromammary "space." This fascia or "space" also allows full mobility of the breast on the deep fascia that is so intimately and tightly bound to the pectoralis major. This deep or muscle fascia investing the pectoralis major muscle, like deep fascia everywhere, sends extensions of its tissue into the substance of the invested muscle to form the perimysium of the muscle fasciculi that compose the muscle in question. Thus, deep fascia, or muscle fascia, is secured to the surface of the muscle and must move in unison with the movements of the muscle. The mammary gland, although loosely adherent to the deep fascia or pectoralis major, is not forced to follow closely the movements of the underlying deep fascia. However, when carcinoma has led to firmer adherence of the glandular tissue to the deep fascia, the muscular action leads to associated displacements of the overlying mammary gland.

The breast shows varying amounts of fat in its substance because it is a branching epithelial duct system that developed by invading the subcutaneous connective tissue (the superficial fascia). The age and state of nutrition of the individual influence the amount of fat in the superficial fascia generally, as well as in the breast itself. The influence of racial, ethnic, and familial growth patterns are also seen in the size and contour of the breast. Certain generalities pertaining to the size and position of the breast may be stated. At the level of the fourth costal cartilage the transverse dimension of the visible breast is from the ipsilateral sternal margin to approximately the midaxillary line. In the midclavicular sagittal plane the vertical extent is approximately from the second to the sixth ribs. The existence of the axillary tail of Spence (Fig. 1-1) may extend the vertical dimension higher than this around the lateral border of the pectoralis major, and upward into the axillary fossa. However, the axillary tail normally is not identifiable on palpation unless swollen. Neither, of course, are the extreme extensions of the gland proper manifest as they pass horizontally across the serratus anterior, or inferiorly across the costal margin.

If the full extent of the mammary gland proper, as demonstrated by Hicken (Fig. 1-2),[1] is taken as the peripheral limit of the breast, it is evident that the breast is applied to some part of the deep fascia of several muscles. These muscles are the pectoralis major, the serratus anterior, the latissimus dorsi (occasionally), the external oblique (occasionally), the pectoralis minor (occasionally, and it is only the axillary tail that relates to this muscle), and the rectus abdominis. In fact, the relationship is to the upper part of the rectus sheath beneath which the muscle lies.

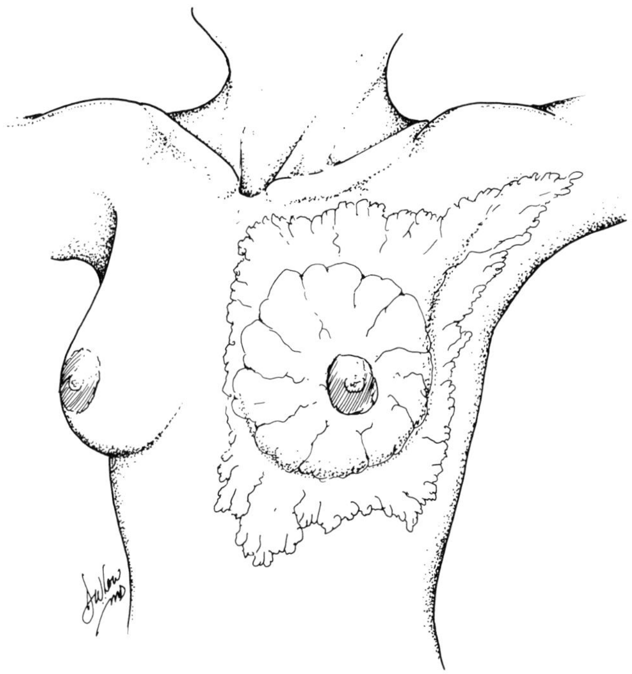

FIGURE 1–1 The left breast shown as stripped of skin. The rounded fatty mass, with areola and nipple centered, indicates the usually recognized locus and limits of the breast. The more extensive sheet of fatty areolar tissue indicates the extremes of outward extension of the glandular elements of the mammary gland, but with those extensions still immersed in fatty connective tissue. The radiating lines or connective tissue sheets that partially isolate the 15 to 20 glandular tracts in the breast are seen as Cooper's retinacular ligaments or septa. The axillary tail of Spence and the epigastric extensions of the lactiferous duct systems or lobes are particularly noticeable.

MUSCLES AND FASCIAE OF THE PECTORAL REGION

The *pectoralis major* arises from the chest wall along a curved line that begins above, along the medial half of the clavicle, and then turns downward along the manubrium and the body of the sternum. This descending line of origin is broad and includes the ipsilateral half of the anterior aspect of the adjacent costal cartilages from the first to the sixth.

The lower part of the pectoralis major has an aponeurotic origin that spreads downward and medialward across the costal margin to blend with the anterior lamina of the rectus sheath. This inferior part of the pectoralis major thus takes its origin chiefly from the abdominal wall and is called the abdominal (costal) part of the muscle. Its degree of development varies from person to person. This portion of the muscles makes up the lower part of the lateral border of the pectoralis major. The abdominal part gradually twists up behind the sternal part to take a higher level of insertion into the lateral tubercular crest of the humerus where all three parts of the pectoralis major take their insertion. This twisting of the sternal and abdominal parts of the muscle upon one another results in essentially a 180-degree turn of these two portions by the time their tendons have reached insertion into the humerus.

The clavicular part, or head, of the muscle forms an anterior lamina of inserting fibers, and is not twisted on itself as it takes its attachment to the lateral tubercular crest of the humerus. Thus the insertion is complicated and essentially trilaminar. This arrangement allows for equalization of the lengths of the fibers of the parts of the muscle as the limb goes from adduction through abduction. Near its origin, the clavicular part may be slightly separated from the sternal part so that a line of cleavage may be found and opened up. The clavicular head is regularly separated from the deltoid muscle along the clavicle by the deltopectoral trigone. Here the cephalic vein of the arm ascends in the crevice between the two muscles to turn deeply into the deltopectoral trigone, and end in the axillary vein. The cephalic vein serves as a guide to the line of cleavage between the clavicular head of the pectoralis major and the deltoid muscle. It has already been mentioned that the pectoralis major is totally invested by a deep fascial sheath (epimysium, or muscle fascia), except where it takes origin and insertion.

The degree of development of the abdominal part of the pectoralis major commonly varies from person to person. This is not correlated with general muscular development, but is intrinsic to this area and may be unilateral or asymmetric. More extensive degrees of agenesis of part of the pectoralis major occur occasionally. It is routinely the lower part of the muscle that is absent, i.e., the abdominal (costal) part and some or all of the sternal part. The clavicular head is usually present in such cases. This can be made very evident in living patients by having them press their hand strongly against their thigh. The missing part is clearly evident on contralateral comparison. This is seen in Poland's syndrome and is the consequence of an early embryonic deficit in the mesoderm (mesenchyme) allotted to the formation of this muscle, and even to other muscles and mesodermal derivatives in this area.

In extreme degrees of this anomalous condition, which go beyond what Poland described in 1845, the pectoralis minor is also absent, and even the ribs and intercostal musculature may be only feebly developed. The wall of the chest is thus thinned and weakened, and paradoxical respiratory movement may occur here. The overlying skin and the breast itself may partake of this inadequate development and there may be obvious underdevelopment of the nipple and areola. It will be recalled that the corium and the fat and connective tissue of the breast are all mesodermal in origin.

The pectoralis minor arises variably from the second, third, and fourth or from the third, fourth, and fifth ribs. The fibers of the muscle project upward and laterally to converge on a tendon that in-

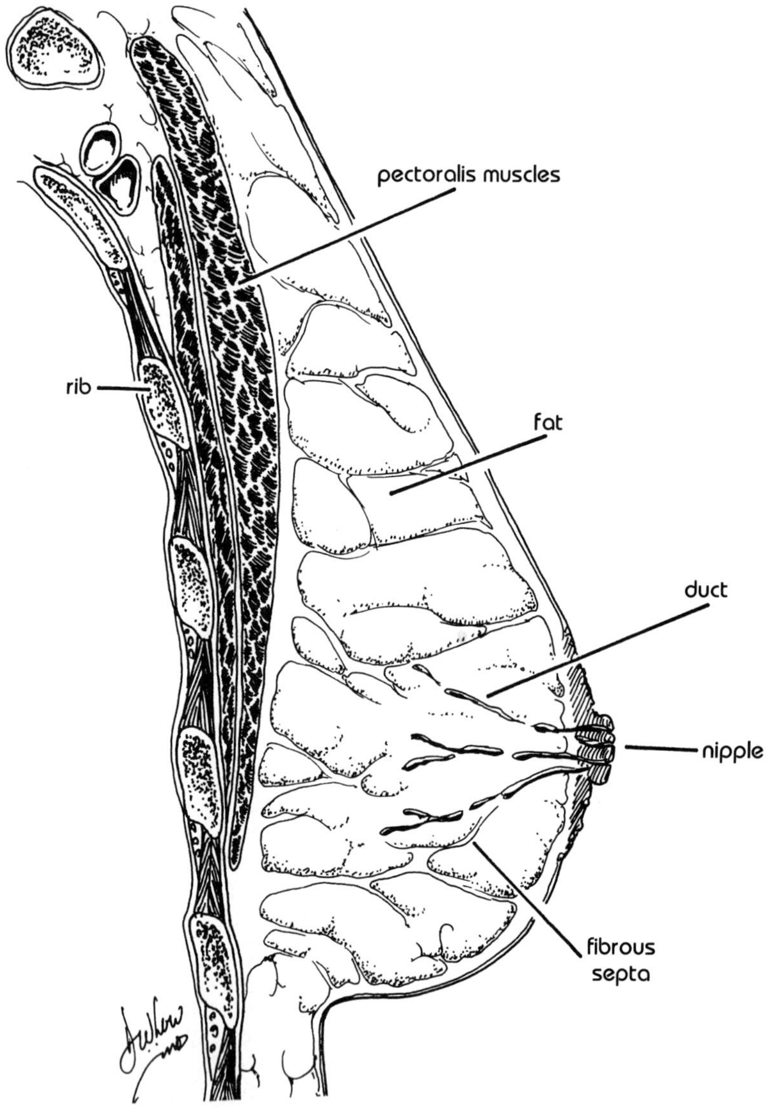

FIGURE 1–2 Sagittal section through the breast, pectoralis major and minor, axillary space and great vessels, and the chest wall. The partial isolation or separation of the lobes (lactiferous duct ramifications) by fibrous septa (Cooper's retinacular ligaments) is seen, as is the so-called submammary space.

serts into the coracoid process. The tip of the coracoid process may be readily felt by placing a forefinger in the infraclavicular fossa, which is the surface expression of the deltopectoral trigone, and then pressing posteriorly and laterally. The three or four slips of the pectoralis minor that spring from the ribs do so just posterior, or lateral, to the junction of the ribs with their costal cartilages. This flat, triangular muscle lies essentially in the coronal plane of the body. The muscle and its fascia is everywhere just deep to the pectoralis major.

The pectoralis minor is encased in deep fascia, which, ascending above the muscle, becomes a single sheet that extends up to the inferior surface of the subclavius muscle. Here this deep fascial sheet splits about the subclavius to reach and fuse with the periosteum of the clavicle. In a similar manner, the anterior and posterior layers of this fascia ensheathing the pectoralis minor fuse along the inferior or lateral border of that muscle, and then proceed as a single layer across the axilla to blend with the brachial fascia where the latter encases the short head of the biceps and the coracobrachialis. Thus, this fascial sheet extends like an opened Japanese fan from the clavicle above (where it ensheathes the subclavius) downward along the anterior chest wall to ensheathe the pectoralis minor, and then proceeds laterally as a single layer to reach the deep fascia of the arm. This fanlike continuous sheet of fascia from clavicle to chest wall to arm is called the *clavipectoral fascia.* The portion of this that lies between the clavicle and the medial border of the pectoralis minor is thickened by additional fibrous tissue, and these bands have led to the terms "costocoracoid ligament" and "coracoclavicular fascia" being applied to this particular portion of the clavipectoral fascia. The surgeon is not truly in the axillary fossa until he has pierced this fascial layer. The pectoral branches of the thoracoacromial axis, or artery, and the medial and lateral pectoral nerves cannot reach the deep surface of the pectoralis major muscle until they have pierced this fascial layer. The inferolateral margin of this clavipectoral fascia bridges across the base of the pyramidal-shaped axillary fossa and is there fused with the upper aspects of the *axillary fascia*. This latter is an ill-defined sheet that spreads from the free border of the pectoralis major (the anterior pectoral fold) to the free border of the latissimus dorsi and teres major (the posterior pectoral fold). Because the clavipectoral fascia fuses with the upper aspect of the axillary fascia and is a relatively inelastic sheet, it may be easily understood how the clavipectoral fascia supports the axillary fascia at a fixed distance from the clavicle. In abduction of the arm the anterior and posterior axillary folds are drawn taut and depressed, while the lateral end of the clavicle is elevated, and the skin of the armpit is arched upward because the clavipectoral fascia is fused with the superior aspect of the axillary fascia. Hence, the French refer to the clavipectoral fascia as the suspensory ligament of Gerdy and recognize it as being responsible for the domelike configuration of the axillary skin during abduction of the arm.

The *serratus anterior* muscle forms the medial wall of the axillary fossa. It arises by digitations from the upper eight or nine ribs. From this expansive area of origin on the surface of the ribs, the digitations blend together as a sheet in such a way as typically to send the major substance of the first and second digitations into an insertion at the superior (medial) angle of the scapula. Digitations from the second, third, and perhaps fourth ribs spread out to insert along the vertebral border of the scapula. This leaves the inferior angle of the scapula free to receive the digitations from the fifth, sixth, seventh, eighth, and sometimes ninth ribs. This arrangement obviously concentrates much of the power of the muscle on the inferior angle where it is most needed for rotation of the scapula during abduction of the arm.

The serratus anterior curves around the lateral aspect of the thorax to reach the medial (vertebral) border of the scapula on its costal or anterior surface. The investing fascia on the lateral surface of the muscle faces the axillary fossa and, in company with the muscle, becomes the medial wall of that fossa. On the medial (or internal) surface of the serratus anterior, the deep fascia of the muscle is separated from the fascial covering of the external intercostal muscles and the ribs by a very loose areolar layer of connective tissue that functions somewhat like a giant bursa in ensuring free play of the serratus anterior muscle, and thus of the entire scapula and the shoulder structures on the side of the chest. This interval between the serratus anterior and the chest wall filled with its loose areolar tissue has been referred to by some as the "scapulothoracic bursa." The axillary fossa itself, with its considerable content of fatty areolar tissue, contributes greatly to the free mobility of the scapula and the shoulder structures on the side of the chest.

The three muscles of the posterior wall of the axillary fossa are the subscapularis, teres major, and latissimus dorsi. It is only a small portion of the latter muscle, however, that enters into the formation of the posterior wall of the axilla and the substance of the posterior axillary (or pectoral) fold. Most of the *latissimus dorsi* is on the posterior aspect of the torso where the muscle arises from the spinous processes of thoracic vertebrae VII to XII, from the spinous processes of all the lumbar vertebrae, from the back of the sacrum, from the posterior part of the iliac crest, and from the lower three or four ribs by small slips. From this extremely expansive origin the muscle fibers converge to form a great triangular muscle. The upper border of this muscle is essentially horizontal, winding around the chest from the level of the tip of the spinous process of the seventh thoracic vertebra, across the lowermost part of the scapula, and then forward along the medial side of the arm to insert as a strong, flat tendon about 1½ inches wide into the medial tubercular crest of the humerus.

Nearing its insertion the latissimus dorsi twists about its own long axis through 180 degrees as it winds about the *teres major* muscle, which also inserts into the medial tubercular crest. The latter muscle, however, is placed farther distally at its insertion into the medial tubercular crest (the lip of the bicipital groove), and therefore it is the teres major that forms the lowest part of the posterior wall of the axilla where these two muscles approach the humerus. These muscles here also form the posterior axillary (pectoral) fold. The teres major takes its origin from the posterior aspect of the inferior angle and lateral border of the scapula, and then, as a thick, ribbon-like muscle, extends laterally and slightly upward to its insertion upon the humerus.

The *subscapular muscle* arises from the medial half of the costal surface of the scapula, and passes across the lateral half of that surface and onward over the anterior aspect of the shoulder joint, where it fuses with the articular capsule. It thus forms the anterior element of the four flattened tendons that are collectively referred to as the rotator cuff of the shoulder joint. The subscapularis insertion is into the lesser tuberosity of the humerus. This muscle and its innervation are vital to the normal function of the shoulder joint. Deep fascia invests each of these three muscles of the posterior wall of the axilla except where they attach to bone. Where they lie adjacent to one another, their fascial coverings blend together and obscure the cleavage planes between these muscles.

It was previously pointed out that the more inferior lactiferous ducts overlie, to varying degrees, the upper part of the external oblique muscle and the upper part of the rectus sheath, within which lies the rectus abdominis muscle. The upper end of the *rectus abdominis* is attached by three slips to the costal cartilages of the fifth, sixth, and seventh ribs in sequence from lateral to medial. Above the costal margin, the anterior wall of the rectus sheath is formed by the full thickness of the aponeurotic tendon of insertion of the external oblique and by one half of the thickness of the aponeurotic tendon of the internal oblique. The full thickness of the transversus abdominis aponeurosis and the posterior half thickness of the aponeurosis of the internal oblique lie behind the rectus. Each of these aponeurotic tendon sheaths carry a film of fascia upon its inner and outer surfaces, just as does the muscle belly of each. Obviously, the posterior wall of the rectus sheath above the costal margin is formed only by the costal cartilages and the intervening intercostal tissue.

The posterior one and one half laminae of the aponeuroses of the three flat muscles of the abdominal wall, which medially form the posterior wall of the rectus sheath, will switch their position to pass in front of the rectus muscle from the semicircular fold (of Douglas) (or arcuate line) downward. This change in the sheath, with all three aponeurotic laminae passing in front of the rectus muscle, occurs typically at a level about halfway between the umbilicus and the upper border of the symphysis pubis. However, it is often only a partial switching of some of the posterior lamina fibers, and thus there may be a duplication of the semicircular fold at another and slightly lower level.

The rectus abdominis is secured within its sheath by the partial fusion of the three tendinous inscriptions to the anterior wall of the rectus sheath (but not to the posterior wall). The inscriptions of the rectus muscle occur typically (1) at about the level of the lower tip of the xiphoid process, (2) at the level of the umbilicus, and (3) about midway between these levels. When a fourth inscription (usually incomplete or partial) occurs, it is equidistant below the level of the umbilicus. This partial segmentation of the rectus is mirrored in the pattern of innervation of the muscle.

The *external oblique* muscle arises by eight digitations from the lower eight ribs (fifth to twelfth ribs). The most superior five slips interdigitate with the serratus anterior, while the lower three or four slips interdigitate with the slips of origin of the latissimus dorsi. The line of attachment to the ribs of these slips of origin of the external oblique parallels the costal margin and is just lateral to the costochondral junctions, or about a hand's breadth lateral to and above the costal margin. The more anterior muscle fibers project downward and medially, becoming converted into a flat, aponeurotic tendon of insertion along a line that coincides roughly with the midclavicular sagittal plane of the body. One or 2 cm medial to this line is the semilunar line marking the lateral border of the rectus muscle and its sheath. The more posterior muscular fibers of the external oblique project downward to attach to the iliac crest.

The posterior border of the external oblique, nearing the level of the iliac crest, forms the anterior border of the *inferior lumbar trigone* (of Petit). The anteriormost fibers of the latissimus dorsi, also arising here from the iliac crest, form the posterior border of that trigone. The floor of the triangle is formed by the internal oblique muscle, but if it does not extend this far posteriorly, the floor will be the aponeurosis of origin of the transversus abdominis. If the latissimus dorsi overlaps the posterior fibers of the external oblique, the inferior lumbar triangle is obliterated and therefore absent, even though the slit between the two overlapping muscles still exists.

Below the twelfth rib another triangle is described: the *superior lumbar trigone* (of Grynfeltt or Lesgaft). It is bounded by the twelfth rib superiorly, by the sacrospinalis (erector spinae) muscle mass medially, and the posterior border of the internal oblique inferolaterally. It is thus seen to be superior and posteromedial to the inferior lumbar trigone. Sometimes the lowest fibers of the *serratus posterior inferior* encroach upon the superomedial corner of the triangle of Grynfeltt, converting it into a quadrilateral space. In any instance, the floor is the aponeurosis of origin of the *transversus abdominis* muscle. This aponeurosis is commonly pierced by the twelfth thoracic nerve and its counterpart subcostal artery. This perforation in the aponeurotic floor of the superior lumbar trigone is a "locus of minor resistance" awaiting the possible development of a hernia adiposa, which will consist of posterior pararenal fat. Such a hernia adiposa usually remains small and flattened, like a beaver tail, owing to the pressure and confinement of the overlying latissimus dorsi. No symptoms result except perhaps occasional ill-defined back pain, probably due to the irritation of the twelfth thoracic nerve by compression at the site of the small hernia. Rarely a larger mass protrudes through and descends deep to the latissimus dorsi, which is stretched across the area like a tight reinforcing bandage. If this mass becomes elongated or enlarged enough to descend and protrude through the inferior lumbar trigone (Petit's), it will become recognizable because it is now subcutaneous. Herniae adiposae the size of a flattened thumb are occasionally seen protruding through Grynfeltt's superior lumbar trigone in laboratory cadavers. Clearly, the overlying latissimus dorsi has suppressed the enlargement of the mass. The unroofing of this area by the use of this portion of the latissimus dorsi as a musculocutaneous flap could promote the development of a hernia here. At least one such case, containing colon, has been reported.[5]

The large herniae said to be through these two triangles, which have been reported through the years, and which are not postsurgical, are probably due to embryologic deficits in the development of the muscular wall of the abdomen in this region, rather than protrusion through normally developed lumbar triangles. Reported cases have been congenital and often bilateral and massive, with the muscular boundaries so ill defined that they were unlikely to be the structures described above.

BLOOD SUPPLY OF THE BREAST AND RELATED STRUCTURES

Arterial Supply

The primary sources of arterial supply to the breast include the anterior perforating branches of the *internal thoracic* (mammary) *artery*, which is a branch of the first part of the subclavian artery; the *lateral thoracic artery*, which arises from the axillary artery; and a third source of lesser importance from the *intercostal* arteries (Fig. 1–3). Intercostal arteries are of two types. There are posterior (or aortic) intercostals, which arise from the aorta, and anterior intercostals, which arise from the internal thoracic artery. These arteries anastomose with each other at an undefinable location in the anterior part of each intercostal space. Accordingly, it is variously stated that these few direct branches to the breast that arise from an intercostal artery (either third, fourth, or fifth) have arisen from the anterior or the posterior intercostal artery. If they arise near the lateral border of the breast, it is probably more accurate to consider them to have arisen from a posterior intercostal artery. Branches from the anterior perforating branches of the internal thoracic artery quite often

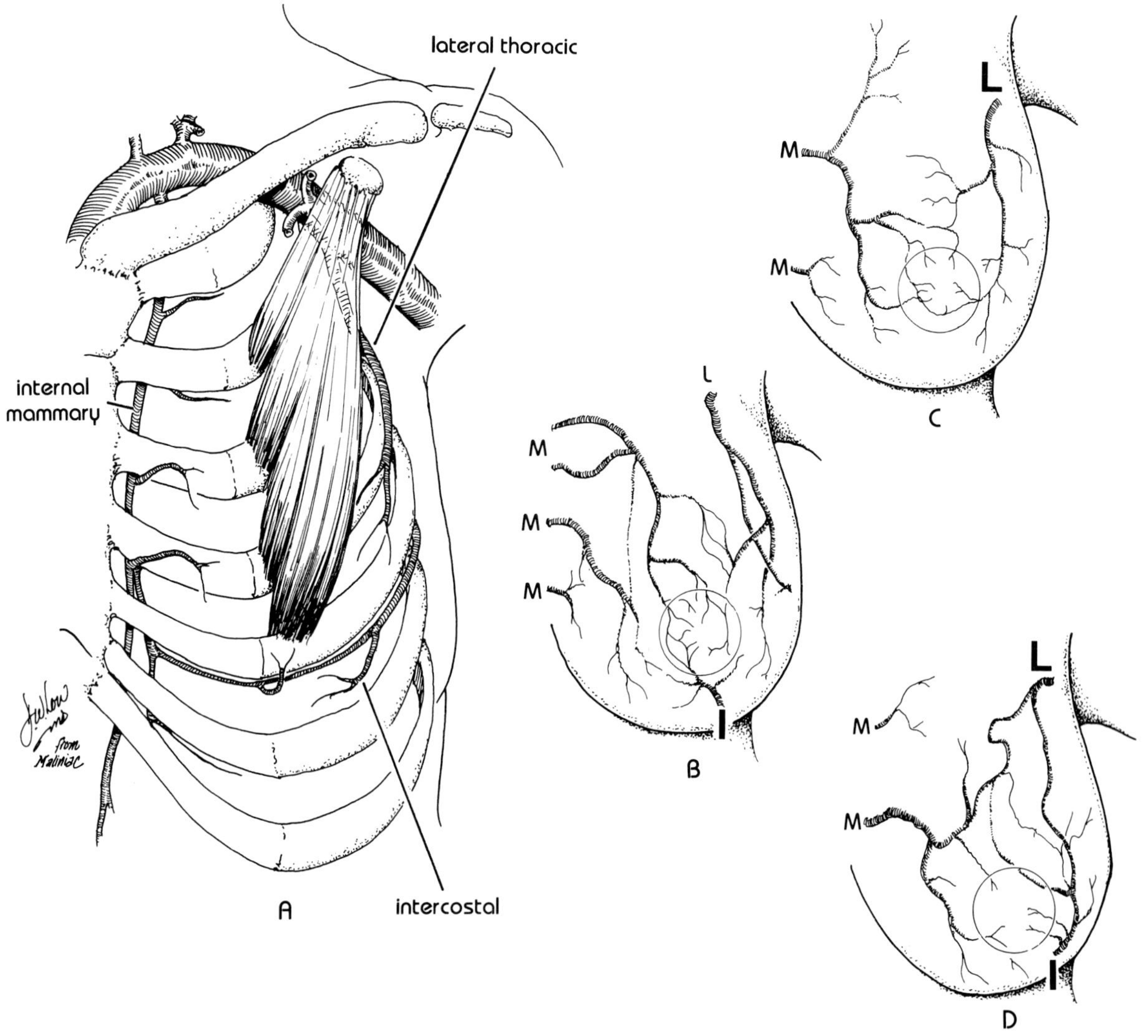

FIGURE 1–3 *A*, Pectoralis minor muscle displayed. Thoracoacromial and lateral thoracic arteries are shown arising from the second part of the axillary artery. The internal thoracic (mammary) artery and the anterior and posterior (aortic) intercostal arteries are seen. *B*, The most common arterial pattern for supply of nipple and areola as seen in about 74 percent of breasts, arranged as a circular, periareolar arterial plexus. Frequency data from Marcus[6] and based on 53 breasts studied by arterial injection, x-ray, and gross dissection. *C*, Loop type of periareolar arterial plexus, seen in about 20 percent of breasts. *D*, Radial type of periareolar arterial plexus, seen in about 6 percent of breasts. In *B*, *C*, and *D* the letter M indicates the anterior perforating branches of the internal thoracic artery, L indicates the lateral thoracic artery, and I indicates a branch from the posterior intercostal artery that penetrates the deep surface of the breast after crossing the retromammary space.

penetrate into the deep aspect of the breast, after piercing through the pectoralis major and then running lateralward from their origin, and are therefore incorrectly identified as intercostal artery branches when they finally penetrate the deep surface of the breast. Direct branches do arise from the intercostal arteries as they lie deep to the breast and penetrate through the intercostal muscles to enter the breast on its deep surface. These vessels are usually small. Still another source of small branches from the intercostal arteries are anterior branches from the lateral perforating branches of the intercostal arteries in the third, fourth, and fifth interspaces. These contribute lateral mammary branches that are primarily for the skin of the lateral side of the breast.

The axillary artery is divisible into three parts by its relationship to the pectoralis minor muscle. The first part extends from the lateral border of the first rib (where the subclavian artery becomes the axillary) to the upper or medial border of the pectoralis minor. The second part is directly behind the pectoralis minor. The third part of the axillary artery extends from the lower or lateral border of the pectoralis minor to the lower border of the tendon of insertion of the teres major as the latter approaches its insertion into the medial tubercular crest of the humerus. Here, the teres major and the latissimus dorsi are forming the contents of the posterior axillary fold. Beyond the teres major the artery is referred to as the brachial artery, for it is now fully within the arm.

There are, in the typical case, six branches from the axillary artery. The first or highest branch, called the *superior thoracic artery*, arises from the first part. Two branches, the *thoracoacromial* and *lateral thoracic*, arise from the second part. Three branches, the *subscapular, anterior circumflex humeral*, and *posterior circumflex humeral*, arise from the third part. Because the axillary artery shifts a little in its relationship to the pectoralis minor muscle as the limb goes from adduction to abduction, it is obvious that these relations of the origin of the two branches from the second part will be modified somewhat by the posture of the limb. In general, however, the thoracoacromial axis (or artery) arises behind the upper border of the pectoralis minor and winds around that border to pierce the clavipectoral fascia, and thereafter approach the deep surface of the pectoralis major.

The *lateral thoracic artery* winds around the lower (lateral) border of the pectoralis minor and thereafter around the lower (lateral) border of the pectoralis major. It supplies twigs to both pectoralis minor and major and to the serratus anterior and adjacent intercostal muscles. It then divides into two or three *lateral (external) mammary* branches that approach the lower lateral aspect of the breast. These last-named branches of the lateral thoracic artery are an important source of arterial supply to the breast, although usually somewhat subordinate to the *anterior perforating branches* of the *internal thoracic artery*, which approach the breast from its medial side and send branches onto the superficial or cutaneous surface of the breast and into its deep surface. The latter branches, because they are continuations of some of the anterior perforating branches, should not be described as branches of the intercostal arteries. These anterior perforating branches turn laterally before they pierce through the pectoralis major, and therefore may be 3 or 4 cm lateral to the sternum before they emerge through the superficial surface of the pectoralis major and its fascia to penetrate the deep surface of the breast after crossing the retromammary space. Thus, they masquerade as having arisen from the anterior intercostal arteries.[7] Arteries piercing through the pectoralis major nearer the lateral border of the breast are truly branches of the intercostal arteries. These penetrate the deep surface of the breast but are usually small and few in number.

As for the distribution of the six branches of the axillary artery, only the lateral thoracic artery provides any significant supply to the breast, and it does so primarily to the lateral half of the breast via its terminal lateral mammary branches. The acromiothoracic artery gives off two or three rather stalwart pectoral branches, some of which penetrate the clavipectoral fascia and some the pectoralis minor itself, supplying the latter, and then penetrating the deep surface of the pectoralis major to irrigate this latter muscle. Occasionally one of these pectoral branches pierces through the pectoralis major and supplies an upper lateral portion of the breast.

Although the other branches of the axillary artery do not usually enter into the supply of the breast, they do supply muscles of the area, and so are of interest. The highest branch, the superior thoracic artery, arises from the first part of the axillary artery, and after a short medial and downward course supplies the muscles of the first and sometimes the second intercostal spaces. It may also contribute twigs to the pectoralis minor.

The thoracoacromial axis is very short and divides into a variable series of branches, which tend to radiate from the hub into some four divergent branches that pierce the clavipectoral fascia and are named, because of their destinations, the *clavicular branch* (to that bone and the subclavius muscle), *the acromial branch* (which also contributes to the deltoid muscle and skin), the *deltoid branch* (which also contributes to the deltoid muscle and skin), and two or three *pectoral branches*, which supply both pectoralis minor and pectoralis major. The branch to the latter muscle is the largest of these branches and is often multiple, or at least branches several times before penetrating the deep surface of the pectoralis major. Another important source of blood supply to the pectoralis major muscle is the series of anterior perforating arteries branching from the internal thoracic artery and arising segmentally along the medial border of the pectoralis major muscle. The lateral thoracic artery also contributes to the pectoralis major muscle. The lateral mammary (external mammary) branches of the lateral thoracic artery not only provide important blood supply to the breast itself, but are the source of a few smaller arterial branches that are primarily cutaneous branches in both males and females.

It is fairly common to find an artery coming around the lateral margin of the pectoralis major to then descend on its anterior surface paralleling the lateral margin. It supplies the zone of skin overlying the lateralmost part of the pectoralis major muscle. This artery is primarily cutaneous in its distribution, but in females it also contributes to the supply of the mammary gland. When present, it is found to arise independently from the axillary artery or to be a very early branch of the lateral thoracic artery. It tends to parallel the course of the latter artery but is more superficially placed, being throughout most of its length on the anterior aspect of the pectoralis major descending near its lateral border. In any event, it warrants a name of its own and is probably best called the *superficial thoracic artery.*[8]

Another variant artery that is commonly found supplying a zone of skin over the most superior part of the lateral margin of the pectoralis major is a purely *cutaneous branch* of either the *acromial* or the *deltoid branch* of the *thoracoacromial artery.* This cutaneous branch escapes from beneath the pectoralis major by emerging through the deltopectoral triangle and turning downward to supply an area of skin roughly the size of one's palm.

From the third part of the axillary artery arises the *subscapular artery,* usually the largest of the branches from the axillary. Some 2 to 4 cm from its beginning the artery divides into its two terminal branches, the *circumflex scapular* and *thoracodorsal* arteries. The latter appears as the continuation of the subscapular artery and continues downward and medialward, paralleling the axillary or lateral border of the scapula, which is concealed behind the axillary border of the subscapularis muscle. The subscapular and thoracodorsal arteries contribute branches to the subscapularis, teres major, and latissimus dorsi, the three muscles that form the posterior wall of the axillary fossa.

Near the inferior angle of the scapula, which commonly corresponds to the seventh intercostal space, the thoracodorsal artery gives terminal branches to the serratus anterior (coating the medial wall of the axilla), a twig or two to the lower end of the subscapularis muscle and to the teres major, and small twigs to the adjacent intercostal muscles, plus an important branch or branches to the lateral border of the latissimus dorsi. These branches penetrate the latissimus dorsi in company with the venae comitantes and the thoracodorsal (or middle subscapular) nerve. After penetrating the muscle, the artery divides into four to five branches that run parallel to the muscle fasciculi and are commonly accompanied by an equal number of twigs of the thoracodorsal nerve. This arrangement allows the latissimus muscle to be split into several segments, each with its own neurovascular supply. The more posterior part of the latissimus dorsi is supplied by medial and lateral dorsal perforating cutaneous branches of the intercostal and lumbar arteries.

A trough is formed between the three muscles forming the posterior wall of the axillary fossa and the serratus anterior forming the medial wall. This trough narrows progressively as it is followed inferiorward, and it is here in the lower end of the trough, where a narrowing wedge or angle is formed between the latissimus dorsi and serratus anterior, that the final branches at the distal end of the thoracodorsal artery are found. These branches and their accompanying venae comitantes anastomose with the intercostal arteries and veins on the medial side and with the periscapular network at the inferior angle of the scapula. This tangle of vessels in the narrowing wedge has been called "the bloody angle."

The circumflex scapular branch of the subscapular artery turns dorsalward immediately after arising and passes through the triangular space bounded medially by the subscapularis and the axillary border of the scapula. The lateral boundary of the triangle is the teres major; the superolateral boundary is the long head of the triceps. The artery curves abruptly medialward between the teres minor and the dorsal surface of the scapula to come to lie in the infraspinous fossa of the scapula, where it supplies the infraspinatus and enters into the periscapular network of anastomosing arteries. Particularly important here as a route of collateral circulation is its anastomosis with branches of the subscapular (transverse scapular) artery, which arises from the first part of the subclavian artery via the thyrocervical trunk.

Two cutaneous branches of the circumflex scapular artery arise from it while it is traversing the triangular space, but before it passes into the infraspinous fossa. These two arterial branches utilize the intermuscular fascia between teres minor and teres major to gain the subcutaneous level. One branch passes medially, paralleling the spine of the scapula but several centimeters inferior to it, and is called the *horizontal branch.* The other descends, paralleling the axillary border of the scapula, and is called the *parascapular branch.* These two arteries often share a common trunk of origin. Sometimes the parascapular branch appears subcutaneously by emerging around the lower or lateral borders of the teres major instead of between the two teres muscles.[9,10]

The two remaining branches of the third part of the axillary artery routinely found are the *anterior circumflex humeral* and *posterior circumflex humeral* arteries. These arise close together from the axillary artery and pass laterally around the surgical neck of the humerus, on the sides thereof, as their names suggest. They anastomose with each other, and both contribute to the supply of the shoulder joint. The posterior circumflex humeral artery passes out of the axillary fossa in company with the axillary nerve by utilizing the quadrilateral space, which is bounded by the subscapularis, the axillary border of the scapula, and the teres minor, all on the medial side; by the long head of the triceps inferiorly; by the teres major laterally; and by the surgical neck of the humerus above. The boundaries as stated are always the same, but their relative positions as given are with the arm in 90 degrees of abduction. This artery and the accompanying axillary nerve both provide a series of branches into the deep surface of the deltoid muscle. There are a number of musculocutaneous perforators from this artery that supply the skin overlying the deltoid muscle. In about 15 percent of body sides the posterior circumflex humeral artery arises from the beginning of the subscapular artery rather than as an independent branch of the axillary.[11] The anterior circumflex humeral gives off an ascending branch that accompanies the long tendon of the biceps, and a descending branch that contributes to the tendon of insertion of the pectoralis major.

It was previously pointed out that the serratus anterior receives branches from the lateral thoracic artery, and at a somewhat lower level it also receives twigs from the thoracodorsal artery. These enter the muscle at about its midlevel along the medial wall of the axilla. A third source of arterial supply to the serratus anterior is from the lateral perforating branches of the aortic intercostals. This latter source is of considerably less importance than the former two, however. The pectoralis minor receives twigs from the thoracoacromial axis, or from the pectoral branches thereof, as these arteries lie along the upper border of the muscle. The pectoralis minor also commonly receives a small branch from the lateral thoracic artery as it lies along the lateral border of the muscle. As occasional variants the muscle may receive a direct twig from the axillary artery and a small branch from the superior thoracic artery.

The arterial supply of the external oblique muscle arises primarily from the lateral perforating branches of the intercostal arteries. These perforators appear as branches from the intercostal arteries in a series emerging along a line parallel with, and some 4 or 5 cm anterior to, the lateral border of the latissimus dorsi (the posterior axillary line). These perforators arise from the sixth to the twelfth intercostal arteries. The lowest intercostal artery is commonly called the subcostal artery. Entering the muscle substances here, for the most part on the deep surface of the external oblique, the many small branches arborize into a network throughout the muscle substance.

The arterial supply of each rectus abdominis muscle is primarily via two arteries, one of which enters the upper end of the rectus sheath and descends, while the other enters the sheath from below and ascends. These two arteries arborize on the deep surface of the rectus and send branches into the substance of the rectus for further branching and network formation. The upper artery is the *superior epigastric artery*, formed as one of the two terminal branches of the internal thoracic at the medial end of the sixth intercostal space. Occasionally the superior epigastric artery immerses itself in the substance of the muscle so quickly that little of it is visible on the posterior surface of the rectus, and it can be identified only on the posterior side of the uppermost 2 or 3 cm of the rectus muscle. The other terminal branch is the *musculophrenic artery*, which continues its course in the costophrenic sinus, offering small anterior intercostal arteries to the seventh, eighth, and ninth spaces and twigs to the diaphragm. The superior epigastric artery pierces the diaphragm through the triangular defect in the diaphragm between the diaphragmatic slip to the xiphoid process and the slip to the costal cartilage of the seventh rib. Between these two slips is a small triangular defect in the muscle of the diaphragm, but this is filled in with a thin layer of fibrous tissue. It is this triangular space, called the costoxiphoid gap (or space of Larrey), that is pierced by the superior epigastric artery and vein and a lymphatic vessel.

The inferior epigastric artery arises as a branch of the external iliac artery just before the latter makes exit from the abdominal cavity to be continued as the femoral artery. The inferior epigastric artery curves upward and medially on the inner side of the abdominal wall, to pass along the medial side of the deep inguinal ring, at the same time forming the lateral boundary of Hesselbach's triangle. The artery enters the rectus sheath by passing upward on the posterior surface of the rectus muscle in front of the semicircular fold of Douglas (or the arcuate line). This latter represents the lower limit of the posterior wall of the rectus sheath. The level of the anastomosis of the superior and inferior epigastric arteries is approximately halfway between the xiphoid process and the umbilicus.

Although it is not the official nomenclature, it is common to call the superior epigastric artery the *deep superior epigastric artery*, and the inferior epigastric artery is then called the *deep inferior epigastric artery*. This is to help differentiate these two arteries within the rectus sheath from the *superficial superior epigastric artery* (which arises, when present, from the deep superior epigastric artery) and the *superficial inferior epigastric artery* (which arises from the femoral artery). These superficial arteries are similar in their courses to the deep ones but lie in the superficial fascia and are purely cutaneous arteries. Manchot[8] appears to have been the first to describe the superficial superior epigastric artery, but he erred in assuming it to be regularly present, when in fact it is present in only about one-quarter of individuals. These two subcutaneous arteries do not effect as abundant an anastomosis with each other as do the two deep arteries. The anastomosis between the two deep arteries (within the rectus sheath) is strong enough to justify the expression "the deep epigastric arcade" and to provide viability to the rectus abdominis flap.

The terminal twigs of most of the intercostal arteries that slant inferomedially through the neurovascular plane of the abdominal wall reach the rectus sheath and pass behind its lateral border to pierce through the posterior wall of the rectus sheath about 1 cm from the lateral border. Thus gaining the interior of the rectus sheath, these several small and segmentally arranged arteries, plus the accompanying intercostal nerves (thoracic nerve, T7 to T12), enter and supply the rectus abdominis muscle. These arterial branches join in the formation of the deep superior and inferior epigastric network. Over the front of the rectus sheath an irregularly placed series of small perforating arteries exit the rectus sheath to become cutaneous arteries. These perforating arteries tend to be more frequently found in the vicinity of the umbilicus.

There is still a further source of arterial supply into the rectus abdominis arterial network (the deep epigastric arcade). This is the entry of small twigs from the lowest anterior perforating branches of the internal thoracic artery (through the fifth and sixth intercostal spaces) into the three slips of upper attachment of the rectus to the fifth, sixth, and seventh costal cartilages. These arterial twigs descend in the muscle and join in the creation of the upper end of the arterial network, which we have identified as the deep epigastric arcade. These small arteries entering the rectus muscle directly are distinct from the (deep) superior epigastric artery, which enters the rectus sheath and lies against the posterior surface of the rectus muscle slightly below this level.

The deep inferior epigastric artery is the dominant artery, but the network of anastomosing arteries, both on the posterior surface of, and to a greater degree in the substance of, the rectus muscle, is so efficient that each of the sources can send its flow of blood throughout the network if the pressure and the volume flow of blood is sufficient. Therefore, each source warrants recognition and consideration, and only experience and the elimination of other adverse factors will allow a reasonable prediction of tissue survival.

Venous Drainage

In general the venous drainage of the breast and the pectoral area parallels the arterial supply. In the breast the veins are single; some of them parallel the arteries closely enough to be called *vena comitans.* By the time the larger veins are reached, there are usually two veins paralleling the artery, and there are commonly cross linkages by short veins that afford multiple anastomoses between these double veins. The latter are, of course, *venae comitantes.* The internal thoracic artery, for example, has venae comitantes accompanying it, and a vein lies on either side of the artery. The veins draining from the breast and pectoral area into the axilla tend to be single veins.

The veins of the breast that are subcutaneous are superficial and can often be seen through the skin. If they are not clearly visible, infrared photography often makes them discernible. Commonly the subcutaneous veins of the female breast are seen to be of either a transverse or a longitudinal looping type. In the former the veins take the simplest and most direct route from the central breast tissue and run as two, three, or four veins medially to turn into the intercostal spaces beside the sternum, and end in the internal thoracic venae comitantes. The laterally running transverse pattern veins parallel the path of the lateral thoracic artery and its lateral mammary branches, and therefore round the anterior pectoral fold to enter the axilla and ultimately join the axillary vein. Before this, however, most of them join what is called the costoaxillary vein or proceed directly into the lateral thoracic vein, which receives the costoaxillary vein as well as the lengthy thoracoepigastric (thoracoabdominal) vein. The lateral thoracic vein empties into the axillary vein. In the longitudinal looping type of superficial venous pattern, there is a predominance of drainage medialward and of course superiorly to end in the internal thoracic veins. A circular to U-shaped vein tends to widely encircle the areola receiving tributaries from the more peripheral portion of the breast. The two limbs of the "U" approach each other, or actually unite, in a teardrop-shaped circle, with the final flow heading by one or several superficial veins to the intercostal spaces anteriorly, where they turn deeply to reach the internal thoracic venae comitantes. In either type some subcutaneous veins disappear at the infraclavicular fossa as these veins pass through the deltopectoral trigone to join the cephalic vein or vena comitans of the pectoral branches of the thoracoacromial axis. Ultimately such veins pierce the upper part of the clavipectoral fascia and drain into the axillary vein. Sometimes these ascending veins from the breast pass above the clavicle to drain into the transverse scapular (suprascapular) vein or to end in the jugulosubclavian venous angle.

Some veins from the deep surface of the breast drain deeply into the subjacent intercostal veins, and thereafter the flow is posteriorly to the azygos system of veins and hence into the superior vena cava. Herein lies the explanation both of hematogenous spread of tumor cell emboli to the lungs and of spread to the bones of the spine and the shoulder girdle; the latter is due to the many venous linkages between the azygos system and the external and internal vertebral venous plexuses. This being a valveless system of veins in the paraspinal area, only the vis a tergo in the vessels determines the direction of flow in these veins, and at times the pressures send blood in the paraspinal or vertebral system of veins into the basivertebral veins, and thus into the interior of the vertebral bodies.

Although the mammary venous plexus drains primarily laterally into the axillary vein and medially into the internal thoracic veins, it has connections with the subcutaneous veins of the abdominal wall that merit comment. Medially, a vein, or a continuous network, lies over the rectus sheath and links the tributaries to the internal thoracic vein with the tributaries to the periumbilical veins dispersed about the umbilicus. This vertical venous channel overlying the rectus sheath corresponds to the occasionally present *superficial superior episgastric artery*, but is more often present than is the artery. However, it usually is too small to be identified unless distended (as it may be in either superior or inferior vena caval obstruction). Laterally, along the flank, there usually are several small venous communications (roughly at the level of the umbilicus) between the tributaries of the superficial epigastric vein and of the superficial circumflex iliac vein (both of which drain downward into the great saphenous vein). They drain as abdominal wall veins and the ascending thoracic wall subcutaneous veins that, collecting into a major trunk, join with the costoaxillary vein and the lateral thoracic vein to empty into the axillary vein. Thus, a continuous subcutaneous venous channel links the axillary vein with the femoral vein. This total channel, which is often more of a network than a single vessel, particularly at the level of the umbilicus, is called the *thoracoepigastric* or *thoracoabdominal vein.* Above the umbilical level the valves direct the flow upward, while below the umbilicus the valves direct the flow downward. In either superior or inferior vena caval obstruction the engorgement of these veins leads to incompetence of the valves, and the flow can go downward with superior caval obstruction or upward with inferior caval obstruction. This laterally placed venous channel may then become remarkably dilated and very visible. The more medially placed venous pathway that links the periumbilical veins and superficial epigastric vein below with the tributaries to the internal thoracic vein also become dilated and visible, although never as much as the thoracoepigastric vein. A thrombophlebitis of some part of the superficial mammary venous plexus has been called Mondor's disease. The thrombosed vein in the breast may be palpable as a cordlike lesion, which may extend out of the breast into the thoracoepigastric vein.[12,13]

The axillary vein, progressing upward and medially toward the apex of the axilla, receives many tributaries, including the venous drainage of the breast, of the muscles of the walls of the axilla, and of the upper limb and the shoulder area. Descriptions of the beginning of the axillary vein are arbitrary. Some authors cite it as commencing at the basilic vein of the arm as it crosses the lower border of the tendon of insertion of the teres major (this is the point taken as the end of the axillary artery and the beginning of the brachial artery). Others require the union of the basilic vein and the brachial venae comitantes before they recognize an axillary vein. Inasmuch as the latter union may be high in the axilla, it is evident that, by such reasoning, the axillary vein will differ markedly in length from person to person. Still others rely strictly on size. When enough tributaries have united to provide a vein of creditable size, they are willing to cite it as the axillary vein. It ends, of course, as it crosses the lateral border of the first rib, becoming the subclavian vein.

A common pattern is for the basilic vein, within a few centimeters after entering the axilla, to receive the brachial venae comitantes and then in quick succession the subscapular vein, the anterior and posterior circumflex humeral veins, and the lateral thoracic vein in a variety of sequences, and often with reduction of the numbers of veins by coalescence before they empty into the axillary vein. Nearer the apex of the axilla, the cephalic vein pierces the clavipectoral (costocoracoid) fascia, along with pectoral veins draining the pectoralis major, to end in the upper part of the axillary vein. A variety of veins draining the muscles of the walls of the axilla end in the axillary vein, either directly or after uniting with others. Thus, the point of entry and the numbers of tributary veins vary a great deal. As the first rib is reached, the axillary vein has entered the neck and is receiving tributaries from the head and neck. Passing medially beyond the lateral border of the first rib, it becomes the subclavian vein. This vein passes in front of the scalenus anterior muscle and, being joined by the internal jugular vein, forms the brachiocephalic (or innominate) vein.

If there is an early coalescence of the many tributaries to the axillary vein, a large vein results, but if some of the tributaries fail to join until high in the axilla, there may be two or three veins of about equal size; the apex of the axilla being obscured, it may then be difficult to be sure which is the axillary vein. In most instances a large vein is identifiable as the axillary vein, lying anterior and somewhat inferior to the axillary artery, thus obscuring the latter and the brachial plexus at surgery. All these structures are embedded in the mass of fatty areolar tissue that fills the axilla. Interspersed throughout this axillary fat mass are the collections of lymphatic vessels and nodes that receive lymph from the breast, the anterolateral thoracic wall skin, the upper limb, and the back of the shoulder area.

INNERVATION OF THE MUSCLES AND SKIN OF THE PECTORAL AND RELATED AREAS

The axillary fossa is routinely described as pyramidal in shape with four walls, a base, and an apex. It is, however, a peculiarly shaped pyramid because, although the anterior, medial, and posterior walls are of about equal dimensions, the lateral wall is very narrow. In fact, it is no wider than the intertubercular (bicipital) sulcus. This is because the three muscles of the posterior wall (the subscapularis, latissimus dorsi, and teres major) insert upon the lesser tuberosity and medial tubercular crest in the order cited from above downward, while the anterior wall muscles extend from the chest to the coracoid process (for the pectoralis minor) and to the lateral tubercular crest (for the pectoralis major). This leaves the narrow intertubercular sulcus for the lateral and third wall.

The medial, and fourth, wall is formed by the ribs, overlaid by the serratus anterior, and extends from the costal attachments of the pectoralis major posteriorly along the rib cage to the vertebral border of the scapula into which the serratus anterior inserts. Actually the space of the axillary fossa is somewhat less than this dimension because the subscapularis muscle is in apposition with the serratus anterior muscle posteriorly, and this pinches off that posteriormost recess of the axillary fossa. By noting the convergence laterally of the anterior and posterior pectoral folds as one looks at the base of the axilla, when the patient's arm is abducted to 90 degrees, it is evident that the dimensions of the lateral wall of the so-called pyramidal space are greatly reduced compared with the other three walls. The lateral wall in fact is no wider than the intertubercular sulcus.

It is a common error to assume that the coracobrachialis and the short head of the biceps are forming the lateral wall, but they are the contents of the axillary fossa, and the tendon of the long head of the biceps is the occupant of that lateralmost interval between the anterior and posterior walls, namely, the intertubercular or bicipital groove. The muscle fascia covering the short head of the biceps and the coracobrachialis is incorrectly taken as the lateral wall, and these structures are not recognized for what they truly are: the contents of the axillary fossa.

The other contents of the axillary fossa are the traditional ones: brachial plexus, great vessels and their branches and tributaries, lymphatics, and a moldable fat mass. The fat encases the other contents, and tethers and protects them as the shape of the axillary fossa changes with the degree of abduction of the arm, and the degree of protraction and retraction and elevation of the shoulder.

The pectoralis minor with its clavipectoral fascia may be thought of as a reinforcement to the pectoralis major, which is the true anterior wall of the axillary fossa. Clearly, however, the axillary fossa is not entered until the clavipectoral fascia is pierced or removed in an anterior approach to the fossa.

The apex of the axillary fossa should not be regarded as a pointed apex, but rather as a truncated apex. The axillary fossa ends above at the triangular interval between the fossa below and the neck above, where the clavicle, first rib, and upper border of the scapula make a kind of passageway between the upper limit of the axillary fossa and the lower limit or root of the neck. It is here in the posterior triangle of the neck, between the scalenus medius and scalenus anterior and the upper aspect of the first rib (scalene triangle), that the brachial plexus begins from the anterior primary divisions of cervical nerves C5 to C8 and thoracic nerve T1. From the same scalene triangle, at its lower limits, there also emerges into the root of the neck the subclavian artery, becoming the axillary artery as it crosses the lateral border of the first rib. The axillary vein, ascending, changes its name to subclavian as it crosses the lateral border of the first rib anterior to the scalenus anterior, and therefore not passing through the scalene triangle, as do the artery and the roots of the brachial plexus.

In descending through the axillary fossa, the axillary artery and vein and the brachial plexus enter the fossa through its truncated apex close to the first rib, but they leave the fossa through its base along the lateral wall of the fossa to pass thereafter into the arm.

The brachial plexus begins as five nerves (the anterior primary divisions of nerves C5 to C8 and T1) and ends as five nerves (musculocutaneous, median, ulnar, radial, and axillary). It is only the anterior primary divisions of the spinal nerves that enter into the formation of the brachial plexus. The posterior primary divisions pass to the muscles and skin of the back. From now on the anterior primary divisions will be referred to simply as spinal nerves C5 to T1. Typically the nerves C5 and C6 unite to form the upper trunk. Nerve C7 continues alone as the middle trunk, and C8 and T1 unite to form the lower trunk. Then the upper, middle, and lower trunks each divide into anterior and posterior divisions. This occurs commonly at the level of the clavicle, or when the brachial plexus is passing through the junction of the root of the neck and the truncated apex of the axilla. The anterior divisions of the upper and middle trunks unite to form the lateral cord. The anterior division of the lower trunk continues as the medial cord of the brachial plexus. The posterior divisions of the upper, middle, and lower trunks unite to form the posterior cord.

At the level of the lateral border of the pectoralis minor, the three cords divide into their six terminal branches. The lateral cord gives rise to the *musculocutaneous nerve* and the lateral head of the *median nerve*. The medial cord gives rise to the medial head of the *median nerve* and the *ulnar nerve.* The posterior cord gives rise to the *axillary nerve* and the *radial nerve.* Because there are two heads to the median nerve, there are only five terminal nerves. These nerves proceed to the lateral wall of the axilla to descend into the arm.

However, the axillary nerve escapes from the axillary fossa by turning posteriorly to pass through the quadrilateral space in company with the posterior circumflex humeral artery and vein, and thereafter to wind about the surgical neck of the humerus on its posterior and lateral side. This nerve gives off a series of branches that supply the deltoid muscle, and some twigs piercing through the muscle supply the skin over the middle third of the deltoid muscle. A small twig supplies the teres minor muscle. A cutaneous branch winds around the posterior border of the deltoid muscle (the lateral brachial cutaneous or upper lateral brachial cutaneous nerve) and supplies a zone of skin over the more posterior and lower part of the deltoid, extending down the posterolateral surface of the arm for a few inches.

The *long thoracic nerve* (once called the external respiratory nerve of Bell) is the nerve supplying the serratus anterior. It arises from the roots of C5, C6, and C7 while still between the scalenus anterior and scalenus medius. These roots unite, and the nerve formed descends down the superficial or external surface of the serratus anterior roughly in the midlateral line. Many branches arise from the nerve, and some digitations of the serratus receive more than one branch of supply. The site of entry of each nerve branch is roughly at the midlength of each digitation.

There are three subscapular nerves, which arise as collateral branches from the posterior cord of the brachial plexus. The *upper subscapular nerve* from C5 to C6 travels downward a short distance to enter the substance of the subscapularis muscle deep (medially) in the axilla. It is commonly accompanied by an arterial branch from the axillary artery directly, or from the subscapular artery. A *lower subscapular nerve* commonly arises from the posterior cord farther down its length (or more laterally). This nerve from C6 to C7 supplies the more lateral part of the subscapularis muscle and is the sole source of supply to the teres major muscle. The *middle subscapular nerve* is commonly called the *thoracodorsal nerve,* because it accompanies the artery of that name. It supplies the latissimus dorsi by a leash by twigs that enter the medial or deep surface of that muscle in a central area between origin and insertion. Here its branches penetrate into the muscle in company with branches of the thoracodorsal artery. The nerve branches and the arterial branches run together in the muscle in a pattern of dividing neurovascular parallel branches radiating from a common source, somewhat as the fingers of a hand radiate from the metacarpus.

The innervation of the pectoralis major and pectoralis minor is via the lateral and medial pectoral nerves (also known as the lateral and medial anterior thoracic nerves). These nerves arise as a root from the lateral cord of the brachial plexus and another root from the medial cord of the brachial plexus. These two roots arch toward each other, and their fibers intermingle in a neural arcade or arch from which the final branches arise and pass forward as one, two, or three branches. Those branches whose fibers arose in the lateral cord are collectively the lateral pectoral nerves, and their fibers will have come from spinal nerves C5, C6, and C7. Another variable branch or branches will arise from the neural arcade, which consists of fibers from spinal nerves C8 and T1. This latter nerve twig or twigs will contain fibers that arise from the medial cord of the brachial plexus. Recall that the elements of the brachial plexus are slanting downward and laterally as they descend through the axilla from the roots in the neck to the five major terminal nerves passing into the arm. The lateral pectoral nerve routinely arises from the lateral cord at a more proximal point, and therefore more medially than does the medial pectoral nerve, which arises more distally from the medial cord and therefore more laterally than the placement of the lateral pectoral nerve. Again, they are named for the cord they arise from, and not for their placement in space as considered on a horizontal plane. Thus, the seeming error or incongruity of their names as medial and lateral nerves is readily understood as being a reference to the brachial plexus cord from which the nerve fibers arose. With this in mind, it becomes evident that the lateral pectoral nerve (or nerves) is/are arising from the higher spinal nerve roots (C5, C6, C7), and the fibers of these nerves pass into the upper part of the pectoralis major muscle, while the medial pectoral nerve (or nerves) is/are arising from the lower spinal nerve roots (C8, T1) and distributed to the lower part of the muscle. Tracing the several pectoral nerves (both medial and lateral) into the substance of the pectoralis major and pectoralis minor suggests that there is a segmental distribution of the nerve fibers in these muscles, so that the higher segments of the spinal cord (and thus the roots of origin of the brachial plexus) are distributed to the upper part of the pectoralis major, while the lower segments of the cervical cord (and thus the lower roots of the brachial plexus) are sending nerve fibers to the lower part of the pectoralis major and to the pectoralis minor. Clinical evidence in terms of nerve root lesions and spinal cord segment lesions corroborates this anatomic data. Thus, there is segmental innervation within the pectoralis major arranged on a plan of C5 to T1 distributed vertically within the muscle. The pectoralis minor is also segmentally innervated, but because of its more vertical orientation its fibers are segmented on a more medial to lateral plan. Spinal nerves represented in the pectoralis minor are probably C6, C7, and C8, but it may be C7, C8, and T1. This variability can be understood if one recalls the frequent variation in the number of slips to the ribs, in the pectoralis minor, sometimes going as low as the fifth or even the sixth rib. The number of spinal nerves contributing to the innervation of a muscle is an expression of the number of somites that contributed to the mesenchyme that formed the premuscle mass out of which that muscle developed. Innervational segmentation in a muscle, however, is never very precise or circumscribed. The peripheral muscle fibers of a portion of a muscle that is predominantly supplied by one spinal nerve are intermingled with the muscle fibers supplied by the next adjacent spinal nerve. This is very much like the intermingling of the peripheral muscle fibers of two or three adjacent motor units. Nevertheless, there is a degree of segmental representation in the innervation of the pectoralis major muscle, so that destruction of the medial pectoral nerve or nerves at surgery will show palsy and atrophy of the lower part of the pectoralis major (the abdominal and sternal part, or the sternocostal part). For example, in the Patey type of modified radical mastectomy, excision of the pectoralis minor and destruction of the medial pectoral nerve twigs that penetrated or were closely associated with the pectoralis minor would cause palsy and ultimate atrophy of the lower part of the pectoralis major (most especially the sternocostal portion). However, the lateral pectoral nerves that arose form the lateral cord of the brachial plexus and are distributed to the upper part (including the clavicular head and uppermost part of the sternocostal head) are out of harm's way as they pierce the upper part of the clavipectoral fascia to reach the deep surface of the upper part of the pectoralis major.[14]

Moosman,[15] in a study of 100 pectoral regions in adult cadavers of both sexes, found that the medial pectoral nerve or nerves had a variety of relationships to the pectoralis minor. The medial pectoral nerve as a single nerve swerved around the lateral border of the pectoralis minor in 38 percent of his cases. The medial pectoral nerve or nerves pierced through the pectoralis minor on their way to the pectoralis major in 62 percent of pectoral regions. The medial pectoral nerve divided into two branches, one branch passing around the lateral border of the pectoralis minor and the other branch piercing the muscle to reach pectoralis major in 32 percent of specimens. The medial pectoral nerve presented as a single nerve that pierced through the pectoralis minor in 22 percent of cases. Moosman found the medial pectoral nerve presenting as two or three branches, all of which penetrated through the pectoralis minor to reach the pectoralis major in 8 percent of cases. Very rarely, he found the medial pectoral nerve passing through the medial margin of the pectoralis minor or remaining entirely to the medial side of the muscle, and therefore piercing only the clavipectoral fascia on the way to the pectoralis major. It must be pointed out that Moosman chose to reverse the names of these nerves to make them conform with their topographic relationship to the sagittal plane, but in these extractions from his report the names have been converted back to the standard anatomic method of naming them for the cord from which they arise.

Other authors contributing anatomic insight into the nerve and blood supply of the pectoralis major and pectoralis minor muscles are Tobin[16] and Morain and colleagues,[17] but their data relate to segmental pectoralis major muscle flaps to be applied elsewhere rather than to the interests and scope of this book. The same applies to the report of Harrison.[18]

The innervation of the skin of the breast comes from the third to the sixth intercostal nerves by two different routes. The anterior ends of those intercostal nerves turn superficially as the anterior cutaneous nerves and, passing through the intercostal space near the sternum, then penetrate through the pectoralis major muscle and divide into short medial cutaneous branches, which go only to the midline of the body and longer lateral branches that extend approximately to the midclavicular or nipple line. These branches reach the breast and, innervating its medial half, are called *medial mammary branches.* A lateral cutaneous nerve arises from each intercostal nerve below the second intercostal nerve. The intercostobrachial nerve is the equivalent branch of the second intercostal nerve. These lateral cutaneous branches arise approximately in the midaxillary or midlateral line, and divide into anterior and posterior branches that appear in the superficial fascia after slipping through the intervals between the digitations of the serratus anterior muscle. The posterior branches run posteriorly over the superficial surface of the latissimus dorsi to approximately the angles of the ribs, where they meet the lateral branches of the cutaneous branches of the posterior primary divisions of their respective thoracic spinal nerve. The anterior branch of the lateral cutaneous branch of the intercostal nerve passes forward over the surface of the serratus anterior to then cross the lateral border of the pectoralis major and extend medially as a lateral mammary branch. This nerve finally meets the previously mentioned lateral branch of the anterior cutaneous branch of the same intercostal nerve. Thus, the innervation of a dermatome has been developed.

A junction line dividing the breast into medial and lateral halves would seem to be formed, but this is too idealized. In a given case the nipple and areola might be supplied solely by either the medial or lateral mammary branch rather than shared by both. The junction line varies from one intercostal level to the next. Only down the midline of the body, ventrally and dorsally, is there any degree of constancy of the line of junction between the fields of distribution between nerves. Thus, it is not possible to predict in any given instance whether the innervation of the nipple and areola comes from the medial or lateral mammary nerves, or is shared by both. At the junction zone of the two approaching nerves, some degree of overlap and mixing inevitably occurs, as with all adjacent nerve fields.

The precise nature of the innervation of the nipple and areola differs somewhat from the innervation of the skin elsewhere over the breast. The nipple and areola are nearly devoid of hairs, whereas the rest of the skin of the breast has many hairs, but they are fine. The nature of the nerve endings and the sensitivity of this hairy skin is comparable with hairy skin elsewhere over the limbs and trunk. The hair and its follicle, with associated nerve fibers, is part of the sensory apparatus itself. The nipple and areola, lacking hairs (almost) and possessed of many specialized nerve endings, seem to be innervated in such a way as to make them sensitive to certain types of stimuli and to be able to respond reflexly in a manner that enhances suckling, but leaves them devoid of or weak in other common types of skin sensitivity.[19]

LYMPHATIC DRAINAGE OF BREAST

The lymphatic drainage of the breast has been described in the literature for many years with varying degrees of detail and, slowly but constantly, changing descriptions and understanding or interpretations. Problems of interpretation arise in (1) the complexity of connections between lymphatic vessels and lymph node groups, (2) the understanding of the volume flow through the various alternative pathways, (3) the variations of pathways from person to person that can be shown to exist with great frequency, and (4) the alterations of pathways that inevitably occur with obstructions of the vessels due to metastatic carcinoma of the breast. For example, if carcinoma of the gland proper has spread by direct extension into the overlying skin, an additional and different pathway of metastasis has been made possible owing to the addition of the purely cutaneous lymphatic drainage routes. Pathways of lymph flow from the breast are multiple in normal circumstances, and the proportionate flow in each pathway has been difficult to judge from cadaver studies or by deduction from an analysis of nodal metastases. Hence, there is much disagreement, confusion, and outright error in the literature. Furthermore, authors often use the nomenclature differently and thus confuse the unwary reader. Injection studies have been done for over 100 years and have introduced errors into the literature due both to interpretation and to technique.

Lymph flow from the mammary gland proper begins in the lobules of the mammary gland and is directed through the multiply valved collecting trunks deeply toward the basal or deep surface of the breast, where the trunks aggregate and follow the axillary tail of breast tissue around the lateral border of pectoralis major. Here they pierce the axillary fascia and extend toward the *pectoral* or *anterior axillary nodes*, which are some four to six in number. However, some of these trunks may pass directly to the *central group of axillary nodes*, which number only three or four but are usually in vague continuity with the other groups. This group warrants its title of "central" nodes not only because it is centrally placed within the axillary fat mass, but because it receives lymph from the *lateral group of nodes*, the *pectoral group*, and the *posterior axillary* or *subscapular nodes* (Fig. 1-4). This latter group of six to eight nodes lies along the subscapular artery at the lateral margin of the subscapularis muscle, and receives the lymphatic drainage of the back of the thorax and shoulder. The pectoral nodes run with the lateral thoracic artery and receive the drainage from the anterolateral thoracic wall skin in general and the mammary gland itself.

The central group of nodes receives lymphatic flow via afferents from both the pectoral and the subscapular groups of nodes and also from the *lateral group of nodes*. This group of five to eight nodes receives afferents from the upper limb, and the nodes lie medial to, and behind or posterior to, the axillary vein. Thus, there is a kind of three-way convergence from the lateral group, the pectoral group, and the subscapular group to reach the central group in the manner of the legs of a tripod. In turn, the central group of nodes send their lymph via afferents that accompany the axillary vein to the *apical group of axillary nodes*. This group of nodes is partly at, but mostly just above or medial to, the upper border of the pectoralis minor, and extends along the medial (costal) surface of the axillary vein to reach the apex of the axilla. At the apex the subclavius muscle and the first rib lie close together, barely permitting the axillary vein to continue through the interval to lie on the upper surface of the first rib as the *subclavian vein*. The apical nodes are also called the subclavian nodes because they are subclavicular, not because they are on the subclavian vein.

The efferent lymph trunk (or trunks) passing from the apical nodes to the jugulosubclavian venous angle (junction) is called the *subclavian trunk*. On the left side it commonly empties into the thoracic duct, which in turn empties into the left jugulosubclavian venous angle. In the axilla, as elsewhere in the body, the lymphatic channels tend to follow arteries, but in a retrograde fashion, as far as flow is concerned. Because of the vena comitans, some authors prefer to relate them primarily to the veins rather than to arteries.

A subsidiary and inconstant (at least, at times undemonstrable) pathway of lymph drainage from the breast is via its deep surface and directly into and through the thickness of the pectoralis major. Lymphatics then emerge from the deep surface of the latter muscle and ascend between the two pectoral muscles, where there are likely to be one or two *interpectoral nodes* (nodes of Rothman and Rotter).

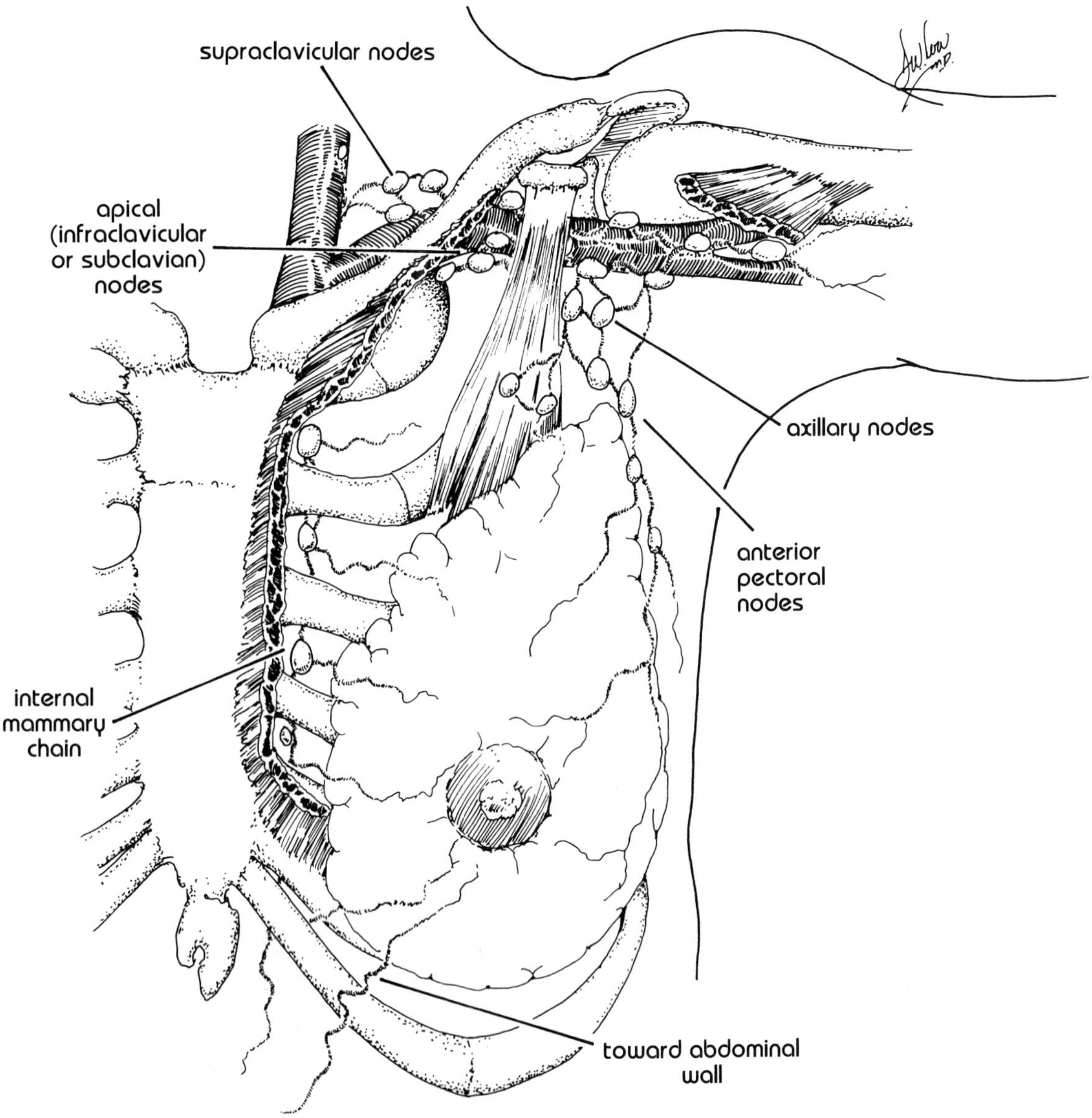

FIGURE 1-4 Lymphatic drainage of the breast illustrating groups of nodes and collecting trunks. Note the axillary tail of Spence and the anterior pectoral nodes draining into the central axillary nodes. The supraclavicular nodes are the lower nodes of the deep cervical or internal jugular chain of nodes. These nodes are sampled in so-called "scalene node biopsy." The two nodes seen on the anterior surface of the pectoralis minor are the nodes of Rotter, or interpectoral nodes.

This lymphatic vessel then pierces the clavipectoral fascia and joins the apical nodes. Its course parallels one of the pectoral branches of the thoracoacromial axis.

Another minor pathway is from the breast superolaterally to the infraclavicular nodes. This pathway parallels the cephalic vein and the deltoid branch of the thoracoacromial axis in the cleft between the deltoideus and the clavicular head of the pectoralis major. This lymph vessel then turns deeply into the deltopectoral trigone, and there, before piercing the clavipectoral fascia, the vessel passes into the one or two *infraclavicular nodes*. The efferents from these nodes then pierce the fascia and join the apical nodes. It is seen that the infraclavicular nodes are, in truth, infraclavicular, but they are not in the axillary fossa, and thus the term "infraclavicular nodes" is not synonymous with apical nodes or subclavian nodes, as is occasionally said.

The *supraclavicular nodes* are actually the *lower nodes* of the *deep cervical* chain, but they do communicate with the apical nodes, and hence metastases from the breast can occur here. These lower nodes of the deep cervical chain also communicate with the bronchomediastinal trunks on both sides and with the thoracic duct on the left side. Thus, the possibility of malignant neoplasms of the mediastinum and abdomen spreading to these lower nodes of the deep cervical chain (supraclavicular nodes) must be born in mind when a lump develops here behind the lower end of the sternocleidomastoid muscle and in front of the lower end of the scalenus anterior muscle, just above the first rib. This metastatic mass is often called Virchow's or Troisier's node, or simply the "sentinel" node.

After the axillary pathway, the next most important pathway of lymphatic spread of breast malignancy is via the *internal thoracic* (*internal mammary*) chain of nodes. Lymph from the more medial portion of the breast (although actually it can come from any portion) flows in vessels that penetrate the medial part of the pectoralis major. Passing into one, two, or three of the intercostal spaces, accompanying the anterior penetrating branches of the intercostal arteries, the lymph vessels then reach the lymph nodes of the *internal thoracic chain of nodes* (*parasternal nodes*). The efferents ascending in company with the internal thoracic artery end by joining the bronchomediastinal trunk, and this carries the lymph to the jugulosubclavian venous angle. Turner-Warwick,[20] studying the flow of lymph from the breast by intravital techniques in human patients, including radioactive colloidal gold (Au^{198}), to determine the pathways, concluded that approximately 75 percent of the total lymph from the breast flowed to the ipsilateral axillary nodes and about 25 percent drained into the ipsilateral internal thoracic chain of nodes. His studies showed that normally there is no drainage of lymph from the breast to the contralateral axillary nodes or to the contralateral internal thoracic nodes. However, in cases of advanced metastases he found patients who did have contralateral metastases, and concluded that it was not due to normally occurring cross-over lymph channels, as Oelsner[21] contended, but to ipsilateral lymphatic blockage by tumor, surgery, or irradiation that forced a contralateral spread via the midline anastomoses of skin and subcutaneous lymphatic vessels.

Turner-Warwick also demonstrated that the posterior intercostal nodes receive a small amount of drainage from the breast. This is a pathway that parallels the anterior cutaneous branch of the lateral perforating artery that arises at the midaxillary line from the posterior or aortic intercostal artery. With the lymph flowing in an opposite direction to the arterial flow, the lymph vessels finally reach the posterior intercostal nodes near the spinal column. Although very little lymph flows along this route, it offers an explanation for metastases in unexpected places. According to Turner-Warwick's findings, the subareolar lymphatic network is not an important outflow pathway from the breast, as has usually been concluded from cadaver injection studies, but is merely a site of anastomosis between skin lymphatic channels and the intrinsic breast lymph channels, which are draining deeply toward the deep surface of the breast rather than outward toward the skin. Turner-Warwick's studies showed that there is no tendency for any particular quadrant of the breast to drain in one direction only. All quadrants can drain to the axillary nodes, the parasternal nodes, or the posterior intercostal nodes. Of course, as previously stated, the volume flow to each of these three sites is very different, but there is no quadrant specificity, as has been so often stated.

References

1. Hicken NF. Mastectomy: A clinical pathologic study demonstrating why most mastectomies result in incomplete removal of the mammary gland. Arch Surg 1940; 40:6.
2. Gershon-Cohen J. Atlas of mammography. New York: Springer-Verlag, 1970.
3. Goldman LD, Goldwyn RM. Some anatomical considerations of subcutaneous mastectomy. Plast Reconstr Surg 1973; 51:501.
4. Goodnight JE Jr, Quagliana JM, Morton DL. Failure of subcutaneous mastectomy to prevent the development of breast cancer. J Surg Oncol 1984; 26:198.
5. Moon HK, Dowden RV. Lumbar hernia after latissimus dorsi flap. Plast Reconstr Surg 1985; 75:417.
6. Marcus GH. Untersuchungen über die arterielle Blutversorgung der Mamilla. Arch Klin Chir 1934. 179:361.
7. Maliniac JW. Arterial blood supply of the breast. Arch Surg 1943; 47:329.
8. Manchot P. The cutaneous arteries of the human body. Republished 1889 edition with translation and historical annotation and commentary by William D. Morain. New York: Springer-Verlag, 1983.
9. Mayou BJ, Whitby D, Jones BM. The scapular flap—an anatomical and clinical study. Br J Plast Surg 1982; 35:8.
10. Gahhos FN, Tross RB, Salomon JC. Scapular free-flap dissection made easier. Plast Reconstr Surg 1985; 75:115.
11. Huelke DF. Variations in the origins of the branches of the axillary artery. Anat Rec 1959; 135:33.
12. Farrow JH. Thrombophlebitis of the superficial veins of the breast and anterior chest wall (Mondor's disease). Surg Gynecol Obstet 1955; 101:63.
13. El Sahy NI. Recurrent Mondor's disease after augmentation mammoplasty. Aesthetic Plast Surg 1983; 7:259.
14. Scanlon EF. The importance of the anterior thoracic nerves in modified radical mastectomy. Surg Gynecol Obstet 1981; 152:789.
15. Moosman DA. Anatomy of the pectoral nerves and their preservation in modified mastectomy. Am J Surg 1980; 139:883.
16. Tobin GR. Pectoralis major segmental anatomy and segmentally split pectoralis major flaps. Plast Reconstr Surg 1985; 75:814.
17. Morain WD, Colen LB, Hutchings JC. The segmental pectoralis major muscle flap: A function-preserving procedure. Plast Reconstr Surg 1985; 75:825.
18. Harrison DH. The pectoralis minor vascularized muscle graft for the treatment of unilateral facial palsy. Plast Reconstr Surg 1985; 75:206.
19. Miller MR, Kashara M. The cutaneous innervation of the human female breast. Anat Rec 1959; 135:153.
20. Turner-Warwick RT. The lymphatics of the breast. Br J Surg 1959; 46:574.
21. Oelsner L. Anatomische Untersuchunger über die Lymphwege der Brust mit Bezug auf die Ausbreitung des Mammacarcinoms. Arch Klin Chir 1901; 64:134.

CHAPTER 2

Embryology of the Breast

STEVEN R. COHEN, M.D.

Breast diseases in the pediatric-aged population are not uncommon. Deformities may be congenital or acquired, and may become manifest at any point during pre- and postnatal development. This chapter is written in order to familiarize the practicing plastic surgeon with the embryology and pathophysiology of congenital breast diseases. Techniques of reconstruction and further discussion of specific derangements are presented elsewhere in this textbook.

The development of the human embryo begins with the establishment of the posterior body wall and ends with the formation of the anterior body wall.[1] The anterior wall is at first represented only by the somatopleure of the overhanging head and tail folds of the embryo, the middle portion being occupied by the body stock and open midgut. Closure proceeds simultaneously from cranial, caudal, and lateral directions, centering on the site of the future umbilical ring (Fig. 2-1).[2] The reduction in size of the body stalk relative to that of the umbilical cord, and the final separation of the cord at birth, completes the development of the anterior body wall.

The anterior thoracic wall and the epigastric portion of the abdominal wall are first represented by the ventral portion of the head fold of the embryo.[3] Most of the primitive wall consists of somatopleure covering the ventral wall of the pericardial cavity. The somatopleure is comprised of a layer of ectoderm and mesoderm. From its ectodermal layer skin will form, but the other components of the definitive body wall will be derived from invading dorsal mesoderm.

During the sixth week, the dorsolateral mesoderm beings to expand into the lateral body wall, forming a sheet obliterating the segmental character of the somites. Extensions of the lateral vertebral processes, the future ribs, accompany the mesodermal extensions, but by the end of the sixth week they lag behind the invading mesoderm from the myotomes. The most cranial elements reach the midline first and the heart moves caudal to this area of fusion to assume its normal thoracic position. The advancing edge of the mesoderm forms a longitudinal rectus thoracis, which corresponds to the rectus abdominis of the lower body wall. It is usually transitory, but occasionally remains on one or both sides as the sternalis muscle.[1] The greater part of the mesodermal sheet splits to form three layers: the external intercostal muscles, the internal intercostal muscles, and an inner layer represented by the transverse thoracic muscle. All of these layers are differentiated by the middle of the seventh week.

The sternum appears during the sixth week as a pair of parallel mesenchymal bands. They begin to chondrify almost at once. During the seventh week the sternal bands join at their cephalic ends and gradually fuse in the midline throughout their length. The fusion progresses with decreasing rapidity to cease during the ninth or tenth weeks, by which time it is usually complete. Often, however, the most caudal portion, the xiphoid process, remains bifid.[1] During the fifth to sixth weeks of human fetal development, before the embryonic wall is completely invaded by dorsolateral mesoderm, two lateral ridges or thickened ectoderm appear between the basis of the anterior and posterior limb buds (Fig. 2-2). In the human embryo, the caudal two-thirds and the most cranial portion of this embryonic milk streak are transitory. In the region of the thorax, the so-called "galactic band" develops to form a mammary ridge, whereas the remaining streak regresses. Incomplete regression or dispersion of the primitive galactic band leads to accessory mammary tissues found in 2 to 6 percent of adult women.[1,3-5]

At 7 to 8 weeks of gestation, a thickening occurs in the mammary anlage. Invagination into the chest wall mesenchyme results in flattening of the ridge by 10 to 14 weeks of gestation. Between 12 and 16 weeks, mesenchymal cells differentiate into the smooth muscle of the nipple and areola. Epithelial buds develop and then branch to form 15 to 25 strips of epithelium. These strips represent the future secretory alveoli. The secondary mammary anlage then develops with differentiation of hair follicles, sebaceous glands, and sweat gland elements.

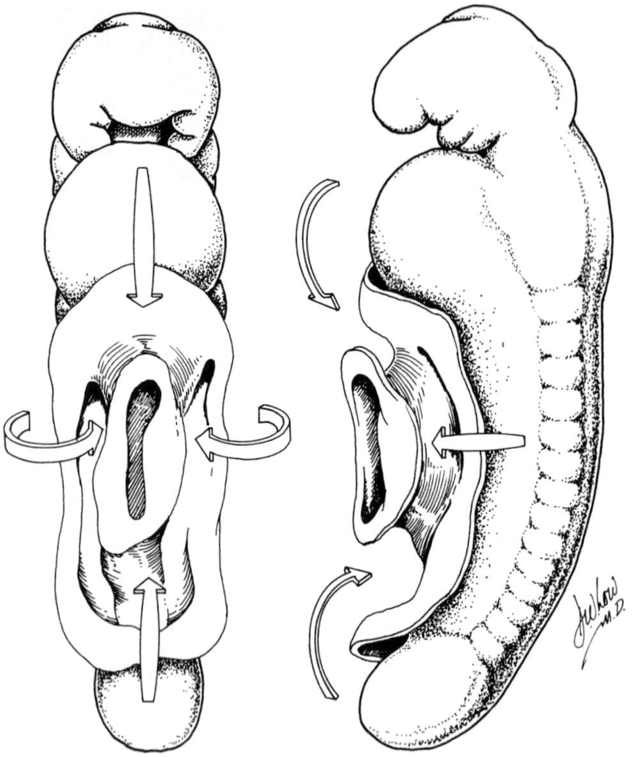

FIGURE 2-1 Direction of closure of the anterior body wall. (From Duhamel B. Embryology of exomphalos and allied malformations. Arch Dis Child 1963; 38:142.)

It is believed that phylogenetically, the breast develops from sweat gland tissue. In addition, special aprocrine glands develop to form Montgomery glands around the nipple. During the third trimester of pregnancy, placental sex hormones enter the fetal circulation and induce canalization of the epithelial tissues.[5] This process continues from the 20th to the 32nd week of gestation. At about term, 15 to 25 mammary ducts are formed, with coalescence of duct and sebaceous glands near the epidermis. Further differentiation occurs at 32 to 40 weeks, leading to the development of lobular-alveolar structures that contain colostrum (witch's milk). There is a fourfold increase in mammary gland mass at this time, and the nipple-areolar complex develops and becomes pigmented. In the neonate, the stimulated mammary tissue secretes colostral milk, which can be expressed from the nipple for 4 to 7 days postpartum in the majority of neonates of either sex. In the newborn, colostral secretion declines over a 3 to 4 week period, secondary to involution of the breast following the withdrawal of placental hormones.[5] During early childhood, under the influence of prolactin and insulin, the end vesicles become further canalized and develop into ductal structures by further growth and branching.

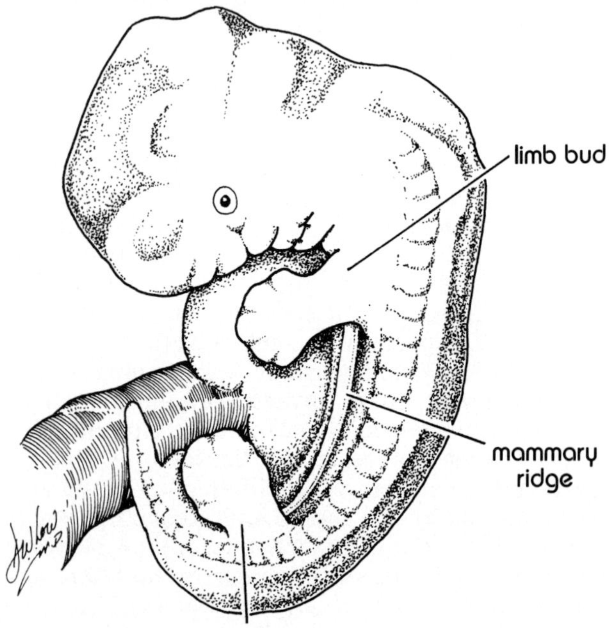

FIGURE 2-2 Depiction of the embryonic milk streak.

TISSUE EPITHELIUM-MESENCHYME INTERACTION IN THE FETAL MAMMARY GLAND

Although descriptive embryology enables surgeons to picture the complex sequence of events that lead to the formation of the breast, tissue combination and organ culture studies have yielded the greatest amount of insight into the mechanisms at work. Development of the embryo depends on cell and tissue interaction. In early stages, inductive interactions between blastemas and tissues are responsible for the diversification of cell types. Later, interaction between already committed cell populations is required for the precise development of the complex structures of vertebrate organs.[13]

Developmental interdependence of these tissues has been demonstrated by means of tissue separation and experimental recombination. In the case of epithelial-mesenchymal organs, such as the breast, studies have shown that in most cases epithelial development depends on the presence of mesenchymal cells.[14] Dependence on the mesenchyme is most obvious during formation of an organ, however, epithelial-stromal interactions probably continue to play a role in the stabilization of adult organ structure. Conversely, disturbance or destabilization of these tissue relationships in the adult may be intimately involved in pathologic processes.[13]

Two special features distinguish the mammary gland from otherwise comparable organs.[13] First, although the development of most epithelial-mesenchymal organs is more or less completed during the embryonic or fetal period, the mammary gland continues to undergo major developmental changes throughout life, suggesting that morphogenetic interaction between epithelium and stroma persists in the adult organ. Second, unlike the situation found in most other glands and gland-like organs, growth and morphogenesis of the mammary gland are regulated by hormones.

Mesenchymal Induction

In most mammals, the epithelium of the mammary gland is derived from the embryonic epidermis.[13] The earliest morphologic indication of breast development is the formation of a band or streak of thickened epithelium referred to as the mammary band (crest) or milk line. In species with numerous pairs of glands, such as the mouse, the milk line runs from the forelimb to the inguinal region. The mammary ridge eventually gives rise to the individual mammary buds. Even those species with only one pair of glands, such as the human, pass through this primitive milkline stage.

To elucidate the possible role of the underlying mesenchyme in the aforementioned developmental sequence, Propper performed tissue combination experiments in the rabbit.[15] Normally, a prominent mammary band forms on day 13. If 12-day-old epidermis from the prospective mammary region is placed on mesenchyme from other areas, no mammary ridge develops. However, when 12-day-old "neutral" epidermis (from the rabbit's head or neck region) is combined with 12-day-old mammary mesenchyme, breast structures develop. From these experiments it seemed that the mesenchyme initiated mammary development, and formation of the mammary crest depended on mesenchymal induction.

The concept of mesenchymal induction and its role in mammary development is supported by the experience derived from analysis of skin development in general. Usually it is the dermal component that determines position, patterning, and type of skin appendages formed in experimental dermis and epidermis combination.[16]

The actual epithelial response to mesenchymal induction is still unknown, but it does not appear to involve a local increase in cell proliferation. Balinsky found reduced mitotic indices in early mammary epithelium as compared to neighboring epidermis.[17] Kratochwil's studies with tritiated thymidine showed even distribution of DNA-synthesizing cells throughout the epidermis during formation of mammary buds in the 11- and 12-day-old mouse embryo.[13]

By day 13, thymidine-incorporating mammary epithelial cells virtually disappeared, yet the mammary buds themselves continued to increase in size. It was proposed that the thickening of the mammary placode and the early growth of the bud was therefore caused by migration of epithelial cells rather than by proliferation.[18]

Sexual Dimorphism

Another unique feature of mammary gland development is that formation of the primordial bud of the mammary anlagen is not immediately followed by outgrowth and branching of the epithelium, as seen in other glands or gland-like organs. Instead, the mammary rudiment passes through an extended period of slow growth with little or no morphogenetic activity (Fig. 2-3). In the mouse gland, the epithelial buds form between days 11 and 12, but outgrowth of the primary sprout does not begin until 16½ days.[13] Similar quiescent periods have been observed in the development of the mammary gland in a variety of other species.[17] Dimorphism in the development of the mouse mammary gland has been extensively reviewed by Kratochwil.[13,19] It appears that in the female mouse embryo the epithelial bud changes very little between days 12 and 16. The mesenchyme under the 11-day placode and around the 12-day bud is morphologically inconspicuous. During the next few days, the nearest mesenchymal cells tangentially orient themselves around the epithelial bud and, by day 14, form a mesenchymal capsule. The most characteristic property of this mesenchyme is its possession of steroid receptors.

Kratochwil goes on to note that the events taking place in the gland of the male mouse fetuses during the "resting phase" are more dramatic.[13] Early development up to day 13 is similar for both sexes. However, in the early hours of day 14 the mammary mesenchyme begins to condense in the male forming a compact capsule around each bud (Fig. 2-4). Later that same day, the mesenchymal condensation slips upward to the stalk of the gland in the first four gland pairs and moves under the bud in the fifth. In the anterior four glands the stalk stretches and eventually ruptures with the gland epithelium becoming permanently separated from the epidermis. The cells of the stalk remaining with the epidermis become necrotic and disappear. This destruction of the male mammary anlagen is caused by testicular androgens as shown by experiments in vivo and in vitro.[21] Apparently this sexual dimorphism in the mouse is not typical for all mammals. However, it does provide insight into the interplay between hormone action and epithelial-mesenchymal tissue interaction.

The Development of Hormone Responsiveness

Tissue interaction in the development of hormone responsiveness has also been discussed by Kratochwil.[13,19] The testosterone-induced destruction of the mammary anlagen in the male mouse fetus takes place on day 14. In vitro experiments have shown that during mammary development, an anlagen-responsive "window" exists for a brief period of time (see Fig. 2-3). The mammary rudiment becomes sensitive to the hormone late on day 13, but is no longer responsive by day 15.[22] The development of hormone responsiveness correlates well with the development of specific anlagen-binding sites.[23] In an experiment performed by Kratochwil, whole mammary rudiments explanted on day 12 became anlagen responsive in vitro over the course of time. It was therefore surmised that the development of testosterone-responsiveness was controlled by processes within the gland rudiment itself.[22] When

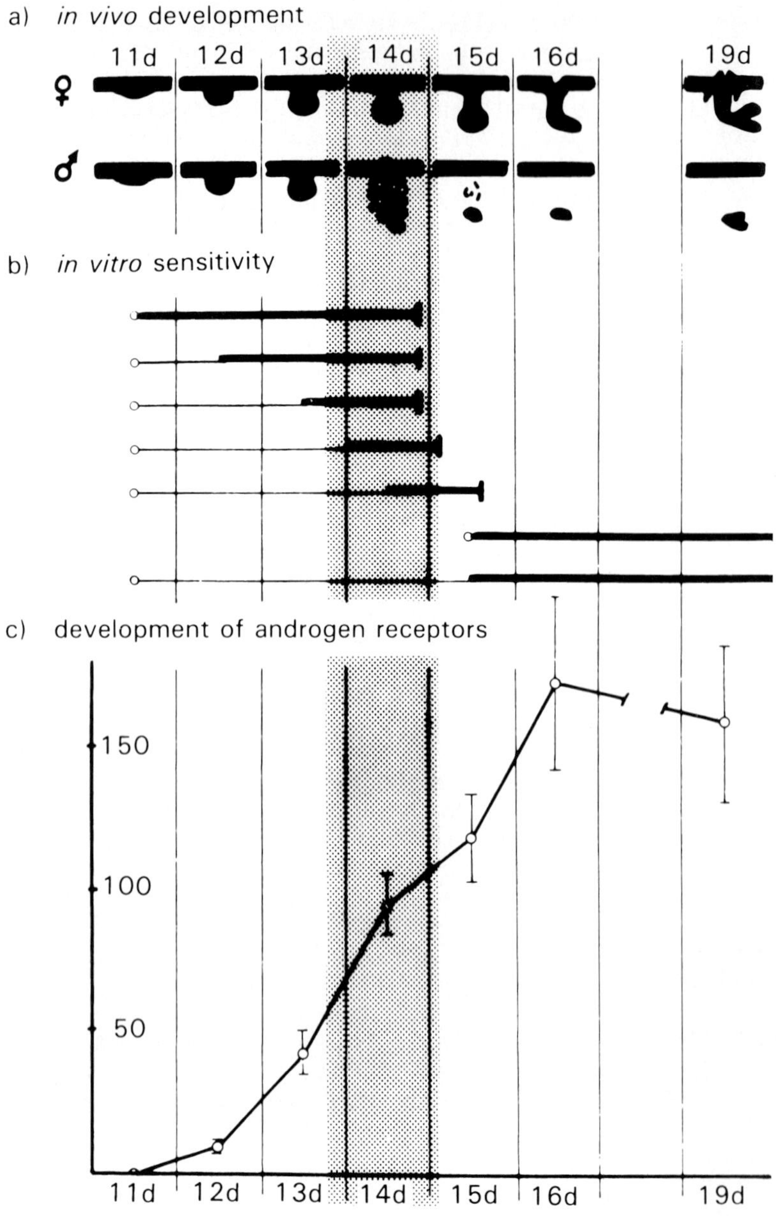

FIGURE 2–3 Schematic representation of experiments demonstrating the androgen-responsive "window" in the embryonic development of the mammary gland, correlating with development of androgen receptors. (a) Morphological stages of gland development in male and female fetuses. Sexual dimorphism becomes apparent on day 14, 36 to 48 hours after differentiation of the gonad. (b) Development of explanted 11-day rudiments exposed to testosterone in vitro. Thin line: Culture in the absence of hormone. Heavy line: Culture in the presence of hormone. When testosterone was present from the beginning (first line), formation and early development of the gland buds was not affected. However, after 3 days in vitro at a stage corresponding to a 14-day embryo, the gland rudiments were destroyed. The time of hormone addition during the first 48 hours in vitro was found to be irrelevant for the time of the response (destruction), indicating that the tissues had not yet become responsive. The first groups of explants showing delayed reaction were those having received the hormone at a stage corresponding to late day 13 (4th and 5th lines), indicating the onset of the sensitive period. Explants of 15-day (female) glands were no longer affected by testosterone (6th line), showing that the organ has again become insensitive to the hormone. The short period of the testosterone-responsive "window," as determined by these experiments, is indicated by the shaded area. Last line: Glands from 15-day embryos and explants of earlier stages cultured for the corresponding period in vitro, lose their sensitivity to testosterone, indicating that both acquisition (top lines) and loss of androgen responsiveness occur in vitro, apparently governed by an intrinsic developmental program of the gland itself.[22] Note that the number of testosterone-binding sites increases markedly with the acquisition of testosterone responsiveness, whereas the loss of hormone sensitivity at day 15 is not at all correlated with a loss or even decrease of receptors.[23] (From Kratochwil K. Tissue combination and organ culture studies in the development of the embryonic mammary gland. In: Gwatkin RBI, ed. Developmental biology. Vol. 4. New York: Plenum Publishing, 1986:315.)

mesenchyme without epithelium was explanted, no testosterone responsiveness was demonstrated.[24] The role of mammary epithelium in the development of hormone responsiveness was revealed by ^{3}H-testosterone autoradiographs on 14-day-old mammary rudiments.[25] Steroid binding was restricted to the first few layers of mesenchymal cells around each gland bud (Fig. 2–5). This distribution was felt to suggest that mammary epithelium had induced the formation of hormone receptors in the immediately adjacent mesenchyme. Thus, Kratochwil goes on to say, "hormone action and epithelium-mesenchyme tissue interaction are interdependent in at least two steps during mammary development. First, an inductive signal from the epithelium causes a synthesis of steroid receptors in adjacent mesenchymal cells. Then in the second step, testosterone-stimulated mesenchymal cells destroy the epithelial anlage in the male fetus. Similarly, outgrowth of the epithelial sprout can be prevented by estrogens acting on the surrounding mesenchyme."[13]

Mammary Ductal Outgrowth

Mammary ductal outgrowth from the primordial mammary bud begins after the previously described, extended period of morphogenetic inactivity (see Fig. 2–3). In the female mouse fetus, outgrowth of a single primary sprout occurs at 16½ days in the thoracic glands and at 17 days in the inguinal glands. The time course of these developments does not appear to be regulated by hormonal changes within the fetus.[26] The outgrowing epithelial sprout breaks through the capsular mesenchyme and enters the

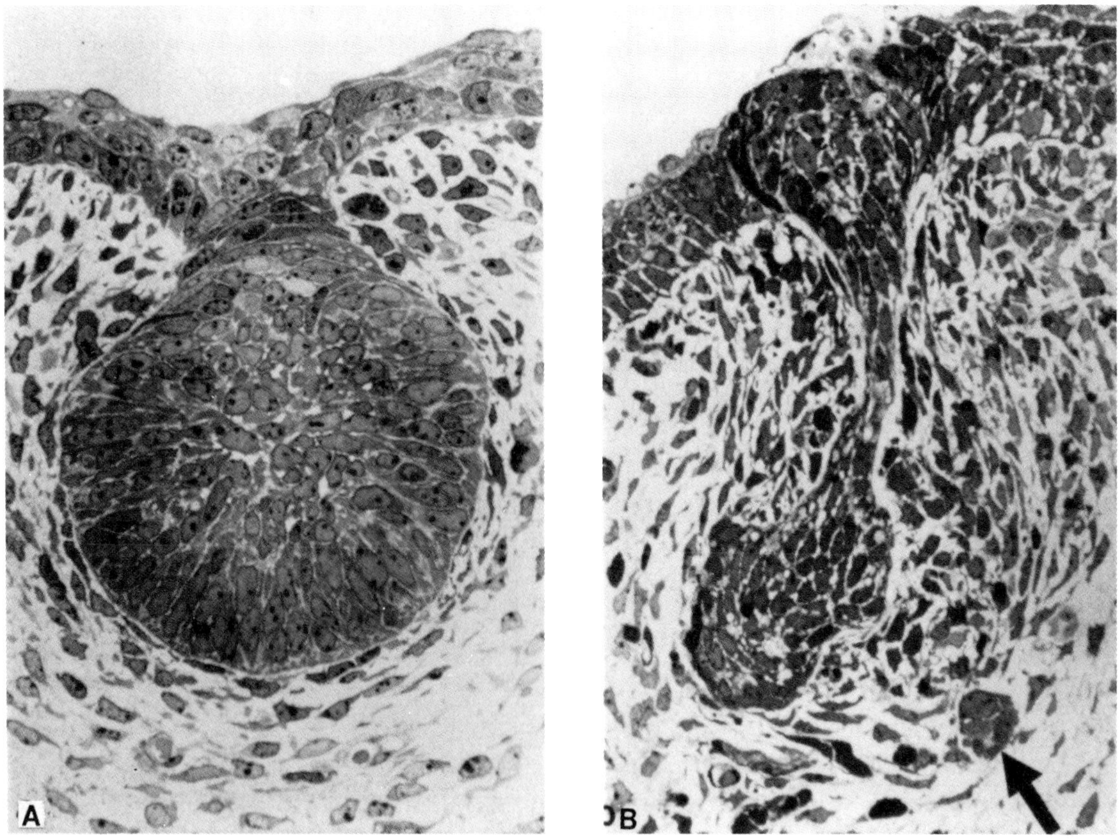

FIGURE 2-4 Histologic sections of 14-day mammary rudiments of a female (A) and a male (B) embryo. In the male, the gland is at an early stage of the androgen-induced destruction. The epithelial bud has become surrounded by dense mesenchyme and is still connected to the epidermis by a narrow "stalk." A few hours later, the lower portion of the gland epithelium will soon break free from the epidermis and become necrotic. (From Kratochwil K. Tissue combination and organ culture studies in the development of the embryonic mammary gland. In: Gwatkin RBI, ed. Developmental biology. Vol. 4. New York: Plenum Publishing, 1986:315.)

mesenchyme of the future fat pad of the breast. All branching activity of the gland takes place in this "second" mesenchymal region.[27] It has been proposed that the fatty mammary stroma arising from the "second" region of mesenchyme eventually determines the characteristic morphology of the adult gland with its widely spaced ducts and branch points.[28]

In summary (Fig. 2-6), the mesenchyme induces formation of the epithelial mammary bud. Then, the young bud induces the development of fibroblastic mammary mesenchyme, characterized by the possession of androgen and estrogen receptors. On day 14 in the male (mouse) fetus, testosterone acts on these mesenchymal cells, which in turn destroy the epithelial anlage. After experimental administration of estrogen, estrogen responsive mesenchymal cells prevent outgrowth of the primary epithelial sprout. In 16- to 17-day-old fetuses, the primary sprout pushes through the fibroblastic mammary mesenchyme and invades the fat pad precursor ("second" region of mesenchyme). The properties of this second area of mesenchyme determine the further growth and branching pattern of the gland epithelium.

CONGENITAL ABNORMALITIES (Fig. 2-7)

Accessory Breasts (Fig. 2-8)

Polythelia

Polythelia, or accessory nipples, is the most frequently observed congenital breast abnormality and is seen in both sexes.[5] Supernumerary nipple tissue may be mistaken for a pigmented nevus, and may occur at any point along the milk streak from the axilla to the groin. Breast tissue found outside of this milk line is said to be ectopic. When true accessory mammary glands (polymastia) develop, they are most often located in the thorax or axilla. In Caucasians, 90 percent of supernumerary breasts are found just below the normal breast.[1] Approximately 5 percent are axillary, and the remaining 5 percent are abdominal.[1] The reverse appears to be the case in Japanese patients, where accessory breasts are found above the normal breast in 95 percent of female cases and 60 percent of male cases.[1] Accessory breast tissue below the thorax is rare. A total of 17 cases of vulvar breast tissue were reviewed by Tow and Shanmuharatnam in 1962.[7] In only two cases was there actual discharge of milk. Breast tissue and oc-

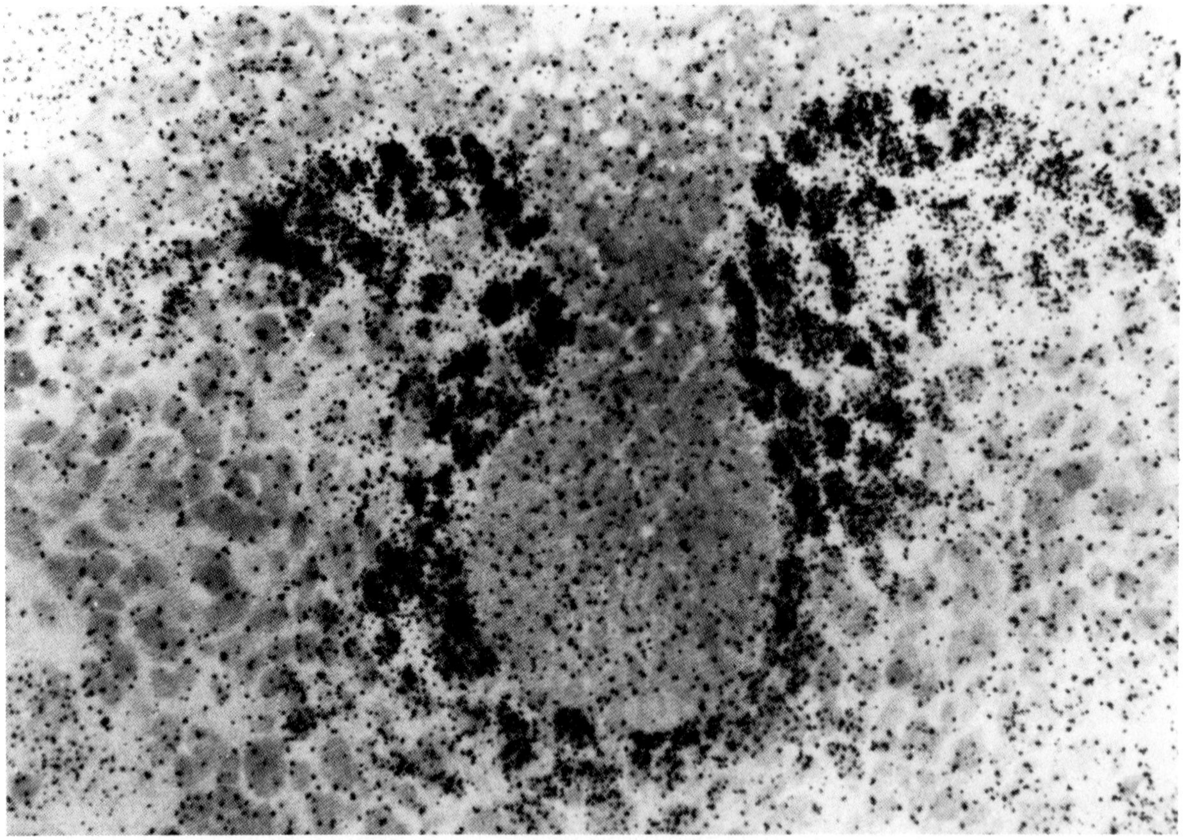

FIGURE 2–5 Distribution of [^{3}H] dihydrotestosterone-binding cells in an autoradiograph of a mammary gland from a 14-day female embryo. Note that hormone binding is restricted to the mesenchymal cells immediately adjacent to the mammary bud. (From Kratochwil K. Tissue combination and organ culture studies in the development of the embryonic mammary gland. In: Gwatkin RBI, ed. Developmental biology. Vol. 4. New York: Plenum Publishing, 1986:315.)

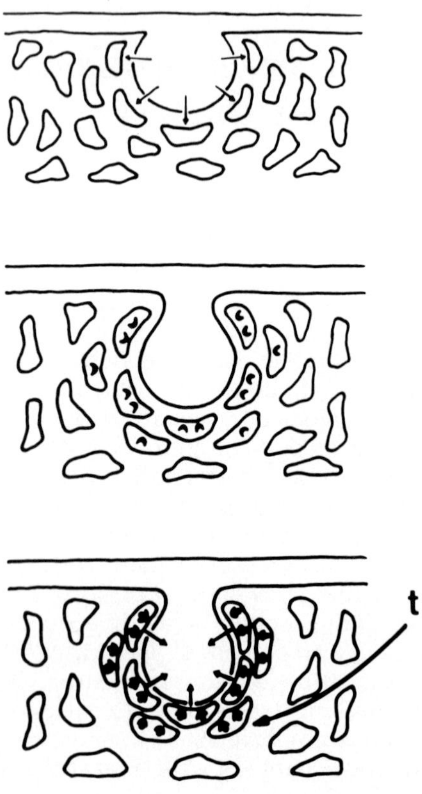

FIGURE 2–6 Schematic illustration of the current concept of epithelial-mesenchymal tissue interaction involved in the development of androgen responsiveness and in the androgen response of the embryonic mammary gland. At an early stage, apparently beginning with the formation of the primordial bud, mammary epithelium acts on neighboring mesenchyme cells and causes them to form androgen receptors. Because the epithelial "signal" is of relatively short range, cells with receptors are only found in the vicinity of the gland bud. Later, at 14 days, testosterone acts on this mesenchymal subpopulation, which then mediates indirectly the effect of the hormone on the epithelium of the gland, causing its destruction by a mechanism that remains unknown. (From Kratochwil K. Tissue combination and organ culture studies in the development of the embryonic mammary gland. In: Gwatkin RBI, ed. Developmental biology. Vol. 4. New York: Plenum Publishing, 1986:315.)

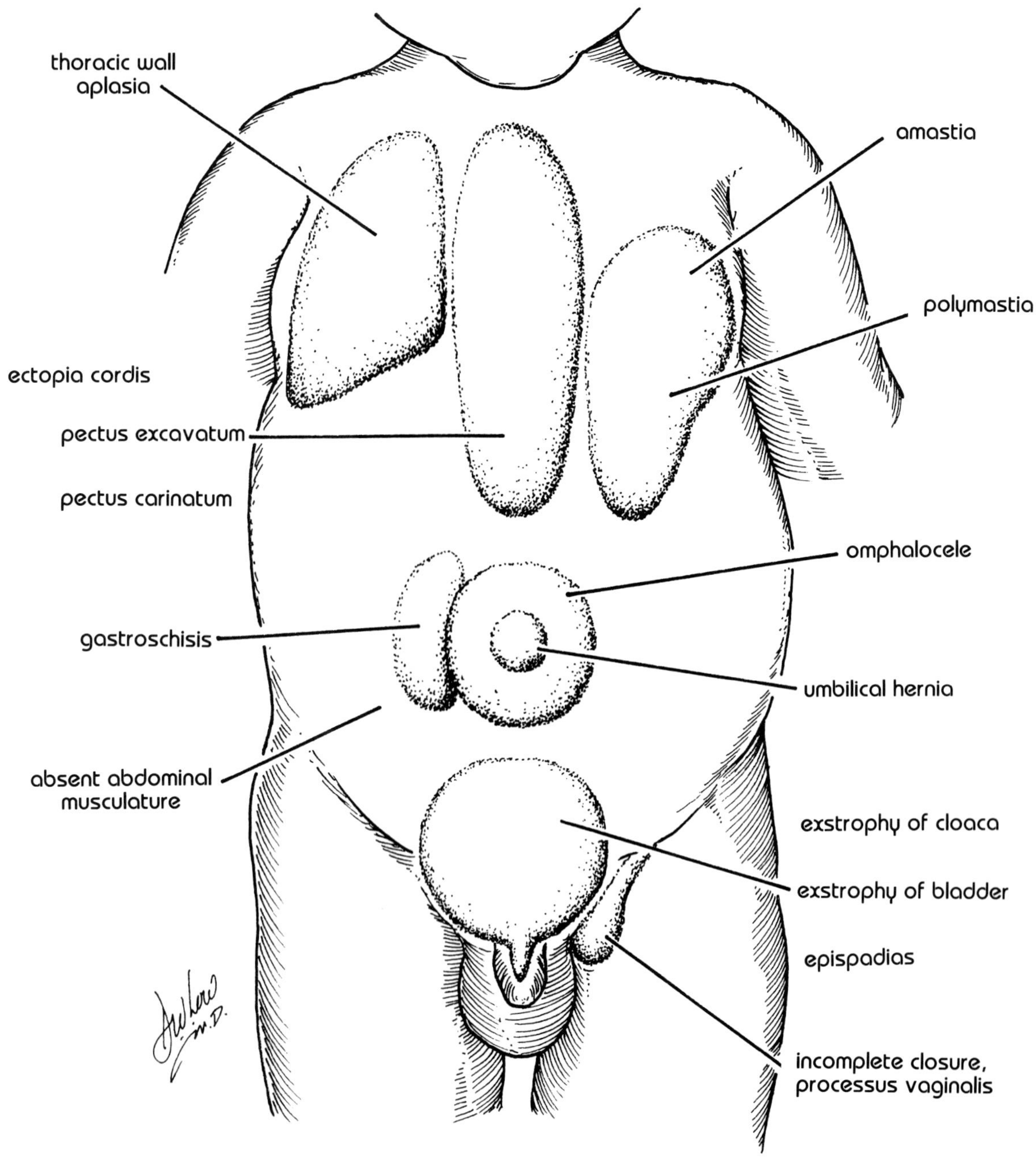

FIGURE 2-7 Range of congenital abnormalities arising secondary to failure of anterior body wall formation.

casionally functional breasts have been reported in a variety of locations outside the embryonic milk line.[1,7,8] Cases have also been reported appearing on the cheek, ear, neck, buttocks, and other locations.[8]

Not all supernumerary mammary structures deserve to be called breasts. Any combination of glandular tissue, areolar or nipple, may be present. Polymastia and polythelia are usually not accompanied by other congenital defects.[8] Unless glandular tissue is present, there are usually no symptoms. When glandular tissue exists, enlargement may lead to diagnosis of polymastia at puberty. More often, swelling during pregnancy is the presenting complaint.[8] If a nipple is present, milk may be secreted. The accessory breast may also become painful during the menstrual cycle. Accessory breasts are sub-

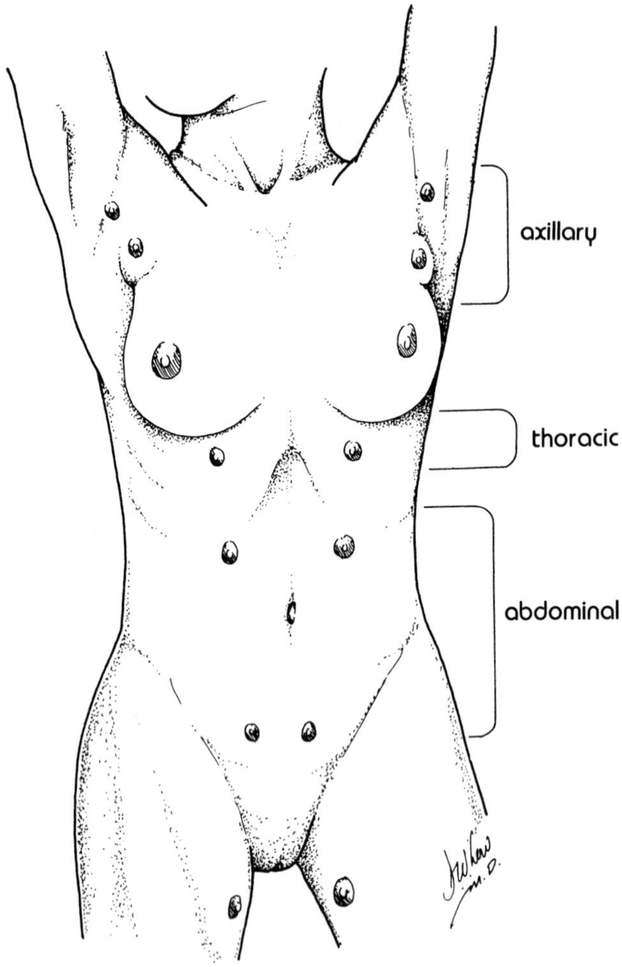

FIGURE 2-8 Locations of accessory breast tissue and/or nipples.

ject to all the diseases that occur in normal breasts.[8] Adenofibromas, cysts, and carcinomas have been reported.[8]

Hypoplasia, Amastia, and Amazia

Hypoplasia is the underdevelopment of the breast, and *amastia* is the congenital absence of the breast. When breast tissue is lacking, but a nipple is present, the condition is termed *amazia.* The wide range of breast abnormalities that have been described may be simply classified as follows:[5] (1) unilateral hypoplasia, contralateral normal; (2) bilateral hypoplasia with asymmetry; (3) unilateral hyperplasia, contralateral normal; (4) bilateral hyperplasia with asymmetry; (5) unilateral hypoplasia, contralateral hyperplasia; and (6) unilateral hypoplasia of breast, thorax, and pectoral muscles (Poland Syndrome).[11]

The majority of these abnormalities are not severe. The most severe deformity, amastia, or marked breast hypoplasia, is associated with hypoplasia of the pectoral muscle in 90 percent of the cases, but the reverse does not apply.[5] In those women with pectoral muscle abnormalities, 92 percent have a normal breast.[9] Congenital abnormalities of the pectoral muscle are usually manifested by lack of the lower third of the muscle and associated deformity of the ipsilateral rib cage. The association between the absence of the pectoral muscle, chest wall deformity, and breast abnormalities was first recognized by Poland in 1841.[10] The original description, however, did not note the concomitant abnormalities of the hand (brachysyndactyly, with hypoplasia of the middle phalanges and central skin webbing), and considerable controversy has evolved concerning the validity of the eponym for this congenital syndrome.[10]

In 1965, Trier was able to collect only 43 cases of amastia in the literature since 1839.[11] In seven of these cases, all males, the absence of breasts was associated with thin, dry, skin, absence of hair and sweat glands, saddle nose, atrophic nasal mucosa, and underdeveloped or missing teeth.[12] These patients appeared to have a generalized defect of ectodermal tissues, (hereditary anhidrotic ectodermal dysplasia) rather than simply amastia. In contrast, most examples of amastia show otherwise normal ectodermal structures, but do have local mesodermal defects, such as absence of the pectoralis muscle and occasionally one or more ribs or costal cartilages. Bilateral absence has been described, but is rare.[11]

References

1. Gray SW, Skandalakis JE. The anterior body wall. In: Embryology for surgeons. Philadelphia: W.B. Saunders, 1972:387.
2. Duhamel B. Embryology of exomphalos and allied malformations. Arch Dis Child 1963; 38:142.
3. Iwai T. A statistical study on the polymastia of the Japanese. Lancet 1907; 2:753.
4. de Cholnoky T. Supernumerary breasts. Arch Surg 1939; 39:926.
5. Osborne MD. Breast development and anatomy. In: Harris JR, Hellman S, Henderson IC, Kinne DW, eds. Breast diseases. Philadelphia: J.B. Lippincott, 1987:1.
6. Seashore JH. Disorders of the breast. In: Welch KJ, Randolph JG, Ravitch MM, O'Neill JA, Rowe MI, eds. Pediatric surgery. 4th ed. Chicago: Year Book Medical Publishers, 1986:559.
7. Tow SH, Shanmuharatnam K. Supernumerary mammary gland in the vulva. Br Med J 1962; 2:1234.
8. Haagensen CD. Anatomy of the mammary glands. In: Diseases of the breast. 3rd ed. Philadelphia: W.B. Saunders, 1986:1.
9. Peers M. Aplasias of the anterior thoracic wall: The pectoral muscle and the breast. Scand J Plast Reconstr Surg Hand Surg 1968; 2:125.
10. Ravitch MM. Congenital deformities of the chest wall. In: Welch KJ, Randolph JG, Ravitch MM, O'Neill JA,

Rowe MI, eds. Pediatric surgery. 4th ed. Chicago: Year Book Medical Publishers, 1986:559.
11. Trier WC. Complete breast absence: Case report and review of the literature. Plast Reconstr Surg 1987; 79:192.
12. Familusi JB, Jacyesimi F, Ojo CO, Attah EB. Hereditary anhidrotic ectodermal dysplasia: Studies in a Nigerian family. Arch Dis Child 1975; 50:642.
13. Kratochwil K. Epithelium-mesenchyme interaction in the fetal mammary gland. In: Medina D, Kidwell W, Heppner G, Anderson E, eds. Cellular and molecular biology of mammary cancer. New York: Plenum Publishing, 1987:67.
14. Grobstein C. Tissue interaction in the morphogenesis of mouse embryonic rudiments in vitro. In: Rudnick D, ed. Aspects of synthesis and order in growth. Princeton, NJ: Princeton University Press, 1955;233.
15. Propper A. Competence de l'epiderme embryonnaire d'Oiseau vis-a-vis de l'inducteur mammaire mesenchymateux. C R Acad Sci (Paris) 1969; 268:1423.
16. Sengel P, Dhouailly D. Tissue interactions in amniote skin development. In: Karkinen-Jaaskelainen M, Saxen L, Weiss L, eds. Cell interactions in differentiation. London: Academic Press, 1977:153.
17. Balinsky BI. On the prenatal growth of the mammary gland rudiment in the mouse. J Anat 1950; 84:227.
18. Balinsky BI. On the developmental processes in mammary glands and other epidermal structures. Trans R Soc Edinburgh 1949; 62:1.
19. Kratochwil K. Tissue combination and organ culture studies in the development of the embryonic mammary gland. In: Gwatkin RBI ed. Developmental biology. Vol. 4. New York: Plenum Publishing, 1986:315.
20. Raynaud A, Raynaud J. La production experimentale de malformations mammaires chez les foetus de Souris, par l'action des hormones sexuelles. Ann Inst Pasteur Microbiol 1956; 90:33, 90:187.
21. Kratochwil K. In vitro analysis of the hormonal basis for the sexual dimorphism in the embryonic development of the mouse mammary gland. J Embryol Exp Morph 1971; 25:141.
22. Kratochwil K. Development and loss of androgen responsiveness in the embryonic rudiment of the mouse mammary gland. Dev Biol 1977; 61:358.
23. Wasner G, Hennermann I, Kratochwil K. Ontogeny of mesenchymal androgen receptors in the embryonic mouse mammary gland. Endocrinology 1983; 113:1171.
24. Durnberger H, Kratochwil K. Specificity of tissue interaction and origin of mesenchymal cells in the androgen response of the embryonic mammary gland. Cell 1980; 19:465.
25. Heuberger B, Fitzka I, Wasner G, Kratochwil K. Induction of androgen receptor formation by epithelium-mesenchyme interaction in embryonic mouse mammary gland. Proc Natl Acad Sci USA 1982; 79:2957.
26. Kratochwil K. Organ specificity in mesenchymal induction demonstrated in the embryonic development of the mammary gland of the mouse. Dev Biol 1969; 20:46.
27. Sakakura T, Sakagami Y, Nishizuka Y. Dual origin of mesenchymal tissue participating in mouse mammary gland embryogenesis. Dev Biol 1982; 91:202.
28. Sakakura T. Epithelial-mesenchymal interactions in mammary gland development and its perturbation in relation to tumorigenesis. In: Rich MA, Hager JC, Furmanski P, eds. Understanding breast cancer. New York: Marcel Dekker 1983:261.

CHAPTER 3

Physiology and Development of the Breast

DAVID N. GOLDBERG, D.O.

ALVIN F. GOLDFARB, M.D.

The breast, although an appendage of the skin, is an endocrine organ. As such, it develops and responds under the control of the same neuroendocrine mechanisms regulating the reproductive system. Without an appreciation of this relationship, it becomes difficult to interpret changes in the breast as being functional or dysfunctional. An adequate clinical comprehension of breast function must be based on an understanding of normal physiologic modification of the breast during growth, development, and lactation.

This chapter reviews the profound changes that occur in the female breast from fetal life, through puberty and the reproductive years, and into the menopause. Special attention is devoted to gestational and postgestational changes, including the physiology and endocrinology of lactation. Finally, the subject of abnormalities of lactation and hyperprolactinemic states is addressed.

GROWTH AND DEVELOPMENT

Fetal and Postnatal

Mammary growth is affected by many factors, including hormones, mesenchyme, diet, environment, and genetics.[1] Mammary development in the early fetus is controlled predominantly by local mesenchymal factors although the gland, even at this stage, is capable of responding to hormonal stimulation. The influence of hormonal substances in the morphogenesis of the breast becomes more important during late gestation, and after birth the gland is stimulated by hormones of the pituitary, ovary, and adrenal gland.

The embryology of the breast is covered in Chapter 2 in this text; therefore, only a general overview is outlined herein. The mammary glands are a specialization of the skin and, therefore, are of ectodermal origin.[2] Beginning around the sixth week of fetal development, epithelial cells, derived from the epidermal layer and destined later to become the areola, migrate into the underlying mesenchyme. About 20 short cords are thus formed which, after developing lumina later in fetal life, become ducts that empty into the nipple.[3]

At the embryonic age of 2 months, the primitive breast bud is well differentiated and little change occurs until about the fifth month of fetal development. At this time a growth phase begins as secondary budding occurs and, as previously mentioned, the cords develop lumina surrounded by two layers of cuboidal cells—an inner secretory layer and an outer layer representing the myoepithelium.[4] A local mesenchymal inhibitory factor ensures that the ducts do not develop too close to each other, thus allowing adequate space for subsequent alveolar development.[5] Coincident with this ductal development, the nipple and areola undergo differentiation.

Just prior to birth, dramatic morphologic changes occur and a small amount of secretory activity is seen. This is evidenced by the formation of "witches milk" by most full-term infants beginning on the fifth or sixth day of life. It is commonly assumed that the breast enlargement and secretion seen at this time is a consequence of the maternal–placental hormonal environment. However, in preterm infants, the secretion of milk often begins some weeks after delivery, long after the maternal hormones have disappeared. The level of prolactin is increased at this time, suggesting that the early development of the breast is influenced more by the infant's prolactin than by the mother's endocrine activity.[6]

Subsequent to a fall in fetal prolactin and placental steroids there is regression of the breast into a resting stage, although breast tissue may be palpable normally, in both sexes, for up to 6 months of life.[3,7] This inactive phase is characteristic throughout childhood until the time of puberty.

Puberty and Adolescence

Near the time of puberty, with increasing amounts of hormones released by the hypothalamus, pituitary, ovaries, and adrenal glands, the mammary gland begins a new growth phase. There is an increase in connective tissue, vascularity, and adipose tissue, and most significantly, there is lengthening and branching of the epithelial ducts with budding of the terminal ends. Alveolar lumen formation occurs and, with deposition of interlobular connective tissue, compartmentalization of the breast occurs.[2]

Endocrinology

The endocrinology of breast development is complex because there are multiple hormonal stimuli and the hormone-receptor actions are interdependent. Because receptors themselves are under hormonal control, numerous feedback loops are established.[5] Overall, the major influence on breast growth at puberty is estrogen. However, the development of estrogen receptors in the breast does not occur without prolactin, and it is estrogen itself that may stimulate the release of prolactin from the pituitary gland. Clinically, optimal development of the breast requires the coordinated action of many hormones including estrogen, prolactin, progesterone, insulin, growth hormone, cortisol, and thyroxine. (Fig. 3-1).[5,3]

In the past, it was thought that estrogen stimulated growth of the duct system and that prolactin and progesterone stimulated lobuloalveolar development.[9] Although this view is obviously oversimplified, it may serve as a functional understanding of pubertal development of the breast. Prolactin is clearly critical to breast control. Prolactin stimulates lobuloalveolar growth but requires estrogen to function optimally. Prolactin also controls much of the process of milk production and secretion. Estrogen is a potent stimulant of mammary growth, but it is inefficient in the absence of prolactin and growth hormone. Similarly, progesterone has little effect in the absence of prolactin and the priming influence of estrogen. Additionally, prolactin receptors in the breast are regulated by estrogen.

Insulin receptors are also present in breast tissue. In vitro studies have demonstrated that, for prolactin to exert its full influence on the breast, insulin must be present.[2,3] Cortisol and thyroxine are probably not inherently essential for breast development but instead play a permissive role. However, endocrinopathies involving either hormone would surely adversely affect mammary growth.[3]

Thelarche is frequently the first sign of the onset of puberty. Breast development occurs in most girls between the ages of 8 and 12 years but there is considerable variation in the timing of onset and rate of development. Absence of breast development by age 13 occurs in less than 1 percent of the girls in the United States.[10] Failure of initiation of breast development beyond age 13 is considered abnormal, as is development prior to age 8.[11]

Tanner Classification

A standard method for classifying breast development has been described by Marshall and Tanner and is divided into five stages (Table 3-1).[12] Some girls pass from stage 1 through stage 5 in only a couple of years, while others may not complete stage 5 until 20 years of age. Early surgical management of abnormal breast development is often inappropriate, because complete growth may not have been achieved.

Briefly, stage 1 is typically prepubertal. Stage 2 occurs in the average girl between ages 10 and 11 and represents the breast bud stage. The diameter of the areola also increases. Between ages 11 and 12 the breasts and areola continue to enlarge. With projection of the areola to form a secondary mound above the level of the remaining breast, stage 4 has begun. This occurs between ages 12 and 13 on the average. Stage 5 is representative of the mature adult breast, where the areola has recessed into the general contour of the breast. This generally occurs between the ages of 13.5 and 15.[12,10]

Developmental and Congenital Abnormalities

Developmental abnormalities of the breast are common and often self-limiting. Isolated premature thelarche is defined as breast development prior to age 8. It is not accompanied by any other sign of puberty and is usually benign. The cause is thought to be increased sensitivity of the breast to the normal low levels of circulating estrogen produced by luteinized or cystic ovarian follicles.[11,13] Spontaneous regression may occur and treatment is unnecessary. Parental reassurance is an important part of management. When other signs of puberty are present (axillary or pubic hair), precocious puberty is evaluated in its entirety. Laboratory evaluation should include baseline steroid as well as thyroid studies. Dynamic testing of pituitary function can further help differentiate precocious puberty from premature thelarche.[13]

Congenital absence of the breast (amastia) or nipple (athelia) is rare and often associated with other congenital abnormalities. Conversely, supernumerary breasts (polymastia) or supernumerary nipples (polythelia) are relatively common, are asymptomatic, and occur along the "milk lines." Polythelia may be found in up to 2 percent of the population. Treatment of congenital anomalies, if necessary, usually requires surgical correction.

Rudimentary breasts that fail to develop at puberty, or that develop only partially, may be asso-

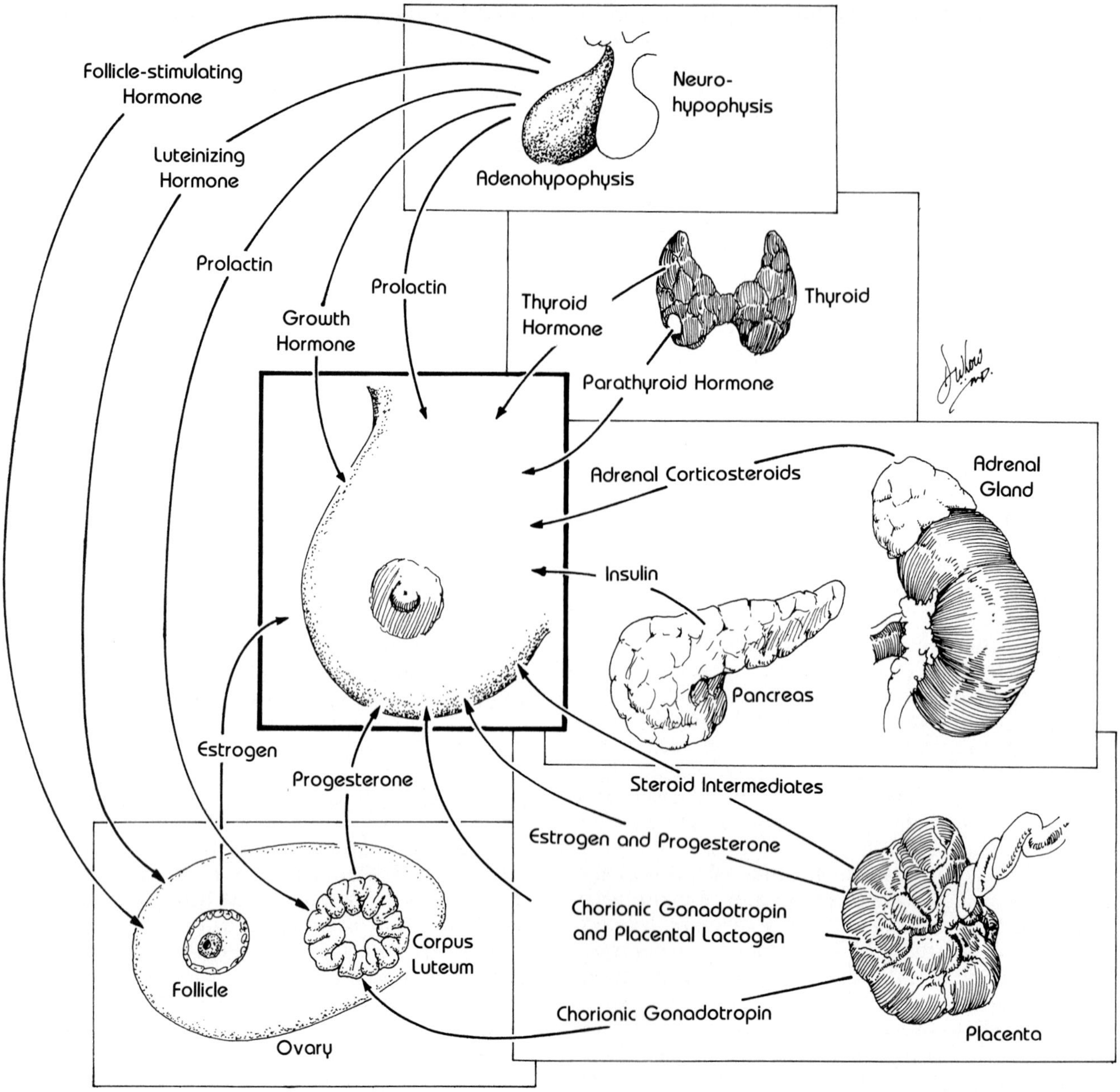

FIGURE 3-1 Breast development depends on multiple hormone stimuli and an interdependence of hormone-receptor actions. Optimal development during puberty requires the coordinated action of estrogen, prolactin, progesterone, insulin, growth hormone, cortisol, and thyroxine. The addition of chorionic gonadotropin and lactogen from the placenta augments breast growth during pregnancy.

TABLE 3-1 Tanner Classification of Breast Development

Stage 1:	No breast development (prepubertal)
Stage 2:	Appearance of breast buds and increased areolar diameter (age 10-11 years)
Stage 3:	Breasts and areola enlarge (age 11-12 years)
Stage 4:	Projection of areola to form a secondary mound above the level of the remaining breast (age 12-13 years)
Stage 5:	Mature adult breast (age 13-15 years)

ciated with gonadal dysgenesis (Turner syndrome) or the syndrome of premature ovarian failure. An elevated gonadotropin level and karyotyping will confirm the diagnosis. Breast growth in these instances can usually be achieved with estrogen replacement therapy.

Occasionally, the breast bud may initially appear on one side only or one breast may grow faster than the other. Asymmetry of the breasts is common during adolescence and usually decreases as development progresses. Whereas exact equality in size is rarely ever obtained, significant asymmetry is correctable only by the reconstructive breast surgeon.

Breast hypertrophy can occur at any time but most commonly occurs during adolescence following a normal pubescence. Unsuspected pregnancy must always be ruled out in these cases. Hypertrophy usually occurs rapidly and is typically bilateral. The etiology is not well understood. Endocrine evaluation of the patient usually demonstrates no abnormalities. The tissue, when studied histologically, demonstrates an increase in connective tissue and fat.[9] Massive enlargement can be associated with pain and skin ulceration. This problem is both a psychologic and a physical burden for the adolescent. Although medical therapy with danazol or bromocriptine has been suggested,[11,3] definitive therapy usually requires reduction mammaplasty. This should be delayed until late adolescence if possible, to allow for complete breast growth, especially if asymmetry exists.

Hypoplasia of the breast can be the result of delayed breast development, secondary to hypogonadism. Most commonly, it is the result of a relative insensitivity of the breast tissue to normal hormonal stimulation. Estrogen replacement, therefore, is often unsuccessful. Augmentation mammaplasty should not be performed until complete breast development has occurred.

Breast atrophy is almost always secondary to nutritional changes and decreased protein intake. This is reversible with adequate nutritional counseling and caloric intake. Inverted nipples may occasionally be seen, and can present a cosmetic problem for the adolescent, correctable only through surgery.[11]

In summary, when treating adolescents with breast abnormalities, a conservative philosophy seems most appropriate. Surgical intervention should be considered only after complete breast development has occurred and appropriate attention has been directed toward the psychologic as well as physical factors involved.

Reproductive Years

Cyclic Menstrual Changes

Complete functional and structural development of the breast is not reached until pregnancy and lactation occurs. Although the time from completion of puberty until pregnancy is generally considered a period of quiescence, definite cyclic changes do occur in the breast in relation to the reproductive cycle.[2] Growth occurs cyclically, with some regression toward the end of each cycle or beginning of the new cycle.

Cyclic engorgement of the breasts may involve an increase in thickness, nodularity, and size. In addition, many women describe an increase in sensitivity of the breast just prior to menses. The increase in size and nodularity, along with the hypersensitivity, usually resolves by the end of the menstrual flow. For this reason, it is commonly recommended to examine the breasts after the flow has ceased. Physiologic nodularity of the breast is usually bilateral and often concentrated in the upper outer portion of each breast. According to Haagensen, breast engorgement is more severe in nulliparous women and women who have never breast-fed.[9] It is less severe during the middle years of menstrual life and begins to increase after age 40, reaching a peak just prior to menopause. Normally, it subsides after menopause.

Mastalgia

Although increased sensitivity of the breast during the premenstruum may be considered physiologic, many women complain of severe pain occurring either cyclically or unrelated to the reproductive cycle. In a study by Preece et al,[14] 232 patients with breast pain were classified into six groups based on clinical, pathologic, and radiologic, features. They were able to group over 90 percent of the patients into six etiologic subgroups. Their study found that the most common reason for breast pain was cyclical pronounced mastalgia and was assumed to have an endocrine basis. Other causes, seen less frequently, included duct ectasia, Tietze syndrome, trauma, sclerosing adenosis, and cancer. In those with cyclical pronounced mastalgia, the discomfort was distinguished from "normal" premenstrual breast discomfort by being more severe and "pronounced." Some of these women experienced pain for more than three quarters of their menstrual cycle. Clinically, these women had diffuse nodularity on palpation with 50 percent demonstrating bilateral involvement. It was therefore concluded that with proper classification of these patients, more effective treatment could be offered.

Others have questioned the efficacy of treatment of mastalgia. The variable response among different patients and the high response rates to placebo therapy cast doubt on many therapeutic strategies utilized in the past. These have included reassurance, local support, diuretics, hormone and antihormone drugs, bilateral oophorectomy, and subcutaneous mastectomy.[15]

Because of the cyclic pattern of most breast pain and its close temporal relation to the hormonal events of the menstrual cycle, it seems likely that mastalgia is often hormone-related. Testosterone has been used in the past; however, virilizing doses were often needed to achieve a clinical response. More recently, danazol has been shown to be more effective than placebo in the treatment of painful nodular benign breast disease.[16] Danazol was able to abolish the midcycle surge of follicle stimulating hormone and luteinizing hormone, and was effective at 200 mg per day. Danazol also exerts its effect by competing with estrogen for its receptor in the breast. Danazol may be effective in relieving discomfort as well as decreasing nodularity. Treatment usually continues for 6 months. Cost and drug-related side effects may limit its usefulness to only those patients with exceptionally severe and persistent symptoms.

Durning et al suggested the usefulness of bromocriptine in the treatment of certain patients with severe cyclical breast pain.[15] No correlation between symptom improvement and prolactin level was found, although there was a statistically significant reduction in pain, tenderness, and nodularity. Improvement has also been reported with the use of vitamin E and abstinence from methylxanthines found in certain foods such as coffee, tea, and chocolate.

Menopause

With the completion of menopause, the cyclic changes of the breast cease and breast size and density diminishes. Histologically, there is atrophy of the lobules with a relatively abundant fibrous matrix. This is accompanied by an increase in the elastic tissue component of the breast postmenopausally.[9] Not uncommonly in today's practice, women given estrogens at menopause have less pronounced changes in their breasts and may even continue having cyclic breast discomfort.

PHYSIOLOGY AND ENDOCRINOLOGY OF LACTATION

Normal Pregnancy, Puerperium, and Lactation

We have only recently begun to understand the endocrinology and physiology of lactation. This understanding is extremely important in light of the fact that breast feeding is still the principal source of infant nutrition in many areas of the world. Orderly secretion of a number of hormones is essential for mammary growth and differentiation during gestation and for subsequent lactation. This section will serve to integrate our current knowledge of the endocrine mechanisms involved in mammary function during gestation, lactogenesis, and lactation.

Gestational Growth and Preparation

Morphologically, a significant increase in mammary ductular-alveolar growth occurs in pregnancy secondary to the steadily increasing amounts of pregnancy hormones. There is intensified ductular sprouting and branching occurring as early as the first month of pregnancy.[6] The growth of early pregnancy is characterized by simple proliferation of the epithelial elements, both the ducts and the acinar systems. They increase in size and complexity, displacing the adipose and connective tissue and thereby establishing a true lobuloalveolar system. As pregnancy proceeds, the alveolar cells become single layered and the lumina begin to dilate. Concurrently, the mammary blood supply increases and new capillaries form around the mammary lobules. Around mid-pregnancy, the mammary proliferative processes are replaced by differentiation and secretory activity. During the third trimester and approaching term, colostrum has been formed and to some degree secreted into the mammary alveoli. In addition to water and minerals, colostrum contains fat droplets, white blood cells, and desquamated alveolar cells.

On a more clinical level, each breast gains approximately three-quarters of a pound in weight during a full-term gestation. The subcutaneous veins become dilated and more prominent. The augmentation of the milk ducts, hypertrophy of connective tissue, increased fat deposition, and retention of water all contribute to the well-known increase in breast size.[17] The areolar skin glands become more prominent and the areolar skin darkens. The nipples often enlarge and become more erect.

During pregnancy, prolactin levels rise from a normal level of 10 to 25 ng per milliliter to concentrations in the 200 to 400 ng/ml range at term. This increase in prolactin is coincident with, and probably stimulated by, the increased secretion of estrogens in pregnancy. In vitro, prolactin causes swelling of the Golgi membranes and induction of synthesis of casein, lactalbumin, lactose, and milk fat. However, high circulating levels of sex steroids may suppress prolactin activity in the mammary tissue, thereby delaying lactogenesis until the peripartum period.[18]

Circulating levels of estradiol and progesterone increase 10 to 100-fold at term.[19] Estrogen stimulates the pituitary gland to secrete prolactin and probably causes the proliferation of pituitary lactotrophs during pregnancy.[20] It contributes to breast growth and differentiation during pregnancy and at the same time inhibits milk production. Estrogen, along with progesterone, stimulates an increase in prolactin binding sites, but progesterone antagonizes the positive action of prolactin on its own receptor.[8] This progesterone inhibition is the primary reason why only colostrum is produced during gestation.

Human placental lactogen is made by the placenta and actively secreted into the maternal circulation beginning around the sixth week of pregnancy. Levels rise steadily and reach a peak at term, falling off precipitously after delivery. The action of placental lactogen is mediated via the prolactin receptor. However, because its binding affinity is relatively low and because of the inhibition of the receptor by progesterone, placental lactogen is probably not truly lactogenic in humans. The functions of insulin, cortisone, and thyroxine have been elucidated mostly by in vitro models, and appear to have a permissive role in mammary gland function during pregnancy (See Fig. 3-1).

Endocrinology of Lactogenesis

The process by which the mammary epithelium differentiates and acquires the ability to secrete milk is called lactogenesis. By the end of pregnancy, the mammary gland is functionally and structurally prepared for the process of lactation. Active lactation begins shortly after parturition, coincident with the precipitous decrease in estrogen and progesterone after delivery of the placenta. Breast engorgement and milk secretion begin approximately 3 days post partum, when these sex steroids have been cleared from the circulation.[8] Thus, lactation begins when the maternal breast, primed by long exposure to estrogen, progesterone, and prolactin, suddenly experiences withdrawal of the two female sex hormones.[3] Quantities of milk produced are extremely variable, especially in early lactation. By 3 weeks post partum, approximately 800 cc of milk is produced daily.[21]

It has been known for years that hypophysectomy during pregnancy suppresses subsequent lactation, and pituitary hormones are therefore necessary for lactogenesis to occur. Minimal requirements for lactogenesis in ovariectomized, hypophysectomized, and adrenalectomized rats are prolactin and a corticosteroid.[18] We now know that prolactin is the primary hormone involved in milk biosynthesis. Without prolactin, the enzymatic steps necessary for the synthesis of casein will not occur, and true milk secretion will be impossible. Specific prolactin binding sites are present on the epithelial cells of the mammary gland. Shiu and Friesen have demonstrated unequivocally that these membrane receptor sites mediate the lactogenic response of prolactin in the mammary gland.[22]

Cortisol induces differentiation of the rough endoplasmic reticulum and Golgi apparatus of mammary tissue, and this appears to be essential for the subsequent prolactin-induced synthesis of casein. Therefore, the current concept is that cortisol is required along with prolactin to initiate lactogenesis.[18]

As mentioned previously, progesterone inhibits lactogenesis by one of several possible mechanisms. Progesterone saturates the glucocorticoid receptor and thereby blocks the effects of cortisol. Progesterone also reduces estrogen binding and may reduce the ability of prolactin to up-regulate its own receptor. This may also explain the fact that prolactin receptor concentration increases significantly after parturition.[23] Finally, prostaglandin F_2 alpha stimulates the release of prolactin and glucocorticoids and concentrations of prostaglandin F are seen to increase coincident with lactogenesis.[18]

GALACTORRHEA AND THE HYPERPROLACTINEMIC STATES

Definition

Galactorrhea refers to the inappropriate secretion from the mammary gland of milk or milk-like fluid in the non-nursing individual. Although usually white or clear, the discharge may be yellowish or even green in color. Nonmilky types of nipple discharge can exist, such as purulent or bloody, and in these cases local lesions of the intraductal epithelium must be ruled out.[24] The amount of milky discharge in true galactorrhea can range from a few drops to an unrelenting flow. The amount of flow has no relation to the pathologic severity of the underlying cause. Any galactorrhea warrants investigation in a nulliparous woman, and beyond 1 year after delivery (or weaning) in a parous woman.[8]

Etiology

The association between galactorrhea and amenorrhea has been appreciated for many years. However, only recently, with the development of a sophisticated radioimmunoassay for prolactin and the availability of computed tomography and magnetic resonance imaging of the pituitary gland, have we come to understand this dynamic relationship with the associated hyperprolactinemic conditions.

The clinical evaluation of galactorrhea can present a complex problem. Only 50 percent of patients with galactorrhea have an elevated serum prolactin,[25] and conversely, not all patients with hyperprolactinemia suffer from galactorrhea. In a report by Kleinberg and associates of 235 patients presenting with galactorrhea, the largest single group were those with galactorrhea and normal menses. The mean prolactin level of this group was within the normal range (18 ng per milliliter). Another problem that makes prolactin interpretation sometimes difficult is the pulsatile secretion of this hormone as well as the sleep-associated increase in serum levels. Finally, there is evidence that there is more than one type of circulating prolactin molecule (big-big; big; and monomeric), each differing in bioactivity and immunoactivity.[27] Therefore, currently available radioimmunoassay techniques for the detection of prolactin may not necessarily correlate with the biologic activity of the respective prolactin molecule.

Despite these problems, it is conceptually best to think of most cases of galactorrhea as representing some abnormality leading to hypersecretion of prolactin. As mentioned previously, the major factor involved in the production and release of prolactin is the continuous secretion of hypothalamic prolactin-inhibitory factor (PIF), believed to be dopamine. Any medication or disease process causing a depletion or reduction in PIF secretion, or blockage of PIF transport, will result in enhanced prolactin release.

Endocrine

With the advent of assays for serum prolactin and improved radiologic techniques, it has become obvious that pituitary tumors are a relatively common cause of galactorrhea and hyperprolactinemia. If amenorrhea is also part of the symptom complex, the majority of these patients will have a pituitary microadenoma.

The mechanism by which pituitary tumors may cause elevated prolactin is varied. Tumor growth may physically block the transport of hypothalamic prolactin-inhibiting factor, or more commonly, tumor cells may function autonomously and secrete prolactin beyond the control of the hypothalamus. Any parasellar tumor, such as a craniopharyngioma, can cause hyperprolactinemia by extension into the hypothalamus. Galactorrhea may also be seen in patients with the empty sella syndrome, Cushing's disease, or acromegaly.[25,26]

The association of galactorrhea, hyperprolactinemia, and hypothyroidism has been described.[28] It is suspected that the elevated hypothalamic thyroid-releasing hormone seen in primary hypothyroidism causes stimulation of the lactotrophs and elevated prolactin. This association may be seen especially in the postpartum period.[29] Thyroid function should be evaluated in all patients with galactorrhea and hyperprolactinemia.

Drugs

Galactorrhea has been associated with a number of different drugs. Most seem to cause increased prolactin levels by blocking the action of dopamine and thereby releasing the hypothalamic suppression. The phenothiazines are probably the most common group of drugs associated with galactorrhea. Up to 50 percent of patients on this type of medication may have galactorrhea.[8] In addition, reserpine, methyldopa, tricyclic antidepressants, benzodiazepines, and others have been associated with galactorrhea. Estrogens have been implicated in galactorrhea by causing hypothalamic suppression with subsequent reduction in secretion of PIF. This may be the mechanism of galactorrhea associated with the use of oral contraceptives. A local effect of estrogen on the breast may also be involved.

Chest Wall

Manipulations of the breast and lesions of the chest wall have been implicated in some cases of hyperprolactinemia and galactorrhea. Included in this group may be individuals with herpes zoster or patients who have undergone thoracotomy or mastectomy. Also included are those patients who, following augmentation mammaplasty, experience nipple discharge after manual massage of the implant, a technique used in an effort to decrease scar capsule contracture. Presumably, the mechanism involved is stimulation of the afferent neural arc leading to prolactin release. The confusing aspect of this theory is that galactorrhea can be seen postoperatively in patients who have undergone surgery remote from the chest wall (e.g., hysterectomy). This suggests that a major factor involved in this postoperative galactorrhea syndrome may be stress-induced hyperprolactinemia.[20]

Idiopathic

It is important to remember that the majority of cases of galactorrhea are still in the idiopathic group. Kleinberg reported that over 40 percent of all patients had idiopathic galactorrhea.[26] That percentage might have been much lower had the technology of today been available at that time. Idiopathic galactorrhea with normal menstruation was the single largest category of all patients with galactorrhea in that study.[26] In the majority of those patients, galactorrhea began with parturition and persisted despite the return of prolactin to normal levels. This is probably attributed to the greater sensitivity of the breasts to normal levels of circulating prolactin following parturition.[3] Historically, the Chiari-Frommel syndrome has been defined as galactorrhea and amenorrhea persisting more then 6 months post partum without evidence of pituitary tumor. With the more sophisticated diagnostic technology available, some of these patients are found to be harboring small pituitary microadenomas. In addition, undiagnosed subclinical hypothyroidism in the postpartum period may contribute to the incidence of galactorrhea.

Other

Ectopic production of prolactin may result from lung or renal tumors, and possibly uterine fibroids.[8] Bilateral bloody nipple discharge of pregnancy is another phenomenon that has been described. This may result from rapid proliferation of the mammary epithelium during pregnancy.[9]

Management

In recent years, an understanding of prolactin physiology and the associated laboratory and diagnostic techniques have grown considerably. Along with this growth has evolved some difference of opinion regarding the appropriate monitoring and therapeutic approach that should be utilized for those patients with galactorrhea and hyperprolactinemia. Isolated galactorrhea does not necessarily require treatment. If there is no evidence of pituitary adenoma, and the patient is having normal menstrual function, treatment is not imperative. Follow-up of these patients with a yearly prolactin level is appropriate. However, if galactorrhea is emotionally or cosmetically debilitating, treatment with bromocriptine, an ergot derivative, is indicated.[30]

Bromocriptine is extremely effective in lowering prolactin levels, and has been the most widely used ergot drug for this purpose. Suppression of prolactin occurs rapidly, sometimes within hours of the initial dose. In contrast, return of cyclic ovulatory function may take weeks, and resolution of the galactorrhea often takes longer than the return of menstruation.

Galactorrhea is a symptom that should be considered related to a pituitary tumor until proven otherwise. The evaluation of the patient with galactorrhea must be comprehensive, considering the various potential etiologies including tumors, drugs, chest wall lesions, and stress. As our knowledge of the hyperprolactinemic states has evolved, so has our management of this condition. Many issues concerning the clinical management of prolactin-related disorders remain unresolved. Recent advances in diagnostic techniques, trans-sphenoidal surgery, and the availability of bromocriptine provide us with a choice of treatment options that can be utilized depending on the desirability of fertility, the degree of menstrual dysfunction, and the size of the pituitary tumor.

CONCLUSION

Plastic and reconstructive surgery of the breast should be performed within the framework of normal breast physiology. The growth and development of the female breast depends on a group of complex neuroendocrine variables. The reconstructive surgeon should have a working knowledge of the normal physiology of the breast and abnormalities of breast function.

References

1. Ceriani RL. Hormones and other factors controlling growth in the mammary gland: A review. J Invest Dermatol 1974; 63:93.
2. Salazar H, Tobon H, Josimovich JB. Developmental, gestational and postgestational modifications of the human breast. Clin Obstet Gynecol 1975; 18:113.
3. Frantz AG, Wilson JD. Endocrine disorders of the breast. In: Wilson JD, Foster DW, eds. Williams textbook of endocrinology. 7th Ed. Philadelphia: WB Saunders, 1985; 402.
4. Porter JC. Hormonal regulation of breast development and activity. J Invest Dermatol 1974; 63:85.
5. Knight CH, Peaker M. Development of the mammary gland. J Reprod Fertil 1982; 65:521.
6. McKiernan JF, Hull D. Prolactin, maternal oestrogens, and breast development in the newborn. Arch Dis Child 1981; 56:770.
7. McKiernan JF, Hull D. Breast development in the newborn. Arch Dis Child 1981; 56:525.
8. Speroff L, Glass RH, Kase NG. Clinical gynecologic endocrinology & infertility. 4th Ed. Baltimore: Williams & Wilkins. 1989:283.
9. Haagensen CD. Diseases of the breast. 3rd ed. Philadelphia: WB Saunders, 1986:47.
10. Coupey SM, Saunders DS. Physical maturation. In: Lavery JP, Sanfilippo JS, eds. Pediatric and adolescent obstetrics and gynecology. New York: Springer-Verlag, 1985:1.
11. Pietsch J. Breast disorders. In: Lavery JP, Sanfilippo JS, eds. Pediatric and adolescent obstetrics and gynecology. New York: Springer-Verlag, 1985:96.
12. Marshall WA, Tanner JM. Variation in the pattern of pubertal changes in girls. Arch Dis Child 1969; 44:291.
13. Brenner PF. Precocious puberty in the female. In: Mishell DR, Davajan V, eds. Infertility, contraception, & reproductive endocrinology. 2nd Ed. Oradell, NJ: Medical Economics Company, 1986:223.
14. Preece PE, Mansel RE, Bolton PM, et al. Clinical syndrome of mastalgia. Lancet 1976; 2:670.
15. Durning P, Sellwood RA. Bromocriptine in severe cyclical breast pain. Br J Surg 1982; 69:248.
16. Mansel RE, Wisbey JR, Hughes LE. Controlled trial of the antigonadotropin danazol in painful nodular benign breast disease. Lancet 1982; 1:928.
17. Vorherr H. Hormonal and biochemical changes of pituitary and breast during pregnancy. Semin Perinatol 1979; 3:193.
18. Tucker HA. Lactation and its hormonal control. In: Knobil E, Neill JD, eds. The physiology of reproduction. New York: Raven Press, 1988:2235.
19. Mishell DR, Marrs RP. Endocrinology of lactation and the puerperium. In: Mishell DR, Davajan V, eds. Infertility, contraception, & reproductive endocrinology. 2nd Ed. Oradell: Medical Economics Company, 1986:143.
20. Kleinberg DL. Lactation and galactorrhea. In: Gold JJ, Josimovich JB, eds. Gynecologic endocrinology. 4th Ed. New York: Plenum Publishing, 1987:481.
21. Tucker HA. Endocrinology of lactation. Semin Perinatol 1979; 3:199.
22. Shiu RPL, Friesen HG. Mechanism of action of prolactin in control of mammary gland function. Annu Rev Physiol 1980; 42:83.
23. Djiane J, Durand P, Kelly PA. Evolution of prolactin receptors in rabbit mammary gland during pregnancy and lactation. Endocrinology 1977; 100:1348.
24. Urban JA, Egeli RA. Non-lactational nipple discharge. CA 1978; 28:130.
25. Magyar DM. Amenorrhea, galactorrhea, and hyperprolactinemia. Journal of American Osteopathic Association 1985; 85:375.
26. Kleinberg DL, Noel GL, Frantz AG. Galactorrhea: A study of 235 cases, including 48 with pituitary tumors. N Engl J Med 1977; 296:589.
27. Andino NA, Bidot C, Valdés M, Machado AJ. Chromatographic pattern of circulating prolactin in ovulatory hyperprolactinemia. Fertil Steril 1985; 44:600.
28. Heyburn PJ, Gibby OM, Hourihan M, et al. Primary hypothyroidism presenting as amenorrhoea and galactorrhoea with hyperprolactinaemia and pituitary enlargement. Br Med J 1986; 292:1660.
29. Kinch RAH, Plunkett ER, Devlin MC. Postpartum amenorrhea-galactorrhea of hypothyroidism. Am J Obstet Gynecol 1969; 105:766.
30. Badano AR, Miechi HR, Mirkin A, et al. Bromocriptine in the treatment of hyperprolactinemic amenorrhea. Fertil Steril 1979; 32:124.

CHAPTER 4

Silicones and Breast Surgery

GEORGE T. GRACE, M.D.,
I. KELMAN COHEN, M.D.

Although silicones are the major biomaterial used in reconstructive and aesthetic breast surgery since their introduction in 1963, many materials were used for breast surgery before that time. The first breast augmentation was performed in 1895 by Czerny who transplanted a lipoma from a patient's back to replace the successful ablation of a breast adenoma.[1] The first alloplastic material used for breast augmentation was a liquid paraffin injected by Gersunny in 1899.[2] Paraffin remained popular until the introduction of polyvinyl alcohol sponges (Ivalon) by Frindlay and Clagett in 1949[3] and used initially by Pangman in 1951 as the first synthetic implant for breast augmentation.[4] Ivalon was thought to be an inert plastic sponge polymer. It is produced by the action of formaldehyde on polyvinyl alcohol. Pangman and Wallace reported on 400 patients with sponge augmentation in 1955, claiming good results.[5] Unfortunately, over the next 10 years it became evident that the polyvinyl alcohol sponge implants changed by an ingrowth of host connective tissue, producing contracture, distortion, and hardness of the breast.[4,6,7] In fact, there appeared to be a loss in volume of the implant itself secondary to degradation of the polyvinyl alcohol sponge material. Finally, liquid silicone injections for breast reconstruction were reported in the 1950s.[1,8]

Poor results from liquid silicone and liquid paraffin and disenchantment with the Ivalon sponge may have been somewhat responsible for the development of the Cronin silicone implant.[9,10] The first silicone mammary prosthesis was implanted in 1962 by Gerow.[1] The use of a silicone elastomer envelope with an enclosed silicone gel changed the field of breast prosthestic devices up to this very day. Although the Cronin silicone implant provided a reasonable cosmetic result soon after surgery, over the ensuing years asymmetry, scar contracture, and hard, firm, capsular breasts occurred with periodic regularity.[12] The search for a better prosthesis continued.

Next, Arion introduced the Simaplast inflatable silicone shell prosthesis in 1965.[13] The reported advantages included a softer, more natural appearance and feel; better adjustment of symmetry in the asymmetric patient; and ease of insertion.[14] The use of the inflatable silicone implant was enhanced by a report demonstrating that saline-filled breast prostheses allowed a better breast examination than gel-filled implants with xeromammography.[15] The most serious complication rate has been spontaneous deflations with a range from 1.2 to 76 percent.[16,17] The high deflation rate appears to be related directly to the type of silicone used in making the implant shell. "Fold flaw" or friction erosion at the site of the implant shell crease is the apparent cause of most of these inflatable implant deflations. Moreover, the specific type of implant shell appears to be related to the incidence of fold-flaw deflation. Opaque room temperature-vulcanized silicone elastomer shells are resistant to fold-flaw deflation compared with the clear shell platinum-cured silicone shells.[18] Filling the implantable prostheses to the recommended volume and silicone regional cross-linking may also reduce fold-flaw deflation.[18] Only room temperature-vulcanized inflatable implants are currently on the market, and their reported deflation rate is extremely low. The inflatable prostheses have allegedly attained a renewed popularity, possibly because they allow better detection of occult breast masses with mammography and because of their reported low deflation rate with room temperature vulcanization.

Despite these changes in implant design for breast augmentation, capsular contracture resulting in a firm breast remains the leading sequela. The cause of capsule contracture is still unknown. One hypothesis has been "gel bleed," in which silicone polymers in the silicone gel pass through the silicone elastomer shell and into the soft tissues. Low-bleed silicone implants were developed to counteract gel bleed.[19] Early clinical reports soon followed, suggesting a decreased incidence of capsular contracture.[20] However, there are no good long-term studies to document the efficacy of these low-bleed devices.

Another implant designed to prevent the firm breast of capsule contraction was the double-lumen implant introduced by Hartley.[21] He reasoned that the outer lumen filled with saline could be deflated by simple percutaneous needle puncture several months or more after augmentation when and if the breast became firm. This would allow the breast to be restored to softness. Unfortunately, such lowering of implant volume did not halt the process of contraction. However, these double-lumen devices have remained popular for other reasons. Some surgeons use them because they believe there is less gel bleed because of the two elastomer shells, but there are no data to support this reasoning. Others use the outer saline-containing chamber for the slow release of drugs through the silicone elastomer membrane, including corticosteroids, antibiotics, and local anesthetics.

Yet another modification of the silicone breast prosthesis was made by Ashley.[22,23] He devised a breast implant filled with silicone gel enclosed within a silicone elastomer shell, then covered with a layer of polyurethane foam to improve contour and projection.[22,23] Interest in the polyurethane prosthesis slowly increased. Early results suggested a decreased incidence of breast capsular contracture in patients undergoing augmentation mammaplasty[24] and reconstruction.[25,26] However, the fate of the polyurethane and the interaction with the body connective tissue remains unknown.[24]

Over the past few years, textured silicone implants have been marketed. It is postulated that, like the polyurethane-coated implants, the collagen matrix forming the capsule around the textured silicone is laid down in a nonspherical orientation that should decrease the incidence of hard, firm breasts. Plastic surgeons unwilling to use the polyurethane-coated implants, but attracted to the theory that a random collagen matrix is produced, have quickly accepted these implants. However, these devices were marketed without any evidence that they actually result in a softer breast. Although they may be equal to or even better than regular silicone implants, their cost must be weighed against any increased benefit in considering their use.

SILICONES: BASIC CHEMISTRY

Silicon (Si), atomic number 14 and atomic weight 28.6, constitutes about 27.6 percent of the earth's crust by weight, and after oxygen is the second most abundant element on earth.[27] The element does not occur in its natural state on earth but as a component of naturally occurring products such as quartz, sand, and silicate. Polydimethylsiloxane is the most commonly used polymer and is produced in industrial, clear, and medical grades. Depending on the chemical backbone, polydimethylsiloxane is produced as a fluid, gel, resin, or elastomer.

Silicones are structured on a molecular skeleton of alternate silicon and oxygen atoms. The skeleton then has various organic groups added. (Fig. 4-1). The most common groups are the methyl ($-CH_3$), phenyls ($-C_6H_5$), and vinyls ($-C_2H_3$).[28] The addition of these various side chains allows for variability of the final product. Short silicone polymers generally result in a thin, clear fluid. However, as the molecular side chains become longer and branch, the silicone polymer becomes more viscous. The longer the side chain or the greater the cross-linking, the firmer the implant gel will be, ultimately producing a rubber-like material.[29] Using catalysts, the linear chains can branch, increasing their viscosity. Side-bending the branching linear chain results in the oils being vulcanized into various elastomers.[1-8]

Silicones are a combination of organic and inorganic compounds mixed through an intricate chemical process.[30] The inorganic silica backbone is derived from quartz or sand and generates the stability. The flexibility is produced by the organic member, usually a hydrocarbon.[30] In general, silicones have a high resistance to heat and moisture and wide temperature variations, and are considered chemically stable. Their primary importance as a prosthesis is based on their physiologic inertness, flexibility, and stability. In part, this is due to the hydrophobic properties of silicone. A review of the basic technology of silicone for the plastic surgeon has been presented.[18]

A retrospective review on the use of silicones in plastic surgery was presented by Braley in 1973.[10] The basic silicones in use today date to Professor F.S. Kippling's lifelong interest in the chemistry of silicone and carbon.[10] The tremendous technologic explosion during World War II solidified silicones as an important area for civilian use.[10] In 1950 De Nicola reported the first implantation of silicone rubber as a replacement for a urethra.[31] The first paper on the use of silicones in plastic surgery was published in 1953.[30] In 1959 Marzoni and colleagues published an

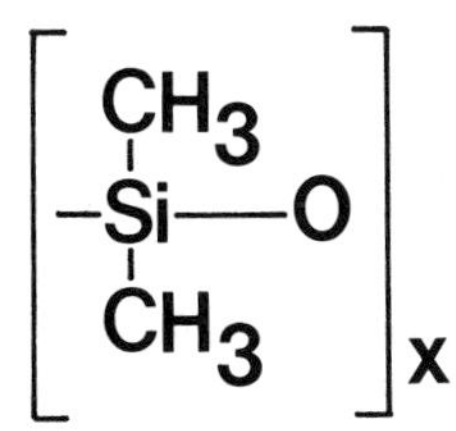

silicone

FIGURE 4-1 Alternate silicon and oxygen atoms combine with methyl groups to form the molecular structure of silicone. Polydimethylsiloxane, the polymer of this structure, is produced in variable lengths that determine the desired viscosity of the final product.

experimental study of silicones as a soft tissue substitute.[32] Finally, the idea of breast augmentation by silicone implantable prostheses was initiated in 1961 when Dr. Frank Gerow, then a resident under Dr. Thomas Cronin, visited Dow Corning to discuss the concept. In 1962, Gerow implanted the first silicone mammary prostheses.[10]

Medical grade polydimethylsiloxane is vulcanized by one of two basic processes. Certain catalysts allow the reaction to occur at room temperature (RTV). High temperatures (HTV) are required for platinum- or peroxide-containing catalysts.[18] In the peroxide-catalyzed process, liquid silicone is produced by the polymerization of dimethylpolysiloxane from elemental silicon.[4] This is then vulcanized with benzoyl peroxide and reinforced with silica to provide a high-strength silicone elastomer.[4] Most of the available mammary prostheses in use today are platinum catalyzed. Their elastomer shell is clear. In contrast, room-temperature vulcanization produces an opaque elastomer shell. It is composed of several distinct types of silicone materials that vulcanize or polymerize at much lower temperatures than peroxide-catalyzed silicone rubber.[28] The room temperature-vulcanized polymers are based on a reactive liquid polysiloxane base that polymerizes over a short time once the catalyst is added. Vulcanization reactions increase both the molecular weight of the silicone polymer and the amount of cross-linking between the siloxane chains. After the catalyst and elastomer are thoroughly mixed, the room-temperature vulcanization becomes an isolated system that undergoes polymerization. Room-temperature vulcanization is used to provide bulk and stability with very little shrinkage.[28]

Silicone rubbers are selectively permeable. This property has been used to explain the concept of gel bleed[18,33] and to make breast implants a drug-delivery system. The yellow color of removed prostheses is due to lipids that easily diffuse into the shell.[18] The implant elastomer shell is very permeable to the lower-molecular-weight fractions of the oils and gels with the resultant "gel bleed."[33] Fluorinated or phenyl-containing silicones with larger side chains and greater cross-linking decrease the permeability and are used in the "low-bleed" implants.[18]

SILICONES: CLINICAL SUMMARY

The widespread use of silicone polymer products in the medical profession documents their safety, success, and usefulness. However, this good clinical record should not make them immune to continued standard safety documentation.

The early favorable results with the injection of liquid silicone into other soft tissue areas led to its widespread use as a breast-enhancing material,[28] especially in Japan and other areas of the Orient. The injection of liquid silicone into the breast parenchyma has never been popular in the United States and should be forbidden. The problems arising from liquid silicone injections for breast augmentation have been well documented,[9,34,35] as have the complications of adulterated silicone fluids.[35-37] Treatment of the silicone-injected breast is troublesome and cosmetically unappealing, usually requiring a total mastectomy.[23,35]

The body's response to silicone gel mammary implants is well known and documented by over 20 years of clinical success and safety. Initially, there is a mild inflammatory reaction with a local inflammatory cell response. This reaction leads to collagen deposition and the formation of a pseudosheath or capsule around the implant.[38] Contraction of this capsule around a soft mammary implant is the most common problem associated with augmentation mammaplasty because it makes the breast firm to palpation.

The issue recently raised by the Food and Drug Administration is whether the silicone-generated inflammatory response and subsequent capsule formation can result in malignancy. Theoretically, this should occur at the silicone gel prosthesis and host interface. Some hypothesize that it is here that mechanical irritation, inflammation, and possible carcinogenesis may occur. Currently, there is no literature to support this hypothesis.

An explanation of possible sarcoma induction in rodents is found in the so-called "Oppenheimer effect." During the course of experiments designed to produce hypertension in rats, Oppenheimer and associates observed the frequent development of sarcomas near the cellophane-wrapped kidney.[39-42] Subsequently, these investigators found that implanting various other foreign body materials into the rats' anterior abdominal wall produced various types of sarcomas.[39-41] Silicone was one of the many materials used that caused sarcomas in the rats.[41] The malignant growths were usually seen 1 to 2 years after surgery and occurred in approximately 35 percent of the rodents who survived surgery at 1 year. Although initial reports failed to demonstrate the development of any soft tissue tumor in the control population,[39,40] subsequent studies confirmed carcinogenesis in the control group as well.[41]

Rees and colleagues injected varying amounts of silicone in several animal species and found no malignancies.[43] Oppenheimer and associates subsequently painted the various polymers on the rodents' skin and were not able to produce tumors.[42] The formation of sarcomas in rodents after the placement of plastic polymers has now been attributed to the Oppenheimer effect, also known as solid state tumorogenesis, and appears to be a characteristic response of rodents to a solid material. The Oppenheimer effect appears to have no bearing on the effects of foreign bodies in humans in the initiation or promotion of neoplasia. One must exercise causation and vigilance, because these effects were seen in rodents 1 to 2 years after implantation.

However, there is no increased incidence of

breast cancer in women after augmentation mammaplasty.[44] There are no studies in humans that associate silicone and malignancy. Likewise, current evidence suggests that silicone does not initiate or promote neoplasia in humans.[45] A recent FDA publication about the risk of carcinoma from silicone breast implants stated that "it is important to bear in mind that not being able to completely rule out the risk doesn't necessarily mean there is one."[46] If such an hypothesis were the foundation for allowing devices to be marketed, there would be no efficacious devices on the market for our patients.

Can silicone have toxic effects? Clearly, there are multiple ways in which silicone comes into contact with body tissues: liquid silicone injections for contour deformities in breast augmentation, silicone gel bleed from gel-filled implants, silicone gel exposure from rupture of the shell. Silicone gel has been reported in axillary lymph nodes,[47] in the fibrous capsule surrounding the implants,[48-50] and associated with granuloma[51] after implant rupture. However, there are no reports of silicone toxicity. Silicone has been injected into several hundred animals, yet no signs of systemic toxicity have been reported.[38,43] Finally, silicone-induced splenomegaly has been reported in a dialysis patient treated by splenectomy. The silicone from the tubing was presumably sheared off by the roller pumps and went to the spleen by a hematogenous route. No systemic toxicity was noted.

In conclusion, although associated with a local inflammatory reaction that ultimately leads to a fibrous capsule, silicone appears to be a biologically inert and nontoxic material when used as a prosthesis.

HUMAN ADJUVANT DISEASE

The evidence that human adjuvant disease exists at all is spurious. In 1954 a condition similar to human polyarthritis was described in rats after an injection of spleen cell homogenate mixed with Freund's complete adjuvant.[53] Ten years later a similar condition in humans called "human adjuvant disease" was described and was characterized by hypergammaglobulinemia following paraffin injection for reconstruction after mastectomy.[54,55] In 1973, Yoshida described seven cases of liquid paraffin or silicone injection for augmentation mammaplasty with the same symptom complex.[56] Removal of these injected materials improved the clinical course in four of the seven patients.[55,56] These initial reports associating paraffin and/or silicone injections with human adjuvant disease were all from Japan. However, in 1982 the first three cases of possible human adjuvant disease after silicone gel implant augmentation mammoplasty were reported in Australia.[57] The first American report followed a year later.[58] Saline-filled silicone implants have also been implicated.[55,59,60]

The mechanism by which silicone may cause human adjuvant disease should be explained. An adjuvant is the substance that increases or alters the immune response to an antigenically unrelated compound. The adjuvant can increase the humoral response and induces a cellular response to the antigen.[55] In human adjuvant disease, it is postulated that silicone is acting in some manner to alter the immune response. Human adjuvant disease is usually considered an autoimmune disorder. Autoimmune disorders are characterized by an immune system reaction to an endogenous antigen with injury to the host tissue. Although scleroderma has been the most common autoimmune disorder associated with possible silicone-induced human adjuvant disease,[60] less common disease processes such as primary biliary cirrhosis and Sjögren's syndrome have also been implicated.[61]

The mechanism of the alleged silicone-induced human adjuvant disease is speculative. The use of injectable silicone for augmentation mammaplasty has been abandoned, but gel-filled silicone implants do "bleed" small quantities of silicone through the elastic envelope.[62] The second method for silicone gel to come into direct contact with tissue is by way of spontaneous rupture or rupture during closed capsulotomy. Silicone from these two sources have been reported to cause a foreign body reaction in axillary lymph nodes,[47] in the fibrous tissue capsule surrounding the implant,[48-50] in the breast parenchyma after rupture,[63] and associated with a granuloma after closed capsulotomy.[51] Finally, the interface of the silicone envelope and breast tissue could theoretically be the stimulus for human adjuvant disease. Accepting that silicone does come into contact with body tissues, the question becomes: does it affect the immune system? The simple placement of a silicone prosthesis has been shown to have an immune effect in rats.[64] The increased cytotoxicity observed in this study returned to normal by the 16th postoperative day.[64] Heggers and colleagues demonstrated an in vivo macrophage inhibition and concluded that silicone can elicit a cellular immune response.[65] The answer is certainly not clear, but evidence suggesting an effect of silicone on the immune system and therefore as the causative agent of human adjuvant disease is based on two different assumptions.

It is interesting that silicone in the breast area has been implicated in human adjuvant disease, even though the exposure is not limited to this area. Silicone is probably present in small quantities throughout the human body. There is probably no human being in the civilized world whose body does not contain small quantities of silicone.[62] Silicone is present as a lubricant in most disposable needles and syringes; in many medications, including antacids; and in processed foods, skin care products, plastic, paper, and upholstery.[62] An insulin-dependent diabetic patient has been estimated to receive several cubic centimeters of silicone from needles and syringes over a lifetime, but no increase in autoimmune or connective tissue diseases has been implicated in this group.[62] Likewise, there are no reports suggesting an association between silicone-containing heart valves, prosthetic finger joints or arteriovenous shunts, and human adjuvant disease.[66] Unless breast tissue has some unique quality, it seems unlikely that the local disposal of silicone alone is sufficient to induce human adjuvant disease.[66]

Most reported cases of human adjuvant disease appear in the Japanese literature and are associated with injectable paraffin, silicone, and other agents. The silicones injected 30 years ago for augmentation mammaplasty (especially outside the United States) and the silicone used for implants today are quite different. Perhaps the human adjuvant disease is secondary to some contaminant that is no longer associated with the silicone gel currently used. A cohort study by Weisman and associates followed patients for a mean of 6.8 years after augmentation mammaplasty with silicone gel implants, and concluded that it does not appear likely that silicone gel prostheses are a significant inducer of inflammatory connective tissue disease.[66] No patient in this cohort study developed an autoimmune-type disease.[66] Likewise, a thorough review of the literature by Sergott and colleagues concluded that at the present time there is no conclusive evidence to implicate the silicone breast implant as inducing an autoimmune disease.[55]

The possible existence of human adjuvant disease as a complication of silicone augmentation mammaplasty remains, but is unlikely. A prospective, double-blind study of patients with and without augmentation mammaplasty followed for many years is needed for a definitive conclusion. However, we believe there is no conclusive evidence associating silicone implants and human adjuvant disease, and that, as Brody stated, these reports are "interesting but probably represent an isolated aberration rather than convincing connection."[62]

SILICONE IMPLANTS AND MAMMOGRAPHY

A long-term epidemiologic study concluded that there was no increased risk of breast carcinoma after augmentation mammaplasty with a silicone gel prosthesis.[44] However, a review in 1984 raised several concerns regarding the safety and efficacy of silicone breast implants following augmentation mammaplasty.[45] Tumor surveillance is one of these major areas of concern. The most important surveillance question is whether the implant obscures the detection of carcinoma in the overlying breast parenchyma by mammography or physical examination.[45]

The incidence of breast cancer is high and the need for early detection great. One in ten women ultimately develop carcinoma of the breast. Mammography is valuable in detecting early breast carcinoma in the nonaugmented breast with about 90 percent accuracy.[67] Women with silicone implants are increasingly entering the age where breast carcinoma is prevalent, because women augmented in the past 20 years are now entering the age group at risk for breast cancer. Therefore, it is important to determine whether augmentation mammaplasty impedes early mammographic detection of breast carcinoma.

The role of mammography in the silicone-augmented breast is controversial.[68–72] Two reports have fostered the opinion that augmentation mammaplasty interferes with reliable mammography.[73,74] Hayes and associates, using solid geometric calculations, suggested that implants obscured 22 to 83 percent of the glandular breast tissue, and questioned the reliability of mammography in making the diagnosis of breast carcinoma in augmented patients.[73] The clinical relevance of these predictions, however, remains obscure. Similarly, Silverstein and associates presented a series of patients following augmentation mammaplasty who presented with a more advanced form of breast cancer compared with a nonaugmented control group.[74] However, this retrospective study represented a biased patient population, and remains unsubstantiated.

Data have been presented by our group from a series of augmented patients in whom the diagnosis of breast carcinoma was made an average of 7.2 years after augmentation mammaplasty. In this population, five out of six patients had a positive mammogram.[75] These patients presented with an early form of breast cancer based on the low number of positive lymph nodes and low rate of recurrence despite a mean follow-up of 32 months.[75] These data led to a suggestion of annual follow-up by the plastic surgeon. Self-examination is also taught and encouraged. There should be a strong emphasis on a cooperative effort with a radiologist who has an interest in mammography. For example, in our center the radiologist reviews the films before the patient leaves the mammography suite. In this manner, additional views as well as sonography can be obtained as needed. Eklund and colleagues described radiologic techniques to improve the yield of mammography in the augmented breast.[76] Additional techniques by others have also added to the armamentarium of the radiologist.[77] A knowledge of these techniques, as together with an interested and committed radiologist, make mammography a valuable screening tool for patients after augmentation mammaplasty.

Although augmentation mammaplasty may obscure visualization of the breast parenchyma during mammography, (1) self-examination; (2) careful and yearly follow-up by the plastic surgeon; and (3) annual mammography after age 35 years in augmented patients by a radiologist with an interest in mammography appear to obviate these problems.

POLYURETHANE-COATED IMPLANTS

Polyurethane is a generic term applied to hundreds of compounds that result from the reaction of disocyanate with a polyol (Fig. 4-2).[78] Along with silicone rubber, polyether-linked polyurethanes are the major group of implanted elastomers. The polyurethane elastomer may be formed by two different cross-linking procedures: (1) polyester that is degradable by hydrolysis and (2) polyether, which has a relatively slow degradation rate. Polyurethane foam with different densities and pore sizes is used as a covering for silicone breast prostheses. The foam undergoes a resorption process over several years with degradation at the interface. The small fragments are phagocytosed while the larger fragments are surrounded by inflammatory cells, fibroblasts, and collagen. This results in a spongelike material of fibrosis with marked adhesions and chronic inflammatory changes.[4,79,80]

Unhappy with silicone gel implants, Ashley designed and implemented a thinned, breast-shaped silicone gel implant covered with a thin layer of polyurethane, known as a Natural-Y Implant.[22] He reported excellent results on short-term follow-up.[22,23] The polyurethane-covered silicone implants used today are manufactured differently. Today's polyurethane is laser cut, resulting in a stronger base and finer foam.[81] In addition, the silicone is more highly cross-linked, giving better shape and decreasing silicone gel bleed.[81]

The theory behind this design was that during the remodeling phase of wound healing, the collagen bundles would be uniformly bound to the fine cell polyurethane oriented in numerous directions, allowing the capsule to remain soft. Thus, a capsule was formed, but because of the multiple orientations of the collagen fibers, a contracture allegedly did not occur.[23] Although this is controversial, Ashley claimed that the interface between the capsule and surrounding tissues could be dissected with a finger.[23]

Modifications of the original Natural-Y polyurethane-coated implants were soon necessary because, despite the low incidence of reported breast capsular contracture, the firm implant was palpable under normal breast tissue.[24] New designs with allegedly excellent clinical results began to appear.[26] The polyurethane-coated implants were popular in reconstructive postmastectomy patients as well.[25] Pennisi claimed excellent results with the polyurethane-covered silicone gel mammary prostheses for successful breast reconstruction and primary and secondary augmentation mammoplasty.[82] He reported that four of 150 breast reconstructions after subcutaneous mastectomy developed a unilateral capsular contracture; follow-up ranged to 8 years. During this same time frame, it was reported by others that microscopic foreign body reactions to the polyurethane were common.[26,80] Soon after their implantation, the polyurethane cover begins to fragment from the silicone capsule and become engulfed by macrophages.[82,83] This intense inflammatory reaction may be related to the erythema not uncommonly seen after polyurethane-coated implants are placed. The degradation and engulfing of the polyurethane is not necessarily a negative comment on polyurethane, because no published reports appear in the literature citing polyurethane as harmful to humans.[82] However, the ultimate fate of the polyurethane remains unknown and therefore is a matter for concern.

The differences in the inflammatory phase of the foreign body reaction between smooth-surfaced silicone implants and polyurethane-coated implants has been defined.[84] The foreign body reaction of the polyurethane-coated implant is characterized by macrophages and giant cells persisting in a state of phagocytic function. This leads to a limited degree of fibrosis, with no single longitudinal capsular band surrounding the implant. The contracting force is dissipated into numerous areas of limited fibrosis with little tension and no linear circumferential contracture around the whole implant. The roughened polyurethane covering thus seems to frustrate the macrophage and maintains the macrophage in a state of prolonged readiness, delaying and inhibiting the fibrogenic action of the fibroblasts.[84] Hester's studies in human tissues show persistence of the intense foreign body reaction for up to 4 years after implant insertion.[85]

The intense foreign body reaction seen with polyurethane-coated implants has been associated with the soft capsule,[82] but this reaction is a source of concern. Pennisi described a patient in whom the polyurethane-covered implant had to be removed shortly after a subcutaneous mastectomy because of exposure secondary to skin necrosis.[82] Large pieces of polyurethane had to be left behind and the breast continued to drain until all these particles were eventually removed.[82] Cocke and associates likewise described difficulty in removing the residual polyurethane when the implant was removed because of infection; one patient was seen 58 times over an 18-month period.[86] Okunski and Chowdary experi-

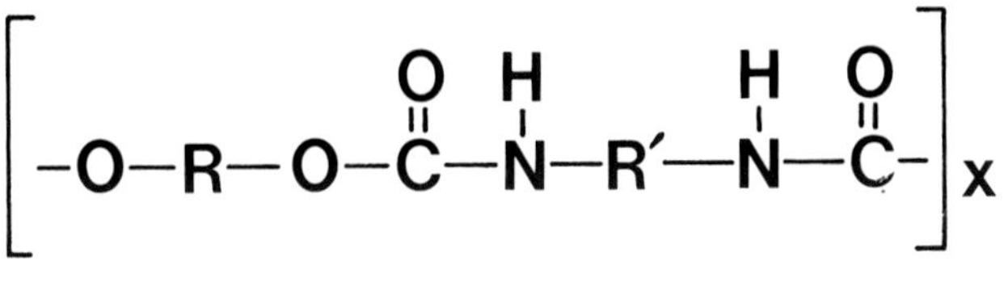

polyurethane

FIGURE 4-2 Polyurethane is a diisocyanate polymer. The foam form of the polymer is used as a covering for silicone breast implants.

enced a *Staphylococcus aureus* infection following a bilateral total mastectomy with insertion of submuscular, polyurethane-coated implants.[87] Three operations were ultimately necessary to remove the polyurethane-coated implants. Salvage reconstruction with smooth-surface silicone implants and bilateral latissimus dorsi myocutaneous flaps were finally required.[87]

If the incidence of capsular contracture is less with polyurethane-coated implants, how does the process work? The alleged clinical absence of contracture around the polyurethane-coated implants may be due to the multiple orientations of the tissue ingrowth into the polyurethane foam.[26,80] As the remodeling phase of wound healing continues, the contracture forces are neutralized by the multiple vectors.[26] Thus, although a capsule as evidenced by a normal inflammatory response is seen, contracture cannot occur because the contracture forces are effectively neutralized. The role of inflammatory reaction following polyurethane-covered implants remains controversial.

Jabaley and Das described two patients with late pain after reconstruction with polyurethane-covered implants.[88] Three aspects were noticeable at operation in these patients: (1) the implant was easily removed; (2) there was only a thin layer of polyurethane remaining on the silicone implant; and (3) polyurethane remained behind in the capsule. These authors speculated that their patients' pain may have developed secondary to a contracture of that portion of the capsule between the engulfed polyurethane and the silicone gel wall. Thus, the process that has been proposed as limiting the incidence of capsular contracture may actually have caused a capsule in these patients. Both of these patients improved when the polyurethane implants were removed. Capsule contracture histology confirms the experience of Jabaley and Das.[88] Brand reported two distinct zones seen on histologic sectioning.[84] One zone is characterized by the typical foreign body reaction seen on the denuded silicone surface; the other is typical of the spongy foreign body reaction normally seen around polyurethane covering. Thus, the smooth silicone surface denuded of the polyurethane surface can be expected to have a typical capsular contracture. In the experience of Hester and associates, this phenomenon has not been identified as a cause of pain, capsular contracture, or other symptoms.[81]

Hester and associates presented the 5-year experience at Emory University with polyurethane-covered mammary prostheses for treatment of capsular contracture, primary augmentation mammaplasty, and breast reconstruction.[81] There were 1,510 total implants and only 18 breasts (1.2 percent) with significant capsule compression (Hester class III).[81] There were 866 prostheses inserted for initial augmentation mammaplasty, with significant class III capsule contracture occurring in two (0.2 percent). Only two capsulotomies were necessary during the 5-year follow-up period. Hester and associates emphasized the importance of recognizing infection early and treating aggressively to minimize infection complications; their 5-year overall infection rate was approximately 1 percent.[81,85]

Clearly, the final answer with the polyurethane implants is not yet known. The increasingly successful clinical results are associated with their rising popularity. However, one must question their efficacy because of the lack of data on the long-term results of polyurethane compared with silicones.

TISSUE EXPANSION

Tissue expansion has been used for centuries in the various tribal customs to stretch lips and ears. Abdominal tissue expansion occurs naturally during pregnancy. Surgical tissue expansion was first performed when Neumann placed a rubber balloon connected to a flexible polyethylene tube in the lateral scalp to expand the scalp skin for reconstruction of an amputated ear.[89] Radovan first expanded with silicone devices and popularized the technique for breast reconstruction.[90-92]

The currently available materials for breast expansion are manufactured from silicone polymers. The prototype temporary expander is the Radovan prosthesis, which is most often used to develop ptosis in the reconstructed breast.[90-92] The Radovan tissue expander is then replaced with a permanent mammary prosthesis. The second category is the "implant/expander" for breast reconstruction. This permanent type of device was first marketed with a design by Becker.[93,94] The saline inner chamber of the Becker prosthesis is filled through a valve, which can be removed under local anesthesia. The Becker device, however, does not result in a distinct inframammary fold and will not provide ptosis to match the opposite breast. These limitations must be considered when selecting a device for reconstruction.

There are a number of other options for breast reconstruction by tissue expansion. Some surgeons are replacing tissue expanders with a permanent polyurethane implant.[95] Customized, textured silicone expanders are being used by some surgeons. Placement of the expander at the inframammary fold is claimed to result in a better inframammary fold because the textured expander will not migrate. These devices are then replaced with permanent polyurethane or silicone implants. Finally, permanent textured silicone implant expanders have now been produced.

Although we believe that reconstruction with autogenous tissue is the gold standard, our approach for breast reconstruction with tissue expansion varies with the needs of the particular patient. The patient with opposite breast ptosis who refuses surgery on the normal breast is reconstructed by placement of a Radovan tissue expander low on the chest, with a change to a double-lumen silicone implant after an appropriate interval. The Radovan tissue expander allows recruitment of abdominal skin to create the desired appearance of ptosis and an inframammary fold. Patients who do not have ptosis of the opposite breast, or who undergo ptosis correction of the opposite breast, are reconstructed with the implant/expander device. More recently, we have found that a textured silicone expander placed at the inframammary fold will create a distinct fold and therefore, moderate ptosis.

IMPLANT ALTERNATIVES

The patient who presents for breast augmentation has a choice of implant types. The surgeon should explain the advantages and disadvantages of each.

Smooth-surface silicone gel implants remain the most popular, and are available as both single- and double-lumen gel implants. These continue to be associated with breast firmness in the range of 30 to 70 percent when placed in a subglandular position, and 15 percent when placed in a submuscular position.[96,97] However, without contraction these implants result in the softest, most natural-appearing augmented breast.

The current silicone saline-inflatable prostheses seem to be associated with a lower spontaneous deflation rate than past products, and may be associated with improved mammographic examination. For these reasons, the silicone-saline inflatable prosthesis seems to be experiencing a resurgence in use.

The textured silicone implants are the latest technologic development for breast augmentation. Although no long-term results are available, there are early enthusiastic reports that are not based on double-blind or controlled studies. The new permanent textured silicone implant expander is an interesting concept, but its effectiveness has not been completely validated.

Finally, polyurethane-coated implants continue to be used with allegedly good results.[95] However, many plastic surgeons are reluctant to use these devices because the fate of polyurethane is unknown and because of the risk of postoperative infection. We have limited our use of these devices to patients who are recalcitrant to standard treatment of breast capsular contractures.

References

1. Lalardrie JP, Mouly R. History of mammoplasty. Aesth Plast Surg. 1978; 2:167.
2. Rees TD. Plastic surgery of the breast. In: Converse JM, ed. Reconstructive plastic surgery. WB Saunders, Philadelphia; 1964:1904.
3. Frindlay JH, Clagett OT. A plastic sponge prosthesis for use after pneumonectomy: A preliminary report of an experimental study. Mayo Clin Proc 1949; 24:538.
4. McGrath MH. Capsular contraction in the augmented breast. In: Rudolph R, (ed.). Problems in aesthetic surgery. Biologic causes and clinical solutions. St. Louis: CV Mosby, 1986:405.
5. Pangman WJ, Wallace RM. The use of plastic prosthesis in breast plastic and other soft tissue surgery. WJ Surg Obstet Gynecol 1955; 65:503.
6. Arons MS, Sabesin SM, Smith RR. Experimental studies with Etheron sponge. Plast Reconstr. Surg 1961; 28:72.
7. Edgerton MT, McClary AR. Augmentation mammoplasty with special reference to polyvinyl alcohol sponge (Ivalon). Plast Reconstr Surg 1958; 21:279.
8. Uchida J. Clinical application of cross-linked dimethyl polysiloxane; restoration of breast, cheeks, atrophy of infantile paralysis, funnel-shaped chest, etc. Jpn J Plast Reconstr Surg 1961; 4:303.
9. Parsons RW, Thering HR. Management of the silicone injected breast. Plast Reconstr Surg 1977; 60:534.
10. Braley S. The use of silicones in plastic surgery. A retrospective review. Plast Reconstr Surg 1973; 51:280.
11. Cronin TD, Gerow FJ: Augmentation mammoplasty: A new natural feel prosthesis. Excerpta Medica International Congress Series No. 66, 1963.
12. Terino EO. Essential concepts in prosthetic breast surgery. Aesth Plast Surg 1982; 6:25.
13. Tabari K. Augmentation mammoplasty with Simaplast implants. Plast Reconstr Surg 1969; 44:468.
14. Worton EW, Seifert LN, Sherwood R. Late leakage of inflatable silicone breast prostheses. Plast Reconstr Surg 1980; 65:302.
15. Cohen IK, Goodman H, Theogaraj SD: Xeromammography—a reason for using saline-filled breast prostheses. Plast Reconstr Surg 1977; 59:886.
16. Rees TD, Guy CL, Coburn RJ. The use of inflatable breast implants. Plast Reconstr Surg 1973; 52:609.
17. Williams JE. Experience with a large series of Silastic breast implants. Plast Reconstr Surg 1972; 49:253.
18. Brody GS. Silicone technology for the plastic surgeon. Clin Plast Surg 1988; 15:517.
19. Barker DE, Retsky MI, Schultz S. The new low bleed mammary prosthesis: An experimental study in mice. Aesth Plast Surg 1981; 5:85.
20. Price JE, Barker DE. Initial clinical experience with low bleed breast implants. Aesth Plast Surg 1983; 7:255.
21. Hartley JH. Specific applications of the double lumen prosthesis. Clin Plast Surg 1976; 3:247.
22. Ashley FL. A new type of breast prosthesis. A preliminary report. Plast Reconstr Surg 1970; 45:421.
23. Ashley FL. Further studies on the Natural-Y breast prosthesis. Plast Reconstr Surg 1972; 49:414.
24. Herman S. The Meme implant. Plast Reconstr Surg 1984; 73:411.
25. Eyssen JE, Von Werssowetz AJ, Middleton GD. Reconstruction of the breast using polyurethane-coated prostheses. Plast Reconstr Surg 1984; 73:415.
26. Capozzi A, Pennisi VR. Clinical experience with polyurethane-covered gel-filled mammary prostheses. Plast Reconstr Surg 1981; 68:512.
27. Encyclopedia Americana. Danbury, CT: Grolier, 1988: 814.
28. Ashley FL, Braley S, Rees TD, Goulian D, Ballantyne DL. The present status of silicone fluid in soft tissue augmentation. Plast Reconstr Surg 1967; 39:411.

29. Adams JS. Grafts and implants in nasal and chin augmentation—a rational approach to material selection. Otol Clin North Am 1987; 20:913.
30. Brown JB, Freyer MP, Randall P, Lu M. Silicone in plastic surgery. Laboratory and clinical investigations, a preliminary report. Plast Reconstr Surg 1953; 12:374.
31. De Nicola RR. Permanent artificial (silicone) urethra. J Urol 1950; 63:168.
32. Marzoni FA, Upchurch SE, Lambert CJ. An experimental study of silicone as a soft tissue substitute. Plast Reconstr Surg 1959; 24:600.
33. Brody GS. Fact and fiction about breast implant bleed. Plast Reconstr Surg 1977; 60:615.
34. Edgerton MT, Wells JH: Indications for and pitfalls of soft tissue augmentation with liquid silicone. Plast Reconstr Surg 1976; 58:157.
35. Ortiz-Monasterio F, Trigos I. Management of patients with complications from injections of foreign materials into the breasts. Plast Reconstr Surg 1972; 50:42.
36. Braley S. Silicone fluids with added adulterants. Plast Reconstr Surg 1970; 45:288.
37. Braley S. The status of injectable silicone fluid for soft tissue augmentation. Plast Reconstr Surg 1971; 47:343.
38. Rees TD, Jobe RP, Ballantyne DL. Inorganic implants. In: Converse JM, ed. Reconstructive plastic surgery. Philadelphia: WB Saunders, 1977:392.
39. Oppenheimer BS, Oppenheimer ET, Stout AP. Sarcomas induced in rats by implanting cellophane. Proc Soc Exp Biol Med 1948; 67:33.
40. Oppenheimer BS, Oppenheimer ET, Stout AP. Sarcomas induced in rodents by embedding various plastic films. Proc Soc Exp Biol Med 1952; 79:366.
41. Oppenheimer BS, Oppenheimer ET, Stout AP, Danishefsky I. Malignant tumors resulting from embedding plastics in rodents. Science 1953; 118:305.
42. Oppenheimer BS, Oppenheimer ET, Danishefsky I, Stout AP, Eirich FR. Further studies of polymers as carcinogenic agents in animals. Cancer Res 1955; 15:333.
43. Rees TD, Ballantyne DL, Hawthorne GA. Silicone fluid research. A follow-up study. Plast Reconstr Surg 1970; 46:50.
44. Deapen DM, Pike MC, Casagrande JT, Brody GS. The relationship between breast cancer and augmentation mammoplasty: An epidemiologic study. Plast Reconstr Surg 1986; 77:361.
45. McGrath MH, Burkhardt BR. The safety and efficacy of breast implants for augmentation mammoplasty. Plast Reconstr Surg 1984; 74:550.
46. Food and Drug Administration Bulletin. Rockville, MD, 1989; 16:57.
47. Hausner RJ, Schoen FJ, Pierson KK. Foreign body reaction to silicone gel in axillary lymph nodes after an augmentation mammoplasty. Plast Reconstr Surg 1978; 62:381.
48. Wickham MG, Rudolph R, Abraham JL. Silicone identification in prosthesis-associated fibrous capsules. Science 1978; 199:437.
49. Gayou RM. A histological comparison of contracted and non-contracted capsules around silicone breast implants. Plast Reconstr Surg 1979; 63:700.
50. Baker JL, LeVier RR, Spielvogel DE. Positive identification of silicone in human mammary capsular tissue. Plast Reconstr Surg 1982; 69:56.
51. Apesos J, Pope TL. Silicone granuloma following closed capsulotomy of mammary prosthesis. Ann Plast Surg 1985; 14:403.
52. Bommer J, Ritz E, Waldherr RR. Silicone-induced splenomegaly. N Engl J Med 1981; 305:1077.
53. Stoerk HC, Bielinski TC, Budzilovich T. Chronic polyarthritis in rats injected with spleen in adjuvants (abstract). Am J Pathol 1954; 30:616.
54. Miyoski K, Miyamura T, Kobayashi Y, et al. Hypergammaglobulinemia by prolonged adjuvanticity in man. Disorders developed after augmentation mammoplasty. Jpn Med J 1964; 2122:9.
55. Sergott TJ, Limoli JP, Baldwin CM, Laub DR. Human adjuvant disease, possible autoimmune disease after silicone implantation. A review of the literature, case studies and speculation for the future. Plast Reconstr Surg 1986; 78:104.
56. Yoshida K. Post-mammoplasty disorder as an adjuvant disease of man. Shikoku Acta Med 1973; 29:318.
57. Van Nunen SA, Gatenby PA, Basten A. Post-mammoplasty connective tissue disease. Arthritis Rheum 1982; 25:694.
58. Baldwin CM, Kaplan EN. Silicone-induced human adjuvant disease? Ann Plast Surg 1983; 10:270.
59. Byron MA, Venning VA, Mowatt AG. Postmammoplasty human adjuvant disease. Br J Rheumatol 1984; 23:227.
60. Spiera H. Scleroderma after silicone augmentation mammoplasty. JAMA 1988; 260:236.
61. Okana Y, Nishikai M, Sato A. Scleroderma, primary biliary cirrhosis, and Sjögren's syndrome after cosmetic breast augmentation with silicone injection: A case report of possible human adjuvant disease. Ann Rheum Dis 1984; 43:520.
62. Brody G. Scleroderma after silicone augmentation mammoplasty (letter). JAMA 1988; 260:3008.
63. Argenta LC. Migration of silicone gel into breast parenchyma following mammary prosthesis rupture. Aesth Plast Surg 1983; 7:253.
64. Schuler FA, Rosato FE, Miller E, Horton CE. Silicone prostheses and antitumor immunity: An in vitro rat study. Plast Reconstr Surg 1978; 61:762.
65. Heggers JP, Kossousky N, Parsons RW, et al. Biocompatability of silicone implants. Ann Plast Surg 1983; 11:38.
66. Weisman MH, Vecchione TR, Albert D, Moore LT, Mueller MR. Connective tissue disease following breast augmentation: A preliminary test of the human adjuvant disease hypothesis. Plast Reconstr Surg 1988; 82:626.
67. Lung JA, Hart NE, Woodbury R. An overview and critical analysis of breast cancer screening. Arch Surg 1988; 123:833.
68. Rintala AE, Svinhufvud UM. Effect of augmentation mammoplasty on mammography and thermography. Plast Reconstr Surg 1974; 54:390.
69. Brody GS, Deapen DM. Breast cancer diagnosis in the augmented patient (letter). Arch Surg 1988; 124:256.
70. Wolf JN. On mammography in the presence of breast implants (letter). Plast Reconstr Surg 1978; 62:286.
71. Snyder RE. Xeromammography: A reason for using saline-filled breast prostheses (discussion). Plast Reconstr Surg 1978; 61:107.
72. Pennisi VR. Xeromammography: A reason for using saline-filled breast prostheses (discussion). Plast Reconstr Surg 1978; 61:107.

73. Hayes H, Vandergrift J, Diner WC. Mammography and breast implants. Plast Reconstr Surg 1988; 82:1.
74. Silverstein MJ, Handel N, Gramagami P, et al. Breast cancer in women after augmentation mammoplasty. Arch Surg 1988; 123:681.
75. Grace GT, Roberts C, Cohen IK. The role of mammography in detecting breast cancer in augmented breasts. Presented at the American Society for Aesthetic Plastic Surgery, Orlando, FL, April 1989.
76. Eklund GW, Busby RC, Miller SH, Job JS. Improved imaging of the augmented breast. Am J Roentgenol 1988; 151:469.
77. Mitnick JS, Harris MN, Roses DF. Mammographic detection of carcinoma of the breast in patients with augmentation prostheses. Surg Gynecol Obstet 1989; 168:30.
78. Lynch W. Implants reconstructing the human body. New York: Van Nostrand Reinhold, 1982.
79. Lilla JA, Vistnes LM. Long-term study of reactions to various silicone breast implants in rabbits. Plast Reconstr Surg 1976; 57:637.
80. Smahel J. Tissue reactions to breast implants coated with polyurethane. Plast Reconstr Surg 1978; 61:80.
81. Hester TR, Nahai F, Bostwick J, Cukic J. A 5-year experience with polyurethane-covered mammary prostheses for treatment of capsular contracture, primary augmentation mammoplasty, and breast reconstruction. Clin Plast Surg 1988; 15:569.
82. Pennisi VR. Polyurethane-covered silicone gel mammary prosthesis for successful breast reconstruction. Aesth Plast Surg 1985; 9:73.
83. Brand KG. Polyurethane-coated silicone implants and the question of capsular contracture. Plast Reconstr Surg 1984; 73:498.
84. Brand KG. Foam-covered mammary implants. Clin Plast Surg 1988; 15:533.
85. Hester TR. The polyurethane-covered mammary prosthesis: Facts and fiction. Perspect Plast Surg 1988; 2:135.
86. Cocke WM, Leathers HK, Lynch JB. Foreign body reactions to polyurethane covers of some breast prostheses. Plast Reconstr Surg 1975; 56:527.
87. Okunski WJ, Chowdary RP. Infected Meme implants: Salvage reconstruction with latissimus dorsi myocutaneous flaps and silicone implants. Aesth Plast Surg 1987; 11:49.
88. Jabaley ME, Das SK. Late breast pain following reconstruction with polyurethane-covered implants. Plast Reconstr Surg 1986; 78:390.
89. Neumann CG. The expansion of an area of skin by progressive distention of a subcutaneous balloon. Plast Reconstr Surg 1957; 19:124.
90. Radovan C. Reconstruction of the breast after radical mastectomy using a temporary expander ASPRS. Plast Surg Forum 1978; 1:41.
91. Radovan C. Tissue expansion in soft tissue reconstruction. Plast Reconstr Surg 1984; 74:482.
92. Radovan C. Breast reconstruction after mastectomy using the temporary expander. Plast Reconstr Surg 1982; 69:195.
93. Becker H. Breast reconstruction using an inflatable breast implant with detachable reservoir. Plast Reconstr Surg 1984; 73:687.
94. Becker H. The expandable mammary implant. Plast Reconstr Surg 1987; 79:631.
95. Artz JS, Dinner MI, Sampliner J. Breast reconstruction with a subcutaneous tissue expander followed with a polyurethane covered silicone breast implant. Ann Plast Surg 1988; 20:517.
96. Scully SJ. Augmentation mammoplasty without contracture. Ann Plast Surg 1981; 6:262.
97. Mahler D, Hauben DJ. Retromammary versus retropectoral breast augmentation—a comparative study. Ann Plast Surg 1982; 8:370.

CHAPTER 5

Diagnostic Breast Imaging in Plastic Surgery of the Breast

G.W. EKLUND, M.D.

Women who have undergone cosmetic or reconstructive breast surgery are at no lower risk for the development of breast cancer than their nonoperated sisters. Ten percent of American women develop breast cancer. Advances in surgical, radiation, and chemotherapeutic management of breast cancer notwithstanding, we have achieved disappointingly little reduction in the breast cancer mortality rate in the past 50 years. Well-controlled studies have shown that death from breast cancer can be reduced by more than one third by early detection and treatment. Early detection is best accomplished by regular screening mammography, yet there is less than 15 percent compliance by American women with the recommended guidelines for mammography.[1-6] Clinicians play the crucial role in promoting compliance with recognized guidelines for screening mammography. In surveys conducted during breast cancer screening projects by the American Cancer Society, the most common reason given by women for not having undergone previous mammography has been: "My doctor never ordered one."[4-6] Treatment of clinically apparent breast cancer has been unsuccessful in achieving significant reduction in mortality rates, and prevention remains unlikely in the foreseeable future. *Mammography is the only diagnostic study capable of reliably identifying clinically occult, curable breast cancer.* Early detection of breast cancer remains the only realistic hope for cure.

Editor's Note: The ideal mammary implant would not only be totally biocompatible with human tissues but would also be radiolucent, allowing mammographic detection of breast lesions and small microcalcifications. The techniques described by Eklund, as well as the use of high quality mammography, are great steps forward in the search for the ideal method to detect small, non-palpable breast carcinomas in women who have had augmentation mammaplasty. Studies on the relative radiodensities of various breast implants have demonstrated that silicone shells filled with silicone gel and/or saline and polyurethane-covered silicone gels have equal radiodensity, completely obscuring phantom artifacts placed in mammography studies. Silicone shells that were filled with gelatin proved intermediate in radiodensity, allowing limited resolution of microcalcifications, but obscuring most soft tissue masses. When silicone shells were filled with peanut oil, visualization of microcalcifications and soft tissue masses greater than 1 mm in diameter were seen. Polyurethane shells filled with peanut oil allowed visualization of microcalcifications and soft tissue masses greater than 3 mm in diameter.[1]

Although a significant improvement from the standpoint of radiolucency, silicone implants filled with peanut oil have not been subjected to human biocompatibility studies especially designed to demonstrate the reactive effect of free peanut oil adjacent to breast tissues, should rupture of the silicone gel occur.

The search should continue for the ideal implant material, which would be nonreactive when exposed in the free state to breast tissue, biocompatible with human tissues, and totally radiolucent on standard film mammography techniques. (RBN)

1. Gumucio CA, Pin P, Young PL, et al. The effect of breast implants on the radiographic detection of microcalcification and soft tissue masses, Plast Reconstr Surg 1989; 84:772.

BREAST CANCER RISK AS A GUIDE TO SCREENING

All women are at risk for the development of breast cancer. Some, however, have identifiable factors that place them at significantly higher risk than other women. It is not enough to focus attention on only those women with "added" risk, because *75 percent of breast cancers develop in women with no identifiable risk factors.*[7]

Many factors contribute some added risk for the development of breast cancer; however, most of these are of either minor or controversial significance and should not be overemphasized.[8,9] Unnecessary anxiety is often the result of enumerating and emphasizing such risk factors, and all too often anxiety is iatrogenic. Anxiety can be a significant form of morbidity.

Risk factors, although they do not predict who will develop breast cancer, do provide a mechanism for identifying women at significantly higher risk. Risk factors that may alter protocols for follow-up or management of a given patient, deserve the designation "significant" and should be understood. In our practice, we have narrowed these "significant" factors to three:

1. *A previous history of breast cancer.* Patients who have had breast cancer are clearly at added risk for development of breast cancer in the contralateral breast and recurrence on the ipsilateral side.
2. *A first-line relative (mother, sister, or daughter) with breast cancer.* The risk is greater still if the relative had premenopausal or bilateral disease.
3. *Previous biopsy diagnosis of one of the "high-risk" benign lesions (atypical ductal hyperplasia or multiple intraductal papillomas).* These lesions are described by some pathologists as premalignant.[8,9]

The presence of any of these "significant" factors deserves careful notation in the patient record and should alert the clinician to the need for vigilance and a more aggressive screening protocol for early breast cancer detection. Women who have a first-line relative (mother or sister) with breast cancer tend to develop cancer about 10 years earlier than women without this history.[10,11] Thus, we have adopted a routine of beginning breast cancer screening 10 years earlier for women in the three "significant" risk factor categories listed above. For these higher-risk patients we recommend baseline mammography at age 25 and annual mammograms beginning at age 30.

There is no evidence to show that the small or "reduced" breast is at any lower risk for the development of breast cancer.

Women are becoming better informed regarding current standards for breast imaging and the medical profession's ability to achieve early detection of breast cancer. However, many wait until their physician orders a mammogram, rather than ask for or independently obtain a mammogram. Although some argue that guidelines should not be used to establish the standard of care, history shows that guidelines followed by a majority of physicians soon become the accepted standard of care. The American Cancer Society recommends baseline mammography for women between ages 35 and 39, mammograms at 1- to 2-year intervals between ages 40 and 49, and annual mammograms after age 50.[1] These guidelines are based on the well-recognized increasing incidence of breast cancer with advancing age. There is a growing consensus among mammographers and others concerned with breast disease that a more aggressive annual screening between ages 40 and 50, and a more flexible schedule of 1 to 3 years for women over 50, may be more appropriate.[11-13] These latter recommendations are based on three factors:

1. *The natural behavior of breast cancer in different age groups.* Women in the younger age group tend to have more aggressive, rapidly growing breast cancers than their older, postmenopausal counterparts.
2. *The character of breast parenchyma in different age groups.* Younger women tend to have more dense parenchyma with a greater potential for masking subtle abnormalities. Fatty involution of glandular breast tissue, occurring with advancing age, renders the breast less radiopaque and therefore less likely to mask a subtle lesion.
3. *The consequences of a delayed diagnosis in the different age groups.* The socioeconomic implications and likelihood of death resulting from a delay in diagnosis are vastly different in the two age groups.

There is no scientifically based consensus on which protocol or guidelines are most appropriate for high-risk patients. Conventional wisdom, however, suggests it is prudent to follow high-risk women more carefully with a more aggressive screening program. The missed diagnosis of breast cancer has become a leading cause of litigation in many states. Surgeons involved in any type of breast surgery must recognize the importance of mammographic screening and its appropriate role in their practices, if the goal of achieving significant reduction in breast cancer mortality is to be realized.

PREOPERATIVE MAMMOGRAPHY

Women being considered for breast surgery should have no less screening consideration than is recommended for all women. Whether women younger than the recommended age for baseline mammography should have mammography before undergoing cosmetic surgery remains controversial. It has been our policy to recommend mammograms for any patient 25 years of age or older who is contemplating cosmetic breast surgery, unless she has had a mammogram within the previous year. The purpose of preoperative mammography is twofold. First, it may identify any abnormality that might alter the procedure; e.g. the discovery of an unsuspected carcinoma or an area of concern that should be histologically resolved before or at the time of surgery. Second, it establishes a baseline for future comparison. *Preoperative mammography must be distinguished from screening mammography* (commonly advocated for asymptomatic women in whom there are no breast findings of clinical concern).

A woman about to have breast surgery is going to develop postoperative symptoms and possible architectural alterations of breast tissue resulting in radiographic findings that may mimic malignant disease.[14,15] Discomfort and areas of palpable induration are common occurrences after any surgical procedure on the breast, including simple needle aspiration. These symptoms or signs may develop immediately after surgery or may not be apparent for weeks or months postoperatively. Similarly, discomfort and induration may be the only presenting sign or symptom of a developing carcinoma requiring a careful diagnostic work-up. The decision to follow postoperative patients clinically can be made more comfortably, and perhaps more justifiably, if a preoperative mammogram shows no radiographic abnormality. A mammographic abnormality, such as a small nodule discovered before reduction or augmentation mammoplasty, should alert the surgeon to the need for inclusion of that area of concern in the resected tissue, or perhaps a separate excisional biopsy before the planned surgery.

Preoperative localization of clinically occult lesions is becoming a routine procedure in most institutions. This is a simple procedure, performed by the radiologists, using a hookwire, blue dye, or a combination of wire and dye to mark the areas of radiographic concern. Radiography of the resected specimen assures the surgeon that the area of concern is contained in the resected tissue. The specimen can be marked by the radiologist to direct the pathologist to the exact area of interest. If the pathologic findings do not adequately explain the radiographic findings, and if the area in question is known to have been removed, the radiologist should request an opportunity to radiograph the paraffin blocks and all remaining tissue for evidence of an overlooked lesion.

DIAGNOSTIC BREAST IMAGING

The term "diagnostic breast imaging" (DBI) may be more appropriate to and descriptive of services provided by the mammographer in a comprehensive diagnostic breast service. *Mammography will be only one of the diagnostic tools utilized.* Ultrasonography, galactography (ductography), cyst aspiration, pneumocystography, and fine needle aspiration biopsies are becoming important components of the complete diagnostic breast service.[16] Although early detection of breast cancer remains the most laudable goal for DBI, it is certainly not its only function. Providing security for the patient and her physician and averting unnecessary biopsies are other important DBI functions.

Radiographic Signs of Breast Carcinoma

To appreciate the capabilities of DBI, the clinician should understand those findings that lead the mammographer to suspect malignancy. Similarly, it is helpful to understand the factors that lead the mammographer to conclude that a radiographic or sonographic finding is benign or of insufficient concern to require biopsy. The clinician should also understand the radiologic alterations that can occur as a result of surgery. Trauma to the breast, including the effects of the surgeon's needle or scalpel, can leave parenchymal changes indistinguishable from mammographic findings associated with breast carcinoma.

Mammographic signs of breast cancer have been grouped into primary and secondary signs (Table 5-1). The discussion below is limited to primary signs.

Microcalcifications. Microcalcifications may be the most important mammographic sign of malignant breast disease, because they represent the earliest identifiable clue to the presence of noninvasive breast carcinoma (intraductal carcinoma or ductal carcinoma in situ, DCIS). It is important to note that lobular carcinoma in situ, LCIS, is not included. There are no clinical or radiologic findings of LCIS. The diagnosis of LCIS is a serendipitous, incidental finding in pathology specimens.[17]It is equally important to note that a histologic diagnosis of LCIS cannot be accepted as the explanation for a radiographic finding that led to biopsy. If the only pathologic finding is LCIS, one should ask whether the area of radiographic concern has been removed, and if so, whether it has been examined by the pathologist.

Calcifications are common in most mature breasts. Benign-type calcifications are typically larger than malignant calcifications. When smaller or punctate, they are more uniformly round and of simi-

TABLE 5-1—Radiographic Signs of Breast Cancer

Primary Signs	Secondary Signs
Mass	Skin thickening
Microcalcifications	Skin or nipple retraction
Parenchymal distortion*	Parenchymal asymmetry
	Abnormal lymph nodes
	Edema

*Considered by some to be a secondary sign

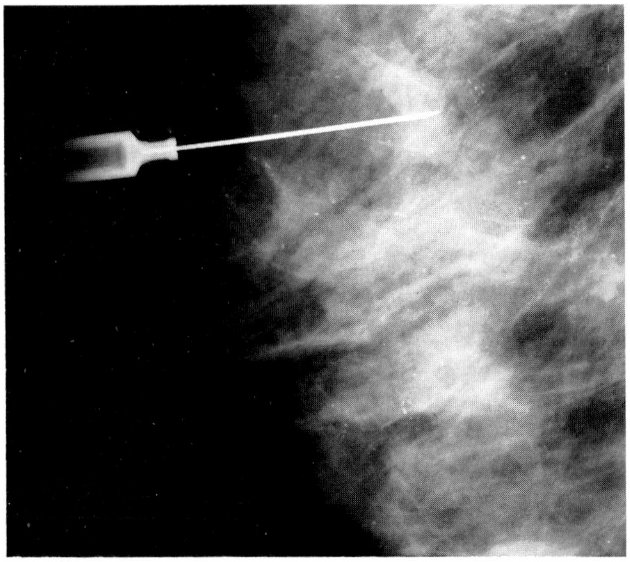

FIGURE 5-1 Multiple punctate, loosely distributed microcalcifications that are typically benign in character. One cluster of calcifications (near the tip of the localizing needle) showed slight pleomorphic features. Biopsy showed the clustered calcifications to be associated with a small noninvasive (intraductal) carcinoma (DCIS). The other benign calcifications were associated with diffuse scleosing adenosis.

lar density (Fig. 5-1). Benign calcifications may also present as smooth castings within the ductal lumina (Fig. 5-5). Malignant-type calcifications, on the other hand, are generally punctate, irregularly rod-shaped or pleomorphic, and of varying density (Figs. 5-1 to 5-4).[18,19] When such calcifications present in small clusters or with ductal orientation, the suspicion of ductal carcinoma may be very high.

Although calcifications that are the direct result of surgery are usually not confused with malignant-type calcifications, some postsurgical calcifications

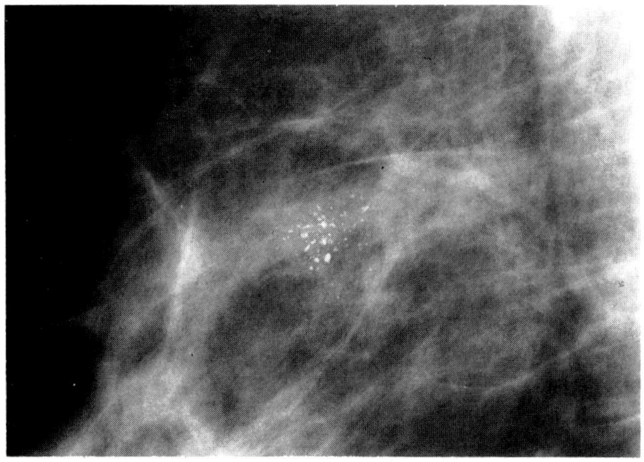

FIGURE 5-3 Small cluster of pleomorphic microcalcifications (magnified image). Pathologic diagnosis: DCIS.

may resemble malignant calcifications and require very close surveillance or re-excision. The more common, larger, benign "dystrophic" calcifications develop in devitalized tissue, or in association with oil cysts (Fig. 5-6).

Masses. By the time breast carcinoma presents as a clinically palpable or radiographically defined mass, it is an invasive cancer.[21] "Doubling time" refers to the time required for a tumor to double its volume, and although doubling times vary considerably, 100 days is accepted as average for breast carcinoma. By the time a tumor has grown to 1 cm in diameter, it has gone through approximately 30 doubling times. Only three doubling times are needed for a tumor to grow from 1 to 2 cm in diameter.[20] A diameter of 1 cm is the generally accepted threshold for palpability of breast masses. Early detection of small, clinically occult, invasive carcinomas is important in order to achieve a realistic opportunity for cure.[17,18,22] At least a 93 percent 20-

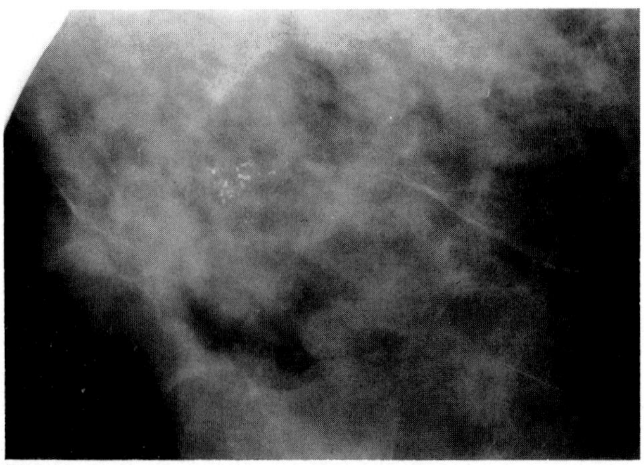

A

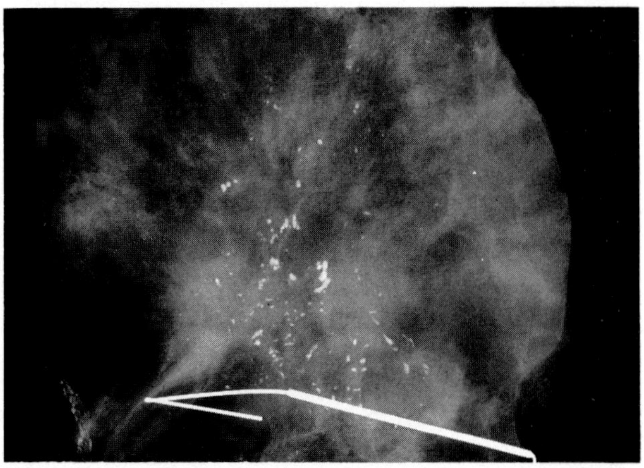

B

FIGURE 5-2 *A*, Small group of pleomorphic punctate calcifications. First screening mammogram in a 40-year-old asymptomatic patient. *B*, Surgical specimen radiograph (magnified image) shows many more calcifications than were suspected on the preoperative mammogram. Pathologic diagnosis: DCIS.

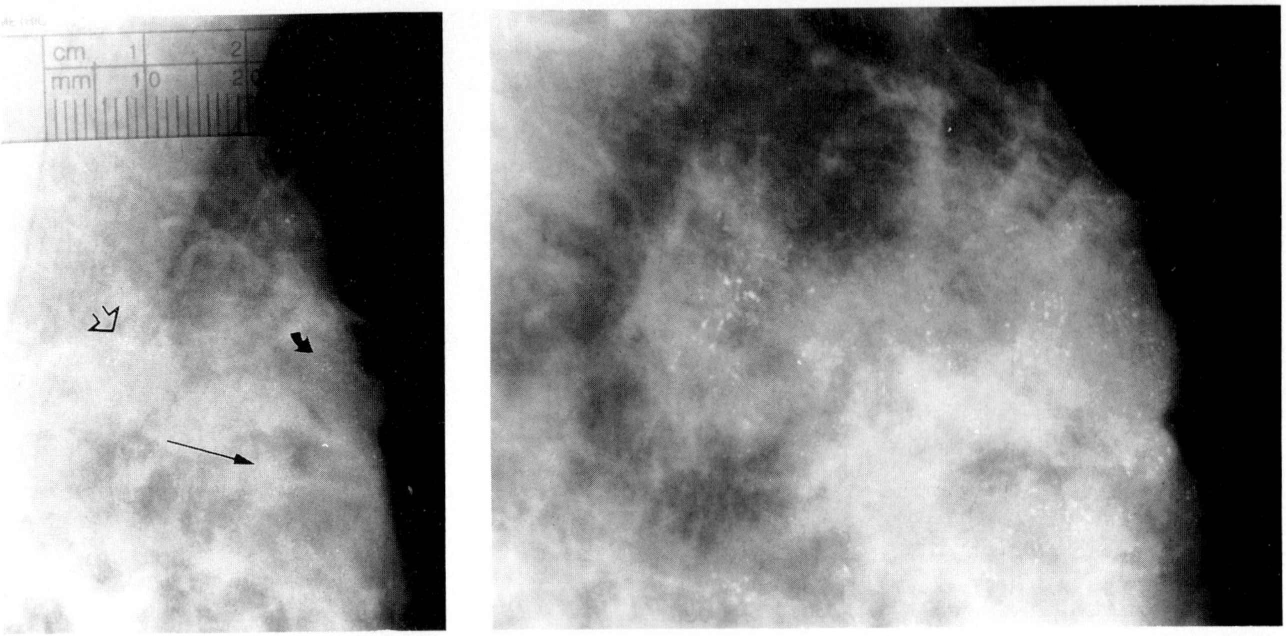

A B

FIGURE 5-4 *A*, Mediolateral-oblique view showing the axillary tail of the breast containing a subtle cluster of microcalcifications. *B*, Magnified image (1.85 ×) of the same area. Note the numerous calcifications, which were not seen with the standard, nonmagnified, image. These are pleomorphic and highly suspicious for carcinoma. Pathologic diagnosis: Diffuse ductal carcinoma in situ (DCIS). There is no evidence of invasion.

year survival rate can be expected with early diagnosis of the in situ stage, or if there is only minimal invasion and the tumor is less than 5 mm in diameter.[23-25] A direct relationship exists between the extent of axillary node involvement and the size of an invasive lesion at the time of diagnosis.[26-28] Five-year survival rates for all breast carcinomas show a drop from 85 percent without nodal involvement to 35 to 45 percent with nodal involvement.[26-28]

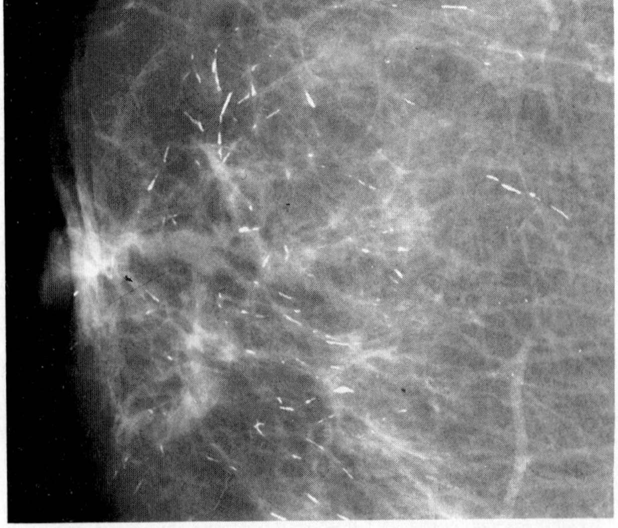

FIGURE 5-5 Large, benign, casting-type calcifications.

Although masses under 1 cm in diameter are rarely palpable clinically, they are often discernible mammographically. Many carcinomas less than 5 mm in diameter can be detected by high-quality mammography (Figs. 5-7, 5-8). Stellate masses may present as mammographically malignant lesions requiring no further evaluation before biopsy (Figs. 5-9, 5-10). Rounded or lobulated masses that appear well marginated can be either cystic or solid. Sonography then becomes a valuable adjunctive imaging tool to differentiate between solid and cystic masses (Figs. 5-11, 5-12). Small cysts are very common in the breast and can usually be left alone. Solid nodules, on the other hand, may be benign or malignant, and although echographic features may strongly suggest a lesion to be benign or malignant, definitive diagnosis requires histologic examination. Many sharply marginated solid nodules with homogeneous echo patterns can safely be followed with mammography, ultrasonography, or both to assure stability, and thus avoid biopsy. Solid masses with mammographically defined irregular margins, or with irregular walls and mixed echo patterns, are of greater concern and may be appropriately biopsied. The age of the patient and identified risk factors may aid the decision to follow or biopsy lesions. A young woman under age 25 with a small, well-circumscribed nodule, showing a homogeneous echo pattern on sonography, almost certainly has a benign fibroadenoma. A similar lesion in a 65-year-old woman with two sisters who developed premenopausal breast cancer should be biopsied.

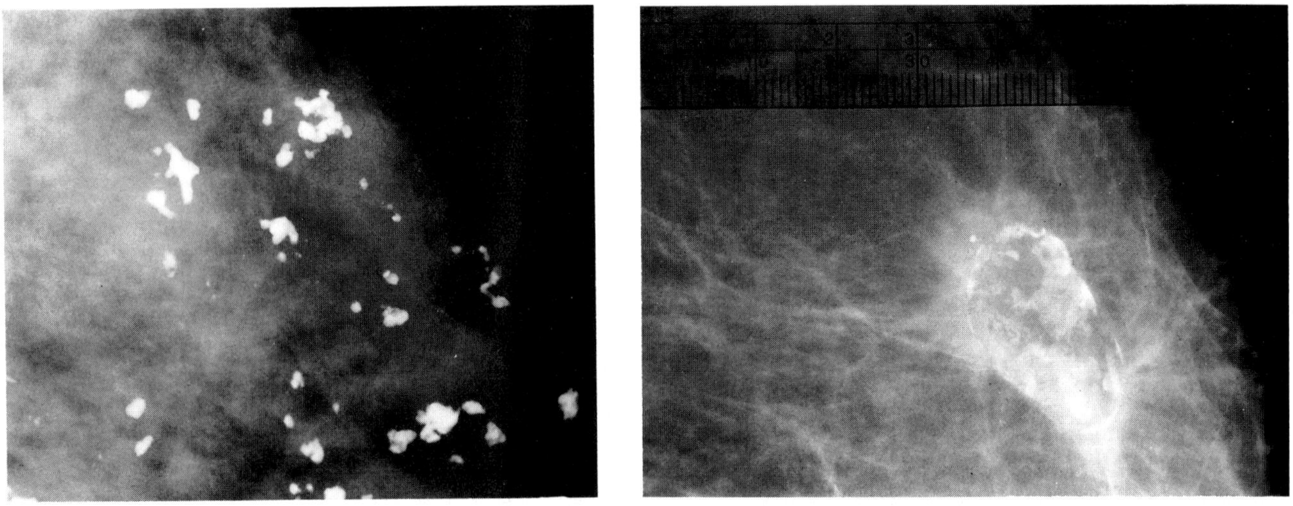

A B

FIGURE 5-6 *A*, Large dystrophic calcifications developing in devitalized tissue, probably in degenerating fibroadenomas. *B*, Calcified hematoma with an oil cyst in the operative site 6 years after biopsy. The spiculated mass effect surrounding the area of calcifications appears sinister, but is all due to fat necrosis.

Postoperative masses may mimic carcinoma (see Fat Necrosis and Scarring, p. 54).

Architectural Distortion. Areas of architectural distortion or conspicuous asymmetry, compared with similar areas in the contralateral breast, are frequently a dilemma for the mammographer. Although listed as one of the primary signs of breast cancer, this finding is more often an indication for further imaging studies. The trained eye of the mammographer develops a threshold level of tolerance for parenchymal irregularity, accepting most such areas as benign tissue. Findings perceived to exceed this benign threshold alert the mammographer to pursue further analysis. The mammographer must first determine whether the area in question is real or an artifact of positioning or superimposition. Additional views with focal compression spot film techniques or magnification may provide sufficient further information to complete the diagnosis or establish an appropriate level of concern.

Postoperative architectural distortion and scarring are common and can be a dilemma for the mammographer (see Fat Necrosis and Scarring, p. 13).

Changing Architecture. The breast is normally a fibrofatty organ with varying degrees of density and nodular-like glandular parenchyma. When an area of parenchymal irregularity appears to have

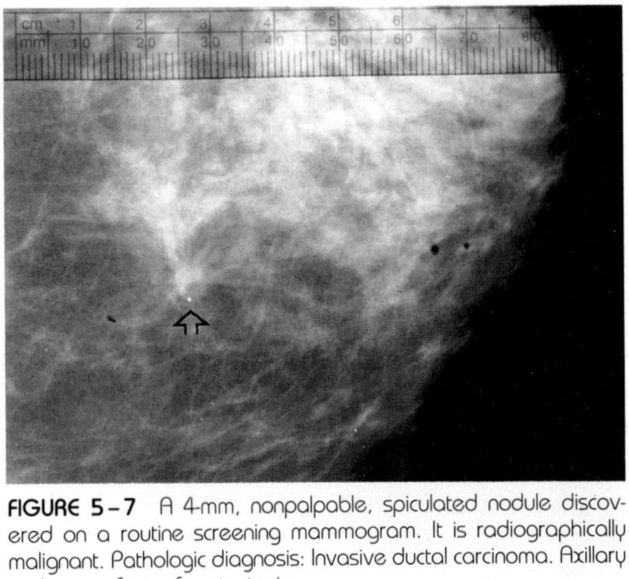

FIGURE 5-7 A 4-mm, nonpalpable, spiculated nodule discovered on a routine screening mammogram. It is radiographically malignant. Pathologic diagnosis: Invasive ductal carcinoma. Axillary nodes are free of metastasis.

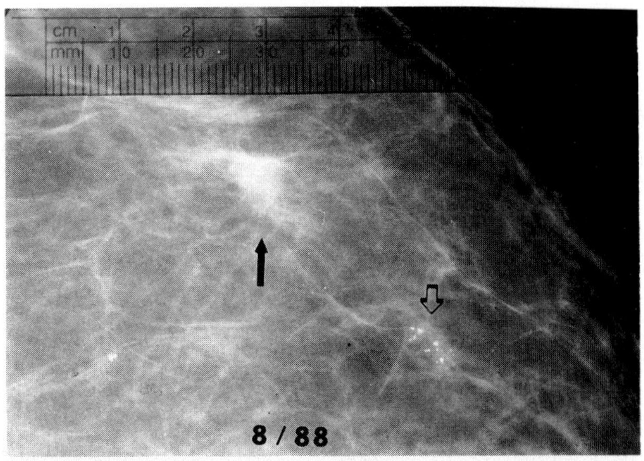

FIGURE 5-8 Two areas of concern: 7-mm density (*black arrow*) and 5-mm cluster of pleomorphic calcifications (*open arrow*). In comparison with the previous year's mammogram, the nodule was slightly larger and the calcifications slightly more numerous. There were no palpable abnormalities. Pathologic diagnosis: Both lesions showed invasive ductal carcinoma. Lymph nodes were free of metastases. Multifocal disease renders the patient an unsuitable candidate for breast-conserving surgery.

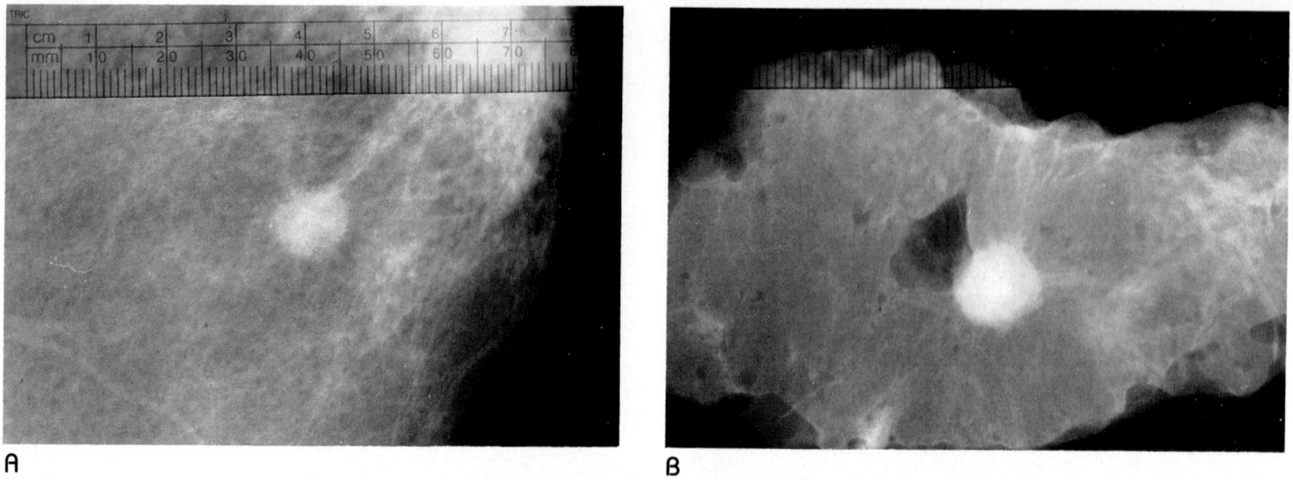

FIGURE 5-9 *A*, An 11-mm nodule with spiculated margins. Such a lesion is radiographically malignant. *B*, Radiograph of biopsy specimen. Spiculated margins are more obvious and seen with sharper detail.

changed since the previous mammograms, the mammographer is once again faced with the need to determine whether the area of concern is real or an artifact of composite densities. By employing the tools of spot compression, magnification, and sonography, or combining careful physical examination with the imaging techniques, the analysis can be completed and a conclusion reached regarding the need for biopsy or continued clinical or radiographic follow-up. Changing architecture is best identified and followed with interval mammography.

Postoperative changing architecture can best be understood when preoperative architecture has been compared.

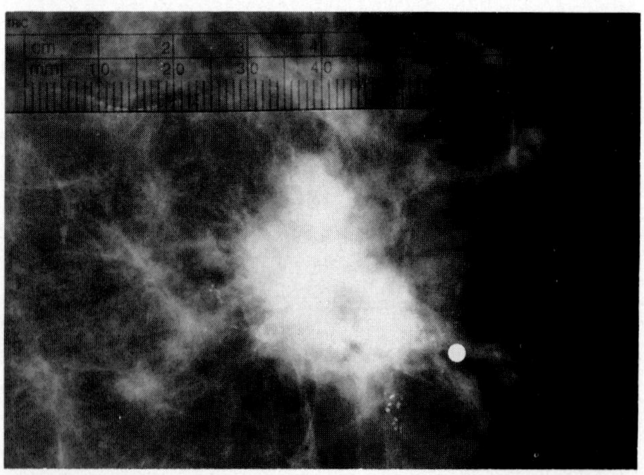

FIGURE 5-10 A 2.5-cm mass with shaggy borders and some spiculation. Note the pleomorphic calcifications. It is radiographically malignant. The bright round dot is a lead "BB" placed over the clinically palpable lump. Pathologic diagnosis: Invasive ductal carcinoma. Four of 11 nodes were positive for metastasis.

COMPARISON MAMMOGRAPHIC STUDIES

The purpose of screening patients at regular intervals is to detect interval change. Short-interval (usually 6-month) follow-up studies may occasionally be recommended to provide added reassurance that an area thought probably to be benign is stable.

Comparison with previous mammographic films is an important part of any breast imaging study. Clinicians can greatly facilitate this part of the evaluation by requesting that previous mammograms be sent to the breast imaging facility. Arrangements can often be made to have the patient obtain and carry the previous study with her when she presents for her new examination.

POSTOPERATIVE CHANGES AFFECTING THE MAMMOGRAM

Fat Necrosis and Scarring

The initial response to trauma is hemorrhage and/or edema (Fig. 5-13). Depending on the degree of containment or diffusion of blood at the site of trauma, the immediate mammographic findings can vary from a definable mass to an area of asymmetric parenchymal density. Contained blood initially organizes but eventually undergoes fibrinolysis (Fig. 5-14). If fibrinolysis occurs in a well-contained area, it may leave a lipid-filled radiolucent mass or "oil cyst." This lesion has distinguishing radiographic features and can be accurately diagnosed by the mammographer. An oil cyst can develop after any surgical procedure on the breast, including cyst aspiration and needle or open biopsy (Figs. 5-15, 5-16).[29] It may be seen as early as a few weeks after

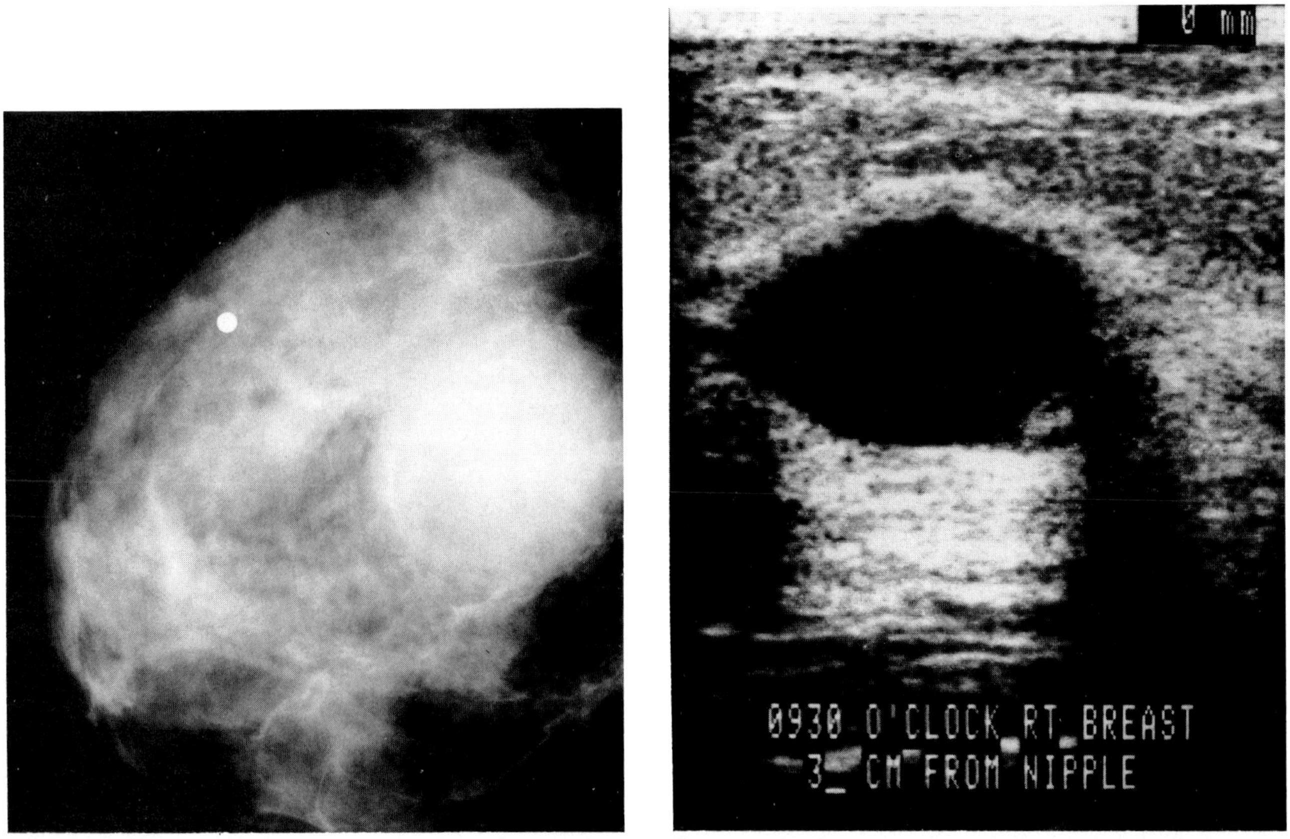

A B

FIGURE 5-11 *A*, Large mass with somewhat irregular margins. It is not possible to differentiate between solid and cystic mass on the basis of the mammogram. *B*, Sonography of the mass seen mammographically in *A*. An echo-free mass with a bright band of acoustical enhancement is seen posteriorly. This is the typical echographic appearance of a fluid-filled mass or cyst.

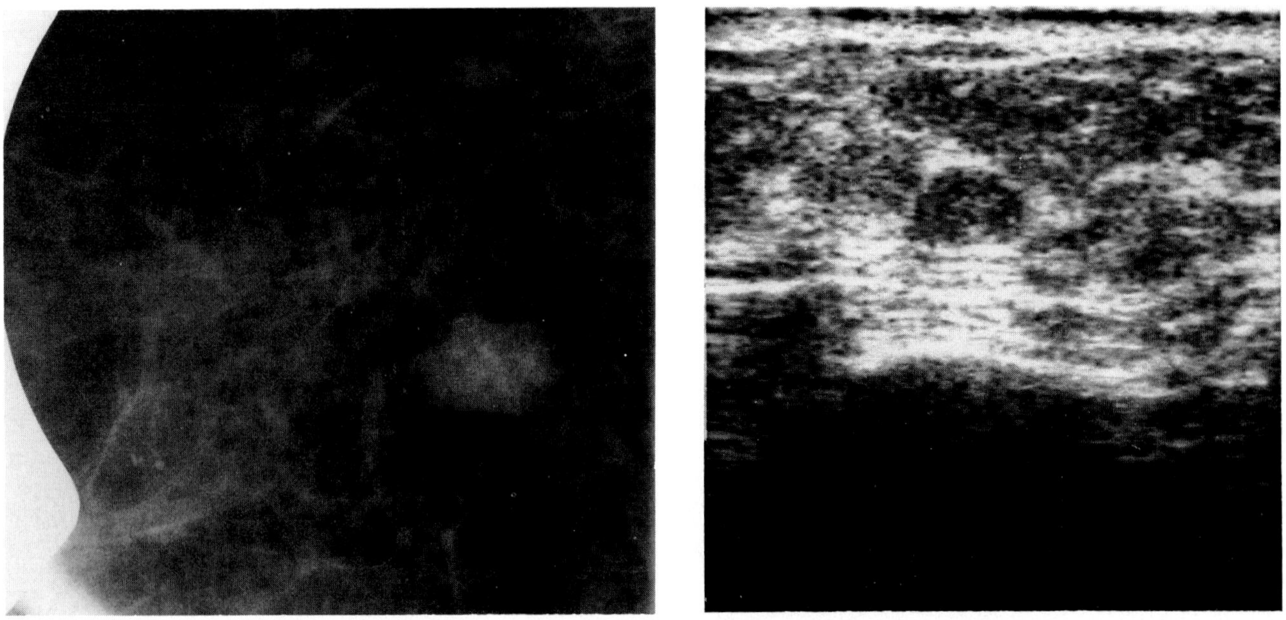

A B

FIGURE 5-12 *A*, Slightly irregular mass. It is not possible to differentiate between solid or cystic mass mammographically, although knobby margins are more characteristic of a solid lesion. *B*, Sonography of the mass seen mammographically in *A*. Internal echos indicate a solid structure. The uniform internal echo pattern is most consistent with a fibroadenoma, which was confirmed histologically.

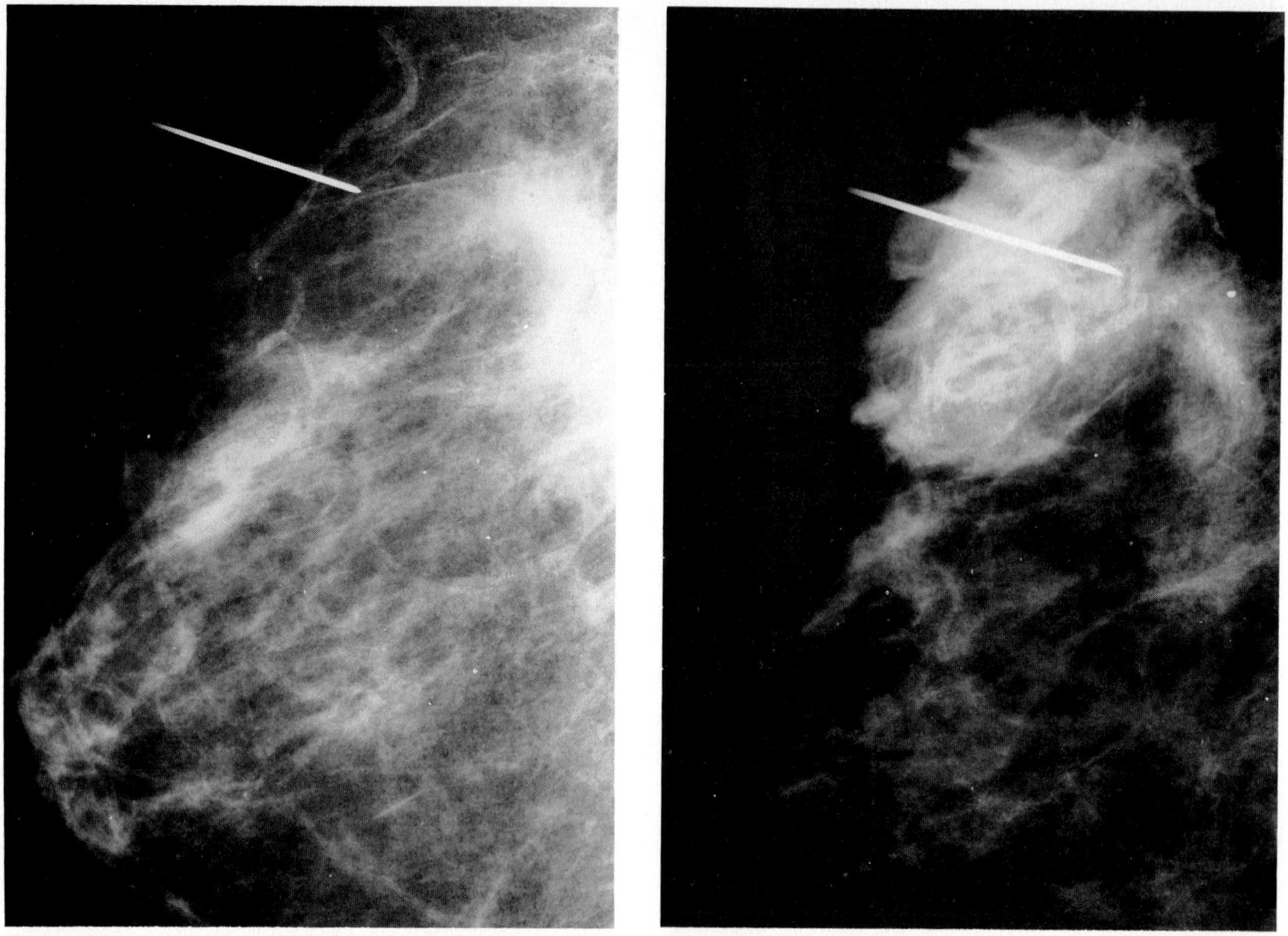

A B

FIGURE 5–13 *A*, A needle was placed preoperatively to localize a small group of microcalcifications. Note the calcified artery. The needle was not long enough to reach the calcifications. *B*, The needle was replaced with a longer one, the tip positioned at the calcifications. Note the large white mass surrounding the needle. This represents a 6-cm hematoma caused by the needle's passage through the artery seen in *A*. Any needle placed in the breast can result in a hematoma, which may or may not be apparent clinically.

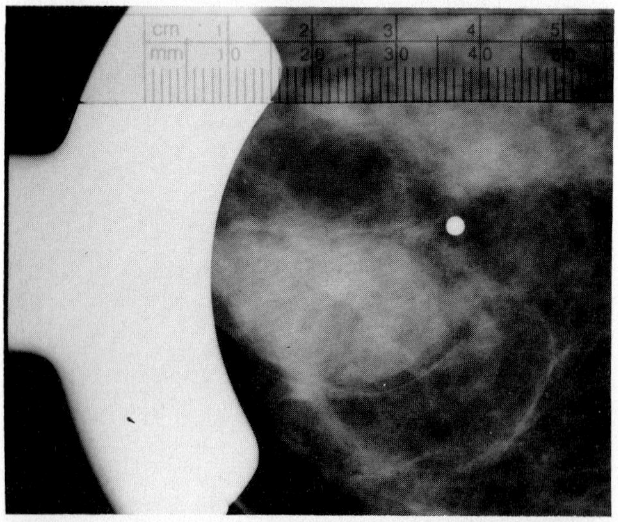

FIGURE 5–14 A 3-cm mass developed in a breast that had been struck by a car door 1 week earlier. Note the central mass is surrounded by a thin radiopaque (white) capsule. Just inside the capsule is a 2- to 4-mm radiolucent band representing the fat density of lipid material surrounding the hematoma undergoing fibrinolysis. The white dot is a lead "BB" placed by the technologist over the palpable mass.

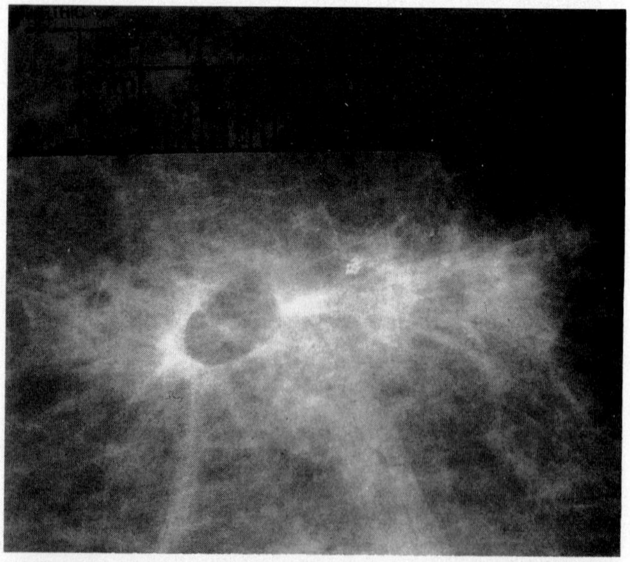

FIGURE 5–15 Spiculated area of radiographic density containing a 5- by 10-mm ovoid radiolucent area. The patient underwent a biopsy in this site 3 months earlier. The spiculated area represents scarring and fat necrosis. The ovoid radiolucent area is an oil cyst within the area of scarring.

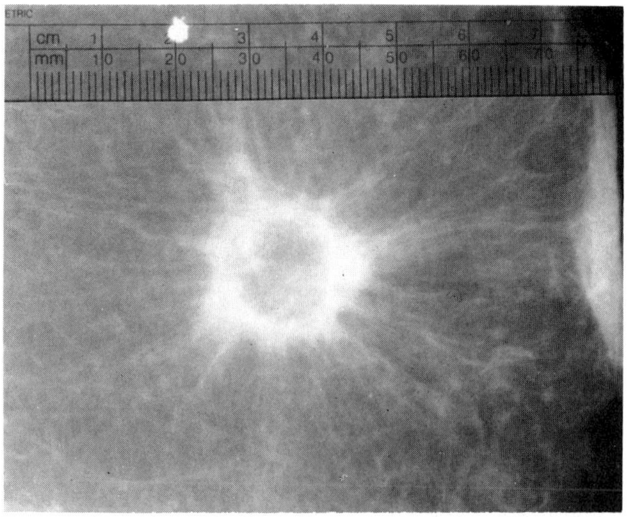

FIGURE 5-16 Spiculated mass containing a central area of radiolucency. This is an area of fat necrosis containing an oil cyst at the site of a biopsy for benign disease 4 years earlier.

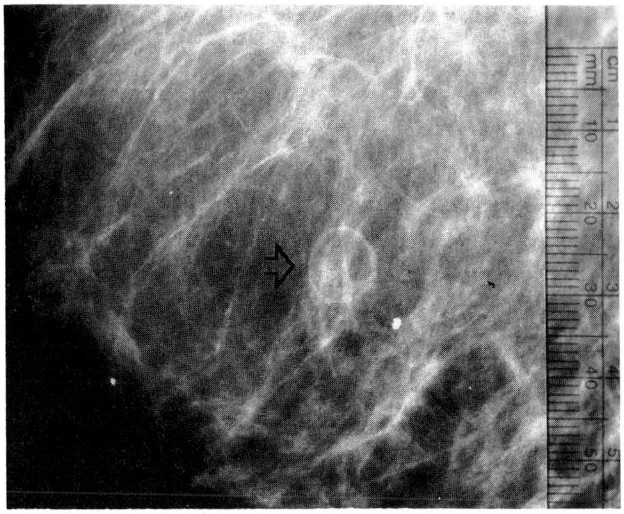

FIGURE 5-17 Faint calcified ring representing calcification in the wall of an oil cyst. The patient had undergone a biopsy in this site many years earlier.

trauma and may remain for years, if not indefinitely. Calcification may develop in the wall of an oil cyst (Fig. 5-17). Large or superficial oil cysts may be palpable. Lipid material that is not contained can incite fibrosis and scarring. This type of desmoplastic reaction can mimic the radiographic characteristics of invasive carcinoma (Figs. 5-16, 5-18). Post-traumatic desmoplastic reactions usually reach their peak within the first 6 months after trauma and may completely resolve over the next few months; however, they may persist indefinitely as scarring. Because of surgical skills, and perhaps the benevolence of mother nature, post-traumatic mammographic findings often resolve with no apparent residual mammographic abnormality. However, some residual architectural distortion may persist as permanent scarring. Postoperative architectural changes that appear to increase after 6 months should be

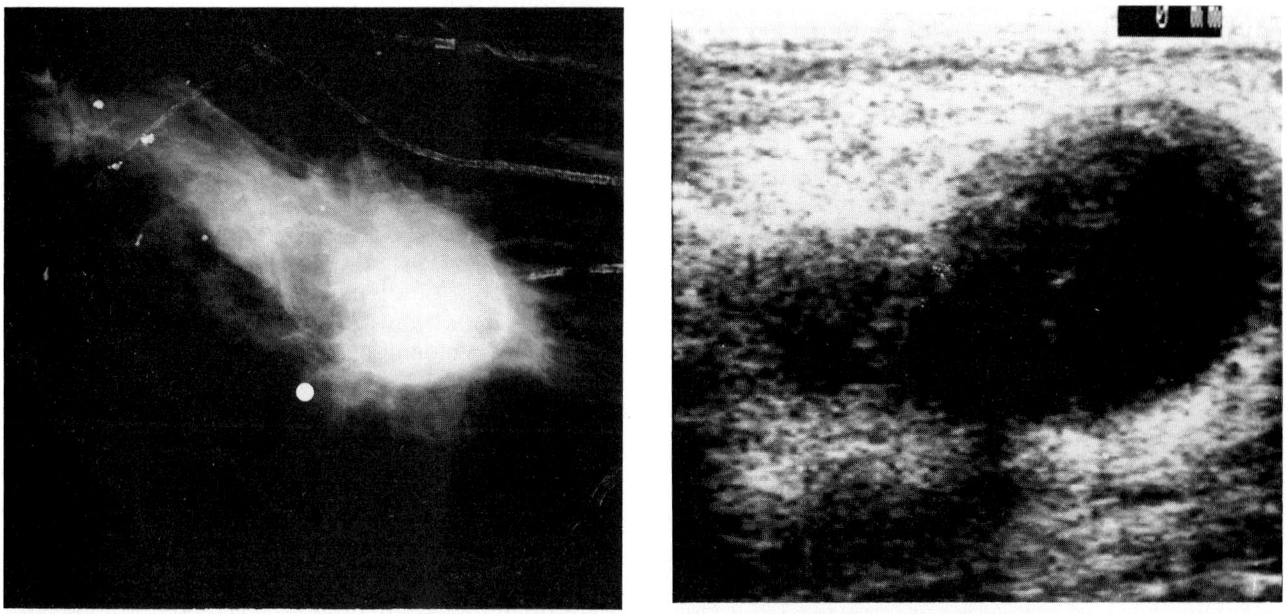

A B

FIGURE 5-18 *A*, Large palpable mass with poorly defined margins. The patient developed a mass in the biopsy site the day after the biopsy. This film is taken 9 months after biopsy for a benign nodule. The mass has not changed in size since first discovered. *B*, Sonogram of the mass in *A* shows a 2- by 4-cm mass with low-level internal echoes, consistent with the clinically suspected hematoma. Fine needle aspiration yielded necrotic material consistent with the radiographic and clinical impression. The lesion was biopsied because of the patient's anxiety. Pathologic diagnosis: Hematoma with fat necrosis.

viewed with suspicion, especially after surgery for malignant disease.

The following case study illustrates the importance of anticipating post-traumatic changes. A 38-year-old woman was biopsied for what proved to be benign calcifications, but was incidentally found to have a focus of LCIS. The excisional biopsy was accepted as the only treatment. The patient was examined every 6 months by the surgeon, but no follow-up mammogram was obtained until 18 months after the biopsy. A 1-cm spiculated mass was detected mammographically in the operative site. The dilemma facing the mammographer was in differentiating benign postoperative fat necrosis from invasive carcinoma. Knowing that patients with LCIS are at added risk for the development of either invasive lobular or ductal carcinoma, and aware of the risk of delaying biopsy of a 1-cm invasive carcinoma, the mammographer felt compelled to recommend biopsy. The pathologic diagnosis was fat necrosis. Had a mammogram been obtained 6 months after the biopsy, a mass with a high probability of being fat necrosis would have been identified, making a decision to follow more reasonable. A short-interval follow-up would be expected to show involutional changes, supporting the benign character of the lesion. Without the benefit of these earlier postoperative studies, the mammographer cannot risk delay in diagnosis of invasive carcinoma, and must recommend biopsy.

A similar scenario can be applied to all types of breast surgery except mastectomy. Thus, our recommendation has been for a 6-month postoperative mammogram in any woman aged 35 or older, to establish, or re-establish, a baseline for future comparison (Fig. 5-19). This is especially important for patients already designated as "high risk." A 6-month postoperative baseline mammogram is appropriate in such women, regardless of age.

There are characteristic patterns of scarring that suggest the type of surgical procedure responsible. Thickened bands of fibrous stranding may be seen radiating caudally from the areola in patients who have undergone reduction mammaplasty. There may be associated skin thickening and/or retraction. Scarring may appear across the lower half of the breast, depending on the particular reduction procedure, the extent of dissection, and postoperative complications such as hematomas or seromas (Figs. 5-20, 5-21). Similar scarring can be seen after mastopexy. It has been our policy to recommend 6-month postoperative mammograms if the patient is 35 years or older, followed by annual mammograms. If the patient is identified as "high risk" by history or pathologic findings, e.g. atypical hyperplasia, in the resected tissue, a 6-month postoperative follow-up with annual mammograms are initiated regardless of age.

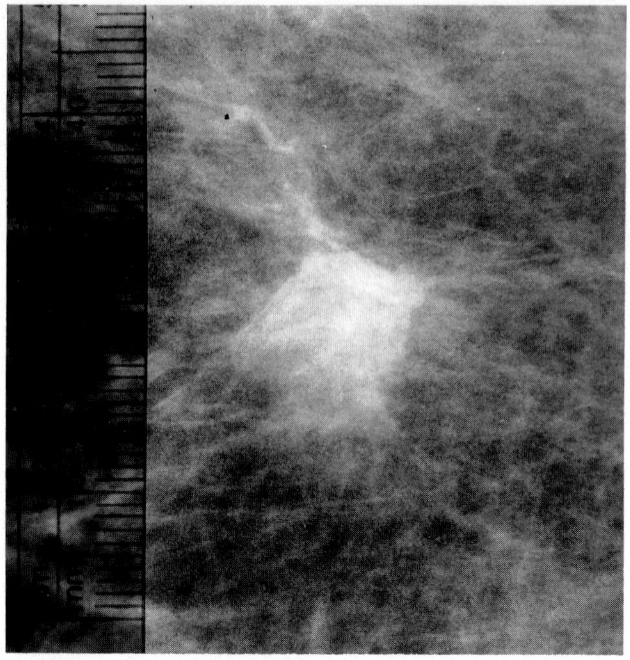

FIGURE 5-19 Irregular mass at the site of lobular carcinoma in situ (LCIS), treated with lumpectomy only 5 months earlier. The radiologic diagnosis was probable fat necrosis. A repeat mammogram in 3 months was recommended to ensure stability or further involution of the process. Biopsy was preferred by the patient and surgeon. Pathologic diagnosis: Fat necrosis with an incidental finding of another LCIS. LCIS is often multifocal, and thus not an unusual finding in such a case.

Calcifications

Typically benign-appearing macrocalcifications often develop in an operative site. They may occur after simple biopsies or cosmetic surgery. They develop in areas of fat necrosis or as dystrophic calcifications in areas of devitalized tissue.[15] The development of microcalcifications may be associated with benign or malignant disease.[19,20] Careful analysis will determine the appropriate level of suspicion and the possible need for biopsy. Magnification imaging is especially important in this analysis (see Fig. 5-4). High-quality mammographic equipment, with a micro-focal spot x-ray tube, is essential to achieve magnified image quality, sufficient to resolve or optimally characterize microcalcifications.

To avoid unnecessary concern or indecisive reporting by the mammographer, the clinician should inform the breast imaging facility about any previous breast surgery and postoperative complications. This important history can be relayed at the time the appointment is scheduled. Some facilities provide their referring physicians referral forms that include check-off lists requiring only seconds to complete by someone familiar with the history.

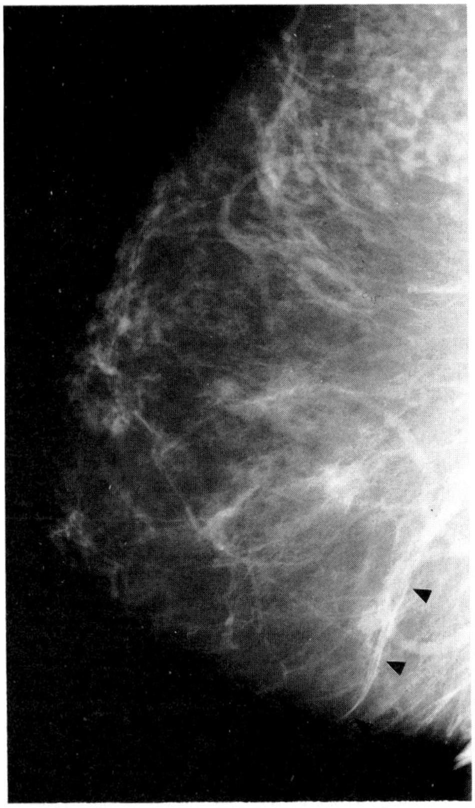

FIGURE 5-20 Typical lower posterior scar from previous reduction mammoplasty (*arrowheads*). Mediolateral oblique view. The patient had breast reduction several years earlier. Such scars can be seen as early as 8 weeks after breast reduction surgery.

Inflammatory Changes

An inflammatory process can present mammographically as a mass or area of asymmetric density, with or without other parenchymal or skin changes. Again, it is of utmost importance for the mammographer to be informed of such clinical concerns and related surgical history. Sonography can be very useful in evaluating and following inflammatory masses. Abscesses typically present with thickened walls, mixed internal echoes, and posterior shadowing. Sonography is useful in assessing the extent of suppuration, and may provide direction for needle aspiration to confirm the diagnosis or obtain material for culture and sensitivity.[30-33]

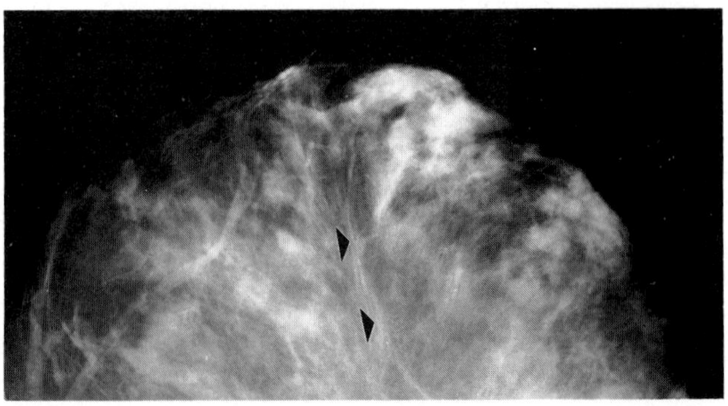

FIGURE 5-21 Typical postreduction mammoplasty scar as seen in the craniocaudal view (*arrowheads*). Breast reduction surgery was performed 2 years earlier.

MAMMOGRAPHIC INTERPRETATION

In reporting conclusions about a breast imaging study, mammographers should be as definitive as possible regarding their level of concern and follow-up recommendations. It is appropriate to make specific recommendations regarding radiographic findings, especially when there are no correlating clinical findings. The decision to biopsy a clinically occult lesion is primarily a radiographic one. Certainly, overriding clinical considerations may influence the decision to proceed with radiologic recommendations. Indecision and ambiguity in mammographic reporting can lead to unnecessary patient anxiety, frustration for the clinician, loss of confidence in the mammographer's role and abilities, unnecessary biopsies, or damaging delays in treatment. The problem of ambiguous and indecisive reporting can often be avoided by a close working relationship and active interaction between the clinician and mammographer regarding clinical and mammographic findings.

Despite efforts to be decisive and offer definitive opinions and recommendations for follow-up, mammographers must occasionally admit they are not sure. At this point they must explain the basis of their uncertainty and recommend careful clinical evaluation with either biopsy or close mammographic follow-up to identify interval change, or determine that the area in question is stable, permitting continued conservative follow-up. Correlation of clinical and mammographic findings is often essential in order to determine the next appropriate action. The mammographer who has interpreted the mammogram without examining the patient and obtaining a complete breast history, and has not been given pertinent clinical information, cannot be as definitive in mammographic conclusions or recommendations and must rely on the clinician for such correlation and conclusions; the mammographer's role has thus been needlessly compromised and left unfulfilled.

THE AUGMENTED BREAST

Mammography of the augmented breast has been the subject of controversy, misunderstanding, confusion, and significant frustration for patients, cli-

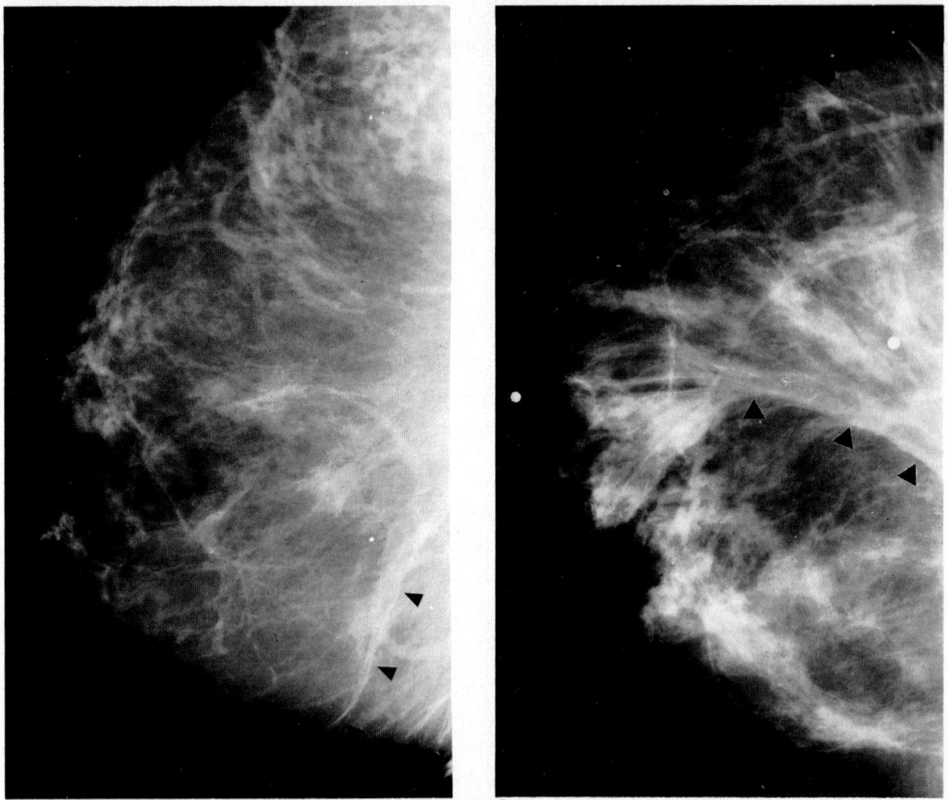

A B

FIGURE 5-22 *A*, Oblique view. *B*, Craniocaudal view. More prominent postreduction scarring in a patient who had undergone reduction surgery approximately 5 years earlier.

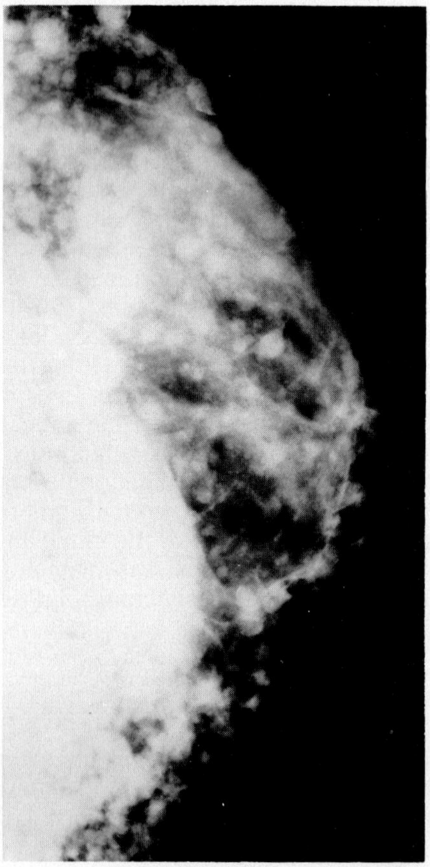

FIGURE 5-23 Silicone injection. The patient had had silicone injections for purposes of augmentation approximately 10 years before. The large, dense mass in the lower portion of the breast represents the largest deposit. Multiple smaller nodular densities represent multiple silicone granulomas. Such a mammographic appearance renders the examination almost useless for excluding early signs of breast cancer.

nicians, and mammographers.[34,35] It has also been the object of significant interpretive indecision and applied disclaimers. Suboptimal imaging has been accepted as an unavoidable consequence of breast implants.[36-40] The early "community" frustration with mammography for the augmented breast took root from the old intramammary silicone injections (Fig. 5-23).[41,42] This procedure, now prohibited in the United States, resulted in deposits of free silicone and development of silicone granulomas throughout the injected breast tissue. Mammographically, nodular densities consisting of silicone deposits or silicone granulomas can occupy large areas or even fill the breast, creating significant potential for masking breast carcinoma and contributing to delayed diagnosis.[41] Native breast tissue can be almost totally obscured. The host response of granuloma formation and fibrosis renders the tissue firm, immobile, and unresponsive to any modified imaging technique. If the silicone deposits spare sections of breast tissue, the spared areas can be evaluated mammographically. It has been our practice to recommend a baseline mammogram for all silicone-injected patients. The extent to which mammography will be useful in such patients can only be determined after evaluating the mammogram. If the breast is essentially filled with silicone, leaving little if any "open" breast tissue, routine follow-up mammograms may not be indicated. These patients should be advised of the mammographic limitations imposed by silicone and encouraged to practice regular breast self-examination (BSE) and have periodic physical examinations. These are the only remaining tools for identifying interval changes that might dictate a need for further evaluation. Changing patterns of texture, or new areas of nodularity, deserve careful evaluation. Armed with knowledge of specific areas of concern, the mammographer may be able to provide meaningful information with spot compression views with or without magnification. Sonography has not been helpful in evaluating these patients.

Although silicone, implanted in the breast tissue of mice, has been associated with an increased incidence of breast cancer,[43] there is no evidence that this also occurs in humans.[44]

Fortunately, we are seeing fewer and fewer of these silicone injected patients and more of the enclosed implants, either intramammary or subpectoral. Standard positioning techniques used for nonaugmented breasts have significant limitations when used for imaging augmented breasts, and frequently result in suboptimal images and frustration in interpretation.[34-38,40] Compression of breast tissue is essential for high-quality mammography. Implants impose a significant limitation to compression. As the compression paddle is brought down on the breast containing an implant, the implant is flattened and forced to expand peripherally (Fig. 5-24). The net effect of this peripheral expansion is to make breast tissue between the implant and skin more compact and radiographically dense. Tissue between the compression paddle and the implant, or between the film and the implant, will be obscured by the radiopacity of the implant.[36,37] Imaging techniques that "see through" the implant have been promoted for imaging patients with implants.[45] The use of saline rather than silicone gel for breast implants has been proposed because saline is less radiopaque than silicone.[45] It is important to understand that the early radiographic signs of small or noninvasive breast carcinoma, e.g. subtle microcalcifications or tiny masses, will still be masked in most cases by the superimposed implant, regardless of its location in reference to the pectoral muscle or its composition.[35-37] These small early lesions are the "curable" carcinomas to which we must direct our finest and most sensitive search efforts. There is no substitute for visualizing the maximal amount of well-compressed breast tissue possible, free of the implant. The ideal scenario would be a mechanism allowing temporary removal of the implant, permitting optimal positioning and compression of breast tissue. With a soft, compressible, and mobile implant, this ideal can be closely approximated. By pushing most of the implant out of the field of view, flattening the remaining implant against the chest wall while pulling breast tissue forward and in front of the implant, excellent compression of breast tissue, free of the implant, is possible (Figs. 5-24 to 5-27).[35-37] An additional 3 to 5 cm of compression is possible with this technique. Most, and in some cases all, of the breast tissue can be well visualized with this modified imaging technique in patients with soft and compressible implants, but in most cases, some degree of compromise to "complete" breast imaging is imposed by the presence of an implant. Surgeons should not convey the impression that new positioning techniques eliminate all previous limitations stemming from an implant.

Submammary Versus Subpectoral Implants

The modified compression technique described is equally applicable to submammary and subpectoral implants (Fig. 5-27). In our experience, we have seen no difference in the ability to achieve optimal modified positioning in patients with saline, silicone, or double-lumen implants. Generally, in patients with subpectoral implants, more complete visualization of breast tissue is possible. However, a freely movable, soft, submammary implant can often be completely excluded from the field of view, allowing excellent mammographic images. Views taken with standard compression to include the implant are less well tolerated by patients with subpectoral implants because of the discomfort associated with direct compression on the muscle. We have observed fewer firm encapsulations with subpectoral implants.

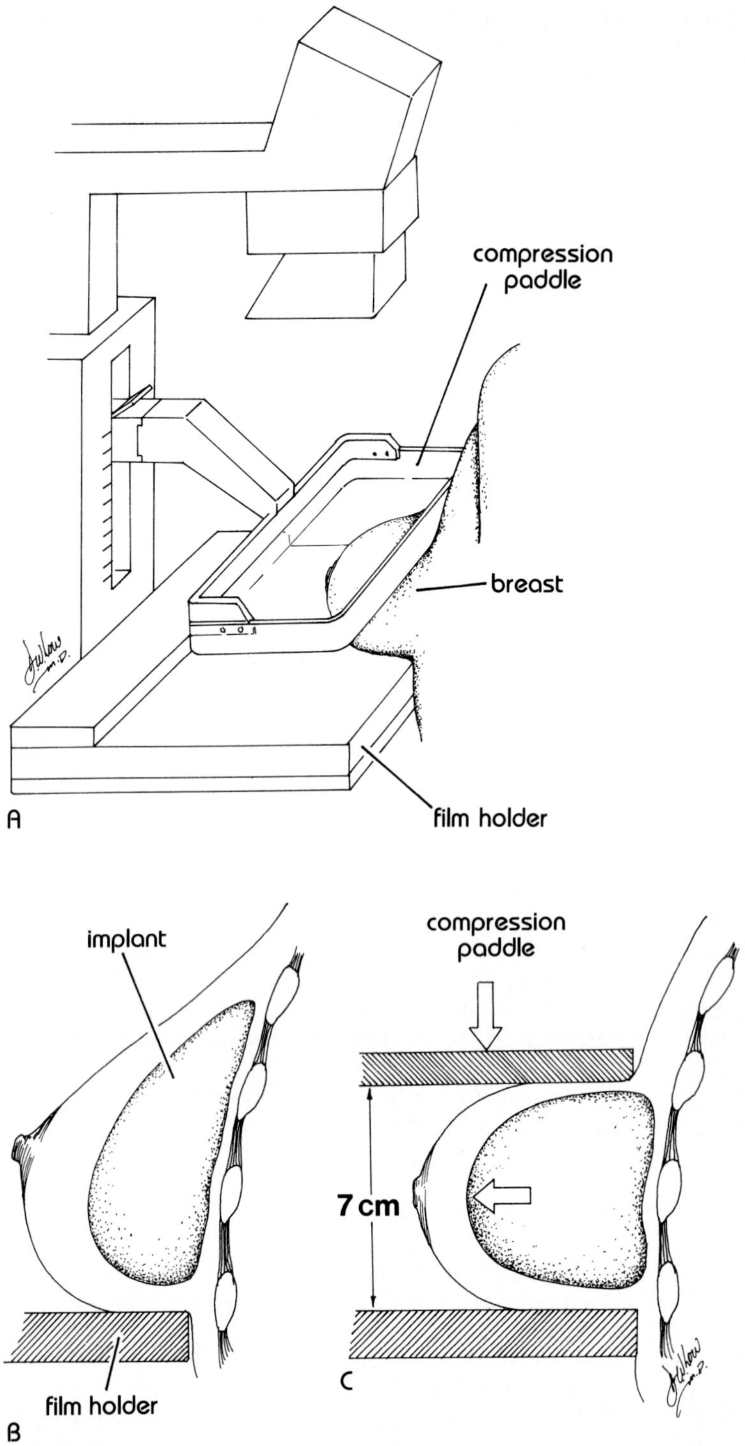

FIGURE 5-24 *A* to *F*, Modified compression technique for imaging the augmented breast. *A*, The breast is placed on the film holder and is compressed with the paddle. *B,C*, Compression of the breast with implant included. As the compression paddle is brought down on the implant, the implant partially flattens while expanding peripherally. Breast tissue is made more compact as it is compressed between the skin and expanding implant. Breast tissue between the skin and the implant is poorly compressed owing to the limitation imposed by the implant. *D*, Breast tissue is pulled over and in front of the implant, while the implant is pushed back against the chest wall and out of the field of compression. The compression paddle is brought down over the anterior convexity of the implant, and helps to force the implant posteriorly. *E*, The hand holds breast tissue that has been brought forward over the implant, while the compression paddle is brought further down to compress breast tissue without the limitation of the implant. *F*, The compression paddle takes the place of the hand to complete the compression process, with marked improvement in the degree of compression and resultant image quality.

Fibrous Encapsulation

With fibrous encapsulation, the implant becomes less compressible and less displaceable. Although firm encapsulation imposes a significant limitation to optimal breast imaging, the modified techniques that pull breast tissue over and in front of the implant enable markedly improved imaging of more breast tissue with good compression (Fig. 5-28*A*, *B*). The greater the degree of encapsulation, the greater are the limitations described.

It has been our practice to include a 90-degree lateral view of the breast if there is fibrous encapsulation of the implant. This provides better visualiza-

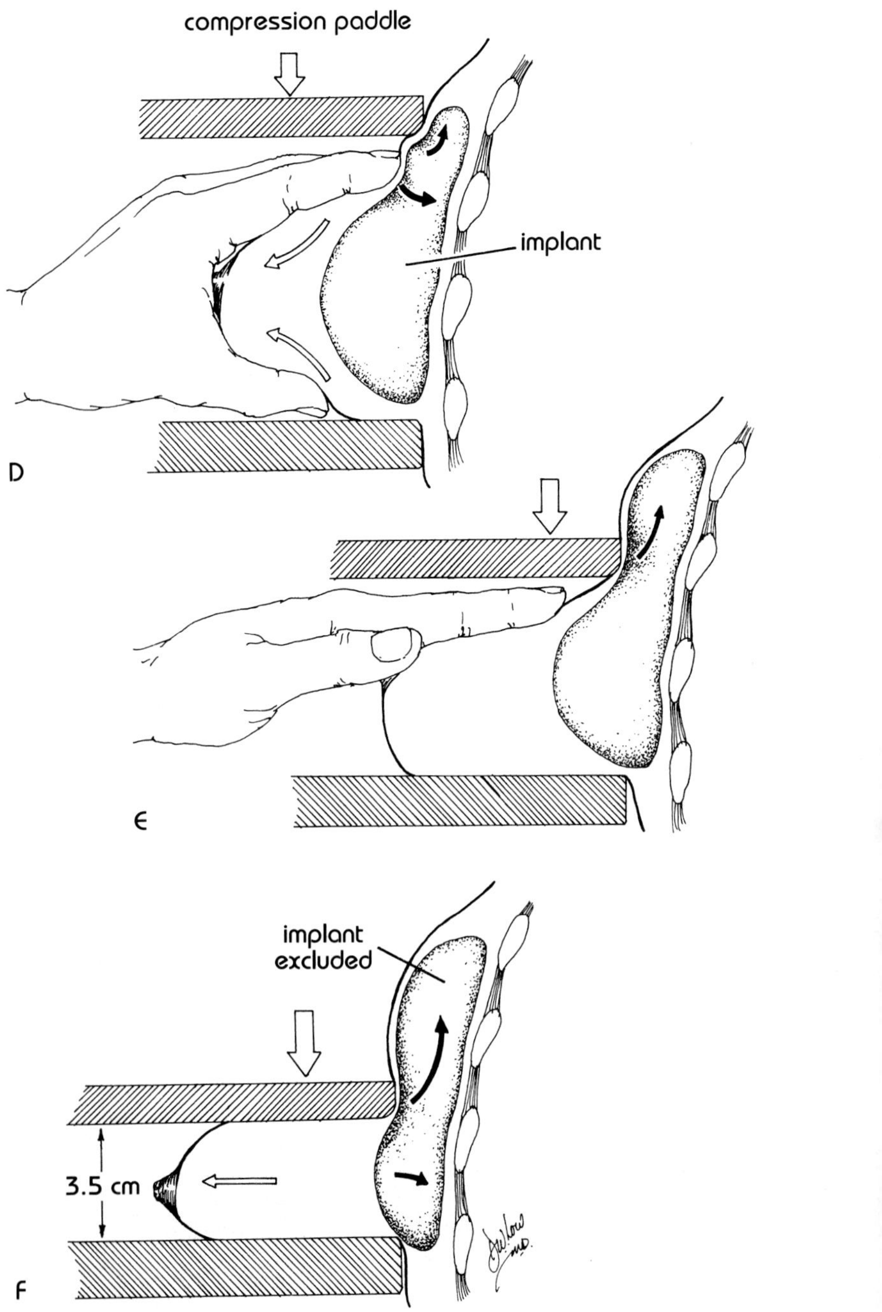

Figure 5-24 *Continued*

tion of breast tissue above and below the implant, which is not visualized with the standard craniocaudal and mediolateral oblique projections (Fig. 5-29).

Although calcification within the fibrous capsule can usually be identified mammographically (Fig. 5-28*C*, *D*), the capsule itself most often is not radiographically identified. The most common radiographic finding suggesting fibrous encapsulation is the round or ovoid shape of the implant as seen in the lateral or oblique projection (Fig. 5-28*A*, *B*). A soft implant without encapsulation usually assumes a teardrop shape with these views (Figs. 5-24 to 5-27). Fibrous encapsulation may not occur symmetrically. Occasionally, fibrous bands form, producing characteristic constrictions of the implant.[46,47] Care must be taken not to misinterpret these bulges as tumor masses.[46] Herniation of an implant through a rupture in the fibrous capsule can present mammographically as a fibrous constriction band (Fig. 5-30).[48] This mammographic appearance should not be misdiagnosed as rupture of the implant.[48] Patients should understand that development of fibrous encapsulation may alter the effectiveness of mammography in early breast cancer detection. This limita-

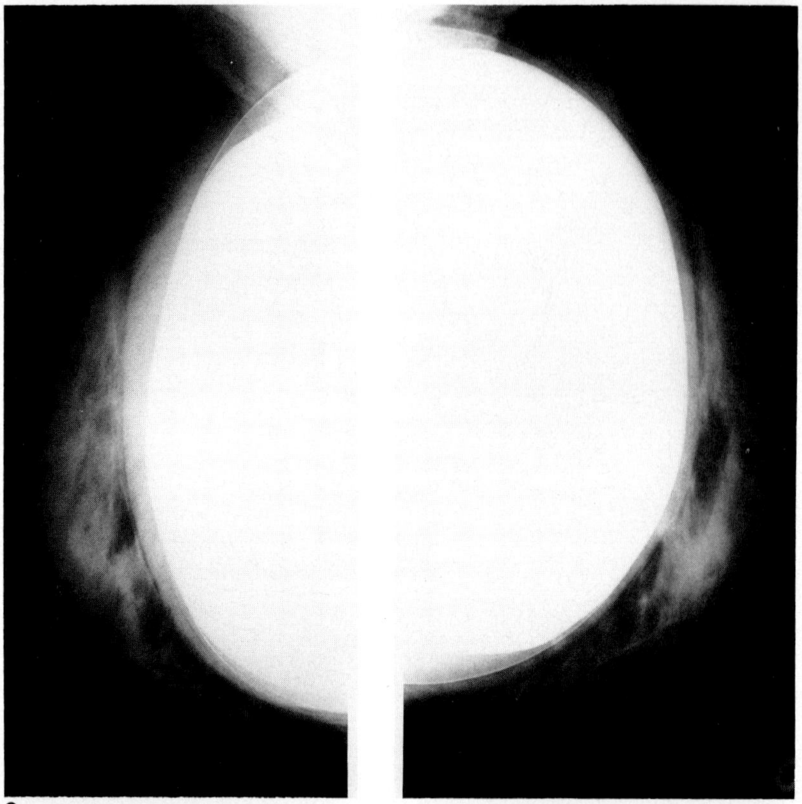

A

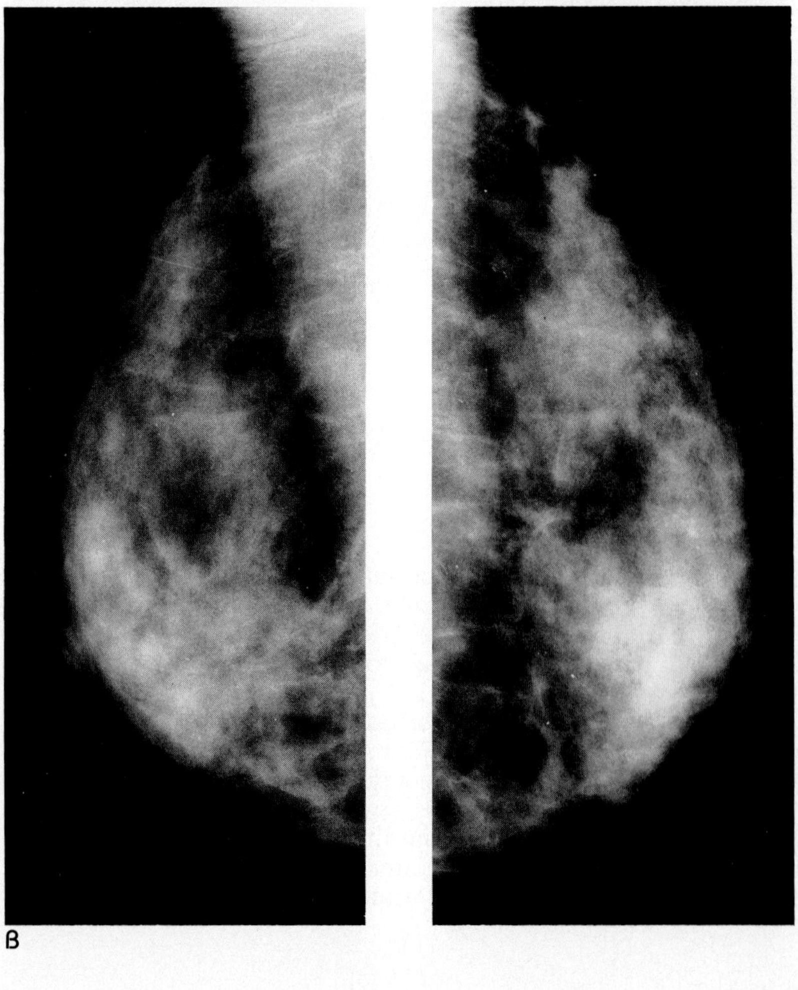

B

FIGURE 5-25 Subpectoral, double-lumen implant. *A*, Mediolateral oblique view with standard compression, including the implant. The implant obscures a significant portion of the breast tissue. Poor compression of breast tissue anterior to the implant results in poor image quality. *B*, Modified compression, mediolateral oblique view taken after breast tissue has been pulled over and in front of the implant and the implant flattened against the chest wall. In this patient the implant was quite mobile, and was partially displaced cephalad and medially out of the field of compression. There is marked improvement in the amount of breast tissue visualized. The greater degree of compression significantly improves image quality.

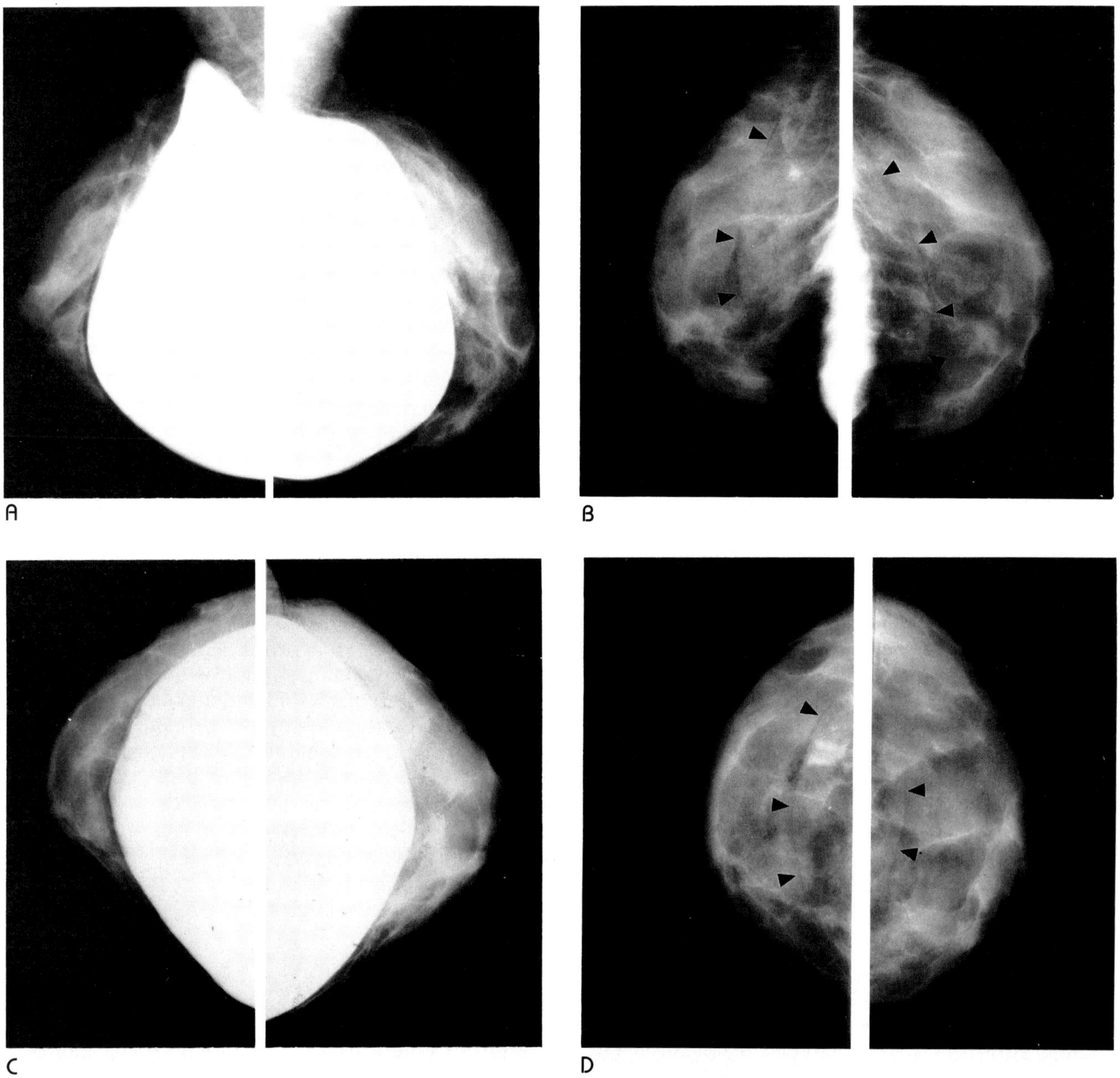

FIGURE 5-26 Submammary polyurethane implant. *A*, Standard compression view with implant included. *B*, Modified compression view with the implant mostly excluded and more breast tissue visualized with better compression. The faint, arching radiolucent line (*arrowheads*) represents the anterior wall of the implant. The author assumes that the firm bond between native breast tissue and the meshlike surface of this implant makes it less displaceable. Because the silicone within the implant can be displaced, leaving only the "empty envelope," there is no significant compromise of image quality. In this case there was no firm fibrous encapsulation that might limit the degree to which the implant could be compressed. *C*, Standard compression craniocaudal view with implant included. *D*, Modified compression craniocaudal view with silicone displaced and the breast with the remaining implant "envelope" well compressed. The anterior wall of the implant is marked with arrowheads.

tion may strengthen the argument for subpectoral placement of implants, with the reported lower incidence of encapsulation.[49] Patients in whom there are high risk factors should be carefully advised of possible limitations imposed by the implant, and perhaps encouraged to consider subpectoral implants if the decision is made to proceed with augmentation.

Breast Ultrasonography

Breast ultrasonography to evaluate patients with submammary implants has been advocated as a useful adjunctive imaging tool.[30-33, 50-52] We have found sonography of no greater or lesser value than in nonaugmented breasts. Breast ultrasound is useful

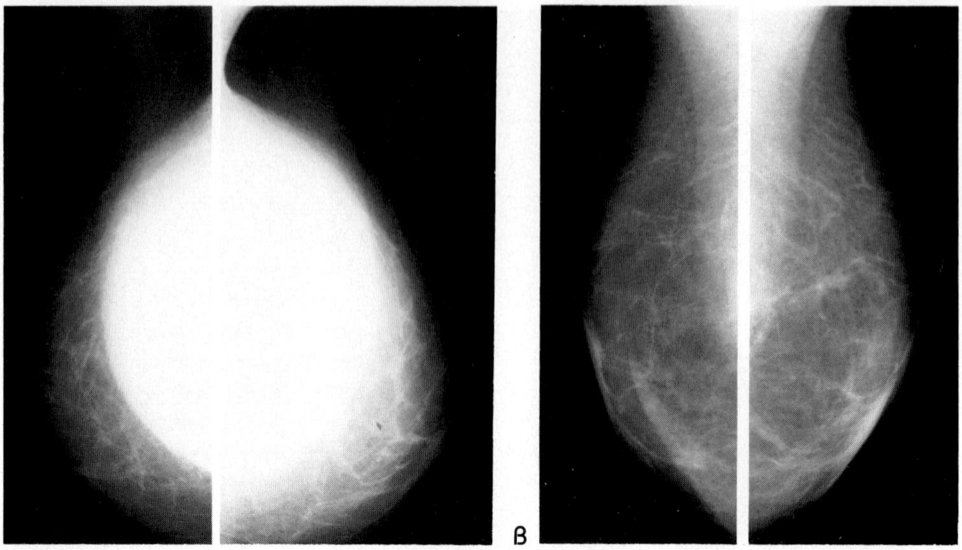

A B

FIGURE 5-27 A, Standard compression mediolateral oblique view with implant included. B, Modified compression mediolateral oblique view with implant excluded.

for differentiating solid and cystic masses, to provide better detail of masses obscured by dense parenchyma on the mammogram, and for following areas of fat necrosis or inflammatory masses. Sonography is not useful in detecting noninvasive breast carcinoma.

Subcutaneous Mastectomy

Subcutaneous mastectomy remains an option for high-risk patients seeking prophylactic treatment. With some techniques, breast tissue must be left in the subareolar region in order to preserve blood supply and viability to the nipple and areola. The subareolar tissue remains at risk for development of breast carcinoma and can be imaged mammographically. The procedure is performed in much the same manner as when imaging patients with firm fibrous encapsulation. No attempt is made to displace the implant. Breast tissue is pulled over and in front of the implant, compression being limited to breast tissue without inclusion of the implant (Fig. 5-31).[36,37]

Patient Anxiety and Fear of Implant Damage

The referring clinician should advise the patient with implants that special "modified" techniques are required to image the augmented breast properly. Four to six images of each breast are usually obtained. Patients should also be reassured that compression of the breast with an implant does not harm the implant when the procedure is properly performed. We have had one experience of an inadvertent capsulotomy performed during the compression process, resulting in immediate asymmetry of the breasts. The patient was referred to a plastic surgeon, and within an hour underwent a closed capsulotomy of the contralateral breast, with an excellent result.

The importance of proper compression during mammographic imaging cannot be overemphasized. Simply stated, compression can make the difference between finding or missing breast cancer. Overlapping structures are separated by compression. The radiation dose to breast tissue is proportionally reduced with the degree of compression. Compression does not damage breast tissue, nor does it damage augmentation implants when properly applied.

Implant Rupture

Implant rupture can occur following trauma. Automobile steering wheels and seat belts pose a risk to the implant at the time of the accident. Mammography can play a useful role in confirming implant disruption by identifying extraluminal silicone.[53] With minor disruption, silicone appears as rounded opaque droplets or nodules outside the implant; however, with greater disruption, there may be complete collapse of the implant and widespread distribution of silicone. Droplets of silicone may migrate along fascial planes to other areas of the body.[54,55]

CONCLUSION

Clinicians play an important role in encouraging the participation of patients in breast cancer screening programs, and thus can be a major factor in changing breast cancer mortality statistics. Plastic surgeons are often perceived by patients for whom they have performed breast surgery as their primary care physician for breast-related problems. Recogni-

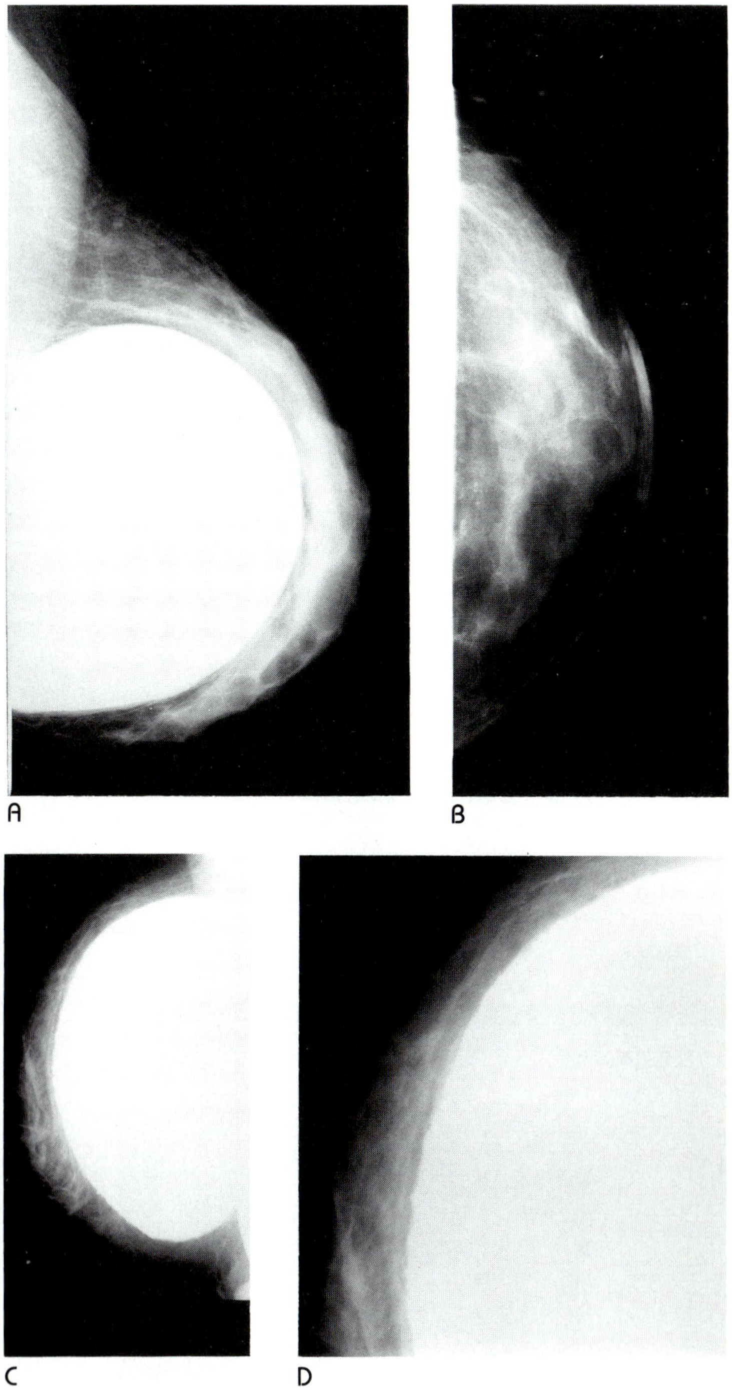

FIGURE 5–28 *A, B,* Firmly encapsulated implant; fibrous encapsulation without calcification. *A,* Standard mediolateral oblique view with implant included. Note the round contour of the implant as opposed to the more teardrop shape of the implant seen in Figure 5–27. This round shape is characteristic of firm fibrous encapsulation. *B,* Modified compression mediolateral oblique view. Although the implant could not be flattened against the chest wall or displaced, it was possible to pull additional breast tissue over and in front of the implant to allow breast compression without limitation of the implant. It is important to appreciate the significantly limited amount of breast tissue that can be well seen when the implant is encapsulated. *C, D,* Calcified implant capsule. *C,* Note the rough and irregular contour of the implant surface. *D,* Magnified view of the implant surface, showing irregular calcification. It is important to note that firm encapsulation can occur without evidence of calcification.

tion of the capabilities, limitations, and appropriate role of diagnostic breast imaging is essential if the full potential for DBI in early breast cancer detection is to be achieved. With this understanding, clinicians can direct a reasonable protocol for breast cancer screening. The patient is reassured to know that someone aware of her concerns and needs is in command. An assurance that current standards of care have been provided is important for the patient as well as the physician.

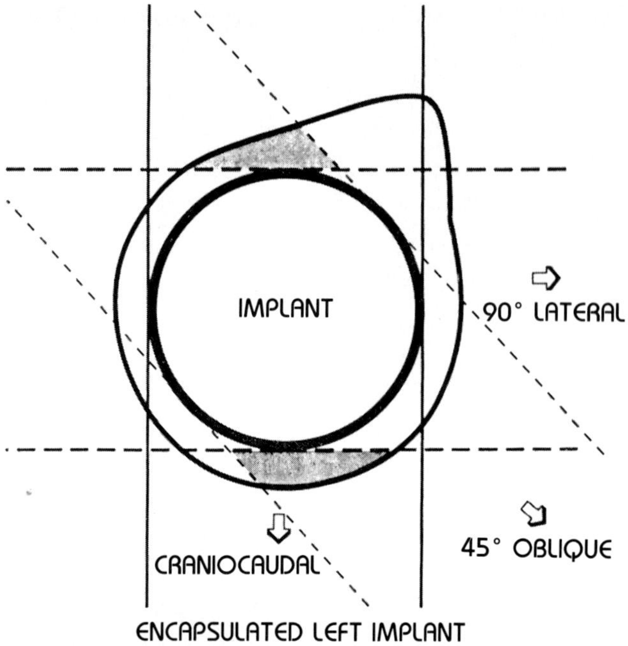

FIGURE 5-29 Illustration of left breast containing an implant. The shaded area represents breast tissue above and below the implant that will be excluded from view on standard craniocaudal and mediolateral oblique images. When the implant is firmly encapsulated and cannot be flattened or displaced, a 90-degree lateral view is added to provide visualization of this tissue.

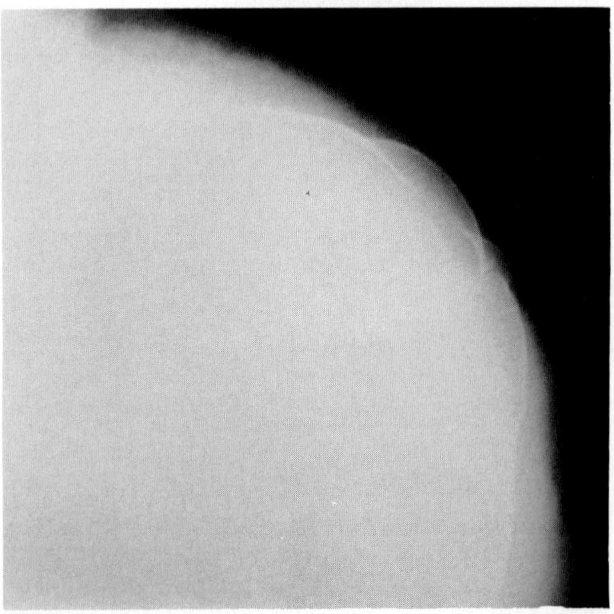

FIGURE 5-30 Herniation of implant through a rupture in the fibrous capsule. The patient developed a soft, palpable mass on the side of a firmly encapsulated implant. The tangential view shows folds in the wall of the implant bulging through the disrupted fibrous capsule.

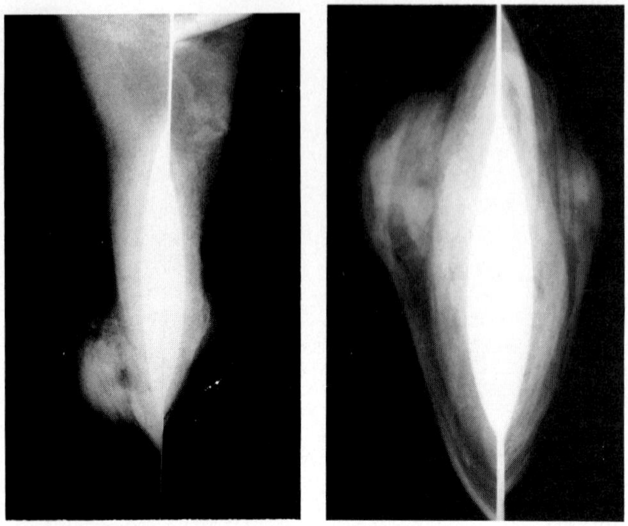

A B

FIGURE 5-31 Modified compression views of a patient with a bilateral subcutaneous mastectomy. *A*, Mediolateral oblique view. *B*, Craniocaudal view.

References

1. American Cancer Society. Mammography guidelines. New York: American Cancer Society, 1986.
2. Cohen DI, Littenberg B, Wetzel C, Neuhauser DVB. Improving physician compliance with preventive medicine guidelines. Med Care 1982; 20:1040-1045.
3. Gallup Poll. 1983 survey of public awareness and use of cancer detection tests. Princeton, NJ: Gallup Organization, 1984.
4. American Cancer Society. Survey of physicians' attitudes and practices in early cancer detection. CA 1985; 35:197-213.
5. Fox S, Baum JK, Klos DS, Tsou CV. Breast cancer screening: the underuse of mammography. Radiology 1985; 156:607-611.
6. Bassett LW, Bunnell DH, Cerny JA, Gold RH. Screening mammography: A survey of 4,200 referring physicians (abstract). Radiology 1985; 157:53.
7. Seidman H, Stellman SD, Mushihski MH. A different perspective on breast cancer risk factors; some implications of the nonattributable risk. 1982; CA 32:301.
8. Schwartz GF. Clinical implications of breast cancer risk factors. In: Feig SA, McLelland R, eds. Breast carcinoma—current diagnosis and treatment. New York: Mason (ACR), 1983: 89-98.
9. Schwartz GF. Lump in the breast versus lumpy breast—a diagnostic dilemma. In: Feig SA, McLelland R, eds. Breast carcinoma—current diagnosis and treatment. New York: Mason (ACR), 1983:385-389.
10. Metlin C. Breast cancer risk factors. In: Breast cancer—diagnosis and treatment. New York: McGraw-Hill, 1986:35-44.
11. Moskowitz M, Gartside PS. Evidence of breast cancer mortality reduction: aggressive screening in women under age 50. AJR 1982; 138:911-916.
12. Moskowitz M. Mammography to screen asymptomatic women for breast cancer. AJR 1984; 143:457-459.

13. Tabar L, Faberberg G, Day NE, Holmberg L. What is the optimum interval between mammographic screening examinations? An analysis based on the latest results of the Swedish two-county breast cancer screening trial. Br J Cancer 1987; 55:547-551.
14. Sickles EA, Herzog KA. Mammography of the postsurgical breast. AJR 1982; 136:585-588.
15. Sickles EA, Herzog KA. Intramammary scar tissue: A mimic of the mammographic appearance of carcinoma. AJR 1980; 135:349.
16. Logan WW. The radiologist's expanded role in breast carcinoma diagnosis. In: Feig SA, McLelland R, eds. Breast carcinoma—current diagnosis and treatment. New York: Mason (ACR), 1983:403-415.
17. Frykberg ER, Santiago F, Betsill WL, O'Brian PH. Lobular carcinoma in situ of the breast. Surg Gynecol Obstet 1989; 164:285-300.
18. Sickles EA. Breast calcifications: Mammographic evaluation. Radiology 1986; 290:289-293.
19. Homer MJ, Marchant DJ, Smith TJ. The geographic cluster of microcalcifications. Gynecol Obstet Surg 1985; 161:532-534.
20. Wertheimer MD, Costanza ME, Dodson TF, et al. Increasing the effect toward breast cancer detection. JAMA 1986; 255:1311-1315.
21. Holland R, Hendricks JHCL, Mravunac M. Mammographically occult breast cancer; a pathologic and radiologic study. Cancer 1983; 52:1810-1819.
22. Rosenberg AL, Schwartz GF, Feig SA, Patchefsky AS. Clinically occult breast lesions: Localization and significance. Radiology 1987; 162:167-170.
23. Gallagher HS, Martin JE. An orientation to the concept of minimal breast cancer. Cancer 1971; 28:1505-1507.
24. Moskowitz M. Breast cancer; age specific growth rates and screening strategies. Radiology 1986; 161:37-41.
25. Frazier TG, Copeland EM, Gallagher HS, et al. Prognosis and treatment in minimal breast cancer. Am J Surg 1977; 133:697-701.
26. Norris HJ, Austin RM. Overview of prognostic factors in mammary carcinoma. Breast 1985; 11:9-17.
27. McSweeny MB, Egan RL. Prognosis of breast cancer related to intramammary lymph nodes. Recent Res Cancer Res 1984; 90:166-172.
28. Lindfors KL, Kopans DB, McCarthy KA, Koerner KC, Meyer JE. Breast cancer metastasis in intramammary lymph nodes. AJR 1986; 146:133-136.
29. Bassett LW, Gold RH, Mira JM. Non-neoplastic breast calcifications in lipid cysts: Development after excision and primary irradiation. AJR 1982; 138:335-338.
30. Hackeloer BJ, Duda V, Lauth G. Ultrasound mammography. Berlin: Springer-Verlag, 1986.
31. Kopans DB, Meyer JE, Lindfors KK, Bucchianeri SS. Breast sonography to guide cyst aspiration and wire localization of occult solid lesions AJR 1984; 143: 489-492.
32. Pearce RB. Ultrasound, a useful adjunct to breast mammography. Diagn Imaging 1986; 8:114-117.
33. Hilton SvW, Leopold GR, Olson LK, Wilson SA. Realtime breast sonography: Application in 300 consecutive patients. AJR 1986; 147:479-486.
34. News from the world of medicine. Reader's Digest 1987; Nov: 63.
35. Jensen R, Mackey JK. Xeromammography after augmentation mammoplasty. Am J Radiol 1985; 144: 629-633.
36. Eklund GW, Busby RC, Miller SH, Job JS. Improved imaging of the augmented breast. Am J Radiol 1988; 151:469-473.
37. Eklund GW. Mammographic imaging of the augmented breast. Admin Radiol 1988; 12:42-43.
38. Parsons RW, Thering HR. Management of the silicone-injected breast. Plast Reconstr Surg 1977; 60:534-538.
39. Koides T, Katayama H. Calcification in augmentation mammoplasty. Radiology 1979; 130:337-340.
40. Silverstein MJ, Handel N, Gamagami P, et al. Breast cancer in women after augmentation mammoplasty. Arch Surg 1988; 123:681-685.
41. Minagi H, Youker JE, Knudson HW. The roentgen appearance of injected silicone in the breast. Radiology 1968; 90:57-61.
42. Timberlake GA, Looney GR. Adenocarcinoma of the breast associated with silicone injections. Surg Oncol 1986; 32:79-81.
43. Dow Corning Corp. Study linking carcinoma of the breast to silicone implanted in rat breast tissue. New York Times, Nov 10, 1988.
44. FDA. Safety of silicone breast prosthesis. FDA Drug Bulletin, February, 1989:2-3.
45. Cohen IK, Goodman H, Theogaraj SD. Xeromammogaphy: A reason for using saline-filled breast prosthesis. Plast Reconstr Surg 1977; 59:886-888.
46. Grant EG, Cigtay OS, Mascatello VJ. Irregularity of Silastic breast implants mimicking a soft tissue mass. AJR 1978; 130:461-462.
47. Burkhardt BR. Fibrous capsular contracture around breast implants: The role of subclinical infection. Infect Surg 1985; June:469-474.
48. Smith DS. False-positive radiographic diagnosis of breast implant rupture: Report of two cases. Ann Plast Surg 1985; 14:166-167.
49. Hipps CJ, Raju DR, Straith RE. Influence of some operative and postoperative factors on capsular contracture around breast implants. Plast Reconstr Surg 1978; 61:384-389.
50. Rosenbaum JL, Bernadino ME, Thomas JL, Wigley KD. Ultrasonographic findings in silicone augmented breasts. South Med J 1981; 74:455-458.
51. Cole-Beuglet C, Schwartz G, Kurtz AB, Patchefsky AS, Goldberg BB. Ultrasound mammography for the augmented breast. Radiology 1983; 146:737-742.
52. Harper P. Ultrasound mammography. Baltimore: University Park Press, 1985:103-104.
53. Argenta LC. Migration of silicone gel into breast parenchyma following mammary prosthesis rupture. Ann Plast Surg 1983; 7:253-254.
54. Capozzi A, Dubou R, Pennisi VR. Distant migration of silicone gel from a ruptured breast implant. Plast Reconstr Surg 1976; 62:302.
55. Delage C, Shane JJ, Johnson FB. Mammary silicone granuloma: Migration of silicone fluid to abdominal wall and inguinal region. Arch Dermatol 1973; 108:104.

SECTION 2

DEVELOPMENTAL DEFORMITIES

CHAPTER 6

Breast Problems in Children

DON LA ROSSA, M.D.

Many problems that affect the adult breast may be encountered in the preadolescent and adolescent population. However, some afflictions are peculiar to the infant, neonate, and prepubertal child. Plastic surgeons become aware of these when the child or the parents seek a consultation for physical or psychological symptoms that have developed.

DEVELOPMENTAL BREAST MASSES

It is normal to palpate a nodule beneath the areola of a neonate, and this is a measure of gestational age. The breast bud continues to enlarge in approximately 60 percent of infants, primarily owing to the accumulation of a colostrum-like material (witch's milk) that can be expressed from the ducts. Indeed, galactorrhea can be noted as late as 2 months postpartum in 1.8 percent of neonates, and a nodule is easily palpable in many infants of both sexes during the first 6 months of life.[1,2] Maternal hormones are thought to provide the stimulus that may result in an enlargement of the gland to several centimeters in diameter, particularly in nursing infants.[3] In the absence of continued stimulation from either maternal or infant hormones, the breast bud decreases in size over several months and remains dormant until puberty.

Breast development usually heralds the onset of puberty, and is followed by the appearance of secondary sexual characteristics. The mean age for puberty is 12.5 years for North American children.[4] Thelarche may begin as early as age 8 years. It is at this time that concerned parents may explore remedies for developmental abnormalities that are becoming evident in their maturing children (see Chap. 4).

CONGENITAL ABNORMALITIES

Amastia

Total absence of the breast, amastia, is true agenesis and a rare condition. It is usually associated with Poland's syndrome in which moderate to severe unilateral hypoplasia is frequently seen. Amastia is usually unilateral and results from complete regression of the milk streak.[5] *Athelia*, complete absence of the nipple, is extremely rare. The diagnosis of simple amastia is made in the absence of the typical findings of Poland's syndrome—absence or hypoplasia of the pectoralis major muscle, often with associated ipsilateral rib, costal cartilage, and upper extremity anomalies. In an affected child with absence of the breast, the nipple-areola complex is usually located too far cephalad, making an accurate restoration of the breast more difficult. The disparity becomes more marked with the development of the normal contralateral breast, which causes gradual downward displacement of its nipple-areola complex. Reconstruction of the affected breast with implants or tissue expanders provides some correction, although this is usually insufficient (see Chap. 7).

Treatment of amastia is begun either at the onset of puberty in bilateral cases, or when the development of the normal breast is sufficient to become a source of concern to the maturing adolescent. Tissue expanders inserted beneath the skin and/or pectoralis muscle, can be gradually inflated to keep pace with the young woman's development. When breast growth is complete, the expander is replaced with a permanent mammary prosthesis. Gel-inflatable permanent expander implants are particularly useful in managing these growing patients, since the device is often left in place for several years. Thus, the risk of deflation seen with shell-type expanders is avoided. In addition, if the implant position and the appearance of the reconstructed breast is acceptable, the gel-inflatable expander may serve as a permanent prosthesis by removal of the filler valve.

Polythelia

The most common congenital anomaly is polythelia, which occurs in 1 to 5 percent of the population. Accessory nipples may appear anywhere along the milk streak. (Fig. 6-1).[3] They are occasionally of concern and embarrassment to teenagers, prompting consultation with pediatricians and plastic surgeons. Excision of the papilla may be a compromise solution, avoiding the larger scar that would result from removal of the entire nipple and areola.

Polymastia

Likewise, polymastia, accessory breasts, may occur wherever the milk streak fails to regress, and is much less common than polythelia. It arises with equal frequency in both sexes and is estimated to affect 1 to 2 percent of the population. There are some racial differences in the incidence, with a more frequent occurrence in Japanese people. It apparently occurs more commonly above the normal nipple in Japanese than in Caucasians, where it is more commonly seen below the nipple. Supernumerary breasts may be unilateral or bilateral and usually occur along the milk line, although atypical locations have been described.[5] It is difficult to explain their presence on the basis of normal embryologic aberrations. It has been suggested that they result from a reversion of ancestral characteristics called atavism, according to the Geoffroy-Saint-Hilaire-Darwin theory. As many as eight separate breasts in a male and ten in a female have been reported by Wiedersheim and Graham-Campbell.[5] There also seems to be a hereditary component to their occurrence. The supernumerary breast is most commonly seen in the axillary region where, in addition to aesthetic concerns, it presents a source of discomfort to the patient, especially at times of premenstrual and gestational enlargement. Growth to full size and lactation has been reported. Excision at the time of earliest diagnosis is indicated to reduce the ultimate size of the scar (Fig. 6-2).

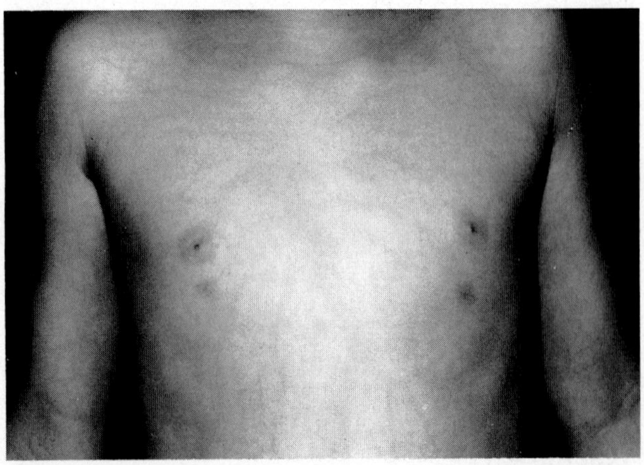

FIGURE 6-1 Polythelia in an 11-year-old male. The accessory nipple may occur anywhere along the milk line.

DEVELOPMENTAL ABNORMALITIES

Breast enlargement can occur at any age and in either sex. Hormonal stimulation from exogenous sources such as accidental ingestion of estrogen compounds, cutaneous absorption from estrogen-containing creams, or consumption of estrogen-contaminated food may be responsible.[6] Endogenous sources may also be a cause, although endocrine studies are not usually helpful. Conflicting reports as to estrogen effect, plasma gonadotropin levels, and luteinizing hormone-releasing hormone (LHRH) are noted in the literature.[6] It has been suggested, although not proved, that breast growth in these situations is a result of increased sensitivity of the breast tissue to normal levels of estrogen. However, a careful history taking and physical examination are warranted to exclude abnormal sources of estrogen stimulation. The pediatrician should note whether there has been an increase in growth velocity, and search for other signs of sexual development. Ovarian enlargement should be determined, along with a screening test for adrenal disease and a determination of bone age to rule out precocious puberty. If these studies are all normal, a presumptive diagnosis of premature thelarche may be made and the patient followed carefully to ensure that the other signs of puberty do not appear.[6]

Gynecomastia

Gynecomastia, breast growth in the male, is discussed in Chapters 8 and 9.

Premature Thelarchy

Breast growth in females below the age of 8 years in the absence of other signs of precocious puberty is referred to as premature thelarchy. It is commonly seen in infants and toddlers and is benign and self-limited when not associated with the findings of precocious puberty. Premature breast development may occur by 12 months of age and may persist for as long as 5 years in a substantial percentage of patients. Since many cases persist, the clinician should be cautious about assuming that the en-

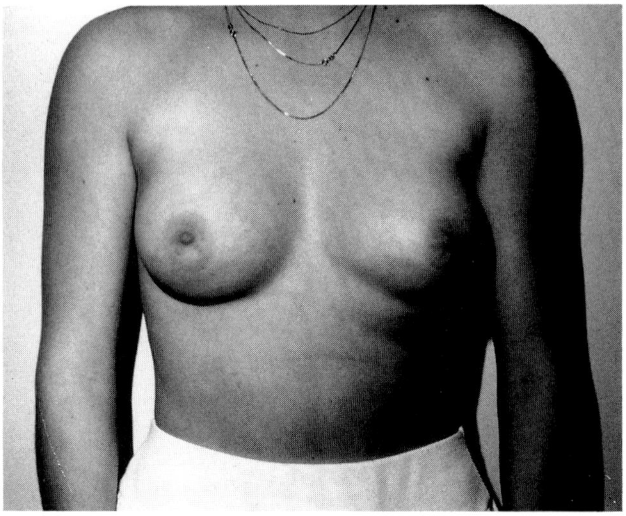

A

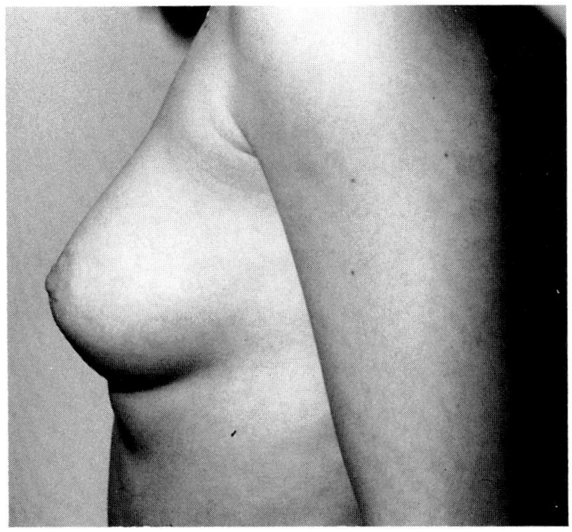

B

FIGURE 6-2 *A, B,* A Supernumerary breast is located inferior and adjacent to the normal left breast. Resection resulted in a scar in the inframammary fold. The accessory breast tissue was delineated from the normal breast by normal intervening tissue planes.

larged breasts will eventually disappear. However, it is safe to predict that the growth is unlikely to progress, particularly if the appearance of the developing breast was not noted until after the neonatal period.[6] Breast size can vary from being barely noticeable to full development. More commonly, however, gradual growth occurs throughout childhood and into adolescence. The condition is usually synchronous and bilateral, resulting in a breast with normal texture and consistency. Biopsy is contraindicated in the absence of a mass because of the potential for distortion of the developing breast. Rather, close follow-up and observation is warranted, particularly in children in whom asynchronous development may occur.

Precocious Puberty

Precocious puberty, conversely, refers to the constellation of signs of puberty, including breast development, in the child or prepubertal female. Although most cases are idiopathic, some derive from abnormal hormone production from an intracranial, ovarian, or adrenal source. Approximately 20 percent have adnexal tumors.[7,8] Computed tomographic (CT) scans can be extremely useful in evaluating idiopathic cases. In one study of 15 females with precocious puberty, 33 percent were found to have hamartomas and other hypothalamic lesions that were treatable by surgical resection.[9] In true idiopathic cases, medroxyprogesterone acetate (Depo-Provera) suppresses ovulation. Cyproterone acetate, an LHRH analog, has been used experimentally in a group of five females with favorable short-term results. However, upon cessation of the drug, all hormonal values and the vaginal maturation index had returned to normal.[10] In cases in which tumors are the cause, removal of the tumor stops sexual maturation and may result in regression of the changes that have already occurred. With the onset of puberty, sexual development once again proceeds normally. In the absence of another identifiable source, precocious puberty is associated with polyostotic fibrous dysplasia in the McCune-Albright syndrome, presumably from a central origin.

Juvenile Hypertrophy

Breast growth presages the onset of puberty and is considered normal as early as age 8 years. The breast evolves in a relatively predictable way in most females, but in rare individuals a rapid and explosive growth pattern known as juvenile hypertrophy can occur. The size increase is primarily due to growth of the periductal connective tissue stroma rather than ducts and parenchyma, resulting in heavy, nodular, firm breasts. Proliferation and branching of the ductal tissues are seen, but lobule formation is not. The histologic picture is similar to that seen in gynecomastia and is essentially an exaggeration of the pattern noted in a normal developing breast.[3,11] The process is not related to measurable hormonal imbalances and is not malignant. Geschickter proposed that it results from an exaggerated response of a hypersensitive breast to the intense hormonal stimulation of normal puberty.[3] The breasts can reach gigantic size and may compromise the skin circulation, resulting in ulceration. Breasts weighing 25 to 30 pounds and reaching to the patient's knees have been reported.[3,12,13] In addition there are the psychological effects. The condition may be unilateral or bilateral (Fig. 6-3). Breast reduction can be per-

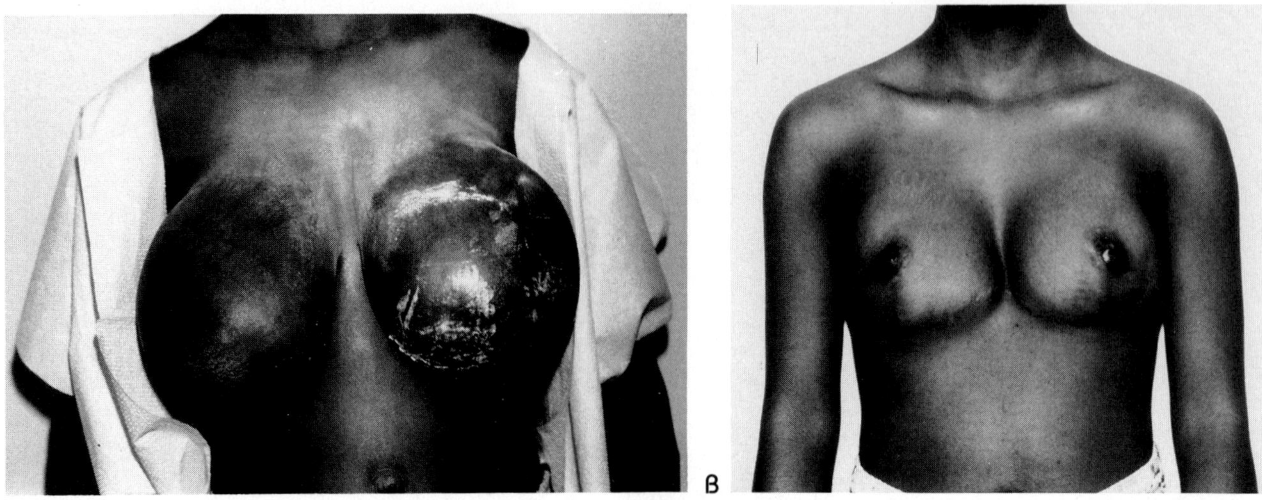

FIGURE 6-3 *A*, This 10-year-old female developed virginal hypertrophy, presenting as rapid and progressive breast enlargement. Skin breakdown occurred prompting surgical treatment by reduction mammaplasty. *B*, After reduction mammaplasty, breast growth recurred, leading to subtotal mastectomy and immediate reconstruction with implants. The resected breast tissue was estrogen and progesterone receptor negative. This illustrates the patients' appearance 7 years after the definitive procedure.

formed but may be technically difficult and bloody. Furthermore, regrowth can occur immediately or with later hormonal stimulation, as with pregnancy, necessitating further surgery. In patients in whom regrowth appears, dydrogesterone (Gynorest) therapy is indicated. This agent is a pure and potent progesterone, does not interfere with ovulation, does not cause masculinization of the fetus, has not shown evidence of teratogenic effect, has rare side effects, has no reported carcinogenic effect, and can be easily taken during 21 days of the menstrual cycle in a 10-mg daily dose.[14] Medroxyprogesterone acetate has also been used after a second reduction mammaplasty to prevent recurrence.[15] However, dydrogesterone is less likely to cause menstrual abnormalities and is as effective, in addition to being an oral medication.[14] When this approach fails, total mastectomy with nipple preservation or free nipple grafting, along with prosthetic reconstruction with implants, is indicated.[14] Patients who have had less than total mastectomy should be cautioned about the risk of recurrence during periods of hormonal stimulation such as pregnancy. The author has seen one patient who had a subtotal mastectomy at age 14 and developed exophytic masses protruding from the surgical scars during a subsequent pregnancy. (Fig. 6-4). When reduction mammaplasty is selected as the form of treatment, free nipple transfer techniques may be needed because the enormous size of the breast may not lend itself to standard pedicle techniques of nipple preservation.

Macromastia

Macromastia is a generic term that describes benign enlargement of the breasts to a degree that symptoms are produced. Back and shoulder pain, grooving of the shoulders, intertrigo, and poor posture are common complaints. Breast reduction is often helpful in relieving symptoms. The indications and techniques for reduction mammaplasty are discussed in detail in subsequent chapters in this text.

ACQUIRED DEFORMITY DURING BREAST DEVELOPMENT

Trauma to the breast bud may result in distortion and maldevelopment of the breast. Therefore, breast masses in children should be approached conservatively, particularly in infants when a palpable breast bud is normal. Destruction of the breast

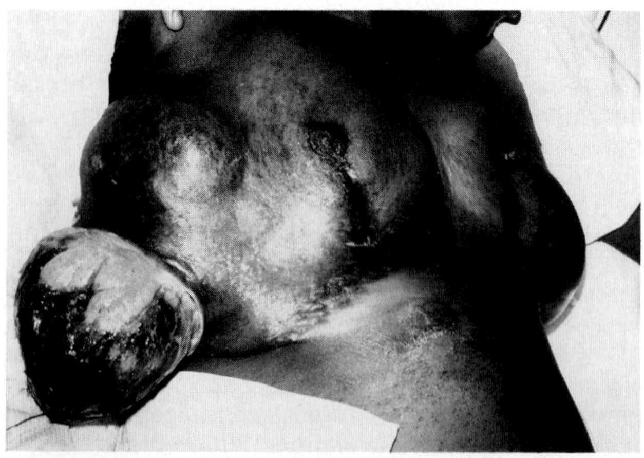

FIGURE 6-4 Exophytic breast masses presented during pregnancy in this 22-year-old woman who had a less than total mastectomy at age 14 for virginal hypertrophy. The masses were excised, and breast tissue involuted after pregnancy.

anlage from infection (mastitis neonatorum) may result in abnormal breast development, although the incidence is not known. Normal breast buds may be red and somewhat tender, but mastitis neonatorum is characterized by a hard, tender, warm mass that may go on to develop fluctuance, making the diagnosis evident. Failing treatment with antibiotics and incision and drainage, generalized sepsis may occur.[16]

Hemangiomas and lymphangiomas may also be seen in children. Again, caution should be exercised in treating these surgically because of the risk of injuring the breast bud.

Burns of the chest skin during childhood can result in late distortion of the developing breast. Complete destruction of the breast bud and subsequent amastia would be unusual. However, surgical release of heavy or constricting scars and contractures, and the addition of skin grafts to accommodate the enlarging breast, may be needed.

The placement of thoracotomy incisions in the young female child can injure the breast anlage or result in a constricting scar that may impair normal breast growth. Surgeons operating in this area must be alert to this danger, and design the incisions to fall below the eventual inframammary fold, thus allowing for subsequent breast development.[17]

BREAST MASSES IN THE CHILD AND ADOLESCENT

Any of the mass lesions that occur in the mature adult breast can be seen in the developing breast of adolescents and children. *Fibroadenomas* are the most common tumor of the breast in this group, representing up to 95 percent of excised breast masses.[16,18] They are probably hormonally dependent tumors, because their peak incidence is later than the age of attainment of adult estrogen levels (17 years). It has been suggested that extended hormonal exposure is required for their development.[19] Fibroadenomas are most often seen in the upper outer quadrant, although they can occur anywhere in the breast, and may be multiple and bilateral in 10 to 23 percent of patients. In one series they were more commonly multiple in blacks.[20] On rare occasions, youngsters may develop several lesions per year (fibroadenomatosis), presenting a difficult management problem. The condition usually becomes quiescent after adolescence; thus, careful follow-up and biopsy is warranted only of very rapidly enlarging lesions.[11] The lesions are most commonly seen in young adult women, but have been reported as early as 2 years before menarche.[21] The tumors are characteristically firm and "slippable" and are generally asymptomatic, although they may be tender. Growing slowly, they can reach sizable proportions. They may appear to have skin involvement, with tenseness of the overlying skin. However, they never involve the skin or the pectoral fascia, which distinguishes them from cystosarcoma phylloides. Their assymetric nature differentiates them from juvenile hypertrophy.[16,20,21] *Giant fibroadenomas* can be large enough to cause a size discrepancy between the breasts after removal. In such cases a reconstruction can be made with an implant. In younger individuals, tissue expanders can be used until full growth has been achieved, at which time an implantable mammary prosthesis can be used to provide permanent correction.

Cystosarcoma phylloides occurs in adolescent females and is usually benign. It is the second most common cause of massive breast enlargement in adolescents.[22] On the basis of the histologic pattern of the stromal element, the condition may be classified benign, intermediate, or malignant.[18] However, it can undergo malignant change in the connective tissue, assuming the histologic characteristics of a fibrosarcoma. Some cases show transition from a benign to a malignant stromal pattern in the same histologic section. Tumors that have metastasized have done so primarily by the hematogenous route; only rarely have lymph node metastases been noted.[13,23] Hoover and coworkers reported 34 cases in females under 20 years of age, four being malignant.[22] Only one patient died of widely metastatic disease, the other three having been cured by surgical excision. Cystosarcoma phylloides may grow very rapidly in adolescent females, producing tumors up to 45 cm in diameter.[24-26] Treatment depends on the histologic picture of the tumor. Because so few of the tumors are malignant in adolescents, conservative resections are recommended. Iverson and Hegg reported 26 cases of benign or intermediate cystosarcoma phylloides in females 11 to 18 years of age; the average age was 15. The patients were all treated with wide local excision, and only two (8 percent) showed evidence of local recurrence. However, women over 18 have a recurrence rate of up to 30 percent with benign disease.[22,27] Therefore, in adolescents under 18 years of age, a wide local excision should suffice. After 18 years of age, a cuff of normal breast tissue should be included to reduce the risk of local recurrence.[23,24,27] Total mastectomy may be indicated, especially if the tumor occupies a significant portion of the breast.[23] Malignant cystosarcoma phylloides should be treated with total mastectomy, including an axillary node dissection if nodes appear involved. A radical mastectomy is indicated if there is invasion of the pectoralis muscle. Major resections of breast tissue may require breast reconstruction to restore symmetry.[28] However, because of the high risk of local recurrence, reconstruction should be delayed for 5 years.[27]

Other *benign lesions* that afflict the adult breast may be seen in children. Bloody nipple drainage and a palpable subareolar mass may be indicative of an intraductal papilloma.[20] Excision is indicated and should cure the condition. Lipomas, skin cysts, and granular cell myoblastomas of the breast skin may be seen in children. The last-named lesions may present a confusing clinical and histologic picture; treatment should be conservative until permanent sections have been obtained.[16,29]

Breast cysts, mastopathies, and fibrocystic disease can afflict the developing breast. Most cysts are solitary, in contrast to those found in adults. Fibrous mastopathy, periductal mastitis (nonsuppurative), fibroadenomatoid mastopathy, sclerosing adenosis, and lobular hyperplasia have been reported in postpubertal adolescents. The symptoms were absent or relatively mild.[20] Management is guided by the same principles as in adults. Inflammatory lesions also occur, notably fat necrosis and abscesses. Although the condition is undoubtedly related to trauma, a definite history is frequently absent. Despite the rarity of carcinoma of the breast in youngsters, these firm, sometimes fixed lesions often come to biopsy.[16,20] In addition to mastitis neonatorum, abscesses may occur, presumably from ductal obstruction, cysts, or ductal ectasia. Incision and drainage is indicated.[16]

Carcinoma of the breast is a rare condition in children, approximately 43 cases having been reported in the world literature. It constitutes about 1 percent of all childhood cancers and less than 0.1 percent of all breast cancers; 0.09 percent or less of all mammary carcinomas occur under age 20.[11,30,31] Only one case has been seen at the Children's Hospital of Philadelphia. A watershed of tumor type and outcome is noted at about age 11. Most children below that age have juvenile secretory carcinomas, originally called juvenile carcinoma by McDivitt and Stewart in 1966.[34] These tumors have a distinctive histologic pattern, with large amounts of intracellular and extracellular secretions, and granular eosinophilic cytoplasm of the cells. The lesions also occur in adults, in whom they have a more aggressive behavior, with axillary metastases in 21 percent and death from disseminated disease in 5 percent of 19 patients reported by Tavassoli and Norris.[32] However, the tumors are much less aggressive in children and respond well to simple or total mastectomy; all but one patient survived in the long term. In none of the reported patients have estrogen or progesterone receptors been positive. In adults over age 20, a more adult pattern of behavior is noted, so that more traditional methods of treatment are recommended. In children older than age 12, breast carcinomas appear to have more adult histologic patterns and behavior. Surgical treatment in this age group has been more "adult-like," although the overall experience is limited because of the small cohort, especially with regard to the use of lumpectomy and irradiation.[16,31,33,34] There may be a difference in the disease as noted in the Japanese, in whom 32 cases have occurred in patients under age 19. Only two cases have occurred under age 10, and the prognosis seems different.[35] Primary sarcomas are even more rare than carcinomas, about 20 cases having been reported in children.[36,37] They tend to be bulky, slow-growing tumors. Treatment consists of wide local excision, the results being better in children than in adults.[11] Pre- and postadolescent patients who have had total or modified radical mastectomies become candidates for breast reconstruction. We have treated one patient with tissue expansion since thelarche at the age of 12. She currently has a permanent expander in place at age 16, and requires periodic inflation to keep pace with continued breast development.

References

1. Madlon, Kay DJ. "Witch's milk." Galactorrhea in the newborn. Am J Dis Child 1986; 140:252-253.
2. McKiernan JF, Hull D. Breast development in the newborn. Arch Dis Child 1981:525-529.
3. Geschickter CF. Diseases of the breast. 1st ed. Philadelphia: JB Lippincott, 1943.
4. Haagensen CD. Diseases of the breast. Philadelphia: WB Saunders, 1986:59.
5. deCholnoky T. Supernumerary breast. Arch Surg 1939; 39:926-941.
6. Mills JL, Stolley PD, Davies J, et al. Premature thelarche. Am J Dis Child 1981; 135:743-745.
7. Drop SLS, Bruining GJ, Visser HKA, et al. Prolonged galactorrhea in a 6-year-old girl with isosexual precocious puberty due to a feminizing adrenal tumor. Clin Endocrinol 1981; 15:37-43.
8. Lack EE, Perez-Atayde AR, Murthy ASF, et al. Granulosa theca cell tumors in premenarchal girls. Cancer 1981; 48(8):1846-1854.
9. Cacciari E, Frejaville E, Cicognani A, et al. How many cases of true precocious puberty are idiopathic? J Pediatr 1983; 102:357-360.
10. Comite F, Cutler GB Jr, Rivier J, et al. Short-term treatment of idiopathic precocious puberty with a long-acting analogue of luteinizing hormone-releasing hormone—a preliminary report. N Engl J Med 1981; 305:1546-1550.
11. Seashore JH. Disorders of the breast. In: Welch KJ, Randolph JG, O'Neill JA, Rowe MI, eds. Pediatric surgery. Chicago: Yearbook, 1986:559-563.
12. Durston W. Concerning a very sudden and excessive swelling of a woman's breasts. Phil Trans, Vol IV, for Anno 1669, Royal Society, London, 1670:1047-1049.
13. Hinderer UT, del Rio JL. An unusual case of gigantomasty. Aesth Plast Surg 1985; 9:91-92.
14. Mayl N, Vasconez LO, Jurkiewicz MJ. Treatment of macromastia in the actively enlarging breast. Plast Reconst Surg 1974; 54:6.
15. Sperling RL, Gold JJ. Use of an anti-estrogen after a reduction mammaplasty to prevent recurrence of virginal hypertrophy of the breast. Plast Reconstr Surg 1973; 52:439.
16. Seashore JH. Breast enlargements in infants and children. Pediatr Ann 1975; 8:542-564.
17. Cherup LL, Siewers RD, Futrell JW. Breast and pectoral maldevelopment after anterolateral and posterolateral thoracotomies in children. Ann Thorac Surg 1986; 41:492-497.

18. Bower R, Bell MJ, Ternberg JL. Management of breast lesions in children and adolescents. J Pediatr Surg 1976; 11:337.
19. Stone AM, Shenker IR, McCarthy K. Adolescent breast masses. Am J Surg 1975; 134:275-277.
20. Farrow JH, Ashikari H. Breast lesions in young girls. Surg Clin North Am 1969; 49:261.
21. Seashore JH. Breast lesions in children. In: Gallagher HS, Leis HP Jr, Snyderman R, Urban JA, eds. The breast. St Louis: CV Mosby, 1978:499-507.
22. Hoover HC, Testiorenau A, Ketcham AS. Metastatic cystosarcoma phylloides in an adolescent girl. Ann Surg 1975; 181:279.
23. Treves N, Sunderland DA. Cystosarcoma phylloides of the breast: A malignant and a benign tumor. Cancer 1954; 4:1286.
24. Amerson JR. Cystosarcoma phylloides in adolescent females. Ann Surg 1970; 171:849.
25. Lee BJ, Pack GT. Giant intracanalicular fibro-adenomyxoma of the breast. The so-called cystosarcoma phylloides mammae of Johannes Mueller. Am J Cancer 1931; 11:2583.
26. Wulsin JH. Large breast tumors in adolescent females. Ann Surg 1960; 152:151.
27. Iverson RE, Hegg SI. Cystosarcoma phylloides presenting as massive unilateral breast hypertrophy in an adolescent. Ann Plast Surg 1980; 4:315-322.
28. Orenstein A, Tsur H. Cystosarcoma phylloides treated by excision and immediate reconstruction with silicone implant. Ann Plast Surg 1987; 18:520-523.
29. Umansky C, Bullock WK. Granular cell myoblastoma of the breast. Ann Surg 1968; 168:810.
30. Ferguson TB Jr, McCarty KS Jr, Filston HC. Juvenile secretory carcinoma and juvenile papillomatosis: Diagnosis and treatment. J Pediatr Surg 1987; 22:637-639.
31. Hammar B. Childhood breast carcinoma: Report of a case. J Pediatr Surg 1981; 16:77-78.
32. Tavassoli FA, Norris HJ. Secretory carcinoma of the breast. Cancer 1980; 45:2404-2413.
33. Massi SR, Rioux A, Beauchessone C. Juvenile carcinoma of the breast. Hum Pathol 1981; 12:1044.
34. McDivitt RW, Stewart FW. Breast carcinoma in children. JAMA 1966; 195:338.
35. Tanimura A, Konaka K. Carcinoma of the breast in a 5 year old girl. Acta Pathol Jpn 1980; 30:157-160.
36. Herman JB. In: Ariel IM, Pack GT, eds. Cancer and allied diseases of infancy and childhood. Boston: Little, Brown, 1960.
37. Torres V, Ferrer R. Cytology of fine needle aspiration biopsy of primary breast rhabdomyosarcoma in an adolescent girl. Acta Cytol 1985; 29:430-434.

CHAPTER 7

Developmental Deformities of the Breast

A. JAY BURNS, M.D.
FRITZ E. BARTON, JR., M.D.

Like any developmental abnormality, congenital breast deformities cover a wide spectrum of anomalies. At one extreme, there is total absence of the breast, amastia; at the other extreme, there is polymastia, with multiple breasts arranged along the primitive milk line. Such quantitative defects clearly fall into the domain of this chapter, but qualitative defects are more difficult to define; at some point, they are simply regarded as variations on the normal. This chapter deals with the classification, diagnosis, and treatment of the more severe developmental breast anomalies. Simple mammary hypoplasia treated by standard augmentation procedures, and mammary hyperplasia treated by standard reduction mammaplasty, are not addressed here, because they are discussed elsewhere in this text.

NORMAL MAMMARY EMBRYOGENESIS

The human mammary gland is regarded as a modified apocrine sweat gland. It first appears during the sixth week of intrauterine life and is noted as a thickened ridge of ectoderm, the milk line or mammary ridge (Fig. 7-1*A*), which extends between the bases of the limb buds on either side of the trunk. As the embryo grows the ridge becomes more distinct, but it is normally confined to the pectoral area, where it thickens and pushes into the mesoderm.

Groups of cells proliferate and become globular, and by the fifth month 15 to 20 cords of cells penetrate into the dermal connective tissue. As branching of these cords occurs, acini are formed. In the remaining months in utero, the cords become hollow and empty into a developing pit, which elevates at birth into the nipple.

The areola surrounding the nipple contains the glands of Montgomery, which are sebaceous secretors. These enlarge and rise above the plane of the skin at puberty in response to hormonal changes.

QUANTITATIVE ABNORMALITIES

Quantitative breast defects arise from developmental abnormalities occurring along the mammary ridge. For example, abnormal persistence of portions of the mammary ridge account for ectopic mammary tissue, *polymastia* or *polythelia*, whereas absence of the breast results from failure of the pectoral portions of the mammary ridges to develop (Fig. 7-1*B*).[1]

Absence of the Breast

Amastia or *amazia* has been defined as developmental absence of the mammary gland; *athelia* is absence of the nipple. To avoid confusion when using these terms, one should remember that amastia must meet the requirement of both an absent mammary gland and an absent nipple. Congenital absence of the breast with persistence of the nipple is more precisely called hypoplasia of the breast.[1]

In 1907 Hubert[2] undertook an extensive review of amastia, and cited Louzier as the first to report congenital absence of the breast in 1802. Unfortunately, Louzier did not comment on the presence or absence of the nipple; therefore, Hubert credited Froriep with the original description in 1839 of true absence of the breast. Since that time, fewer than 50 cases of amastia have been reported worldwide.

Trier[1] identified three distinct categories of amastia:

1. Absence of both breasts with congenital ectodermal defect (Fig. 7-2). In addition to bilateral amastia, these male patients have thin, dry

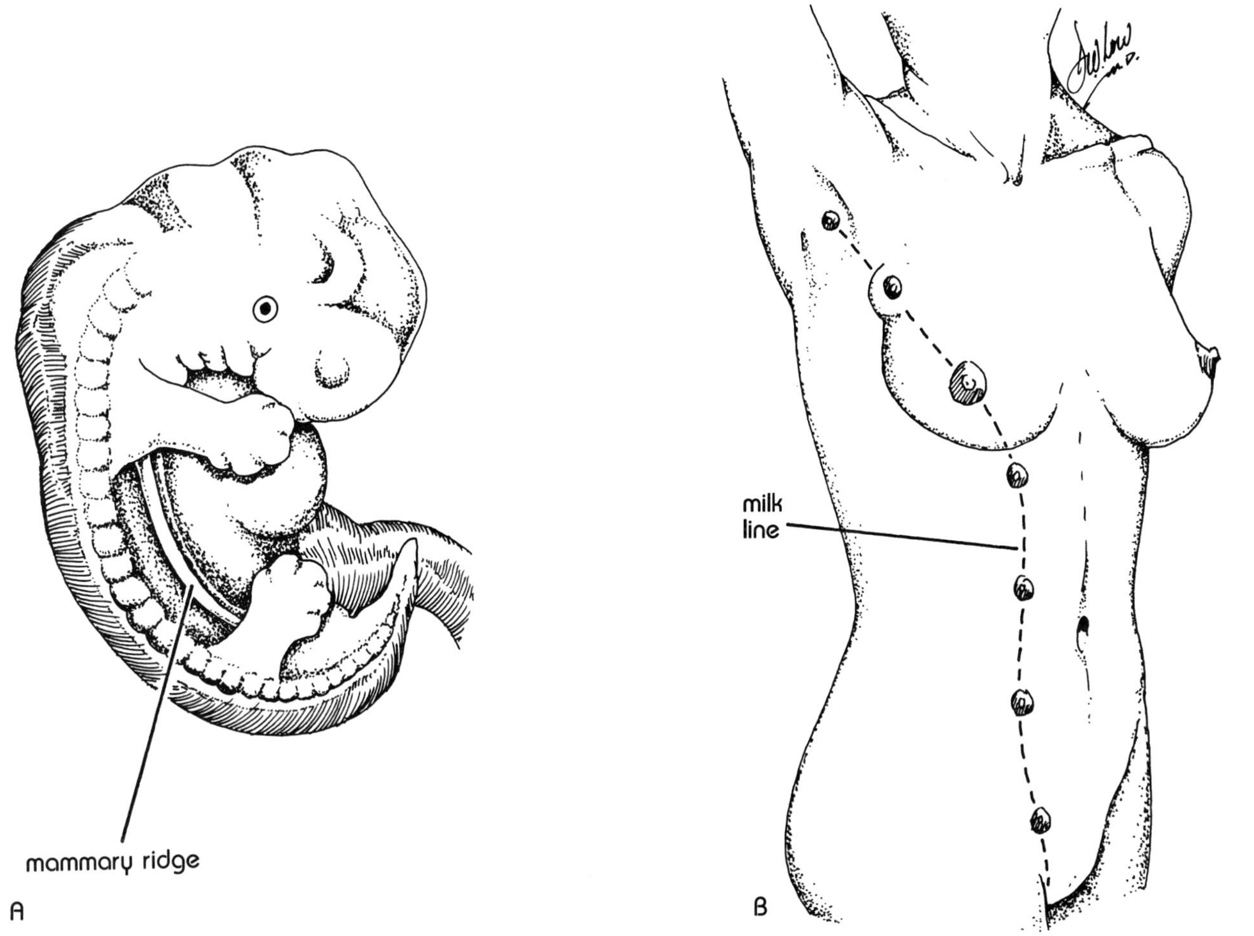

FIGURE 7–1 *A*, The mammary ridge extends between the bases of the limb buds on either side of the trunk in the 13-mm embryo. *B*, The primordial milk line corresponds to the mammary ridge location. Polymastia or polythelia may occur along this line.

skin and cannot perspire; show alopecia to various degrees (except for lanugo-type hair); exhibit a saddle nose and atrophic nasal mucosa; and typically have underdeveloped or missing teeth. These are the phenotypic manifestations of a congenital ectodermal defect said to be transmitted by a recessive sex-linked gene that passes from the mother to a male child.

2. Unilateral absence of the breast. Fewer than 24 cases are recognized in the literature. Approximately 90 percent of these children lack the corresponding pectoral muscles. The condition most closely resembles Poland's syndrome, but in the latter there is always a nipple, even though it may be rudimentary. The presence of glandular tissue without a nipple is difficult to explain. There have been anecdotal reports, but no histologic documentation of this condition is available. Occasionally, ectopic glandular tissue may be seen without a nipple, e.g., in the axilla, but this most likely represents the separated tail of a normal breast.
3. Bilateral absence of the breast (Fig. 7–3). Gilly[3] in 1882 was the first to describe this condition in a 33-year-old woman who also had atrophy of the right pectoral muscles with ipsilateral absence of the ulna and ulnar side of the hand. Other reports followed[4,5] that described women who were normal in other respects and bore normal children, but who had bilateral absence of the breasts.

Multiple Breasts

The opposite of amastia is polymastia, or the condition characterized by multiple breasts on one or both halves of the trunk. Although the extra breast is usually found somewhere along the primordial milk line, it has also been reported in other locations such as the back.[6] Polythelia is usually recognizable at birth, but it is necessary to wait until puberty or pregnancy to determine where there will be breast growth under the supernumerary nipple. The supernumerary breast should be treated by simple excision and primary closure. A common location of a supernumerary breast is the axilla, where it may represent a separate and hypertrophic tail of Spence (Fig. 7–4).

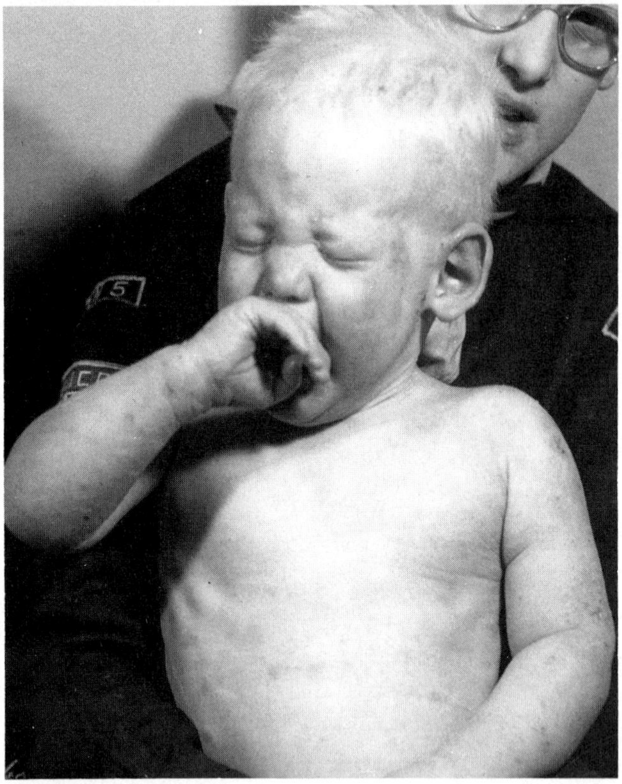

FIGURE 7-2 Boy with congenital ectodermal defect and complete breast absence. (Patient of Raymond A. Osbourn, M.D. Photograph published with permission of Medical Society of the District of Columbia.)

QUALITATIVE DEFORMITIES

Poland's Syndrome

In a review of the literature dealing with Poland's syndrome, it becomes clear that there is much confusion as to which specific findings make up the syndrome.

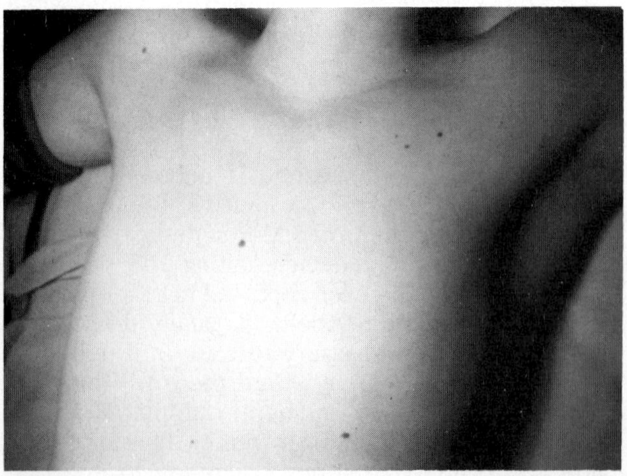

FIGURE 7-3 Child with total absence of both breasts. Note the lack of both nipple and areola. (From Trier WC. Complete breast absence. Plast Reconstr Surg 1965; 36:430-439.)

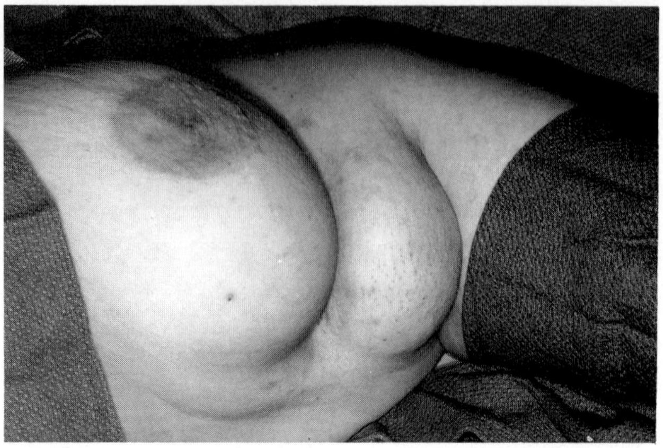

FIGURE 7-4 A common location of supernumerary breast is the axilla. This most likely represents extension of the axillary tail of Spence or a separate, hypertrophic growth of the axillary tail.

In 1841 Alfred Poland described a patient aged 27 who was found at autopsy to have an absent sternocostal portion of the pectoralis major with an intact clavicular origin to the muscle on the left side.[7] In addition, there was an absent pectoralis minor and severely hypoplastic serratus anterior and external oblique muscles. The autopsy also disclosed absence of the middle phalanges of the left hand, in conjunction with syndactyly. Poland titled his report "Deficiency of the pectoral muscles" and apparently failed to recognize the hand deformities as part of the symptom complex. Six years before Poland's report, Sir Charles Bell[9] had described a similar instance of congenital absence of the pectoral muscles, and subsequently more than 300 case reports appeared in the literature. It is therefore intriguing to wonder why Clarkson[8] chose to name the syndrome he described in 1962 after Poland, who, despite reporting the upper extremity abnormalities, did not associate them with the chest wall anomalies. In fact, it was a Dutch student named Bierens deHaan[10] who first linked the skeletal deformities of the trunk and hand in the title of his doctoral thesis (1902). Despite the historical evidence to the contrary, we are nevertheless compelled to continue using Poland's name to describe the syndrome consisting of unilateral absence of the sternocostal head of the pectoral major muscle and ipsilateral syndactyly, because it seems entrenched in the literature. Any change at this point would only add to the confusion. For the purpose of this chapter, we consider Poland's syndrome as hypoplasia of the breast in conjunction with absence or hypoplasia of the ipsilateral pectoral musculature. Progressing from this minimal requirement, patients can present with any one of a number of clinical pictures, up to and including the more severe classic defect consisting of at least partial absence of the pectoralis major (usually the sternocostal head) and absence of the pectoralis minor, with variable degrees of deformity of the serratus anterior, infraspinatus, supraspinatus, latissimus dorsi, and external oblique muscles (Fig. 7-5). In the ipsilateral chest wall the deformity varies from costal flattening up to total absence of the anterolateral ribs with herniation of the lung. In addition, both pectus carinatum and pectus excavatum have been reported in conjunction with Poland's anomaly. Scoliosis is a common finding in the more severe presentations of the syndrome.

A wide range of developmental anomalies of the hand and upper extremity have been recorded in association with Poland's syndrome. The most common deformity is symphalangism with syndactyly

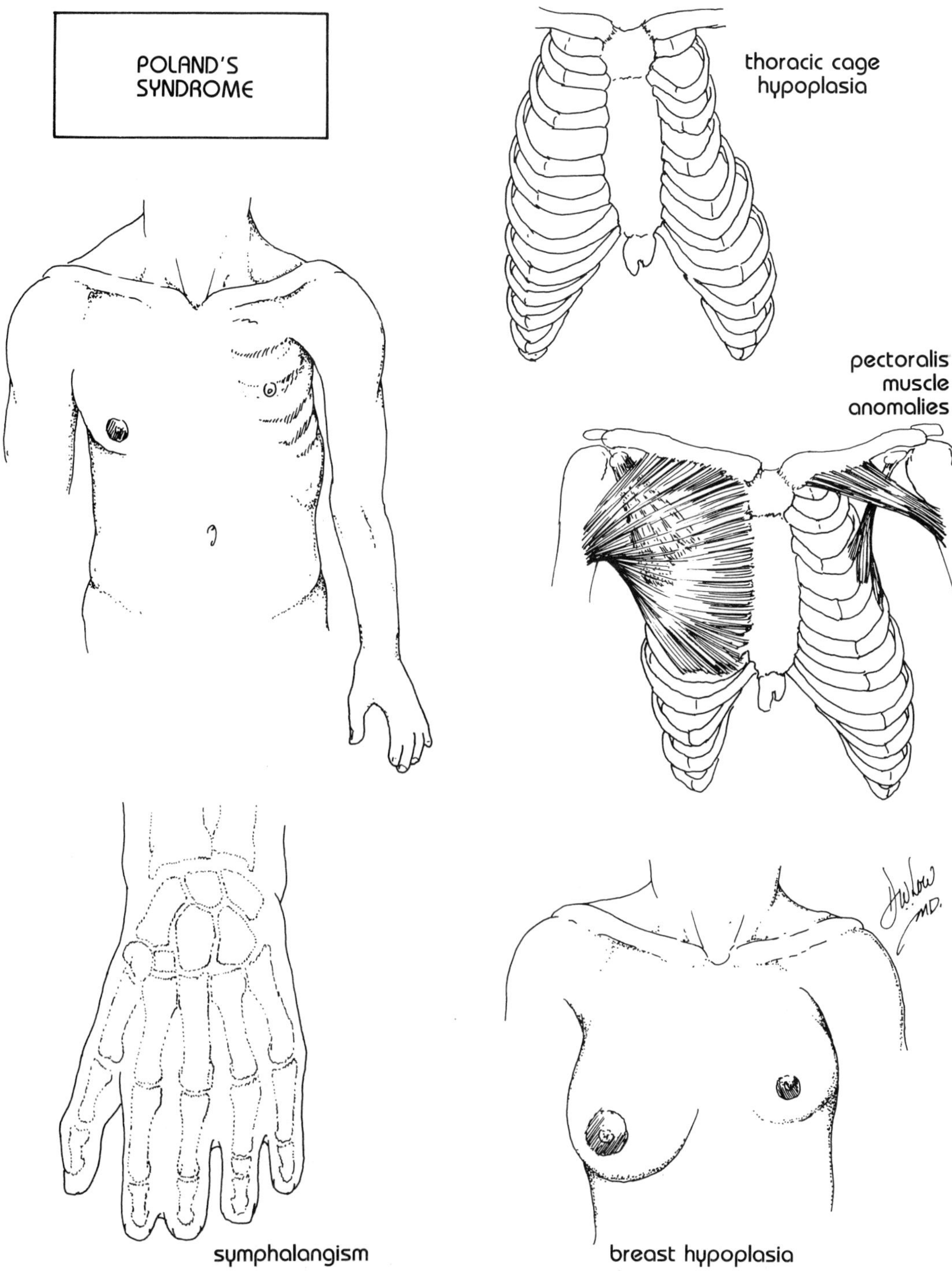

FIGURE 7-5 Poland's syndrome may be exemplified by any number of possibilities: partial absence of the pectoralis major muscle, absence of the pectoralis minor with variable degrees of deformity of the serratus, infraspinatus, supraspinatus, latissimus dorsi, and external oblique muscles. Various chest wall defects are seen as well as obvious hypoplasia or absence of the breast with superior displacement of the nipple. Arm and hand anomalies are common.

and hypoplasia or complete absence of the middle phalanges. The entire limb may be foreshortened, with most of the hypoplasia in the forearm, the upper arm above the elbow being of near-normal size. A detailed discussion of the multiple hand anomalies and their treatment can be found in any textbook on congenital hand surgery.

Epidemiology

Because of the above-mentioned discrepancy over the constituents of Poland's anomaly, we lack a universally accepted definition of the syndrome, and the epidemiologic data are unreliable. A frequently quoted incidence is one in 30,000 births. This is based on the work of Freire-Maia and colleagues,[11] who in 1973 surveyed 60,000 birth from a small area in Brazil and detected only two cases of Poland's syndrome. A review of other published sources suggests the incidence of the syndrome to be somewhere between 1:10,000 and 1:100,000.

The right side is affected almost twice as often as the left. Some large series report a clear male predominance[12,13] whereas others just as convincingly show a female majority.[14,15] Pooling the literature, it is apparent that males and females are affected with the same frequency, the gender difference being explained by a bias in data collection. The cases reported in the plastic surgery literature are mostly of women seeking breast reconstruction; those seen in orthopedic surgery practice tend to be male patients requesting correction of hand problems (Tables 7-1, 7-2).

Etiology

The cause of Poland's syndrome is unknown, but there are several interesting hypotheses. At the present time, the most widely entertained theory proposes a vascular origin.

Vascular Hypothesis. Bouvet and colleagues[16] detailed the evidence to support their argument, which holds that hypoplasia of the ipsilateral subclavian artery gives rise to the malformations known collectively as Poland's syndrome. The authors compared eight patients affected with the deformity, some of whom also had ipsilateral hand anomalies, with ten normal children. Vascular studies showed marked asymmetry between the involved arm and the normal arm of affected children. The abnormal findings included statistically significant differences in mean velocity of blood flow, even after correction for the discrepancies in limb volume.

From the vantage point of considerable knowledge of normal human embryology, Bouwes Bavinck and Weaver[17] suggested a vascular etiology for Poland's and other related anomalies. The authors theorized that during or around the sixth week of gestation, certain loci within the subclavian arteries, vertebral arteries, or other branches become occluded, giving rise to predictable patterns of defects. During this rapid growth phase, the subclavian artery is forced into a U-shaped configuration as the

TABLE 7-1 Poland's Syndrome Without Arm Anomalies

Authors/Year	M:F	R:L
Krause et al, 1969[29]	0:2	2:0
Amoroso and Angelats, 1981[34]	0:1	1:0
Hester and Bostwick, 1982[31]	4:7	No Data
Urschel et al., 1984[32]	0:2	1:1
Haller et al., 1984[33]	3:1	3:1
Argenta et al., 1985[14]	0:6	3:1
Santi et al., 1985[35]	0:2	1:1
Holmstrom et al., 1986[26]	0:1	1:0
Seyfer et al., 1988[15]	8:25	21:12
TOTALS	**15:47**	**33:16**

TABLE 7-2 Poland's Syndrome With Arm Anomalies

Authors/Year	M:F	R:L
Baker and Mara, 1976[30]	0:1	1:0
Anderl and Kerschbaumer, 1986[37]	2:0	2:0
Sackey et al., 1984[23]	6:4	8:2
Pisteljic et al., 1986[24]	0:1	0:1
Gausewitz et al., 1984[13]	8:2	6:4
Senrui et al., 1982[12]	4:0	2:2
Parker et al., 1981[22]	1:0	0:1
Suzuki et al., 1983[27]	7:0	4:3
Trosev et al., 1966[19]	3:1	1:3
TOTALS	**31:9**	**24:16**

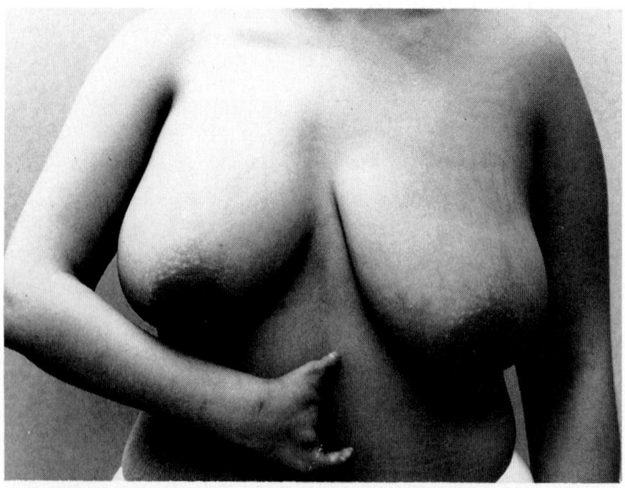

FIGURE 7-6 A 19-year-old presented for treatment of breast asymmetry. Note the right axillary deformity caused by hypoplasia of the pectoralis muscles, relative hypoplasia of the right breast, and the upper extremity anomaly. Hypoplasia or absence of the middle phalanges is seen as a component of Poland's syndrome. (Photograph and case courtesy of R. Barrett Noone, M.D.)

ribs grow forward and medially, with the vertebral artery at the center of this curve (Fig. 7-7). Distortion of either vessel at such a critical time could lead to kinking of the arterial wall and partial-to-total occlusion of the lumen. Bouwes Bavinck and Weaver[17] called this process the "subclavian artery supply disruption sequence" (SASDS), and outlined specific sites of blocks that culminate in Klippel-Feil, Moebius', and Poland's syndromes. Occlusion along the proximal origin of the subclavian artery leads to the more severe presentations of Poland's with arm, chest, and breast anomalies, whereas a more distal occlusion produces the more common clinical deformity limited to the chest wall.

Although intriguing, these studies fall short of answering all the questions surrounding the etiology of Poland's syndrome. Proponents of the vascular origin hypothesis argue that the convoluted embryology of the human circulatory system on the right half of the body, coupled with the observed right-sided prevalence in the syndrome, bolsters their claim. Poland's anomaly is indeed more common on the right, but approximately one third of known cases have been on the left side, a fact not adequately explained by the vascular origin hypothesis.

It is well to remember that all theories of the etiology of Poland's anomaly are necessarily conjectural. There is no objective evidence that the decreased size of the vessel and reduced blood flow in the affected limb is causal rather than derivative. It is just as easy to suppose that the small artery and low flow are simply an expected by-product of a more basic, underlying pathologic process.

Environmental Trauma Hypothesis. In 1972 David[18] suggested that environmental factors may play a role in the etiology of Poland's syndrome, on the basis of a study of ten cases. There was evidence that the mothers of most of these patients had tried unsuccessfully to abort the fetus. In one case David reported that the mother took an unknown dose of ergonovine maleate, which is a basic structure of lysergic acid that may be a cause of limb deformities in humans. He rightly questioned, however, why the effect should be unilateral. Interestingly, five of these ten children were adopted.

Hereditary Hypothesis. There is little evidence of genetic inheritance of Poland's syndrome. Only in two families reported by Trosev and colleagues[19] were there a manifested familial link consistent with autosomal dominant transmission from parent to child.

Associated Disorders

Poland's syndrome has been associated with several other conditions and systemic disorders.

Moebius Anomaly. Approximately 20 cases of Poland-Moebius syndrome have been reported to date.[20,21] By itself, the Moebius syndrome consists of a variable degree of facial paralysis with inability to abduct the eyes beyond the midpoint.[22] Herrmann and coworkers[21] defined the Poland-Moebius syndrome as any combination of congenital bilateral cranial nerve palsies associated with hypoplastic to absent pectoralis muscle, concomitant chest wall abnormalities, and/or hand defects of the symbrachydactyly type. They estimate a prevalence of one in 500,000 for the combined syndrome.

Hematopoietic Malignancy. Sackey and colleagues[23] reviewed seven previously reported cases of Poland's syndrome associated with leukemia or lymphoma. To these they added three new patients from their own series. They concluded that the incidence of non-Hodgkin's lymphoma in patients with Poland's syndrome is too high to be fortuitous, and that children with Poland's syndrome are at increased risk of developing leukemia and non-Hodgkin's lymphoma.

Isolated cases of rare anomalies in patients with Poland's syndrome are intriguing, but too sporadic to warrant the assumption of an association. Pisteljic and associates[24] reported a 12-year-old girl with signs of Poland's syndrome on the left side and a coloboma of the left optic disc, the so called "morning glory" syndrome. Mace and coworkers[25] described one patient with absence of the right pectoralis major muscle, flattening of the right thoracic

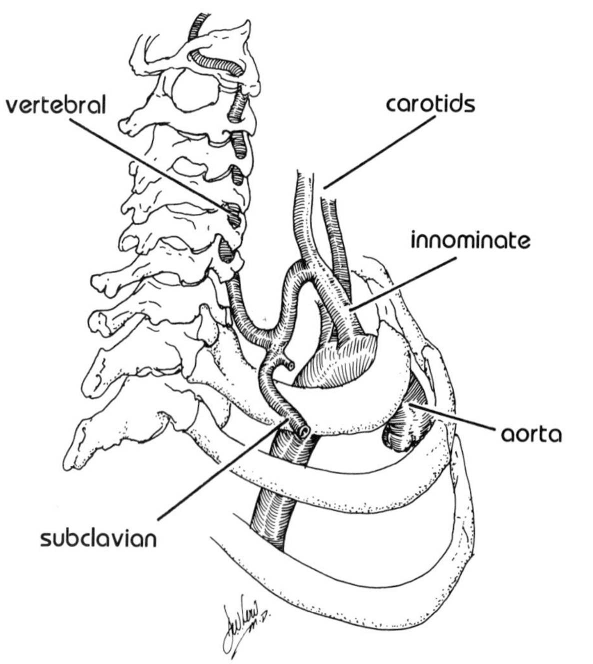

FIGURE 7-7 U-form shape of the right subclavian artery during horizon 18 and later. From Congdon (1922). Stephens (1980) correlates horizon 18 to gestational days 40-42. This U-shaped configuration is thought to lead to kinking and/or occlusion of the artery in individuals affected with Poland's syndrome. (From Bouwes Bavinck JN, Weaver DD. Subclavian artery supply disruption sequence: Hypothesis of a vascular etiology for Poland, Klippel-Feil, and Moebius anomalies. Am J Med Genet 1986; 23:903-918.)

cage, aplasia of the T3 hemivertebra on the right, and absence of the ipsilateral kidney.

Natural History

Seyfer and colleagues[15] reviewed the clinical course and treatment of 33 patients with Poland's syndrome over a 10-year period from 1978 to 1988. Even in severe cases, the functional disability associated with the disorder is mild; one girl with absence of the latissimus dorsi reported difficulty in performing cartwheels and other gymnastic exercises because of poor shoulder strength, but most of the male patients were able to participate in athletics despite some weakness on rope climbing and pull-ups in those severely affected. The hand deformities seemed to cause little subjective complaint, although one would expect major functional impairment with progressive degrees of upper extremity anomalies.

Preoperative Assessment

Initial evaluation begins with a thorough history taking and physical examination, to include accurate prenatal history with specific reference to drug use. The physical examination should pay special attention to the chest wall, shoulder, and hand. The presence or absence of the latissimus dorsi should be noted, because this is important in any future attempt at reconstruction.[26] A head and neck examination is appropriate, and in particular one should look for any changes along the distribution of the sixth and seventh cranial nerves, which would be indicative of Moebius' syndrome.

Laboratory studies should include a serologic search for blood-borne malignancies, i.e., leukemia and lymphoma. Computed tomography (CT) is helpful in delineating the exact aberrant anatomy found with this syndrome[27,28] (Fig. 7–8).

Treatment

Appropriate management of the breast deformities of Poland's syndrome coincided with the introduction of the silicone breast implant in 1965.[29,30] Krause and associates described two patients with concomitant pectoralis major and ipsilateral breast hypoplasia who were treated with breast implants alone. Although insertion of an internal mammary prosthesis was a vast improvement over previous methods of treating the breast defect of Poland's, implantation alone did not address the underlying chest wall deformity or the absent pectoral fold.

Custom-fitted implants were subsequently introduced.[30] These were constructed of various materials such as methylmethacrylate and silicone. Unfortunately, although women treated with mammary implants alone tended to develop capsular contracture with alarming frequency, those patients treated with custom-made chest wall prostheses often experienced displacement of the implants. In short, the long-term results of these procedures were generally unsatisfactory.[15]

Such was the status of thoracic reconstruction in Poland's syndrome until only a decade ago, when Hester and Bostwick[31] pioneered the use of the latissimus dorsi muscle transposition flap to fill the chest wall defect. The authors described operative refinements of the usual latissimus dorsi muscle flap technique, when intended for Poland's patients, to include limited incisions and transferring the insertion of the muscle anteriorly to correct the "double anterior axillary fold deformity" (Fig. 7–9). In women this later modification allows total submuscular placement of a breast implant. Polyurethane implants were used for this condition, but an argument can be made for use of silicone implants, because total muscle coverage is achieved.

There is continued debate in the literature over the perceived necessity to repair the anterior thoracic defect directly. Haller and colleagues[33] proposed stabilization of the chest wall with autologous rib grafts and the use of prosthetic fabric to replace the absent endothoracic fascia. Marlex mesh, Prolene mesh, and synthetic dura mater have all been used to reinforce the thoracic defect. This entire repair is subsequently covered with a latissimus dorsi muscle flap that is rotated into place.[32–34] The controversy stems from the wide array of deformities encountered in the various syndromes and the high degree of variability possible among patients. Seyfer and colleagues[15] believe that repair of the herniated lung with rib grafts or alloplastic material is unnecessary. In men, the latissimus dorsi muscle would largely cover the structural defect, and most mild-to-moderate deformities in patients of either sex can be managed by latissimus muscle transposition and submuscular implant placement alone. Severe manifestations of the syndrome in women, however, may need further skeletal bolstering to achieve a stable base for prosthesis insertion, and to ensure adequate projection and symmetry of the reconstructed breast.

Santi and associates[35] proposed correcting the thoracic anomaly of Poland's syndrome through limited axillary and dorsal shoulder incisions to transpose the humeral attachment of the latissimus dorsi anteriorly and use the muscle to cover the chest defect. The prosthesis is inserted through a curvilinear incision along the new areolar border. Because accurate placement of the muscle and breast implant is critical, we still prefer a lateral submammary incision, as described by Hester and Bostwick,[30] to obtain adequate exposure of the surgical field and proper development of the implant pocket.

The chest wall is the foundation on which the breast reconstruction is to be carried out, so it must be addressed first (Fig. 7–10). In most cases latissimus dorsi muscle transfer alone is adequate, but if the chest wall defect is severe enough, repair with

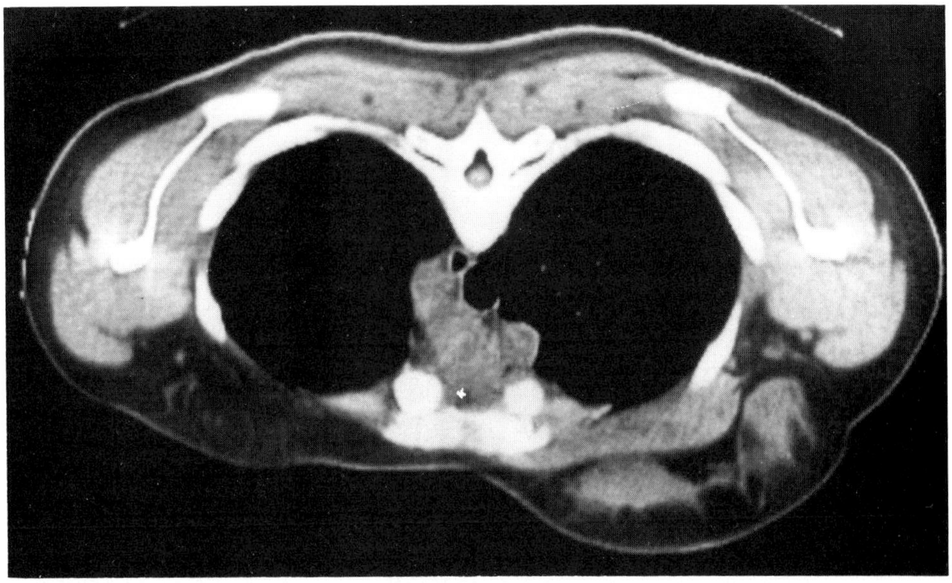

A

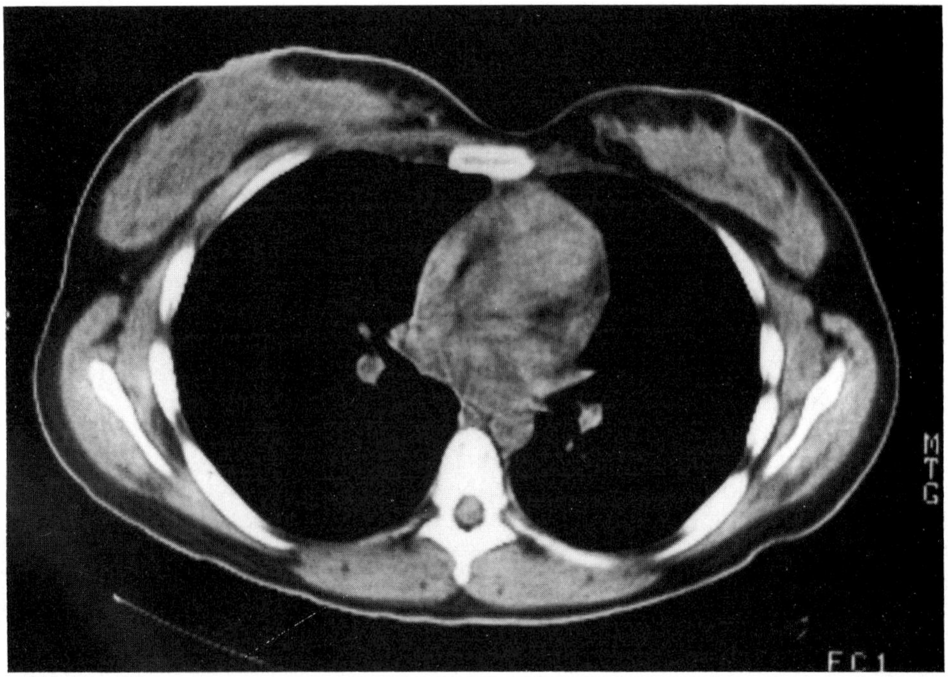

B

FIGURE 7-8 *A*, Computed tomography section at the sternal end of the clavicles. The right pectoralis muscles are normal. The left pectoralis minor is absent. A portion of the clavicular head of the pectoralis major remains. *B*, Two cm caudal, the sternocostal head of the left pectoralis major and the left pectoralis minor are absent. Note the asymmetry of the breasts. (From Demos TC, Johnson C, Love L, Posniak H. Computed tomography of partial unilateral agenesis of the pectoralis muscles. J Comput Assist Tomogr 1985;9:558–559.)

Marlex mesh or rib graft may be necessary before embarking on the soft tissue reconstruction. Anterior transposition of the humeral insertion of the latissimus dorsi also helps in reestablishing the anterior axillary fold. The neurovascular pedicle should be preserved intact to maintain muscle bulk and function.

Nipple Reconstruction. Many patients with Poland's syndrome have nipples that are superiorly displaced and hypoplastic. This is one of the most challenging aspects of the treatment, as discussed by Argenta and colleagues.[14] Tissue expansion is a relatively recent solution and one that offers hope for an aesthetically pleasing result: the expander is placed under the nipple and just superior to it, thus expanding both nipple-areola size and the skin above it. Upon removal of the expander and insertion of the permanent breast prosthesis, the excess skin in the upper pole allows the nipple to drop slightly to its desired position. The newly constructed breast will have a more ptotic, mature look resembling the opposite side in adult women. Argenta and colleagues

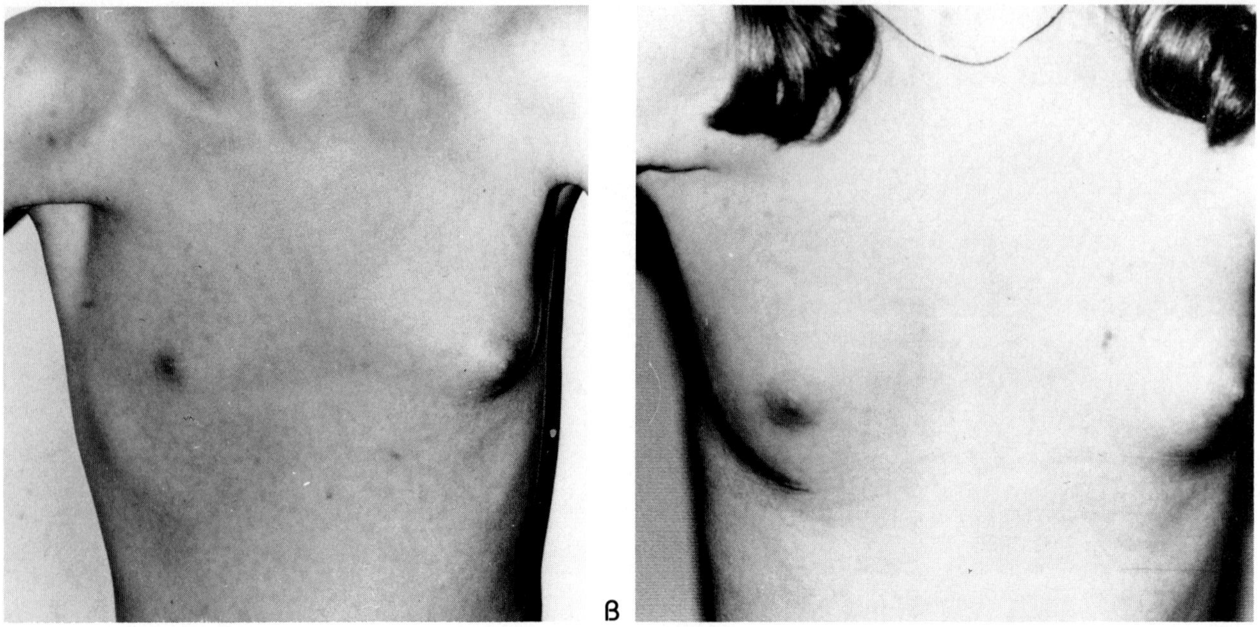

A B

FIGURE 7-9 *A*, Preoperative view of an 11-year-old girl with Poland's deformity. *B*, Double axillary fold resulting from transposition of the latissimus dorsi anteriorly *without* transferring the insertion anteriorly on the humerus. (From Hester TR Jr, Bostwick J III. Poland's syndrome: Correction with latissimus muscle transposition. Plast Reconstr Surg 1982; 69:226–233.)

suggest a program of prolonged tissue expansion throughout puberty, with gradual inflation to correspond with growth of the normal breast. Argenta reported five young women with Poland's syndrome in whom he performed reconstruction before their breasts were fully developed (Fig. 7-11). The expander is inserted through a small incision within the distal axillary hair, and a space is developed on the anterior chest wall by sharp dissection. As the expander beneath the nipple-areola complex is inflated over a period of several years, the skin between the nipple and clavicle also expands, resulting in inferior displacement of the nipple-areola complex. To minimize tension during active exercise and keep up with mammary growth in these girls, Argenta recommended considerable redundancy in the inflation tube.

Progressive tissue expansion through the period of active breast growth in adolescent girls seems a reasonable approach, especially if a permanent expander-implant is used.[36] Slow, gradual enlargement should mimic the development of the normal side and give the reconstructed breast the best chance for symmetry, as long as capsular contracture around the expander does not intervene. Tissue expansion is also a useful technique in the postpubertal female who presents with Poland's deformity. Obviously the expander needs to be in place only until the skin requirements are met (Fig. 7-12).

Timing of Reconstruction. The timing of treatment of the skeletal and soft tissue deformity in Poland's syndrome is also a widely debated issue. Most patients first seek medical attention at puberty, when the defect starts to become obvious with growth of the normal breast in girls or development of the pectoral musculature in boys. As an alternative, Anderl and Kerschbaumer[37] reported early surgical correction in two boys one aged 5 years, and the other aged 8 months. Thirteen years and 10 years respectively, after anterior thoracic reconstruction with a latissimus dorsi muscle flap, the rib cage and overlying musculature appeared grossly normal, the spine was straight and well balanced, and there was no significant deviation from normal skeletal structures in either patient. Orthopedic measurements well documented this improvement.

The dramatic relief seen with this early surgical intervention in Poland's syndrome may force a reevaluation of the best time for treating these patients. Latissimus dorsi muscle flap transposition at a young age theoretically could facilitate the patient's learning to use the muscle in its new position, and might stimulate adjacent skeletal and soft tissue structures to develop and function normally. However, a series with a larger number of patients would help to strengthen these authors' position.

Tuberous Breast

In 1976 Rees and Aston[38] coined the term "tuberous breast" to describe a gland whose base is deficient in both its horizontal and vertical dimensions. A tuberous breast is usually accompanied by an excessively large and prominent nipple and areola. Other features of the tuberous breast include

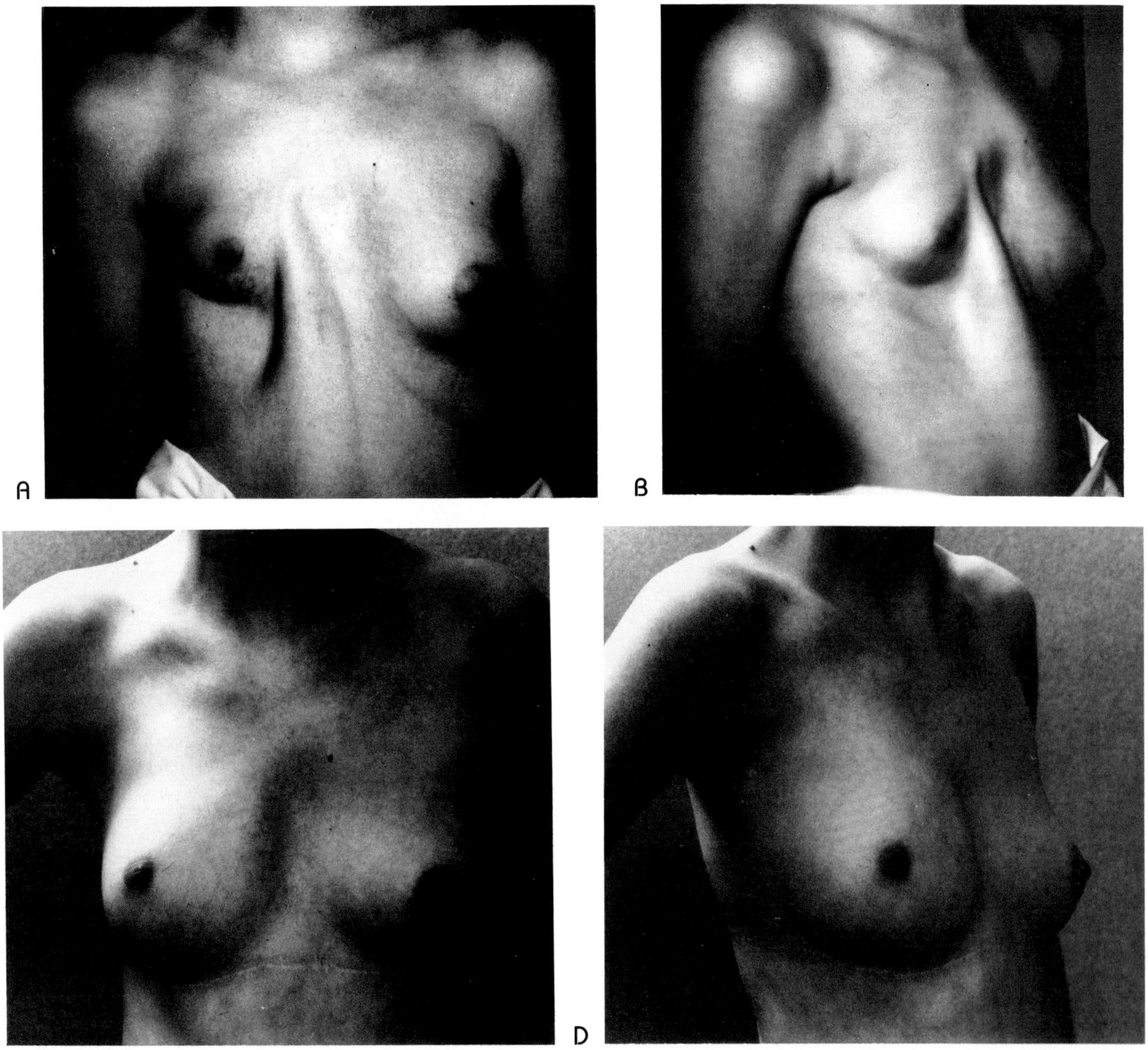

A B C D

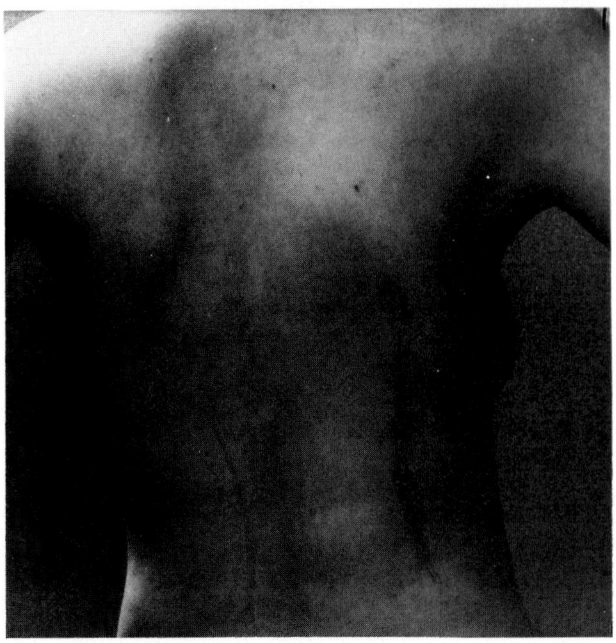

E

FIGURE 7 – 10 *A, B,* A variety of Poland's syndrome with breast hypoplasia, superior nipple displacement, pectus excavation, thoracic cage assymmetry, and abnormal development of thoracic soft tissues. *C, D, E,* Anterior, oblique, and posterior views 9 years after two-stage reconstruction. The skeletal deformity was reversed in the first operation. This was followed by muscle and breast reconstruction with the latissimus dorsi technique. (Case and photographs courtesy of R. Barrett Noone, M.D.)

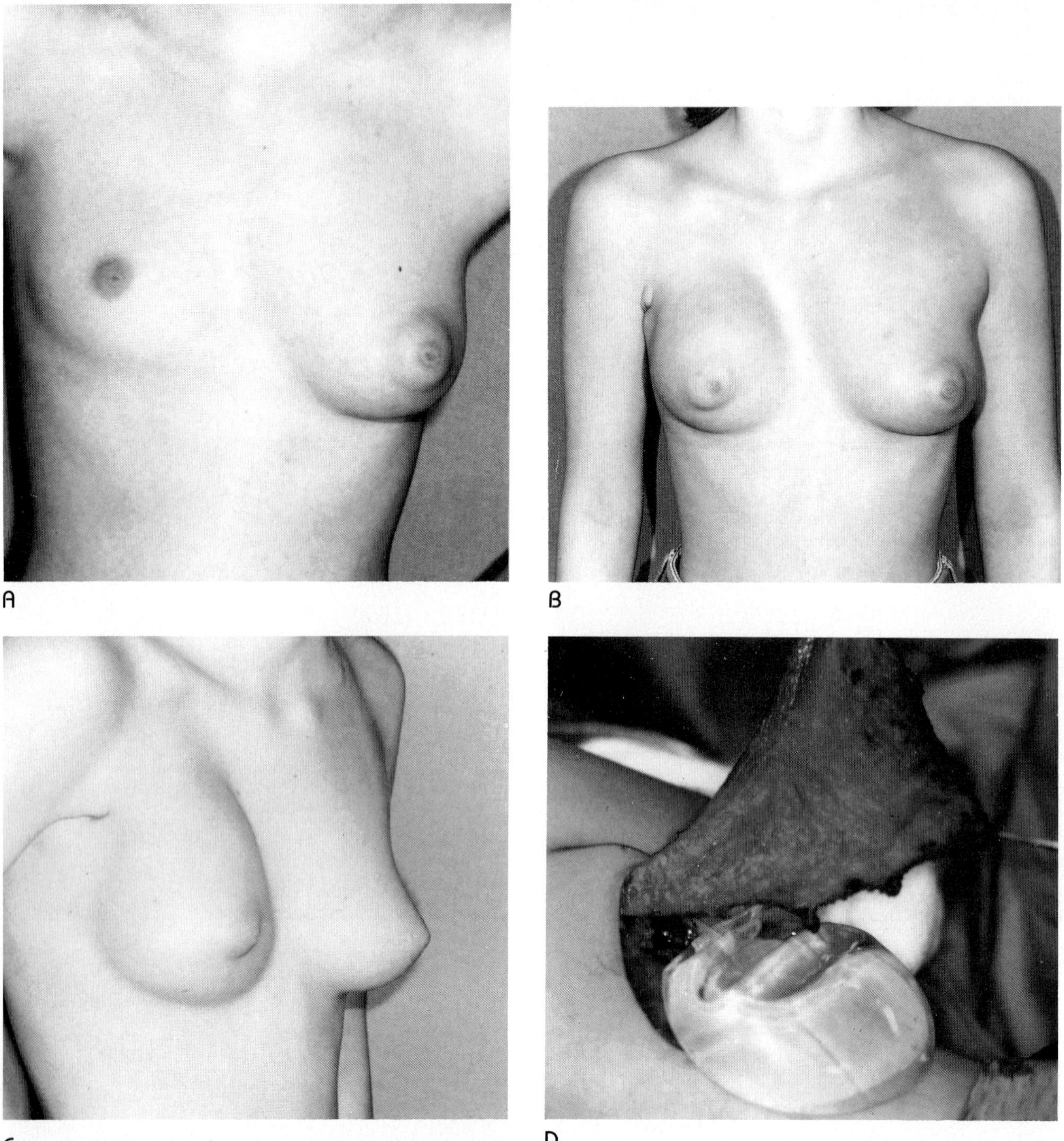

FIGURE 7-11 *A*, A 15-year-old girl with Poland's syndrome of a less pronounced degree. *B*, *C*, The breast was reconstructed at 14 years of age with a transaxillary tissue expander that was left in place for $4\frac{1}{2}$ years. *D*, At $18\frac{1}{2}$ years of age the prosthesis was removed and a latissimus dorsi muscle flap transferred through an incision along the anterior border of the latissimus. *E*, *F*, Five months after muscle transfer and placement of a permanent prosthesis, the patient has excellent asymmetry, projection, and softness. (From Argenta LC, VanderKolk C, Friedman RJ, Marks M. Refinements in reconstruction of congenital breast deformities. Plast Reconstr Surg 1985; 76:73–80.)

glandular hypoplasia, reduced vertical extent, and ptosis. The areolar hypertrophy is thought to be caused by herniation of the breast parenchyma into the nipple.[38]

Management. Routine augmentation mammaplasty of the tuberous breast accentuates the deformity by making the nipple and areola protrude even further. Rees and Aston described correction of the

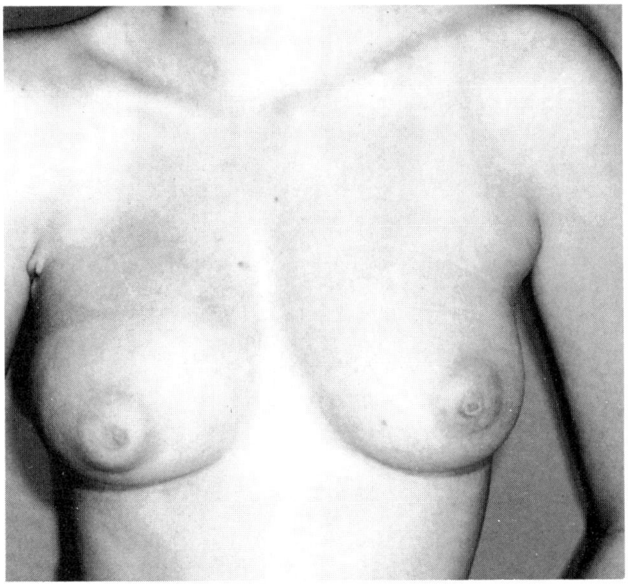

E

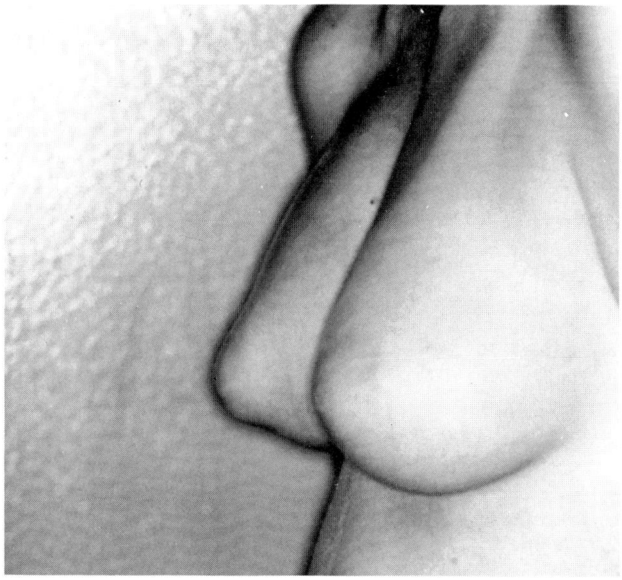

F

Figure 7-11 *Continued*

deformity by proceeding with dissection of the skin envelope away from the breast combined with implant placement for strategic augmentation. A circular incision is made within the enlarged areola to the desired dimensions. The breast parenchyma is then dissected from the lateral pole. The implant is next inserted through an incision at the inferior aspect of the gland between the posterior capsule of the breast and the pectoralis fascia. The breast parenchyma is then reduced and the skin brassiere is tightened to hold it in place (Fig. 7-13).

Many surgeons[3] believe that the true deformity of a tuberous breast lies in the skin deficiency at the base of the envelope, manifested by a narrow transverse diameter and a circumferential constriction. Dinner and Dowden[39] suggested that no real herniation exists and that adequate correction of the malformed breast depends on releasing the constricting ring of skin at the base.

Various techniques have been described to bring additional skin to the tuberous breast. Elliott[40] reported a musculocutaneous transposition flap

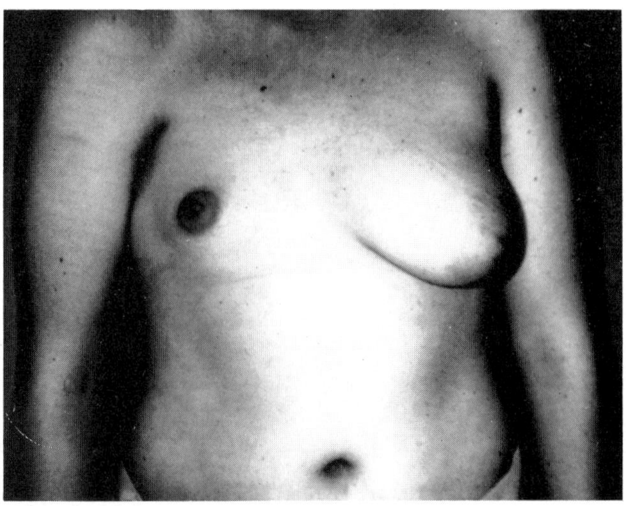

A

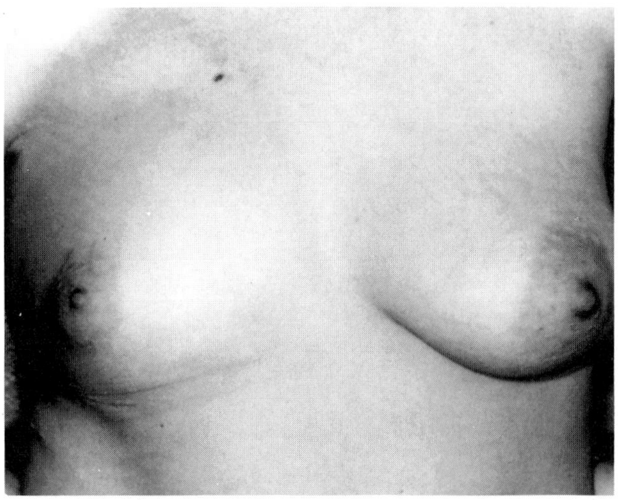

B

FIGURE 7-12 *A*, The breast of a 19-year-old girl with Poland's syndrome was reconstructed by placement of a tissue expander through a midaxillary incision followed by inflation of the expander to 500 ml. After 6 months it was removed and the latissimus muscle transferred over the 300-ml permanent prostheses. *B*, The patient $1\frac{1}{2}$ years postoperatively has a soft, symmetric breast. (From Argenta LC, VanderKolk C, Friedman RJ, Marks M. Refinements in reconstruction of congenital breast deformities. Plast Reconstr Surg 1985; 76:73-80.)

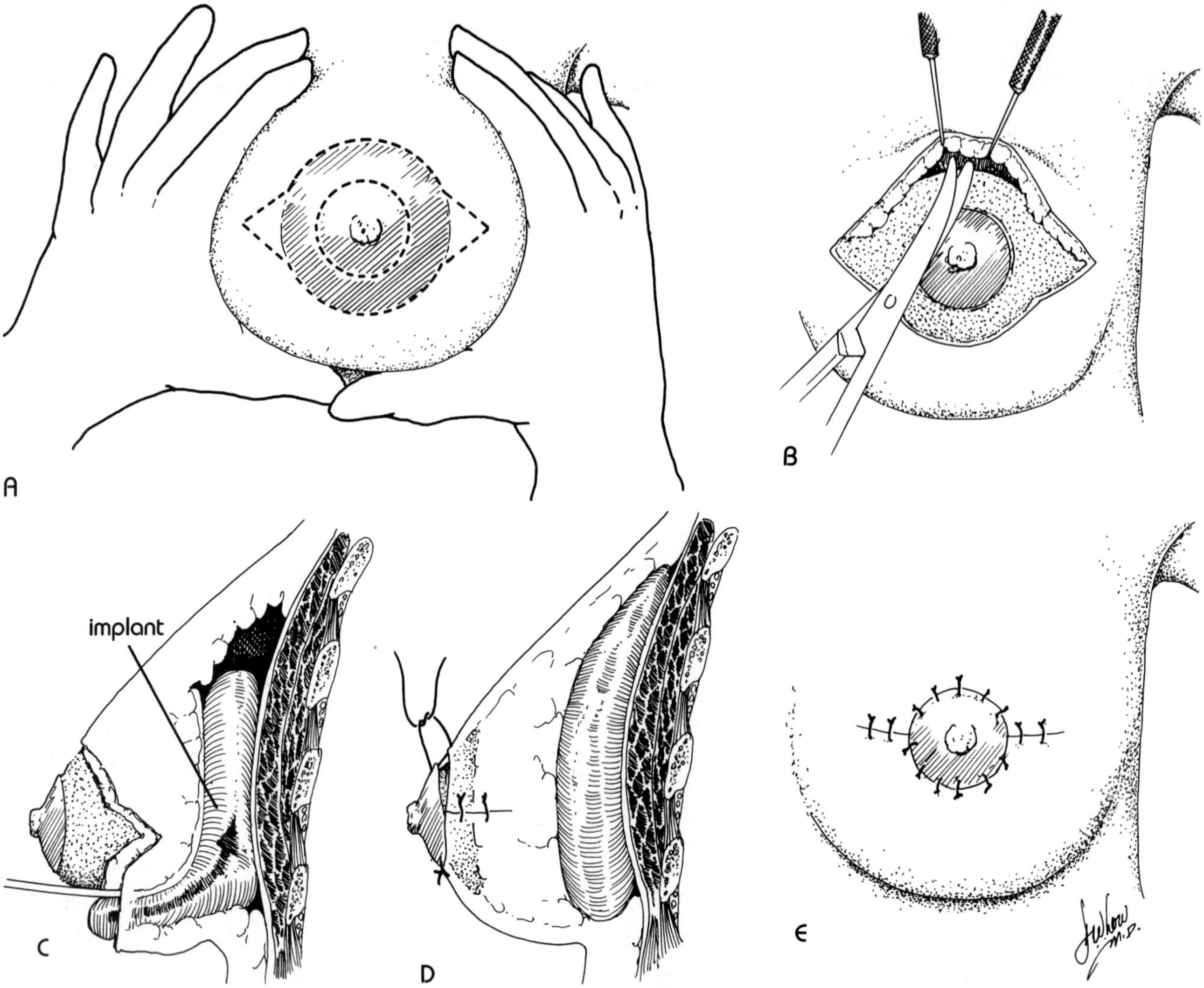

FIGURE 7-13 Telescoping technique for the herniated nipple deformity. *A*, New nipple size and skin incisions outlined. *B*, Breast tissue denuded in the subcutaneous plane. *C*, Prostheses placed under breast tissue on prepectoral fascia. *D*, *E*, Breast tissue telescoped into the new skin brassiere and the incision sutured. (Adapted from Rees TD, Aston SJ. The tuberous breast. Clin Plast Surg 1976; 3:339–347.)

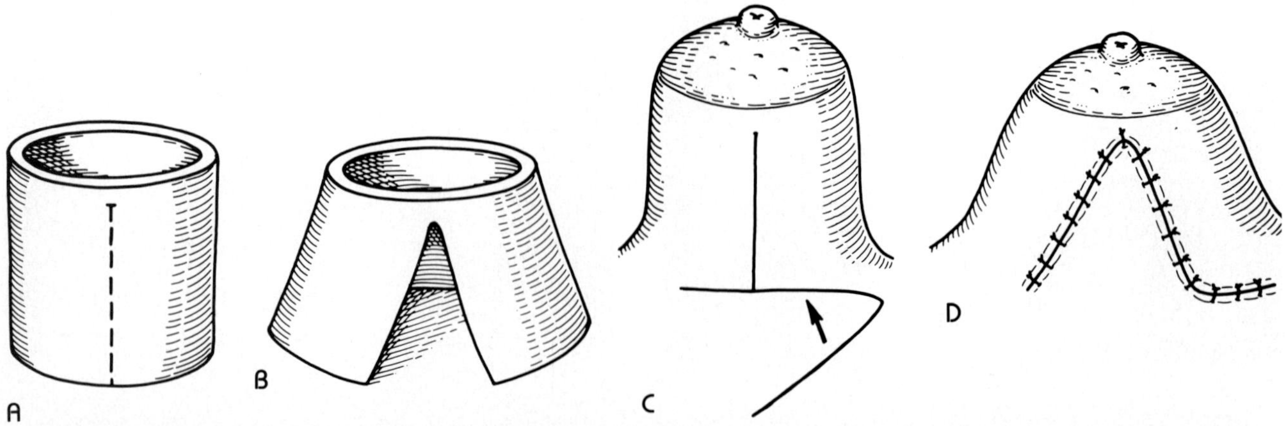

FIGURE 7-14 *A*, Constructed model of the tubular breast. *B*, Incision of the skin from the base of the breast to the areola transforms the breast from a tubular to a conical shape. *C*, *D*, Drawing of the submammary flap used to repair the defect created by vertical release of the constricting defect. (From Dinner MI, Dowden RV. The tubular/tuberous breast. Ann Plast Surg 1987; 19:414–420.)

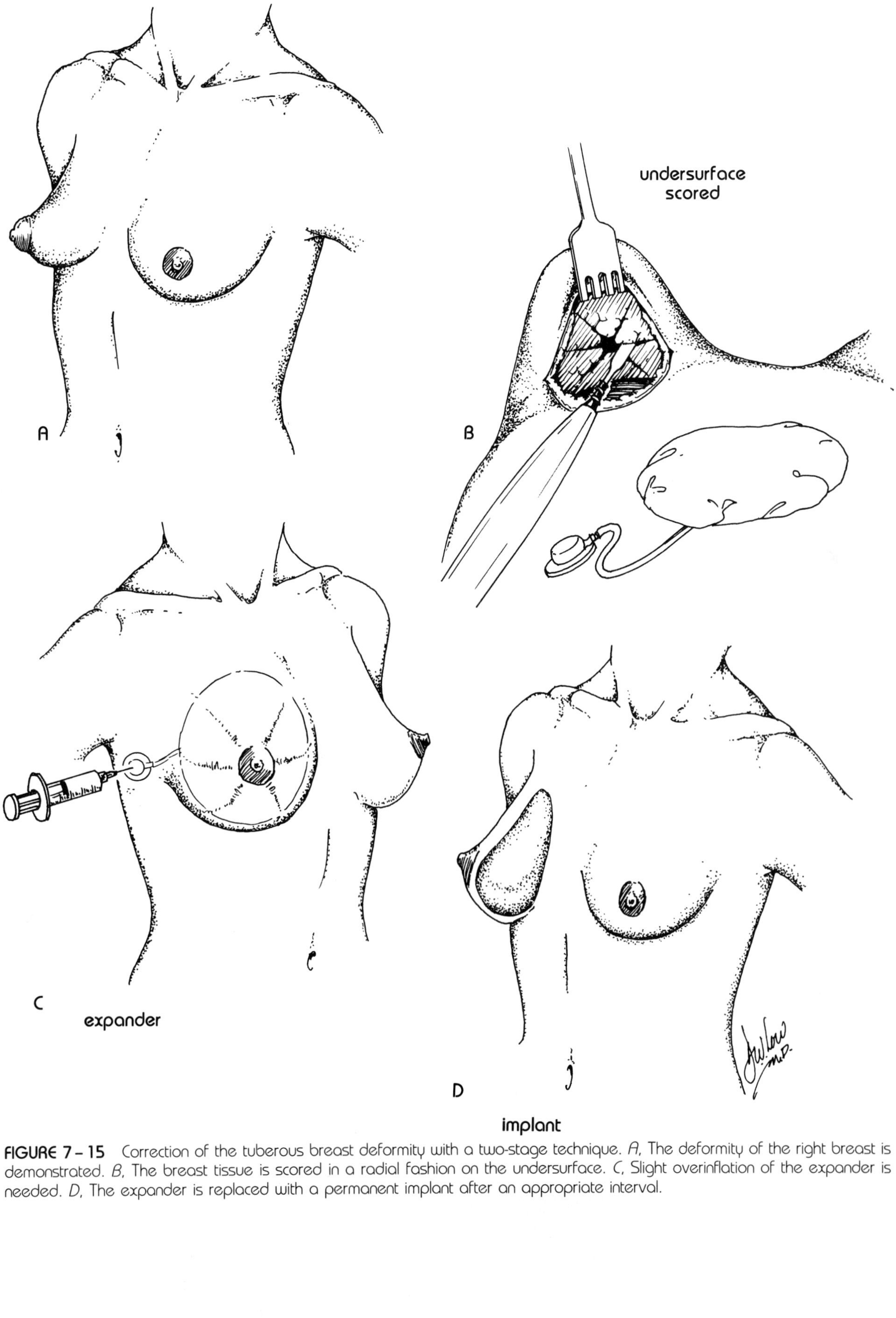

FIGURE 7–15 Correction of the tuberous breast deformity with a two-stage technique. *A*, The deformity of the right breast is demonstrated. *B*, The breast tissue is scored in a radial fashion on the undersurface. *C*, Slight overinflation of the expander is needed. *D*, The expander is replaced with a permanent implant after an appropriate interval.

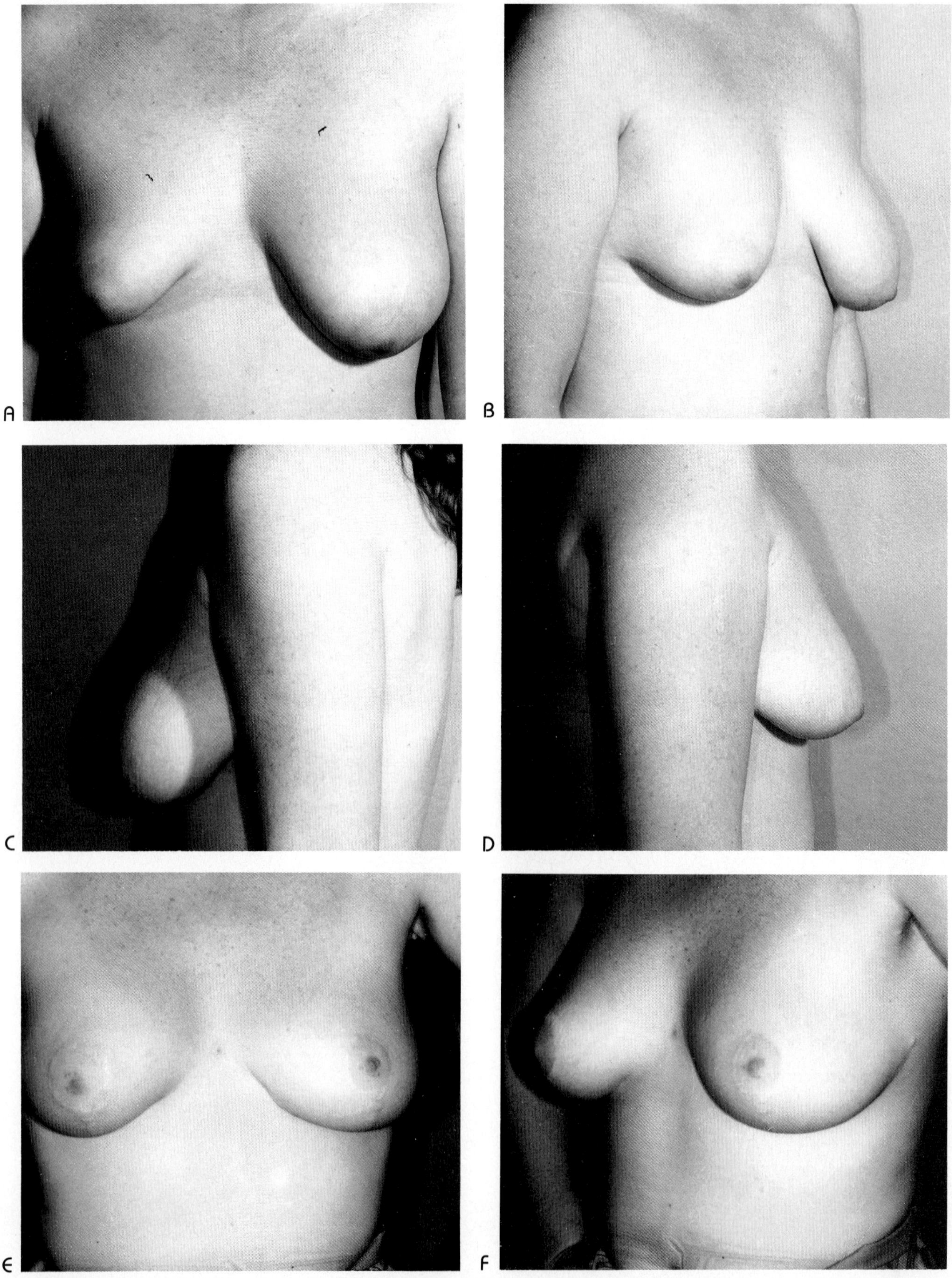

FIGURE 7-16 *A* to *D*, Preoperative anterior, oblique, and lateral photographic views of a patient with nonsyndromic breast asymmetry. *E* to *I*, Two years after right augmentation mastopexy with insertion of a 235-ml polyurethane-covered implant and a left-reduction mammaplasty.

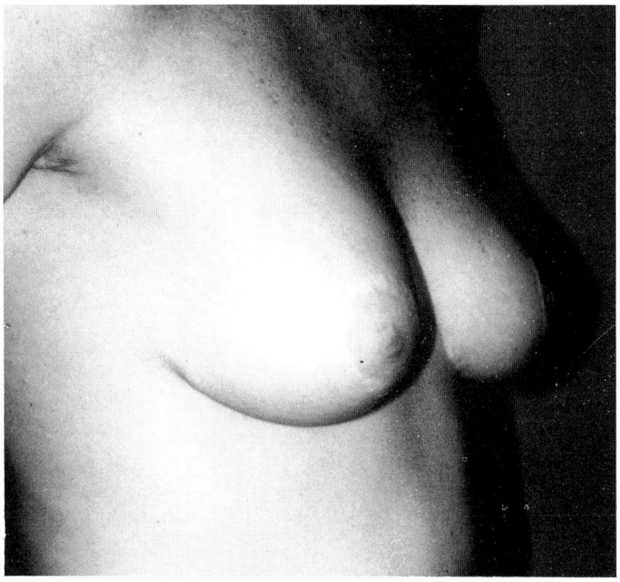
G

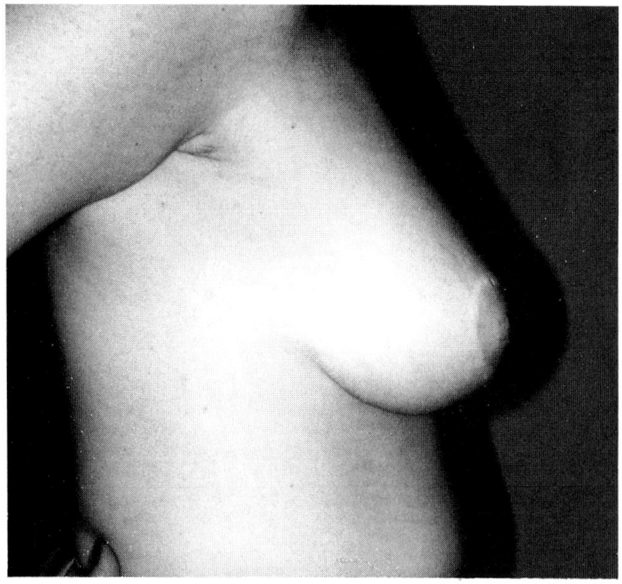
H

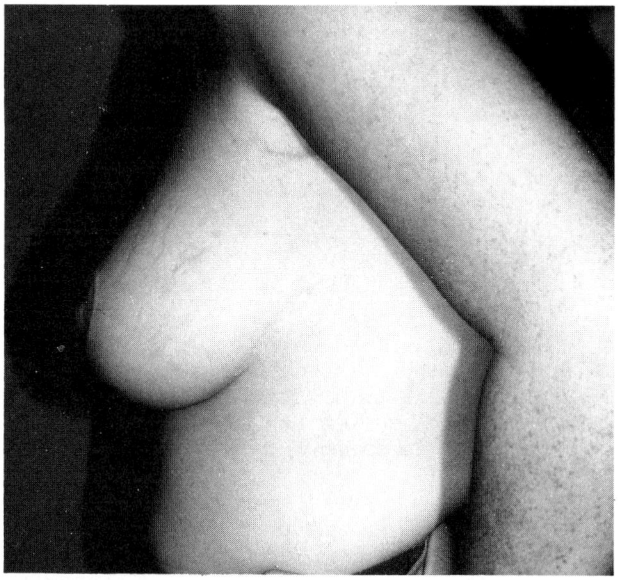
I

Figure 7-16 *Continued*

mammaplasty for correction of the tuberous breast. Dinner and Dowden[39] assessed the extent of skin deficiency after incising the breast. They then designed a local transposition flap to rotate into the defect (Fig. 7-14).

Although these flap techniques allow correction of the tuberous breast in one stage, they add excessive scarring to the repair of a tuberous breast. We prefer to approach the breast through a submammary incision and proceed with radial scoring of the skin around the areola to expand the base. A tissue expander is inserted and inflated to 200 to 300 ml above the desired breast volume. After an appropriate interval, the expander is removed and a breast implant inserted (Fig. 7-15). Although this approach implies a two-stage procedure, we believe it to be justified by a well-concealed scar and an improved aesthetic contour.

Breast Asymmetry

The management of nonsyndromic breast asymmetry is relatively straightforward: the smaller breast can be augmented or the larger breast can be reduced, whichever will achieve the most pleasing effect. A combination of procedures may need to be carried out if neither side is satisfactory (Fig. 7-16). In addition, the use of tissue expansion of the hypoplastic breast, followed by a second-stage replacement of the expander with an implant, may be the procedure of choice (Fig. 7-17).

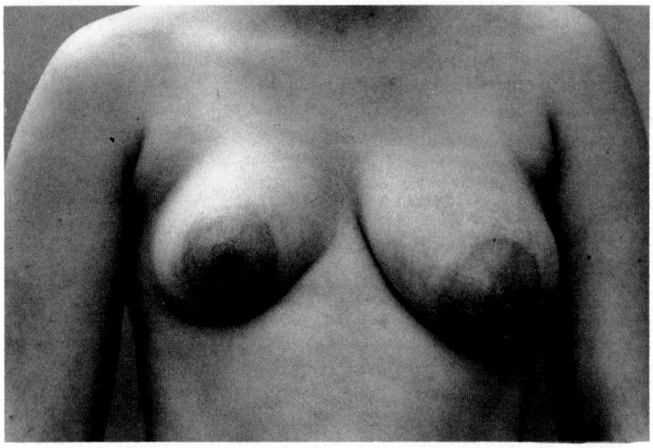
A

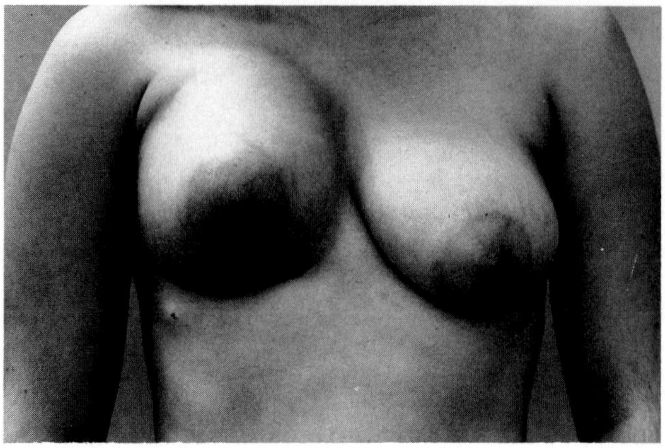
B

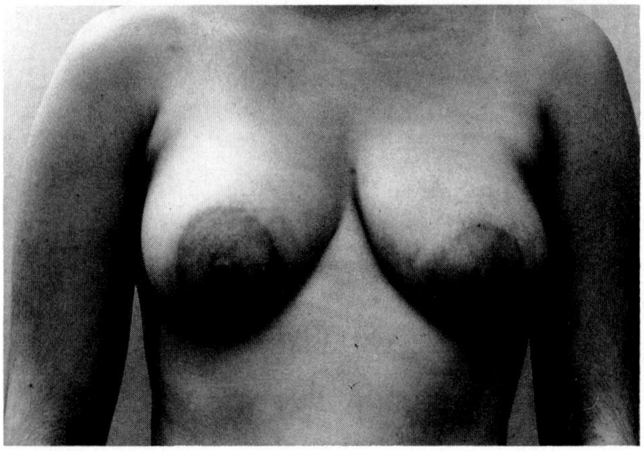
C

FIGURE 7-17 *A*, Hypoplasia of the right breast was treated by the two-stage tissue expansion technique. *B*, After completion of expansion of the temporary breast expander. *C*, After replacement of the expander with a mammary implant. (Case and photographs courtesy of R. Barrett Noone, M.D.)

References

1. Trier WC. Complete breast absence. Plast Reconstr Surg 1965; 36:430-439.
2. Hubert C. Étude sur pamastie. Thése pour le doctorat en médécin. Paris: A Mchalon, 1907.
3. Gilly E. Absence complete de mammelles chez une femme mere. Atrophie de membre supérieur droit. Courrier Med 1882; 32:27.
4. Wylie W. Case of entire absence of both mammae in a female aged 21 years. Br Med J 1888; 2:235.
5. Batchelor HT. Absence of mammae in a woman. Br Med J 1888; 2:876.
6. Schurter M, Letterman G. Breast deformities and their surgical repair. J Invest Dermatol 1974; 63:138-141.
7. Poland A. Deficiency of the pectoral muscles. Guy's Hosp Rep 1841; 6:191-193.
8. Clarkson P. Poland's syndactyly. Guy's Hosp Rep 1962; 111:335.
9. Brown JB, McDowell F. Syndactylism with absence of the pectoralis major. Surgery 1940; 7:599.
10. Bierens de Haan JCJ. Aangeboren ontbreken van de groote borstspier met syndactylie. Herinneringsb., pp. 3-19 (2 pl.), Prof SS Rosenstein. Leiden, 1902.
11. Freire-Maia N, Chautard EA, Opitz JM., et al. The Poland syndrome—clinical and genealogical data, dermatoglyphic analysis, and incidence. Hum Hered 1973; 23:97-104.
12. Senrui H, Egawa T, Horiki A. Anatomical findings in the hands of patients with Poland's şyndrome. J Bone Joint Surg 1982; 64A:1079-1082.
13. Gausewitz SH, Meals RA, Setoguchi, Y.: Severe limb deficiency in Poland's syndrome. Clin Orthop Rel Res 1984; 185:9-13.
14. Argenta LC, VanderKolk C, Friedman RJ, Marks, M. Refinements in reconstruction of congenital breast deformities. Plast Reconstr Surg 1985; 76:73-80.
15. Seyfer AE, Icochea R, Graeber GM. Poland's anomaly. Natural history and long term results of chest wall reconstruction in 33 patients. Ann Surg 1988; 208: 776-782.
16. Bouvet J-P, Leveque D, Bernetieres F, Gros J-J. Vascular origin of Poland's syndrome. Eur J Pediatr 1978; 128:17-26.
17. Bouwes Bavinck JN, Weaver DD. Subclavian artery supply disruption sequence: Hypothesis of a vascular etiology for Poland, Klippel-Feil, and Moebius anomalies. Am J Med Genet 1986; 23:903-918.
18. David TJ. Nature and etiology of the Poland anomaly. N Eng J Med 1972; 287:487-489.
19. Trosev K, Cervenka J, Gerberova E. Congenital dysplasia of the pectoralis muscles associated with congenital malformations of the hand and finger of the ipsilateral upper limb. Acta Chir Orthop Traumat Cechaslovaca 1966; 33:320-327.
20. Hopper KD, Haas DK, Rice MM, et al. Poland-Moebius syndrome: Evaluation by computerized tomography. South Med J 1985; 78:523-527.
21. Herrmann J, Pallister P, Gilbert E, et al. Studies of

malformation syndromes of man. XXXXIB: Nosologic studies in the Hanhart and the Moebius syndrome. Eur J Pediatr 1976; 122:19-55.
22. Parker DL, Mitchell PR, Holmes GL. Poland-Moebius syndrome. J Med Genet 1981; 18:317-320.
23. Sackey K, Odone V, George SL, Murphy SB. Poland's syndrome associated with childhood non-Hodgkin's lymphoma. Am J Dis Child 1984; 138:600-601.
24. Pisteljic DT, Vranjesevic D, Apostolski S, Pisteljic DD. Poland syndrome associated with "morning glory" syndrome (Coloboma of the optic disk). J Med Genet 1986; 23:264-266.
25. Mace JW, Kaplan JM, Schanberger JE, Gotlin RW. Poland's syndrome. Report of seven cases and review of the literature. Clin Pediatr 1972; 11:98-102.
26. Holmstrom H, Suurkula M, Lossing C. Absent latissimus dorsi muscle and anhidrotic axilla in Poland's syndrome. Scand J Plast Reconstr Surg 1986; 20:313-318.
27. Suzuki T, Takazawa H, Kashino T. Computed tomography of the pectoralis muscles in Poland's syndrome. Hand 1983; 15:35-37.
28. Demos TC, Johnson C, Love L, Posniak H. Computed tomography of partial unilateral agenesis of the pectoralis muscles. J Comput Assist Tomogr 1985; 9: 558-559.
29. Krause JL Jr, Crikelair GF, Cosman B. The Cronin implant in the treatment of combined chest wall and breast deformities. Plast Reconstr Surg 1969; 44:536-540.
30. Baker JL Jr, Mara JE. Simultaneous correction of the chest wall deformity and prosthetic augmentation mammaplasty in a case of Poland's syndrome. Br J Plast Surg 1976; 29:347-351.
31. Hester TR Jr, Bostwick J III. Poland's syndrome: Correction with latissimus muscle transposition. Plast Reconstr Surg 1982; 69:226-233.
32. Urschel HC Jr, Byrd HS, Sethi SM, Razzuk MA. Poland's syndrome: improved surgical management. Ann Thorac Surg 1984; 37:204-211.
33. Haller JA Jr, Colombani PM, Miller D, Manson P. Early reconstruction of Poland's syndrome using autologous rib grafts combined with a latissimus muscle flap. J Pediatr Surg 1984; 19:423-429.
34. Amoroso PJ, Angelats J. Latissimus dorsi myocutaneous flap in Poland's syndrome. Ann Plast Surg 1981; 6:285-289.
35. Santi P, Berrino P, Galli A. Poland's syndrome: Correction of thoracic anomaly through minimal incisions. Plast Reconstr Surg 1985; 76:639-641.
36. Becker H. The expandable mammary implant. Plast Reconstr Surg 1987; 79:631.
37. Anderl H, Kerschbaumer S. Early correction of the thoracic deformity of Poland's syndrome in children with latissimus dorsi muscle flap: Long-term follow-up of two cases. Br J Plast Surg 1986; 39:167-172.
38. Rees TD, Aston SJ. The tuberous breast. Clin Plast Surg 1976; 3:339-347.
39. Dinner MI, Dowden RV. The tubular/tuberous breast syndrome. Ann Plast Surg 1987; 19:414-420.
40. Elliott MP. A musculocutaneous transposition flap mammaplasty for correction of the tuberous breast. Ann Plast Surg 1988; 20:153-157.

CHAPTER 8

Gynecomastia

ROBERT W. CHRICHLOW, M.D.
SPENCER W. GALT, M.D.

Gynecomastia is benign enlargement of the male breast. It is not a disease, but a sign of either a relative imbalance of steroid hormones or an absolute increase of feminizing steroids. In certain age groups, gynecomastia is physiologic and ubiquitous, but in others it is rare and may be a sign of occult disease. Because of a greater understanding of the biochemistry and physiology of steroid hormones, the etiology of gynecomastia can now be identified with increasing frequency. Surgery remains the mainstay of therapy, although medical therapy has been effective in certain circumstances. Gynecomastia is a condition that challenges primary care physicians, endocrinologists, and surgeons alike and therefore deserves careful examination.

PREVALENCE

Gynecomastia occurs frequently in neonates and pubertal males. Palpable breast tissue can be identified in 60 to 70 percent of otherwise healthy adolescent males, typically those between the ages of 12 and 15 years.[1] Because the condition is usually asymptomatic in this age group, its presence often goes unnoticed unless brought to the attention of a physician for cosmetic reasons.

Although it has been stated that any palpable breast tissue in the normal adult male is abnormal,[2] palpable asymptomatic gynecomastia is common. In 306 military reserves aged 17 to 58 years, the overall prevalence of breast enlargement was 36 percent. Among men younger than 19 years old, the prevalence was 17 percent, but it increased to 33 percent by age 25 years. In 100 male veterans studied, the overall prevalence was 32 percent, with gynecomastia detected nearly equally in both inpatients and outpatients.[4] An overall prevalence of 65 percent was found in 214 hospitalized adult men aged 27 to 92 years. In this study, gynecomastia was identified in 72 percent of patients aged 50 to 69 years. The prevalence decreased to 47 percent in the 70- to 89-year-old age group, and gynecomastia occurred in 54 percent of men aged 30 to 49 years.[5] Other studies have demonstrated similar prevalence.[6,7] Conversely, prepubertal gynecomastia is distinctly rare; in the few cases reported in the literature, the patients often had demonstrable underlying pathology.[8]

PATHOGENESIS

Knowledge of basic biochemistry and physiology of sex steroid synthesis and control in normal males is essential for understanding the pathogenesis and etiologies of gynecomastia (Table 8–1). Testosterone is the most important and abundant androgen in the systemic circulation. It is primarily responsible for the development and maintenance of male secondary sex characteristics. The Leydig cells of the testes secrete more than 95 percent of circulating testosterone with the remainder secreted by the adrenal glands. The weak androgens dehydroepiandrosterone and androstenedione are also secreted by the testes in small amounts with negligible androgenic effects. The steps in steroid biosynthesis are illustrated in Figure 8–1.

Blood androgens either are in the free (unbound) state or are bound to plasma proteins. Only 3 percent of testosterone is free in the blood; the balance is bound primarily to sex hormone-binding globulin (SHBG) or albumin. Only free testosterone is able to enter cells and exert its metabolic effects. Most circulating testosterone undergoes conversion in the liver into relatively inactive 17-ketosteroid sulfates and glucuronides, which are excreted in the urine. The majority of 17-ketosteroids, however, are formed from the metabolism of adrenal steroids, and therefore urinary 17-ketosteroid determinations do not accurately reflect testosterone secretion.

The control of testosterone synthesis and secretion by Leydig cells primarily depends on luteinizing hormone (LH), secreted by the anterior pituitary in response to the hypothalamic peptide gonadotropin-releasing hormone (GnRH). Increased LH secretion stimulates Leydig cell hypertrophy and increased

TABLE 8-1 Etiologies of Gynecomastia

- Physiologic
- Pathologic
  - Hyperestrogenism
    - Increased Estrogen Secretion
      - Testicular tumors
        - Estrogen-producing: Leydig cell, Sertoli cell
        - hCG-producing: embryonal carcinoma, choriocarcinoma, teratoma, and seminoma (rarely)
      - Carcinoma of the lung and other ectopic hCG producing tumors
      - True hermaphroditism
      - Primary liver neoplasms
    - Increased substrate for peripheral aromatase
      - Adrenal neoplasm
      - Adrenal hyperplasia
      - Liver disease
      - Renal disease
      - Thyrotoxicosis
    - Increased peripheral aromatase activity
  - Androgen Deficiency
    - Congenital anorchia
    - Klinefelter's syndrome
    - Congenital enzyme blocks in androgen synthesis (pseudohermaphroditism)
    - Testicular failure secondary to exogenous causes
      - Viral orchitis
      - Trauma
      - Radiation
      - Castration
      - Cryptorchidism
      - Neurologic diseases (myotonia dystrophica, paraplegia)
      - Granulomatous disease
    - Starvation
    - Androgen resistance (incomplete testicular feminization)
  - Drug-Induced
    - Mimicking or enhancing endogenous estrogen formation
      - Estrogens (DES, oral contraceptives)
      - hCG
      - Clomiphene citrate
      - Digitalis derivatives
      - Marijuana
    - Inhibiting testosterone synthesis or action
      - Ketoconazole
      - Spironolactone
      - Cimetidine
      - Ranitidine
      - Cytotoxic agents
      - Ethanol
    - Unknown mechanisms: busulfan, ethionamide, isoniazid, methyldopa, tricyclic antidepressants, diazepam, penicillamine, reserpine, phenytoin, calcium channel blockers, domperidone, anabolic steroids, metronidazole, amiodarone, theophylline, captopril, amphetamines, and sulindac
  - Associated With Other Diseases: Ulcerative colitis, HIV infection, lymphoma, cystic fibrosis, and hypothyroidism

testosterone secretion. Luteinizing hormone is reciprocally controlled by direct action of testosterone on the anterior pituitary and an inhibitory effect at the hypothalamic level by negative feedback control. The inhibitory effect of androgens on the hypothalamus is mediated principally by estradiol, which is formed locally in the hypothalamus from androgens.

Estrone and estradiol are the important blood estrogens in males. Small amounts of estrogens are secreted from the testes and the adrenal glands. The primary source of blood estrogens is through the peripheral aromatization of testosterone and androstenedione to estradiol and estrone, respectively. Estrogens have trophic and stimulatory effects on the male breast,[9] and estrogen receptors are present on gynecomastic breast tissue.[10] Androgens may inhibit mammary epithelial proliferation, but this phenomenon is less well defined.[11] Normally, there is a tightly controlled ratio of estrogen to androgen in the blood. Increasing this ratio, whether through androgen deficiency or resistance, or estrogen excess, may lead to feminization, including the development of gynecomastia.

PHYSIOLOGIC GYNECOMASTIA

Breast bud enlargement often occurs in otherwise normal newborns. The breast enlargement is stimulated by placental estrogens. There may be an associated secretion of a colostrum-like substance ("witch's milk"). Typically, the swelling recedes over several weeks, although occasionally it may persist.[12]

Gynecomastia is common in adolescent males, with a peak prevalence of 65 percent at 14 years of age,[1] and is regarded as a normal physiologic response to changes in the hormonal milieu during puberty. Although transient hormonal imbalance has been implicated, specific mechanisms of the development of adolescent gynecomastia have not been well elucidated. Some investigators contend that the plasma estradiol concentration in adolescent males reaches the adult level before the adult level of testosterone is attained.[13,14] Others report that increased breast sensitivity to estrogens or an increased conversion rate of weak androgens to estrogens is responsible for the occurrence of adolescent gynecomastia.[15] Relative deficiencies in the androgenic adrenal hormones dehydroepiandrosterone and its sulfate, and androstenedione, with normal testosterone and estrogen levels, have been reported in adolescents with gynecomastia.[16] Changes in breast tissue binding of sex steroids, intracellular aromatization of androgens to estrogens, and levels of SHBG have not been thoroughly investigated and may play a role. Undoubtedly, there is a complex interplay of factors in the development of pubertal gynecomastia.

Any increase in the estrogen-to-androgen ratio may cause gynecomastia in mature men. Physiologic changes associated with aging include increasing plasma estrogen concentrations because of greater peripheral aromatization of androgens. There is a concomitant fall in plasma testosterone level and an increase in SHBG, resulting in a marked decline in

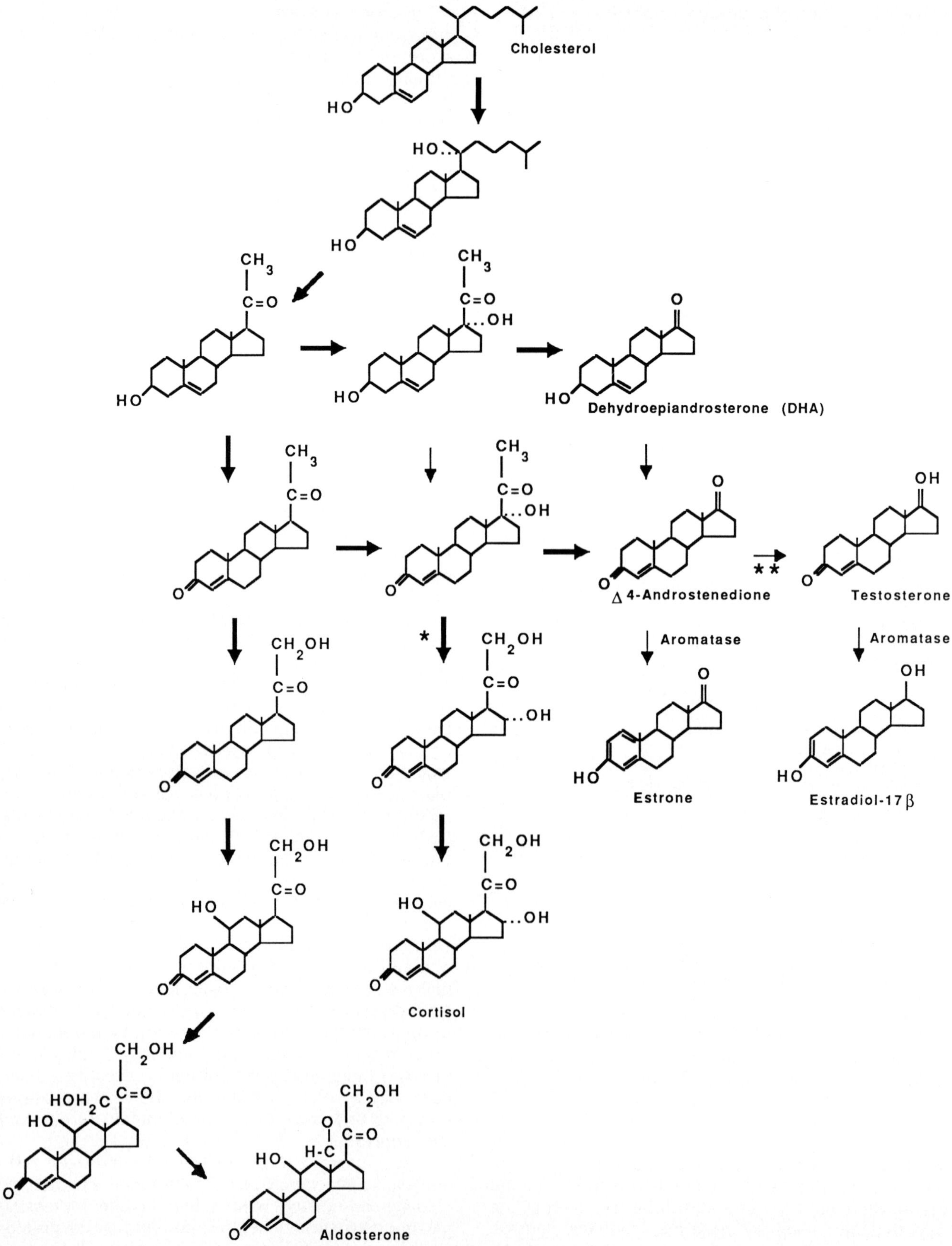

FIGURE 8–1 The biosynthesis of steroids.

the level of unbound testosterone. Finally, there is an increase in plasma LH associated with decreased testosterone, which stimulates further production of testicular estradiol.[17-22] All of these mechanisms may contribute to an increase in the estrogen/testosterone (E/T) ratio in otherwise healthy males.

PATHOLOGIC GYNECOMASTIA

Hyperestrogenism

Testicular Neoplasms

Gynecomastia may be the presenting sign of testicular tumors, both benign and malignant. In two large series of patients with testicular cancer, the prevalence of gynecomastia ranged from 2.5 to 6 percent.[23,24] Testicular neoplasms may induce growth of breast tissue by two mechanisms. Germinal cell tumors, including embryonal carcinoma, choriocarcinoma, teratoma, and rarely, seminoma, may produce human chorionic gonadotropin (hCG), which stimulates Leydig cell estradiol secretion primarily in the uninvolved area of the testis. This appears to occur without a parallel increase in testosterone secretion, which may be because of inhibition of testosterone synthesis by estrogens,[25] or increased aromatization of testosterone to estradiol in the Leydig cell. Additionally, hCG-producing tumors may act like normal trophoblastic tissue, producing estrogens from circulating prohormones.[26]

Stromal (Leydig and Sertoli) cell tumors may autonomously secrete estradiol. Although representing only 1 percent of testicular neoplasms, 10 to 30 percent of Leydig cell tumors are associated with gynecomastia.[27,28] In patients with these tumors, the level of LH is often in the normal range.[29,30] Plasma testosterone level is either normal or decreased, and plasma estrogens are either normal or high, but the E/T ratio is always elevated.[30] Unlike germinal cell tumors, stromal cell tumors do not produce hCG.

Carcinoma of the Lung and Other Ectopic hCG-Producing Tumors

Bronchogenic carcinoma may secrete hCG, causing gynecomastia. As in the case of testicular germinal cell tumors, the hCG stimulates Leydig cells to secrete estradiol. Bronchogenic carcinoma also may act as trophoblastic tissue, converting androgens to estrogens,[31,32] thus increasing the E/T ratio. Any gonadotropin-producing neoplasm may cause gynecomastia in the same manner. Gynecomastia has been detected in patients with choriocarcinoma of the lung,[33] mediastinal choriocarcinoma, and gastric adenocarcinoma,[26] among others.

Primary Liver Cancer

Hepatocellular carcinoma and its variant, fibrolamellar carcinoma, are capable of converting circulating androgenic hormones to estrogens and have been reported as causes of gynecomastia. Although extracts of tumor tissue may show high levels of the beta subunit of hCG, none have been detected in the blood of patients with primary liver cancer. Human chorionic gonadotropin, therefore, is not thought to contribute to the hormonal imbalance in these cases.[34,35]

True Hermaphroditism

When sperm and oocytes are present in one or both gonads (ovotestes), true hermaphroditism exists. Depending on the level of testicular function of the fetal gonads, complete virilization with male phenotype may result, although most true hermaphrodites exhibit anomalous or ambiguous genitalia. In phenotypic males, secretion of excess estrogens by the ovotestes may occur at puberty, causing feminization.[2]

Increased Substrate for Peripheral Aromatase

Adrenal Neoplasms

Feminizing adrenal tumors are rare and usually malignant. The mechanism of the hyperestrogenism caused by these tumors has not been fully explained, although two theories seem plausible: (1) the majority of these tumors are associated with increased androstenedione levels, which may result in hyperestrogenism from peripheral aromatization; or (2) there are also tumors in which estrogens are probably secreted autonomously.[36]

Adrenal Hyperplasia

Although six varieties of congenital adrenal hyperplasia have been described, only the most common cause, 21-hydroxylase deficiency (see Fig. 8-1), is relevant to gynecomastia. Cortisol and aldosterone synthesis are impaired, but in milder forms of the defect, hypersecretion of adrenocorticotropic hormone (ACTH) stimulates the adrenal cortex sufficiently to maintain plasma cortisol and aldosterone levels.[37] Because adrenal androgens do not require 21-hydroxylation, they are hypersecreted from excess ACTH stimulation, resulting in precocious puberty and virilism. Under these conditions, gynecomastia may occur because of peripheral conversion of increased plasma androgens.

Liver Disease (Cirrhosis)

The mechanism by which cirrhosis causes gynecomastia is not entirely clear, partly because ethanol consumption, the most common cause of cirrhosis in the United States, may itself cause gynecomastia. Despite conflicting reports of plasma estrogen levels in patients with alcoholic cirrhosis, elevated E/T ratios have consistently been found. This is most likely a result of the inability of the damaged liver to metabolize testosterone and androstenedione normally, leaving increased available substrate for peripheral aromatization to estrogens. There also appears to be an increase in plasma SHBG, which reduces the fraction of free testosterone, thus compounding the hormonal imbalance. Finally, the testosterone production rate is diminished, although this may not be a consequence of the cirrhosis, but the effect of ethanol on the testes.[38]

Renal Disease

Gynecomastia is common in patients with renal failure. Usually, breast enlargement occurs shortly after the institution of dialysis and spontaneously resolves several months later. A variety of hormonal abnormalities have been noted in patients with renal failure, including depressed testosterone levels, normal to high estradiol levels, and elevated LH levels. The mechanism responsible for these hormonal alterations is unclear. The decrease in plasma testosterone is probably a result of decreased secretion as well as increased clearance. Additionally, some authors have reported normal testosterone levels after the institution of dialysis, although this has not been universally confirmed.[38] It has been postulated that dialysis allows the testes to resume normal hormonal secretion in response to the high plasma LH concentration, effectively causing a "secondary puberty."[2,38,39]

Thyrotoxicosis

As many as 40 percent of men with hyperthyroidism develop gynecomastia. Although levels of both plasma testosterone and estrogens have been found to be elevated in these patients, the testosterone elevation results from an increase in SHBG. However, these patients also have elevated free estrogen levels, resulting in increased E/T ratios.[40] Elevated LH levels also occur, which may be a consequence of supranormal resetting of the hypothalamic-pituitary-gonadal axis.[40] Androstenedione production is enhanced, perhaps in response to LH stimulation.[41] Therefore, increased estrogen production may result from both increased testicular secretion in response to LH, and increased peripheral conversion of androstenedione.[41]

Increased Peripheral Aromatase

Gynecomastia has occasionally been attributed to increased extraglandular aromatase activity.[42-44] Conversion rates of androstenedione to estrone have been found to be 10 times normal in three siblings with gynecomastia and, in one patient with gynecomastia, the conversion rate of testosterone to estradiol was found to be 8 to 10 times normal in vivo.[43] This trait appears to have X-linked or autosomal dominant sex-limited inheritance. Pubic skin fibroblasts, which are known to contain aromatase, were cultured in vitro in an unrelated group of subjects with gynecomastia and compared with cultured pubic skin fibroblasts from a control group of patients without gynecomastia. Increased aromatase activity was found in those patients with gynecomastia. Rapid estradiol oxidative metabolism was also identified, which may in part explain the normal estradiol levels in some patients with no demonstrable hormonal abnormalities.[44]

ANDROGEN DEFICIENCY

Congenital Anorchia

In congenital anorchia, the testes are absent in phenotypically normal 46XY males. Plasma testosterone remains virtually undetectable even after pharmacologic gonadotropin stimulation. Male sexual differentiation is normal in the infant, suggesting that the testes were present and functioning until late in embryonic life. The plasma estradiol concentration in these individuals is low, derived solely from peripheral conversion of androstenedione. About 50 percent of these patients will develop gynecomastia because they have increased E/T ratios despite having low serum estradiol levels.[2,45]

Klinefelter's Syndrome

Individuals with Klinefelter's syndrome are hypogonadal as a result of Leydig cell failure with its accompanying decrease in androgen synthesis. Plasma testosterone concentration in these individuals is usually about one-half normal, although occasionally the level is normal. Plasma estradiol is often elevated, which may be due in part to reduced clearance. Gynecomastia may, therefore, occur in patients with either a normal or decreased testosterone level. The extra X chromosome may predispose these patients to develop gynecomastia for an unknown reason or may be responsible for their increased risk of breast cancer, which may approach 3 percent.[46]

Congenital Enzyme Block in Androgen Synthesis

Several congenital enzyme deficiencies resulting in subnormal testosterone synthesis have been described.[2] Most of these deficiencies result in severely diminished androgen and estrogen synthesis, with neither feminization nor virilization of the male embryo. However, 17-beta hydroxysteroid dehydrogenase (17-ketoreductase) (see Fig. 8-1) deficiency may not be evident at birth. Extreme deficiency or absence of this enzyme results in a phenotypic female at birth. Signs of virilization occur at puberty, often with accompanying gynecomastia.[47] When the deficiency is less pronounced, the phenotype at birth may be that of a normal male. At the onset of puberty, gonadotropin stimulation of Leydig cells occurs normally. However, the conversion rate of androstenedione to testosterone is abnormally slow, leading to the accumulation of androstenedione. The extra androstenedione is available for peripheral aromatization to estrogen. Interestingly, plasma testosterone levels may be normal or nearly so, because the enzyme may undergo substantial product activation. When sufficient testosterone is produced locally in the Leydig cells, the enzyme becomes activated, and the rate of conversion of androstenedione to testosterone increases sharply. When all of the available substrate androstenedione is converted, the enzyme reverts to its former state of low activity.[48]

Testicular Failure

Primary testicular failure results from any process that directly affects the hormonal and spermatogenic potential of the testes. Obvious causes of testicular failure include testicular atrophy secondary to viral orchitis, radiation exposure, trauma, cryptorchidism, and castration. Granulomatous disease, particularly lepromatous leprosy, may also lead to testicular failure.[38] Primary testicular failure may occur in various neurologic diseases, including paraplegia and myotonia dystrophica,[38] although the hypogonadism in these disorders is poorly understood. In all of these conditions plasma testosterone is low, and gonadotropin levels are high.

Starvation

Transient gynecomastia occuring after reversal of severe malnutrition was observed in at least 6 percent of American prisoners of war during World War II.[49] The mechanism leading to gynecomastia in refeeding has not been fully elucidated. It is clear that malnutrition leads to impaired Leydig cell function and decreased testosterone production. It has been postulated that the return of Leydig cell function upon refeeding causes a "secondary puberty."[4] Others have suggested that the gynecomastia seen in these patients may result from liver disease,[2] which occurs commonly in malnourished patients.[49]

Androgen Resistance

Androgen resistance ranges from complete insensitivity of androgen receptors, representing complete testicular feminization, to subtle abnormalities in androgen sensitivity, in which virilization may be nearly complete and affected individuals may be fertile, with gynecomastia the only overt sign of feminization. The gynecomastia is caused at least in part by androgen resistance in breast tissue. Additionally, testosterone negative feedback at the hypothalamic-pituitary axis may be impaired by androgen resistance.[50,51] Hypersecretion of LH causes overproduction of testosterone, which is then available for peripheral aromatization. Androgen resistance syndromes appear to be X-linked, or have an autosomal mode of inheritance with expression limited to males.

DRUG-INDUCED GYNECOMASTIA

Drugs Mimicking Estrogen or Enhancing Endogenous Estrogen Formation

Estrogens may cause severe gynecomastia. The therapeutic application of estrogenic hormones such as diethylstilbestrol (DES) for the treatment of metastatic prostate cancer commonly causes gynecomastia.[52] Inadvertent absorption of estrogens may occur percutaneously through exposure to powders, skin creams, hair lotions, vaginal lubricants, and rarely, embalming compounds.[53] Boys and young men are particularly susceptible to the feminizing effects of estrogenic compounds.[2]

Clomiphene citrate is an estrogen antagonist that has been administered in the treatment of gynecomastia with limited success. However, it may also act as an agonist, inducing gynecomastia in some individuals.[54]

Digitalis preparations have been reported to cause gynecomastia, although not all investigators agree that a relationship exists.[5] Digitoxin reacts with estrogen receptors in human premenopausal uterine cell cytosol, suggesting that it could exert estrogen-like side effects. However, digoxin does not react with estrogen receptors, and therefore it is unlikely that it is an estrogen agonist.[55] In patients debilitated by congestive heart failure, gynecomastia associated with digoxin use may result from an effect comparable to that seen in malnourished patients who have been refed.[4] Furthermore, in patients with compensated congestive heart failure, there is increased peripheral conversion of androgens to estrogens.[56] Therefore, an association between digitalis derivatives and gynecomastia may be coincidental.

Gynecomastia may be seen in men who heavily abuse *marijuana* and *heroin*. Both substances seem to cause depression of testosterone levels.[57,58] Additionally, tetrahydrocannabinol, the compound responsible for the psychotropic effects of marijuana, seems to exert a direct estrogenic effect on breast tissue.[59] It is unclear whether abnormal liver function also plays a role, especially in intravenous drug abusers, in whom hepatitis is common. *Ethanol* may also induce gynecomastia in the absence of liver disease. Acute alcohol intake can lower plasma testosterone levels, and chronic intake may cause testicular atrophy and poor testosterone production. Ethanol may also increase the number of tissue estrogen receptors, causing heightened breast sensitivity to circulating estrogens.[60]

Inhibition of Testosterone Synthesis or Action

Ketoconazole, a potent inhibitor of testosterone and adrenal steroid synthesis, causes depression of both free and bound plasma testosterone levels, with a concomitant but lesser decrease in estrogens, resulting in an increased E/T ratio.[61] *Spironolactone* affects androgen metabolism in two ways: it binds with androgen receptors in target tissues competitively inhibiting testosterone binding,[56] and it inhibits testosterone biosynthesis.[62] The net result is impaired effect and reduced plasma testosterone levels. The relationship between *cimetidine* and gynecomastia is well documented. The overall prevalence is 1 percent,[63] and development is both dose- and time-dependent; gynecomastia has not been observed in patients receiving standard doses of cimetidine for less than 3 months. It appears that the mechanism is blockage of androgen receptors.[64] *Ranitidine*, another H_2 receptor blocker, originally was thought to exhibit no antiandrogenic side effects; as its use has become more widespread, isolated cases of gynecomastia have been reported.[65]

Many *cytotoxic chemotherapeutic agents* cause Leydig cell damage, with consequent hypotestosteronemia. Curiously, gynecomastia develops more often after the cessation of chemotherapy than during treatment. No substantive data explain this observation. The "refeeding phenomenon" has been invoked by some to explain post-chemotherapy gynecomastia, because patients are often in a state of relative malnutrition during chemotherapy. Cytotoxic agents reported to lead to gynecomastia include cyclophosphamide, dactinomycin, vincristine, vinblastine, bleomycin, cisplatin, melphalan, cytosine arabinoside, and adriamycin.[66-69]

A variety of other drugs have been implicated in the development of gynecomastia, although their mechanisms are unclear. These include busulfan, ethionamide, isoniazid, tricyclic antidepressants, diazepam, reserpine, methlydopa, phenothiazines, amphetamines, anabolic steroids, metronidazole, penicillamine, sulindac, calcium channel blockers, domperidone, amiodarone, phenytoin, captopril, and theophylline.[70-78]

HISTOPATHOLOGY

Gynecomastia progresses from an early, active, florid phase to an inactive or senescent phase. The predominant histopathologic features are related to the duration of the gynecomastia, regardless of etiology. Even with continued hormonal stimulation, such as in DES therapy, gynecomastia seems to progress to the inactive phase.[82]

The active stage is characterized by an increased number of ducts, occasionally occurring in pseudolobules. Proliferation of ductal epithelium occurs, as well as periductal stromal hyperplasia with variable degrees of fibroblastic proliferation. Areas of adipose tissue demonstrate stromal replacement.[7,10]

In long-standing, inactive gynecomastia, confluent peri- and interductal hyaline fibrosis predominates. There may be a slight increase in the number of ducts containing atrophic ductal epithelium with occasional limited epithelial proliferation. Small areas of squamous metaplasia are often present, although rarely pronounced.[83] Fibroblastic proliferation is absent or insignificant, and adipose tissue becomes hyalinized.[7,10]

As the florid phase progresses to the inactive phase, breast enlargement recedes. The epithelium of the ducts atrophies, and hyalinized bands form around and between the ducts, which eventually disappear. If gynecomastia is of long duration, fibrosis may become so extensive that complete resolution of breast enlargement never occurs, even if the underlying cause is resolved.[82] Rare cases of lobule and acinus formation have been described. The significance of this is unknown, and it does not appear to be associated with specific etiologies of gynecomastia.[8]

DIAGNOSTIC EVALUATION

In most patients, gynecomastia is easily identified by physical examination. Gynecomastia usually presents as a symmetrical firm button of easily palpable subareolar breast tissue, although in severe cases the breast tissue may extend beyond the subareolar region. This tissue is easily distinguished from surrounding fat, as a discrete mass is absent in simple fatty enlargement. If uncertainty exists regarding whether or not the enlargement is breast tissue, comparison with the subcutaneous fat in the anterior axillary fold may be helpful. Generally, if the breast tissue is greater than 2 cm in diameter, gynecomastia is said to exist.[5]

Differential diagnosis is rarely difficult. Adenocarcinoma, the most common malignancy of the male breast, is more frequently eccentric, ill-defined, and associated with nipple or areolar abnormalities.

If there is uncertainty in the diagnosis, mammography may aid in clarification. The mammograms of men with gynecomastia demonstrate glandular proliferation extending from the nipple into the fatty tissue of the breast. The glandular density is often triangular or flame-shaped, and is usually symmetrically positioned behind the nipple. In men who are receiving exogenous estrogens for metastatic prostate carcinoma, a more diffuse proliferation of ductal and glandular elements, resembling tissue of female breast, may be seen.[84] Sonography has also been advocated as a useful diagnostic modality,[85] although it appears to be less helpful than mammography. If, despite the use of these imaging techniques, the diagnosis remains in question, biopsy is indicated.

A routine history and physical examination often provide information adequate to determine the etiology of gynecomastia. The examiner should note patient age, duration of presence of the gynecomastia, associated breast pain or tenderness, and alcohol or other drug use, both therapeutic and illicit. During the examination, it is paramount that the possibility of breast carcinoma be excluded. The examiner should be aware that gynecomastia may be markedly asymmetric or unilateral. Physical examination of the testes should also be performed. If testes in the adult are small (<4 cm in long axis), testicular hypofunction may exist. If they are asymmetric, or a definite mass is palpable, a testicular tumor may be present.

If the etiology of the gynecomastia is not obvious, a variety of screening tests may be used, including a limited endocrine evaluation and liver function tests. Urinary 17-ketosteroids are often elevated in feminizing adrenal states, but they are not an indicator of testicular function. Plasma hCG may be measured, as it is elevated in various malignant neoplasms. Plasma LH, estradiol, and testosterone may be measured as well. A high serum estradiol concentration suggests a primary source, such as a Leydig cell tumor. The combination of high LH and low or normal testosterone suggest testicular insufficiency, while a high LH and high testosterone suggests androgen resistance. In patients with a gonadotropin-secreting tumor, LH will be elevated, but the testosterone level may vary widely. Further endocrine workup and radiologic studies may be indicated according to the results of the screening tests.

Gynecomastia in adolescents requires only a history and physical examination; further evaluation is unnecessary and will most likely be unrevealing. Similarly, in otherwise healthy patients whose gynecomastia is asymptomatic and of long duration, the condition can usually be ignored. Conversely, gynecomastia in prepubertal boys should be carefully investigated. Despite the rarity of this phenomenon, approximately 50 percent of cases reported have been associated with underlying pathology, often in the adrenal glands.[8] In all other age groups, the recent, sudden onset of gynecomastia is commonly a manifestation of disease and investigation should be undertaken. It is likely that the cause will be drug related, especially in older patients.[4] It should also be noted that the presence of pain or tenderness does not increase the probability that underlying pathology is present.

TREATMENT

The mode of treatment for gynecomastia depends on the underlying cause. If a specific etiology such as feminizing tumors or hyperthyroidism can be identified, the gynecomastia will usually involute rapidly after the underlying pathology is corrected. In pubertal, refeeding, and hemodialysis-induced gynecomastia, reassurance that the breast enlargement is benign and will resolve spontaneously, usually within months, is satisfactory therapy for most patients. However, for causes such as androgen resistance, increased peripheral aromatase activity, and congenital blocks in androgen synthesis, further specific therapy may be necessary. Gynecomastia causes some adolescents to become profoundly distressed. They may be reluctant to attend school or participate in athletics, which may require disrobing in the presence of peers. Other patients may find the condition cosmetically unacceptable and seek active treatment.

Several medical therapies have been advocated, primarily in adolescents with pubertal gynecomastia. Both parenteral[36] and percutaneous[87] dihydrotestosterone administration may be effective, although the specific mechanism by which dihydrotestosterone decreases breast size is unknown. Danazol,[88] a specific gonadotropin inhibitor, has also demonstrated potential benefit. Both compounds, however, suppress the hypothalamic-pituitary-gonadal axis, and the long-term effects of this condition are not fully defined in adolescent males. Testolactone, an inhibitor of aromatase activity, may also be effective, and there appears to be no suppression of the hypothalamic-pituitary-gonadal axis.[89] However, no controlled trials have been performed with any of these drugs; therefore, they cannot be recommended as treatment. Clomiphene citrate has been reported to reduce gynecomastia in some patients, although it may cause gynecomastia as well.[54,90] The antiestrogen tamoxifen has demonstrated efficacy in a controlled trial in adult males and is relatively free of toxicity.[54] Tamoxifen has not been widely tested in adolescents, but a short-term trial in adults may represent a safe approach toward reducing breast size.

Radiation therapy to the breast is an effective means of preventing gynecomastia induced by estrogen hormone treatment in patients with prostate cancer. Radiation must be used prophylactically, because it is well documented that it does not effectively reduce the breast size after breast hypertrophy has occurred.[52]

Because controlled trials in the use of pharmacologic agents in the treatment of gynecomastia are lacking, and long-term effects of these compounds are unknown in the population concerned, the indications for the use of these agents are not fully defined. Additionally, in gynecomastia present for more than $1\frac{1}{2}$ to 2 years, medical therapy is less likely to be effective because substantial fibrosis of the breast tissue will have occurred. For these reasons, surgery remains the mainstay of therapy. However, excision of the breast tissue should not be recommended as a means of prophylaxis against breast cancer, because there is no evidence that gynecomastia is a premalignant lesion.[4,81,91] The patient's decision for excision should be based on improvement of appearance alone.

Gynecomastia typically exhibits excess breast tissue without redundant skin. A periareolar incision is well-suited for the correction because large amounts of breast tissue may be excised, and the incision usually heals well. The planned incision is outlined from the three o'clock position to the nine o'clock position, at the junction of the hyperpigmented areolar skin and the surrounding skin of the chest wall. The areolar skin is then incised, continuing the incision to about 1 cm deep into the breast tissue. The breast tissue is then cut across beneath the nipple to provide a button of breast tissue below it. This prevents a sunken, flat nipple postoperatively.

Dissection is continued concentrically in the plane between the subcutaneous tissue and the breast tissue. After complete separation of the breast tissue from the subcutaneous tissue, the pectoral fascia is exposed either from the inferior pole of the breast, or by an incision through the breast tissue to the pectoral fascia. The breast tissue is bluntly dissected from the underlying pectoral fascia.

At the margins of the breast tissue resection, scissors may be used to bevel the junction of the pectoral fascia and the subcutaneous tissue. Some surgeons prefer to employ suction-assisted lipectomy for peripheral contouring. If no breast tissue but only adipose tissue requires resection, suction may be used exclusively. Breast tissue must be resected sharply.[92]

Careful attention to hemostasis is necessary because hematoma and seroma formation are the most common complications following gynecomastia resection. A small Jackson-Pratt drain may be placed in the dependent portion of the subcutaneous pocket. The wound is approximated with absorbable sutures placed between the subcutaneous tissue beneath the nipple and the inferior skin flap. The skin is approximated with monofilament nonabsorbable sutures. An occlusive dressing should be placed, which may be removed with the drains 48 to 72 hours postoperatively.

References

1. Nydick M, Bustos J, Dale JH Jr, Rawson RW. Gynecomastia in adolescent boys. JAMA 1961; 178:449.
2. Wilson JD, Aiman J, MacDonald PC. The pathogenesis of gynecomastia. Adv Intern Med 1980; 25:1.
3. Nuttall FQ. Gynecomastia as a physical finding in normal men. J Clin Endocrinol Metab 1979; 48:338.
4. Carlson HE. Current concepts: Gynecomastia. N Engl J Med 1980; 303:795.
5. Niewoehner CB, Nuttall FQ. Gynecomastia in a hospitalized male population. Am J Med 1984; 77:633.
6. Ley SB, Mozaffarian GA, Leonard JM, et al. Palpable breast tissue versus gynecomastia as a normal physical finding. Clin Res 1980; 28:24A.
7. Williams MJ. Gynecomastia: Its incidence, recognition and host characterization in 447 autopsy cases. Am J Med 1963; 34:103.
8. Haibach H, Rosenholtz MJ. Prepubertal gynecomastia with lobules and acini: A case report and review of the literature. Am J Clin Pathol 1983; 80:252.
9. Poulsen HS. Demonstration of hormonal sensitivity in gynecomastic tissue by thymidine incorporation in vivo. Acta Pathol Microbiol Immunol Scand 1977; 85A:19.
10. Andersen J, Ørntoft TF, Andersen JA, Poulsen HS. Gynecomastia: Immunohistochemical demonstration of estrogen receptors. Acta Pathol Microbiol Immunol Scand 1987; 95e:263.
11. Terkington RW, Topper YJ. Androgen inhibition of mammary gland differentiation in vitro. Endocrinology 1967; 80:329.
12. Bronstein IP, Cassola EJ. Breast enlargement in pediatric practice. Med Clin North Am 1946; 30:121.
13. Lee PA. The relationship of concentrations of serum hormones to pubertal gynecomastia. J Pediatr 1975; 86:212.
14. LaFranchi SH, Parlow AF, Lippe BM, et al. Pubertal gynecomastia and transient elevation of serum estradiol level. Am J Dis Child 1975; 129:927.
15. Knorr D, Bidlingmaier F. Gynecomastia in male adolescents. J Clin Endocrinol Metab 1975; 4:157.
16. Moore DC, Schlaepfer LV, Paunier L, Sizonenko PC. Hormonal changes during puberty: V. Transient pubertal gynecomastia: Abnormal androgen-estrogen ratios. J Clin Endocrinol Metab 1984; 58:492.
17. Pirke KM, Doerr P. Age-related changes and interrelationships between plasma testosterone, oestradiol, and testosterone-binding globulin in normal adult males. Acta Endocrinol 1973; 74:792.
18. Pirke KM, Doerr P. Age-related changes in free plasma testosterone, dihydrotestosterone, and oestradiol. Acta Endocrinol 1970; 80:171.
19. Vermeulen A, Rubens R, Verdonck L. Testosterone secretion and metabolism in male senescence. J Clin Endocrinol Metab 1972; 34:730.
20. Stearns EL, MacDonnell JA, Kaufman BJ, et al. Declining testicular function with age: Hormonal and clinical correlates. Am J Med 1974; 57:761.
21. Rubens R, Dhont M, Vermeulen A. Further studies on Leydig cell function in old age. J Clin Endocrinol Metab 1974; 39:40.
22. Smals AGH. Gynaecomastia. Neth J Med 1987; 31:47.
23. LeFere RE, Stewart BH, Levin HS, et al. Testis tumors:

Review of 125 cases at the Cleveland Clinic. Urology 1975; 6:588.
24. Kurohara SS, George FW III, Dykhuisen RF, Leary KL. Testicular tumors: Analysis of 196 cases treated at the U.S. Naval Hospital in San Diego. Cancer 1967; 20:1039.
25. Forest MG, LeCoq A, Saez JM. Kinetics of human chorionic gonadotropin-induced steroidogenic response of the human testis. II. plasma 17α-hydroxyprogesterone, Δ^4-androstenedione, estrone, and 17β-estradiol: Evidence for the action of human chorionic gonadotropin on intermediate enzymes implicated in steroid biosynthesis. J Clin Endocrinol Metab 1979; 49:284.
26. Kirschner MA, Cohen FB, Jespersen D. Estrogen production and its origin in men with gonadotropin-producing neoplasms. J Clin Endocrinol Metab 1974; 39: 112.
27. Gabrilove JL, Nicolis GL, Mitty HA, Sohval AR. Feminizing interstitial cell tumor of the testis: Personal observations and a review of the literature. Cancer 1975; 35:1184.
28. Kim I, Young RH, Scully RE. Leydig cell tumors of the testis: A clinicopathological analysis of 40 cases and a review of the literature. Am J Surg Pathol 1985; 9:177.
29. Kuhn JM, Mahoudeau JA, Billaud L, et al. Evaluation of diagnostic criteria for Leydig cell tumors in adult men revealed by gynaecomastia. Clin Endocrinol 1987; 26: 407.
30. Bercovici J.-P, Nahoul K, Tater D, et al. Hormonal profile of Leydig cell tumors with gynecomastia. J Clin Endocrinol Metab 1984; 59:625.
31. Fusco FD, Rosen SW. Gonadotropic-producing anaplastic large-cell carcinomas of the lung. N Engl J Med 1966; 275:507.
32. Becker KL, Cottrell J, Moore CF, et al. Endocrine studies in a patient with gonadotropin-secreting bronchogenic carcinoma. J Clin Endocrinol 1968; 28:809.
33. Whitcomb RW, Schimke RN, Kyner JL, et al. Endocrine studies in a male patient with choriocarcinoma and gynecomastia. Am J Med 1986; 81:917.
34. Kew MC, Kirschner MA, Abrahams GE, Katz M. Mechanism of feminization in primary liver cancer. N Engl J Med 1977; 296:1084.
35. McCloskey JJ, Germain-Lee EL, Perman JA, et al. Gynecomastia as a presenting sign of fibrolamellar carcinoma of the liver. Pediatrics 1988; 82:379.
36. Gabrilove JL, Sharma DC, Wotiz HH, Dorfman RI. Feminizing adrenocortical tumors in the male: A review of 52 cases including a case report. Medicine (Baltimore) 1965; 44:37.
37. Kadair RG, Block MB, Katz FH, Hofeldt FD. "Masked" 21-hydroxylase deficiency of the adrenal presenting with gynecomastia and bilateral testicular masses. Am J Med 1977; 62:278.
38. Morley JE, Melmed S. Progress in endocrinology and metabolism: Gonadal dysfunction in systemic disorders. Metabolism 1979; 28:1051.
39. Schmitt GW, Shehadeh I, Sawin CT. Transient gynecomastia in chronic renal failure during chronic intermittent hemodialysis. Ann Intern Med 1968; 69:73.
40. Chopra IJ, Tulchinsky D. States of estrogen-androgen balance in hyperthyroid men with Grave's disease. J Clin Endocrinol Metab 1974; 38:269.
41. Southren AL, Olivo J, Gordon GG, et al. The conversion of androgens to estrogens in hyperthyroidism. J Clin Endocrinol Metab 1974; 38:207.
42. Hemsell DL, Edman CD, Marks JF. Massive extraglandular aromatization of plasma androstenedione resulting in feminization of a prepubertal boy. J Clin Invest 1977; 60:455.
43. Berkovitz GD, Guerami A, Brown TR, et al. Familial gynecomastia with increased extraglandular aromatization of plasma $Carbon_{19}$-steroids. J Clin Invest 1985; 75:1763.
44. Bulard J, Mowszowicsz I, Schaison G. Increased aromatase activity in pubic skin fibroblasts from patients with isolated gynecomastia. J Clin Endocrinol Metab 1987; 64:618.
45. Edman CD, Wenters AJ, Porter JC, et al. Embryonic testicular regression: A clinical spectrum of XY agonadal individuals. Obstet Gynecol 1977; 49:208.
46. Evans DB, Crichlow RW. Carcinoma of the male breast and Klinefelter's syndrome: Is there an association? CA 1987; 37:240.
47. Balducci R, Toscano V, Wright F, et al. Familial male pseudohermaphroditism with gynaecomastia due to 17β-hydroxysteroid dehydrogenase deficiency: A report of 3 cases. Clin Endocrinol 1985; 23:439.
48. Rogers DG, Chasalow FI, Blethen SL. Partial deficiency in 17-ketosteroid reductase presenting as gynecomastia. Steroids 1985; 45:195.
49. Jacobs EC. Effects of starvation on sex hormones in the male. J Clin Endocrinol Metab 1948; 8:227.
50. Grino PB, Griffin JE, Cushard WG Jr, Wilson JD. A mutation of the androgen receptor associated with partial androgen resistance, familial gynecomastia, and fertility. J Clin Endocrinol Metab 1988; 66:754.
51. Larrea F, Benavides G, Scaglia H, et al. Gynecomastia as a familial incomplete male pseudohermaphroditism Type 1: A limited androgen resistance syndrome. J Clin Endocrinol Metab 1978; 46:961.
52. Chou JL, Easley JD, Feldmeier JJ, et al. Effective radiotherapy in palliating mammalgia associated with gynecomastia after DES therapy. Int J Radiat Oncol Biol Phys 1988; 15:749.
53. Finkelstein JS, McCully WF, MacLaughlin DT, et al. The mortician's mystery: Gynecomastia and reversible hypogonadotropic hypogonadism in an embalmer. N Engl J Med 1988; 318:961.
54. Parker LN, Gray DR, Lai MK, Levin ER. Treatment of gynecomastia with tamoxifen: A double-blind crossover study. Metabolism 1986; 35:705.
55. Rifka SM, Pita JC, Vigersky RA, et al. Interaction of digitalis and spironolactone with human sex steroid receptors. J Clin Endocrinol Metab 1977; 46:338.
56. Edman CD, MacDonald PC. Extraglandular aromatization—primary and extrahepatic metabolic process. Gynecol Obstet Invest (abstract) 1977; 8:50.
57. Mendelson JH, Kuehnle J, Ellingboe J, Babor TF. Plasma testosterone levels before, during and after chronic marihuana smoking. N Engl J Med 1974; 291:1051.
58. Mendelson JH, Mendelson JE, Patch VD. Plasma testosterone levels in heroin addiction and during methadone maintenance. J Pharmacol Exp Ther 1975; 192: 211.
59. Harmon JW, Aliapoulios MA. Marijuana-induced gynecomastia: Clinical and laboratory experience. Surg Forum 1974; 25:423.
60. Boyden TW, Parmenter RW. Effects of ethanol on the male hypothalamic-pituitary gonadal axis. Endocr Rev 1983; 4:389.
61. Pont A, Goldman ES, Sugar AM, et al. Ketoconazole-

induced increase in estradiol-testosterone ratio: Probable explanation for gynecomastia. Arch Intern Med 1985; 145:1429.
62. Caminos-Torres R, Ma L, Snyder PJ. Gynecomastia and semen abnormalities induced by spironolactone in normal men. J Clin Endocrinol Metab 1977; 45:255.
63. Humphries TJ, Myerson RM, Gifford LM, et al. A unique postmarket outpatient surveillance program of cimetidine: Report on phase II and final summary. Am J Gastroenterol 1984; 79:593.
64. Funder JW, Mercer JE. Cimetidine, a histamine H_2 receptor antagonist, occupies androgen receptors. J Clin Endocrinol Metab 1979; 48:189.
65. Tosi S, Cagnoli M. Painful gynaecomastia with ranitidine (letter). Lancet 1982; 2:160.
66. Saeter G, Fossa SD, Norman N. Gynaecomastia following cytotoxic therapy for testicular cancer. Br J Urol 1987; 59:348.
67. Large DM, Jones JM, Shalet SM, et al. Gynaecomastia complicating treatment of myeloma. Br J Cancer 1983; 48:69.
68. Tseng A Jr, Horning SJ, Freiha FS, et al. Gynecomastia in testicular cancer patients: Prognostic and therapeutic implications. Cancer 1985; 56:2534.
69. Trump DL, Anderson SA. Painful gynecomastia following cytotoxic therapy for testis cancer: A potentially favorable prognostic sign? J Clin Oncol 1983; 1:416.
70. Lucas LM, Kumar KL, Smith DL. Gynecomastia: A worrisome problem for the patient. Postgrad Med 1987; 82:73.
71. Reid DM, Martynoga AG, Nuki G. Reversible gynaecomastia associated with D-penicillamine in a man with rheumatoid arthritis. Br Med J 1982; 285:1083.
72. Kapoor A. Reversible gynecomastia associated with sulindac therapy (letter). JAMA 1983; 250:2284.
73. Tanner LA, Bosco LA. Gynecomastia associated with calcium channel blocker therapy. Arch Intern Med 1988; 148:379.
74. Van der Steen M, Du Caju MVL, Van Acker KJ. Gynecomastia in a male infant given domperidone (letter). Lancet 1982; 8303:884.
75. Antonelli D, Luboshitzky R, Gelbendorf A. Amiodarone-induced gynecomastia. N Engl J Med 1986; 315: 1553.
76. Monson JP, Scott DF. Gynecomastia induced by phenytoxin in men with epilepsy. Br Med J 1984; 294:612.
77. Markusse HM, Meyboom RHB. Gynaecomastia associated with captopril (letter). Br Med J 1988; 296: 1262.
78. Dardick KR. Gynecomastia associated with theophylline? J Fam Pract 1984; 18:141.
79. Russi EW. Gynaecomastia in cystic fibrosis (letter). Br Med J 1984; 288:1160.
80. Couderc LJ, Clauvel JP. HIV-infection induced gynecomastia (letter). Ann Intern Med 1987; 107:257.
81. Crichlow RW. Diseases of the male breast. In: Gallagher HS, Leis HP Jr, Snyderman RK, Urban JA eds. The breast. St. Louis: CV Mosby, 1978:508–523.
82. Nicolis GL, Modlinger RS, Gabrilove JL. A study of the histopathology of human gynecomastia. J Clin Endocrinol Metab 1971; 32:173.
83. Gottfried MR. Extensive squamous metaplasia in gynecomastia. Arch Pathol Lab Med 1986; 110:971.
84. Dershaw DD. Male mammography. Am J Radiol 1986; 146:127.
85. Kuhn J-M, Roca R, Laudat M-H, et al. Studies on the treatment of idiopathic gynaecomastia with percutaneous dihydrotestosterone. Clin Endocrinol 1983; 19: 513.
86. Eberle AJ, Sparrow JT, Keenan BS. Treatment of persistent pubertal gynecomastia with dihydrotestosterone heptanoate. J Pediatr 1986; 109:144.
87. Beck W, Stubbe P. Endocrinological studies of the hypothalamic-pituitary gonadal axis during danazol treatment in pubertal boys with marked gynecomastia. Horm Metab Res 1982; 14:653.
88. Jackson VP, Gilmor RL. Male breast carcinoma and gynecomastia: Comparison of mammography and sonography. Radiology 1983; 149:533.
89. Zachmann M, Eiholzer U, Muritano M, et al. Treatment of pubertal gynaecomastia with testolactone. Acta Endocrinol [Suppl] 1986; 279:218.
90. Plourde PV, Kulin HE, Santner SJ. Clomiphene in the treatment of adolescent gynecomastia: Clinical and endocrine studies. Am J Dis Child 1983; 137:1080.
91. van Geel AN, van Slooten EA, Mavrunac M, Hart AAM. A retrospective study of male breast cancer in Holland. Br J Surg 1985; 72:724.
92. Courtiss EH. Gynecomastia: Analysis of 159 patients and current recommendations for treatment. Plast Reconstr Surg 1987; 79:740.

CHAPTER 9

Surgical Treatment of Gynecomastia

EUGENE H. COURTISS, M.D.

BACKGROUND AND HISTORY

Gynecomastia (from the Greek *gyne*, "referring to women," Greek *mastos*, "breast") describes the presence of a female-like breast in a male. Because the presence of the condition is subjective and based on aesthetic grounds, its exact frequency cannot be determined with accuracy. However, it has been estimated to occur in between 40 and 65 percent of males.[1,2]

As detailed in Chapter 8, the etiology of gynecomastia may be physiologic (neonatal, pubertal, or involutional); endogenous (testicular, adrenal, thyroid, or pituitary); or exogenous (hormones or drugs).[3]

Although the process is hormonally related, medical treatment is rarely of benefit and may be contraindicated.[4] As a result, when treatment is advised, surgery is advocated. Originally, surgical techniques were adaptations of methods used for treating females. When the breast was large, surgery included both glandular and skin excision, which left anchor-shaped scars.[5] When the breast was smaller, the approach through the areola incision left less obvious scars.[6] However, it is acknowledged that excision of breast tissue with a knife or scissors is associated with undesired sequelae and complications. A more recently adopted alternative has been the use of suction to remove fat, a method associated with fewer complications.[7] Another advantage of removing breast fat by suction is that the need to excise skin is eliminated. However, the currently designed suction cannulas do not remove breast parenchyma, and therefore suction is not applicable to all patients.

ESSENTIAL PATHOLOGY

The microscopic appearance of the tissue that causes the breast enlargement may be purely fat (Fig. 9-1*A*), purely parenchyma (Fig. 9-1*B*), or a combination of fat and parenchyma (Fig. 9-1*C*). Some pathologists consider that parenchyma must be present for a diagnosis of gynecomastia. As a result, when only fat is present, they do not diagnose gynecomastia. However, gynecomastia is a clinical diagnosis that may be characterized by any of the three microscopic findings (Fig. 9-1).

PATIENT SELECTION

Gynecomastia is treated to make the patient feel better about his appearance. As a result, the patient's expectations are important.

If the onset of gynecomastia was before puberty, the patient should be evaluated to determine whether a tumor is present that may be causing the breast enlargement. In addition, if the gynecomastia is unilateral and firm, carcinoma of the breast, albeit rare, may be present and a biopsy should be performed.

PREOPERATIVE EVALUATION AND CARE

If the testicles are normal on examination, hormonal laboratory studies are unnecessary, being neither cost effective nor medically effective.

The breast should be palpated to determine whether the enlargement is due to fat, parenchyma, or a combination of both. In addition, some patients, particularly body builders, are troubled by a chest contour that is due to muscular development. Such individuals should be evaluated carefully, because surgery removes fat or parenchyma but does not treat muscle hypertrophy.

Because of potential adverse effects on blood

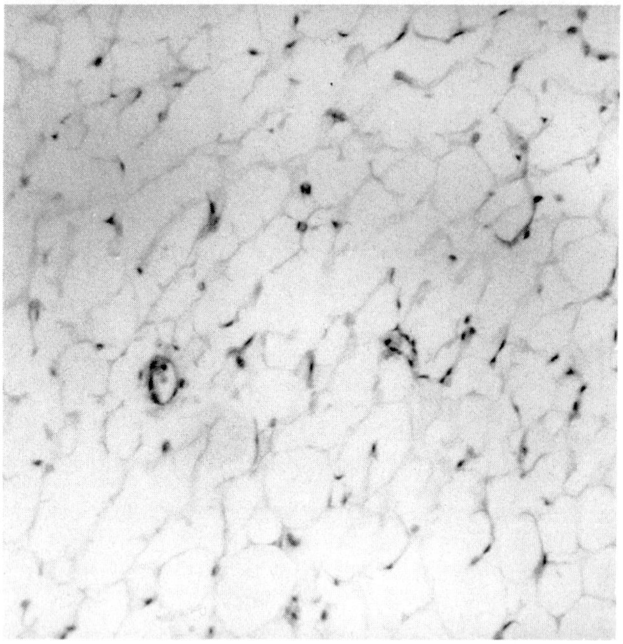

A

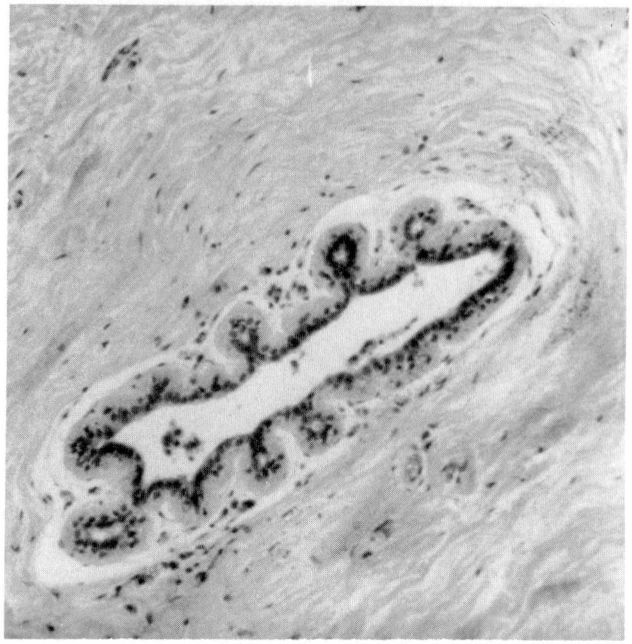

B

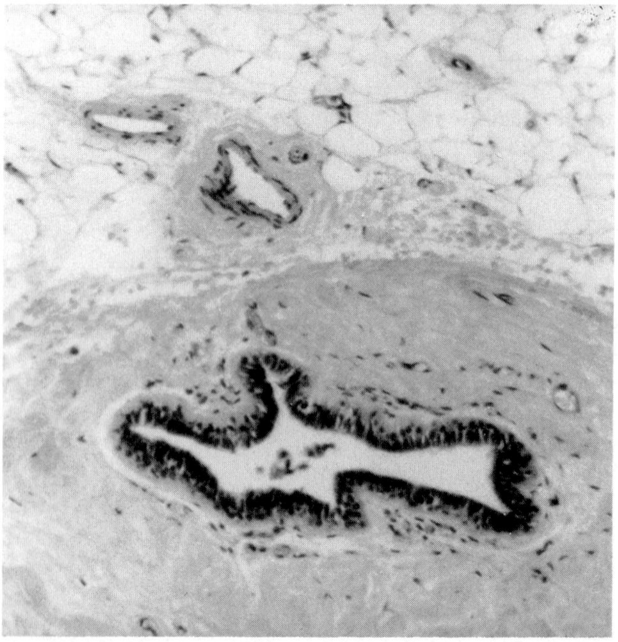

C

FIGURE 9-1 Photomicrographs of material removed during surgery for gynecomastia (H&E, 200X.). *A*, Fat only. *B*, Parenchyma only. *C*, Combination of fat and parenchyma. (From Courtiss EH. Gynecomastia: Analysis of 159 patients and current recommendations for treatment. Plast Reconstr Surg 1987; 79:740.)

coagulation, aspirin should not be taken for 2 weeks before surgery.

SURGICAL TREATMENT

Marking. The patient should be marked while standing, and a contour map should be drawn upon his chest. The point of maximal protrusion should be indicated (Fig. 9-2*A*).

Anesthesia. Local anesthesia (with or without sedation) or general anesthesia may be used. If general anesthesia is chosen, the simultaneous injection of a local anesthetic helps provide hemostasis and postoperative pain control. To that end, 0.25 percent bupivacaine may be given, to which *fresh* epinephrine is added to make a concentration of 1:400,000, plus 300 units of hyaluronidase, or many other solutions. The hyaluronidase helps to reduce swelling, and thus facilitates contour assessment. It also

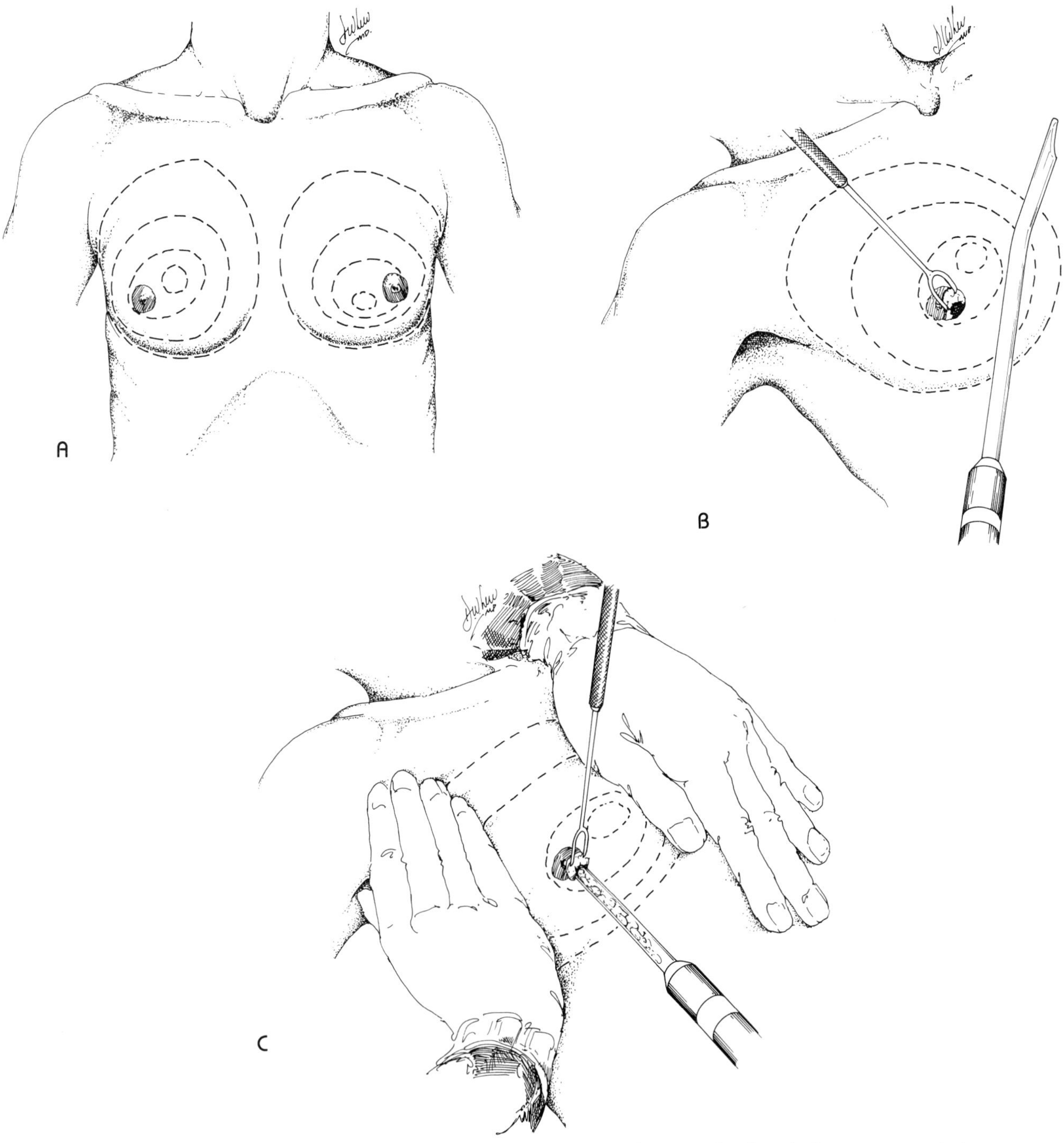

FIGURE 9–2 *A*, A contour map with the point of maximal protrusion is drawn on the chest before surgery with the patient standing. *B*, An areolar incision has been made at 6 o'clock. The plastic cannula is demonstrated. *C*, The cannula is inserted. Note the assistant's hands holding the tissues firmly. *D*, The cannula is redirected into other quadrants of the breast. *E*, Visualization and palpation are used to determine the adequacy of resection. *F*, Scissors are used to remove parenchyma, held in forceps.

allows more rapid penetration of nerves and blood vessels by the anesthetic and the epinephrine. However, the belief that hyaluronidase produces fat lysis is an illusion.

Position. The patient should be placed in a semireclining position with arms akimbo.

Incision. An incision just large enough to allow insertion of a cannula is made in the areola at the 6 o'clock position (Fig. 9–2*B*).

Cannula and Pump Selection. Either plastic (Fig. 9–2*B*) or metal cannulas may be used. If the distal end has multiple holes, a smaller cannula may be used than when a single-hole model is chosen. Any one of many pumps may be used. To remove a

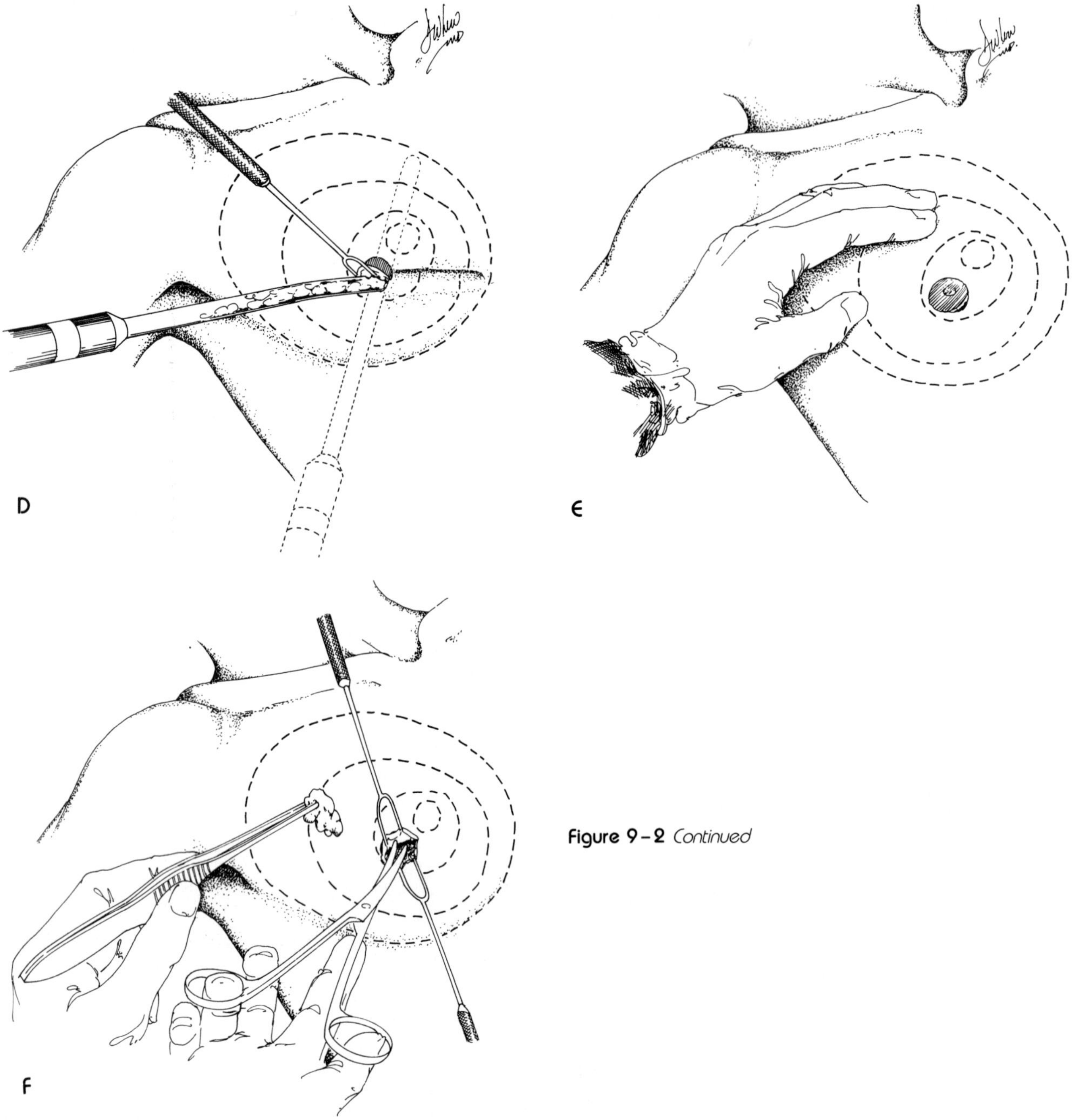

Figure 9–2 *Continued*

given amount of material, smaller cannulas require a greater vacuum than larger cannulas. Conversely, when larger cannulas are used, the vacuum generated by the pump may be turned down lest too much tissue be removed.

Lipectomy with Suction. As in other forms of suction surgery, the cannula is inserted and worked back and forth. Tunnels are not created, but neither is a "windshield wiper" action used. Fat is removed from where the contour is full (Fig. 9–2*C,D*). However, a layer of fat, which is difficult to measure, should be left under the skin (Fig. 9–2*E*). Pinch and feel may be used to determine when enough has been removed, but the appearance is the most important determinant (Fig. 9–2*E*). The volume of tissue removed is unimportant; what is left is crucial: it is easy to remove more, but replacement is almost impossible. Removing fat *before*, rather than after, parenchymal excision may eliminate the need for such excision; if excision *is* needed, it is more easily performed.

If breast ptosis is present, the inframammary fold should be interrupted with the cannula.

Evaluation for Excision. After the fat is removed, the contour should be reassessed. If the problem was due to fat alone, the suction will have provided the desired contour and it is time to close the wound. However, since the cannula does not remove parenchyma, and if the chest contour was due to fat *and* parenchyma, the contour will be improved by suction alone, but parenchyma, which feels like firm tissue under the nipple-areola complex, will remain and must be excised.

Parenchymal Excision. The small incision may need to be enlarged to expose the parenchyma, which should be excised under direct vision with scissors, knife, or cautery (Fig. 9-2*F*). This should be tailored to leave sufficient tissue under the nipple-areola complex to prevent it from becoming depressed, producing a saucer-shaped appearance. In patients in whom the only problem is parenchymal hypertrophy, the preliminary suction does not significantly change the contour, and excision is needed. However, the suction will have removed any fat present and will have broken the breast septa, making the subsequent parenchymal excision easier.

Nipple Excision. If the nipple protrudes excessively, the protruding part may be excised. A knife or

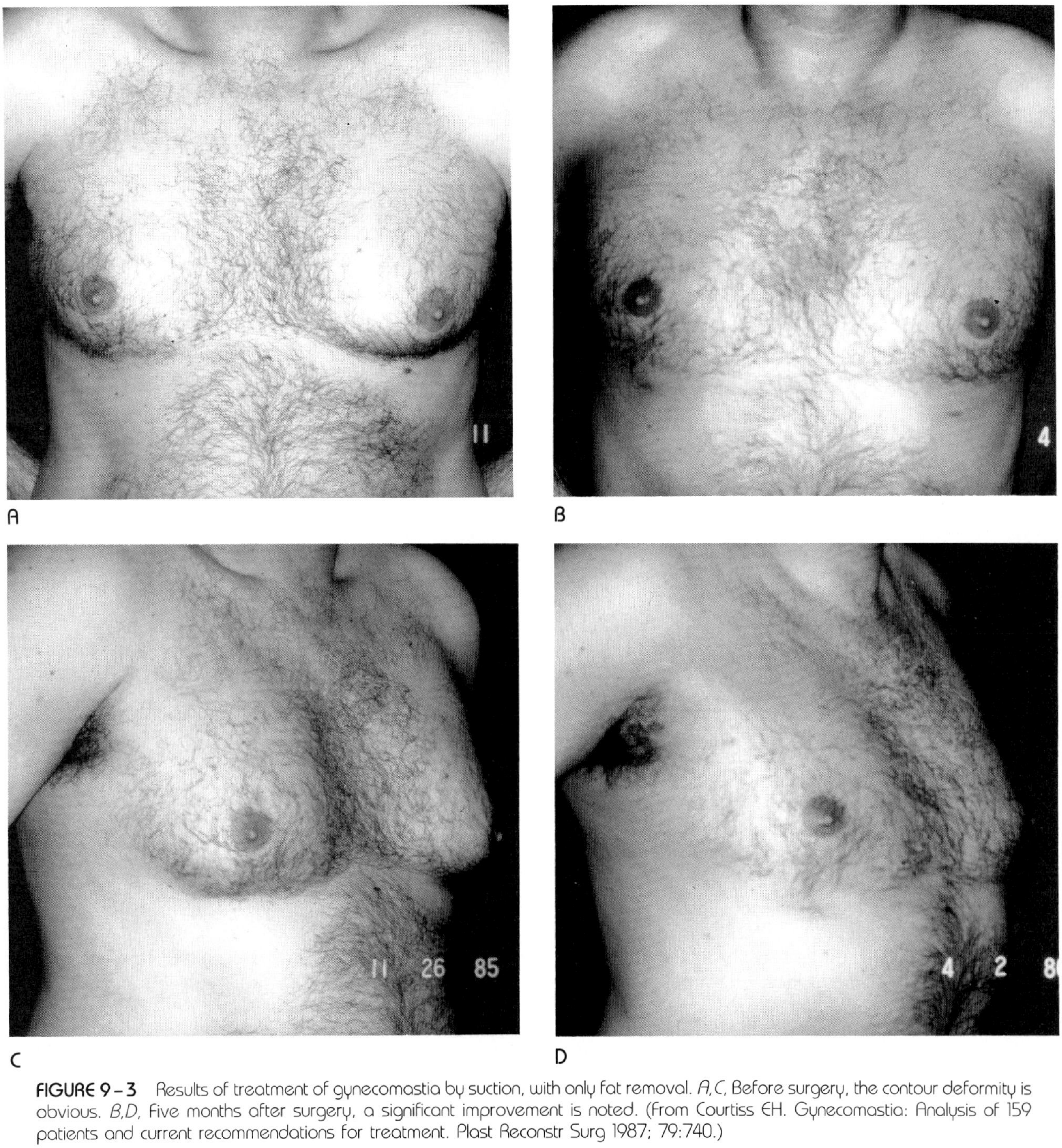

FIGURE 9-3 Results of treatment of gynecomastia by suction, with only fat removal. *A,C,* Before surgery, the contour deformity is obvious. *B,D,* Five months after surgery, a significant improvement is noted. (From Courtiss EH. Gynecomastia: Analysis of 159 patients and current recommendations for treatment. Plast Reconstr Surg 1987; 79:740.)

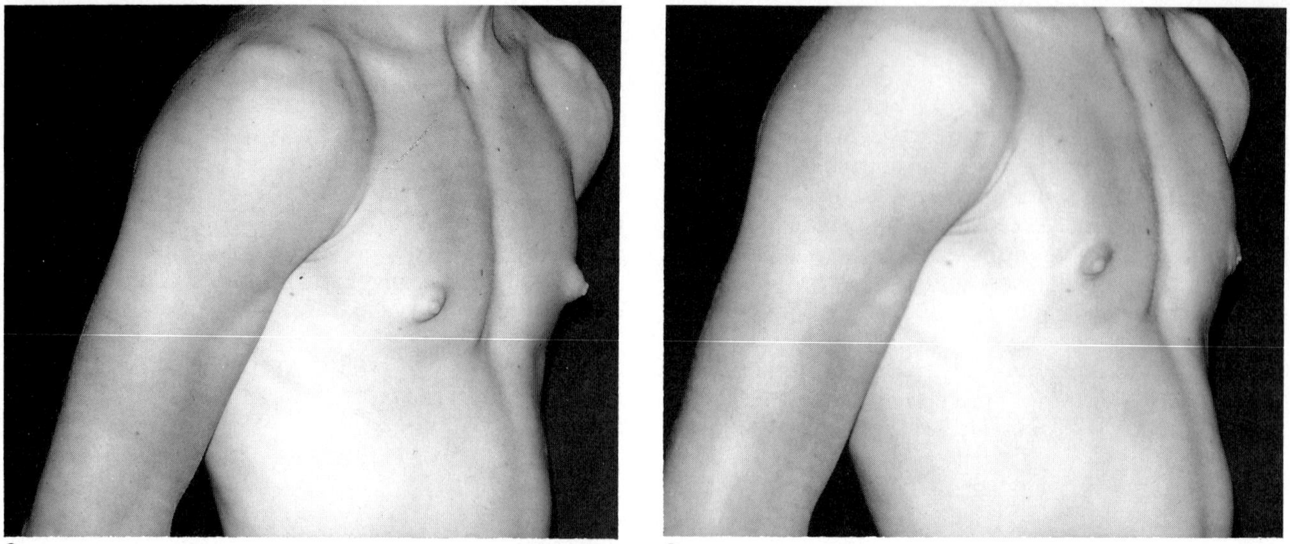

A B

FIGURE 9-4 Results from treatment of parenchymal hypertrophy only. *A*, Preoperative view demonstrates breast parenchyma beneath the nipple-areola complex. *B*, One year after surgery the improved contour is maintained. (From Courtiss EH. Gynecomastia: Analysis of 159 patients and current recommendations for treatment. Plast Reconstr Surg 1987; 79:740.)

scissors horizontally transects the extra tissue, just as if it were being removed as a nipple graft. No sutures are used. The wound is covered with a nonadherent dressing. Of course, the excised tissue should be examined microscopically.

Drains. If a drain is to be inserted, it may be placed through the incision or through a lateral stab wound. As an alternative, neither drains nor sutures may be placed, but the wound instead left open to drain. The wound later heals by contraction and epithelialization, and the scar is indistinguishable from that produced when sutures are used.

Closure. If the wound is closed, the subcutaneous fat and skin should be approximated with appropriate sutures.

Dressing. A dry, absorbent dressing is applied.

Binder. Regardless of whether the wound has been drained, a firm binder, such as a rib belt, is applied over the dressing.

POSTOPERATIVE CARE

The dressing should be removed and the patient examined 1 week after surgery, or sooner if he complains of pain. Except to change it or during a shower, a binder should be worn for 6 weeks, particularly if the reduction was large or ptosis was present. No corticosteroids, antibiotics, ultrasonography, or massage are used.

RESULTS

The results from such methods have been gratifying to both patient and surgeon (Figs. 9-3 to 9-5).

AVOIDANCE OF COMPLICATIONS

Seroma. The most common complication is seroma formation, which often develops and cannot be prevented. When it occurs, it should be treated by aspiration under sterile conditions and continued binder compression. A permanent deformity is unusual.

Undesired Contour. On occasion it may be appropriate to remove additional material at a second operation. This indicates that the surgeon was conservative during the initial surgery. Should removal of more material be indicated, at least 3 months should pass before secondary surgery, to allow any swelling to resolve.

Sensory Changes. Altered sensation is present in most patients, but is usually temporary.[8]

Generic Complications. Certain complications such as hematoma and infection are generic to all surgery, and other complications such as decreased sensation and edema are generic to suction surgery. These have been discussed elsewhere.[9]

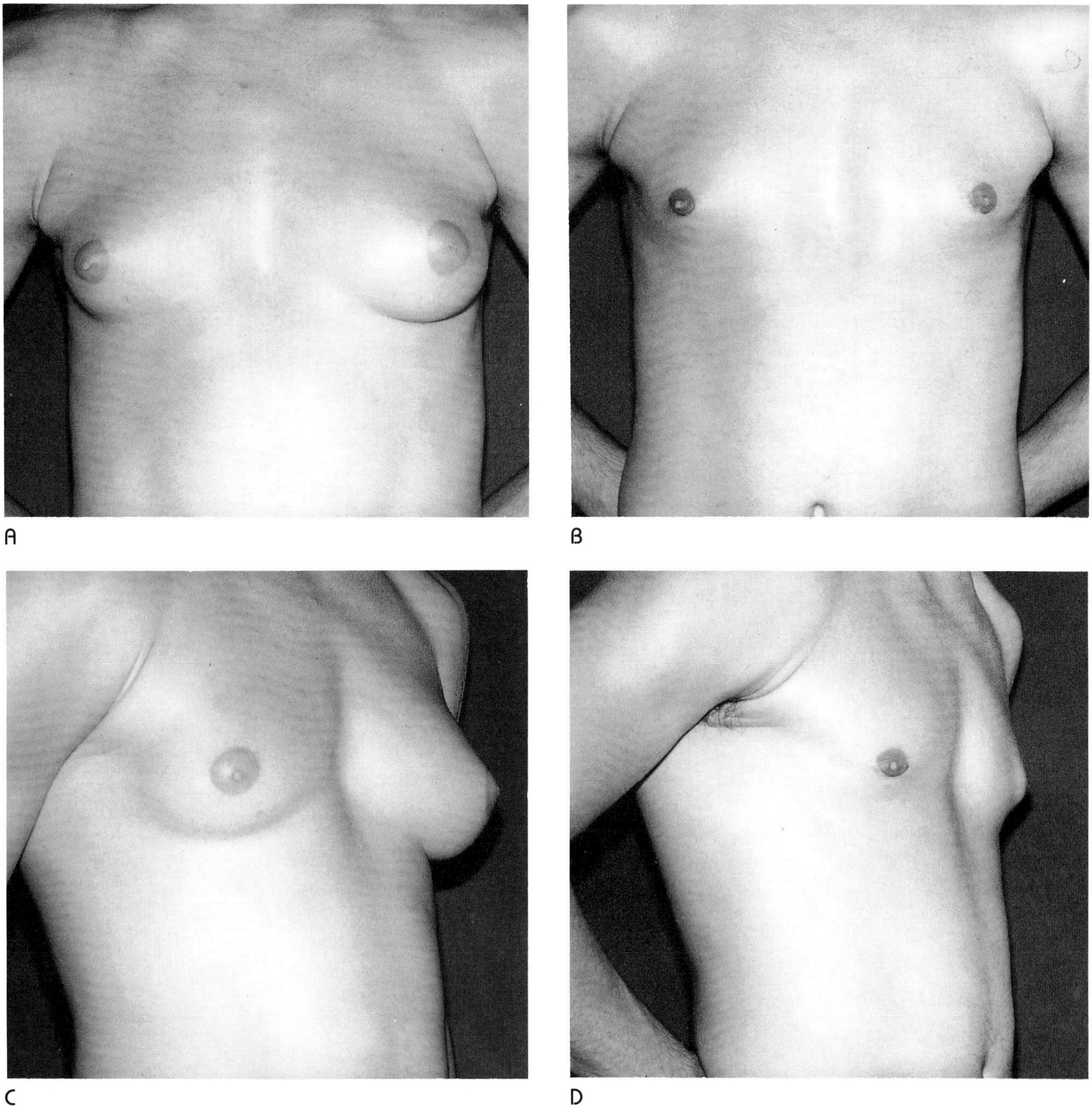

FIGURE 9-5 Results of treatment of the combination of fat and parenchymal hypertrophy. *A,C,* Preoperative views show significant gynecomastia deformity. *B,D,* Nine months after surgery the contour improvement is impressive, without the need for skin excision. (From Courtiss EH. Gynecomastia: Analysis of 159 patients and current recommendations for treatment. Plast Reconstr Surg 1987; 79:740.)

References

1. Williams MJ. Gynecomastia: Its incidence, recognition and host characterization in 447 autopsy cases. Am J Med 1963; 34:103.
2. Nydick M, Bustos J, Dale JH Jr, Rawson RW. Gynecomastia in adolescent boys. JAMA 1961; 178:449.
3. Letterman G, Schurter M. Gynecomastia. In: Courtiss EH, ed. Male aesthetic surgery. St Louis: CV Mosby, 1982.
4. Madaren NK. Gynecomastia. In: Gellis SS, Kagen BM, eds. Current pediatric therapy II. Philadelphia: WB Saunders, 1984.

5. Graham WP III, Miller SH. Reconstructive surgery of the breast. In: Nora PF, ed. Operative surgery. 2nd ed. Philadelphia: Lea & Febiger, 1980.
6. Simon BE, Hoffman S. Correction of gynecomastia. In: Goldwyn RM, ed. Plastic and reconstructive surgery of the breast. Boston: Little, Brown, 1976.
7. Courtiss EH. Gynecomastia: Analysis of 159 patients and current recommendations for treatment. Plast Reconstr Surg. 1987; 79:740.
8. Courtiss EH, Donelan MB. Skin sensation after suction lipectomy: A prospective study of 50 consecutive patients. Plast Reconstr Surg 1988; 81:550.
9. Gargan TJ, Courtiss EH. The risks of suction lipectomy, their prevention and treatment. Clin Plast Surg 1984; 11:457.

SECTION 3

AUGMENTATION MAMMAPLASTY

C H A P T E R 10

Overview of Augmentation Mammaplasty

GARRY S. BRODY M.D.

RATIONALE FOR CURRENT TREATMENT

Homo sapiens is the only species that modifies physical appearance by decoration.[1] The variety of decor in the human experience is almost infinite because of our unique ability to reason, imagine, and prognosticate, which is facilitated by tool-making skills. The functional need for warmth has led to the use of clothing as decor in Northern climes. Those living in warmer latitudes are more likely to use direct skin decoration. The paler skin characteristic of the Northern peoples permitted tattooing and paint as skin decor, whereas scarification was more common in the pigmented races.

Scarification was perhaps the first cosmetic surgery of prehistory. Later, ancient Egyptians bound the skulls of royal children between boards to create an attractive tower-shaped skull. The Chinese bound the feet of infant girls to enhance their beauty until after the revolution of 1912, when the practice was abolished. Although seemingly barbaric to the Western mind, it is no more so than the Western European practice of using corsets on children to produce the wasp-waisted men and women of the last century. The current American fashion of perforating ear lobes and noses for jewelry differs only in degree from the African custom of inserting large lip and ear discs or nasal rings. Can face lifts, liposuction, or breast implants be any more civilized? The difference lies only in the current norm of beauty in any given society.

From a freudian perspective all decor has a sexual connotation either to attract, as in the revealing clothing of the coquette, or to deny, as in the nun's habit. It is the secondary sexual characteristics that are the most powerful human attractants. The greater the difference between men and women, the more these opposites attract.

Because of the overwhelming variety of human decor, it is not surprising that concepts of beauty and sexual attractiveness are learned cultural experiences. The female breast dominates many cultures as a symbol of fertility and sexual attractiveness, but this perception is not universal. The dictates of modesty (another uniquely human characteristic) suggest that the hidden parts of our body are more tantalizing to the opposite sex. Thus, in cultures in which the clothed or semiclothed breast is fashionable, the bosom becomes more enticing and erotic than in those societies in which the breast is exposed. Maeder[2] showed that the artistic representation of the clothed bosom often reflects its idealized form in the nude. Indeed, he was even able to show that one could date a statue by the shape of its breasts, and how this shape would have been achieved in confirmation with the clothing of the time.

Conversely, in a recent visit by the author to the Island of Yap in Micronesia, where topless sarongs and loincloths are the norm, the natives were asked about the erogenous characteristics of the exposed breast. They replied that the breast was "about as sexy as an elbow," but that covered thighs were indeed stimulating. There were also some clues about the concept of breast size from that same community. One matriarch pointed out that all the women in village A seemed to have very small breasts, whereas those in village B had very large bosoms. When asked which was more attractive to the Yapese, they responded after a moment of thought that the women with the small breasts wanted to be larger and the women with large breasts wished to be smaller!

Even in this modern day of free exchange of literature and culture, there are regional differences in the concept of attractiveness of the female breast.

In South America, where large breasts are more common, there is perhaps a greater incidence of breast reduction than in the United States. Similarly, brassiere construction suggests that the ideal South American breast shape is more conical than the rounder North American ideal.

Beginning with the flattened bosom of the American flapper in the 1920s, the idealized breast has become larger and larger with time. Such landmarks as Lana Turner's sweater girl image and Jane Russell's full bosom have represented milestones in this change. Implant manufacturers note that the average implant size has gradually increased over the years. Many plastic surgeons have also noted the steady increase in volume desired by their patients during the 1980s. Regional differences also exist, with a larger average size of implants sold on both coasts than in middle America. Conversely, bra manufacturers sell larger bras in the mid-West, suggesting that population already is naturally larger.

With the infinite variety of learned experience, it is not surprising that each of us develops a unique concept of our own self-image that varies widely within the spectrum of today's norm. How cultural images play upon the inherited physical appearance of each of us becomes an overwhelmingly complex mix of social experience and inherited psyche.

Unfortunately, we are socially ambivalent concerning physical appearance. As much as we admire beauty, attractiveness, and sexuality, it is also often a subject for criticism and titillation. We lack empathy for those whose concepts differ from our personal bias. Thus, the woman who desires to augment her breast will find much private support but public disapproval. The latter even permeates the official statements of the Food and Drug Administration:

> *Because implantation of a breast prosthesis device is discretionary cosmetic surgery, consideration of the total risk to health from implantation of such a device must include the usual risks of the surgery involved and the risks of surgical error that are enhanced by the properties of the device itself.*
>
> An FDA Official

The quality-of-life issues that have sexual overtones are more controversial than those that do not. No woman can escape being aware of some public disapproval, which must generate at least a modicum of guilt to temper her interest and delight in breast augmentation.

As demonstrated by primitive tattooing, Chinese foot binding, and western European corseting, the practice of altering the physical form of the body surgically and otherwise is not new. Modern materials and enhanced surgical and anesthetic safety have permitted a significant extension of techniques available before the second half of the 20th century. If the estimate of 2 million augmented women is anywhere near accurate, it certainly represents a universal interest in larger breasts and must approach the norm of human behavior rather than an aberration. Perhaps it is only those who cannot empathize with women's desire for a fuller bosom who are the cultural outliers.

Owing to its fluidity and mobility, the breast has no constant shape and thus far has defied any anthropometric or anthropomorphic quantification. There are no anthropologic studies of the normal breast nor any scholarly works on the esthetics of that organ, either in art or in life. Perhaps this is because its flexibility permits such a subtle variety in its shape that no baseline can be established.

There has been an increasing interest in breast size over the last 60 years, but it is difficult to know what the future may hold. It would not be surprising to see a reversal of this trend. If so, it is to be hoped that any reversal will occur slowly enough to extend beyond the life expectancy of women currently undergoing the surgery. Although every woman who undertakes this procedure hopes and anticipates that one operative procedure will solve her concerns for a lifetime, we know that complications and unfavorable results often mean multiple procedures for some. Surgery is never comfortable to contemplate, but it also is not improper to consider later revisions if fashion so dictates. Many physical and psychological health issues such as dentistry, joint replacements, and psychotherapy require repetitive procedures or treatments. Revision of a breast implant merely creates a somewhat different equation of the risk:benefit ratio.

HISTORY OF THE IMPLANT

In 1952 Dr. John Pangman of Los Angeles performed what was probably the first breast implant procedure using a modern polymeric material.[3] He hand-carved his prostheses from Ivalon, which was the trade name for a commercially available polyvinyl sponge. With the possible exception of metals in bone, common dogma dictated that the body poorly tolerated foreign materials. "Real" plastic surgeons used autogenous tissue only. However, there were some early favorable reports of the use of polymeric materials for other reconstructive purposes by such respected surgeons as Drs. John Gridley,[4] O.R. Clagett,[5] and J Barrett Brown.[6]

Use of a foreign object in the breast was an even greater anathema, especially for "frivolous" cosmetic enlargement. Prior to the 1950s, aesthetic surgery lacked the status and respect associated with reconstructive procedures. It was carried out by most, but admitted to by only a few brave souls who suffered denunciation by the Establishment. In 1955 Pangman and Wallace published the first paper on alloplastic breast augmentation, reporting on more than 400 patients.[7] As evidenced by Kiskadden's writing, he was heavily criticized by his colleagues:[8]

> *It therefore seems highly dangerous, unscientific, and without valid clinical reasoning or application to introduce a foreign plastic material whose immediate results are so indifferent and whose long term outlook is filled with the potential danger of cancer.*

Pangman's report was a model of thoroughness. He included extensive laboratory data, careful clinical analyses, and concern over potential carcinogenesis. He was aware of Oppenheimer's work[9,10] on solid-state carcinogenesis, predicting that it was probably inapplicable to human biology. He described the breast capsule and honestly reported on the firmness and shrinkage that occurred in almost 100 percent of his patients. His photographs showed results that would be considered excellent today. Pangman was ahead of his time in his understanding of the psychosexual and social significance of the female breast. Describing a survey of his patients, he noted that all but two were pleased with the results and only one would not undergo it again.

This article also described Pangman's first modification. He scooped out the center of an implant and placed the removed material into a polyethylene bag. The bag was then reinserted into the shell to provide a barrier that limited tissue ingrowth and fluid uptake in an attempt to avoid the shrinkage problem. The Plastic Surgery collection at the Countway Museum at Harvard University contains examples of even later experimental modifications, including a silicone inflatable model.

In 1963, Ben Edwards,[11] also of Los Angeles, reported the use of an implant composed of silicone sponge, coated by an impervious layer of silicone adhesive and an outer layer of Teflon felt.

In a survey by Harris[12] published in 1961, 110 of 283 plastic surgeons did not perform augmentations and the remainder estimated that they had carried out 16,660 implants. All used sponge material made of polyurethane, polyvinyl (Ivalon), or polyethylene (Etheron or polystan). In those early years, the implants were hand carved and fabricated by the surgeon himself. In 1967, Hoopes and Edgerton[13] estimated that 40,000 breast implants had been performed.

At the third International Congress of Plastic Surgery in 1963,[14] Drs. Thomas Cronin and Frank Gerow revolutionized breast implant design when they presented their experience with a "New 'Natural Feel' Prosthesis" produced by the Dow Corning company. Their design of a gel-filled silicone device remains the basis of all implants used today, and spawned an industry that at various times consisted of as many as ten different companies. There have been innumerable modifications of this basic design, as follows:

Shape: Round; teardrop; high profile; low profile
Shell: Single; double; septate ("Natural-Y")
Thick; thin
Seamed; seamless
Fixation patches; patchless
High bleed; low bleed
Smooth; textured; polyurethane covered
Fill: Adjustable: saline; dextran
nonadjustable: gel (thick; thin)

All modern implants are made entirely of silicone except for the Natural Y product, which has an outer coating of polyurethane sponge. In 1970 Ashley[15] first reported on a new prosthesis that contained a central Y-shaped partition designed to prevent sag. He covered the outer shell with a thin film of polyurethane foam as a fixation device. This implant did not gain popularity, because at about this time surgeons began to realize that fixation to tissue was not required and probably not desirable. Also, the Y partitions could be felt in women with very little cover. The Ashley style of prosthesis, with and without the partitions, continued to be used by a few surgeons for reconstruction, and they noted serendipitously that these implants stayed remarkably soft. Herman in 1986[16] was the first to report the use of the MEME prosthesis for cosmetic augmentation and noted the remarkable absence of contracture.

Despite these early reports, surgeons continued to resist the use of polyurethane implants for cosmetic augmentation. This was due to skepticism regarding the lack of contracture and the paucity of information concerning the possible risks arising from the fragmenting and dissolving outer coat. It was counter-intuitive to think that the foam structure that led to such hard breasts in the pre-silicone era could be so soft in this configuration. It was also difficult to accept that reactivity and increased scar was a desirable attribute. Eventually, the lack of any evidence of significant toxicity and the reports of reliable softness became so widespread as to be irrefutable. The polyurethane-covered implant now has a solid place in our armamentarium.

GOVERNMENT INVOLVEMENT

In 1906, in response to Upton Sinclair's exposure of abuses in the meat packing industry, Congress passed the first Food and Drug Act. This has been amended many times. The most recent significant addition was the device amendment of 1976 (Public Law 94.295 Medical Device Amendment of Food, Drug and Cosmetic Act May 28, 1976). The law provided for division of all medical devices into three classes:

Class I. Restricted to devices for which no additional regulation other than good manufacturing practices are necessary and generally represent no real risk. For example, tongue blades should not splinter and bedpans should not have sharp edges.

Class II. Devices with more critical functions for which performance standards are required, such as electrocardiograph machines and x-ray units.

Class III. Reserved for life-sustaining or implantable devices that do not automatically fall within Classes I or II. The law specifies that implantable devices are automatically placed in Class III unless sufficient data on safety and efficacy convince the Food and Drug Administration (FDA) that the risk:benefit ratio warrants placement into Class II.

In order to deal with the enormous number of devices that were on the market at the time, advisory committees called Classification Panels were established. These groups had no authority, but their purpose was to advise the FDA concerning classification of the existing devices. They served at the discretion of the FDA and dealt only with devices on which the agency requested their counsel. There were separate panels for different specialties, and general and plastic surgery were combined into one group. Currently, there are five voting members on this panel and multiple additional advisory members from industry, the scientific community, and the lay public. The present panel includes one plastic surgeon, one general surgeon, an epidemiologist, a rheumatologist, and an internist. In 1982 this panel voted to place the breast implant in Class II. Subsequent panels rejected this advice, and in 1988 the FDA published their intention to classify the breast implant as Class III in the Federal Register. This implies that the implant will require essentially the same kind of safety and effectiveness testing and data that a new drug application would require—a complex and expensive process. This law regulates only the importation and sale of these devices in interstate commerce, and has jurisdiction only over manufacturers and distributors. The FDA has no jurisdiction over any device that is custom made, because these are considered as being for one-time use in an individual patient. Surgeons may legally implant anything into the human body without the concern of the FDA.

In November 1988 and January 1989, the Plastic and General Surgery classification panel held hearings with full media coverage to consider public input and make recommendations to the FDA as to what information may be required. The classification panel made several recommendations. First, they advised undertaking an epidemiologic study that would further address the issue of cancer and cancer detection. Although there was no significant evidence of any relationship between the breast implant and cancer, they felt that current studies were not long term enough to be definitive.

Second, they were concerned about outcome and complications in terms of the implant performance and useful life and surgical complications. They were especially concerned about the issue of capsular contracture. Finally, the panel felt that the few reports in the medical and legal literature suggesting a relationship between connective tissue diseases such as "human adjuvant disease" and scleroderma to the implant needed more definitive clarification. The rheumatologist on the panel implied that the evidence for such an etiologic relationship was tenuous at best.

The FDA stated that they had received more complaints concerning the breast implant than about any other medical device. However, this statement was not placed in perspective by weighing it against the fact that the breast implant is by far the most common implanted medical device in the United States.

In an internal review of their complaint files, the FDA concluded that patients were not always adequately informed of the risks of breast implantation. (It is, of course, easy to see how information extracted only from complaint files would lead to this conclusion.) Consequently, there was a strong recommendation from the classification panel that the FDA develop a patient information brochure.

In response to this request, the Office of Communication of the FDA established a large task force consisting of surgeons, manufacturers, radiologists, and consumers to draft such a document. They are divided into three groups: one addressing cosmetic augmentation, a second for reconstruction, and a third dealing with the production and distribution of the booklet. Because of the disparate attitudes toward augmentation among the various participants, there is some concern over whether a consensus is possible.

The Maryland State Legislature mandated the production of a booklet that must be given to every woman in the state who is contemplating implants. The Maryland law requires that the booklet describe all possible risks and hazards but the evidence for benefits is considered insufficiently proved to include.

In considering what information a woman who is contemplating augmentation be given, the consent issues can be divided into three areas:

1. Information that is directly implant related:
   a. Type of implant
   b. Life expectancy of the implant
   c. Silicone bleed
   d. Implant rupture
   e. Granulomas
   f. "Immune disease"
   g. Silicone migration
   h. Degradation of the silicone and/or polyurethane
   i. Rejection
   j. Calcification
2. Issues that are surgically related:
   a. Bleeding
   b. Infection

c. Capsular contracture
d. Asymmetry
e. Malposition
f. Sensory change
g. Cancer risk, detection, and treatment
h. Pregnancy and nursing
i. Breast maturation and aging
j. Ptosis
k. Incisions and scars
l. Supra- or submuscular placement
m. Tissue loss
n. Expected size, shape, and esthetics

3. New disorders that can result from implants:
   a. Fat necrosis
   b. Calcification
   c. Granulomas
   d. Oleomas
   e. Scar
   f. Broken implants with or without silicone spread
   g. Pain

COMPLICATIONS

Certainly, no woman should enter into this procedure without understanding that complications may result. It is an interesting observation that complications seem to arise in groups. Revisions are seemingly performed in the same small percentage of women, often more than once. In the Los Angeles Breast Implant Cancer Study the charts of 3,501 patients were abstracted not only for cancer information but also for outcome. The following list represents any notation of concern to patients that was found in the physicians' records of a patient population dating from 1962 to 1979.[17] There is no information as to the magnitude or significance of any of the complications. Infection might mean anything from a slight inflammation around a suture to septicemia. Hematoma might be a true collection of blood or nothing more than extensive bruising. Therefore, this list should be interpreted only in general terms and not necessarily as representing truly significant complications. The rates are probably low, because the records varied significantly in their completeness.

Capsular contracture:	24.8%*
Hematoma:	4.6%
Size change:	2.9%
Seroma:	2.6%
Wrinkling or displacement:	2.3%
Associated breast disease:	2.6%
Infection:	2.2%
Implant rupture:	2.1%
Gel .46%	
Saline 8.14%	
Scar revision	.8%
Wound separation	.4%
Unacceptable shape	.2%
Numbness	.2%
Thinning of skin	.1%

1.4% underwent removal and replacement of the implant.

*Judgment of the reliability of this data must take into account the fact that the recorded incidences varied among surgeons between 0 and 65 percent, even between two plastic surgeons who were partners in the same office. Of this group of patients, 13.5 percent had closed capsulotomies, 8.4 percent had open capsulotomies, and 3.6 percent were untreated.

A reasonable perspective for any woman is to consider that the implant represents a new body part. Even nature cannot produce a totally trouble-free organ, and the complications may be considered illnesses or injuries to this new component.

CANCER

The single most common and significant disorder of the female breast is cancer. There is no evidence in the current literature to suggest that the breast implant in any way increases the risk of cancer. In fact, all the information suggests that the incidence of cancer, at least for the 27 years that implants have been available, is less than might be expected.[17,18] These data are not statistically significant, but they do demonstrate a strong trend.

One possible explanation of the decreased incidence of cancer in this population is that small or involuted breasts have a lower incidence of cancer than in larger ones. However, the relationship of cancer to breast size has never been studied, nor is the normal spectrum of breast size known. In an attempt to obtain some rough estimates of the range and incidence of breast size in the United States, a mail order brassiere company was contacted. Because the cup size of bras sold across the counter are not standardized, the retail outlet information was considered unreliable. It was thought, however, that mail order bras must have some standardization, as they are bought without a fitting. Size information from this source was thought to be dependable. We were advised, however, that contrary to our expectations this information would indeed be inaccurate, because small-breasted women tended to use padding and large-bosomed women tended to stuff themselves into cups that were too small. The only solid information that one could glean from this cooperative firm was that they sold larger sizes in the mid-West than at either coast. This is not inconsistent with the implant manufacturers' obverse experience.

Some information is available from the American Cancer Society concerning external prostheses ordered by women after undergoing mastectomies. It is assumed that the prostheses would be approximately the same size as the uninvolved breast. The following list of size ranges sold over an 8-month period in 1981 was provided by the California branch of the American Cancer Society:

A-cup	46
B-cup	133
C-cup	107
D-cup	45

Although this follows the expected bell-shaped curve, it is not meaningful without a knowledge of the normal population distribution of breast size.

After 27 years of use, the silicone implant continues to increase in popularity with no sign of saturation. It appears to be relatively safe, and despite a variety of outcomes continues to enhance the quality of life for over 2 million women. Thus far its popularity has resisted the concern of governments and attacks of those who have no empathy for the needs of others. Dissatisfaction to the point of implant removal remains very rare. Everyone has the right to control his or her own body and mind after duly considering the social pressures and the physical and psychological risks. As plastic surgeons, our responsibility is to provide balanced information and to assess the physical and psychological indications for the surgery in our patients. The perfect breast enlargement or reconstruction will probably not be achieved by implants, but must await further advances in genetic engineering. In the meantime, currently available implants remain relatively safe and effective substitutes.

References

1. Brain R. The decorated body. New York: Harper & Row, 1979.
2. Maeder E. Breast aesthetics in art and fashion. Presented at the first annual Plastic Surgery Educational Foundation Breast Symposium, Santa Fe, NM, September 1985.
3. Pangman J. Personal communication.
4. Grindlay JH, Clagett OR. A plastic sponge prosthesis for use after pneumectomy: Preliminary report of an experimental study. Proc Staff Meet Mayo Clin 1949; 24:538-539.
5. Grindlay JH, Clagett OR. Plastic sponge which acts as a framework for living tissue: Experimental studies and preliminary report of use to reinforce abdominal aneurysms. Arch Surg 1951; 63:288-297.
6. Moore AM, Brown JB. Investigation of polyvinyl compounds for use as subcutaneous prosthesis. Plast Reconstr Surg 1952; 10:453-459.
7. Pangman WJ, Wallace RM. The use of plastic prosthesis in breast plastic and other soft tissue surgery. West J Surg 1955; 63:503-512.
8. Kiskadden WS. Operations on bosoms are dangerous. Plast Reconstr Surg 1955; 15:79-80.
9. Oppenheimer BS, Oppenheimer ET, Stout AP. Sarcomas induced in rodents by implanting cellophane. Proc Soc Exp Biol 1948; 67:33.
10. Oppenheimer BS, Oppenheimer ET, Stout AP. Sarcomas induced in rodents by implanting various plastic films. Proc Soc Exp Biol 1952; 97:366.
11. Edwards BF. Teflon-silicone implants. Plast Reconstr Surg 1963; 32:519-526.
12. Harris HI. Survey of breast implants from the point of view of carcinogenesis. Plast Reconstr Surg 1961; 28:81-83.
13. Hoopes JE, Edgerton MT. Organic synthetics for augmentation mammaplasty: Their relation to breast surgery. Plast Reconstr Surg 1967; 39:263-270.
14. Cronin TD, Gerow FJ. Augmentation mammaplasty: A new natural feel prosthesis. Transactions of the IIIrd Congress of Plastic Surgery, 1963:41-49.
15. Ashley FL. A new type of breast prosthesis. Plast Reconstr Surg 1970; 45:421-424.
16. Herman S. The MEME implant. Plast Reconstr Surg 1984; 73:411-414.
17. Deapen DN, Pike MC, Casagrande JT, Brody GS. The relationship between breast cancer and augmentation mammaplasty: An epidemiologic study. Plast Reconstr Surg 1986; 77:361-367.
18. Deapen DN, Brody GS. The Los Angeles breast implant-cancer study: A five year follow up. In preparation.

CHAPTER 11

Selection of Technique for Augmentation Mammaplasty

JACK FISHER, M.D.
G. PATRICK MAXWELL, M.D.

In any surgical procedure, there are two critical events. First is the intellectual, decision-making component: planning the surgical procedure for a particular patient on the basis of previous experience and knowledge. Second is the performance of the surgical procedure. Augmentation mammaplasty may be considered a simple or routine surgical exercise, but this attitude may be due to oversimplification of the procedure.

Problems can occur with augmentation mammaplasty because of a failure to analyze properly the first phase of patient or procedure selection. The oft-quoted phrase "when your only tool is a hammer, the world is a nail" is relevant discussing augmentation mammaplasty, because no single procedure is appropriate for all patients. Although the plastic surgeon may prefer a particular procedure, a type of implant, or an anatomic location, the surgeon should be familiar with all potential variables in order to execute this operation properly. It may be easier to teach someone to perform the technical aspects of the various procedures than it is to teach selection of the best operation for a particular patient.

In discussions among plastic surgeons, one may hear "this is how I do my augmentations" when it may be more appropriate to say "this is how I select a particular procedure for this type of patient."

This chapter is not specifically about surgical technique, but rather is a discussion on the thought processes behind patient selection for augmentation mammaplasty. If surgeons examine their results critically, with a sharp aesthetic eye, judgment and selection of the proper surgical procedure becomes a critical component in successful breast augmentation.

PATIENT EVALUATION

One of the first steps in proper selection of technique for augmentation mammaplasty is a thorough and full discussion with the patient. Both positive and negative aspects of breast augmentation must be discussed. The patient must be presented with potential negative issues, especially those that periodically appear in the lay literature. A proper history of any previous breast pathology should be taken. Results of previous mammography are important, and preoperative mammograms are obtained in most patients. Family history must be considered as well as previous breast biopsies.[1] In patients with a marked family history of breast cancer, other options may be considered. Currently, a variety of implants and surgical approaches are available and should be thoroughly discussed with the patient. In particular, the combination most appropriate to the individual situation should be stressed. Obviously, a discussion of the risks and complications of breast augmentation is mandatory, including scars, changes in nipple sensation, bleeding, and infection.[2]

Patients often have preconceived ideas of augmentation mammaplasty. This is especially true today, because many women have undergone breast augmentation, and a significant number of potential patients have friends or family members with experience of this procedure. It is common for a patient with a ptotic breast to assume that mere placement of implants will provide an ideal result, or for a patient with chest wall deformity or breast asymmetry to be unaware of their presence. A thorough discussion brings these issues to light.

Another problem arises when a patient compares her breasts with those of another and does not understand some of the anatomic relationships or problems that may be associated with her particular breast anatomy and configuration. The limitations of the procedure, especially for a woman who is relatively small and wants to have large breasts, should be made clear. The patient must be given a realistic appraisal of what can be accomplished. With the development of intraoperative rapid expansion, increased sizes are feasible, but the limitations of available tissue will always be there.

A thorough examination is performed in order to select the appropriate surgical technique. Breast development is variable from patient to patient and largely determines the technique selected and the results of the operation. Analysis of breast mound, shape, and contour and of the underlying bony, muscular, and soft tissue anatomy is critical, especially in patients with unrecognized deformities or asymmetries (Fig. 11-1).

To ensure a proper analysis of the patient, the surgeon must understand the different components that make up the breast and its contour. First, the amount and location of glandular tissue should be assessed. Many patients seeking augmentation mammaplasty, especially after pregnancy, complain about the lack of breast tissue in the superolateral portion of the breast mound.

Next, any potential anatomic differences or variables of the pectoralis major muscle should be evaluated, especially in patients in whom subpectoral or submuscular augmentation is considered. Irregularities or abnormalities of the subcutaneous fat and tissue should also be evaluated at this time. In some patients there are significant differences in the amount of skin between one side and the other, especially after pregnancy and nursing.

The location of the nipple areola-complex with any potential asymmetry, as well as differences in areola or nipple size, should be identified and pointed out to the patient. It is extremely important to make the patient aware of any breast asymmetry or abnormalities (Fig. 11-2).

Many areas may also be overlooked and unsuspected by the surgeon, leading to postsurgical problems and patient dissatisfaction. Among these are unrecognized tight or high inframammary folds, scoliosis, components of the tubular breast, and breast ptosis. The anatomy and location of the inframammary fold is frequently overlooked; this is an important area, especially in a woman with a tight and high inframammary fold who wants a full breast mound. Disruption of the fold can lead to an unsightly result if care is not taken. The tubular breast may be worsened by an augmentation, if it is unsuspected and an incorrect procedure is performed. Also, unrecognized chest wall deformities may be exaggerated after an augmentation mammaplasty, if symmetric implants are put in and the component of the chest wall deformity is unappreciated. Because all these variables can affect the result, a careful examination with these possibilities in mind is crucial to the outcome of surgery and patient satisfaction.

Obviously, preoperative and postoperative pho-

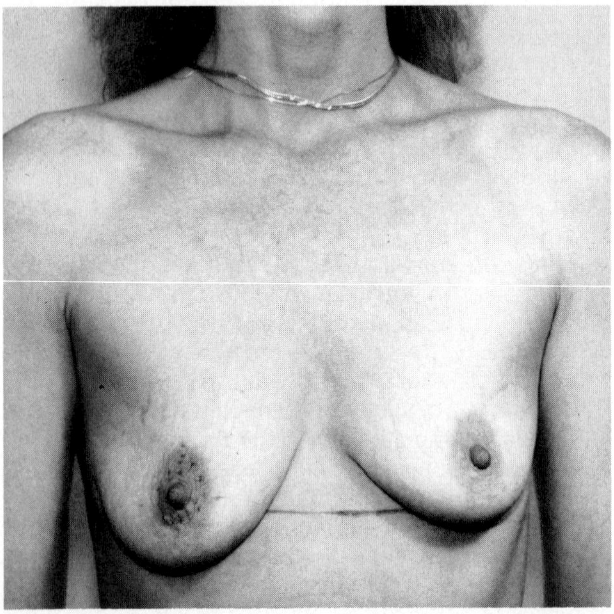

A

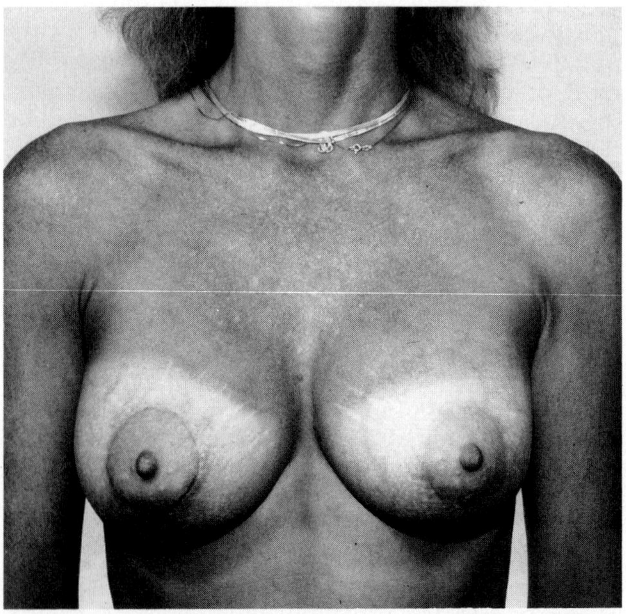

B

FIGURE 11-1 *A*, A 34-year-old patient with breast asymmetry. She was unaware of the significance of the asymmetry and requested a bilateral augmentation mammaplasty. *B*, After a thorough discussion the patient underwent augmentation of the left breast by means of a periareolar incision and a mastopexy with augmentation of the right breast. Even marked asymmetry can be unrecognized by some patients.

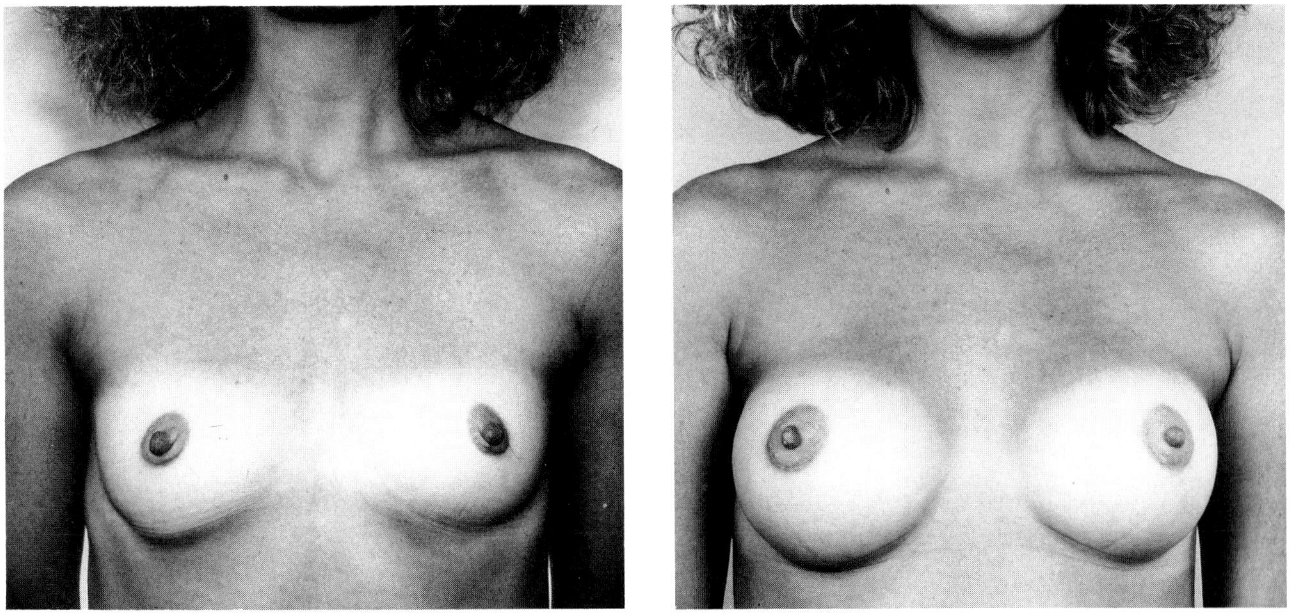

A B

FIGURE 11-2 *A*, A 29-year-old patient with asymmetry of the inframammary folds. Although the difference does not seem great preoperatively, postoperative views after augmentation showed the difference to be more noticeable. *B*, After breast augmentation the distance between the areola and inframammary fold is more exaggerated on the patient's right side. Preoperative views help demonstrate these differences to both patient and surgeon.

tographs are important in the evaluation process for both surgeon and patient. A photograph is often more critical than the eye in evaluating patients. Preoperative views may also demonstrate to the patient the presence of anatomic variations or existing abnormalities (Fig. 11-3).

SELECTION OF INCISION

All plastic surgeons have their own preference as to the location of the incision for augmentation mammaplasty. There are three major approaches: periareolar, inframmamary, and transaxillary. It is not the author's intention to select the "best" approach; this must be determined by each surgeon according to individual preference. Also, with the changes in types of implants used today, especially in view of the textured surfaces, certain surgical approaches are more applicable than others.

Periareolar

In our experience, certain concepts and generalizations can be made about each of the incisions. In the periareolar approach, it is a common experience that the scar should be within the pigmented areola tissue in most individuals, to give a better pigment and color match, and less risk of thick scarring.

In black women it may be more appropriate to stay just outside the areola, depending on the relationship of areola pigmentation with that of the surrounding skin. For example, in the case of an extremely black areola, because the scar will often be lighter, it is best to plan the incision outside the areola in the lighter pigmented skin. For the periareolar incision, care must be taken to preserve the branches of the fourth intercostal nerve.[3]

Inframammary

For the inframammary incision, one should stay just above the inframammary fold to provide a better location of the scar. If the scar is directly at the inframammary fold, there may be some inferior displacement or the scar may be visible in some types of clothing. With the incision in the inframammary fold, the resultant scar may be too low if capsular contracture develops. Staying above the fold is therefore preferable. The inframammary incision can vary from 3 to 5 cm in length, depending on the type of implant used. As a general rule the incision is placed slightly lateral in relationship to the areola, thus preventing a visible scar medial to the vertical plane of the areola. In patients receiving polyurethane or textured silicone implants, the larger incision dimension may be necessary. In the case of polyurethane implants it is critical to place them in the proper position initially, and adequate exposure is necessary.

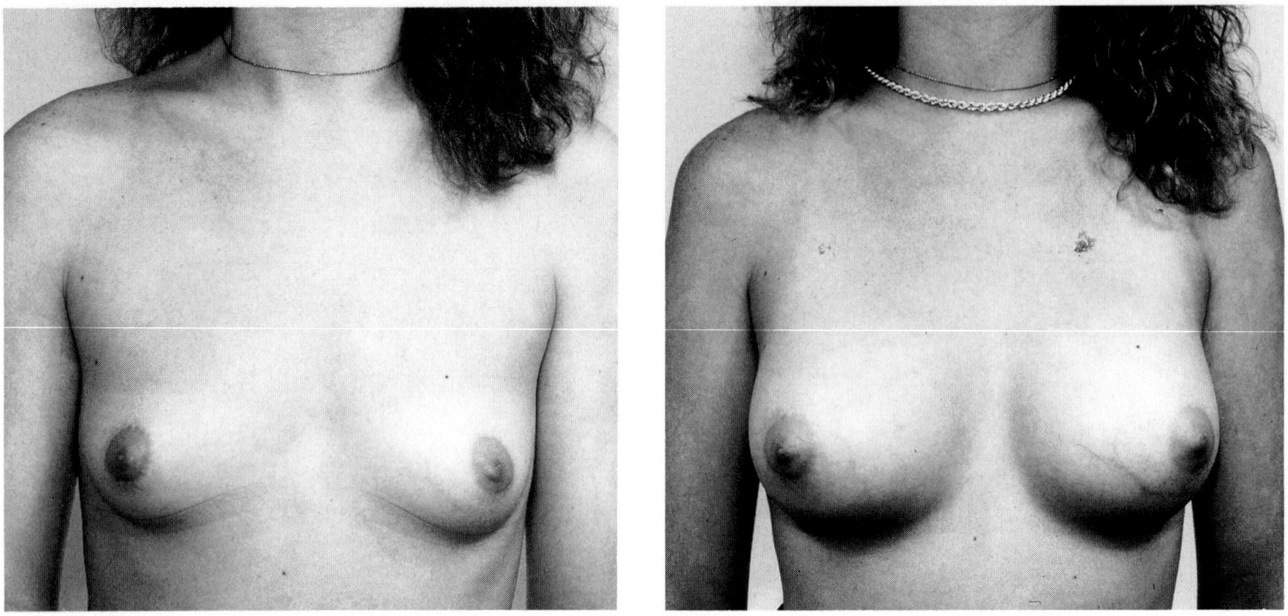

A B

FIGURE 11–3 *A,* A preoperative view of a 23-year-old woman whose areolae are slightly displaced laterally. *B,* Postoperative view demonstrates significant lateralization of the nipple-areola complex (NAC) after breast augmentation. The patient was pleased with the result and not aware of the NAC relationship. These subtle changes are often more detectable in photographs than upon clinical examination.

Transaxillary

The benefits of the axillary incision have been well documented.[4] This procedure places the scar at a distance from the breast mound, with obvious aesthetic benefit. The scar must be positioned in the correct location to give the ideal result.[5] The transaxillary subpectoral augmentation has the combined advantage of an axillary scar with retropectoral location of the prosthesis, which is considered by many to reduce the incidence of capsular contracture with smooth-walled implants. Other benefits of the transaxillary subpectoral augmentation are preservation of nipple sensation; a reported lower incidence of periprosthetic space infection, because contact of the prosthesis with the breast tissue is minimized; and, with smooth-walled implants, a reduced incidence of capsular contracture.[5] However, there are certain situations in which the transaxillary approach is less useful. These include potential difficulties in positioning textured implants, and problems with glandular ptosis and tubular or tuberous breasts, resulting in a "Snoopy" or double-bubble appearance.

Finally, for secondary complications such as capsular contracture, malposition of the implant, or inframammary fold problems, the transaxillary approach may not be feasible, and the inframammary or periareolar approach may be a better choice.

IMPLANT POSITION: SUBGLANDULAR OR SUBMUSCULAR

The issue of subglandular versus submuscular placement of implants is discussed in two separate chapters. However, a thorough discussion of selection of technique for augmentation mammaplasty requires a brief presentation of this topic. There are two primary issues relating to the virtues or drawbacks of submammary as opposed to subpectoral augmentation. The first is aesthetic; the second concerns capsular contracture. The first issue relates to the preoperative appearance of the breast. In the patient with minimal to moderate ptosis, it may be possible to obtain a satisfactory result with a subglandular augmentation, especially with a large implant, while placing it submuscularly (Fig. 11–4). However, the patient with essentially no breast tissue, in whom an implant outline may be noticed in the subcutaneous position, may be better served with an implant in the subpectoral plane. Thus, the location of the implant may be determined by the anatomic site that provides the best breast contour, aside from the issue of capsular contracture.

A patient who desires to continue a strenuous exercise program must understand that subpectoral placement of an implant may cause noticeable changes during exercise. She needs to be aware of the appearance of the subpectoral implant and the

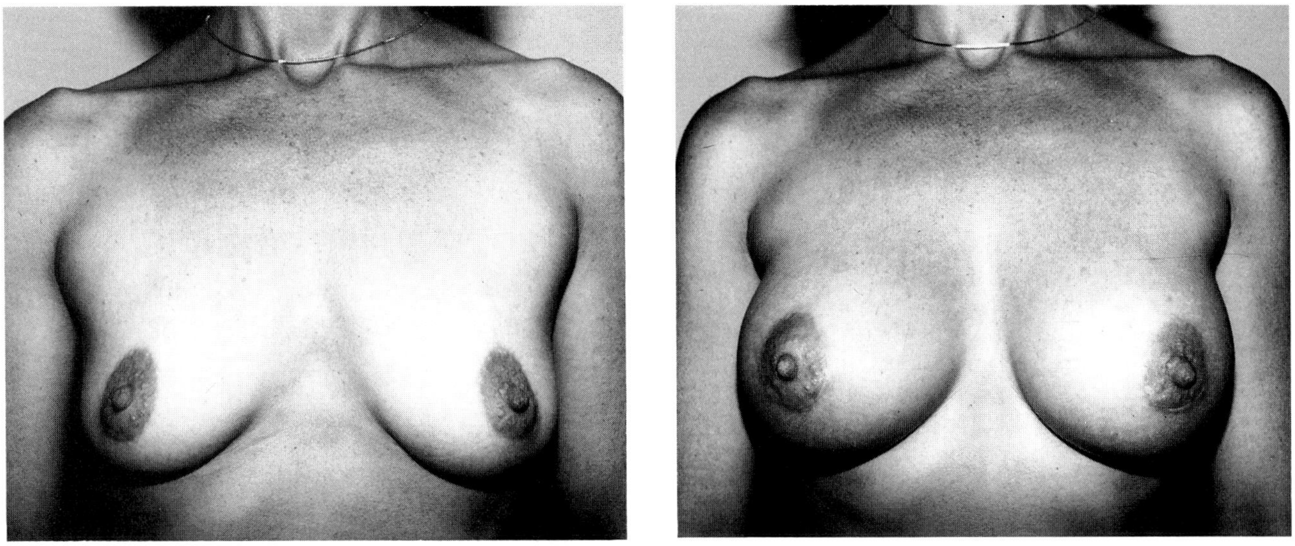

A B

FIGURE 11-4 *A,* A 39-year-old patient with glandular ptosis. *B,* Placement of implants in the subglandular space improves the relationship of the nipple-areola complex to the breast mound. Submuscular placement in this patient may not have been ideal.

possibility of distortion during muscular contracture. One area that should be obvious is the avoidance of total submuscular coverage in a patient with minimal to moderate ptosis in whom the breast tissue will roll off the implanted submuscular mound, leading to the obvious "Snoopy" deformity. The pros and cons of subpectoral versus submammary augmentation will be further discussed later. With smooth-walled implants, many surgeons have noticed a significant decrease in capsular contracture when implants are placed submuscularly.[6-8] However, with the development of the textured implants, both silicone and polyurethane, this issue may be less clear-cut. It has been shown that in patients with polyurethane implants the capsular contracture rate is low regardless of whether submuscular or subglandular placement is used.[8,9]

The decision whether to place the implant submuscularly or subglandularly in primary augmentation may be based on the best anatomic site for the patient in relation to aesthetic appearance and not necessarily to the capsular contracture rate. Subglandular placement may be best in patients who have a degree of ptosis, who have adequate tissue, and who are concerned about their appearance during exercise. However, a patient who is thin, nonptotic, and not athletic may be best suited with submuscular placement of the implant. Finally, in a patient with adequate breast tissue and no ptosis, either anatomic site is appropriate for the resultant aesthetic appearance.

Many of the issues concerning placement of the implant, whether submuscular or subglandular, may be less critical as more experience and knowledge is gained about textured implants, and the anatomic location may be based primarily on aesthetics rather than on any concepts of capsular contracture.

SELECTION OF IMPLANT

Just as the choice of surgical procedure requires a knowledge of the individual approach appropriate for the patient, so does the choice of implant. Implants vary in relation not only to their projection, but also to their base diameter. Attempts to place an implant with a significantly greater base diameter than the available space on the chest wall, especially in the case of polyurethane implants, can lead to obvious problems of wrinkling and folds.

Many implant types are available to the plastic surgeon today. They vary not only in contour and shape, but also in surface. Both smooth-walled and textured silicone surfaces are available, as well as polyurethane-covered silicone implants. The implants themselves can be filled with either saline or silicone gel.

In selecting the implant it is important to be aware of both the dimensions of the prosthesis and the volume. There is a tendency to oversimplify and look only at implant volume. It is obvious that implants are available in different width to height and projection ratios, and varying the type of implant may be important in patient management. A broad-based style of implant may be more appropriate in correcting a specific problem such as a tubular breast. This exemplifies how measurement of the base diameter of the breast is important in helping to select the proper implant. It is critical for the surgeon to become familiar with the subtleties of the implants, especially the base diameter.

The final selection of proper implant size and contour is best made on the operating table. It is our practice, after making the appropriate pocket through the incision that has been selected, to insert several different types of temporary implants and place the patient in the upright position. No single preoperative procedure can provide the same quality of result as this intraoperative decision-making process. Subtle differences or abnormalities that may not have been noticed preoperatively become apparent at this stage.

One dilemma relates to the choice of implant size. It is not unusual for a patient to say "don't make me too large," only to wish postoperatively that a larger implant had been used.

Becker demonstrated a significant incidence of patient dissatisfaction with implant size.[10] Of his patients with inflatable implants, 50 percent desired a larger volume than predicted preoperatively. Adjustable implants have the benefit of size modification in the postsurgical period, and for this reason may gain wider acceptance.

ADJUNCTIVE SURGICAL OPTIONS

The simplest procedure that can give the patient the desired result is the best. Often, however, the goals of the patient and of the surgeon may require additional measures to give the ideal result. This is where adjunctive procedures play an important role in augmentation mammaplasty. Four such procedures are (1) intraoperative expansion, (2) use of adjustable implants, (3) rotating or stacking polyurethane implants, and (4) altering the inframammary fold.

In a patient with tight skin and tissue, immediate intraoperative expansion has been found to be a very useful procedure (Fig. 11–5). After the appropriate pocket is created a temporary implant is inserted,

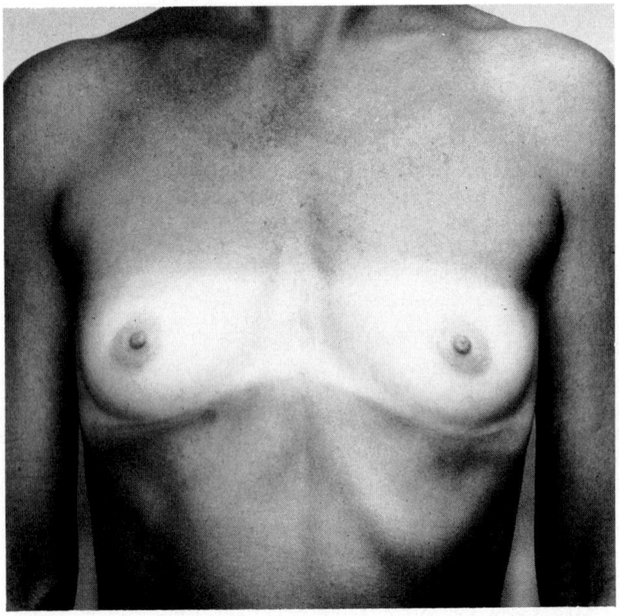

A

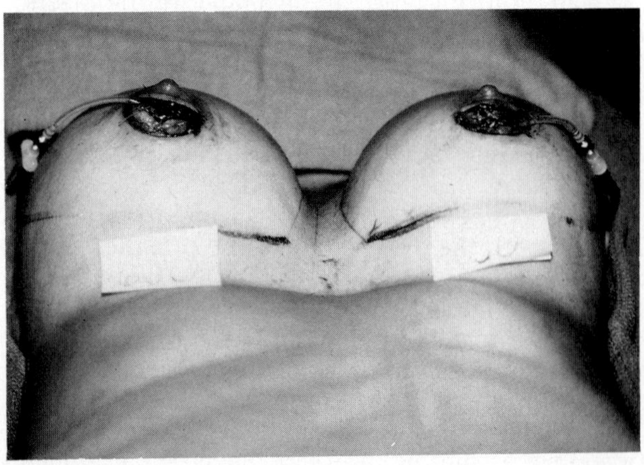

B

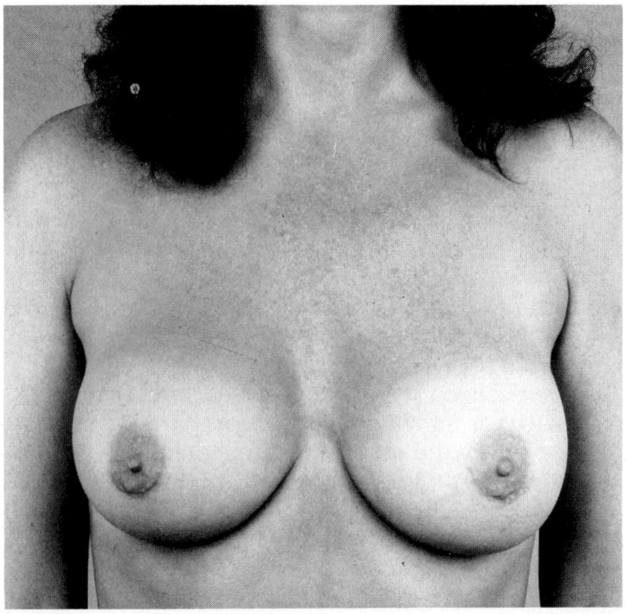

C

FIGURE 11–5 *A*, A 24-year-old patient with minimal breast tissue who desired large breast implants. *B*, Subglandular pockets were created through periaerolar incisions. Initially, 250-ml implants were inserted with difficulty. Tissue expanders were inserted into the subglandular pockets and filled to 650 ml for several minutes and three cycles. *C*, Final implants of 350 ml were inserted without difficulty, and the patient is seen 3 years after breast augmentation.

and tightness documented. Temporary tissue expanders are then placed and inflated, usually to 500 to 700 ml. We use a three-way stopcock and expand with air; avoiding the need for saline. Typically a 50 to 100 percent increase in breast implant size is obtainable with this technique.

In selected patients, adjustable implants can be another useful tool in breast augmentation. Advantages of the expandable mammary implant include the ability to alter the size of one or both breasts. This offers obvious benefits in dealing with asymmetry, and may also be useful in improving contour in patients with tubular breasts.[11]

Another adjunctive procedure involves rotation or stacking of polyurethane implants. It is possible to rotate or stack these in such a way that the area of maximal projection of the implants can compensate for either a deformity or an abnormality of the chest wall or breast tissue.

The fourth adjunctive procedure relates to the

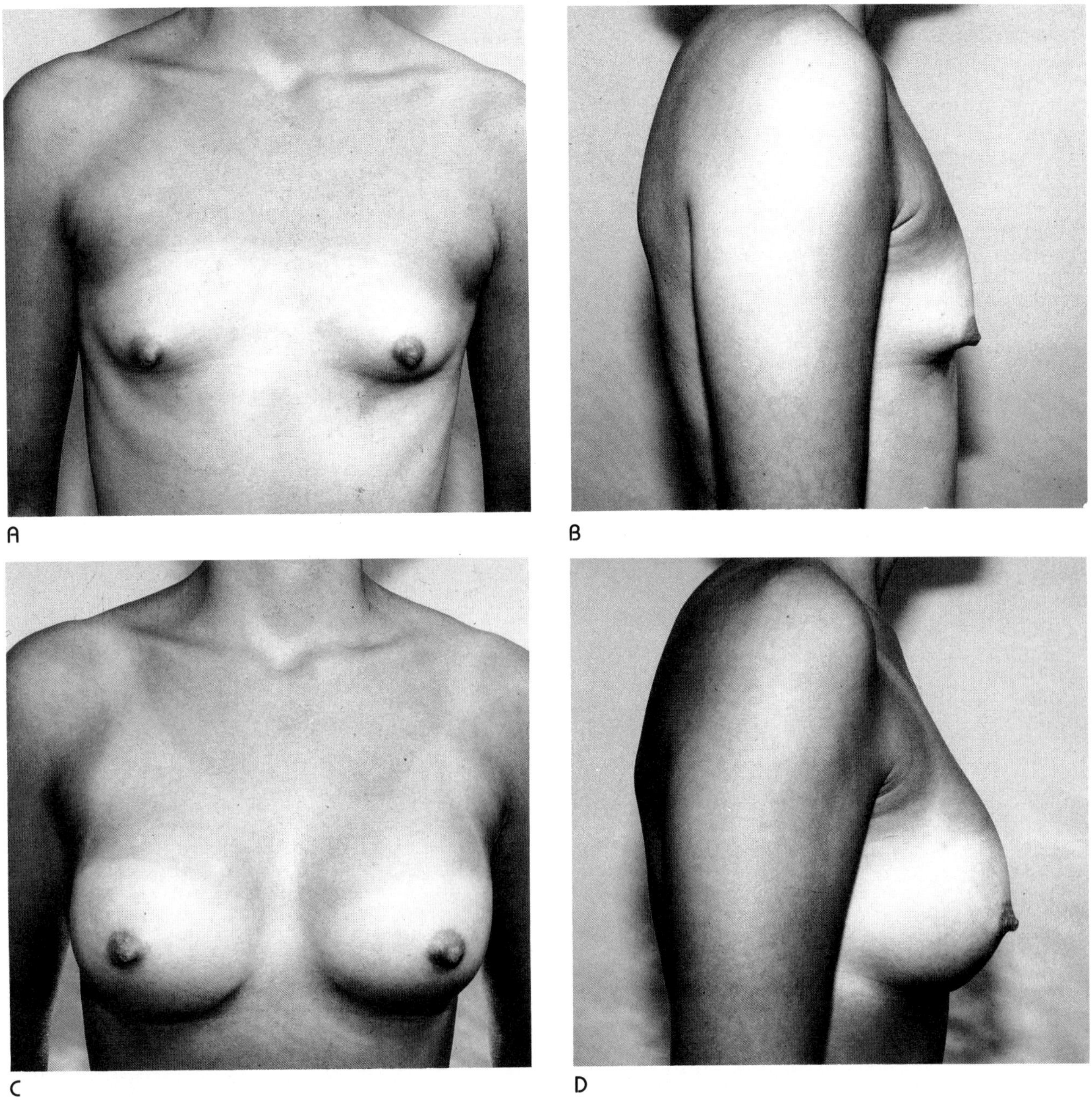

FIGURE 11-6 *A, B,* A 27-year-old patient with high, tight inframammary folds with minimal breast tissue. Approximately 5 cm below the areola, the proposed inframammary folds were marked and incisions made slightly above this line. Radial incisions were made in lower breast tissue to release the fold. *C, D,* Appearance of the patient after augmentation with low-profile 310-ml polyurethane implants.

inframammary fold. In selected patients, lowering or altering of the inframammary fold is an important part of the procedure. Preoperative recognition of the patient with a high, tight fold is critical to avoid problems (Fig. 11-6). Physical examination and photography before surgery, and intraoperative assessment with implants in place and the patient upright, are all crucial factors in properly managing such patients.

CONCLUSION

It is important for the surgeon not to consider breast augmentation a repetitive or blueprint procedure to be methodically performed in the same way in every patient. An individualized analysis of the patient, including her wishes and anatomic configuration, is important in formulating the proper procedure. The procedure clearly differs from patient to patient with regard to the location of the incision, the type of implant used, and the anatomic site selected. Therefore, an honest appraisal must be made of the patient's goals in order to ensure proper selection of the surgical procedure.

References

1. Dupont WD, Page DL. Risk factors for breast cancer in women with proliferative breast disease. N Engl J Med. 1985; 312:146.
2. Cole NM. Informed consent: Considerations in aesthetic and reconstructive surgery of the breast. Clin Plast Surg 1988; 15:541.
3. Farina MA, Newby BG, Alani HM. Innervation of the nipple-areola complex. Plast Reconstr Surg. 1980; 66:497.
4. Tebbetts JB. Transaxillary subpectoral augmentation mammaplasty: Long-term follow-up and refinements. Plast Reconstr Surg 1984; 74:636.
5. Tebbets B. Transaxillary subpectoral augmentation mammaplasty: A 9-year experience. Clin Plast Surg 1988; 15:557.
6. Biggs TM, Yarish RS. Augmentation mammaplasty: Retropectoral versus retromammary implantation. Clin Plast Surg 1988; 15:549.
7. Puckett CL, Croll GH, Reichel CA, et al. A critical look at capsule contracture in subglandular versus subpectoral mammary augmentation. Aesthetic Plast Surg 1987; 11:23.
8. Vazquez B, Given KS, Houston GC. Breast augmentation: A review of subglandular and submuscular implantation. Aesthetic Plast Surg 1987; 11:101.
9. Hester T Jr, Nahai F, Bostwick J, Cukic J. A 5-year experience with polyurethane-covered mammary prostheses for treatment of capsular contracture, primary augmentation mammaplasty, and breast reconstruction. 1988; 15:569.
10. Becker H. Expansion augmentation. Clin Plast Surg 1988; 15:587.
11. Becker H. Breast augmentation using the expander mammary prosthesis. Plast Reconstr Surg 1987; 79:192.

CHAPTER 12

Subglandular Augmentation Mammaplasty with Polyurethane-Covered Implants

T. RODERICK HESTER, JR. M.D.

In the early years of augmentation mammaplasty, the vast majority of prostheses were placed in the subglandular position. However, the extent of the problem of capsular contracture associated with smooth-walled silicone mammary implants placed in the subglandular position after augmentation mammaplasty or in the subcutaneous position after breast reconstruction, has now been well documented.[1,2] Up to 75 percent of patients undergoing such procedures have been reported to develop clinically significant contracture. Beginning in the late 1970s, reports of lowered contracture rates when smooth-walled silicone prostheses were placed in the submuscular position[3-11] resulted in an enthusiasm for that approach by many surgeons, including this author. However, despite these favorable reports, there are two problems with submuscularly placed, smooth-walled implants that have not been addressed adequately by the plastic surgery community. First, it is becoming increasingly apparent that the rate of occurrence of clinically significant capsular contracture with submuscular placement of smooth-walled silicone mammary prostheses increases significantly if patients are followed for 5 or more years after surgery.[12-15] Second, there are anatomic situations in which subglandular placement of a mammary prosthesis represents a distinct aesthetic advantage over placement in the submuscular space.

Unlike the smooth-walled silicone implant, the polyurethane-covered mammary prosthesis does not require submuscular placement to lower capsular contracture rates.[15,16] This important fact allows the surgeon to place polyurethane-covered prostheses in the anatomic space best suited to the patient.

The polyurethane-covered mammary prosthesis was introduced by Ashley in 1970.[17,18] Although his reports of very low capsular contracture rates generated some interest, the implant remained controversial and not widely used throughout the 1970s. In the early 1980s, technical improvements in manufacture of the foam and silicone center of the implant were accomplished, evolving to the modern Meme and Replicon varieties of the prosthesis.* Since 1982 a growing number of plastic surgeons have used the polyurethane-covered implant as the magnitude of the capsular contracture problem associated with the use of smooth-walled prostheses has become more apparent. Reports of up to 6 years' experience with modern versions of polyurethane-covered im-

*Surgitek Medical Engineering Corporation, 3003 Rollie Gates Drive, Paso Robles, CA 93446.

plants have been consistent in reporting low capsular contracture rates following their use.[15,16,19-25] Also, results from the increasingly large clinical experience have shown no evidence that polyurethane of the type used in modern mammary implants represents a danger to the patient in terms of carcinogenicity or toxicity.[15]

The Meme and Replicon implants are the updated versions of the original Ashley prosthesis, and according to the manufacturer they incorporate improvements in foam texturing and stability. Also, a thicker gel is now used that allows shaping for projection without the need for the stiff internal septum used in the earlier implants.

Polyurethane foam appears to work by inhibiting the occurrence of circumferential concentric fibrosis characteristic of the capsule around standard smooth-walled silicone implants. The histologic response of the tissue to polyurethane is characterized by deposition of collagen in a diffuse and sporadic manner around the interconnecting strands of the polyurethane foam, resulting in dispersion of the vectors of contracture.[15,26]

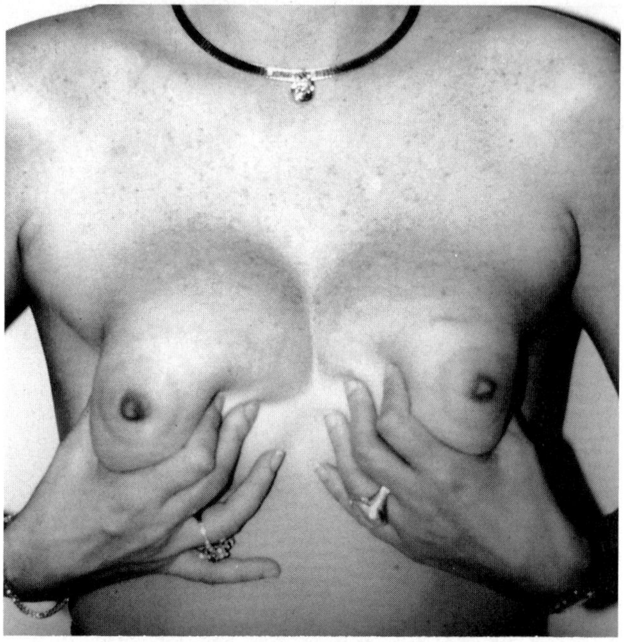

FIGURE 12-1 Appearance 30 months after subglandular augmentation with 325-ml Replicon implants. Class I breast compressibility is demonstrated.

CLINICAL EXPERIENCE

Definition of Capsular Contracture with Polyurethane-covered Prostheses

As previously reported,[15,16] a simplified three-class system is used to describe capsular contracture as it occurs when polyurethane-covered prostheses are used for augmentation mammaplasty. This system, described in Table 12-1, is based on digital implant compressibility between the thumb and digits.

Figure 12-1 is illustrative of patients with Class I breasts after augmentation mammaplasty with polyurethane-covered implants. The implants are totally compressible between the thumb and digits without any perception of firmness by either patient or surgeon.

Patients with Class II resistance to implant compression do not perceive significant firmness, and surgical intervention is rarely indicated. Patients with Class III resistance to implant compression have obviously firm breasts and require surgical intervention for correction.

TABLE 12-1 Classification of Breast Compressibility with Polyurethane-covered Mammary Implants Using Digital Pressure

Class I	No resistance to implant compression (0-2 cm)
Class II	Minimal resistance to implant compression (2-4 cm)
Class III	Significant resistance to implant compression (>4 cm)

Patient Experience: Submuscular versus Subglandular Placement of Polyurethane-covered Implants

In the past 6 years 1,076 implants were placed in 568 patients for augmentation mammaplasty. Adequate follow-up was available in 72 percent of patients. Twenty-six percent of prostheses were placed in subglandular pockets and 74 percent in partially submuscular pockets.

A summary of capsular contracture data related to prosthesis site placement gleaned from review of this group is presented in Tables 12-2 and 12-3. As seen in Table 12-2, the overall rate of occurrence of capsular contracture was 4.8 percent for Class II and 0.4 percent for Class III. Table 12-3 shows that there was no difference in capsular contracture rate of either the Class II or III variety related to implant site.

Approximately two thirds of the prostheses were placed in the partially submuscular space. The

TABLE 12-2 Augmentation Mammaplasty with Polyurethane-covered Mammary Implants: 6-Year Experience

Occurence of Capsular Contracture	
Class II	52 (4.8%)
Class III	4 (0.4%)
Revisions	6 (0.6%)

TABLE 12–3 Augmentation Mammaplasty with Polyurethane-covered Mammary Implants: 6-Year Experience

Occurrence of Capsular Contracture Related to Implant Site		
Class II Contracture		
Subglandular	15/280	(5.3%)
Submuscular	37/796	(4.6%)
Class III Contracture		
Subglandular	1/280	(0.4%)
Submuscular	3/796	(0.4%)

preponderance of implants placed in the submuscular space was due partially to the author's belief that this approach protected the patient from capsular contracture. However, it soon became apparent that there was no significant difference in contracture rates with polyurethane-covered prostheses placed in either the submuscular or subglandular position. This principle has been confirmed in the overall 6-year experience summarized in Table 12–3. Unlike the smooth-walled silicone prosthesis, the ability of the polyurethane-covered prosthesis to resist capsular contracture in the subglandular as well as the submuscular pocket has allowed use of the approach best suited to the individual aesthetic needs of the patient.

The author has published guidelines used to help in deciding whether to place polyurethane-covered implants in the submuscular or subglandular space. These are summarized in Table 12–4.

Tissue Thickness

Patients who are thin, with very little glandular tissue and subcutaneous fat in the upper pole of the breast, generally have a perceptibly better aesthetic result with at least partial submuscular implant placement. This is true because of the benefit thin patients derive from the presence of the pectoralis major over the upper pole of the implant, resulting in more natural contour and texture as healing occurs.

In patients with a more reasonable thickness of fat and glandular tissue (especially in the supra-areolar area), the subglandular space can be chosen for implant placement with confidence if a polyurethane-covered prosthesis is being used. With adequate tissue thickness, excellent aesthetic results will accrue with subglandular or submuscular placement, and the choice of space in this group of patients depends on the surgeon's prejudices and the patient's wishes.

TABLE 12–4 Factors Considered in Choosing Site for Placement of Polyurethane-covered Prostheses

Subglandular Placement of Polyurethane-covered Implants	1. Sufficient gland and subcutaneous fat 2. Ptosis 3. Athletically active patient
Submuscular Placement of Polyurethane-covered Implants	1. Insufficient gland and subcutaneous fat 2. No ptosis 3. Athletically inactive patient

Ptosis

In the presence of ptosis of any degree, implant placement in the subglandular space is generally preferred. In this anatomic setting, submuscular placement of the prosthesis often results in prolonged to permanent unattractive supra-areolar fullness, especially if a mastopexy is not performed. Also, when there is ptosis, the unattractive distortion of the breast with flexion of the pectoralis major is often magnified.

The degree of ptosis is important in deciding whether or not a mastopexy is required. If the nipple is level with or no lower than 2 cm below the inframammary fold, a generous-sized implant in the subglandular space will lift the breast sufficiently that acceptable contours accrue and a formal mastopexy can be avoided. As the nipple falls farther below the inframammary crease, a mastopexy is more likely to be needed to achieve acceptable form. However, a distinct advantage of subglandular implant placement is that greater degrees of ptosis can be corrected without mastopexy with contours acceptable to the patient than can be done with similar-sized implants placed in the submuscular position.

At this point a note of caution is in order. In patients with the severest degrees of ptosis and in whom the nipple-areola will be elevated 8 to 10 cm or more, the author places the implant in the submuscular position. In this anatomic setting, the combined release of the nipple-areola complex to allow adequate elevation and the division of chest wall muscular perforating blood vessels necessary for subglandular prosthesis placement could result in vascular compromise of the central breast cone and nipple-areola. Furthermore, in very thin patients with severest degrees of glandular involution, one might choose the partially submuscular pocket and carry out the necessary skin envelope modification in order to obtain more soft tissue coverage of the prosthesis.

Athletic Activity

Patients who engage in vigorous physical activity on a regular basis are theoretically better served by subglandular prosthesis placement. Subglandular placement avoids the unpleasant distortion of the upper breast that can occur with pectoralis flexion in such activities as swimming, tennis, and weight lifting.

The patient in Figure 12–2 has polyurethane-covered implants in the submuscular position. She was very active athletically and was disturbed by the breast distortion that occurred with pectoralis major flexion as illustrated. The problem was corrected by replacement of the prostheses in the subglandular space with resuturing of the pectoralis major to the chest wall.

However, as a practical matter, the minimal distortion that occurs with pectoralis major flexion in most patients without ptosis is not significant. Certainly many patients with submuscular implants engage in many forms of athletic activity without significant problems. However, if a patient is active athletically and has sufficient glandular tissue and subcutaneous fat, the author prefers to place the implant in the subglandular position.

A special case is the female weight lifter who desires augmentation. These patients have minimal subcutaneous fat and often glandular atrophy. They also have strenuous objections to submuscular placement of the prosthesis. In this setting the author prefers a smaller (180 to 250 ml) Meme implant placed in the subglandular space. The Meme is chosen over the Replicon because one is less likely to be able to palpate the edge of the implant after healing. The patient is warned, however, that because of the thin cover of tissue over the implant, some compromise in breast shape and texture may occur and that she may be able to palpate the peripheral edge of the prosthesis.

TECHNIQUE

Preoperative Evaluation

All patients requesting augmentation mammaplasty should be completely informed about the potential negative sequelae of the procedure. Important items to be covered in the informed consent discussion should include the topics of capsular contracture, decreased sensitivity of skin and nipple, and infection. Also, concerns regarding breast physical examination and mammography with breast implants in place make it important that the patient have yearly examinations by the plastic surgeon, and that any indicated mammography take place in a unit familiar with the implant compression technique.

Anatomic evaluation should include careful examination of the breasts to rule out significant breast pathology and to make careful note of the levels of inframammary folds and any degree of asymmetry. The amount of glandular tissue and subcutaneous fat and any degree of ptosis is noted. After considering the important anatomic factors mentioned, one may choose the subglandular space as best suited to a

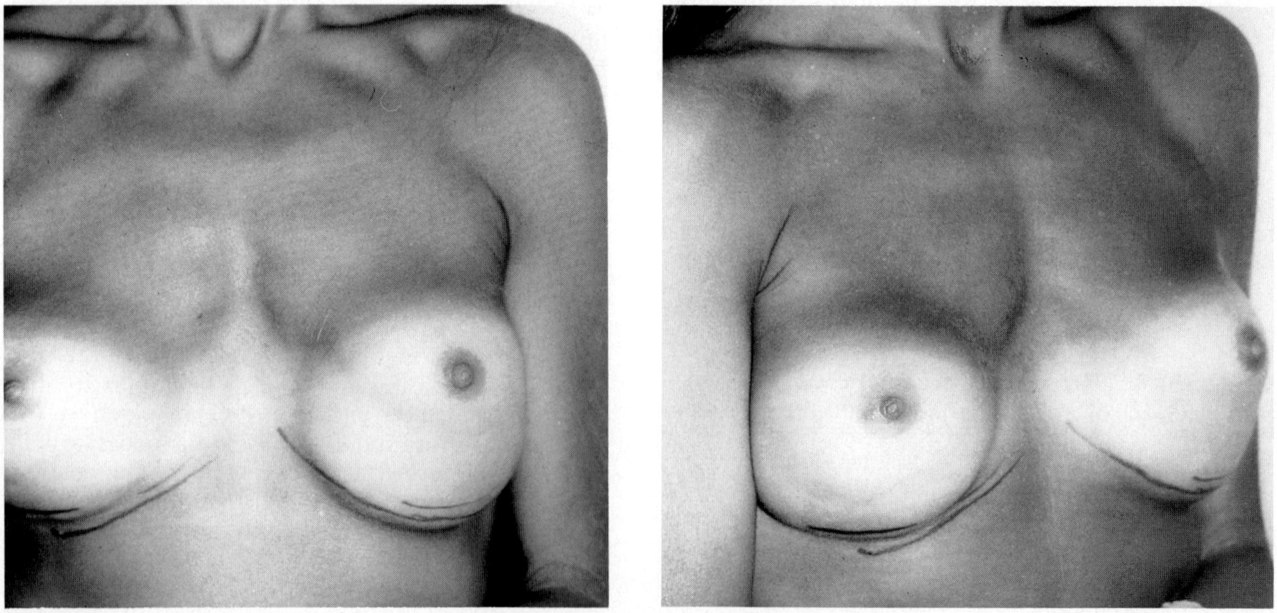

A B

FIGURE 12–2 *A, B,* Distortion of the breast with pectoralis flexion after submuscular augmentation mammaplasty. Preoperative markings indicate the proposed location of the implants with conversion to a submammary position.

given patient. In the author's opinion, a polyurethane-covered prosthesis should be used if the subglandular space is chosen.

Choice of Implant

For augmentations requiring a prosthesis size of up to 250 ml, the Meme implant is usually selected. For augmentations requiring larger implants, the Replicon is generally used because of its narrower base diameter and greater forward projection. The ideal size of implant for an individual patient depends on chest wall dimensions and the availability of mammary skin.

Incision

An incision 5 to 6 cm in length is ideal for polyurethane-covered implants, although shorter incisions can be made as the surgeon gains experience. The inframammary approach has been used most often by the author, but the infra-areolar and axillary approaches can be employed by surgeons experienced in the techniques of insertion of polyurethane-covered implants (Fig. 12–3).

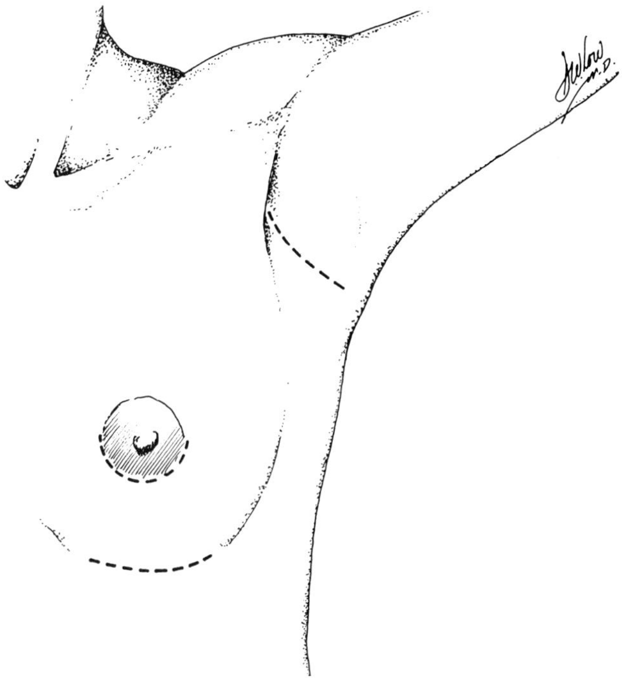

FIGURE 12–3 Although the inframammary incision is the one most frequently used, polyurethane implants may be introduced through infra-areolar or axillary incisions.

Pocket Dissection

Dissection of the pocket begins at the inframammary fold and extends superiorly, medially, and laterally. Superior dissection should extend to a point 2

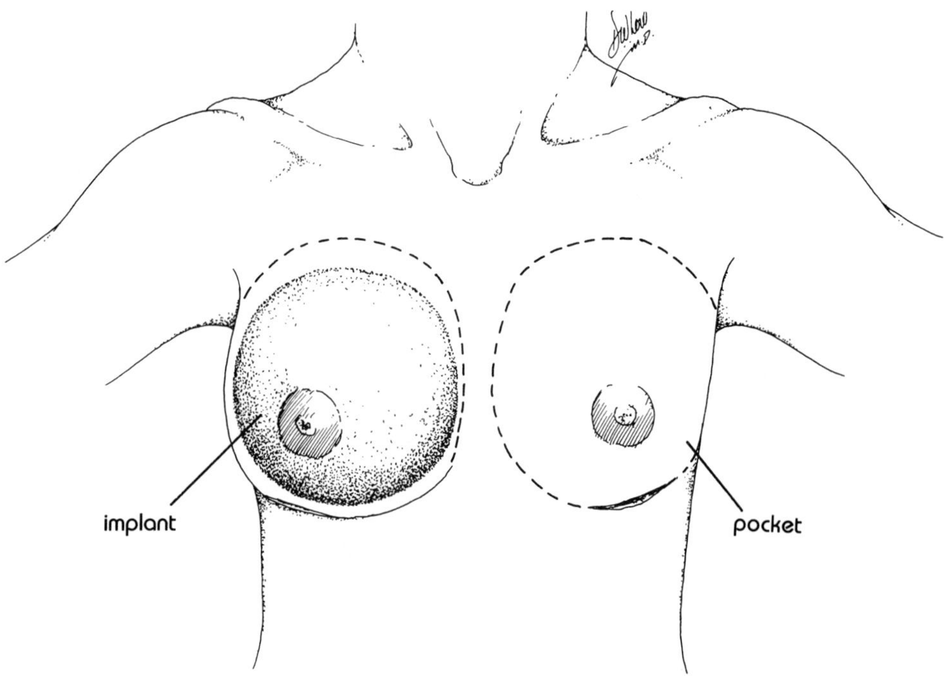

FIGURE 12–4 The submammary pocket should be slightly larger than the dimensions of the implant to prevent buckling or wrinkling of the implant.

to 4 cm beneath the clavicle, depending on the base dimensions of the implant chosen. Medially, the dissection extends to the lateral sternal border. Overzealous medial dissection can result in symmastia or palpation of the implant edge under the very thin skin directly overlying the body of the sternum. The lateral dissection should extend to the lateral border of the pectoralis major, or slightly farther if a larger implant is to be used. Finally, the dimensions of the pocket should be slightly larger than those of the implant, to permit atraumatic placement of the prosthesis without buckling or wrinkling (Fig. 12–4).

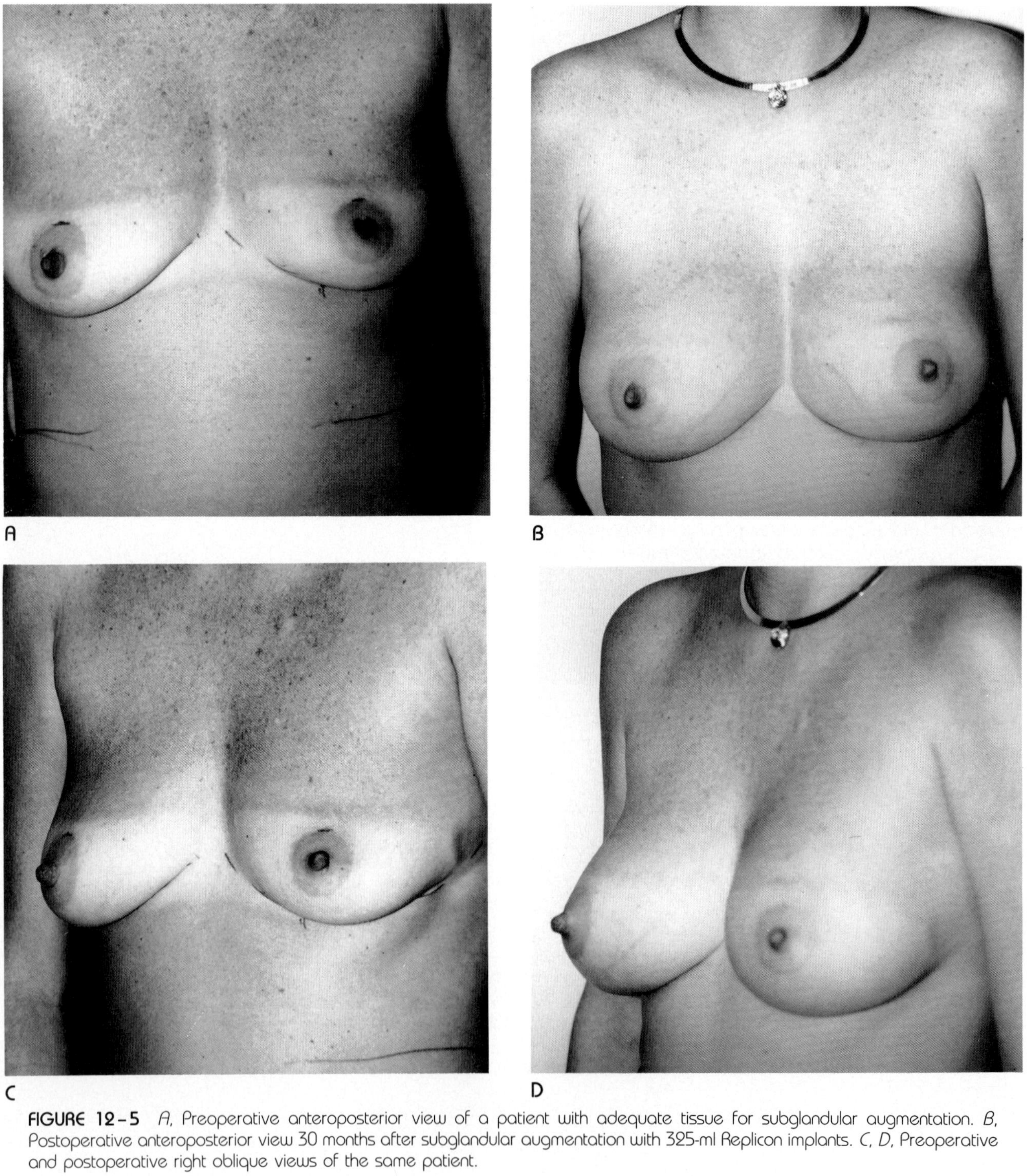

FIGURE 12–5 *A*, Preoperative anteroposterior view of a patient with adequate tissue for subglandular augmentation. *B*, Postoperative anteroposterior view 30 months after subglandular augmentation with 325-ml Replicon implants. *C*, *D*, Preoperative and postoperative right oblique views of the same patient.

Implant Insertion

After adequate pocket dissection, the implant is inserted by gentle digital pressure, with or without a Silastic sleeve. It is important that the implant lie perfectly flat in the pocket to prevent buckling and wrinkles, which might be palpated through the skin later. Proper implant placement is ensured by digital palpation and smoothing of both the posterior and anterior surfaces of the prosthesis.

Results

As noted previously, results in terms of very low rates of capsular contracture through at least 6 years can be expected when polyurethane-covered implants are used for subglandular augmentation mammaplasty. The patients described below illustrate the excellent aesthetic results to be expected.

Figure 12–5 is illustrative of a standard patient with adequate subcutaneous fat and glandular tissue who is an excellent candidate for subglandular augmentation with polyurethane-covered implants.

Figure 12–6 illustrates the patient with minimal ptosis and postpartum glandular involution who can expect excellent results without mastopexy with subglandular polyurethane-covered implants.

The patient in Figure 12–7 had a more severe degree of ptosis and was treated with mastopexy and augmentation. She maintained excellent contours and supra-areolar fullness 3 years after surgery.

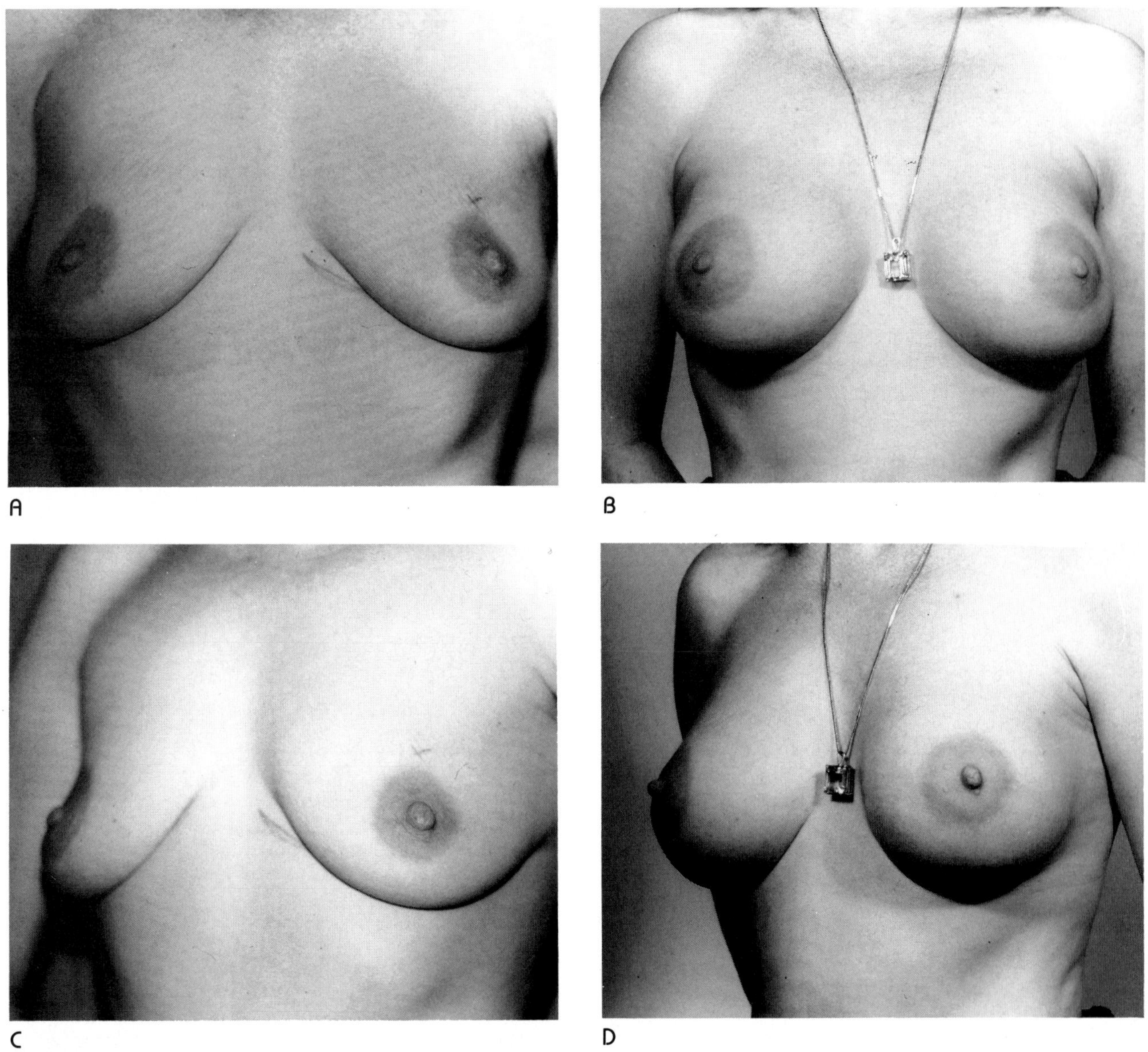

FIGURE 12–6 *A*, Preoperative anteroposterior view of a patient with mild ptosis. *B*, Postoperative anteroposterior view 18 months after subglandular augmentation with 325-ml Replicon implants. *C*, *D*, Preoperative and postoperative right oblique views of the same patient.

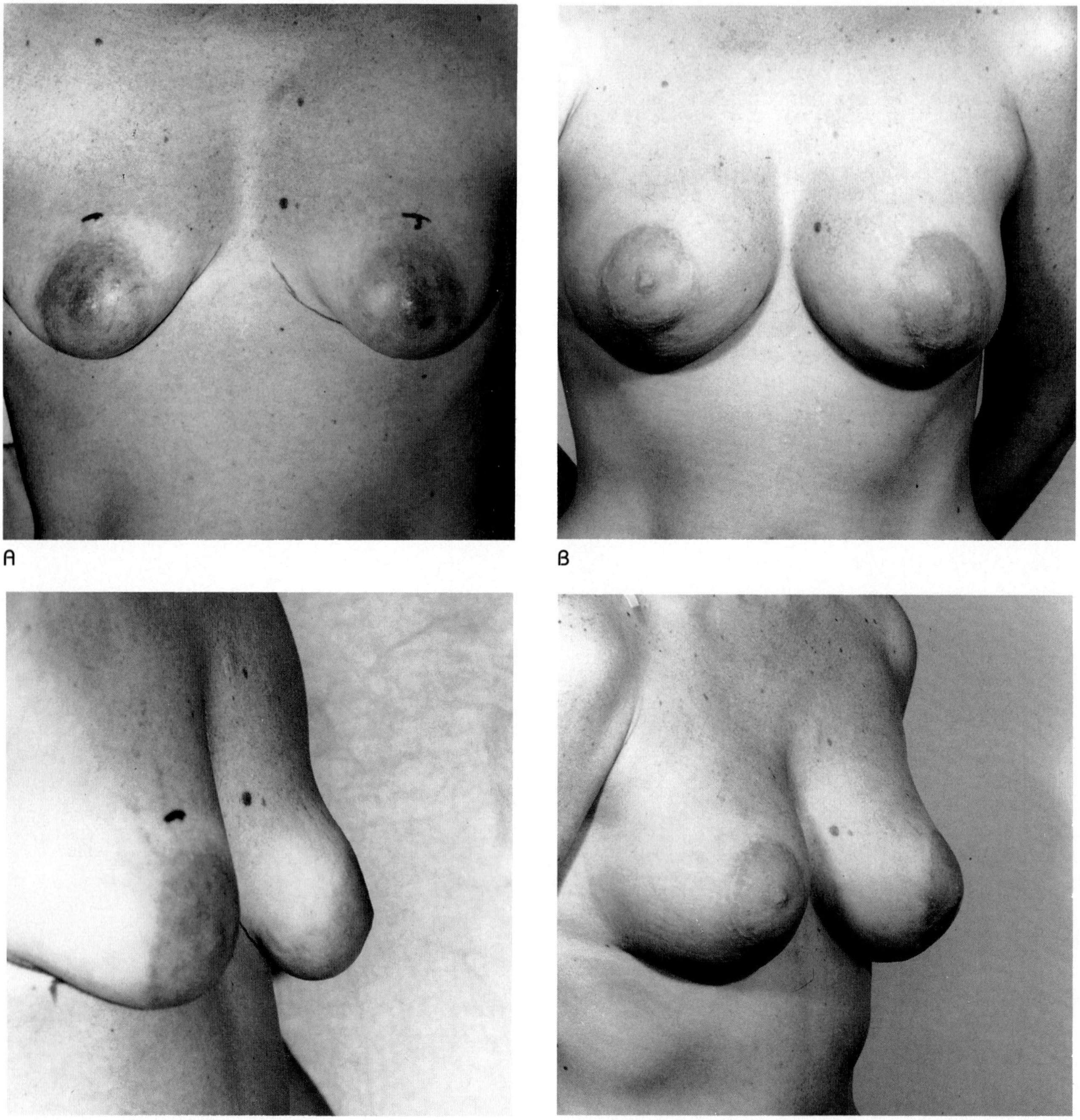

A B C D

FIGURE 12–7 *A*, Preoperative anteroposterior view of a patient with ptosis. An augmentation mastopexy is planned and the new nipple location is marked. *B*, Postoperative anteroposterior view 3 years after mastopexy and subglandular augmentation with 295-ml Replicon implants. *C*, *D*, Preoperative and postoperative left oblique views of the same patient.

COMPLICATIONS

Infection

Infection from polyurethane-covered prostheses used for augmentation mammaplasty is distinctly rare. The very rare severe periprosthetic infection requires implant removal, which should be done as soon as the diagnosis is made, before significant implant-tissue bonding has occurred. Antibiotic prophylaxis includes preoperative administration of a cephalosporin and 3 days oral use after surgery. The implant pocket is also irrigated with Neosporin G.U. Irrigant before prosthesis placement.

Cutaneous Rash

A patchy, erythematous rash rarely occurs in very thin patients. The rash can be differentiated from infection by the lack of systemic signs and itching. Usually the eruption occurs on the third to fifth postoperative day and can persist for 7 to 10 days. Symptoms of itching are controlled by topical corticosteroid cream applications. Occasionally systemic corticosteroids may be necessary.

Hematoma

Hematoma is rare but should be treated by open surgical evacuation, including temporary removal of the prosthesis. Cleansing of the fibrin and clot material from the surface of the implant must be done before replacement. In the author's experience, remnants of the hematoma left in the periprosthetic space represent a distinctly increased risk of capsular contracture.

Implant Malposition

It is important that polyurethane-covered mammary implants be placed accurately in relation to the inframammary fold and other anatomic markers. Because of the high friction coefficient between the implant surface and surrounding tissue and early tissue bonding with the prosthesis, one cannot expect spontaneous correction of any significant degree of implant misplacement. The correction of significant implant malposition with polyurethane-covered mammary prostheses usually requires open adjustment of implant position, and should be done in the first 7 to 10 days after insertion before tissue bonding complicates the situation further.

CONCLUSION

Compared with smooth-walled implants, the polyurethane-covered mammary prosthesis offers the patient the distinct advantage of low capsular contracture rates when placed in the subglandular space. Awareness of this allows the surgeon the option of subglandular placement in patients in whom this technique represents an aesthetic advantage.

References

1. Imber G, Schwager RG, Guthrie RH, Gray GF. Fibrous capsule formation after subcutaneous implantation of synthetic materials in experimental animals. Plast Reconstr Surg 1974; 54:183.
2. McGrath MH, Burkhardt BR. The safety and efficacy of breast implants for augmentation mammaplasty. Plast Reconstr Surg 1984; 74:550.
3. Jarret JR, Cutler RG, Teal DF. Aesthetic refinements in prophylactic subcutaneous mastectomy with submuscular reconstruction. Plast Reconstr Surg 1982; 69:624.
4. Dalton EW, Silverstein P, and Kelly JM. Subcutaneous mastectomy by extended peri-areolar incisions. Am J Surg 1978; 136:719.
5. Woods JE, Irons GB, Arnold PG. The case for submuscular implantation of prosthesis in reconstructive breast surgery. Ann Plast Surg 1980; 5:115.
6. Pickrell KL, Puckett CL, Given KS. Subpectoral augmentation mammaplasty. Plast Reconstr Surg 1977; 60:325.
7. Truppman ES, Ellenby JD. A 13-year evaluation of subpectoral augmentation mammaplasty. In: Owsley JQ Jr, Peterson RA, eds. Symposium of aesthetic surgery of the breast. St Louis: CV Mosby, 1978:293–298.
8. Dempsy WC, Latham WD. Subpectoral implants in augmentation mammaplasty. Plast Reconstr Surg 1968; 60:325.
9. Scully SJ. Augmentation mammaplasty without capsular contracture. Ann Plast Surg 1981; 6:262.
10. Mahler D, Hauben DJ. Retromammary versus retropectoral breast augmentation. Ann Plast Surg 1982; 8:370.
11. Hagerty RF, McIver FA. Subcutaneous mastectomy with delayed subpectoral reconstruction. South Med J 1978; 71:525.
12. Perrin ER. The use of soluble steroids within inflatable breast prostheses. Plast Reconstr Surg 1976; 57:163.
13. Ellenberg AH, Braun H. A three and one-half year experience with double-lumen implants in breast surgery. Plast Reconstr Surg 1980; 65:307.
14. Burkhardt BR, Fried M, Schnur PL, Tofield JJ. Capsules, infection, and intraluminal antibiotics. Plast Reconstr Surg 1981; 68:43.
15. Hester TR. The polyurethane-covered prosthesis: Facts and fiction. Perspect Plast Surg 1988; 2:135.
16. Hester TR, Nahai F, Bostwick J, Cukic J. A 5-year experience using polyurethane-covered mammary prostheses in the treatment of capsular contracture, primary augmentation mammaplasty, and breast reconstruction after mastectomy. Clin Plast Surg 1988; 15:569.
17. Ashley FL. A new type of breast prosthesis: Preliminary report. Plast Reconstr Surg 1970; 45:421.
18. Ashley FL. Further studies on the Natural-Y breast prosthesis. Plast Reconstr Surg 1972; 49:414.
19. Eyssen JE, von Werssowetz AL, Middleton GD. Reconstruction of the breast using polyurethane-coated prostheses. Plast Reconstr Surg 1984; 73:415.
20. Schatten WE. Reconstruction of the breasts following mastectomy with polyurethane-covered, gel-filled prosthesis. Ann Plast Surg 1984; 12:147.
21. Herman S. The Meme implant. Plast Reconstr Surg 1984; 73:411.
22. Dolsky RL. Polyurethane-coated implants. Plast Reconstr Surg 1985; 76:974.
23. Whidden PG. Augmentation mammoplasty. Transplantation/Implantation Today 1986; 3:43.
24. Melmed EP. Polyurethane implants: A 6-year review of 416 patients. Plast Reconstr Surg 1988; 82:285.
25. Shapiro MA. Smooth vs. rough: An 8 year survey of mammary prostheses. Plast Reconstr Surg 1989; 84:449.
26. Brand GK. Foam covered mammary implants. Clin Plast Surg 1988; 15:533.

CHAPTER 13

Submuscular Augmentation Mammaplasty

RONALD P. GRUBER, M.D.
GARY D. FRIEDMAN, M.D.

Submuscular augmentation mammaplasty came about because the major problem in breast enlargement was, and still is, capsular contracture. Over the years, capsular contracture rates after subglandular augmentation mammaplasty have been reported as from 1 to 75 percent, indicating how difficult it is to establish accurate figures for the incidence of this problem. However, no one has ever questioned the fact that contracture was the leading problem. Beginning in the late 1960s, however, it became apparent that placing a silicone implant beneath the muscle during the course of augmentation mammaplasty resulted in a significantly softer breast.[1] Gradually it became an accepted fact that a quantum leap in the improvement of results was produced simply by placing the implant beneath the muscle.[2-4] Since that time, the popularity of such placement has increased to the point at which at least half the nation's plastic surgeons place the implant beneath the pectoral muscle on a routine basis.

In this chapter the various techniques used to perform submuscular or subpectoral augmentation mammaplasty are described and discussed. Particular emphasis is given to the authors' preferred procedure, the periareolar subpectoral approach, and the reasons for it. Modifications of this approach are also discussed. In addition, other types of subpectoral implantation, e.g., the transaxillary approach, are discussed. Complications are presented and discussed in terms of both treatment and prevention. The various types of implants available for submuscular implantation are discussed, along with the rationale for their use in the subpectoral space. Finally, a discussion is devoted to the reasons why submuscular implantation has enjoyed such success.

DEVELOPMENT OF THE AUTHORS' PREFERRED TECHNIQUE, PERIAREOLAR SUBPECTORAL AUGMENTATION

A number of subpectoral augmentation procedures were performed by the authors using an inframammary incision, and proved to be successful; however, they left something to be desired in terms of the scar of the inframammary fold. Before this time, Hoehler had described the transaxillary subpectoral approach,[5] and the authors also found this to be successful in minimizing capsular contracture. However, there seemed to be much less control during development of the subpectoral pocket, and there was concern about potential bleeding from what is, in essence, a blind dissection. Consequently, there was a search for a new modified approach.

In 1979, the benefits of the periareolar approach used in subglandular augmentation mammaplasty were combined with the known benefits of subpectoral insertion. Consequently the authors' first patient was chosen. Her breasts on examination were of a satisfactory size and shape, but she wanted them to be larger. The risk of capsular contracture had to be absolutely minimized, as did the scar, because this patient's overall breast appearance could not be improved except by the requested increase in size. After surgery, the result of the periareolar scar was excellent, and the breasts were soft and natural. From that time, the periareolar subpectoral approach became the authors' technique of choice for routine augmentation mammaplasty.[5a]

During that first operation, one of the most difficult problems was visualization. The opening to the subpectoral space was small, and even though a headlight was used it was very difficult to see, particularly when any small bleeding occurred. At that time, the lateral edge of the pectoralis muscle was retracted to enter the subpectoral space, and it became apparent that this was not the best site of entry into the subpectoral cavity. It was clear later that the muscle should be split, and that formal muscle closure of the cavity would be preferable.

Subsequent experience with other patients made it easier to visualize the dissection. By paying great attention to hemostasis, a dry field was maintained at all times, and by observing the anatomy and noticing the natural plane that develops between the pectoralis major and minor, it was possible to avoid entering the pectoralis minor muscle inadvertently. This minimized additional bleeding. It also became apparent that the dissection in the inferior aspect of the pocket should be carefully visualized, especially the edge of the fascia of the rectus abdominis muscle, in order (1) to remain in the least vascular plane and (2) to avoid entry into the rectus and serratus muscles (in the lower outer quadrant).

During these early procedures it also became clear, however, that the surgeon had full control of the operation. Hemostasis was controlled because the periareolar incision was directly above and central to the entire cavity, allowing access to every corner. With proper hemostasis it was possible to search for and avoid nerve fibers. It was also evident that the size of the cavity could be well controlled. For example, if the pocket was inadvertently made too large, as indicated toward the end of the operation, the surgeon had easy access to repair those portions of the pocket that were overdissected. Finally, it was noted that dissection was easier if the pectoralis muscle was split for a sufficient distance (7.5 to 10 cm), and larger implants could be inserted than had been anticipated.

PREOPERATIVE EVALUATION

The usual factors obtained in the history are acquired, including a family history of cancer as well as the patient's breast history (whether there had been previous biopsies or symptoms of fibrocystic disease). The patient's reason for augmentation mammaplasty is discussed and her general psyche evaluated. At physical examination the size and shape of the breasts are noted, particularly the presence and degree of ptosis, and whether there is a need to make a new inframammary fold. The old criterion that ptosis is a deterrent to augmentation if the nipple is below the level of the inframammary fold is used only as a general guideline. The areolar size is noted, for obvious reasons. The breast itself is examined for possible masses, and axillary adenopathy sought. A mammagram is obtained preoperatively on all patients over age 35 years, and on all patients of any age with a history of breast disease.

The patient is allowed to try on sizer implants of various volumes in her existing bra. By placing the sizers beneath the breast within the bra, the patient can get some idea, especially on a profile view, of the size she desires. When in doubt, she is encouraged to choose the larger of the two sizes. Retrospective evaluations of patients who were dissatisfied with their postoperative breast size indicated that almost all wished that they had been augmented to a slightly larger size than that initially requested.

Various options are given to the patient: the type of anesthesia (local versus general), the types of implants that are available and their respective advantages and disadvantages, and whether the implant should be placed above or below the pectoralis muscle. Invariably, patients ask the surgeon's opinion, and usually the subpectoral approach is recommended. Patients comply with the authors' recommendations in almost all instances. Some patients have a friend or relative who had an augmentation mammaplasty performed in a certain manner that gave a successful result. In these cases, when patients specifically request a type of procedure, their wishes are granted in the absence of any medical contraindication.

INDICATIONS FOR AND CONTRAINDICATIONS TO PERIAREOLAR SUBPECTORAL AUGMENTATION

The indications obviously include common breast hypoplasia where there is no gross abnormality of the breast shape. The thin-skinned patient is also an excellent candidate for periareolar subpectoral augmentation simply because there is more soft tissue between the skin and the implant. A small degree of ptosis is considered acceptable, certainly if the nipple is not below the level of the inframammary fold, and some patients whose nipple is below this level are considered candidates. This is done by determining whether a postoperative "double-bubble phenomenon" (when the breast is distinct from the underlying implant, creating two mounds) is likely to develop. The examining hand lifts the ptotic breast and moves it away from the chest wall. If, as a result of this maneuver, the breast has a reasonable shape, i.e., is not tubular, subpectoral augmentation is considered.

There are definite contraindications. One is noted in the patient with moderate to severe ptosis, in whom mastopexy, with or without augmentation, is recommended. The "Snoopy" deformity, in which the base of the breast is narrow and expands suddenly into a globular appearing breast, is certainly a contraindiction to a routine periareolar subpectoral approach alone. Any breasts that are of a small, globular type (i.e., a small-diameter base and wide separation between the breasts) are considered for skin reduction in conjunction with augmentation. Moreover, the augmentation must usually be submammary as opposed to subpectoral, so that the skin envelope (and parenchyma) can be filled. Small nipples are an occasional contraindication to periareolar subpectoral augmentation. This is particularly noted in some Asian patients. In these patients, a decision is usually made to use a transaxillary rather than inframammary approach because of the occasional conspicuous nature of the inframammary scar. The athletic ability of the patient and her frequent use of the pectoralis muscle is seldom a contraindication, even if she is an avid sports enthusiast; transecting the lower half of the medial aspect of the pectoralis muscle is not considered a significant deterrent to athletic activities. The exception is made in the case of women actively involved in body building, in whom there is so much use of the pectoralis that distortion of the implant poses a potentially serious problem.

THE OPERATION (PERIAREOLAR SUBPECTORAL AUGMENTATION FOR ROUTINE BREAST HYPOPLASIA)

The position and preparation for surgery involves setting the operating table so that it can be tilted to approximately 45 degrees during the procedure. Tape is used to stabilize the knees, and a footboard is added to the operating table. Armboards are attached to the table, with the patient's elbows padded and palms up to prevent ulnar nerve palsy. By placing the hands down at the sides on the armboard rather than at 90 degrees, the pectoralis muscle is easier to elevate during the process of dissection, and it is easier to appreciate the lie of the breast immediately postoperatively after the implants have been inserted.

The surgical equipment includes a head light, various-sized Deaver and Army-Navy retractors, and peanut dissectors (Fig. 13-1). General anesthesia is generally used because it is not easy to perform extensive dissection of the subpectoral plane under local anesthesia, even when ketamine is added. However, local anesthesia is used on occasion. This involves a mixture of lidocaine hydrochloride (Xylocaine) with epinephrine and bupivacaine hydrochloride (Marcaine) with epinephrine following premedication consisting of meperidine hydrochloride (Demerol), midazolam hydrochloride (Versed), and diazepam (Valium). The usual breast field block, as employed for submammary augmentation, is given. Additional local anesthesia is placed in the subpectoral region once that area is reached surgically. At the time that subpectoral dissection is necessary, ketamine hydrochloride (Ketalar) (30 to 50 mg) may be added. The use of ketamine hydrochloride with local anesthesia is confined to patients who are psychologically and emotionally stable enough to endure this type of agent. Ketamine can produce significant adverse psychological effects during surgery, including hallucinations, particularly in patients with a history of emotional stress or instability. Intercostal nerve block is the third option for the surgeon, but in the authors' experience has been difficult to achieve, time consuming, and often not totally effective.

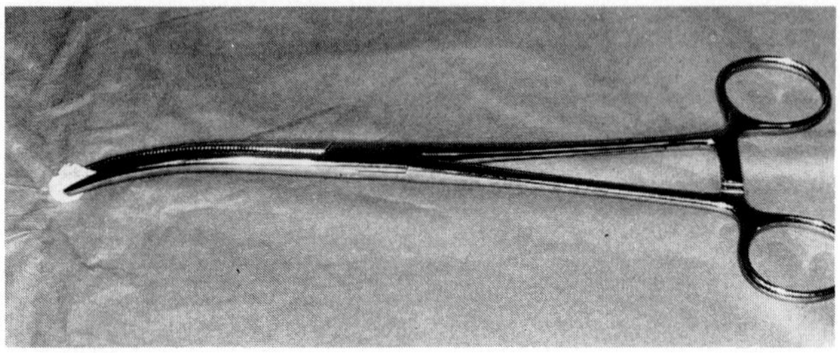

FIGURE 13-1 The peanut dissector facilitates development of the subpectoral pocket.

When general anesthesia is employed, local infiltration of a mixture of lidocaine and bupivacaine with epinephrine is given into the periareolar area and parenchyma leading down to the pectoralis muscle. Additional infiltration is made along the medial pectoralis border, along the inframammary fold, and laterally in an effort to obtain vasoconstriction and early postoperative pain relief. No attempt is made to infiltrate the subpectoral region because of the risk of pneumothorax.

Preoperatively the patient is given 500 mg of vancomycin hydrochloride intravenously. The rationale for the use of this antibiotic is not just the prevention of infection, but specifically the eradication of *Staphylococcus epidermidis*. Although it is not completely proved, the theory that *S. epidermidis* is an etiologic factor in capsular contracture seems sufficiently well founded to warrant the use of this antibiotic. *S. epidermidis* is known to be a cause of infection in cerebrospinal fluid shunts and prosthetic cardiac valves. Although the organism does not necessarily cause a purulent infection in hip prostheses, it is known to be responsible for loosening prostheses. Of all the antibiotics, vancomycin hydrochloride is virtually 100 percent effective against this organism.[6,7] Cephalosporins are slightly less effective, although acceptable. Erythromycin has been used by the author for patients allergic to penicillin, but it is less effective than either vancomycin or cephalosporins.

Hydrocortisone (100 mg) is given intravenously during the course of the operation for three reasons: (1) it tends to minimize edema, (2) it has a slightly euphoric effect, and (3) it may play a small role in preventing thromboembolism. This small dosage is not considered to be a threat to the immune system's ability to ward off infection. It is not given for the purpose of preventing capsular contractures.

The patient is prepared with Povidone-iodine (Betadine) scrub followed by Betadine solution, which is effective against *S. epidermidis.* Surgery by the right-handed surgeon is begun on the left breast because it is easier to dissect the cavity in the inferior and lateral quadrants. Familiarity with the patient's anatomy gained during the first breast procedure makes it easier for the surgeon to operate on the contralateral right breast.

The periareolar incision is made from 3:00 to 9:00 o'clock. It is often helpful to place the incision 1 mm peripheral to the areola-breast skin junction, to preserve the normally feathered edge of the areola. Various other periareolar incisions have been tried and abandoned; these are discussed later. For some years dissection was taken straight down through the parenchyma to the pectoralis muscle, but this approach has recently been altered. It appears that the plane of dissection through the parenchyma should be in a somewhat inferior direction so as to avoid branches of the nerves to the nipple and breast. It is not necessary to circumvent the entire parenchyma (by staying subcutaneously) until the pectoralis is reached; if this were done, one would not necessarily end up in the center of the pectoralis major, but rather in the lower outer quadrant of the breast. Therefore, by angling somewhere between a straight-down and a completely subcutaneous course, the surgeon can reach the central pectoralis muscle and still minimize transection of small nerve branches that innervate the nipple (Fig. 13-2).

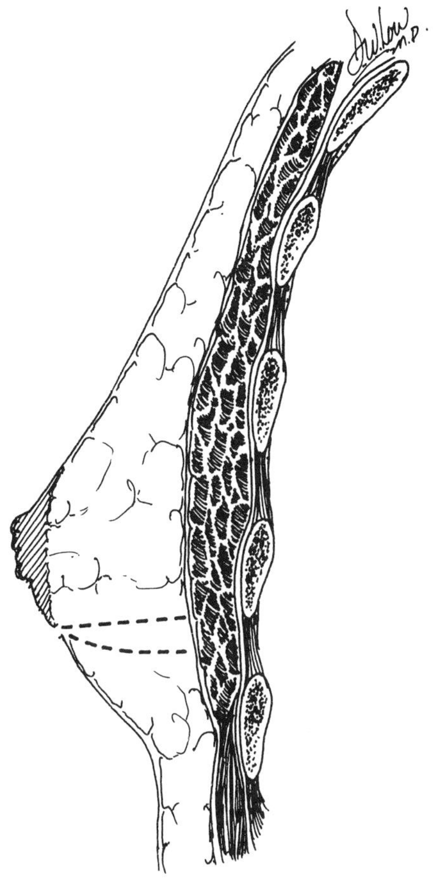

FIGURE 13-2 The periareolar incision can be made to extend directly down (perpendicular) to the muscle. However, to preserve small nerve fibers to the nipple, it may be helpful to angulate it somewhat inferiorly.

Once the fascia is reached, retractors are used to expose a large area superficial to the pectoralis fascia. The novice is likely to dissect too small an area superficial to the pectoralis fascia, resulting in inability to split the muscle adequately. Therefore, an area of 2.5 by 7.5 to 10 cm is cleared off the pectoralis fascia to provide a good deal of exposure. No dissection is made laterally and inferior to the lateral edge of the pectoralis major. Using a tooth forceps and electrocautery, the muscle is split over a distance of 2 to 3 cm initially. Incisions in the pectoralis muscle can result in much bleeding. By using electrocautery to get started, bleeding is minimized. The deeper portion of the muscle can then be gently spread with Metzenbaum scissors until the white, glistening ribs are visible. At that point, an Army-Navy retractor is inserted along with the surgeon's finger to spread the fibers of the pectoralis major. The spreading should continue for a length of 7.5 to 10 cm (Fig. 13-3*A*). There is a tendency to make this muscle opening too small. This could compromise the ability to visualize the subpectoral cavity and make the dissection more difficult.

Once under the muscle, the peanut dissector is used to free the pectoralis major from the ribs in the superior quadrant where dissection is virtually bloodless. Any bleeding is handled immediately, because blood from an ignored blood vessel stains the field and makes subsequent dissection more difficult. The dissection is continued from the superior quadrant into the upper outer quadrant, staying between the pectoralis major and minor. One invariably sees a small fat pad on the undersurface of the pectoralis major, and this serves to distinguish the pectoralis major from the minor. A downward pushing action with the peanut dissector allows the surgeon to peel the pectoralis minor away from the pectoralis major rather than vice versa. After the upper outer quadrant is completed, the lateral aspect of the cavity is developed. Using the peanut again in a downward pushing fashion, the serratus is pushed away to expose and enlarge the cavity. This type of sweeping motion with the peanut dissector is in an essentially bloodless area.

It becomes apparent that there is a limit to the size of the cavity beyond which further pushing with a peanut meets great resistance. Sometimes it is helpful to use the Metzenbaum scissors to spread the tissues in a perpendicular fashion in an attempt to open this part of the cavity slightly more. Having enlarged the superior, upper outer portion and the lateral portion of the cavity, the surgeon's attention

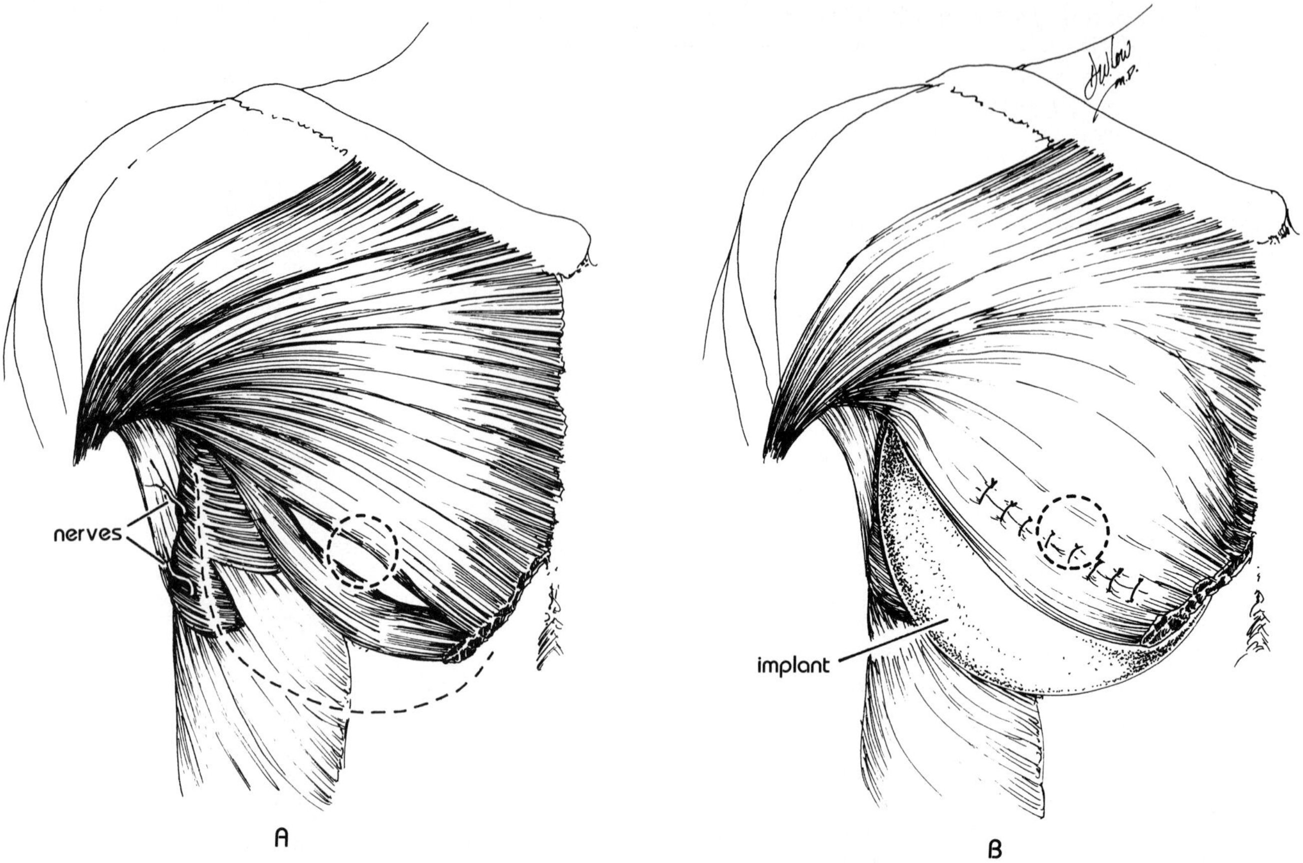

FIGURE 13–3. *A*, The pectoralis is split medial to the lateral edge for a distance of 7.5 to 10.0 cm. The muscle is totally released inferiorly and medially to the level of the nipple. Nerves in the inferolateral quadrant are easily visualized. *B*, After the implant is inserted, the muscle is closed to provide a rich vascular barrier against potential invading organisms.

is turned to the inferolateral quadrant. This, too, is a relatively bloodless area. By using the peanut dissector, the serratus can be pushed away from the overlying roof of the cavity. Nerve fibers come into view, although usually the major fourth intercostal nerve, which is responsible for most of the sensations of the nipple, is not seen. If possible, these smaller branches coming through the serratus between the ribs should be preserved. Occasionally a branch is located just lateral to the lateral edge of the pectoralis major and cannot be preserved, but this is not clinically significant. Another reason for developing the lateral portion of the cavity as well as the inferolateral quadrant is that up to this point there is essentially no bleeding and it is easy to see the nerves and to develop this plane of dissection with good visualization.

After completion of the lower outer quadrant, the peanut dissection is continued along the inframammary area, beginning laterally and moving toward the central and medial aspects of the inframammary fold. The lateral aspect of the rectus fascia is seen, and every attempt is made to keep the dissection plane just superficial to the rectus fascia, exposing approximately 2 cm of it. By using the peanut dissector to make a small subcutaneous tunnel superficial to the rectus fascia, one also remains just deep and inferior to the origin of the pectoralis major. It is now time to transect the origin of the pectoralis major from the ribs with the electrocautery. Perforators bleed briskly and require coagulation. After the muscle fibers are released from the ribs, further dissection and release of the muscle is made in the medial aspect of the cavity as one approaches the sternum.

In previous years, electrocautery was used to transect the muscle fibers all the way to within 2 cm of the midline, but the peanut dissector now is also used. There are branches of the internal mammary neurovascular bundles that provide sensation to the medial aspect of the breast. To reduce injury to the perforators and minimize loss of sensitivity in the medial breast, the peanut is used to stretch the muscle fibers and rupture them from their origin. This medial release is made up to the level of the nipple. In fact, the muscle will be seen to retract slightly as the medial-most fibers are released. So doing bilaterally will not cause the cavities to communicate. It will, however, allow the pectoralis to be somewhat displaced laterally. Upon adequate muscle release, the examiner's finger should be able to pull the muscle anteriorly, right into the parenchyma (Fig. 13-4).

It should also be noted that because the lateral dissection is limited by the tightness of the fusion of the fascia of the serratus with the subcutaneous tissue (and also by the presence of nerves), pocket enlargement is best obtained by medial rather than more lateral dissection. Having this extensive muscle release is perhaps one reason why the authors have not experienced problems with muscle banding and lateral migration. This is in contradistinction to the original subpectoral procedures in which minimal muscle origin release was made and the implant was placed beneath a pectoralis muscle that was so taut as to force the implant laterally.

If the pocket is made too large, as may occasionally occur in the inferior aspect of the cavity, it can easily be closed with interrupted 3-0 nylon sutures. Because there is so much control of the medial aspect of the pocket, there has also been a temptation to overexpand this area, and it too may sometimes need to be closed with interrupted 3-0 nylon sutures.

The type of implant the authors have employed over the years has generally been the silicone gel. Of the various types of silicone, the low-profile implant, which is easy to insert, is generally used because the shape of the breast is more determined by the cavity that has been developed and the gravitational effect on the implant than by the shape of the implant. The choices of implant are discussed in more detail later in the chapter.

Once the cavity has been adequately made on both sides, symmetry is estimated by sweeping the finger around it and comparing one side with the other. Inserting the implant is not usually difficult when the nipple-areola complex is of normal size. Difficulty of insertion, when it occurs, is often due to (1) inadequate splitting of the pectoralis muscle fibers and (2) failure to elevate the posterior wall of the cavity (using retractors). It often is not so much the size of the periareolar incision that prevents the implant from being inserted, but the failure adequately to retract the breast tissue anteriorly to create a cavity into which the implant can be pushed.

At this time, a test of the adequacy of the pocket and the extent of undermining is made by pressing on the upper half of the breast to see if essentially most of the implant can fit into the lower half of the cavity. Because of the tendency for breast cavities to close in the inferior aspect more than in the (subpectoral) superior aspect, every attempt is made to ensure that the inferior cavity is adequate.

No intraluminal antibiotics or intraluminal corticosteroids are used. Intraluminal corticosteroids, in particular, are contraindicated because of the problems they have caused in eroding the inframammary area. However, the pocket itself is irrigated with Betadine solution before the implant is inserted.

No drains have been employed by the authors in recent years, although at one time Jackson-Pratt silicone drains were used routinely and passed through a separate stab wound incision in the lateral inframammary fold area. It was found that these drains caused patients much discomfort, and that in view of

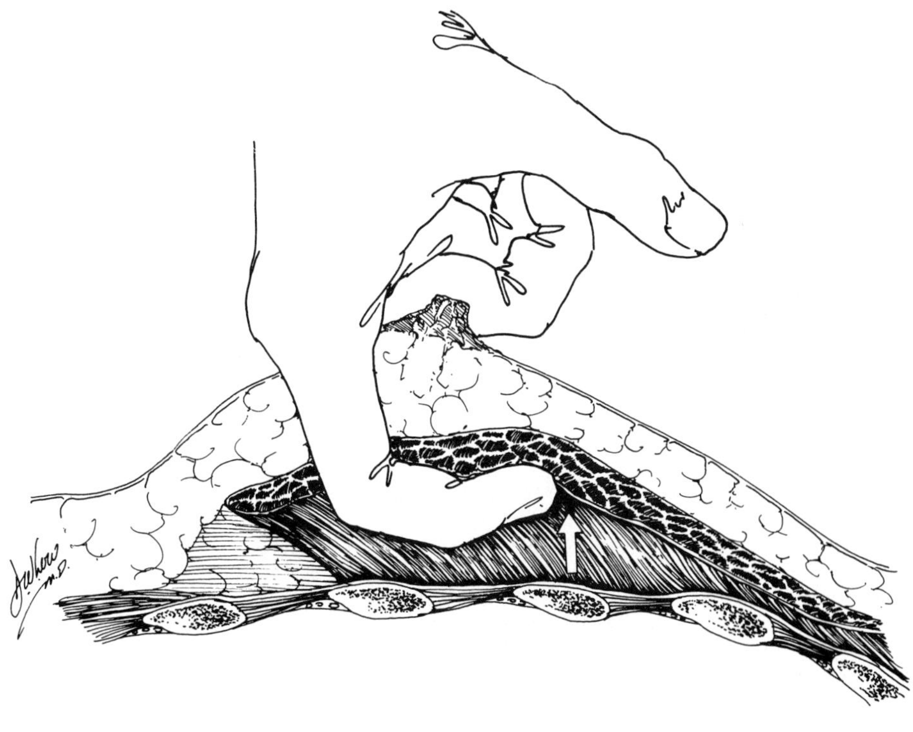

FIGURE 13-4 Inadequate muscle release is a cause of lateral displacement and excessive muscle banding. The muscle should be completely released from its medial attachments up to the level of the nipple. A test of adequacy of release is made by pulling the muscle with one finger and noting the desired laxity.

the proper hemostasis obtained during surgery, there was little need for this type of drainage; other authors have confirmed this.[8] Closure of the wound is with Dexon or Vicryl 3-0 and 4-0 sutures to the muscle layer as well as the parenchyma and subcutaneous layer (Fig. 13–3*B*). The areola is closed with interrupted and running 5-0 nylon sutures.

The potential for the banding effect is most apparent at the time of closure of the muscle, because if there is inadequate release of the medial aspect of the origin of the pectoralis, the implant is flattened and closure of the muscle layer is difficult owing to compression of the muscle against the implant. If there is any doubt regarding the aesthetic appearance of the breast, the operating table is tilted, and in difficult cases a polaroid picture is taken to obtain a two-dimensional perspective of the appearance of the breast. Finally, it should be remembered that if the breasts do not appear satisfactory at the time of surgery, they are not likely to improve during the postoperative course. Therefore, every attempt should be made to ensure that the appearance is satisfactory at the completion of the operation before the patient recovers. The total time in surgery is typically 2 hours: longer than for other types of augmentation mammaplasty, but well worth it.

The "double-bubble" phenomenon is an occasional problem in a subpectoral augmentation mammaplasty of any kind. It is usually caused by an attempt to lower the inframmary fold in patients with ptosis. The old inframammary fold is held away from the chest wall by the implant, and the implant is located inferior to the level of the old inframammary fold (Fig. 13–5*A*). The old inframammary fold does not stretch, causing the patient to appear as if she has one breast sitting on top of another mound, the mound being nothing more than the implant below the inframammary fold. This problem tends not to occur after submammary augmentation because the implant fills the breast envelope. However, filling the breast envelope (and parenchyma) can be a great disadvantage, particularly in patients with ptosis (Fig. 13–5*B*). Filling the parenchyma (or breast envelope) tends only to make the breast more globular

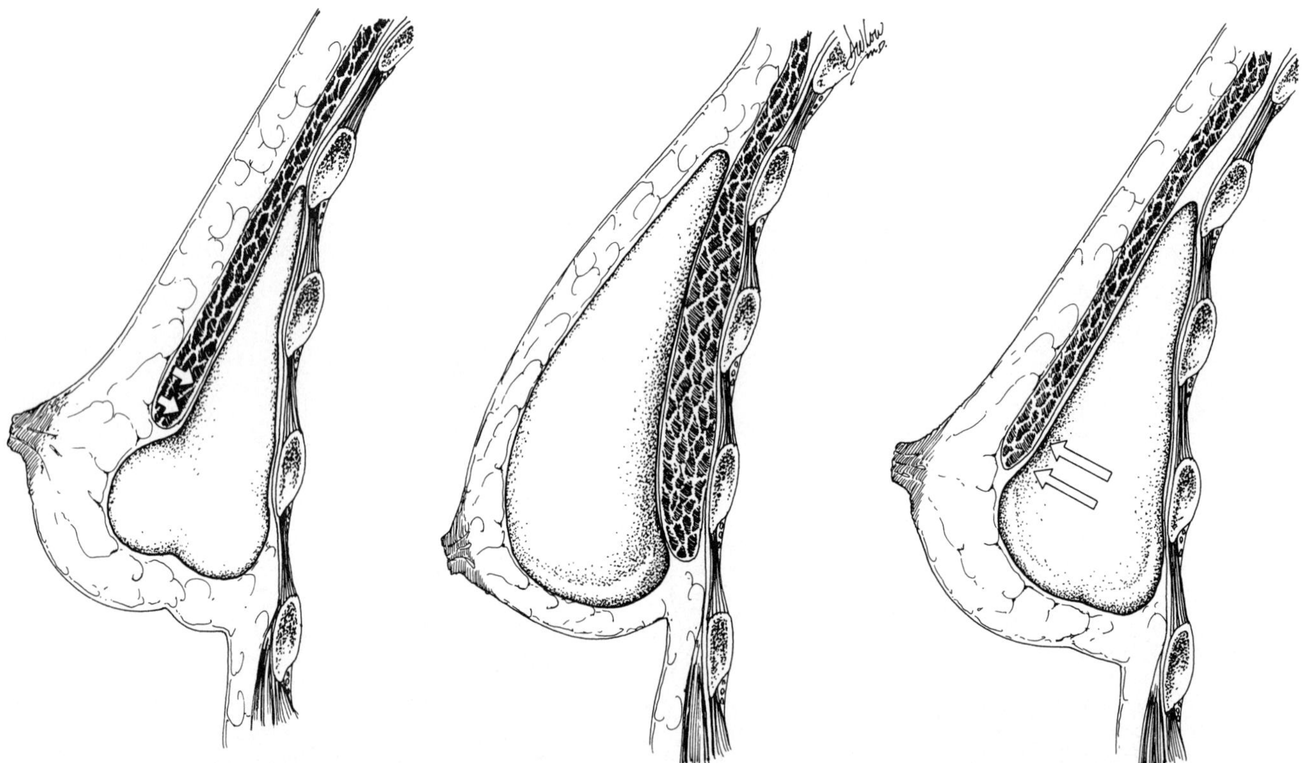

A B C

FIGURE 13–5 *A*, The "double-bubble phenomenon" may be seen after subpectoral augmentation when attempting to correct ptosis by lowering the inframammary fold. It is due to (1) lowering the fold too much; (2) inadequate pectoralis release, preventing the implant from filling the breast envelope; or (3) too large an implant. *B*, Correcting ptosis by subglandular augmentation is not likely to give a "double-bubble phenomenon." However, the implant tends to fill the breast envelope completely and not put pressure in the area of the newly intended inframammary fold. Consequently, the breast still has some ptosis and an inferiorly pointing nipple. Also, the upper half of the breast profile tends to be convex because the pectoralis is not superficial to the implant to maintain the more desirable straight profile. *C*, The "double-bubble phenomenon" is minimized by adequate release of the muscle. This allows the muscle to be pushed anteriorly into the parenchyma by the implant. The implant can then fill some of the envelope of the breast, but at the same time put pressure on the old inframammary fold to obliterate it.

and the nipple point more inferior. If, however, the implant is forced to stay near, at, or just inferior to the inframammary fold, as can be made to occur following subpectoral implantation, the implant can actually expand the area of the inframammary fold. The implant has the potential to improve the ptosis by stretching out the fold (and the inferior half of the breast) and causing the nipple to point more superiorly.

A mild degree of "double-bubble" phenomenon is acceptable at the time of surgery and will subside in time, giving an overall improved appearance to the breast with better correction of the ptosis. To prevent a conspicuous "double-bubble" phenomenon that will not subside with the passage of time, it is essential for the surgeon to evaluate the patient intraoperatively (by elevating the table if necessary) and carefully noting whether the inferior aspect of the cavity has been overdeveloped. If so, it should be closed with interrupted 3-0 nylon sutures. Also, the adequacy of the muscle release should be evaluated as described previously. Releasing the muscle allows more of the implant to fill the parenchyma (Fig. 13-5*C*). Finally, the implant may be too large, having nowhere to go except in the easily distensible tissues inferior to the level of the old inframammary fold. This can be detected at surgery and corrected before closure.

The patient is instructed on discharge to be alert for any unusual pain or swelling of one breast. The usual pain medications given are either hydromorphone hydrochloride (Dilaudid) or oxycodone (Percocet). The pain and discomfort from subpectoral augmentation mammaplasty is distinctly greater than that of submammary augmentation mammaplasty for the first 48 hours, and the patient needs to be warned of this. Postoperatively the patient is given cephalexin (Keflex) 250 mg tid for a total of 5 days. Because the initial bolus of vancomycin has been given, oral Keflex suffices for the remaining several days.

On the first postoperative day, the patient is seen for three purposes: (1) to reinforce the postoperative instructions, (2) to evaluate nipple sensitivity and confirm that the patient is doing well, and (3) to check for any unusual problems that were not recognized during surgery, such as hematoma or malposition of the implant. Sometimes the implant tends to migrate superiorly despite adequate pocket dissection inferiorly; if so the patient is asked to wear an Ace bandage superior to the level of the nipple-areola complex to prevent this type of migration. This particular problem occurs only in a small percentage of patients and is due to the pressure of the inframammary fold against that part of the implant that was placed just at the level of the inframammary fold. If needed, the Ace bandage is worn for 1 to 3 weeks.

No massage is recommended for a periareolar subpectoral augmentation mammaplasty; at least one report indicated that massage may be harmful.[9] Instead, at 48 hours the patient is allowed to wear a bra provided it does not contain a metal or wire stay. If implants tend to rise, a bra is not recommended. If the patient feels better wearing a bra, it is cut along the bottom so that the implants are not pushed superiorly.

Results after almost 10 years of periareolar subpectoral augmentation are such that the typical case is a soft, natural breast. The slope of the breast from the clavicle to the nipple is generally in the form of a straight line. The profile from the nipple to the new or old inframammary fold is an arc of a circle. The result is a natural contour. Figure 13-6 demonstrates a patient with breast hypoplasia who underwent periareolar subpectoral augmentation mammaplasty. Two years after surgery she exhibits a normal contour, adequate softness, and no significant periareolar scar.

MODIFYING THE OPERATION

Capsular contracture following subglandular augmentation is one of the major indications for the periareolar subpectoral approach. Many of these patients have had either an inframammary or a periareolar scar. Although it might appear that if the patient has an inframammary scar from the first operation, any correction should be made through the same scar, it is the authors' opinion that it is still preferable to perform the second corrective surgery through a separate periareolar approach. This does result in two scars, but the periareolar approach, as discussed later, has two distinct advantages over an inframammary subpectoral approach: (1) better control of pocket dissection and (2) more important, complete muscle closure, which helps prevent bacterial entry into the cavity. Small suture reactions that have the potential to work their way down to the implant can be avoided if the patient undergoes a complete muscle repair to protect the underlying implant.

Thus, at surgery for capsular contracture after subglandular augmentation, the implant is removed through the periareolar incision, and the posterior wall of the capsule is incised to enter the muscle. In most cases the anterior and posterior capsule walls can be sutured together with interrupted 3-0 nylon sutures. Usually, a portion of the capsule is excised to allow the cavity to adhere. When it is necessary to reoperate on these patients years later, e.g., to insert a larger implant at their request, it has been found that most of these cavities have closed. Taping of the breasts postoperatively also helps prevent ptosis of the glandular tissue. Usually, no attempt is made to perform a capsulectomy unless the cavity is so large that breast parenchyma tends to become ptotic. One of the main reasons for not performing a complete capsulectomy is the increased morbidity of the pro-

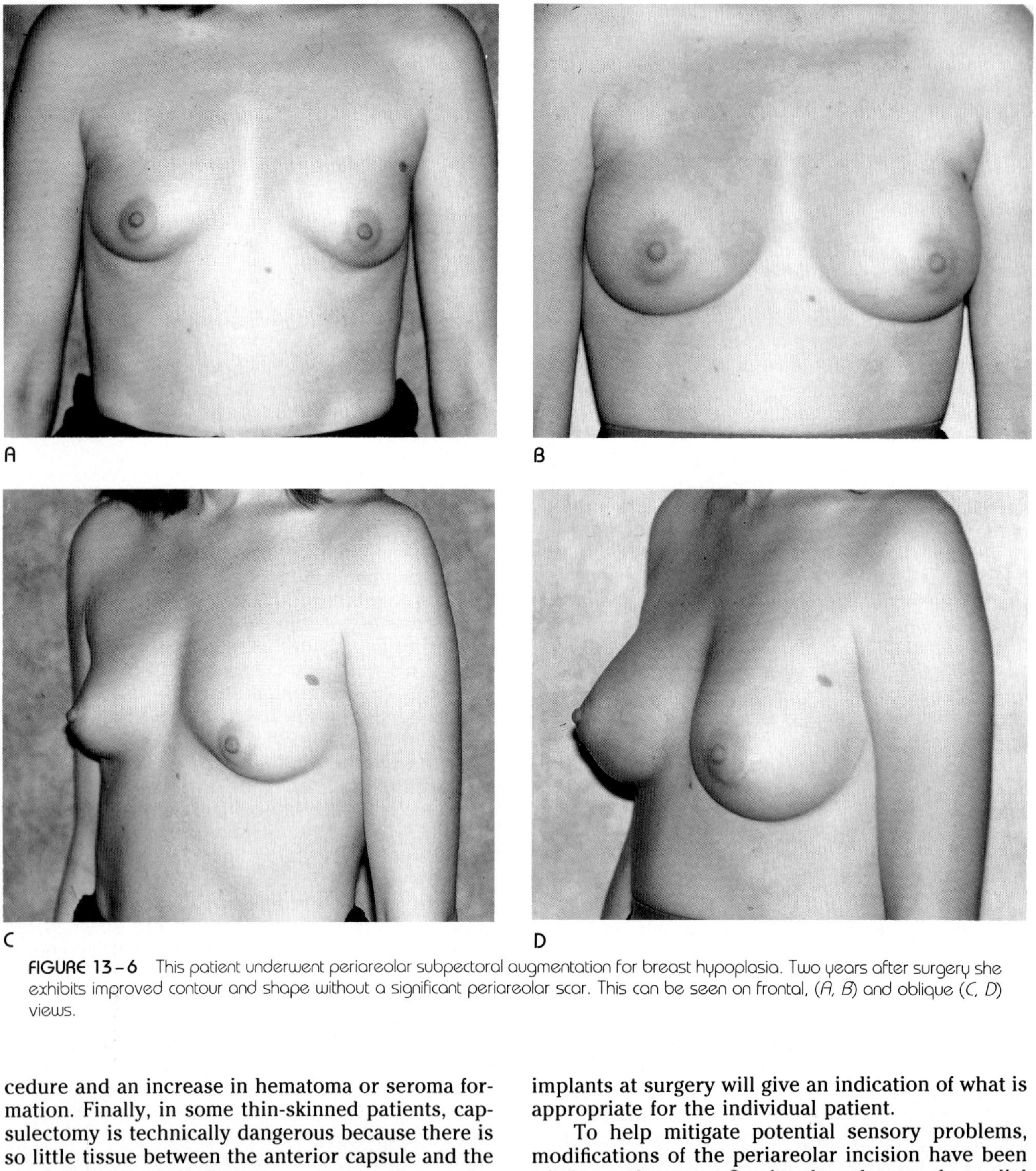

FIGURE 13–6 This patient underwent periareolar subpectoral augmentation for breast hypoplasia. Two years after surgery she exhibits improved contour and shape without a significant periareolar scar. This can be seen on frontal, (*A*, *B*) and oblique (*C*, *D*) views.

cedure and an increase in hematoma or seroma formation. Finally, in some thin-skinned patients, capsulectomy is technically dangerous because there is so little tissue between the anterior capsule and the overlying skin of the breast.

After the pectoralis muscle is opened, a completely separate subpectoral pocket is developed. Even in the area inferior and lateral to the pectoralis, there is substantial tissue between the old cavity and the serratus anterior muscle that forms the anterior wall of the new (subpectoral) cavity. Frequently an implant of a different size from that used in the subglandular space is necessary. A larger one generally gives the proper contour. Only trial of different-sized implants at surgery will give an indication of what is appropriate for the individual patient.

To help mitigate potential sensory problems, modifications of the periareolar incision have been tried over the years. One involves the use of a medial incision from the 6:00 to 12:00 o'clock positions, as suggested by Spear and colleagues.[10] The rationale is that most of the nerve fibers to the nipple-areola complex come from the inferolateral quadrant. When this part of the parenchyma is not violated, there is less sensory loss. For similar reasons, the authors in previous years have attempted to minimize sensory changes by using a superiorly located incision that extended from the 9:00 to 3:00 o'clock positions.

However, the superiorly located scar poses a small problem when even slightly noticeable, and it appears important that the patient should not see any portion of the scar from her perspective. More important is the fact that the superiorly located areolar incision does not in fact improve the sensory changes. It is only when the traditional infra-areolar incision is extended through the parenchyma at an oblique angle to the chest, so as to circumvent most of the parenchyma, that most of the minor sensory difficulties abate.

Some pectus carinatum and excavatum problems are well handled by the periareolar subpectoral approach; other surgeons have also used it with great success.[10] The periareolar incision allows total access in order to reduce the cartilaginous portions of the ribs. An osteotome and mallet are all that are necessary to make these corrections (Fig. 13–7). In addition, by elevating the muscle off the sternum with the peanut elevator and electrocautery, the soft tissues and implants tend to partially fill the sternal area. Great care must be taken not to enter the contralateral breast region or transect internal mammary neurovascular bundles.

Another advantage of the periareolar approach to subpectoral augmentation is that any area that coincidentally needs biopsy is easily accessible through this approach. The same cannot always be said of the inframammary or transaxillary approach.

An uncommon but difficult complication that is very responsive to the periareolar subpectoral approach is skin wrinkling, with or without capsular contracture. This is seen in thin-skinned patients who have undergone subglandular augmentation mammaplasty and who, being middle-aged, develop wrinkling and in some cases folds of the skin. Figure 13–8 is an example of one such patient with skin wrinkling. At surgery the implant that was superficial to the pectoralis muscle was removed. The space between the capsule and the skin was too thin to allow a safe capsulectomy; instead, a subpectoral pocket was developed that provided adequate padding in the sternal area where the skin was wrinkled. In patients who have skin wrinkling but no capsular contracture, it may seem difficult to justify periareolar implant relocation, but the authors have found no better solution to the problem of wrinkling than placing the implant beneath the muscle. Other procedures have been tried over the years, such as imbricating capsule tissue on itself and trying to obliterate portions of the cavity where the wrinkled skin is located, but these have not been nearly as successful.

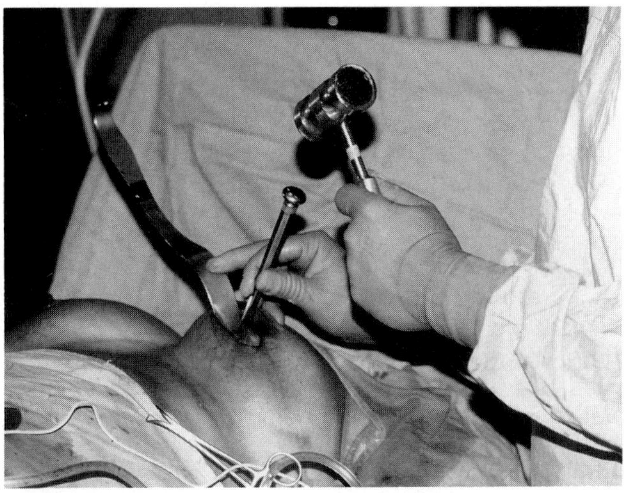

FIGURE 13–7 The osteotome is used to improve pectus carinatum deformities.

Finally, some of the undesirable results following transaxillary procedures have responded best to the periareolar subpectoral approach. This includes the problem of inadequate cleavage, which tends to be the case with transaxillary augmentation when the surgeon has not adequately released the muscle medially. Capsular contracture itself after transaxillary augmentation has responded to the periareolar approach because the capsulotomy or capsulectomy is very difficult to perform from the axillary approach. Also, any malpositioning that occurs after the transaxillary subpectoral approach is more difficult to correct in the authors' hands by going back into the axilla. The one great advantage of the periareolar approach is complete visualization and accurate development of the cavity, with complete hemostasis.

A small areola is a distinct disadvantage to the periareolar approach. With experience, smaller and smaller areolae can be approached and successful subpectoral augmentation carried out. However, areolae smaller than 3 cm tend to be difficult. The operation has been modified on occasion in order to stay with the periareolar approach and avoid an inframammary incision; this has involved extending the incision radially for about 1 cm, which definitely makes the operation easier. At this time, however, the scar from such a lateral extension is seldom considered worth producing because the radial component of the scar can be conspicuous. An alternative solution is to extend the periareolar incision from the 2:00 to 10:00 o'clock positions, which permits better exposure without additional sensory loss. For the patient with small areolae, either the transaxillary or the inframammary approach is the best solution.

INFRAMAMMARY SUBPECTORAL AUGMENTATION

The inframammary approach to a subpectoral augmentation was one of the first reported.[1,2] The capsular contraction rate appeared to be more favorable than that following submammary augmentation.

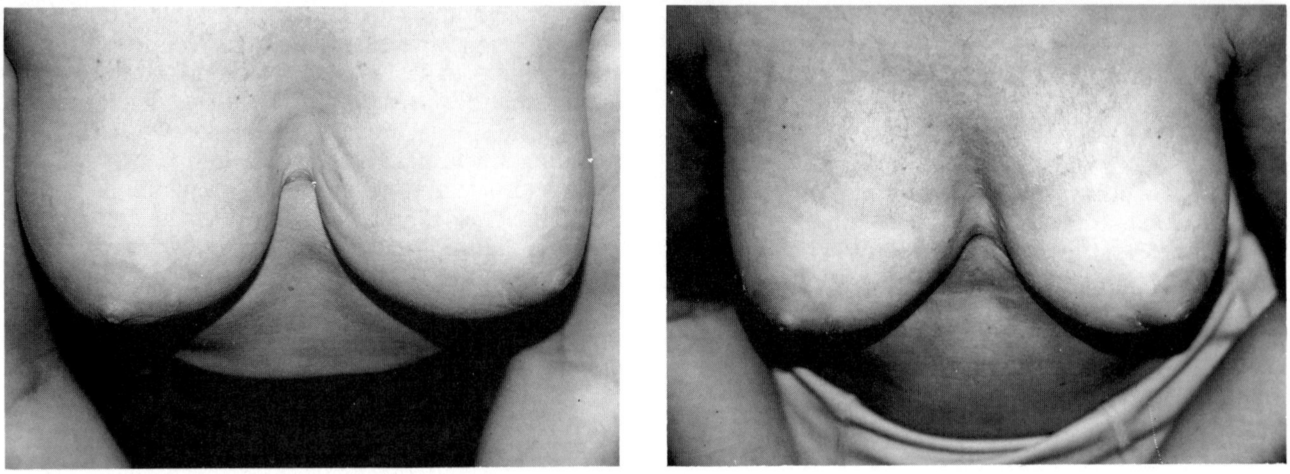

A B

FIGURE 13-8 Skin wrinkling may be seen after submammary augmentation (*A*). It is exaggerated when the patient leans forward. Treatment involves subpectoral relocation of the implant. In this case the periareolar subpectoral approach was used. After surgery skin condition is improved (*B*).

Other authors have since reported the success of their series.[11] The indications for the procedure are similar to those for the periareolar subpectoral approach. The one factor that tends to favor the use of the inframammary fold is a patient who has a distinct inframammary crease on preoperative evaluation. Obviously, small-breasted women who do not show a substantial inframammary increase are likely to produce an exposed scar. If that scar proves unfavorable, it will be a disappointing feature of the operation.

Some surgeons who use the inframammary subpectoral approach ask patients to refrain from using birth control pills during the month before surgery. The reasoning is that there may be less breast engorgement and that therefore the breast size can be better evaluated. Another reason to discontinue birth control pills is the possible reduction of hormone-associated venous thrombosis. Some surgeons also prefer to avoid surgery during the last two weeks of the menstrual cycle when swelling or engorgement of the breasts is noted.

One of the more commonly utilized techniques involves an inframammary incision made on the breast itself just superior to the inframammary fold. It can be made in the midinframammary fold or in the lateral aspect. In the authors' opinion, scars in the midinframammary fold are slightly less noticeable. Dissection begins in the inferolateral quadrant, taking the dissection down to the fascia of the serratus anterior. The peanut elevator is used to sweep the tissues off the fascia of the serratus and help avoid injury to any nerves. The lateral edge of the pectoralis fascia is incised to permit entry into the compartment just deep to the pectoralis major. The subpectoral space is immediately visualized. Perforators are cauterized and the inferomedial aspect of the muscle is released, as described for the periareolar subpectoral approach. Care is taken not to enter the pectoralis minor muscle. Sweeping tissues off the pectoralis rather than sweeping the pectoralis major off the ribs (and pectoralis minor) helps avoid this problem. After the implant is inserted and the pocket size and position are determined to be sufficient, closure of the wound is made in layers. Absorbable sutures such as Vicryl or Dexon are used. Closure must be meticulous because (1) there is no muscle just deep to the incision and (2) an excellent inframammary scar demands it.

A variation of this technique was described by Bostwick.[12] An incision approximately 3.5 to 4 cm long is made slightly above the inframammary crease. Bostwick makes a point of dissecting between the superficial and deep fascia so as to lift the breast off the deep fascia, over the serratus and external oblique muscles. Using finger dissection, the pectoralis major is lifted off the ribs, care being taken to separate it from the pectoralis minor. The blunt dissection continues over the ribs beneath the fascia of the serratus anterior. This causes some muscle fiber elevation of the serratus. In the authors' experience a true elevation of the fascia off the serratus can be a bloody dissection and is generally reserved for reconstruction of postmastectomy deformities. Nonetheless, Bostwick finds fascia elevation a useful addition and continues the surgery by elevating the fascia along with the adjacent fascia of the external oblique. After the appropriate-sized pocket is developed, the implant is inserted. The patient is then placed in the sitting position so that symmetry may be evaluated. Closure is made in multiple layers after preplacing sutures between the fascial edges to prevent damage to the implants.

Postoperative treatment is similar to that after

the periareolar subpectoral approach. Variations in care are frequent, depending on the surgeon's choice, and include a different choice of antibiotics. Many surgeons also employ vitamin E postoperatively (1000 units twice daily for 4 weeks) in an attempt to minimize the likelihood of capsular contracture.

Results are generally satisfactory with the inframammary subpectoral approach, and may be superior to those from the subglandular approach. Biggs and Yarish reported a retrospective analysis of approximately 1000 patients, in whom the rates of capsular contracture for retromammary and retropectoral augmentation were 17 and 9 percent, respectively.

TRANSAXILLARY SUBPECTORAL AUGMENTATION

The transaxillary approach has become popular in the placement of the implant beneath the pectoralis muscle, largely because the resultant scar is in an essentially inconspicuous location and because the blunt technique of developing the cavity does not require a meticulous search for bleeders. Thus, this approach usually decreases operating time. One of the indications for transaxillary subpectoral augmentation, in the authors' opinion, is a patient with a small nipple-areola complex. Others have found that no matter what the size of the complex, the transaxillary approach is good because it allegedly produces the same results as the periareolar subpectoral approach without the potential for a conspicuous periareolar scar and without the need for meticulous dissection through the periareolar approach, as has been described.

Our second indication for using the transaxillary approach is when a small-to-modest enlargement of the breast is the only objective. It has been difficult in our hands to achieve a substantial enlargement from a transaxillary approach because of the uncertainty of what is being torn by the blunt method of dissection, particularly in the medial and lateral aspects of the cavity. Third, for patients who are absolutely insistent that there be no visible scar whatsoever on the breast itself, the transaxillary approach is the operation of choice.

A technique described elsewhere[13-15] is similar to that summarized here (Fig. 13-9). It involves marking the axilla with an incision approximately 5 cm within one of the skin folds in such a way that when the patient's arms are at her sides, the marking will not be seen. The operation is done under general anesthesia for the reasons mentioned in the periareolar subpectoral approach. The arm is positioned at 90 degrees to the long axis of the body, and great care is taken in proper positioning of the extremity

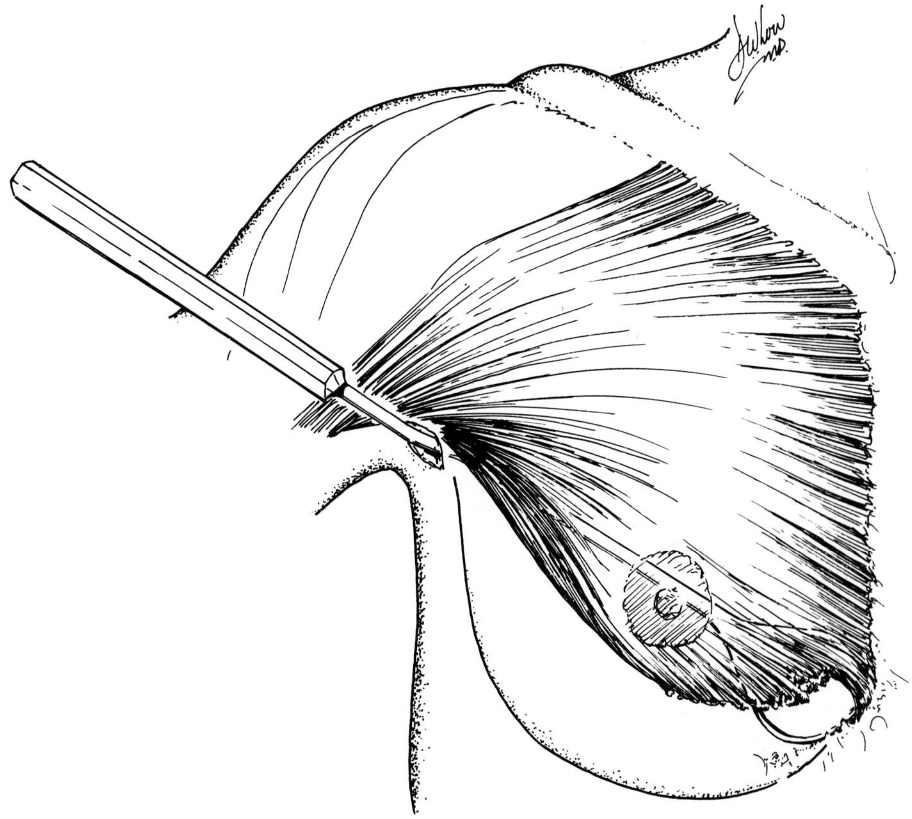

FIGURE 13-9 Transaxillary subpectoral augmentation requires stripping of the origin of the pectoralis major muscle with a blunt urethral sound or dissector. The operation is especially well suited for patients with small areolae.

to avoid potential damage to the brachial plexus and ulnar nerve. Local epinephrine infiltration for the purpose of hemostasis is made both in and around the breast area and all the way up to the axilla. Dissection is taken down through the subcutaneous tissue, extending in an inferior direction toward the palpable edge of the pectoralis major muscle. It is at the inferior aspect of the subcutaneous axilla that entry is made into the subpectoral space beneath the edge of the pectoralis major. The pectoralis minor is not fused with the pectoralis major at this location, allowing ease of dissection. This approach allows one to avoid sensory nerve branches to the arm. By blunt dissection with the finger and with the aid of an Army-Navy retractor, it is possible to place a finger beneath the pectoralis and then spread a small cavity that allows one to enter the subpectoral space without any bleeding. Once the proper plane has been entered, the cavity is developed with the aid of a No. 34 urethral sound or one of the commercially available instruments. The sound or dissector can be used to avulse the muscle fibers medially by pushing in the direction of the sternum rather than pulling or pushing in a superior/inferior direction along the sternum, which would otherwise injure branches of the internal mammary vessels. In the lateral aspect of the cavity, the instrument is used to push laterally in an attempt to separate tissues away from the posterior wall of the developing cavity. Here, too, the temptation to pull and push in a superior/inferior direction is avoided because this may cause damage to nerve branches exiting between the ribs and through the serratus. The inferior aspect of the cavity is likewise developed. Great care is taken to avoid overdissection of the inferior pocket because this cannot be corrected easily. A warm laparotomy pad is inserted into the cavity after it has been developed, and attention is turned to the development of the cavity of the contralateral breast. It is our observation that there is less bleeding than during the periareolar subpectoral approach. This is partly because one cannot see the blood that is developing, and partly because there is a tendency not to elevate as much muscle owing to the force required and the fear of avulsing neurovascular bundles. Various-sized implants are used in an attempt to obtain the best overall aesthetic appearance. The cavity is irrigated with Betadine solution before final closure of the pocket. The patient is given vancomycin and hydrocortisone intravenously, as in the subpectoral periareolar approach. Closure consists of 3-0 and 4-0 Dexon for the edge of the pectoralis major as well as the subcutaneous tissue, followed by interrupted or running 4-0 nylon sutures for the skin. Postoperative treatment for the transaxillary approach is identical to that for the periareolar subpectoral approach.

There are a few disadvantages to the otherwise useful transaxillary approach. It may not be possible to insert as large an implant as requested by the patient or required by the type of breast. This is due to an inability to dissect as large a pocket with the sound or elevator as can be done with the aid of the electrocautery and peanut dissector under direct vision though the periareolar approach. As mentioned, there is a reluctance to avulse muscle in the region of the perforators of the internal mammary neurovascular bundles and lateral branches of the nerve to the nipple-areola complex. During transaxillary dissection, the exact extent of the pocket is not fully controllable with the dissector or sound. Thus, when cleavage is a particularly desirable feature of the augmentation mammaplasty, the periareolar approach is preferred. Because of the reluctance to release the pectoralis fully, muscle banding tends to be more severe following the transaxillary approach. It is true that the "double-bubble" phenomenon tends to occur less often because of the reluctance to overdevelop the inferior aspect of the pocket. However, although the transaxillary approach may produce fewer "double-bubble" phenomena, in the authors' experience it may allow the implant to migrate superiorly.

The possibility of not obtaining proper hemostasis is a theoretical objection to the transaxillary approach, but in fact gross bleeding after the blunt dissection of the cavities during the transaxillary approach has not been a significant problem in our hands. It is always possible that small amounts of blood do accumulate following a transaxillary approach and may contribute to capsular contracture. However, this may be more theoretical than empirical because (1) some reports have indicated that hematoma may not be a factor in capsular contracture[16] and (2) many studies dealing with transaxillary augmentation mammaplasty show a hematoma rate comparable with that of the periareolar and inframammary approach.

COMPLETE SUBMUSCULAR AUGMENTATION MAMMAPLASTY

When submuscular breast implant insertion is performed for mastectomy patients, they undergo elevation of the pectoralis major and serratus anterior and in some cases of the rectus abdominis muscle in an attempt to provide a complete muscle coverage for the implant. This is also important in cases of subcutaneous mastectomy because the overlying skin can not be depended on to protect the implant. In general, favorable results are achieved, although in many instances the breasts are somewhat flattened in appearance, causing a retreat to simple subpectoral implantation. A compromise has been developed by many authors whereby the complete thickness of the serratus is not elevated, but instead a superficial (and thereby more distensible) portion. This avoids flattening the implant and yet provides an additional thin layer of muscle coverage. The concept of total muscle coverage for aesthetic augmentation mammaplasty was not considered practical until Spear and colleagues[17] decided to use it in a large series of patients. These authors found that the capsular contracture rate can indeed be kept remarkably low, that flattening is not necessarily a problem, and that other complications (such as the bleeding that might be expected from elevation of the serratus external oblique and rectus abdominis) are not significant. More recently, Haggerty and colleagues[18] described total submuscular coverage in aesthetic augmentation mammaplasty. They use the inframammary approach, and the implant is placed beneath the pectoralis major, serratus anterior, and portions of the rectus abdominis muscles. Their theory is that in complete muscular coverage there is no interference with the breast parenchyma and/or its lymphatics. Should breast carcinoma occur later in these patients, the breast implant will be remote from the pathologic process.

CHOICE OF IMPLANT FOR THE SUBMUSCULAR SPACE

A discussion of the various types of implants is warranted. For periareolar subpectoral augmentation the gel implant has been the authors' implant of choice, mostly because there is no leaking, which is known to occur with the saline-filled implants. Low-profile implants are preferred to round and high-profile implants because they are easier to insert into a small nipple-areola complex and because the shape of the breast is not significantly determined by the shape of the implant. Whether the implant has a round, ovoid, or double-density configuration, it takes on a natural tear-shape appearance due to the force of gravity when the patient is in an upright position.

The double-lumen implant is occasionally used as an alternative; the original total saline-filled implant is no longer used. Any leaking that occurs poses a minimal problem. As long as most of the implant is gel and not saline, the sensation of fluid movement that was occasionally noted with total saline implants is also not a significant problem. Thus, if the patient specifically requests a double-lumen implant, it is used for the periareolar subpectoral approach. However, there is no significant difference between the capsular contracture rate of double-lumen implants and that of silicone gel implants (for the periareolar subpectoral approach described above); the importance of the double-lumen implant when used in the submammary space may be much greater.

The polyurethane implant has undergone a revival of interest, particularly in the form of Meme and Replicon. It was of course devised for the submammary approach in the hope that the capsular contracture rate could be substantially reduced from that seen after submammary insertion of silicone gel, saline-filled, and double-lumen implants. Several reports over the years have suggested that the capsular contracture rate, at least for the submammary insertion of polyurethane implants, is reduced to a level below that obtained by any other implant. The polyurethane implant is not generally used for the subpectoral approach, but some discussion is indicated.

Several concerns have been raised by those who do not favor the polyurethane implant. First, some cases of infection have been reported, which was not a major problem with the silicone implant. Some of this potential problem with infection may be more theoretical than empirical, however, because bacteria has proven to grow better on surfaces that have interstices. Hester reviewed a large series of submammary augmentation mammaplasties in which the polyurethane implant was used.[19] In these patients the infection rate was noted to be 0.3 percent (much lower than that in most studies). Moreover, the capsular contracture rate was as good as or better than even some of the best results from silicone studies: 1.8 percent. Others found results to be more mixed, although the danger of infection has not been as severe as the literature first suggested.[19a] However, in comparison to most of the studies done using silicone gel or double-lumen implants under the muscle, the infection rate is still slightly higher. Assuming that the polyurethane capsular contracture rate is significantly lower than that obtained with silicone implants, the question is whether it is better to have a slightly higher risk of infection with a slightly lower risk of capsular contracture, or a slightly higher risk of capsular contracture with a lower risk of infection. Dealing with an infection following augmentation mammaplasty is much more difficult, in the authors' view, than having to cope with a class III capsular contracture.

Another objection to the polyurethane implant, however, is that if it has to be removed it may pose a greater problem surgically. It has been known for some time that if the polyurethane has not been dissolved from the surface of the implant, as tends to occur over time, it can be a laborious task to remove the fragments of polyurethane. This process of removal adds to the overall morbidity of the operation. Perhaps, as Hester contends, if infection should occur, it will be detected early at a time when the polyurethane has not had a chance to become deeply imbedded into the tissues, so that implant removal will not be that difficult.

Another potential problem with the polyurethane is the fact that the toxic potential has not been fully established. Burns and colleagues[20] found that there appears to be minimal activation of the immune system. Obviously there must be some immune response, as indicated by the fact that 5 percent of patients with polyurethane implants experience a rash. Nonetheless, this may or may not be any more significant or frequent than the types of immune response seen with silicone, including the human adjuvant syndrome.

A potential technical problem with polyurethane is that it is not distensible enough to insert routinely through the periareolar or transaxillary approach. Even with the use of sterile Lacri-Lube, as suggested by Schlesinger,[21] it is seldom that the polyurethane implant can be placed through anything other than an inframammary incision. It will not be surprising if in the near future a polyurethane implant is devised that is inflatable. This would allow it to be inserted via either the periareolar approach or the transaxillary approach in the subpectoral space. This might permit the advantage of the lower contracture rate from the submuscular approach to be combined with the alleged lower contracture rate due to the use of the polyurethane surface.

One other type of implant deserves discussion because it is being used with greater frequency: the textured silicone implant. Since the advent of the irregular-surface polyurethane implant, an innovative approach has been developed whereby the surface of an otherwise smooth silicone implant is constructed so that it has the surface irregularities similar to, but not exactly like, polyurethane. Thus, if the success of the polyurethane implant is due to the manner in which the scar tissue surrounding it is deposited (in an irregular fashion rather than in long, straight fibers), it appears that the textured silicone implant might have the advantages of the polyurethane without the potential disadvantages (toxicity of the breakdown products of the polyurethane, and potential infection). It is also easier to insert through a small incision (such as the periareolar or transaxillary incision). Ersek championed the use of the textured implant.[22] Studies to date are incomplete but look promising in that the capsular contracture rate is as good as that with the polyurethane implant. Only time will tell if the textured implant will be the implant of choice.[23]

A Becker expander implant has been used principally for the submammary approach.[24] It has the distinct advantage of allowing the patient and surgeon to adjust the size of the implant postoperatively. The fact that it can also be used to treat capsular contracture is another positive feature. However, no significant experience has so far been acquired with this type of implant in the retropectoral space.

POSSIBLE REASONS FOR SUBMUSCULAR SUCCESS

Since its inception, the most prominent theory as to why the submuscular implant has resulted in a low capsular contracture rate is that the muscle itself acts to massage or press on the capsule surrounding the implant, keeping it soft. This has never been definitively proved, but it is one of the reasons why so many surgeons have found it unnecessary to massage the patient's breasts postoperatively. The better hemostasis obtainable through the periareolar subpectoral approach has been claimed to be one of the reasons for the low capsular contracture rate. However, as mentioned, this is in conflict with the study in which a "second-look" operation was undertaken.[16] Small amounts of blood were found in the cavity, but these were not associated with a higher incidence of capsular contracture.

At one time it was thought that the reason for the success of the subpectoral approach was that the subpectoral space may be alymphatic. If capsular contracture is due to a specific or nonspecific immune response to silicone molecules, and if the subpectoral space is alymphatic, one would expect less capsular contracture from the subpectoral location of the implant. To answer this question, we performed a study in which a radioisotope (99m-technetium-antimony-chloride, which is picked up by lymphatics) was inserted into the subpectoral space of one breast and the submammary space of the contralateral breast. Lymphoscintigraphy (axillary lymph node scanning) was then performed to detect the degree of uptake. Although in many patients uptake by the axillary nodes was not seen on the side in which the isotope was placed subpectorally, but *was* seen on the side in which it was placed in the submammary space, the finding was random when statistically reviewed. The study turned out to be negative, and thus the possibility that the better results seen with subpectoral implant placement are due to the alymphatic (immunologically privileged) aspect of the subpectoral space is considered unlikely.

Another possible reason for better results with subpectoral implants may be that the tissue in the subpectoral space is of an areolar quality. It is known that areolar tissue generally tends to be associated with a less vigorous scar response. An example of this is eyelid skin, which has a component of areolar tissue immediately deep to it: this skin tends to form very little scarring both on its surface and subcutaneously. Even though only half of the "subpectoral space" contains this areolar tissue (located deep to the muscle), it may play a significant factor quantitatively in that approximately half the space, because of its areolar nature, may be less prone to scar deposition than the other half. It would also account for the fact that the inferolateral aspect of the pocket is what generally contracts during capsular contracture, causing the implant to ride superiorly.

Perhaps a more likely factor responsible for a lower capsular contracture rate in subpectoral and submuscular augmentation mammaplasty is the muscle closure itself. In the periareolar approach the muscle opening is the only access for any bacteria that arise from the skin or ducts of the parenchyma. Presumably muscle, because of its better blood supply, is better able to guard against bacteria. This suggests that the inframammary incision used for subpectoral implantation, and the transaxillary approach used for subpectoral implantation, are at somewhat of a disadvantage. In fact, the authors consider this a distinct possibility. There have been a few cases of small sinus formations in the axillary wounds after transaxillary subpectoral augmentation that communicated directly with the subpectoral space. This type of sinus formation and drainage extending down to the subpectoral cavity is almost nonexistent when there is proper muscle closure during the periareolar approach. It also suggests that the periareolar approach should specifically encompass a splitting of the pectoralis muscle rather than incision of its lateral edge when developing a cavity for the implant. The lateral edge closure is not a muscle-muscle closure.

References

1. Dempsey MC, Latham WD. Subpectoral implants in augmentation mammoplasty: Preliminary report. Plast Reconstr Surg 1968; 42:515-521.
2. Regnault P. Partially submuscular breast augmentation. Plast Reconstr Surg 1977; 59:72-76.
3. Vasquez B, Given KS, Houston GC. Breast augmentation: A review of subglandular and submuscular implantation. Aesthet Plast Surg 1987:101-105.
4. Puckett CL, Croll GH, Reichel CA, Concannon MJ. A critical look at capsule contracture in subglandular versus subpectoral augmentation. Aesthet Plast Surg 1987; 11:23-28.
5. Hoehler H. Breast augmentation, the axillary approach. Br J Plast Surg 1973; 26:272-276.

5a. Gruber RP, Friedman GD. Subpectoral augmentation mammaplasty through a periareolar incision. Plast Reconstr Surg 1981; 67:453.

6. Aldridge KE. Topics in clinical microbiology. Infect Contr 1982; 3:161-165.
7. Lowy FD, Hammer SM. *Staphylococcus epidermidis* infections. Ann Intern Med 1983; 99:834-839.
8. Colon GA. The reverse double lumen prosthesis: A preliminary report. Ann Plast Surg 1982; 9:293-297.
9. Marshall WR. Amelioration of capsular contracture by motion restriction. Ann Plast Surg 1986; 16:211-219.
10. Spear SL, Matsuba H, Little JW III. The medial periareolar approach to submuscular augmentation mammaplasty under local anesthesia. Presented at the A.S.A.P.S. Meeting, Los Angeles, 1987.
11. Biggs TM, Yarish RS. Augmentation mammaplasty: Retropectoral versus retromammary implantation. Clin Plast Surg 1988; 15:549-555.
12. Bostwick J III. Aesthetic and reconstructive breast surgery. St Louis: CV Mosby, 1983:67-136.
13. Tebbetts JB. Transaxillary subpectoral augmentation mammaplasty: A 9-year experience. Clin Plast Surg 1988; 15:557-568.
14. Peterson R. TASPMA (Transaxillary subpectoral mammary augmentation). In: Georgiade NG, ed. Aesthetic breast surgery. Baltimore: Williams & Wilkins, 1983:63.
15. Brink R. Transaxillary subpectoral augmentation mammaplasty: A personal approach. Video presented at the A.S.A.P.S. Meeting, Orlando, FL, 1989.
16. Caffee HH. The effect of hematoma on implant capsules. Ann Plast Surg 1986; 16:102-105.
17. Spear SL, Romm S, Hakki A, Little JW III. Costal cartilage sculpturing as an adjunct to augmentation mammaplasty. Plast Reconstr Surg 1987; 79:921-926.
18. Haggerty RC, Vaughn T, Cathcart RS. Augmentation mammaplasty via the transrectus route. Presented at the A.S.A.P.S. Meeting, Orlando, FL, 1989.
19. Hester TR. The polyurethane-covered mammary prosthesis: Facts and fiction. Perspect Plast Surg 1988; 2:135-163.

19a. Caffee HH, Hathaway C. The effects of polyurethane foam covering on implant capsule contracture. Presented at the A.S.A.P.S. Meeting, Orlando, FL, 1989.

20. Burns J, Lipsky PE, Cush J, Barton FE. Immunologic alterations after implantation with polyurethane breast implants. Presented at the A.S.A.P.S. Meeting, Orlando, FL, 1988.
21. Schlesinger SL. Transaxillary subglandular augmentation mammaplasty. Presented at University of California, San Francisco, Grand Rounds, February 1989.
22. Ersek RA, Beisang AA. Misty. Molecular impact surface textured implant. Presented at the A.S.A.P.S. Meeting, San Francisco, 1988.
23. Stuart JD, Morgan PF. Evaluation of capsule formation in response to traditional and textured silicone implants. Plast Surg Forum 1988; 11:95-96.
24. Becker H. Expansion augmentation. Clin Plast Surg 1988; 15:587-594.
25. Gruber RP, Perkins PJ, Chafen LT, Shrago GG. Augmentation mammaplasty in the submuscular space—an immunologically privileged site? Unpublished data, 1984.

CHAPTER 14

Mastopexy with Augmentation

PAULE REGNAULT, M.D.

The results of simple mastopexy, on a long-term basis, are often disappointing, especially when the tissues are not firm. The mere resection of skin and the various means of trying to anchor the gland have given good results only on a temporary basis. The ptotic part of the gland always migrates back down, sooner or later, and the upper part appears flat or even depressed.[1-4]

To avoid this evolution, the author uses a resection of the lower pole of the breast with the VOQ or B techniques, which are described in this chapter. A somewhat similar technique was described for the first time in 1966 by the author.[5] In the past it was purposely used to increase the volume at the same time as to elevate the breast; now the idea is to remove the lower, pendulous pole and to change the volume according to the case, the implant being used to keep the breast mound elevated.[6-8]

DEFINITION AND CLASSIFICATION OF BREAST PTOSIS

It is essential to define the various degrees of breast ptosis in order to classify and clarify the various problems seen and plan adequate treatment (Fig. 14-1).[6]

An aesthetic breast has a volume in proportion to the body and is pleasingly rounded. The nipple is *above* the level of the inframammary fold.

The *first degree* of ptosis, or *minor* ptosis, exists when the nipple is at the level of the inframammary fold, while some part of the areola remains above the fold.

The *second degree*, or *moderate* ptosis, is present when the nipple is below the fold but above the lower contour of the breast.

The *third degree* or *major* ptosis, exists when the nipple is at the lower contour of the breast.

In addition to these three most frequent kinds of ptosis, two others are occasionally seen in practice. *Pseudoptosis* appears similar to minor ptosis, but consists of a flat and somewhat flabby breast with a nipple above the fold. This is merely a hypotrophic breast, easily corrected by a simple augmentation mammaplasty. *Partial ptosis* is usually a secondary deformity consisting of a glandular ptosis, with the nipple-areola complex above the fold, sometimes abnormally high, the glandular tissue elongated downward, and a long vertical scar. It is usually seen after inverted-T techniques of reduction mammaplasty.

LOWER POLE REDUCTION-MASTOPEXY WITH AUGMENTATION: INDICATIONS AND CONTRAINDICATIONS

This technique is mainly used for cases of moderate, major, and partial ptosis, with or without volume augmentation.[4,6] It is obvious that when a volume reduction is desired and the lower pole of the breast is removed using the B technique, the risk of recurrence of ptosis is reduced and no implant is useful. The most successful candidates for mastopexy with augmentation are flabby soft tissues and flat upper poles. Results are usually excellent with these patients.

The patient's acceptance of either periareolar or subareolar scarring is essential. Refusal to accept general anesthesia, or contraindications for such, do not rule out this technique, because local anesthesia has been used many times. Patients who have already had an augmentation and have acquired ptosis may present various problems, but may very well be candidates for this technique; fibrosis or unsatisfactory size is dealt with at the same time. A previous breast reduction or mastopexy is also an excellent indication. The technique *is* contraindicated if patients refuse to accept the possibility of visible scars or refuse to accept silicone implant augmentation.

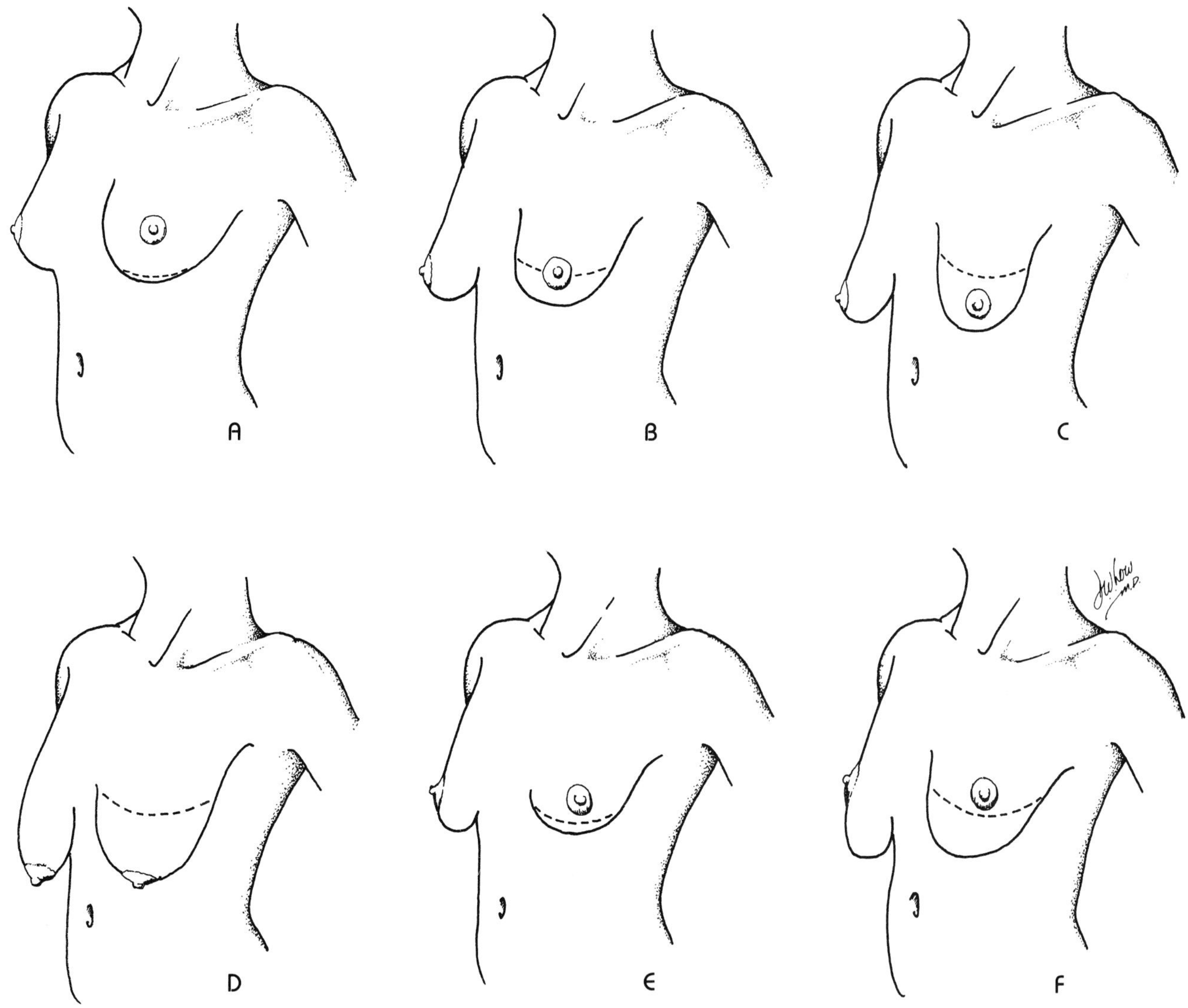

FIGURE 14–1 The degree of ptosis is determined by the relationship of the nipple to the inframammary fold. *A*, Normal breast with nipple above the inframammary fold. *B*, Minor ptosis with nipple at the level of the fold. *C*, Moderate ptosis with nipple below the fold but above the lower breast contour. *D*, Major ptosis with nipple at the lowest point on the breast. *E*, Pseudoptosis creates the impression of a ptotic breast, but the nipple remains above the inframammary fold. *F*, Glandular ptosis is usually associated with a previous reduction mammaplasty. It is denoted by descent of the gland and nipple elevation.

EXAMINATION AND PREOPERATIVE EVALUATION

After history taking to eliminate any contraindications for surgery, the breast is carefully examined.[4,6,9] A search is made for any pathologic breast condition. The presence of fibrocystic disease is a contraindication only when it is severe and involves recurrent painful episodes, which might be exacerbated by augmentation. These symptoms remain unchanged, or may be improved by a simple mastopexy and lower pole reduction.

After elimination of pathology, some measurements are made with the patient standing. The actual breast size, which the patient knows according to her brassiere size, may be verified by measuring the thoracic periphery at the inframammary fold level and at the nipple level with the brassiere on, so that the nipple is at its nonptotic location. The patient is asked whether she desires some change in breast size. The hip contour is measured to obtain an idea of the ideal size to aim for. If she is unsure of the best size, a B cup brassiere size is best advised, because this is a standard size for readymade clothing and also the most aesthetic. This is easily understood by any patient.

The skin and breast tissues are examined to verify the absence of skin or breast disease and evaluate the quality of the tissue as regards firmness, flabbiness, and elasticity. This helps to determine the importance of the breast and skin resections to be done.

The *location of the inframammary fold* is verified and marked lightly on the skin. The patient is asked to recline and the location of the fold is also marked in this position to observe its change in these two different positions. A young, aesthetically pleasing breast is limited by an inframammary fold located at approximately the sixth rib level when its volume is that of a B cup. With aging, the fold goes down, more or less, according to the tissue quality and weight of the breast.

The *nipple location* is then measured in relation to the sternal notch and its position in relation to the inframammary fold is checked, in order to determine the degree of ptosis. The size and shape of the *areolae* are also checked, so that their modifications can be discussed. The nipples may present some minor deformities such as hypertrophy or invagination, which may be documented and treated at the same time as the breast.

Breast symmetry is verified in case one side requires a larger reduction of the lower pole or a different-sized implant.[7] Experience has shown that it is preferable to perform a different volume reduction rather than use different sizes of implants. (Editor's note: I share this experience and opinion.)

EXPECTATIONS

Once the examination and measurements are completed, it is easy to discuss the case with the patient and to agree on the best surgical procedure. When the patient refuses scars or implants, she takes her own responsibility for the result, but she should not be pressured in the choice of technique. She has come to the consultation with the hope of obtaining a permanently beautiful breast, with no complications, and may be disappointed to learn that there may be scars or capsule formation. It is often wise to ask her to take time before deciding on the procedure.

The surgeon's expectations should always remain completely realistic when explaining the various possible techniques and the possible complications and disadvantages of surgery. According to the quality of the patient's tissues and the amount of skin to be removed, the extent of the scars and the durability of the results will vary. The young patient, in whom pregnancy may be expected, should be advised that she will be able to breast feed but that it is better to avoid such distention, which may be followed by a degree of atrophy.

It is useful to show some photographs illustrating the scars. This is a good way to learn the patient's opinion about the volume to be obtained. Implants may also be shown to the patient and the advantages of the different kinds explained.

At the conclusion of the examination and the discussion, the *choice of anesthesia* is discussed, because local infiltration alone is possible with the method described below. It is easier when the patient herself asks for it or when there is a contraindication to general anesthesia. She should never be influenced about the choice, but when she is uncertain, the surgeon is free to choose and to explain the reasons. The surgeon is in a position to accept or reject the patient for surgery. The best candidates for the technique of mastopexy with augmentation are patients with major or moderate ptosis, who ask for a reasonable change of volume or the same volume, and who accept some scarring.

TECHNIQUE

The operation is usually performed in an outpatient facility, but some patients may be hospitalized.

Routine preoperative laboratory tests are performed. The date chosen for surgery is preferably after the menstrual cycle. Aspirin is forbidden for 1 month before surgery, and the patient is asked to shower or bathe twice daily for a few days with any mild soap disinfectant.

Preoperative measurements and planning are carried out immediately before surgery, with the patient standing or sitting, shoulders straight and on the same level (Figs. 14–2, 14–4).[10]

1. The *new upper limit of the areola* is marked with a heavy felt pen. This mark (point V in the illustrations) is located at a varying distance from the sternal notch, usually between 15 and 22 cm. This distance should be verified by putting one finger horizontally at the inframammary fold; point V should be about 3 cm above the fold level.
2. The vertical midline of the sternum is marked, which aids in locating other marks and in symmetric planning.
3. The areolar axis, vertical and horizontal, is marked.
4. The inframammary fold is marked at its actual location. The patient is then asked to recline, so that she may be given more sedation or general anesthesia. The drawing is continued with the patient in the recumbent position.
5. The distance from the midline to the *new limit of the areola* (points M to M′) is the next step of the drawing.
6. The new submammary fold is marked when it is to be at a higher level (cases of major ptosis or breast reduction.) It should be parallel to the previous fold and 1 to 4 cm higher.
7. In a case of *minor ptosis* (Fig. 14–2), an oval is drawn using the points V and M′. This oval is vertical and symmetric, in relation to the ver-

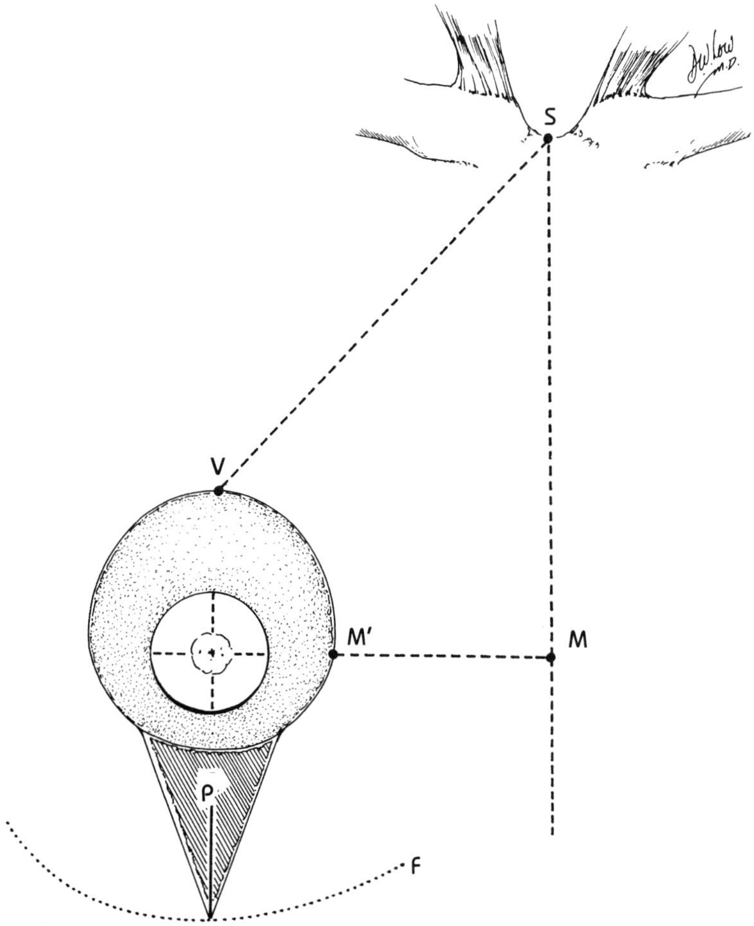

FIGURE 14-2 Preoperative measurements are made with the patient standing or sitting. S to V, Sternal notch to the upper limit of the new areola location; M to M', midline to the new medial limit of the areola (usually half of SV); P, vertical incision through the gland to approach the subglandular or subpectoral spaces; F, inframammary fold, unchanged. The stippled (shaded) area denotes epidermal removal; the oblique lines, full-thickness skin removal.

tical axis of the areola. The lower limit of the oval is 1 cm below the new contour of the areola.

8. By pinching the subareolar tissues vertically, it is possible to estimate the amount of resection to be done; a triangle is drawn, with the summit at the inframammary fold level.
9. In a case of *moderate or major ptosis* (Fig. 14-4), after the oval is drawn around the areola, point T is marked on the oval 1 cm lateral to the vertical tangent of the oval medial contour and about 1 cm below the new areola. From this point T is drawn a curve, down to the new inframammary fold, tangent also to the vertical of the oval medial contour. The upper and lower curves give the medial limit of the excisions. Between the two curves, a small angle is formed at T, giving the appearance of the letter B.
10. By pinching the tissues between the lower medial curve and the lateral part of the breast, it is then possible to estimate the approximate width of tissue to be resected. A lateral curve is drawn temporarily until it is time to reevaluate the resection, after the medial lower flap has been dissected from its upper, medial, and lower limits, and when the implant is in its pocket.

The drawing is then terminated and anesthesia is induced, followed by routine skin preparation. I favor the use of local anesthesia when the patient is a suitable subject. Good analgesia is obtained by the use of 0.5 percent lidocaine (Xylocaine) with 1/200.000 epinephrine. The intercostal blocks are done first, at the third, fourth, and fifth intercostal spaces, followed by an infiltration of the submammary area, the deep submuscular area, and the incision lines. When using *general anesthesia* the intercostal blocks are not done, but the deep and superficial infiltrations of anesthetic are used.

SURGICAL PROCEDURE

Minor Ptosis (Fig. 14-2)[11]

The periareolar circle is incised superficially as well as the oval and subareolar triangle, as previously planned. The epidermis is dissected and removed from the same areas. The incision is then continued through the dermis all along the periphery.

A vertical incision (P) is made through the dermis and gland down to the pectoralis major muscle. The lower fibers of the muscle are severed at the inframammary fold level and a blunt dissection is made behind the muscle, superficial to the costal grill at the lower part and superficial to the pectoralis minor at the upper part.[12] The pocket size is made larger than the implant base. Caution should be taken that the medial insertions of the pectoralis major are well detached; these are very strong in some patients. Careful hemostasis is always verified with direct illumination. The implant is easily introduced, since the incision and approach are fairly large.

Approximation of the skin is tested, and if there is any redundancy or tension at closure, part of the subareolar triangle may be reduced. In such an event the removal is quantitatively evaluated, in order to obtain symmetric breasts.

Absorbable 2-0 suture material is used to close the glandular tissues.

When the triangular area has been left intact, it is plicated so that it releases skin tension. A few separate sutures are placed at the four areolar quadrants and a subcuticular continuous suture of 4-0 absorbable material completes the closure. (Fig. 14-3).

The dressing is light: paper Steri-Strips and a few gauze pads. The patient is asked to wear a sport brassiere to maintain the dressing night and day for about a week, until the postoperative examination. At that time all separate sutures are removed. Other paper strips are used for a few days.

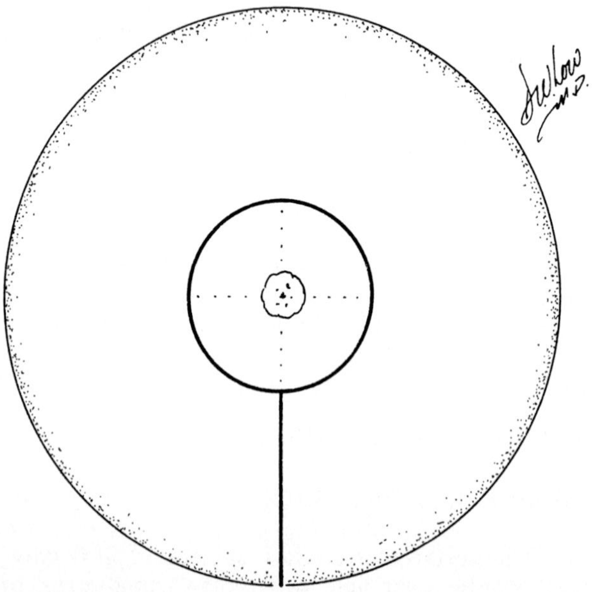

FIGURE 14-3 The final suture line, periareolar and vertical. The large circle represents the implant.

Moderate and Major Ptosis (Fig. 14-4)

The general principles of the surgical procedure for moderate or major ptosis are the same as for minor ptosis, but the epidermal excision is larger.[13,14] Glandular resection of the lower pole of the gland is always performed and is much larger.

Local anesthesia alone may also be used, but for the larger excisions it is easier to use general anesthesia in the absence of any contraindication. Local infiltration is always used concomitantly.

The epidermis is removed from the upper part, all around the areola. The incision of the dermis and the full skin incisions are made all along the drawing except at the lateral part of the subareolar drawing.

The glandular incisions are made from under the areola, horizontally continuing at the angle T and lower curve C, down to the new inframammary fold. This forms a flap of full-thickness skin and gland, which remains attached laterally at C′. In performing the dissection of this flap, one should be careful to leave a little more breast tissue than skin medially at C, but on the opposite side to remove more breast than skin between the new and the previous inframammary folds.

The flap is completely elevated from the pectoralis major. The lower fibers of the muscle are severed obliquely, following approximately the direction of the inframammary fold, and a blunt elevation of the muscle is made. The pocket obtained should be somewhat larger than the implant base.

In such cases, the approach is quite wide, providing easy visibility of the pocket for adequate hemostasis.

Once the implant is in position, the flap of breast and skin is pulled medially under moderate tension so that its optimal resection may be judged. The estimated resection is drawn on the flap. Most of the time, this drawing corresponds to the one done before surgery (C′), but it may be a little different when the elasticity of the tissue appears greater after dissection. The resection is made perpendicular to the skin or may be intentionally modified according to the quality of the tissues. To provide for closure of the deep tissues of the flap, the implant is temporarily removed. A few absorbable 2-0 sutures permit approximation of the gland. The implant is then placed back in its location. The lower part of the implant is not covered by the pectoralis major, which is left open.

For suturing (Fig. 14-5), the maximal convexity of the flap should come into the maximal concavity of the lower curve C. Some minor resections of skin may be made to obtain a smooth suture line.

A few deep sutures may be placed at the inframammary fold to keep it in position and prevent any slipping down of the implant.

Some superficial separate sutures are placed in the skin, and minor periareolar skin modifications

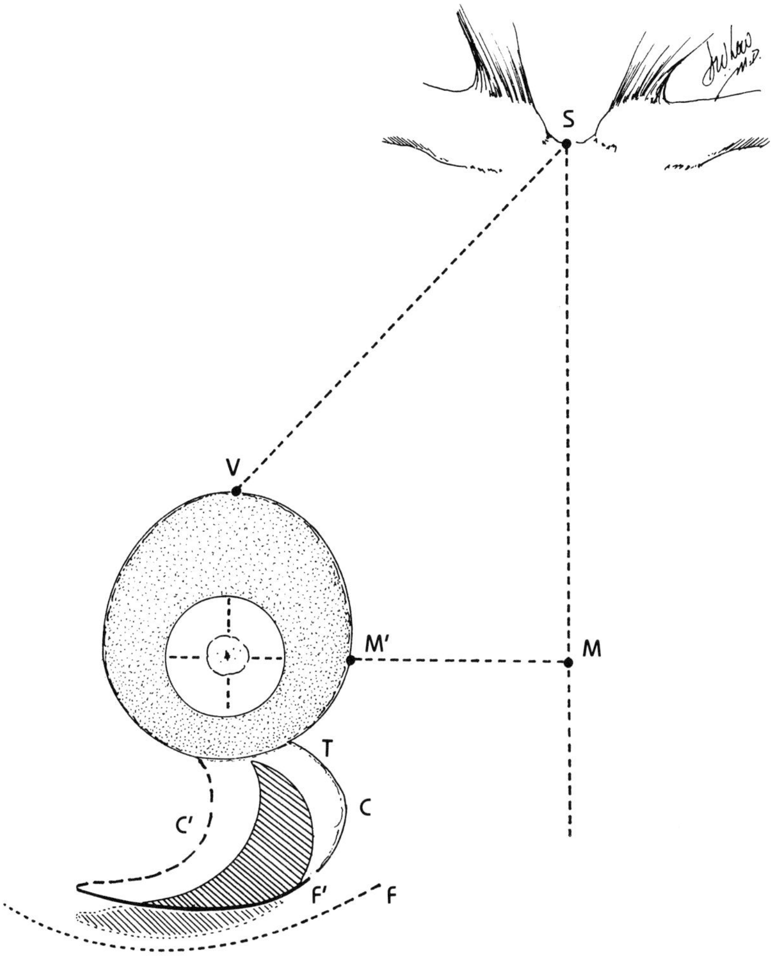

FIGURE 14-4 In moderate or major ptosis the deepithelialized (shaded) area is larger. S to V, New distance from the sternal notch to the upper limit of the areola; M to M', midline to the medial limit of the areola (usually half of SV); T, triangular flap, about 1 cm wide and located 1 cm below the areola; C, lower curve, tangent to a vertical line from M'; F, previous inframammary fold; F', new inframammary fold; C', lateral resection of the flap, the last step before suturing. The stippled (shaded) area denotes epidermal removal; the lower oblique lines, the area of gland and fat removal, down to F.

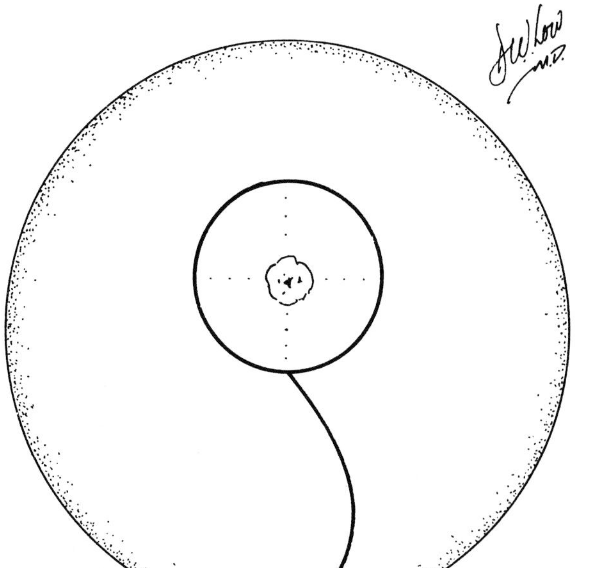

FIGURE 14-5 The final suture line, periareolar and vertical, with the curve to the inframammary fold. The large circle represents the implant.

may be made if appropriate. The suturing is terminated with a subcuticular continuous 4-0 material.

If there is any doubt about the adequacy of the hemostasis, a drain may be left for 24 to 48 hours at the declivity of the pocket.

Dressing is accomplished with paper tapes on the scars, gauze pads, and a well-fitted sport brassiere. If drains have been used, an elastic adhesive bandage is applied instead of the brassiere.

POSTOPERATIVE CARE

The patient may be discharged a few hours after surgery with postoperative instructions to restrict shoulder strain and sport activities for about 3 weeks, and to sleep on the back for about 2 weeks. A prescription is given for a narcotic analgesic for 48 hours, followed by milder pain medication. A broad-spectrum antibiotic is prescribed to be taken for 1 week after surgery.

If drains have been used, the patient should be seen the following day or after 48 hours for removal. When no drain is left, the patient is seen about 1 week after surgery. Separate stitches are removed. Paper tapes may be replaced for a few days.

Pain normally has almost disappeared a week after surgery. If not, some complication must be sought.

FINAL RESULTS (Figs. 14–6, 14–7)

Normally the *scars* remain visible for a few months and then progressively fade, leaving only a small well-located line.

The *shape* of the breast is very much improved. Sagging has disappeared. The nipple-areola complex is now above the level of the inframammary fold and altogether the breast appears more youthful and pleasingly rounded.

The *size* may be the same as before surgery if the breast tissue removed has been of the same volume as the implant, as discussed with the patient before surgery. In my practice, patients with fairly pendulous breasts request a slightly larger breast, which may have a more youthful appearance as well as being more comfortable.

COMPLICATIONS

At the Time of Surgery

Excessive bleeding should not occur when there has been careful preoperative interrogation and when laboratory tests are normal, and aspirin has been discontinued for 4 weeks. However, bleeding may occur even after the use of local anesthesia with epinephrine. In such an event, the insertion of an implant should be postponed until the end of the operation, when bleeding is under control, and drains should be used.

Excessive tension and difficulty in approximating the tissues is noted after temporarily inserting the implant before sectioning the lower pole flap, if the excision has not been carefully evaluated. In such an event, it is necessary to use a smaller implant or remove some deep glandular tissue, medially or laterally, taking care not to create a breast deformity.

In the Early Postoperative Period

Inordinate pain may present in the very sensitive woman who may require higher doses of analgesics. In any case of abnormal pain, a verification of the local conditions is safer in order to eliminate a complication.

Hematoma is rare but always possible. It is necessary to evacuate the blood as soon as the diagnosis is made and to leave a drain for 1 or 2 days. In order to evacuate an hematoma completely, it may be necessary to open the inframammary scar and to remove the implant temporarily, replacing it immediately after drainage.

Infection at the site of the implant is an excep-

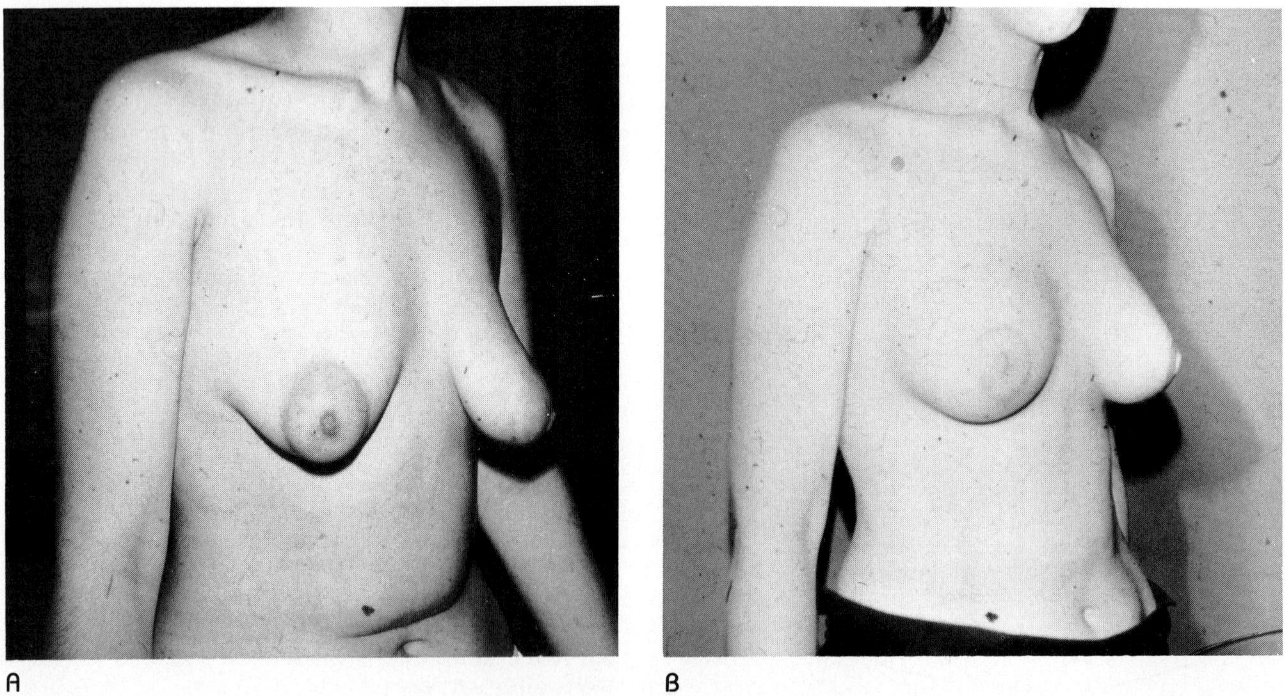

A B

FIGURE 14–6 *A*, This 29-year-old patient with major ptosis was treated with the B reduction technique and subpectoral augmentation. Resection of 150 g of breast tissue was needed to correct the ptosis. An implant size of 180 ml was used for augmentation. *B*, Result 2 years after surgery.

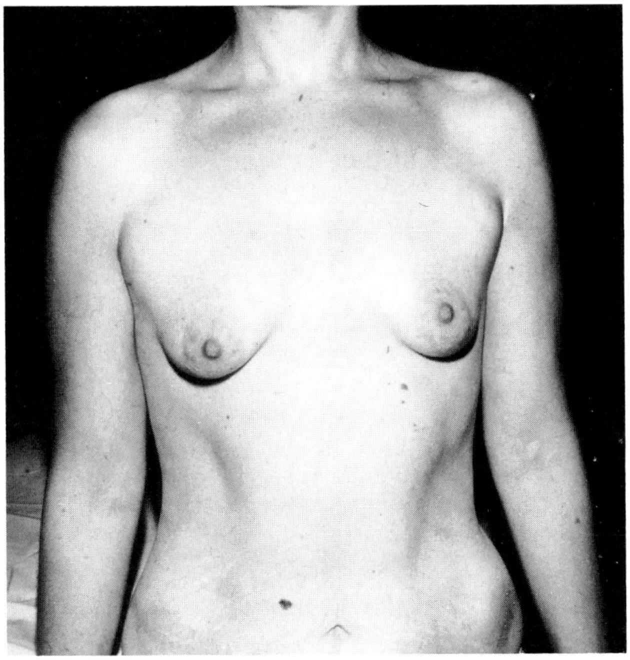

A

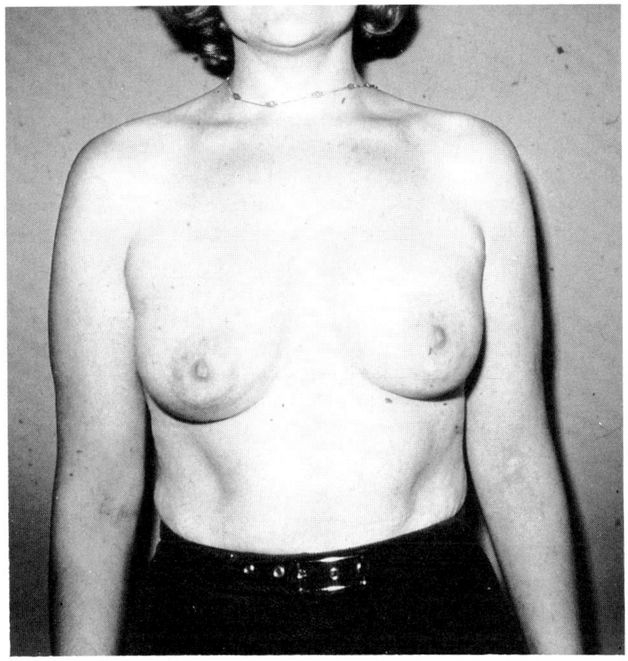

B

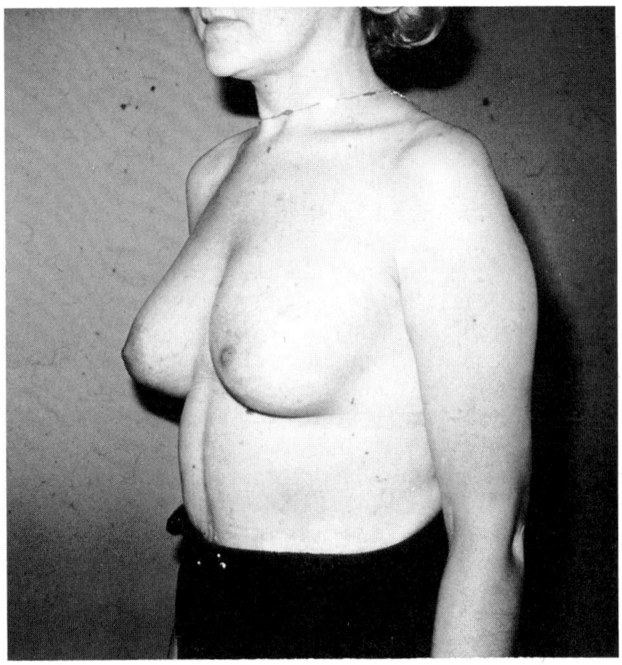

C

FIGURE 14-7 *A*, A 34-year-old female with moderate ptosis. *B*, Frontal view of the same patient 3 years after 70 g reduction of the lower pole of the breast by the B technique, and 260-ml subpectoral augmentation. *C*, Appropriate nipple position and breast fullness is demonstrated on this three-quarters view photograph.

tion, but some reactions of mild inflammation may occur at the sutures. These are treated by topical antibiotics and suture removal as soon as wound healing allows. Infection at the site of the augmentation is a rare but serious complication. The use of local and systemic antibiotic therapy may not be sufficient, and the implant may need to be removed. It can be replaced after an appropriate time.

Necrosis occurs only when excessive tension has been used to close the suture lines, or when a hematoma has not been evacuated early enough. Serious infection may also cause necrosis. Necrosis is treated by surgical cleaning, at least once a week, and the wound is allowed to heal by secondary intention. The poor scarring that may result will be corrected after a few months.

Late Complications

Sensory loss of the nipple-areola complex is very rare with the B technique of mastopexy. Diminution of sensitivity may be due to the augmentation, but also is most often temporary, lasting 1 or 2 years at the most. The desensitized area may decrease with time.

Capsular contracture does not happen more frequently in such cases than in any augmentation mammaplasty, and the treatment is the same. Closed capsulotomy is possible when the capsule is seen early. When this is not possible, an open capsulotomy is performed. It is routine in such cases to infiltrate the capsule wall with 5 ml of 10 percent triamcinolone. In a case of recurrent fibrosis, the implants may be changed for implants with a polyurethane coverage.

Scars may be temporarily hypertrophic. If they last more than a year, they may be revised, the skin being undermined widely enough to close without any tension. Hypotrophic scars should be corrected using the method of island flap plication.[12]

Unaesthetic breast shape may be due to capsular contracture or to uneven removal of breast tissue and misjudgment of the appropriate excisions. The nipple-areola complex may not be well located at the center of the breast mound. This happens only when the preoperative measurements have not been correct. Secondary corrections should be made after a few months.

Asymmetry is noted only when preoperative measurements in the sitting or standing position have not been made carefully enough, or, in a case of preoperative asymmetry, not well compensated for. A secondary revision is always possible and should not present any difficulty.

Secondary ptosis should be seen only when there is important weight loss, or when the patient breast feeds, after surgery. A secondary revision following the same scars is possible.

Adhesions of the implants to the pectoralis major happen rarely and are noticed at muscular contraction. They may be due to capsule formation and should be treated by open capsulotomy. If a serious psychological problem is thereby created, the implants are changed from the submuscular pocket to the subglandular space.

CONCLUSION

Mastopexy with augmentation is a procedure that requires careful preoperative evaluation and planning. The surgical procedure is more lengthy than a simple mastopexy or a simple augmentation, but its result is more aesthetically pleasing and longer lasting.

The technique described in this chapter has been used by the author for many years in a large number of patients. It is currently used exactly as described.

References

1. Hinderer UT. Mammaplasty: The dermal brassiere technique. Aesthetic Plast Surg 1978; 2:1.
2. Letterman G, and Shurter M. History of surgical correction of mammary ptosis. In: Owsley JQ, Peterson R, eds. Symposium on aesthetic surgery of the breast. St Louis: CV Mosby, 1978:183.
3. Pousson M. De la mastopexie. Bull Soc Chirurgie 1897; 13:507.
4. Regnault P. Unfavorable results after mastopexy. In: Goldwyn R, ed. Unfavorable results in plastic surgery. 2nd ed. Boston: Little, Brown, 1984:703.
5. Regnault P. The hypoplastic and ptotic breast: A combined operation with prosthetic augmentation. Plast Reconstr Surg 1966; 37:31.
6. Regnault P. Breast ptosis: Definition and treatment. Clin Plast Surg 1976; 3:193.
7. Regnault P. Ptosis, asymmetry, tubular breast and congenital anomalies. In: Owsley JQ, Peterson R, eds. Symposium on aesthetic surgery of the breast. St Louis: CV Mosby, 1978:107.
8. Regnault P, Daniel R. Depressed scars and soft tissues. Ann Plast Surg 1983; 10:427.
9. Regnault P, Daniel RK. Mastopexy. In: Regnault P, Daniel RK, eds. Aesthetic Plastic Surgery. Boston: Little, Brown, 1984: 539, 559.
10. Regnault P. Reduction mammaplasty by the B technique. Plast Reconstr Surg 1974; 53:19.
11. Aries G. Una nueva tecnica de mastoplastia. Rev Latinoam Cirurgia Plast 1957; 3:23, 38.
12. Regnault P. Breast augmentation. In: Strombeck JO, Rosato FR, eds. Surgery of the breast. New York: G Thieme Verlag, 1986:312.
13. Dufourmentel C, Mouly R. Évolution de la méthode oblique latérale de plastie mammaire pour hypertrophie et ptose. Collection Méd-chirurg. Paris: Flammarion, Mise à jour 1971:1978.
14. Strömbeck JO. Reduction mammaplasty. In: Strömbeck JO, Rosato FE, eds. Surgery of the breast. New York: Georg Thieme Verlag, 1986:277.

CHAPTER 15

Unfavorable Results of Augmentation Mammaplasty

ROSS RUDOLPH, M.D.

Augmentation mammaplasty is a cosmetic surgical procedure with a high rate of patient satisfaction.[1] As with any operation, however, unfavorable results and complications can occur. The greatest attention has been paid to capsular contracture, a little understood scar formation and tissue hardening around the implants, which can lead to a firm and uncomfortable breast. However, other better understood complications can also occur.

Significant improvements have occurred in the manufacture of implants since their introduction in 1962. These have included thinner-walled implants with a lower gel viscosity, resulting in a more natural feeling augmented breast, and the elimination of Dacron fixation patches. This chapter focuses on complications and unfavorable results that are (1) commonly seen; (2) occasionally seen; and (3) rarely seen, using the most modern types of implants. Each problem will be discussed with suggestions for both prevention and treatment.

COMMON UNFAVORABLE RESULTS

Capsular Contracture

Nothing in plastic surgery has generated so much confusion, glib opinion, and sheer "malarkey" as the problem of capsular contracture after silicone breast augmentation. The literature is confusing and contradictory.[2] Few good, controlled studies have been done, largely because of the peculiarities of cosmetic surgery practice.[3] Competition for patients is fierce and therefore, there is a natural reluctance on the part of aesthetic surgeons to ask them to participate in controlled studies. These patients are looking for perfection and are often not amenable to participating in such studies. Those surgeons who do a great number of cosmetic breast augmentations, are not inclined to do controlled studies because they are often happy with their individual methods and they wish to maintain their busy practices. Nevertheless, occasional controlled studies have been done.

The *pathologic process* of capsular contracture is well understood regarding gross anatomy, although its causes are less certain.[4] Both patients and surgeons often speak of "implants becoming hard", but in fact the implants remain perfectly soft and pliable. Instead, the normal fibrous capsule that forms around a smooth silicone implant, rather than remaining soft, pliable, and larger in size than the implant, shrinks and contracts in some patients. This appears to be a modification of the body's response to a foreign body, attempting to enclose and extrude the foreign material. The contracting capsule tries to compress and extrude the implant which, being liquid or gel filled, is not compressible. Instead, the shrinkage of the capsule converts the flat pancake-shaped implant to the smallest surface area per volume, which is a sphere (Fig. 15-1*A* and *B*).[4]

Contracture can either be relatively mild or, less commonly, severe and causing symptoms. Most surgeons currently use the Baker classification which, although subjective, is straightforward and easily communicated from surgeon to surgeon and easily compared from study to study.[5] This classification is as follows.[4,5]

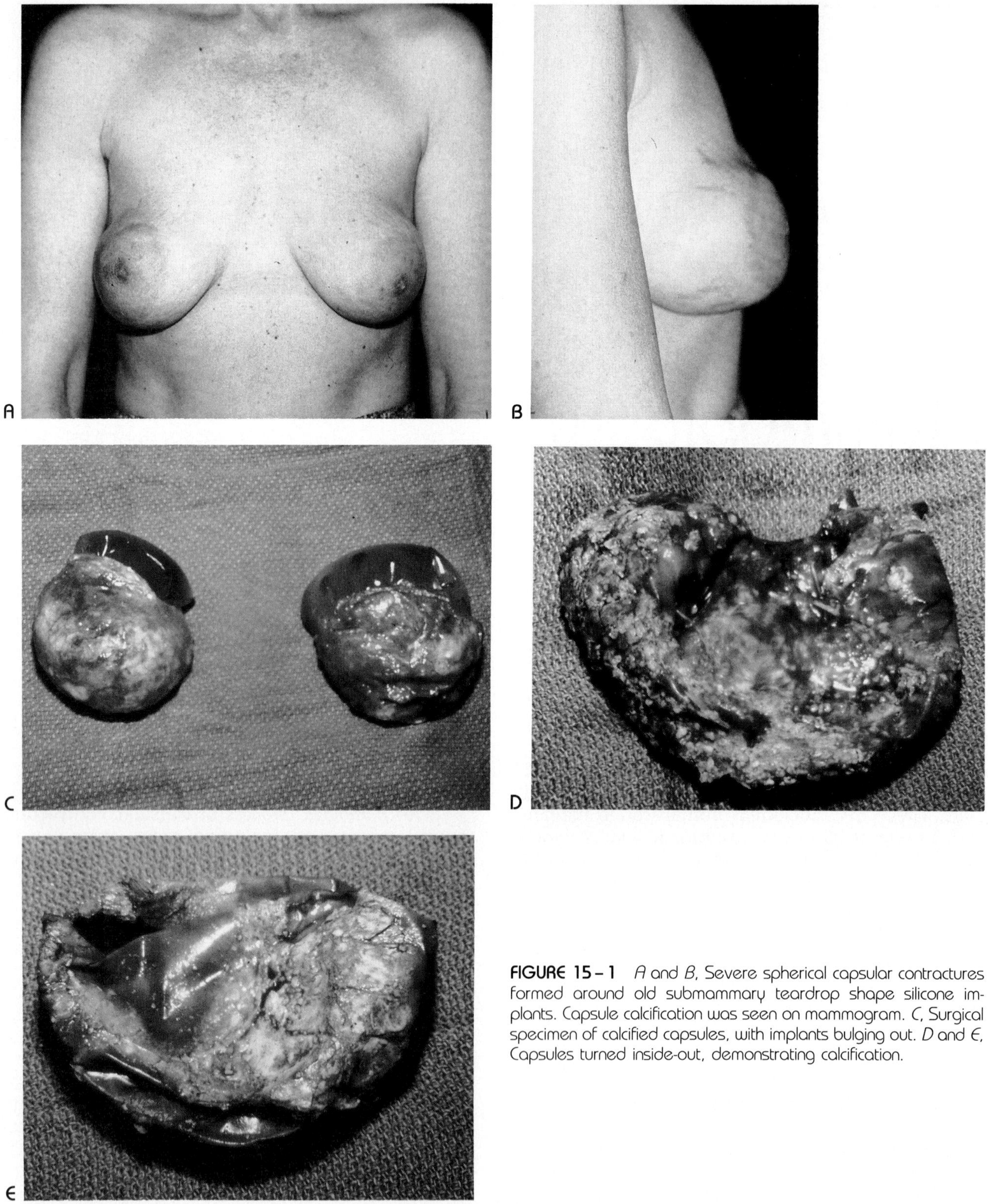

FIGURE 15–1 *A* and *B*, Severe spherical capsular contractures formed around old submammary teardrop shape silicone implants. Capsule calcification was seen on mammogram. *C*, Surgical specimen of calcified capsules, with implants bulging out. *D* and *E*, Capsules turned inside-out, demonstrating calcification.

I. The augmented breast is as soft as the unoperated one
II. The breast is less soft; the implant can be palpated but is not visible
III. The breast is firm; the implant can be palpated easily, and it, or distortion from it, can be seen.
IV. The breast is hard, tender, and painful; distortion is pronounced.[4]

Capsular contracture is most common within the first 6 months after surgery, but can occur at any time after the procedure.[4,6] Reported incidence varies widely, ranging from 0 to 75 percent![6] Late capsular contracture may be preceded by a viral or bacterial infection elsewhere.[7] For reasons *totally* not understood, one breast may develop capsular contracture while the other breast remains soft, a puzzle that has confused surgeons and made theories of explanation exceedingly difficult.[2,6] In capsular contracture that is longstanding, often more than 10 years, calcification can develop in the collagenous capsules, making the capsule even firmer and more rigid (Fig. 15-1 *C-E*). This process appears to be similar to that which can develop in collagen-fabricated prostheses.[8] The other large implant placed superficially in the chest—a pacemaker—can also develop symptomatic contracture.[9]

Histologically, the peri-implant capsule is a smooth fibrous structure composed of layered collagen interspersed with flattened fibroblasts. Most contracted capsules are thicker than normal, uncontracted capsules, although contracted capsules may also be thin-walled. Under the electron microscope, myofibroblasts can be seen in recently contracted or operated-on capsules. These cells, which share the electron microscopic appearance of fibroblasts and smooth muscle cells, are probably the contractile mechanism of capsular contraction,[10,11] similar to that of wound contraction processes elsewhere such as burn scar contracture, cirrhosis, and Dupuytren's contracture of the palmar fascia.[12,13] Alternate theories have suggested that mobile fibroblasts pulling on the surrounding stroma, rather than contraction of fibroblasts themselves, cause the force of capsular and wound contraction.[14] Regardless of which of these theories is correct, all agree that the active fibroblasts affecting the surrounding collagenous stroma and perhaps being influenced by that stroma, are the motor force for peri-implant capsular contraction and consequent contracture.

Baker and Penn have pointed out that a soft breast, with a collagen-lined bursa larger than the implant, is almost an anomaly.[15] The body's natural reaction to a foreign body is compression and extrusion; and the question has been asked why not all implants undergo this type of compression. Fortunately the great majority do not, because the body is also capable of responding to a smooth foreign body by producing a smooth nonreactive bursa which, while containing the foreign body, allows it mobility. This smooth, large bursa is the sought-after state of a natural appearing breast following smooth silicone implantation.

Various implant modifications have been introduced to attempt to change the contraction process. Both electron microscopy[12,16] and chemical analysis[17] have shown microscopic amounts of silicone in capsules surrounding gel implants. However, no connection was found between the presence of such gel leak and capsular contracture.[12,18] Nevertheless, saline-filled and "low-bleed" implants have been designed and used based on the theory that silicone leak is responsible for contracture. Although some decrease in contracture has been found with saline-filled implants,[1,19,20] neither type of implant (saline or low-bleed) has met with wide acceptance because of problems with saline leak[20] and the lack of convincing studies showing definitive reduction of capsular contracture.

Recently introduced are implants that have a rough coating, either of polyurethane matting[21] or textured, rough, silicone. These implants are designed to allow tissue ingrowth into the implant, thereby modifying the contraction process.

What is not understood clearly is the *initiating* event for most capsular contractures around a silicone breast implant. The majority of capsular contractures appear spontaneously, although some causes are obvious. For example, both clinically and experimentally, the presence of an undrained hematoma appears to incite both thickening of the capsule and possibly a higher rate of capsular contracture. This may be because of the irritating effect of hematoma via production of free radicals.[22]

A frank infection, even if controlled by antibiotics, often leads to a severe capsular contracture. Less clear-cut is the suggestion of "sub-clinical" infection,[23] in which there are no obvious signs of infection. The presence of relatively small numbers of bacteria, particularly *Staphylococcus epidermidis*,[24] is theorized to cause a contractile reaction in the surrounding tissue. The theory of subclinical infection is based on the finding of positive cultures for *S. epidermidis* in surgical exploration of contracted breasts, and by the reduction in capsular contracture using topical antibacterials and antibiotics.[25,26] Electron microscopy of contracted capsules does not show significant numbers of bacteria,[27] which are expected if true infection exists. Experimental study of infected implants in animals has shown increased contracture.[28] As an infectious disease consultant has pointed out, theories of "subclinical infection" are at this point speculation, and could be subjected to a randomized controlled study.[29] To date, such a study has not been accomplished with antibiotics that do not in themselves potentially modify the wound healing process.[30]

The great majority of capsular contractures simply seem to occur without an obvious cause, which has been a source of great frustration to both surgeons and patients. It would seem that the most logical explanation is that capsular contracture is multifactorial, i.e., there may be a genetic predisposition triggered by one or more as yet unidentified events.

Prevention

Because the etiology of capsular contracture is obscure, there have been many suggestions on how to prevent such contracture.[4] We are all aware of "the fad of the year" in which almost annually a new suggestion is made by someone claiming to have developed the elixir of capsular contracture prevention (Table 15-1).

From this list of suggested remedies, a number have met with moderate success.[4] They have been discovered empirically and have not been developed from a sound scientific basis.

Avoidance of Dacron Fixation Patches. As Williams pointed out, the use of Dacron fixation patches is associated with a higher chance of capsular contracture.[31] The initial rationale for these patches was to avoid implant displacement, which proved unnecessary. Hence, fixation patches have been universally discontinued with an apparent decrease in capsular contracture.

Massage of Implants. Most plastic surgeons instruct their patients who have smooth silicone implants to massage and compress the breast after surgery; this is, in essence, a physical therapy.[2] Such massage is designed to move the implants around in the capsule, to keep the developing capsule stretched into a smooth bursa larger than the implant.[32] However, not all plastic surgeons agree, and some feel that immobility is best.[33] No convincing scientific studies absolutely document the efficacy of massage,[34] which is thus prescribed on a common sense basis. Because early capsules contain new, immature collagen, implant massage may stretch and mold their shape, as with physical therapy of new scar elsewhere in the body.

Use of Glucocorticoids (Steroids). Because glucocorticoids inhibit collagen synthesis and wound contraction, as well as reduce experimental capsular contracture and thickness,[35] their prophylactic use in breast augmentation was initially greeted with great acclaim.[36] However, use of glucocorticoids in high dosage led to tissue atrophy in the breasts with occasional exposure of the implants (see later), markedly inhibiting the surgeons' enthusiasm. Use of steroids in lower doses still meets with favor from some plastic surgeons, particularly in difficult or recurrent contraction. For example, Gruber has injected Kenalog into the capsule at the time of surgical capsulotomy.[37] Caffee has suggested the use of small amounts of soluble steroids such as Solumedrol in double-lumen implant outer envelopes with submuscular placement.[38,39] Less than 20 mg/100 ml of Solumedrol appears to be a safe dose that may inhibit capsular contracture.[39,40] Others have used methylprednisolone (Solumedrol) or less soluble triamcinolone (Kenalog) in the implant pocket, but there is a concern about this material pooling at the bottom of the wound and leading to atrophy. Both Baker and Penn[15] and Brody[39] pointed out the potential medical legal hazards of placing any material within an implant itself, as the implants are classified as devices rather than as drugs. At this time, some competent authorities still suggest steroids for prevention of capsular contracture, but in lower doses than previously used and with great circumspection, while others feel steroids should not be used (especially in implants).[39] Oral vitamin E has been used empirically by some surgeons for its (possibly) weak, systematic steroid-like effect.[41] The side effects of systemic steroids have prevented their use in treating capsular contracture.

Rough-Coated Implants. The rough-coated implant represents a radically different approach to capsular contracture. Whereas the standard smooth silicone implants are designed to move around in the pseudo-bursa, which remains larger than the implant, the rough implants are designed to allow tissue ingrowth. Polyurethane-coated implants have been available for many years, and do appear to reduce the rate of capsular contracture. Some plastic surgeons have used them with great enthusiasm for initial augmentation. Studies have shown, however, that the polyurethane coating incites a significant tissue reaction and disappears with time causing uncertainties about the fate of the polyurethane coating.[42,43] Most plastic surgeons currently use such implants as a last resort for the patient with recurrent, difficult capsular contracture.

An implant was recently introduced that has a closed-cell, rough outer silicone coating that theoretically should eliminate some of the concerns about polyurethane coating changes. Studies are only preliminary; therefore there are insufficient data at present to recommend rough-coated implants as the universal answer to capsular contracture.

Subpectoral (Submuscular) Implantation. An increasing trend nationally is the placement of implants underneath the pectoralis major muscle

TABLE 15-1 Control of Breast Capsular Contraction "The Fad of the Year"

1. Avoidance of Dacron patches
2. Inflatable implants
3. Steroids
4. Massage
5. Large pockets
6. Different implant shells (gel barrier)
7. Subpectoral position
8. Antibiotic foam
9. Antibiotics in implants
10. Different implant shells (rough-coated)

rather than in the initially described submammary or subglandular (i.e., on top of the muscle)[4, 44-46] locations. This subpectoral approach is based largely on increasing numbers of reports that suggest that capsular contracture is less likely to occur.[4, 44-46]

The author initially greeted these reports with considerable skepticism. In fact, I reviewed my practice statistics at a time (1985) when my practice contained equal numbers of postmastectomy and cosmetic augmentations.[47] All of the postmastectomy reconstructions were performed in the submuscular position; two-thirds of the cosmetic augmentations were submammary and one-third were submuscular. All implantations were performed by myself with similar saline/silicone implants and techniques. Statistics at that time, in 73 reconstructive patients with submuscular implants, showed 27.4 percent developing Baker class III or class IV hardness. Cosmetic patients numbered 68; 21 were submuscular with a hardness rate of 38.1 percent, and 47 had submammary placement with a hardness rate of 38.3 percent. Breast implants were also analyzed by numbers of breasts augmented. For reconstructive submuscular implantations, 25.0 percent became hard. In cosmetic implantations 33.3 percent of submuscular and 25.0 percent of submammary breasts became hard. If surgery for recurrent contracture was deleted, this left a primary contracture rate for cosmetic surgery of 30.0 percent for submuscular implantations and 22.2 percent for submammary implantations. Looking at all augmentations for all purposes, 25.0 percent of 88 submammary augmentations became hard compared with 27.4 percent of 146 submuscular augmentations. These data suggested that submuscular silicone implantation did not confer major protection against capsular contracture as compared to the submammary approach.

Reluctant to accept these numbers as appearing to fly in the face of increasing opinion, I conducted a national survey of plastic surgeons who promoted the use of submuscular implantation. Although many factors such as the size and the type of implant varied from surgeon to surgeon, I found a number of constants. These were: (1) use of general anesthesia; (2) use of periareolar rather than inframammary incision; and (3) use of antibacterials either in the implant pocket or in the implant itself.[26] In discussions with the plastic surgeons who had provided this information, it became apparent that use of general anesthesia (or high dose ketamine hydrochloride) allowed the surgeon more leeway in doing dissection properly to allow a generous pocket, and to control hemostasis better than could be done under local anesthetic with sedation. Submuscular anesthesia may be difficult to obtain using local anesthesia, which may reduce the surgeon's ability to do an extensive dissection. Use of the periareolar approach allows the surgeon to avoid the serratus muscle substance, which reduced bleeding.[45] Finally, use of antibiotics and antibacterials, at least the commonly used half-strength povidone-iodine (Betadine) or cephalosporins, does have potential effects on the coagulation cascade and on fibroblast growth and function, both of which could influence contraction.[30]

I now do most breast augmentations using the subpectoral approach, general anesthetic, the periareolar approach whenever possible, and irrigation of the surgical pocket with half-strength Betadine solution. Although it is too early to evaluate with certainty, I recently reviewed my statistics for the last 2 years and found a contracture rate of only 9 percent. Hence, my personal experience mirrors that of the literature, in that capsular contracture is less likely when a subpectoral approach is used.

Treatment

In the patient with developing capsular contracture, increased massage and use of oral vitamin E is commonly suggested. An occasional patient may achieve some softening of the newly developed capsular contracture with this treatment. This approach is worth trying but more often than not the capsule contracture persists and develops a steady state of firmness.

Manual capsulotomy has been used commonly as treatment for capsular contracture when the implant is in the submammary position. This somewhat medieval but effective procedure is accomplished by applying direct pressure to the breast to "pop" the contracted capsule thereby softening the breast. Ideally this should be done in a circumferential fashion to produce a smooth, uniform release. Potential problems include acute bleeding, tear of the implant, or asymmetric tear of the capsule, producing an unusually shaped breast, any one of which may lead to the need for acute or scheduled surgical capsulotomy. When performing manual capsulotomy on a patient operated on by another surgeon, try to obtain information about the type of implant used, in case acute surgery is required. Vigorous massage can be used soon after, within a day or two of the manual capsulotomy, possibly accompanied by use of vitamin E by mouth. Manual capsulotomy is difficult if not impossible to do in the patient with subpectoral implants, in the patient with dense calcification, or in the patient with severe capsular contracture. A submuscular position prevents a good application of the rupturing force, whereas the severely contracted or calcified capsule may be softened but a pleasing shape often cannot be achieved.

Open capsulotomy is the next step for treating the severely contracted or submuscular contracted breast. Once the pocket is opened surgically, a number of options exist. For the patient with a submammary implant, use of general anesthesia allows submuscular placement of that implant, with closure of the prepectoral pocket to prevent the implant from displacing anteriorly.

If the implant is already submuscular, circumferential and radial capsulotomy will produce a larger space with careful attention paid to producing a smooth, uniform, and symmetric appearance. Sitting the patient up during surgery is often useful for achieving this goal. Even with submuscular implants, capsular release can often be done under a local anesthetic with sedation. Some plastic surgeons have suggested replacement of a contracted submammary implant by a rough-coated implant accompanied by circumferential and radial capsulotomy, or by capsulectomy, as an alternative to subpectoral placement. If an implant is being replaced into the same pocket, Gruber has suggested injection of triamcinolone (Kenalog) around the periphery.[37]

Unfavorable Shape and Position

Implants may be placed too high, too low, too lateral, too medial, or may displace anteriorly if a submammary implant was being placed submuscularly.

High Implant. A high implant can occur if there is not enough dissection inferiorly. This is especially a problem in the subpectoral implantation if the inferior attachments of the pectoral muscle to the ribs are not adequately freed. The pectoral muscle inserts into the fifth rib, which is one interspace too high for the normal appearing breast. If these fibers are not adequately detached, the implant will sit high.

Novice plastic surgeons should be careful with the concept of "total submuscular cover," as therein lays a trap for the unwary. Inferior to the fifth rib attachment of the pectoral muscle is a tight band of fascia and serratus muscle which, if dissected under but *not* adequately released, will push the implant too high. Many plastic surgeons solve this problem by staying on top of the serratus muscle and the rectus abdominus fascia.[45] This means that the "submuscular" implant is not completely covered by muscle. If the surgeon chooses to place an implant *completely* underneath the serratus and rectus fascia, he or she must be sure there is adequate release; otherwise the implant will tend to ride high.

A too high implant may also occur after capsular contracture, even if initial placement was correct (Fig. 15-2*A and B*). Although the reason for the directional force is not known, if capsular contracture does cause implant displacement, it is almost always upward.

Low Implant. This defect can occur when dissection of the inframammary crease extends lower than intended. Right-handed surgeons have a tendency to make the left breast slightly lower than the right because of the greater ease of dissection, when the periareolar, submuscular approach is used. Inframammary incisions are less likely to lead to low implants, possibly because the incisional scar supports and defines the inframammary line.

Lateral Implant. Lateral implant position can occur if excessive dissection is done laterally, usually with blunt dissection not done under direct vision.

Medial Implant. Medial implant position can occur if the patient has a prominent sensory nerve that lies more medial than normal, preventing the surgeon from creating an adequate lateral pocket for the implant selected. It can also happen if dissection is directed past the costo-sternal junction.

Anterior Displacement. Anterior displacement may occur if a smooth silicone implant is surgically moved from the submammary to the subpectoral position, but the original smooth pocket is left intact and unsutured. The implant can slip inferiorly under the muscle edge and back into the anterior pocket.

Prevention

Implant Too High or Too Low. Proper and symmetric location of the implant and the inframammary crease can be obtained by marking the sitting patient immediately prior to anesthesia and surgery. The new crease is usually 1 to 2 cm lower than the visible preoperation inframammary crease. The actual amount of difference depends on the size of the breast, the size of the implant, and the contour of the patient's chest. At surgery, prevention of the too high implant can be accomplished by adequate dissection of the pectoralis muscle, dividing all muscle until whitish-yellow tissue is seen, and staying on top of the serratus muscle and rectus fascia. The too-low implant can be guarded against by carefully marking and adhering to the appropriate level of dissection. If there is a question, the patient can be placed in the sitting position, even under general anesthesia (with the cooperation of the anesthesiologist), to establish the inframammary crease.

Implant Too Lateral. This can be avoided by careful measurement and dissection under direct vision, taking into account the intended width of the implant and the width of the patient's breast and chest.

Implant Too Medial. Avoidance of a too medial implant can be accomplished by placing a smaller implant or possibly by dissecting the sensory nerve laterally through the serratus, which may be a bloody procedure.[37] A very medially placed sensory nerve may occasionally be divided if there is no other choice, understanding that this may cause some sensory loss.

Anterior Displacement of an Implant. This can be prevented by suturing the submammary pocket closed at surgery, to avoid anterior displacement of the newly placed submuscular implant.

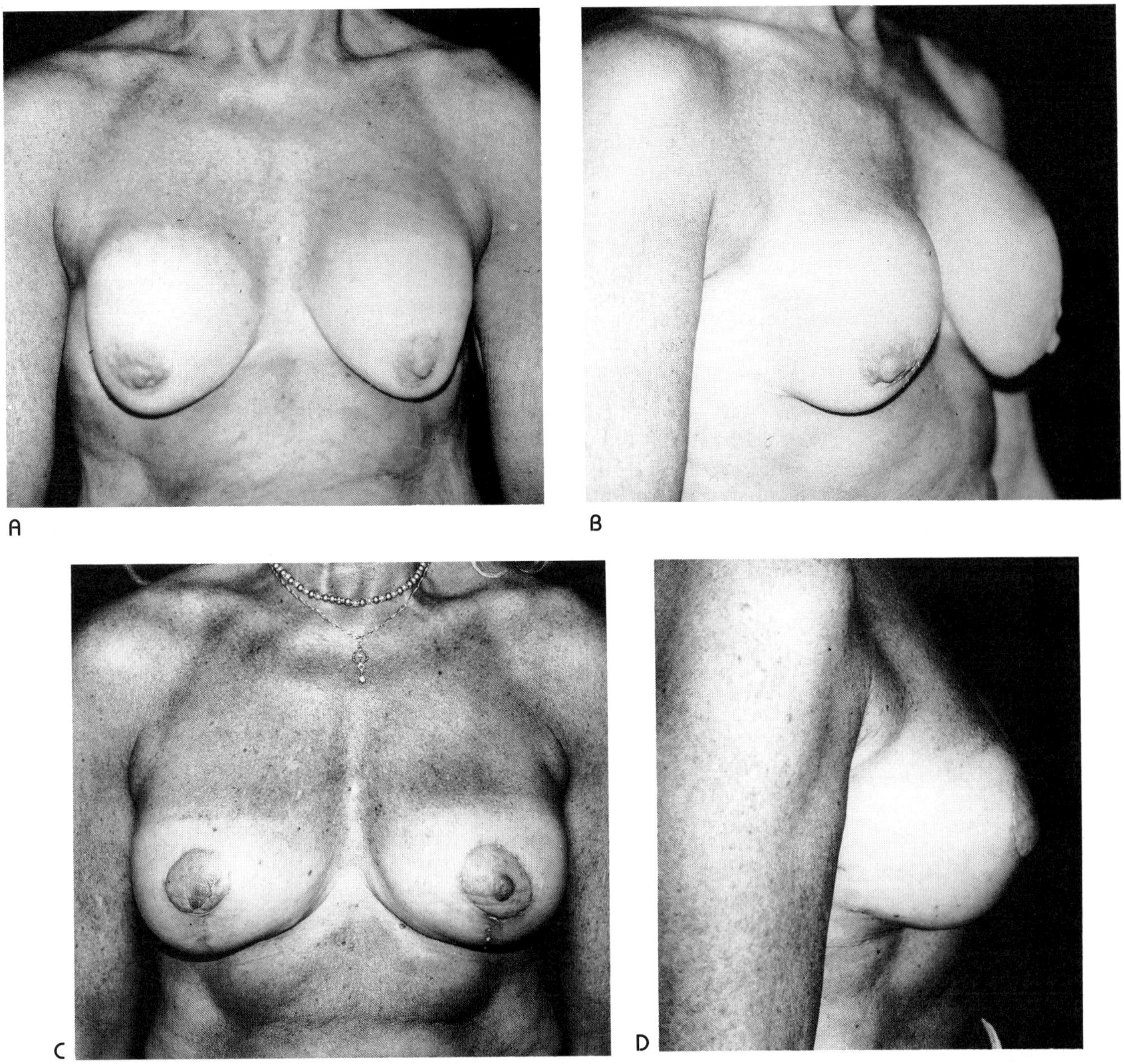

FIGURE 15–2 *A* and *B*, Severe capsular contracture produced superiorly displaced implants and ptosis, many years after submammary silicone implantation. *C* and *D*, Postoperative photographs after subpectoral placement of rough-coat silicone implants (McGhan Biocell) and mastopexy.

Treatment

Implant Too High. In the immediate postoperative period, some surgeons have tried to use an Ace bandage compression to force the implant downward, but this is generally unsuccessful, as excessively high implant position results from retained muscle attachment of the pectoralis major muscle, or to a tight band of serratus muscle, rectus fascia, and inferomedial pectoralis fascia near the sternum.

Surgical capsulotomy is required for correction, with dissection both radially and circumferentially to allow the implant to drop into the ideal position (Fig. 15–2*C* and *D*). Patients should be marked while in the upright sitting position, prior to anesthesia, to allow localization of the dissection extent.

After release, marking the proper bra position on the patient's chest will prevent the bra from closing the newly-dissected, inferior pocket; the patient can place and keep the bra in the ideal location.

Implant Too Low. In contrast to the high implant, a low implant can usually be elevated in the immediate postoperative period by application of a tape dressing. If left for 2 to 3 weeks, and supplemented by a tightly worn bra properly placed at the intended inframammary crease location, often the inframammary pocket will close and the implant will remain elevated. If postoperative massage is used, it must be done upward, medially, and laterally only, and not in a downward direction. Vitamin E should probably be avoided during this time. If taping is not successful, surgical tailoring of the capsule is required later.[48]

Implant Too Lateral. This correction requires surgical capsulorrhaphy with closing of the pocket by excision of capsule and suturing in layers. Although some have recommended nonabsorbable sutures, the author has found that 2-0 polyglactin (Vicryl) sutures work just as well. In the postoperative period, pressure that would push the implant laterally needs to avoided.

Implant Too Medial. Surgical capsulotomy and lateral dissection can be performed to correct this problem. The sensory nerve must be sought and avoided. If the nerve is more medially placed than normal, a smaller implant may be placed instead of performing further surgical capsulotomy.

Anteriorly Displaced Implant. The only solution to this is surgical replacement of the implant back under the muscle. This should be done soon after diagnosis to avoid loss of the submuscular dissection pocket.

Residual Ptosis

Residual ptosis after breast augmentation is common if the nipple position is initially too low.[49] If, when the patient is standing or sitting, the midportion of the nipple lies well below the inframammary crease, then augmentation alone is not likely to correct the ptosis. The implant then sits higher than the breast tissue, which droops over the implant. Ptosis can also occur if capsular contracture elevates the implant but soft breast tissue remains low (Fig. 15–2*A* and *B*).

Prevention

Postoperative ptosis can be prevented by performing mastopexy at the time of augmentation if the patient has a pre-existing ptosis. If the nipple position is borderline, implantation can be either submammary or subpectoral, with some correction of ptosis. Rough-coated implants in the submammary position may be particularly effective. The greater likelihood of submammary capsular contracture with smooth implants suggests that submuscular implantation be done, with extensive release of the muscle attachments to the fifth rib and of the inferior fascia to allow the implant to drop adequately. If an attempt is being made to correct borderline ptosis, the implant may need to be placed lower than would be normally the case.

Treatment

Treatment of residual ptosis is by mastopexy (see Fig. 15–2*C* and *D*). In the case of borderline ptosis, patients may be told that secondary mastopexy could be needed if adequate correction is not accomplished by the breast augmentation.

Double-Bubble Deformity

Gruber has called attention to the undesirable crease that can result from subpectoral augmentation because of the necessary elevation of the inframammary crease from the chest wall when a large implant is placed.[37] Two bulges may be seen, with the first from the nipple to the previous inframammary crease, and the second from the old inframammary crease to the new inframammary crease. This can also be seen following submammary dissection but tends to be more common with periareolar submuscular dissection. The crease can persist, although it does tend to relax and lessen with time. A constricted, "tubular" breast may be especially prone to a double-bubble contour.

Prevention

Prevention of the "double-bubble" deformity is facilitated by surgical release of the banding structure from within, especially of the medial pectoralis major muscle as it attaches to the sternum. If the patient has a tubular breast,[7] where there is a true horizontal deficiency of tissue, introduction of a triangular-shaped flap may be necessary to avoid a severe double-bubble deformity.[50] Some double-bubble effect may persist despite all surgical maneuvers. A minor crease is usually well tolerated by most patients, especially because it tends to improve with time.

Treatment

In the immediate postoperative period, occasional success with taping or bra elevation of the breast is found. More often surgical correction is required that may involve closing of the inferior pocket and placement of a smaller implant as well as release of muscle.[37] Minor mastopexy with nipple elevation may be needed in an augmented tubular breast, if nipple and breast droop over the double-bubble crease.

OCCASIONAL UNFAVORABLE RESULTS

Major Permanent Sensory Changes

Minor sensory changes are common after breast augmentation, and are not correlated with the incision site.[51] Patients often have patchy areas of sensory loss in the lower portion of the breast. These losses are generally temporary, with sensation returning over 6 to 12 months. Courtiss and Goldwyn noted that as many as 15 percent of patients may have decreased sensation 2 years after surgery.[51] Major sensation loss of the nipple is less common and can occur if the sensory nerve to the nipple is divided as lateral dissection is being done. Such complete sensory loss to the nipple may be permanent although, even with complete division of a sensory nerve, some sensation often returns. Patients for whom nipple sensation is an important part of sexual stimulation may find a diminished orgasmic capacity if complete numbness of the nipple occurs.[37] *Hypersensitivity* of the nipple can also occur postoperatively, possibly because of the nipple being thrust out against clothing and bra by the underlying implant. Hypersensitivity almost always resolves within 3 months.[51]

Prevention

The only way to prevent major sensory loss is by preserving the main sensory nerve to the nipple. In most cases, this nerve can be seen in the lateral extent of the dissection at about T4, because the nerve comes out of the serratus muscle and passes into the breast substance.[52,53] The nerve in many patients is a relatively large structure measuring approximately 2 to 3 mm in diameter. The surgeon should avoid extensive blind dissection or tearing of bands laterally, and this dissection should be done under direct vision using a fiberoptic light. Some patients will have multiple nerves and vessels rather than a single large nerve, and dissection ideally should be between the bundles that appear to be nerves. It is occasionally difficult to distinguish multiple nerves from blood vessels. A rare patient will have an apparent large sensory nerve coming from chest wall to breast tissue almost within the middle of dissection, preventing placement of an implant. Under these circumstances, nerve division may be necessary. If the nerve is more medially placed than normal, it can often be stretched and the implant placed nevertheless. This is a satisfactory solution as long as the implant is not unduly displaced, although patients may for some time complain of burning pain in the nipple after this maneuver. Gruber and Friedman have suggested dissecting the nerve back through the serratus muscle as another way of obtaining greater length;[37] this can be a bloody and technically difficult maneuver. Farina et al suggested modifying the periareolar incision so that it is more superomedially turned, possibly preserving small sensory nerves.[53]

Treatment

Prevention is the only treatment for sensory loss caused by mammary augmentation. Patients can be reassured, however, that even major sensory changes are likely to improve somewhat with time.

Hypersensitivity can often be treated by gentle padding. Soft and fluffy nursing pads sold for use by nursing mothers are often helpful. A rare patient with nipple sensitivity may have a neuroma, particularly if a periareolar incision was used. A trigger point can sometimes be located. Injection with local anesthetic and/or steroids, or even excision may be appropriate if a specific tender point can be consistently identified.

Hematoma

As with any surgical procedure that involves dissection of a large space, excess bleeding can lead to a hematoma. Numerous series have shown that in breast augmentation, hematoma occurs in about 2 percent of all cases.[15] In the immediate postoperative period, this is manifested by acute pain, tense, swollen skin with asymmetric size, and later, bruising. Fortunately, overlying necrosis of the skin, as can occur if a hematoma develops in a facelift, is almost unheard of. Hematomas usually occur within the first 24 hours but have been seen as late as 4 to 5 days later if a patient engages in vigorous and unwise physical activity. Clinically, small undrained hematomas often result in capsular contracture, although experimental evidence is conflicting.[54,55]

Prevention

Meticulous hemostasis at the time of surgery is essential. Electrocautery, irrigation, and good lighting are used. Saline irrigation is helpful in identifying specific bleeding points. The commonly used povidone-iodine (Betadine) irrigation may slightly increase punctate bleeding and such bleeding must be looked for. If the patient appears to have a slow persistent ooze of blood, placement of drains through the incision may be useful, to be removed in 1 or 2 days. Some surgeons place drains in all patients. The periareolar incision helps the surgeon avoid the bloody serratus muscle during the submuscular dissection and allows better visualization of bleeding vessels. Patients need to be educated to reduce their activity significantly for the first 4 to 5 days.

If a patient gives a significant history of past bleeding, hematologic studies should be obtained. Patients should also avoid drugs that affect platelet function. The most common of these, which patients may take unknowingly, are salicylates and nonsteroidal anti-inflammatory agents. Platelet effect from aspirin may last as long as 10 days, whereas the nonsteroidal anti-inflammatory agents appear to clear their effect on platelets within 2 to 3 days. The author has found it useful to include in the printed preoperative instructions to the patient, advice to avoid aspirin and similar drugs for 10 days prior to surgery. If there is a question regarding ingestion of drugs, the most useful test is the *bleeding time.* More complicated tests such as prothrombin time, partial thromboplastin time, and platelet counts, *will not* detect the most common cause of postoperative bleeding, which is aspirin ingestion and consequent interference with platelet function.

Treatment

Evacuation of a symptomatic hematoma as soon as possible is probably best to reduce tissue reaction. General anesthesia is often wise because it is difficult to obtain complete hemostasis under local anesthesia. Patients may be reluctant to have evacuation of a hematoma with general anesthesia because of costs. It would be appropriate for the surgeon to charge no fee under these circumstances, but often anesthesia charges and hospital charges must be incurred. Fortunately, many insurance companies, even though they exclude cosmetic surgery, may pay for the cost of a complication such as a major hematoma. Ellenberg has noted that if hematoma evacuation is delayed a few days, there will be less bleeding and local anesthetic will suffice.[49] Small hematomas absorb but may lead to increasing capsular contracture, especially if steroids have not been used in the implant.[49]

After evacuation of a hematoma, it is often wise to place drains as well as a compression dressing. Coagulation studies should be done to detect previously unsuspected bleeding syndromes. These should include a complete blood count with platelet count, prothrombin time, partial thromboplastin time, and bleeding time.

Hypertrophic and Widespread Scars

The presence of hypertrophic and widespread scars is the primary objection to the inframammary incision, which would otherwise be satisfactory because the patient is unable to see that scar on a routine basis. An inframammary incision that becomes a fine hairline scar is acceptable but the not uncommon spreading or hypertrophy of a scar is a cosmetic deformity more obvious as it sits in the middle of otherwise intact skin (Fig. 15-3). Fortunately, inframammary scars generally ride slightly up onto the breast and are therefore hidden under the usual clothing. There is no obvious relationship of the occurrence of such scars to patient ethnicity, although a history of keloids or hypertrophic scars developing elsewhere should raise suspicions.

Prevention

Periareolar incisions are less likely to develop hypertrophy or spread, and are less visible because of the natural disguise of the juxtaposition of pigmented and nonpigmented skin. If an inframammary incision is chosen, leaving subcuticular polypropylene (Prolene) or nylon sutures for approximately 3 weeks may make scar spreading less likely but may not prevent hypertrophy.[56]

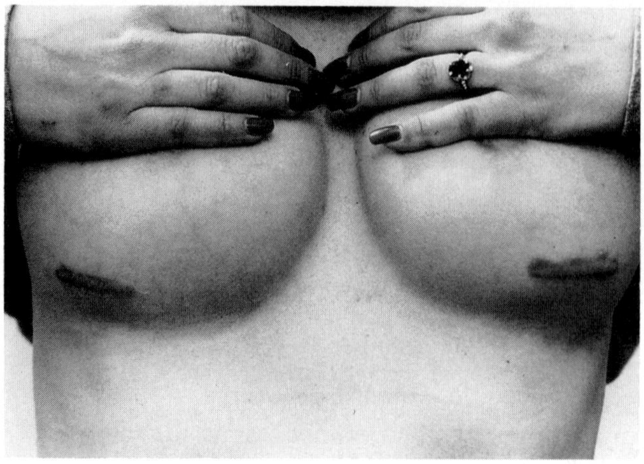

FIGURE 15-3 Hypertrophic scars are more common following the inframammary approach to augmentation mammaplasty than following other incisions.

Treatment

The hypertrophic or spread scars can be excised and resutured, and this maneuver often produces a thinner, smaller scar. Triamcinolone (Kenalog) injection can be used either at the time of surgical revision, or as injection treatment of hypertrophic scars.[49] This injection will lead to less red pigmentation and itching, and will flatten the hypertrophic scar, but will not narrow that scar.[57] Kenalog injection has not been used by the author at the time of primary breast enlargement with an inframammary incision because of concerns of potential wound dehiscence.

Asymmetry Caused By Implant Mismatch or Incorrect Implant Size

Asymmetry after implantation is rarely a problem if a patient has symmetric breasts, but can be more common if she has asymmetry of size and in particular of shape. Symmetric augmentation of a normal breast, when the other breast has been reconstructed after mastectomy, is often particularly difficult because of significant differences in shape. In the patient with symmetric breasts, an occasional patient may complain that the implants are too small. Although in theory patients can complain that implants are too large; in practice and with careful patient selection, this almost never occurs.

Prevention

A good estimate of the implant size required to produce symmetry can usually be achieved by having the patient try on breast implant sizers in a bra. Different sizers are placed into the bra and the patient is asked to look in a mirror and judge the appropriate volume. This method is not infallible but it does provide the range of implants satisfactory to the patient. Patients commonly say that they wish to have their implants "proportional to the rest of the body and not too big." Experience suggests that patients generally want to be proportional plus some extra volume and so patients are encouraged to go slightly on the larger side of the implant that they initially considered. Patients are often concerned that coworkers and friends will find their augmentation obvious. In fact, small breasted women often wear baggy, loose clothing, and so placing conservatively sized implants rarely produces an effect that is glaringly obvious.

Selection of implants for matching with mastectomy reconstruction can also be achieved with sizers. The use of a tissue expander may also allow the patient to choose the desired size; as the implant is gradually expanded, a range of volumes can be experienced.

Treatment

Although some change in breast size will occur with normal postoperative decrease in swelling, obvious disparities in breast size secondary to implants persist. After an appropriate amount of time has elapsed to allow wound maturation, surgical capsulotomy and appropriate implant size change can be performed. The Becker combination tissue expander and implant can allow for changing of implant size without the need for total implant replacement.

Implant Deflation or Rupture

Saline-filled implants have been used because of a reported reduced rate of capsular contracture.[19] Early saline-filled implants had relatively thin walls and were subject to a moderate rate of total deflation because of leakage of saline filling solution.[31] Such deflation could occur rapidly or, more likely, slowly over a number of days. Folds in implants led to knuckles of silicone that slowly folded and thinned, allowing leakage through the implant shell. Occasional leaks occurred because of defective valves, but this was less common.[2]

Deflation of saline-filled implants has become less of a problem because of the use of thicker-walled implants. Aston and Rees have noted a deflation rate using saline-filled implants of 1 to 2 percent.[7] Double-lumen implants, with the majority of the volume composed of silicone and a relatively small amount of saline, would undergo minimal changes even if the saline envelope were to deflate. A rare cause of deflation of saline implants is traumatic puncture of an implant at surgery, which is usually obvious and requires immediate implant replacement.

Rupture of a gel implant is more difficult to detect. This may rarely occur spontaneously or after manual capsulotomy. Nonsymptomatic ruptures probably occur and are not detected unless mammography is done. Occasionally, asymmetric shape or chronic pain can result from rupture, as can local gel migration (Fig. 15-4 *A* and *B*).[49]

Prevention

Use of the newer, thicker-walled implants appears to have reduced the rate of saline implant deflation substantially. Implants should not be significantly underfilled, a situation that could form knuckles and folds. At surgery, suturing should be done under direct vision to avoid puncturing the implant when closing. If a subpectoral implantation is used, grasping the cut edges of the muscle with Allis clamps and everting them, and placing a malleable retractor over the implant allows easy suturing of the muscle with minimal risk to the saline-filled implant. Rupture of gel-filled implants at manual capsulotomy is minimized by careful technique.

Treatment

Deflated saline implants require replacement. Double-lumen implants allow the benefit of an outer envelope of saline without the risk of total deflation. Ruptured gel implants, when symptomatic, should be replaced. No statistics exist about the need to replace a ruptured gel implant that is asymptomatic and found only on mammography. The patient should be informed of the discovery and replacement discussed with her.

Breast Distortion Caused by Muscular Action

While rarely a problem in submammary implantation, distortion caused by active contraction of the pectoralis major muscle can be bothersome in subpectoral augmentation. Distortion may occur as a superior displacement and bunching of the breast soft tissue, or as a visible line at the lower two-thirds of the breast where the muscle edge is present. Most patients with this condition accept it willingly as a minor cost in reduction of capsular contracture. Occasional patients, however, are very troubled by this transient distortion, and may require further surgery (Fig. 15-5 *A* to *I*).

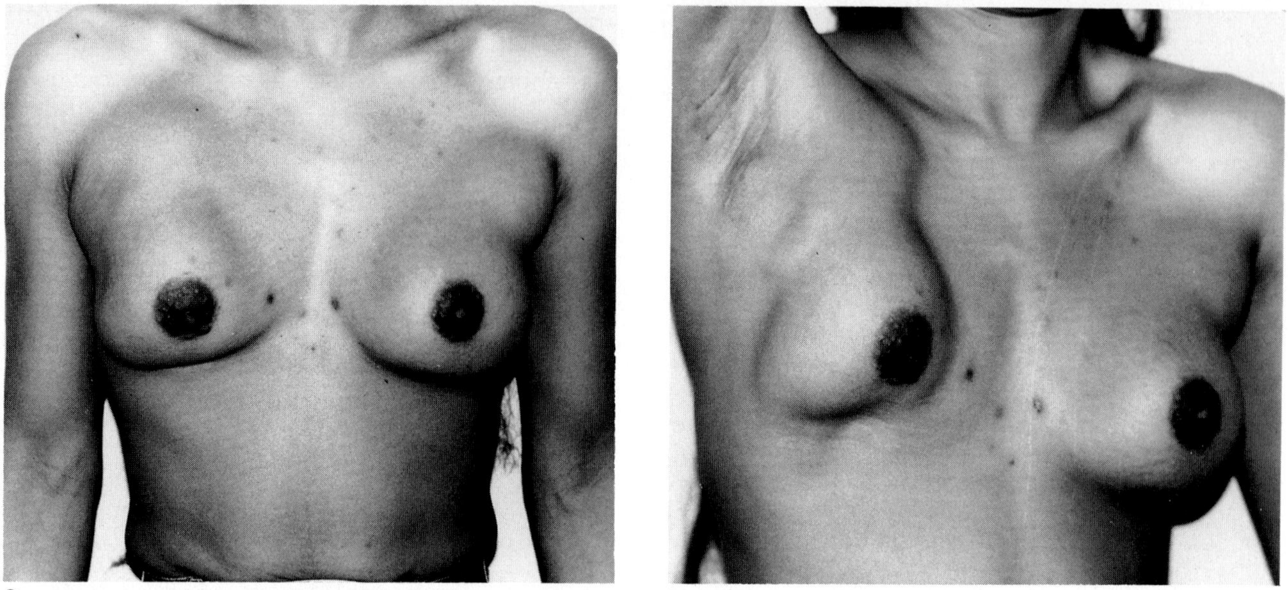

A B

FIGURE 15-4 *A* and *B*, Rupture of gel-filled silicone implant can produce breast distortion and migration of gel into local tissues. (Photographs courtesy of R. Barrett Noone, M.D.)

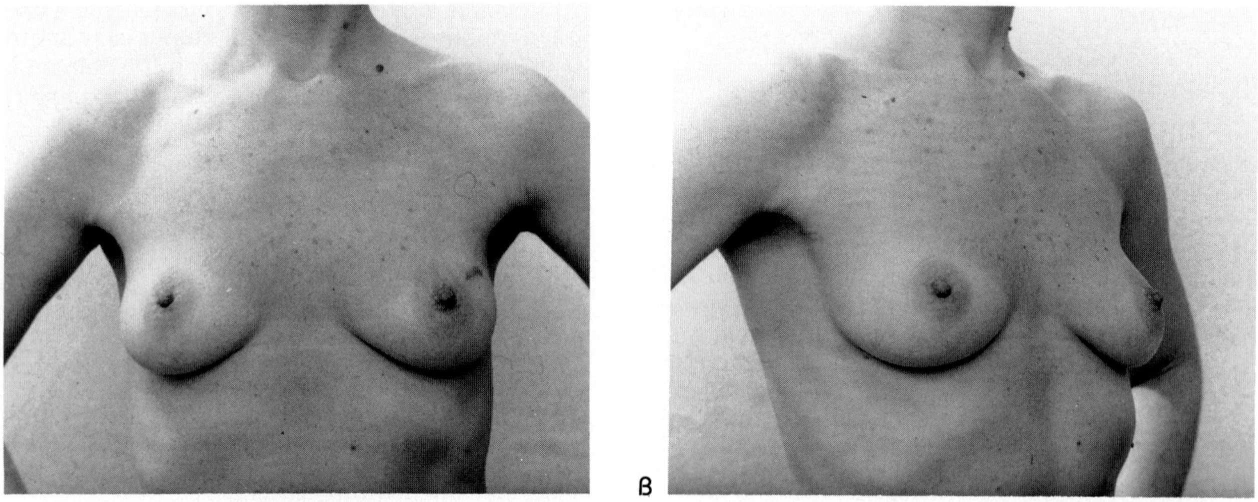

A B

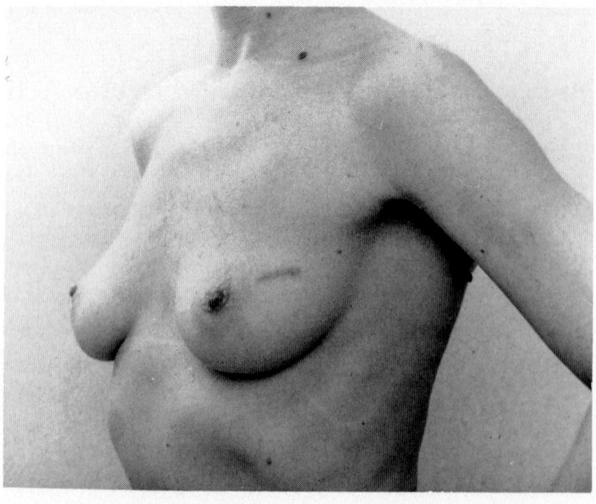

C

FIGURE 15-5 *A* to *C*, Preoperative photographs of a 41-year-old athletic female requesting augmentation mammaplasty. *D* to *F*, Following subpectoral augmentation, lateral distortion of the implants is seen with contraction of the pectoralis muscles. *G* to *I*, Bilateral capsulotomy and lateral capsulorrhaphy resulted in symptomatic improvement and a satisfactory aesthetic result. (Case and photographs courtesy of R. Barrett Noone, M.D.)

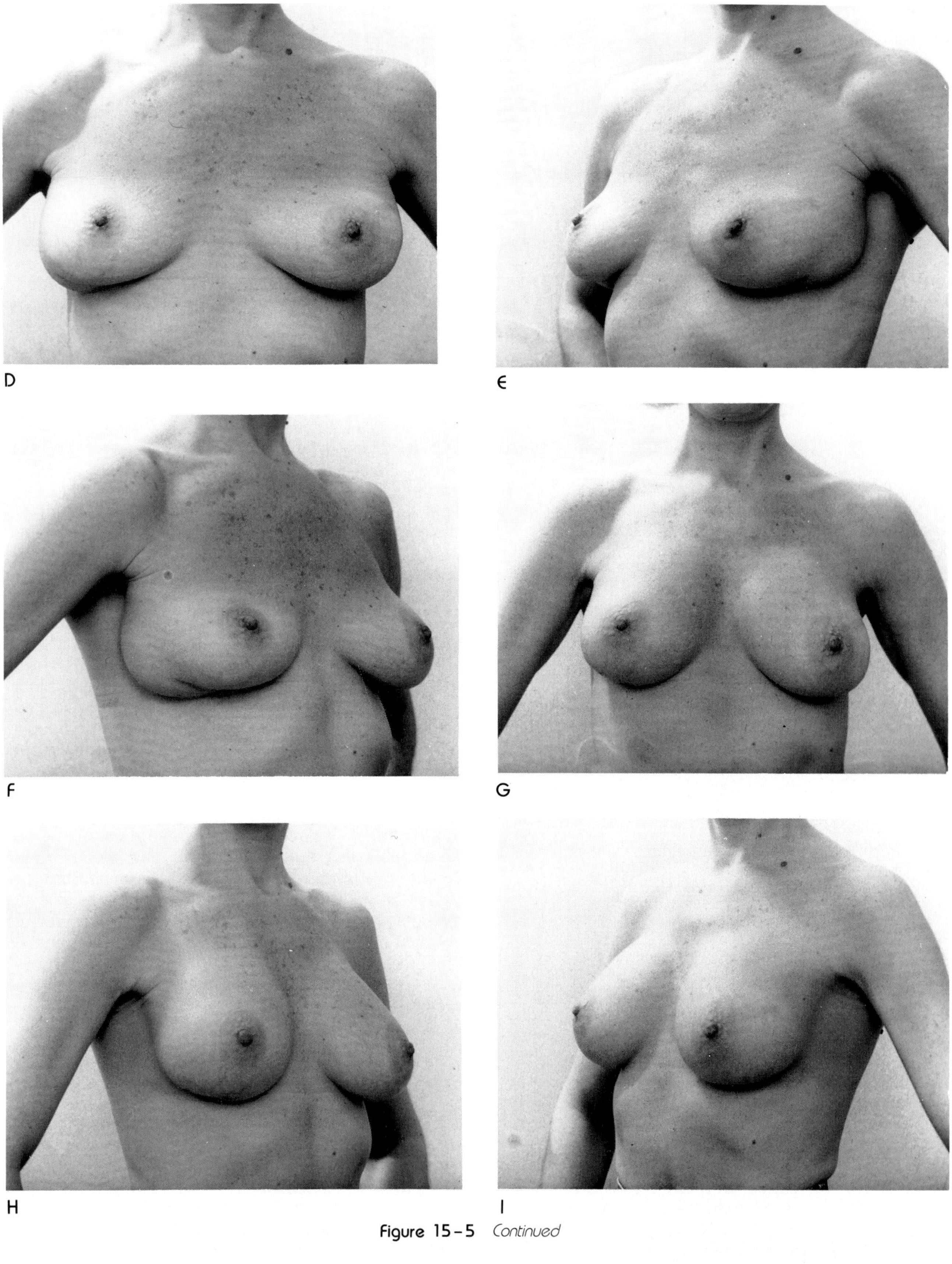

D E F G H I

Figure 15–5 *Continued*

Prevention

Generous release of muscle inferiorly and medially, formation of an adequately large pocket, and avoiding an overly large implant may make this condition less likely. At surgery, palpation and release of the occasional tight band at the lower edge of the pectoralis major should be performed to avoid this undesired result.

Treatment

Further release of muscle banding by open capsulotomy may be useful. Some surgeons have recommended neurectomy and myomectomy in the pectoralis muscle. In theory, the implant could be placed in the submammary rather than subpectoral position at a second surgery, or a lateral capsulorrhaphy may be performed.

RARE UNFAVORABLE RESULTS

Infection

As opposed to the "subclinical infection", which is theorized as being the cause of capsular contracture and problematic at best, the pathology of an obvious infection of a silicone implant is well understood. The true clinical infection of a smooth silicone implant is fortunately rare, in the range of 1 percent.[7] Initial reports concerning polyurethane covered implants suggested a higher rate of infection with *Staphylococcus epidermidis* in these rough-coated implants,[58] but subsequent larger series have suggested that this is not the case. Clinically, infection around a breast prosthetic implant is manifested as it is elsewhere in the body with significant redness, pain, warmth, swelling, and asymmetry. Because the implant pocket is a closed space and the organism is usually *S. aureus*, toxic shock syndrome is a rare complication that has been reported.[2]

Prevention

Meticulous surgical technique is the key to prevention of infection. Whereas most plastic surgical operations, especially those in the facial area, enjoy a certain ability to accept breaks in sterile technique, the placement of a silicone implant is not as forgiving. Surgeons and assistants should be willing, at the slightest question of a break in surgical technique, to take appropriate measures such as changing gloves and adding draping as necessary. Antibiotics are used by most plastic surgeons and are generally broad spectrum. Antibiotics are most effective if given intravenously just before the surgical incision is made.[29] The antibiotics given within the implant lumen or into the surgical pocket for control of "subclinical" infection also help to prevent clinical infection. If an obvious and significant break in sterile technique occurs, thorough irrigation with saline as well as with topical antibacterial solutions will reduce the likelihood of infection.

Treatment

In the case of an obvious infection, most implants need to be removed and the implant pocket drained. The pocket will slowly close and the implant can be replaced at a later date. A 4 to 6 month wait is probably best, although authors such as Gruber and Friedman have suggested reimplantation as soon as 4 to 8 weeks.[2,37] Because of the inflammation following an acute infection, this appears to be too short a time, and a longer time frame is suggested to allow maturation of scar tissue as well as to be sure that there is no infection present (Fig. 15-6*A* and *B*).[49]

Courtiss and his co-workers suggested that the occasional use of antibiotics, for 4 to 6 weeks with careful observation, will suppress an infection without the need for implant removal.[59] Regrettably, even if the implant infection is cured, typically a significant and severe capsular contracture develops. Antibiotic usage with observation is most helpful when there is a question as to whether there is a true infection, particularly if the patient is afebrile and does not have an elevated while blood cell count. Of note is that the coated implants, both polyurethane and rough silicone, may incite an inflammatory reaction that can mimic a low-grade, clinical infection. Antibiotics, as well as Atarax, can be administered for 2 to 3 weeks, with the expectation that the majority of these reactions will subside and are in fact not caused by true bacterial infection.

Although the overwhelming majority of true clinical infections are caused by *Staphylococcus aureus*, other organisms may be implicated. When the implant is removed, culture and sensitivities should be obtained and appropriate antibiotics should be given. While awaiting culture, the use of cephalosporin antibiotics is common. Complete removal of polyurethane fragments in infection may be difficult. Ellenberger et al have suggested an indium-III, oxide-labeled leukocyte scan to locate residual fragments.[60]

Implant Exposure and Extrusion

This rare complication primarily occurs through a nonhealing incision.[61] However, a severe capsular contracture can lead to progressive thinning of the overlying skin and protrusion of an implant through the capsule with eventual exposure (Fig. 15-7*A* and *B*). High doses of glucocorticoids in implants or surgical pockets have led to significant thinning of capsules and overlying skin.

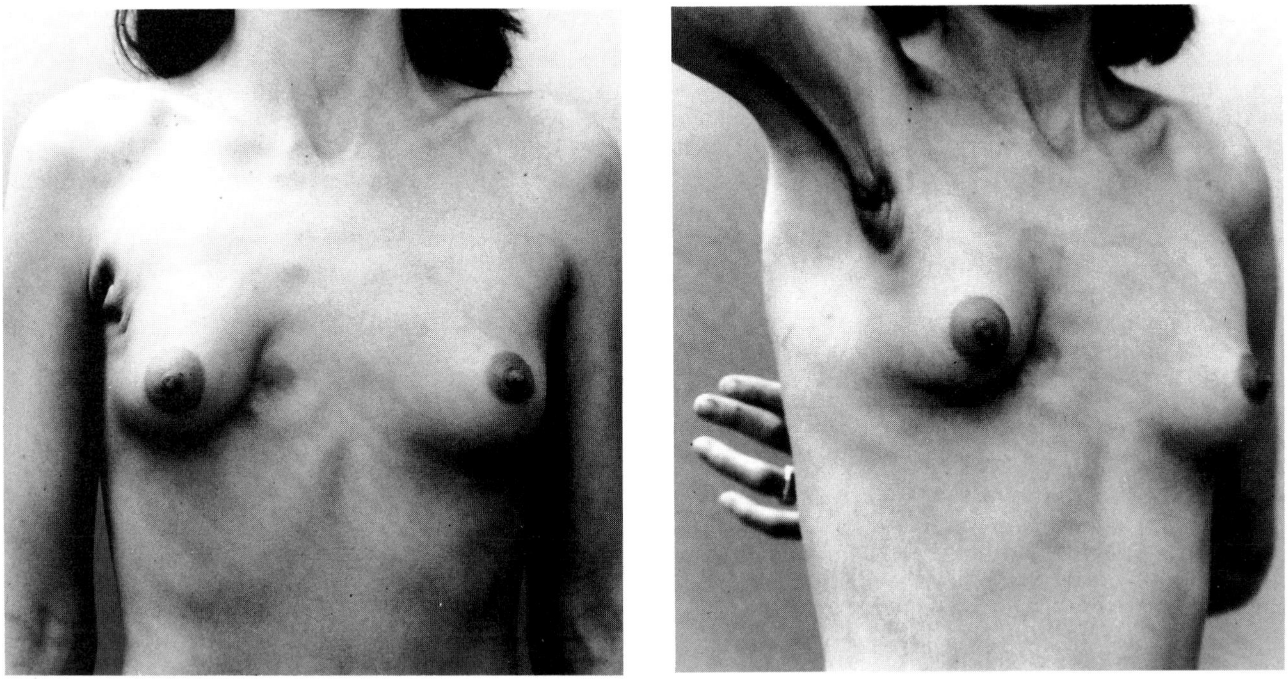

A B

FIGURE 15-6 *A* and *B*, Infection following augmentation mammaplasty performed through axillary incisions resulted in implant removal. The severe inflammatory response caused axillary and chest wall scar contracture. (Photographs courtesy of R. Barrett Noone, M.D.)

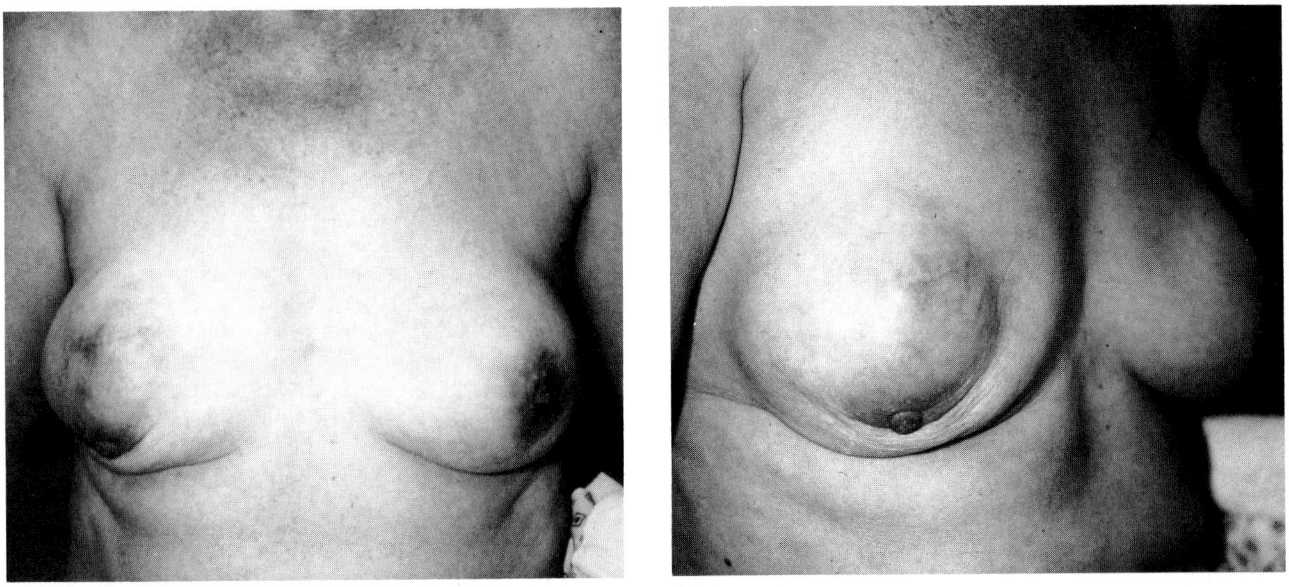

A B

FIGURE 15-7 *A* and *B*, Capsular contracture exerting so much force that silicone implant extrusion is imminent. This patient had undergone prior subcutaneous mastectomy.

Prevention

Placement of the implant in a submuscular position and use of a periareolar approach appear to have obviated this complication. Avoiding the use of steroids in the surgical pocket and avoiding large doses of steroids in the implant lumen will contribute to a lower incidence of this complication.

Treatment

An implant in the submammary position that is gradually eroding through the skin can be placed in the subpectoral position. Ideally, this should be done prior to any visible erosion of the implant through the skin. On rare occasions, the prompt surgical closure of an exposed implant using capsulotomy, antibiotics, drainage, and a sterile implant can salvage the implant,[61] although such exposure may often lead to repeated breakdown and infection. An exposed, rough-coated implant may be more difficult to enclose because of the greater likelihood of persistent infection of the rough surface.

Steroid-Caused Atrophy

The use of high doses of glucocorticosteroids, either in the implant itself or in the surrounding pocket, leads to gradual thinning of the skin and capsule over the implant, as well as striae in the skin.[62,63] This is especially a problem with submammary incisions, submammary placement of the implant, and use of particulate, low-soluble glucocorticoids such as triamcinolone (Kenalog),[64] which can pool in the inferior portion of either the implant or the pocket because of the force of gravity. Steroid atrophy can lead to abnormally low implant position, to a visible implant with obvious wrinkles in the skin, and less commonly, to exposure of the implant.

Prevention

Prevention is obvious—*use no steroids.* If steroids are used, as possibly in a difficult recurrent capsular contracture problem, the use of soluble rather than particulate steroids avoids the pooling that could concentrate the atrophic effect of the steroids. Lower doses of steroids and lower concentrations of steroid per volume are safer.[49,62,64] Recommended dosages of methylprednisolone (Solumedrol) are less than 20 mg per 100 ml of saline placed into the implant, keeping in mind that in double-lumen implants, the concentration for a given drug amount will be higher than in a totally saline-filled implant. In some patients, however, even small amounts of steroids can still cause problems, although at a lower rate.[62]

Treatment

If the steroid atrophy is minimal, support of the breast with a good bra, without surgical intervention, may allow dissipation of its effect over 3 to 6 months. However, progressive atrophy and impending rupture through the skin requires immediate treatment. The author has on one occasion used vitamin A orally, resulting in an immediate visible inflammatory reaction in the skin scar and an apparent reversal of the progressive steroid atrophy. Vitamin A is known to be an antagonist of steroid effect and has been used to reverse that effect in other wound healing situations.[65]

Progressive atrophy and impending skin thinning suggest the need for surgical capsulotomy with placement of the implant in the subpectoral position. Numerous procedures have been performed using the thinned capsule to reinforce the anterior thinned skin, but it seems wiser simply to place the implant beneath the muscle and thereby protect it.

Galactorrhea

The physical act of breast augmentation may stimulate milk production. The milk may drain from breast ducts, in which case it is called galactorrhea. On rare occasions, a large collection of milk may form around the implant itself, causing a galactocele. The galactocele can mimic a seroma or infection.

Prevention

There is no known prevention that would be used on a regular basis in all patients. The author has on one occasion used bromocriptine mesylate prophylactically in a patient who had augmentation 5 months after she finished breast feeding; collections of milk in the breasts had been found at surgery.

Treatment

Treatment of galactorrhea consists of hormonal manipulation to suppress prolactin. Gruber has recommended bromocriptine mesylate (Parlodel) at 1.2 to 2.5 mg/day.[37] This will suppress prolactin in the same manner as milk production can be suppressed after childbirth. Discontinuing massage and breast manipulation may also help. Should the milk production continue, Goldwyn has suggested obtaining the help of an endocrinologist to evaluate the possibility of hormone-producing tumors.[15]

Mondor's Disease

Mondor's "disease" is the spontaneous occurrence of breast vein thrombosis underneath the surface of the skin. This is manifested by firm, tortuous, and slightly tender cords, and is usually seen near or slightly below the inframammary fold.

Prevention

There is no known method to prevent the rare occurrence of Mondor's disease.

Treatment

Supportive care with warm moist compresses and salicylates may be used for treatment. Spontaneous resolution is the natural course of this event.

Tense Seroma (Pseudocapsular Contracture)

On rare occasions, a seroma in the subglandular pocket may produce a tense fullness suggestive of hematoma or of contracture.[37] This appears most often when a subglandular implant has been placed submuscularly, and fluid accumulates in the remaining subglandular pocket. Tense seroma can also occur around submuscular implants and may even mimic infection with tenderness and redness, and yet yield negative cultures upon drainage.

Prevention

Theoretically, removing the submammary capsule during conversion to the submuscular position may help to prevent seroma. Capsulectomy should be used in a patient with recurring seroma.

Treatment

Usually the seroma must be drained and the patient treated with antibiotics. The surgeon may be forced to remove the implant if the clinical course suggests infection, even though negative cultures may be found.

Thin Skin Breast Syndrome

In submammary augmentation, an occasional patient with thin skin will exhibit a visible implant edge with wrinkling of the skin. Wrinkling of the implant can be seen both with smooth silicone, and with polyurethane and silicone rough-coated implants.

Prevention

In patients noted to have thin skin during preoperative evaluation, subpectoral augmentation will provide a layer of padding between the implant and the thin skin and lessen this problem. If an inflatable or double-lumen implant is placed in the sub-glandular position, selection of a size that will allow maximum saline filling may make wrinkling less likely.

Treatment

Replacement of the submammary implant into the subpectoral position, or use of a fully inflated implant will be helpful.

UNFAVORABLE RESULTS CAUSED BY MANUAL CAPSULOTOMY

Manual capsulotomy is most commonly performed for capsular contracture when the implant is in the submammary position. This manipulation can produce acute problems such as implant rupture, silicone migration (particularly toward the axilla), and acute hematoma. There is no absolute prevention other than careful application of uniform force, avoiding excessive sudden force. Treatment of acute bleeding or implant tear generally involves evacuation of the implant pocket and replacement of an implant in the subpectoral position. Potentially a ruptured implant without symptoms could be left untreated and carefully observed.[37]

Another potential problem is a misshaped breast because of incomplete rupture of the capsule. This can be prevented by trying to complete the manual capsulotomy with circumferential careful application of pressure in all quadrants of the breast. If the asymmetric rupture persists, open capsulotomy and revision are required.

POTENTIAL LONG-TERM PROBLEMS AFTER BREAST AUGMENTATION

Recent attention has been paid to long-term potential problems of breast augmentation.[66] These are: (1) potential difficulty obtaining complete mammography; (2) possible carcinogenesis caused by the implants; and (3) possible autoimmune diseases.

Mammography

Mammographers have noted difficulty in visualizing the entire breast with silicone-containing implants placed in the submammary position, particularly if capsular contraction has developed.[67] Recent techniques by Ecklund et al, which involve pulling the breast substance away from the implant,[68] have improved the visualization of breast tissue although there still may not be as much breast tissue visualized as in the nonaugmented patient. However, even the authors most critical of breast augmentation as an inhibitor of mammography[67] agree that implants placed in the subpectoral position are not likely to interfere with mammography.[69] The improving techniques of mammography added to the gradually increased use of subpectoral augmentation, will probably reduce the obscuring of mammographic findings to a minimum.

Carcinogenesis

Patients commonly ask whether breast implants can cause breast cancer. In a large study by Deapen et al of over 3,000 patients,[70] the data suggested that patients are less likely to develop breast cancer if they have had silicone implants. This finding does not suggest implants reduce cancer but probably represents a degree of self-selection among the patient population.

Recent publicity has been given to the development of fibrosarcoma in a percentage of rats injected with liquid silicone by the Dow Corning Corporation. Publicity by consumer groups questioned whether this meant that breast implants were contraindicated. In fact this is not the case for a number of reasons.[66] Rats are subject to a phenomenon known as solid-state carcinogenesis, in which any smooth surface will induce fibrosarcoma (not breast adenocarcinoma). The phenomenon of solid-state tumor generation does not appear to occur in humans. The closest that anyone has come to this experiment being performed in humans is the past injection of liquid silicone into breasts and faces for purposes of augmentation. Although significant wound healing problems and inflammatory reactions led to lack of general clinical usage of this material, tumor generation was not a problem. If a solid-state carcinogenesis finding were to be applied to humans, this would suggest that no smooth implant of any sort would be ever placed in humans, including breast implants, cardiac pacemakers, cerebrospinal fluid shunts, and joint implants. At present, the consensus is that silicone breast implants in humans do not cause cancer.[66] The extended history of breast implants, in use since 1962, suggests that if silicone were a carcinogen, malignancies would have developed and would have been studied by this time.[66]

Autoimmune Disease

Scattered anecdotal reports of patients developing collagen autoimmune diseases, specifically scleroderma and rheumatoid arthritis, have raised the question of whether autoimmunity develops in response to silicone implants.[71] Small amounts of silicone do "bleed" from the implants into the surrounding tissues and may be found in regional lymph nodes.[16] However the tissue reaction to this silicone material appears minimal.[12] A recent study by Weisman et al has suggested that in a well-defined, studied population, silicone breast implants do not cause autoimmune disease.[72] The Food and Drug Administration, while calling for further study, has found no convincing connection between implants and autoimmune disease.[66]

Acknowledgment

I am grateful to Ronald P. Gruber, M.D. for his suggestions in the organization and preparation of this manuscript.

References

1. Hetter GP. Satisfactions and dissatisfactions of patients with augmentation mammaplasty. Plast Reconstr Surg 1979; 64:151.
2. McGrath MH, Burkhardt BR. The safety and efficacy of breast implants for augmentation mammaplasty. Plast Reconstr Surg 1984; 74:550–560.
3. Brody G, Latts JN. Discussion of Burkhardt BR, et al. Plast Reconstr Surg 1981; 68:48.
4. McGrath MH. Capsular contracture in the augmented breast. In: Rudolph R, ed. Problems in aesthetic surgery. St. Louis: CV Mosby 1986:405.
5. Baker JL. Classification of spherical contractures (Abstract). Presented at Aesthetic Breast Symposium, Scottsdale, Arizona.
6. Gayou R, Rudolph R. Capsular contracture around silicone mammary prostheses. Ann Plast Surg 1979; 2:62.
7. Aston SJ, Rees TD. Mammary augmentation, correction of asymmetry, and gynecomastia. In: Rees TD, ed. Aesthetic plastic surgery. Philadelphia: WB Saunders 1980:954.
8. Strates B, Lian J, and Nimni ME. Calcification in cardiovascular tissues and bioprostheses. In: Nimni ME, ed. Collagen, Volume III, Biotechnology, Boca Raton: CRC Press, 1988:273.
9. Rudolph R, Utley J, Woodward M. Contractile fibroblasts (myofibroblasts) in a painful pacemaker pocket. Ann Thorac Surg 1981:31.
10. Baker JL, Chandler ML, LeVier RR. Occurrence and activity of myofibroblasts in human capsular tissue surrounding mammary implants. Plast Reconstr Surg 1981; 68:905.
11. Gabbiani G, Ryan GB, Majno G. Presence of modified fibroblasts in granulation tissue and their possible role in wound contraction. Experientia 1971; 27:549.
12. Rudolph R, Abraham J, Vecchione T, et al. Myofibroblasts and free silicon around breast implants. Plast Reconstr Surg 1978; 62:185.
13. Rudolph R. Capsule contraction around silicone breast implants. In: Rubin I, ed. Biomaterials in reconstructive surgery. St. Louis: CV Mosby, 1983:576.
14. Rudolph R, Ehrlich HP, VandeBerg J. Wound contraction and scar contracture. In: Cohen IK, Diegelmann RF, Lindblad WJ, eds. Wound healing: Biochemical and clinical aspects. Philadelphia: WB Saunders, 1989.

15. Baker JL Jr, Penn JG. Augmentation mammaplasty (Comments: RM Goldwyn, pp. 734-737. In: Goldwyn RM, ed. The unfavorable result in plastic surgery. Boston: Little, Brown, 1984:719.
16. Wickham MG, Rudolph R, Abraham JL. Silicone identification in prosthesis-associated fibrous capsules. Science 1978; 199:437.
17. Baker JL, LeVier RR, Spielvogel DE. Positive identification of silicone in human mammary capsular tissue. Plast Reconstr Surg 1982; 69:56.
18. Rudolph R, Abraham JL. Tissue effects of new silicone mammary-type implants in rabbits. Ann Plast Surg 1980; 4:14.
19. Asplund O. Capsular contracture in silicone gel and saline-filled breast implants after reconstruction. Plast Reconstr Surg 1984; 73:270.
20. McKinney P, Tresley G. Long-term comparison of patients with gel and saline mammary implants. Plast Reconstr Surg 1983; 72:27.
21. Brand KG. Letter to the editor: Polyurethane-coated silicone implants and the question of capsular contracture. Plast Reconstr Surg 1984; 73:498.
22. Angel MF, Narayanan K, Swartz WM, et al. The etiologic role of free radicals in hematoma-induced flap necrosis. Plast Reconstr Surg (In press).
23. Burkhardt BR. Fibrous capsular contracture around breast implants: The role of subclinical infection. Infect Surg 1985; 4:469-474.
24. Lowy FD, Hammer SM. Staphylococcus epidermidis infections. Ann Intern Med 1983; 99:834.
25. Shah Z, Lehman JA, Stevenson G. Capsular contracture around silicone implants: The role of intraluminal antibiotics. Plast Reconstr Surg 1982; 69:809.
26. Burkhardt BR, Fried M, Schnur PL, Tofield JJ. Capsules, infection, and intraluminal antibiotics. Plast Reconstr Surg 1981; 68:43.
27. Rudolph R, Woodward M. Absence of visible bacteria in capsules around silicone breast implants. Plast Reconstr Surg 1983; 72:32.
28. Shah Z, Lehman JA, Tan J. Does infection play a role in breast capsular contracture? Plast Reconstr Surg 1981; 68:34.
29. Richman DD. Infectious disease problems in cosmetic surgery. In: Rudolph R, ed. Problems in aesthetic surgery. St. Louis: CV Mosby, 1986:181.
30. Rudolph R. Letter to the editor: Antibacterials and breast capsule contracture. Plast Reconstr Surg 1986; 78:830.
31. Williams JE. Experiences with a large series of Silastic breast implants. Plast Reconstr Surg 1972; 49:253.
32. Foerster DW. "False bursa" concept in augmentation mammaplasty. Aesthetic Plast Surg 1978; 2:419.
33. Marshall WR. Amelioration of capsular contracture by motion restriction. Ann Plast Surg 1986; 16:211.
34. Caffee HH. External compression for the prevention of scar capsule contracture: A preliminary report. Ann Plast Surg 1982; 8:453.
35. Ksander GA. Effect of diffused soluble steroid on capsules around experimental breast prostheses in rats. Plast Reconstr Surg 1979; 63:708.
36. Perrin ER. The use of soluble steroids within inflatable breast prostheses. Plast Reconstr Surg 1976; 57:163.
37. Gruber RP, Friedman GD. Periareolar subpectoral augmentation mammaplasty. In: Georgiade N, ed. Aesthetic breast surgery. Baltimore: Williams & Wilkins, 1990 (In press).
38. Caffee HH. The effects of intraprosthetic methylprednisolone on implant capsules and surrounding soft tissue. Ann Plast Surg 1984; 12:348.
39. Brody G, Caffee HH, Spear SL. Letters to the editor. Winter/Spring. Aesthetic Surg. 3-4, 1989.
40. Ellenberg AH, Braun H. A 3-1/2 year experience with double-lumen implants in breast surgery. Plast Reconstr Surg 1980; 65:307.
41. Baker JL, Jr. The effectiveness of alpha-tocopherol (vitamin E) in reducing the incidence of spherical contracture around breast implants. Plast Reconstr Surg 1981; 68:696.
42. Smahel J. Tissue reactions to breast implants coated with polyurethane. Plast Reconstr Surg 1978; 61:80.
43. Lilla JA, Vistnes LM. Long-term study of reactions to various silicone breast implants in rabbits. Plast Reconstr Surg 1976; 57:637.
44. Dempsey MC, Latham WD. Subpectoral implants in augmentation mammoplasty: Preliminary report. Plast Reconstr Surg 1968; 42:515.
45. Gruber RP, Friedman GD. Subpectoral augmentation mammoplasty through a periareolar incision. Plast Reconstr Surg 1981; 67:453.
46. Mahler D, Hauben DJ. Retromammary versus retropectoral augmentation—A comparative study. Ann Plast Surg 1982; 8:370.
47. Rudolph R. Submuscular versus submammary placement of breast prosthesis. (Abstract). Presented at Plastic Surgery Research Council, Portland, Oregon, 1985.
48. Clarendon CCD. Implant descent: A complication of augmentation mammaplasty and its correction. Ann Plast Surg 1988; 21:452.
49. Ellenberg AH. Basic principles in the management of complications following augmentation mammaplasty. In: Georgiade NG, et al eds. Essentials of plastic maxillofacial and reconstructive surgery. Baltimore: Williams & Wilkins, 1987:688.
50. Elliott MP. A musculocutaneous transposition flap mammaplasty for correction of the tuberous breast. Ann Plast Surg 1988; 20:153.
51. Courtiss EH, Goldwyn RM. Breast sensation before and after plastic surgery. Plast Reconstr Surg 1976; 58:1.
52. Fisher JC, Rudolph R. Augmentation mammaplasty. In: Fisher JC, Guerrerojantos J, Gleason M, eds. Manual of aesthetic surgery. New York: Springer-Verlag, 1985:13.
53. Farina MA, Newby BG, Alani NM. Innervation of the nipple-areolar complex. Plast Reconstr Surg 1980; 66:497.
54. Caffee HH. The effect of hematoma on implant capsules. Ann Plast Surg 1986; 16:102.
55. Williams C, Aston S, Rees TD. The effects of hematoma on the thickness of pseudosheaths around silicone implants. Plast Reconstr Surg 1975; 56:194.
56. Elliot D, Mahaffey PJ. The stretched scar: The benefit of prolonged dermal support. Br J Plast Surg 1989; 42:74.
57. Rudolph R. Widespread scars, hypertrophic scars, and keloids. Clin Plast Surg, 1987; 14:253.
58. Umanski C. Letter to the editor. Infection with polyurethane coated implants. Plast Reconstr Surg 1985; 75:925.
59. Courtiss EH, Goldwyn RM, Anastasi GW. The fate of breast implants with infections around them. Plast Reconstr Surg 1979; 63:812.

60. Ellenberger P, Graham WP, Manders EK, Basanab NR. Labeled leukocyte scans for detection of retained polyurethane foam. Plast Reconstr Surg 1986; 77:77.
61. Weber J Jr, Hentz RV. Salvage of the exposed breast implant. Ann Plast Surg 1986; 16:106.
62. Carrico TJ, Cohen IK. Capsular contracture and steroid-related complications after augmentation mammaplasty: A preliminary study. Plast Reconstr Surg 1979; 64:377.
63. O'Neal RM, Argenta LC. Late side effects related to inflatable breast prostheses containing soluble steroids. Plast Reconstr Surg 1982; 69:641.
64. Ellenberg AH. Marked thinning of the breast skin flaps after the insertion of implants containing triamcinolone. Plast Reconstr Surg 1977; 60:755.
65. Hunt TK, Ehrlich HP, Garcia JA, Dunphy JE. Effect of vitamin A on reversing the inhibitory effect of cortisone on healing of open wounds in animals and man. Ann Surg 1969; 170:633.
66. FDA Drug Bulletin. February 1989:2-3.
67. Silverstein MJ, Handel N, Gamagami P, et al. Breast cancer in women after augmentation mammoplasty. Arch Surg 1988; 123:681-685.
68. Eklund GW, Busby RC, Miller SH, Job JS. Improved imaging of the augmented breast. Am J Radiol 1988; 151:469-473.
69. Silverstein MJ. Reply, letter to the editor. Arch Surg 1989; 124:257.
70. Deapen DM, Pike MC, Casagrande JT, Brody GS. The relationship between breast cancer and augmentation mammoplasty: An epidemiologic study. Plast Reconstr Surg 1986; 77:361-367.
71. Endo LP, et al. Silicone and rheumatic diseases. Semin Arthritis Rheum, 1987; 47(2):112-118.
72. Weisman MH, Vecchione TR, Albert D, et al. Connective tissue disease following breast augmentation: A preliminary test of the human adjuvant disease hypothesis. Plast Reconstr Surg 1988; 82:626-630.

SECTION 4

REDUCTION MAMMAPLASTY

CHAPTER 16

Surgery for Mammary Hypertrophy

SCOTT L. SPEAR, M.D.
GREGORY A. ANTOINE, M.D.

To define mammary hypertrophy, Lalardrie and Jouglard quantified breast size on the basis of frontal projection and height, thus placing patients in one of five categories (Table 16-1).[1] Breast enlargement has both physical and psychological consequences with common physical abnormalities, including chronic neck and back pain, irritating shoulder grooves from brassiere straps, and occasional maceration and dermatoses in the inframammary fold area. Among the psychosocial and psychosexual aspects of the excessively enlarged breast is limitation of physical and social activities, particularly among younger patients, because of discomfort, embarrassment, or unsympathetic attitudes and remarks.[2] Bilateral enlargement may often require reduction for its correction, but unilateral asymmetric enlargement is an even more compelling reason for surgery to relieve the psychological and physical burdens associated with the awkward imbalance of one-sided hypertrophy. Although not an absolute indication for breast reduction or mastectomy, the inability to examine carefully the breast that is massively enlarged must also be considered, especially in patients with a strong family history of breast carcinoma. This is especially so during planning for immediate or delayed unilateral breast reconstruction, for which preoperative discussions should often include consideration of the "normal" breast for reduction or mastectomy to achieve symmetry.

Although breast reduction is best performed in a young, healthy female with no medical problems who has essentially completed her breast development, this unfortunately may not always be possible. Very young patients and those whose breasts are still enlarging may be operative candidates when the possibility of reoperation is outweighed by the physical, social, and emotional burdens of continuing with enlarged breasts.

Despite an extensive search for the underlying etiology of breast hypertrophy and gigantomastia, these remain poorly understood problems of end-organ hormonal response, genetic background, and overall body weight.[3] Surgery is best performed in the young, but advanced age is not a contraindication to surgery. Elderly women may benefit just as much as younger women from resolution of a lifelong physical and emotional problem. Although obese patients should be encouraged to undergo planned weight reduction preoperatively, they often do not succeed, and a successful breast reduction may prove to be the impetus they need to pursue weight reduction with greater enthusiasm and success.

As for any medical problem, a thorough history taking and physical examination must be performed in patients seeking elective reduction mammaplasty, in particular bearing in mind the risk of malignancy, breast cancer being currently the leading cause of cancer death among American women.[4] The physical examination should include evaluation of the regional lymph nodes as well as inspection of the breast in both the sitting and recumbent positions. Fibrocystic disease, recurrent mastitis, and previous breast biopsies are not absolute contraindications to reduction mammaplasty, although previous scars may pose some challenging technical problems. All patients 35 years of age and older should receive preoperative mammography, to be repeated within 1 year of surgery as a baseline for future comparison. Patients should be questioned regarding nipple sensation, and informed that it may be diminished after surgery with a pedicle technique and likely will be lost after a free nipple graft procedure. Depending on the magnitude and technique of the proposed reduction, collection of autologous blood preoperatively may prove to be prudent. Finally, professional-quality, standardized preoperative photographs are extremely useful for both planning and documentation purposes.

TABLE 16-1 DEFINITION OF MAMMARY HYPERTROPHY*

Ideal	250-300 cm^3
Moderate hypertrophy	400-600 cm^3
Rather significant	600-800 cm^3
Significant	800-1,000 cm^3
Gigantomastia	>1,500 cm^3

*Based on frontal projection and height of the breast, according to Laxardrie and Jouglard[1]

HISTORICAL ASPECTS OF REDUCTION MAMMAPLASTY

The first modern communication about breast reduction was in 1897 by Pousson of Paris.[5] Later, during the early part of the 20th century, Morestin, also of Paris, incorporated lessons learned from ablative techniques on the breast into practical aesthetic techniques (Fig. 16-1).[6] At about the same time, Guinard, in 1903, described his operation for correction of mammary hypertrophy. Morestin was the first to report on reduction for unilateral breast hypertrophy in 1909.[7] None of these early operations, however, corrected ptosis or removed much of the breast gland itself. Transpositioning of the nipple was the turning point in refining the technique of reduction mammaplasty by allowing the correction of ptosis, and Aubert is generally credited as the first to describe such a technique performed at the time of reduction mammaplasty.[8]

During the subsequent decades, inconsistent survival of the nipple-areola complex remained the major dreaded complication associated with these various procedures. To avoid this calamity, Thorek enthusiastically endorsed free nipple grafting rather than nipple transposition as his preferred technique (Fig. 16-2). This remains valid and is still commonly used in reductions of generous proportions.[9] Biesenberger proposed an approach in which skin flaps were widely undermined from the breast tissue with excision of the entire lateral parenchyma of the breast (Fig. 16-3*A*).[10] The remaining portion of the breast with its attached nipple-areola was rotated laterally and superiorly to transpose the nipple. The skin was then redraped over the remaining tissue and the excess skin excised and closed. This operation remained popular for over 20 years despite a

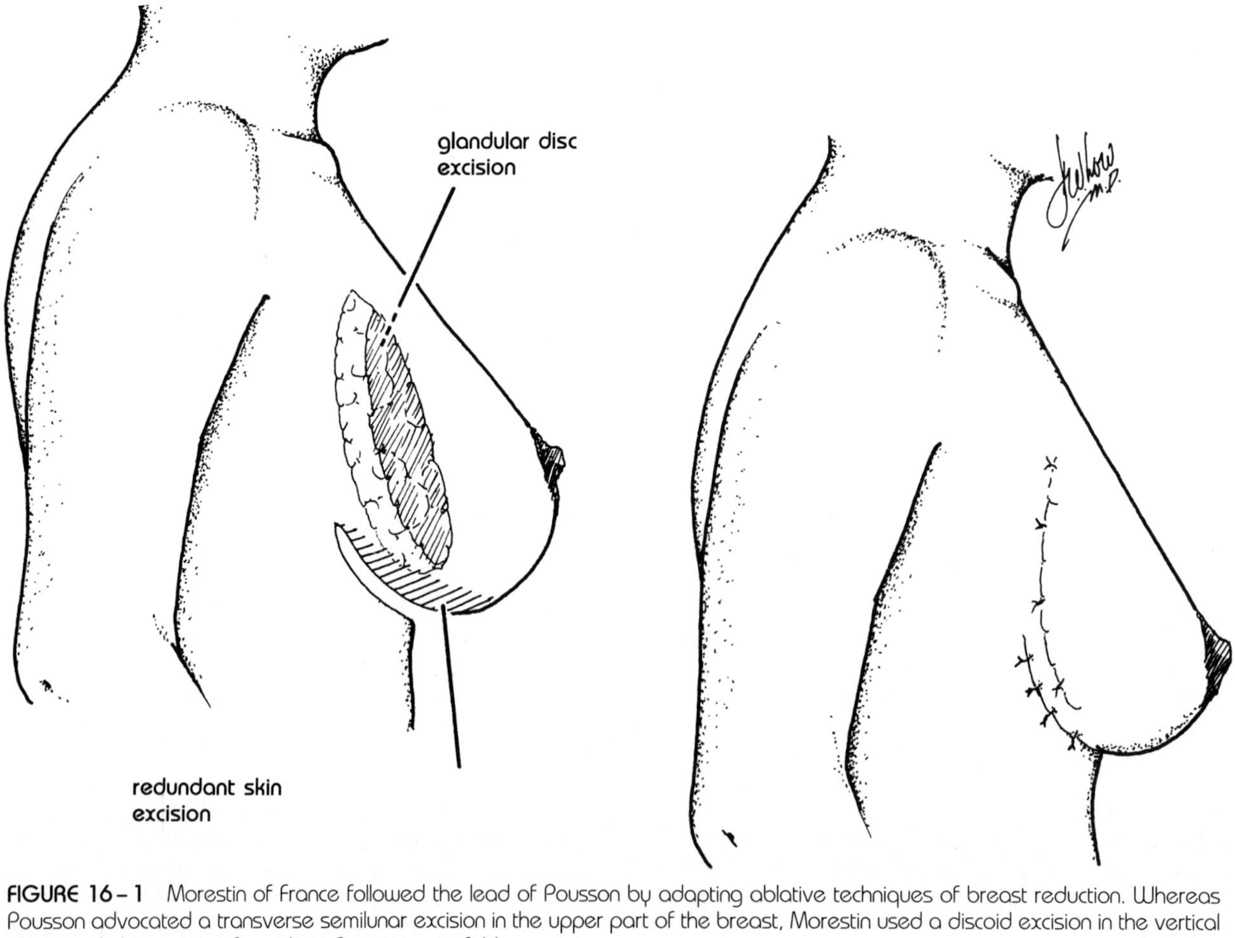

FIGURE 16-1 Morestin of France followed the lead of Pousson by adapting ablative techniques of breast reduction. Whereas Pousson advocated a transverse semilunar excision in the upper part of the breast, Morestin used a discoid excision in the vertical plane and skin excision from the inframammary fold.

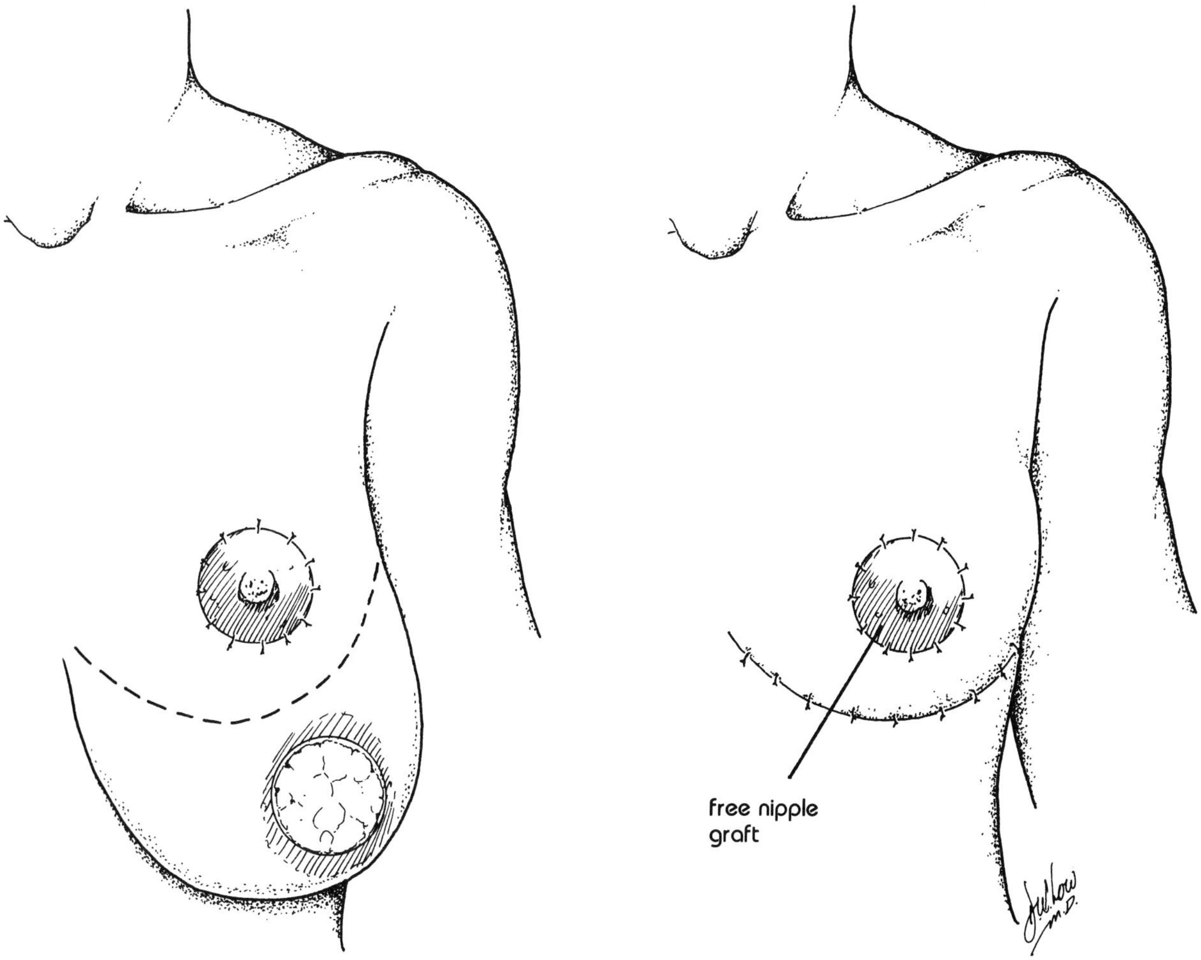

FIGURE 16-2 Thorek introduced the free transplantation of nipple and areola with ablation of the inferior ptotic portion of the gland.

high incidence of skin necrosis, flap ischemia, and nipple necrosis. Schwarzmann, in 1930, described a superiorly based dermal pedicle to vascularize the nipple-areola complex.[11] He believed that the skin and its dermal plexus rather than the breast parenchyma were primarily responsible for the vascular supply to the nipple.

Thirty years later, in 1960, Strömbeck introduced the modern era of breast reduction with his horizontal dermoglandular pedicle, directed toward more reliable nipple survival.[12] This is illustrated in a subsequent chapter in this textbook. This procedure combined the ideas of Biesenberger and Schwarzmann to produce reliable skin flaps and increased nipple-areola survival. The major problem with this technique was excessive flatness across the inferior aspect of the breast after reduction in the extremely large breast. Dufourmentel and Mouly popularized the lateral resection technique, transposing the nipple and areola on a dermal pedicle (Fig. 16-4).[13] In 1972, McKissock described a vertical dermoglandular bipedicle flap that enfolded on itself.[14] This technique has proved safe and reliable, giving predictable results in breasts up to at least 1,000 g in size. Subsequently, Ribeiro's early description of transposition of the nipple on an isolated inferior pedicle was modified by Courtiss and Goldwyn and Georgiade and colleagues to produce a procedure that reliably safeguards nipple sensation and survival (see Chap. 20).[15-17] More recently, the superior pedicle has been refined by Weiner and colleagues for effective nipple transposition in selected patients.[18] At about the same time, Balch described a central mound technique without a dermal pedicle that still allows breast reduction with reliable nipple survival.[19]

PATIENT SELECTION

Surgery for mammary hypertrophy today is directed toward preservation of sensation, continua-

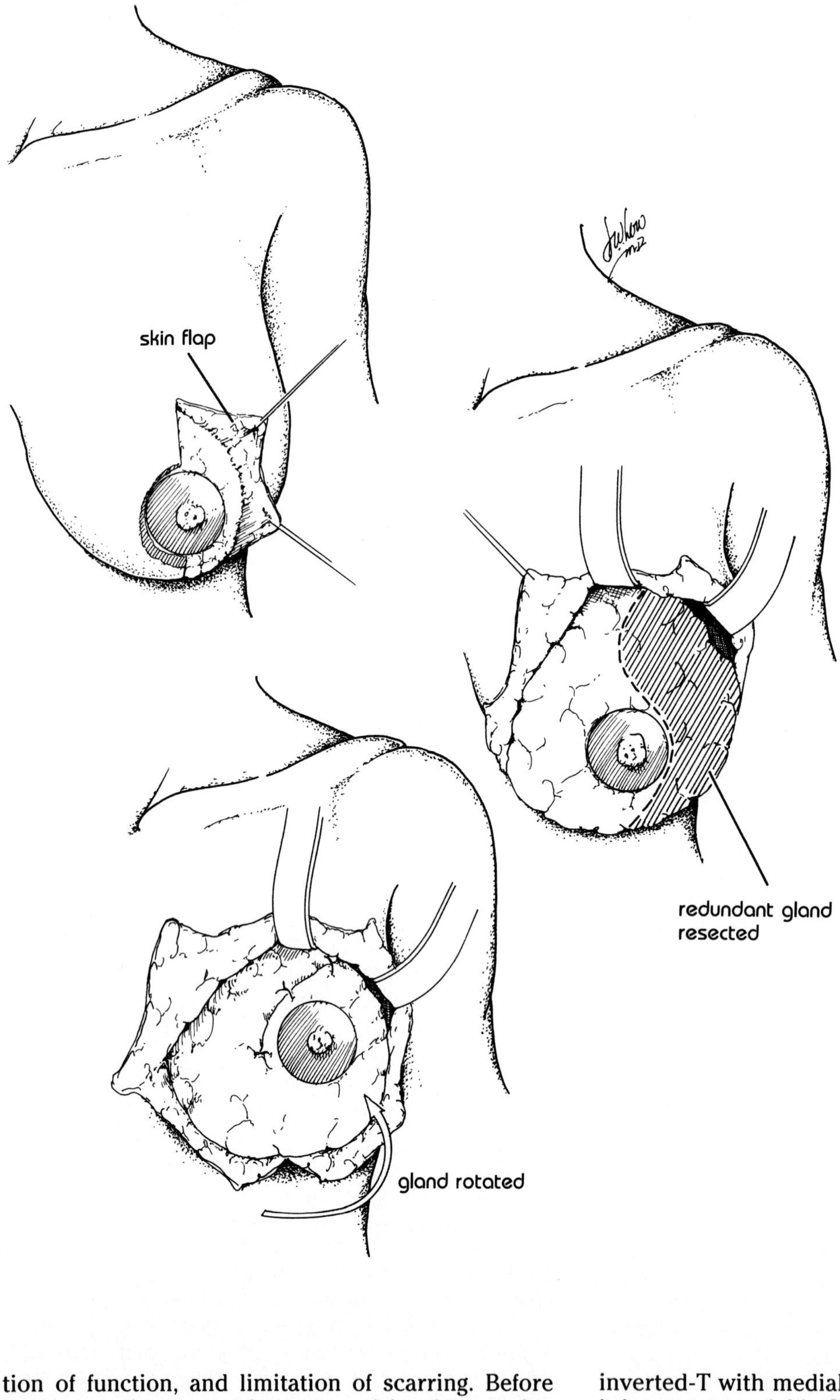

FIGURE 16–3 The Biesenberger technique was introduced in 1928. It involved wide undermining of skin flaps, generous lateral breast parenchymal resection, and rotation of the remaining portion of the breast to transpose the nipple.

tion of function, and limitation of scarring. Before surgery, patients must be prepared for the scarring that is inevitable in this procedure, no matter what technique is chosen. Selecting the correct procedure for a given patient requires that the surgeon be familiar with several techniques. Current techniques can be differentiated by their pattern of scarring and skin resection. With most methods, the final scar is in an inverted-T with medial and lateral extensions in the inframammary fold. Other methods may leave the scar laterally and obliquely to the areola without a medial component. The design that produces an inverted-T scar is compatible with the inferior pedicle, vertical bipedicle, central mound, superior pedicle, and other techniques.

The authors generally prefer the McKissock

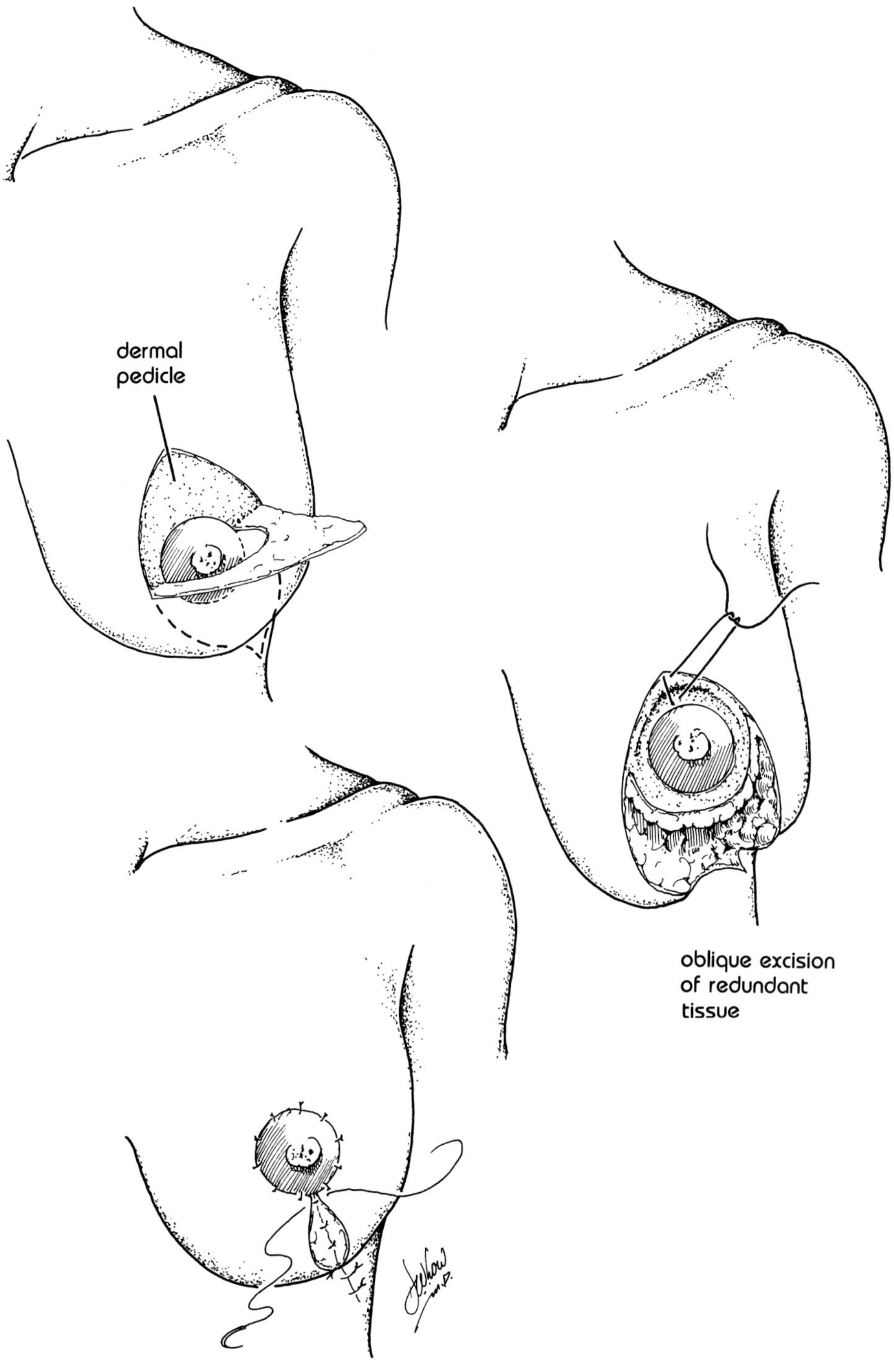

FIGURE 16–4 The lateral wedge reduction mammaplasty, popularized by Dufourmentel and Mouly, avoids scarring in the medial and lateral inframammary fold and involves superomedial transposition of the nipple.

technique for most patients, reasoning that this offers not only the greatest versatility, but also the greatest reliability in terms of nipple and flap survival. The inferior pedicle technique, although similar, should preferably be used in more moderate-sized reductions in younger, healthier patients. The central mound and superior pedicle technique likewise can be used effectively in small to moderate reductions or in patients with contralateral breast cancer when minimal superior or pedicle dissection is desirable. Free nipple graft techniques are advocated primarily for the very large breast, or for patients in whom rapid, simple resections are preferable in terms of safety, speed, or cancer surveillance.

Despite our preference for the vertical bipedicle technique, the inferior pedicle technique can be safely used in young healthy patients when a modest amount of parenchyma reduction and nipple elevation is anticipated. In such low-risk patients the slightly greater technical risk of the inferior pedicle may be sufficiently compensated by the increased speed and efficiency in the development of the inferior pedicle compared with the bipedicle.

When the volume of the reduction is small and little or no nipple elevation is planned, a superior pedicle or central mound technique may actually be preferable to a McKissock or inferior pedicle reduction in order to reduce the extent of dissection in the central and upper regions of the breast. This situation is commonly found in unilateral reduction for congenital asymmetry or in unilateral reduction contralateral to a breast reconstruction, whether by implant or flap. Avoiding unnecessary dissection in the central and upper breast has special appeal in patients under close surveillance for the development of breast cancer, e.g., those who have already undergone unilateral mastectomy.

Although many surgeons prefer to avoid reduction with a free nipple graft, we find it useful in several situations. When the extent of the reduction is truly impressive or the viability of the transferred nipple is in doubt, transposition of the nipple as a free graft is safer, as well as quicker and simpler. Speed and simplicity are great advantages in elderly patients or when technical issues complicate the procedure. In patients undergoing substantial reduction opposite a mastectomy or reconstruction, the limited dissection and guillotine nature of the free nipple technique could be desirable features during monitoring for pathology in the reduced breast.

Although it is true that the mastering of one technique for reduction mammaplasty is paramount, it is equally true that skill with several techniques is important in dealing with a variety of situations. The authors recommend that others interested in this area develop experience and expertise with several methods including free graft, inferior or bipedicle, superior, and central mound techniques.

References

1. Lalardrie JP, Jouglard JP. Plasties mammaires pour hypertrophie et ptose. Paris: Masson, 1973.
2. Goin MK, Goin JM, Gianini MH. The psychic consequences of a reduction mammaplasty. Plast Reconstr Surg 1977; 59:530.
3. Ryan RF. Virginal hypertrophy. Plast Reconstr Surg 1985; 75:737.
4. CA-A Cancer Journal for Clinicians: A Journal of the American Cancer Society. Jan/Feb 1990.
5. Pousson M. De la mastopexie. Bull Mem Soc Chir Paris 1897; 23:507.
6. Morestin H. Bilateral mammary hypertrophy corrected by discoid resection. Bull Mem Soc Chir Paris 1907; 33:201.
7. Morestin H. Hypertrophie mammaire unilateral corrigée par la resection discoide. Bull Mem Soc Chir Paris 1909; 35:996.
8. Wise RJ, Gannon JP, Hill JR. Further experience with reduction mammaplasty. Plast Reconstr Surg 1963; 32:12.
9. Thorek M. Possibilities in the reconstruction of the human form. NY Med J 1922; 116:572.
10. Biesenberger H. Eine neue Methode der Mammaplastik. Zentrabl Chir 1928; 55:2382.
11. Schwarzmann E. Die Technik der Mammaplastik. Chirurgie 1930; 2:932.
12. Strömbeck JO. Mammaplasty: Report of a new technique based on the two-pedicle procedure. Br J Plast Surg 1960: 13:79.
13. Dufourmentel C, Mouly R. Plastie mammaire per la methode oblique. Ann Chir Plast 1961; 6:45.
14. McKissock P. Reduction mammaplasty with a vertical dermal flap. Plast Reconstr Surg 1972; 49:245.
15. Ribeiro L. A new technique for reduction mammaplasty. Plast Reconstr Surg 1975; 12:110.
16. Courtiss E, Goldwyn RM. Reduction mammaplasty by the inferior pedicle technique. Plast Reconstr Surg 1977; 59:500.
17. Georgiade NG, Serafin D, Morris R, Georgiade G. Reduction mammaplasty utilizing an inferior pedicle nipple-areola flap. Ann Plast Surg 1979; 3:211.
18. Weiner DL, Aiache AE, Silver L, Tittiranonda T. A single dermal pedicle for transposition in subcutaneous mastectomy, reduction mammaplasty, or mastopexy. Plast Reconstr Surg 1973; 51:115.
19. Balch C. The central mound technique for reduction mammaplasty. Plast Reconstr Surg 1981; 67:305.

CHAPTER 17

Reduction Mammaplasty with Horizontal Pedicle Techniques

JAN OLOF STRÖMBECK, M.D.

Preserved circulation of both the mammary gland and the nipple is of paramount importance for a successful reduction mammaplasty.

On the basis of the work on breast circulation by Salmon, Ragnell in 1946 described a technique that took into account the main arterial blood supply to the breast from the internal mammary and lateral thoracic arteries (Fig. 17-1).[1] A similar technique was described by Maliniac in 1945.[2] In their 1939 paper, Gillies and McIndoe mentioned the possibility of upper and lower resection, even though their main interest was the Biesenberger procedure, which relies on a medial vascular pedicle only.[3,4]

My own experience with the Ragnell procedure, which in many cases was a two-stage operation, led me to design a two-pedicle operation without undermining of the skin.[5]

The areolar region was based on a horizontal pedicle, preserving the dermal part of the pedicles as well as the main vessels medially and laterally. Maintenance of the vascular supply could be demonstrated with arteriography before and after the operation.[6]

Further experience with reduction mammaplasty has shown that the circulation of the areolar region can also be sufficient if the areola-carrying pedicle is based caudally,[7,8] laterally,[9] medially,[4,10] or superiorly.[11] The importance of the dermal and subdermal circulation for the areola has been demonstrated particularly by Skoog[9] and by Weiner and associates.[11]

DEVELOPMENT OF THE AUTHOR'S TECHNIQUE

A pattern is used to design the size of the skin envelope preoperatively (see Fig. 17-5). The basic principle includes resection of breast tissue above the areola and from the lower part of the breast, leaving the areolar region on a deepithelialized double glandular pedicle between the vertical incision lines of the skin pattern (Fig. 17-2). When the skin incisions are closed, the areola is automatically transposed to its new position in the opening outlined by the pattern (Fig. 17-3). The operation is performed without any undermining of the skin.

In my first report on this technique, I claimed the advantages to be (1) a one-stage procedure even in large hypertrophies; (2) technically a simple operation; (3) good circulation in the remaining gland and nipple; (4) no risk of skin necrosis; (5) no sutures in fat or gland, reducing the risk of necrosis; and (6) cosmetically good and safe results.[5]

Further experience has shown that a ptotic, fibromatous breast is easy to operate with this original technique, but the fat and tense breast gives greater difficulties. This has resulted in some modifications of the original technique, and I have found it most instructive to describe the technique used today in order to show how difficulties can be managed.

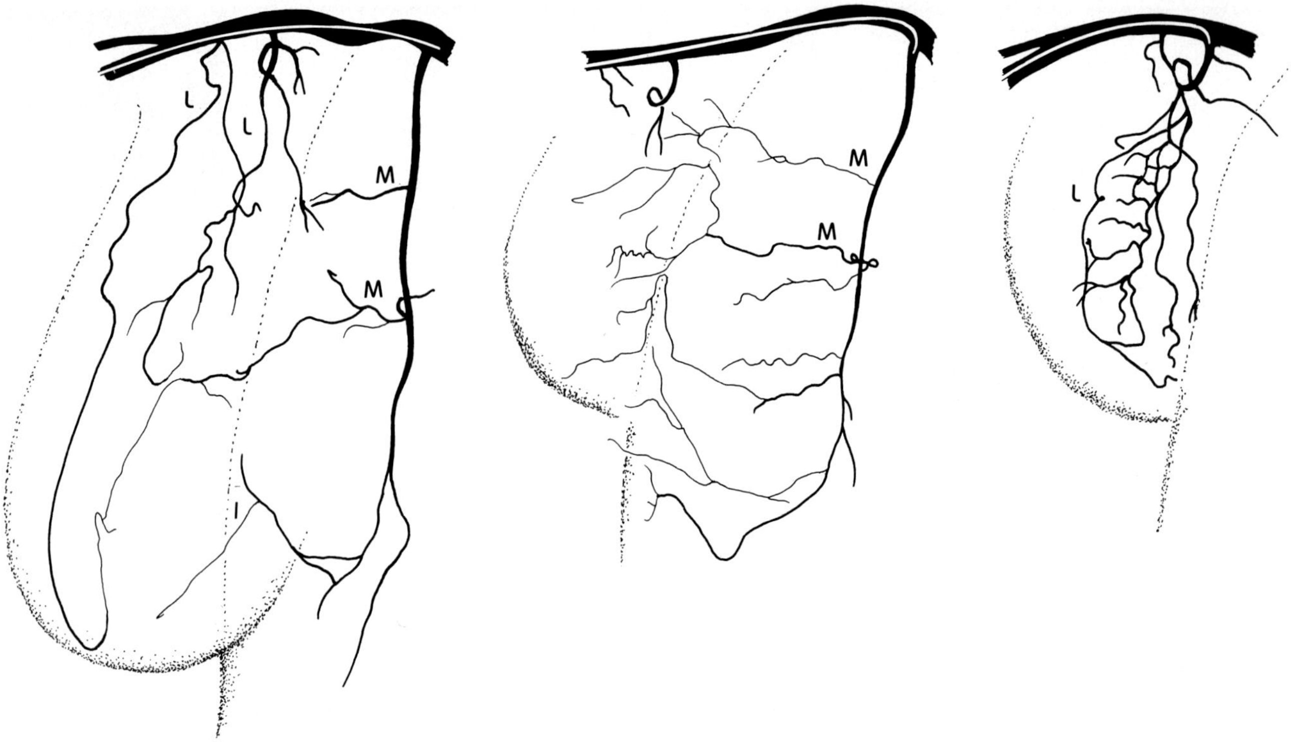

Preoperative **Postoperative**

FIGURE 17–1 Blood supply to the mammary gland was examined angiographically both before and after operation. Main vessels from the internal mammary artery are marked M, branches to the breast from intercostal vessels I, and lateral mammary branches L. The broken lines indicate the contours of the mammary gland and the thoracic wall. (From Edholm P, Strömbeck JO. Influence of mammaplasty on the arterial supply to the hypertrophic breast. Acta Chir Scand 1962; 124:521.)

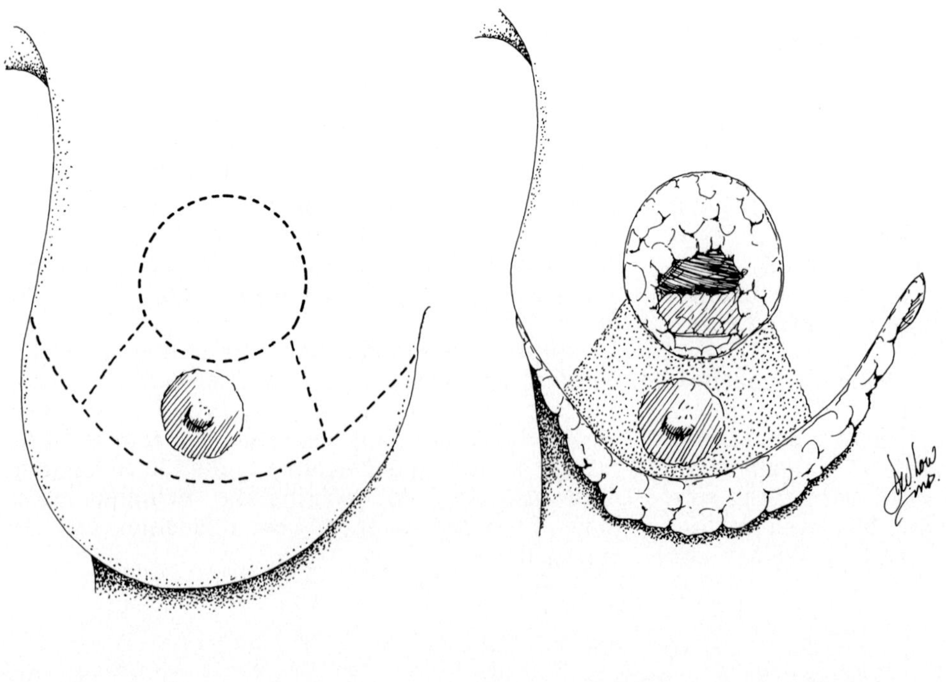

FIGURE 17–2 The areola-carrying horizontal pedicle technique was Strömbeck's original procedure described in 1960.

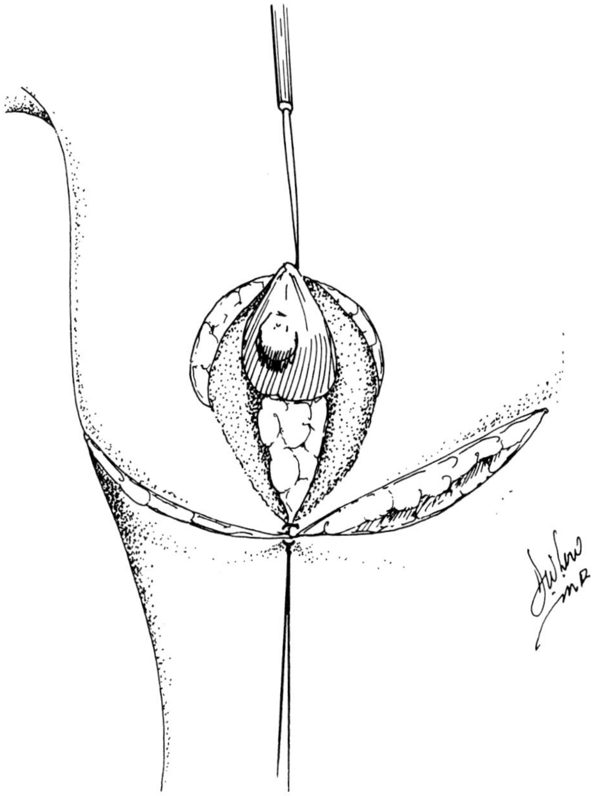

FIGURE 17-3 Closure of the skin flaps directs the areola into its new position.

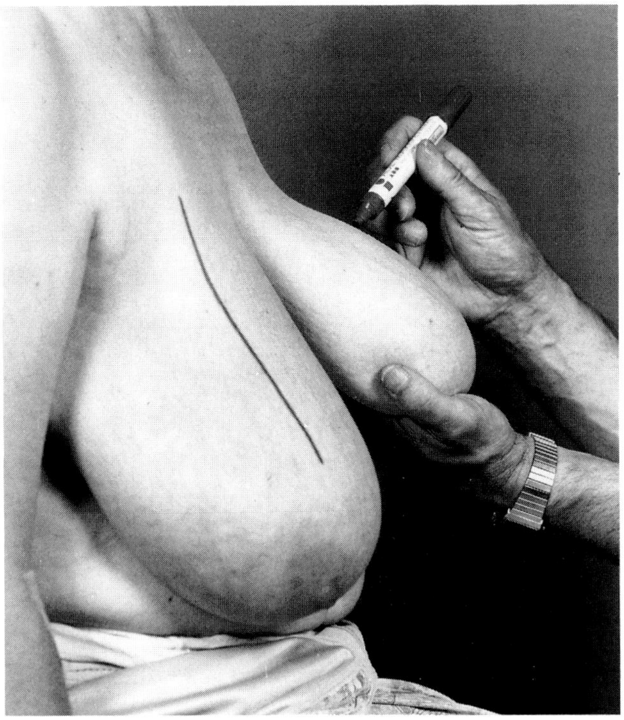

FIGURE 17-4 The projection of the submammary fold is used to determine the new level for the nipple on the breast meridian.

THE AUTHOR'S PRESENT TECHNIQUE

Preoperative Planning

The markings are made with the patient in the sitting position. A line is drawn dividing the breast into two equal halves. On this line the new position of the nipple should be at the level of the submammary fold (Fig. 17-4). The pattern is placed on the breast (Fig. 17-5). The lower resection is designed, keeping in mind that the horizontal incision in the submammary fold should be as short as possible and never extend outside the breast either medially or laterally (Fig. 17-6). This means that the length of this horizontal incision may be shorter than the sum of the horizontal parts of the skin flaps, which have to be gathered when suturing. Moving the breast laterally (Fig. 17-7) and then medially makes it possible to check that the skin flaps are large enough to allow closure without tension (Fig. 17-8). If necessary, the skin flaps (most often the lateral) are elongated. It must be stressed that the pattern is not ideal for all patients, but is used as a guide to help achieve good symmetry (Fig. 17-9).

Part of the preoperative planning is directed toward estimating differences in size between the two breasts.[12] This must be done with the patient in the sitting or standing position because it is almost

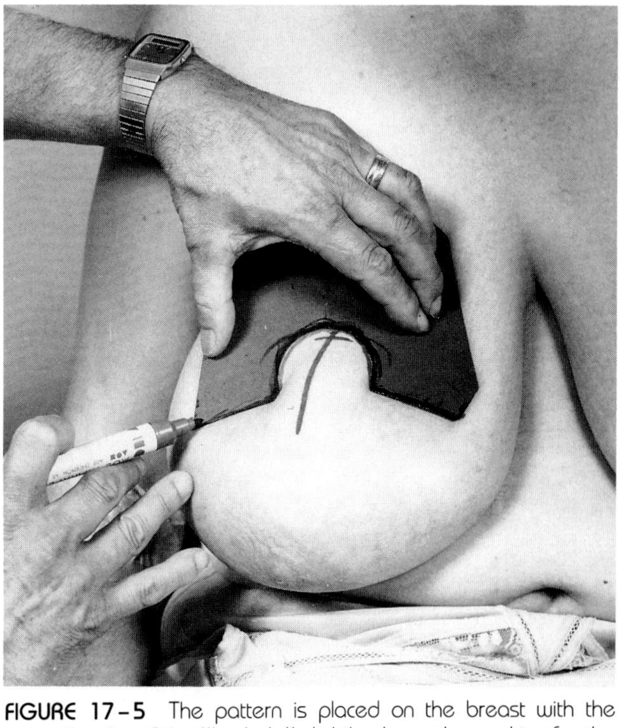

FIGURE 17-5 The pattern is placed on the breast with the upper border of the "keyhole" slightly above the marking for the nipple. The borders of the pattern are marked on the skin.

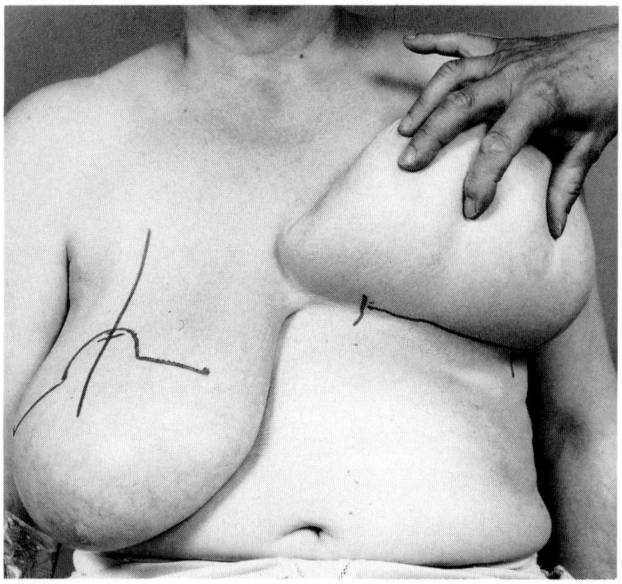

FIGURE 17–6 The length of the submammary incision is marked.

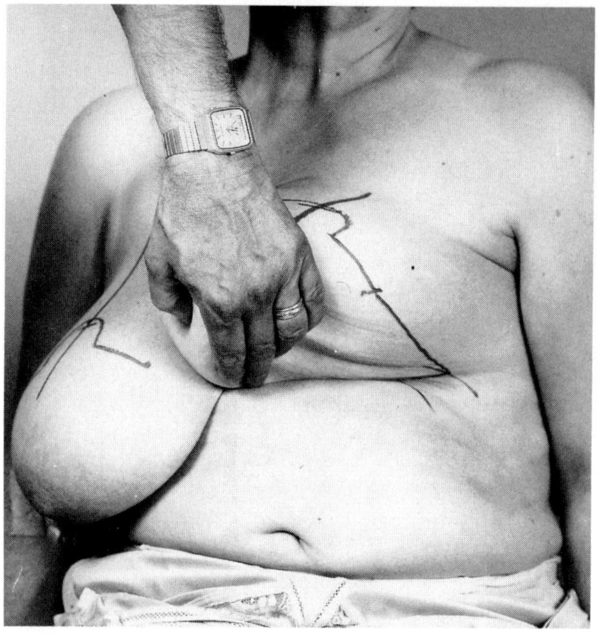

FIGURE 17–8 The lower border of the lateral skin flap is marked.

impossible to judge difference in size when the patient is lying on the operating table.

Anesthesia

The operation is performed with the patient under general anesthesia and in the supine position. Additional lidocaine with epinephrine is infiltrated along the incision lines and above the pectoral fascia. We use a solution of 0.25 percent lidocaine with 2.5 μg epinephrine per ml. About 50 ml on each side is sufficient. This reduces the bleeding considerably and also allows for a more superficial anesthetic level (Fig. 17–10).

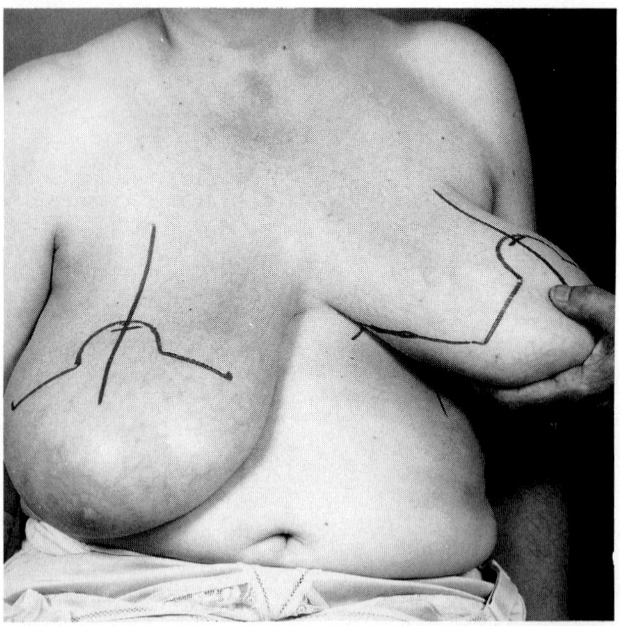

FIGURE 17–7 The point at which the medial skin corner is to be sutured is marked on the submammary fold as well as the lower border of the skin flap.

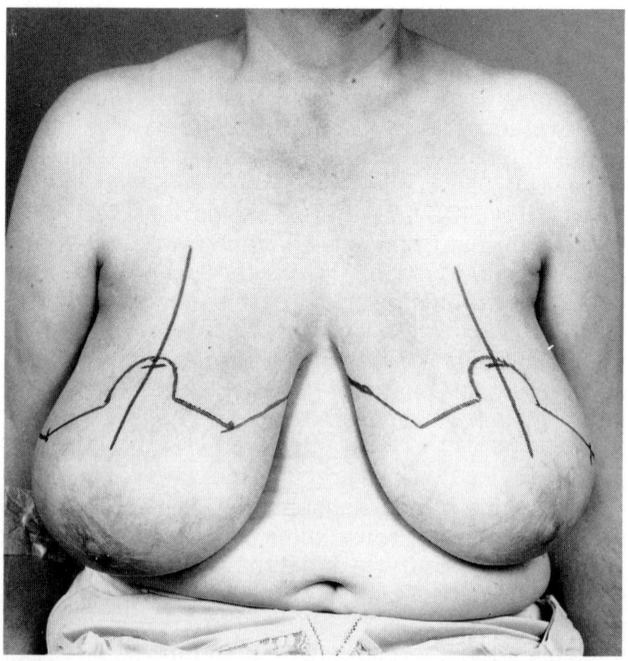

FIGURE 17–9 The preoperative planning is completed. Size differences, if any, must be estimated in volume preoperatively while the patient is in the erect position.

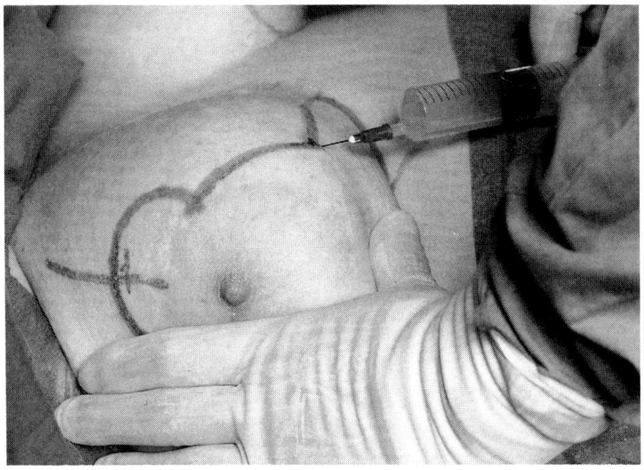

FIGURE 17-10 Local anesthesia (0.25 percent lidocaine with epinephrine 1:400,000) is infiltrated along the incision lines and above the pectoral fascia.

Surgical Procedure

The breast is distended by a rubber tourniquet placed around the base of the breast. A large Penrose drain serves this purpose well. The areola-carrying pedicle is designed. In my early experience, this was made between the skin flaps (see Fig. 17-2). However, the folding of this two-pedicle glandular flap may sometimes be difficult when the pedicles are short or in fat breasts, in which the areola transposition may become tense. To avoid this problem, I have attempted to cut part of the dermis where the tension lies, but have found it better to sacrifice the lateral pedicle completely, relying only on a medial pedicle. This means that I currently design the areola-carrying pedicle with one broad medial pedicle (Fig. 17-11).

The resection is then made by cutting along the borders of the skin flaps, glandular pedicle, and submammary fold, all the way through skin and gland to the pectoral fascia (Figs. 17-12, 17-13).

By approximating the skin edges, the breast is shaped and the areola transposed to its new position (Fig. 17-14). *It is imperative that the areola should be sutured without any tension.* If tension should occur, it can be easily released by cutting part of the dermis and, if necessary, into the fat. A suction drain is introduced through a separate incision laterally.

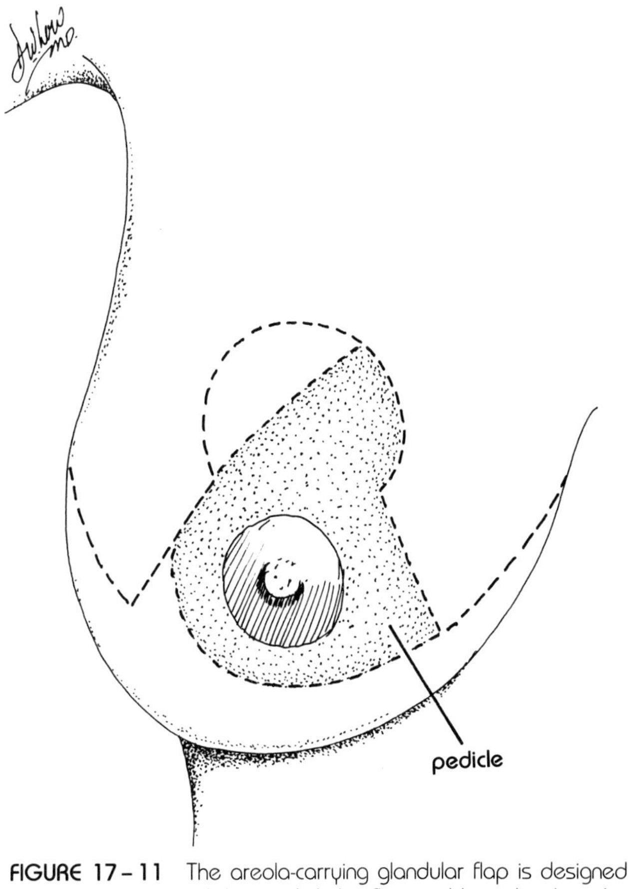

FIGURE 17-11 The areola-carrying glandular flap is designed with its base toward the medial skin flap and broader than the vertical part of the skin flap. The skin in the pedicle is deepithelialized.

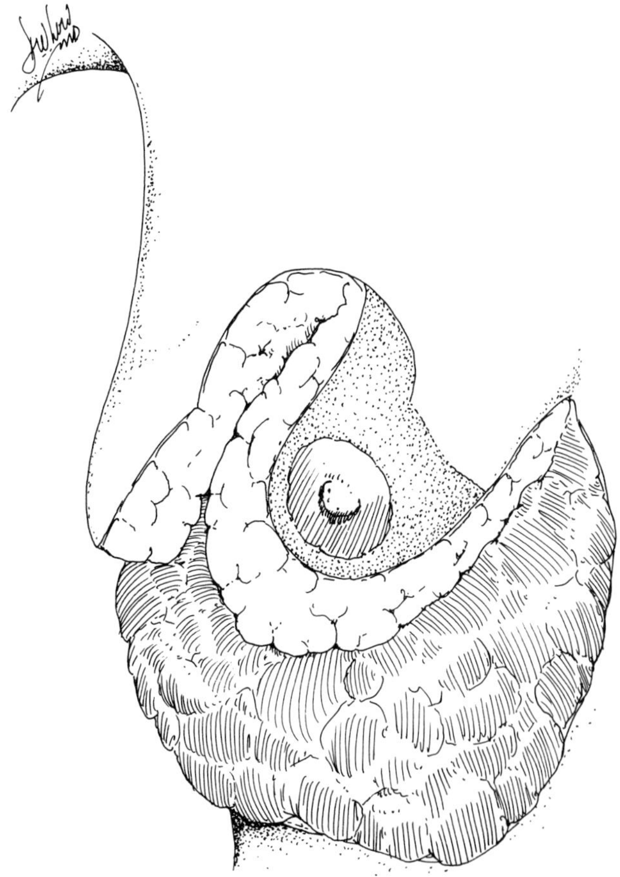

FIGURE 17-12 The incision is made through the glandular tissue along the skin marking from the upper lateral corner of the deepithelialized pedicle to the lateral corner of the marking in the submammary groove. The next incision is made along the areola-carrying pedicle and extended to the medial corner of the submammary marking.

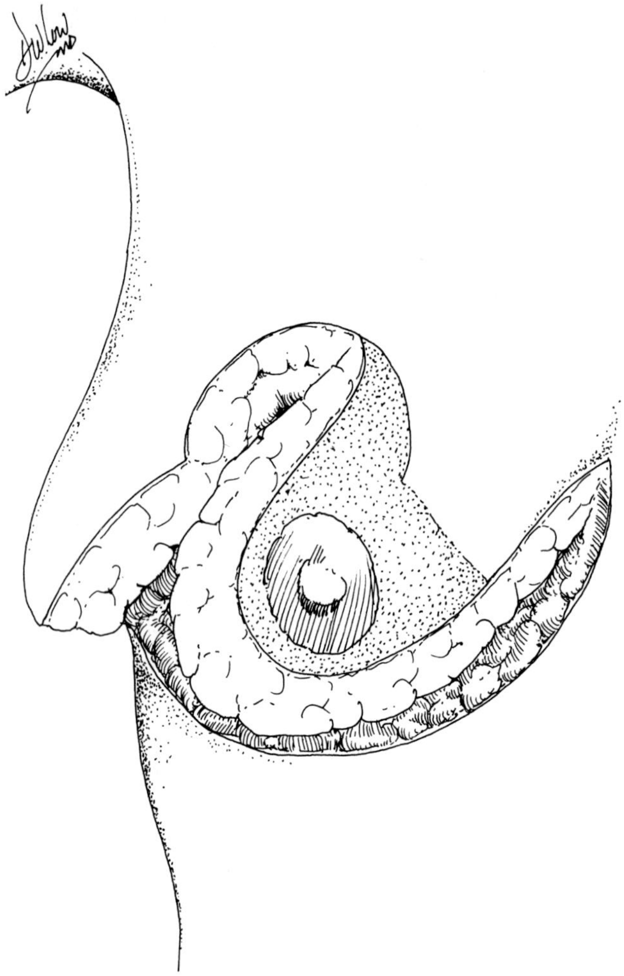

FIGURE 17-13 Through an incision in the submammary groove the resection is completed.

After completion of the intracutaneous suture, I apply Micropore tape (Fig. 17-15).

When local anesthesia with epinephrine is used, the bleeding seldom exceeds 200 ml and blood transfusion is never necessary.

Postoperative Care

The patient remains in the hospital for one or two nights after surgery. The sutures are removed after 2 weeks. The patient is instructed to wear a brassiere day and night for the first 2 weeks after surgery.

Younger patients are recommended to have their scars taped with Micropore for at least 3 months.

PERSONAL SERIES OF REDUCTION MAMMAPLASTY

During the 30-year period 1959 to 1988, I have performed the reduction mammaplasty operation on 1,473 patients (2,788 breasts). Of these, 1,104 (2,125 breasts) were operated on with the technique described above (Figs. 17-16, 17-17, 17-18), 326 patients (570 breasts) with a lateral technique that I have described,[13,14] and 43 patients with other techniques.

Material Operated with the Author's Technique

Of the 1,104 patients operated on with the above technique, 96 were operated on unilaterally, 51 because of congenital asymmetry and 45 because of

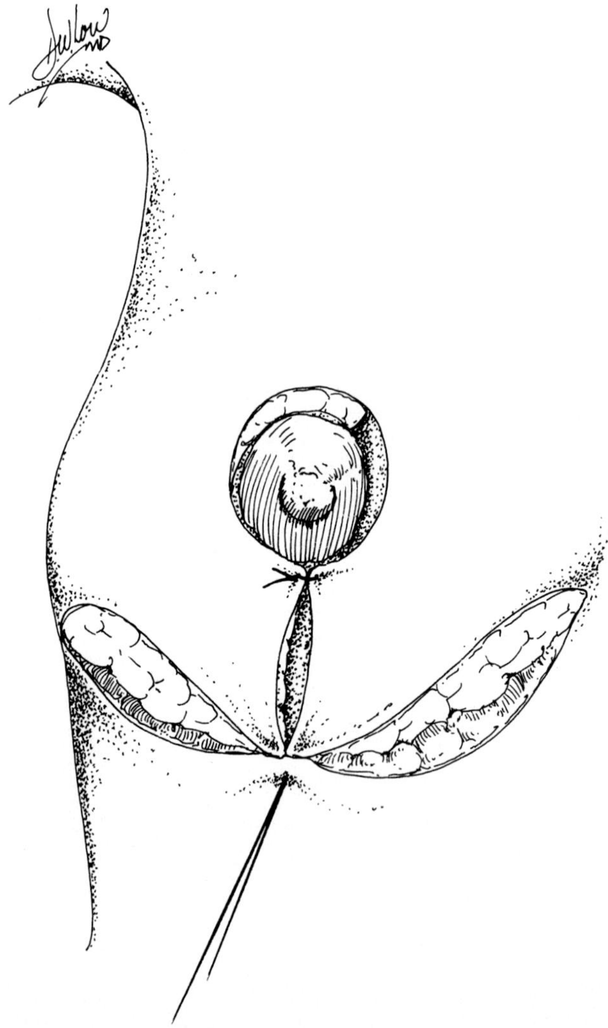

FIGURE 17-14 Skin closure begins with suturing of the corners of the skin flaps.

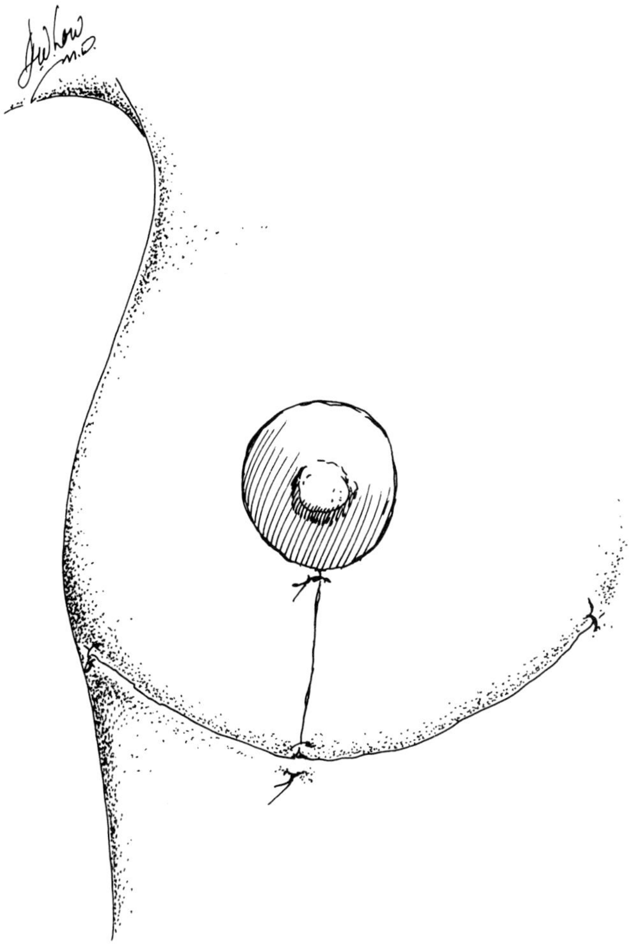

FIGURE 17-15 After completion of the skin closure, the suture lines are reinforced with Micropore tape.

contralateral mastectomy for carcinoma. Thirty-four patients had a mastopexy with resection of less than 100 g per breast. The mean resection weight was 501 g per breast (Fig. 17-19) and the mean age 37 years (Fig. 17-20).

Of the 2,125 breasts, 1,363 were operated on with double pedicles (mean resection weight 480.5 g) and 762 with one medial pedicle (mean resection weight 537 g).

Complications

Hematoma. Twenty-three patients (2.08 percent) developed postoperative hematoma in a total of 25 breasts (1.18 percent). Of these, six patients (seven breasts) were reoperated and four patients (four breasts) had their hematomas evacuated without operation. Thirteen patients (14 breasts) with diffuse hematomas required no intervention.

Fat Necrosis. Fat necrosis with signs of circulatory disturbances of the areola occurred in 11 patients (12 breasts). One patient with complete nipple necrosis on one side developed an infection with beta-hemolytic streptococci. The others healed spontaneously, leaving various areas of depigmentation.

Fat necrosis without involvement of the areola but which required drainage was seen in 14 patients (15 breasts).

Smaller, localized areas of fat necrosis, which did not complicate the healing, but which led to a need for excision of the residual lump at a later date, was seen in 11 patients (11 breasts). These cases were not included when the incidence of fat necrosis was calculated.

The total number of patients with significant fat necrosis was 25 (2.26 percent) in 27 breasts (1.27 percent). If the occurrence of fat necrosis is correlated to the patient's weight and resection weight, it is found that this complication is more common in overweight patients in whom large resections were made (Table 17-1).

Delayed Skin Healing. The number of patients requiring more than four postoperative visits for wound care was 22 (1.99 percent).

Reoperated Patients. Secondary operations including additional reduction or shaping procedures were needed in eight patients and secondary scar revision in five. Operations for inverted nipples were performed in three patients and postoperative augmentation (mammaplasty with mastopexy) in one. Mastectomy to treat carcinoma was necessary in three patients.

PATIENT SELECTION

On principle, all patients requiring reduction mammaplasty or mastopexy can be operated on with the above technique. Personally, I use it in most cases. However, in smaller reductions and mastopexies, especially in younger patients, I often prefer to use the lateral technique with L-shaped scars.[13,14] In very large, fat breasts, I also consider an inferiorly based pedicle.[7,8]

ADVANTAGES AND DISADVANTAGES OF THE TECHNIQUE

It is a simple technique, easy to teach, and once mastered gives reliable results.

The main disadvantage is the length of the submammary incision. However, if the surgeon is aware of this and avoids extending the incisions outside the new-shaped breast medially or laterally, this ceases to be a problem.

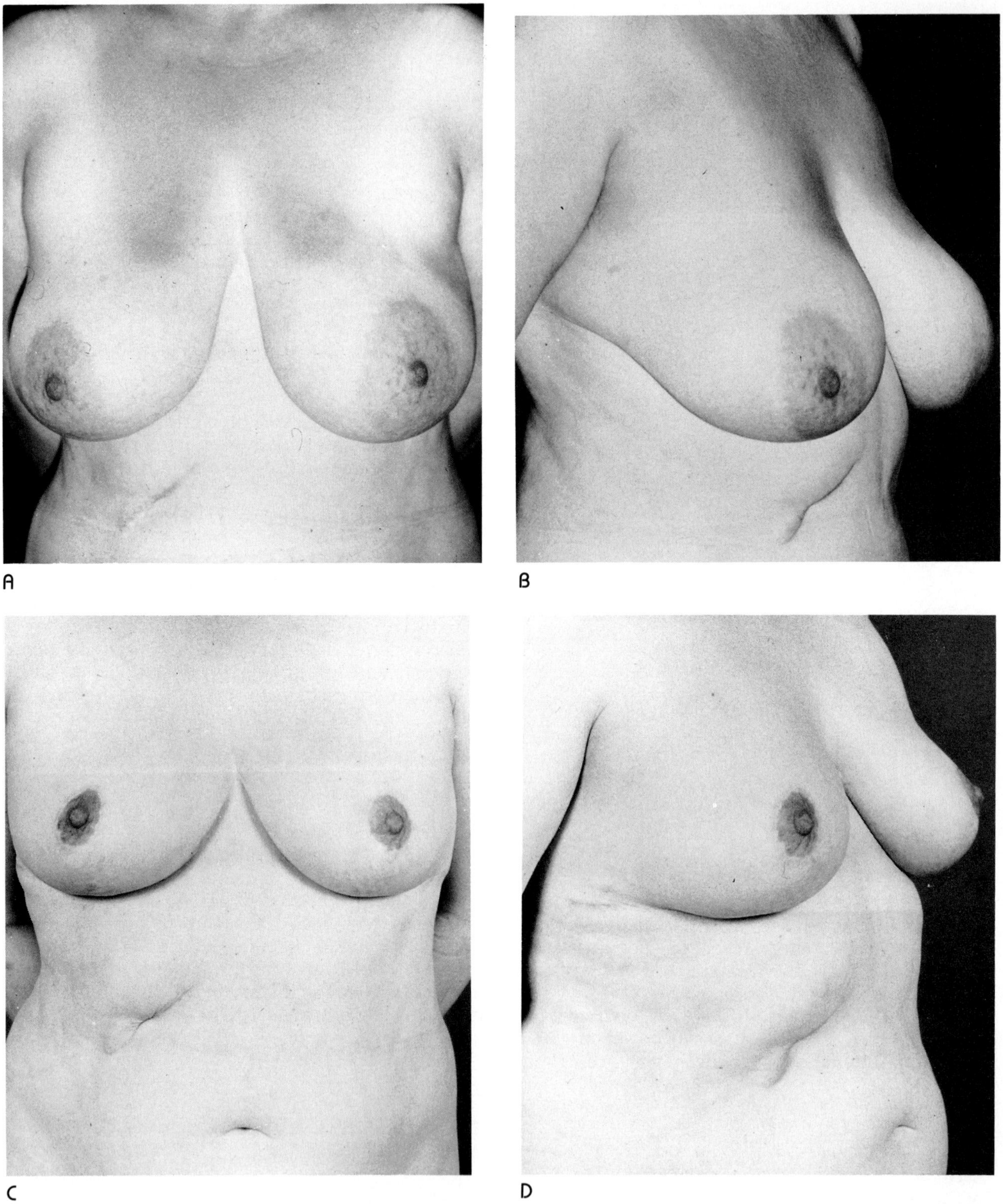

FIGURE 17–16 *A, B,* A 46-year-old patient before surgery. *C, D,* Five years after resetion of 550g of breast tissue from the right breast and 620g from the left. The nipple position is maintained and the breasts remain symmetric.

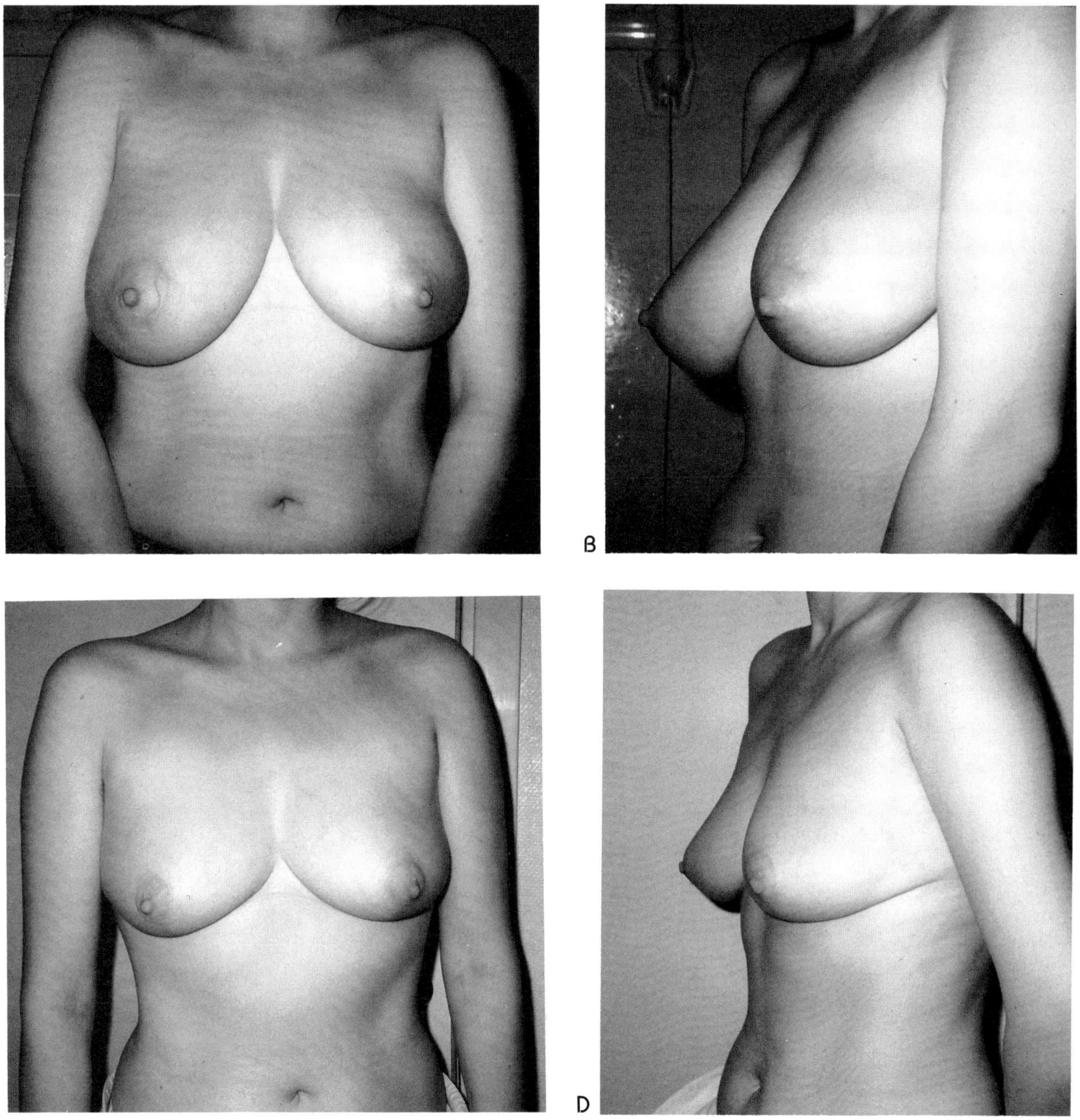

FIGURE 17–17 *A, B,* A 30-year-old patient before surgery. *C, D,* One year after resection of 450g from the right breast and 325g from the left breast.

EVALUATION OF RESULTS BY THE PATIENTS

Over the years, I have conducted follow-up studies using questionnaires to discover the patients' subjective views of the result.[14-17] The results from three studies were summarized in 1986.[18]

The scars and the breast size seem to be of greatest importance for the satisfaction of the patient. Nipple sensitivity does not seem to be as important. An evaluation of age at the time of operation revealed that younger patients, above all those below the age of 20, and to a lesser extent those between 20 and 24, were less satisfied than those over age 25. Asked "If you had a second choice, would you like to have the operation?", 95 percent of women above the age of 20 answered "yes" as compared with 76 percent of those younger than age 20 years.

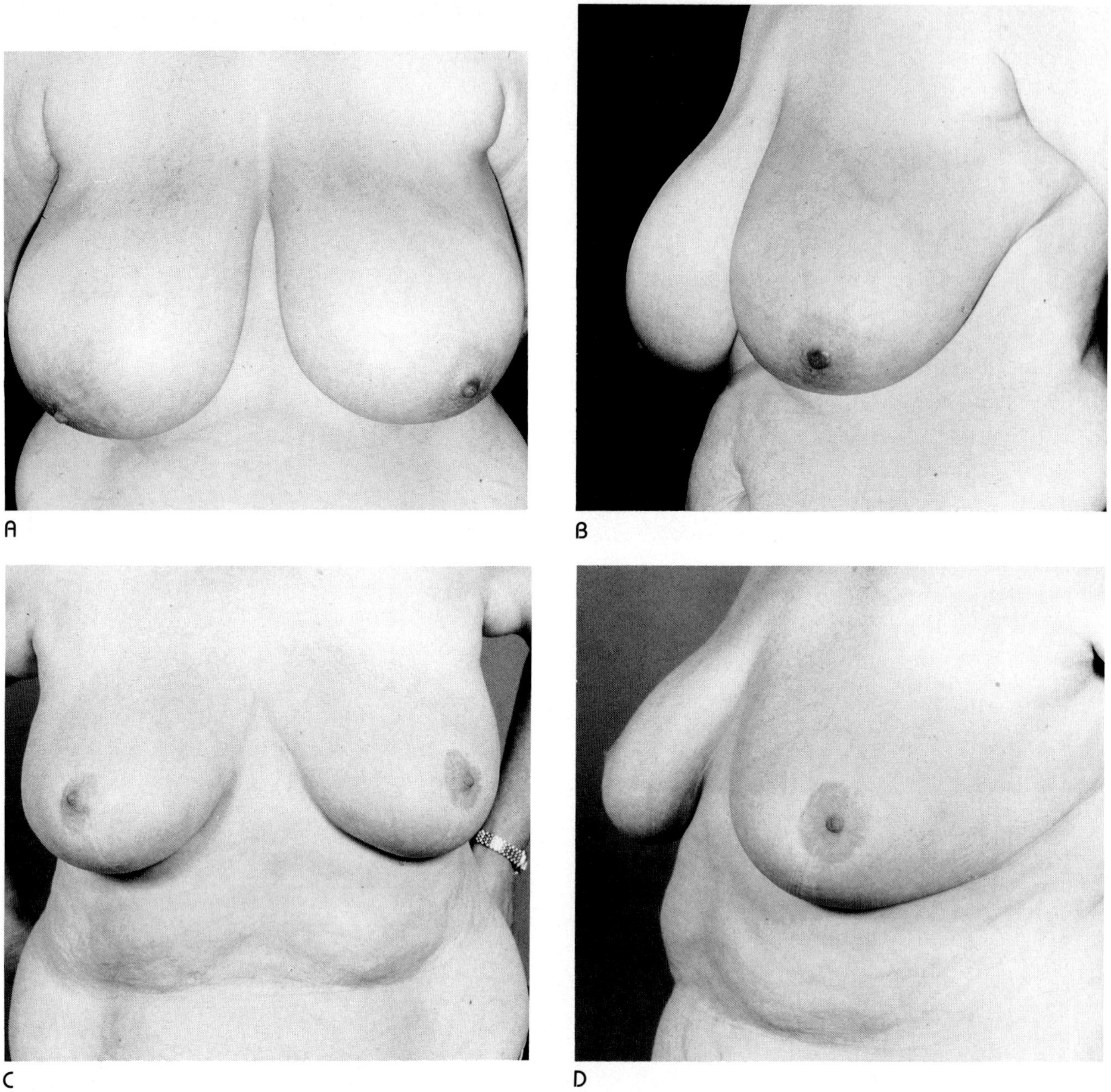

FIGURE 17–18 *A, B,* A 42-year-old patient before surgery. *C, D,* Eighteen years after resection of 1,140g from the right breast and 960g from the left by the medial pedicle technique.

When 375 patients were asked to grade their degree of *satisfaction,* 60 percent claimed to be extremely satisfied, 25 percent satisfied, 14 percent fairly satisfied, and 1 percent dissatisfied. The *scars* were regarded as almost invisible by 56 percent, somewhat disturbing by 33 percent, and ugly by 11 percent. The postoperative *breast size* was considered satisfactory by 83 percent, too large by 13 percent, and too small by 4 percent. *Nipple sensitivity* was claimed to be the same as preoperatively by 53 percent, somewhat reduced by 31 percent, and poor by 16 percent.

As the main part of the remaining gland has connection with the nipple, *lactation* is possible. The outcome differs, however, and I tell my patients that they have a 50 percent chance of being able to breast feed. The actual probability is most likely somewhat higher.

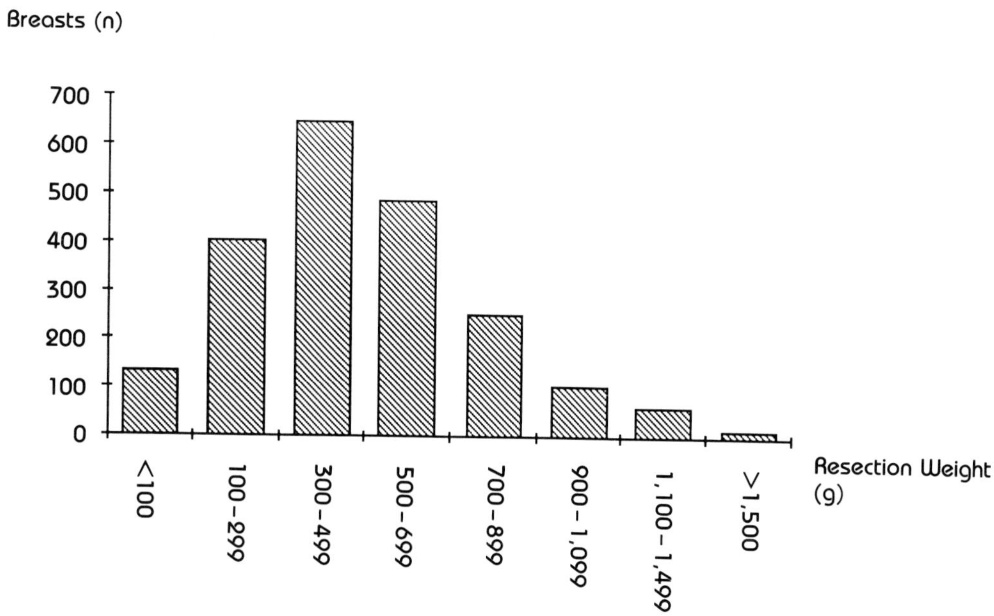

FIGURE 17-19 Resection weight.

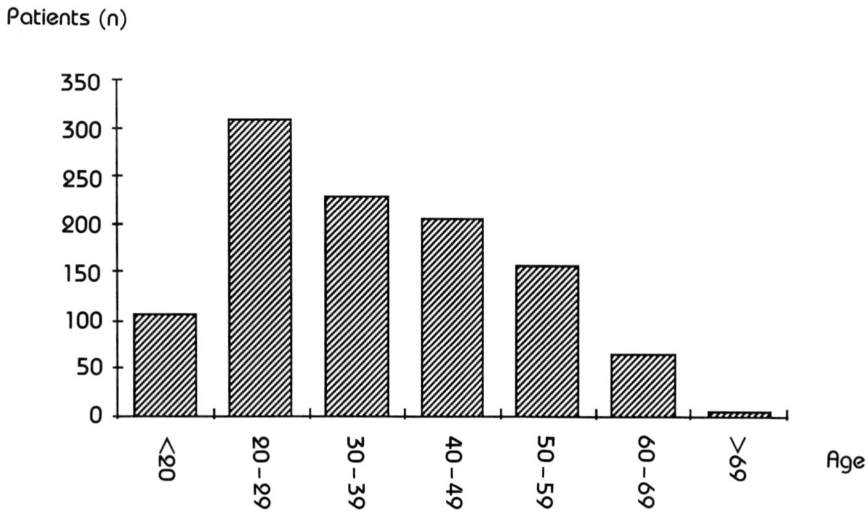

FIGURE 17-20 Age distribution.

TABLE 17-1 Overweight Correlated to Resection Weight

	<500	500-999	>1,000	Total
< + 6 kg	0/872	1/295	0/7	1/1174
	0%	0.3%	0%	0.1%
+6−+15	2/281	3/331	2/36	7/648
	0.7%	0.9%	5.6%	1.1%
> + 15 kg	0/41	9/178	10/84	19/303
	0%	5.1%	11.9%	6.1%
Total	2/1194	13/804	12/127	27/2,125
	0.2%	1.6%	9.4%	1.6%

HOW CAN THE RESULTS BE IMPROVED?

The most important consideration, as in all types of aesthetic surgery, is to be sure of what the patient expects from the operation. It is also important to discuss her wishes in detail regarding size, and to explain what scars she will have and all possible drawbacks, such as reduced nipple sensitivity and lactation capacity. The overweight patient should be encouraged to reduce weight before the operation so that she will have the weight she believes she will be able to keep in the future. Reduction mammaplasty is a beneficial operation, but a strict selection of patients is essential, especially on cosmetic grounds.

References

1. Ragnell A. Operative correction of hypertrophy and ptosis of the female breast. Acta Chir Scand 1946; Suppl 113.
2. Maliniac JW. Two-stage mammaplasty in relation to blood supply. Am J Surg 1945; 68:55.
3. Gillies H, McIndoe AH. The technique of mammaplasty in conditions of hypertrophy of the breast. Surg Gynecol Obstet 1939; 68:658.
4. Biesenberger H. Deformitäten und kosmetischen Operationen der weiblichen Brust. Vienna: W Maudrich, 1931.
5. Strömbeck JO. Mammaplasty: Report of a new technique based on the two-pedicle procedure. Br J Plast Surg 1960; 13:79.
6. Edholm P, Strömbeck JO. Influence of mammaplasty on the arterial supply to the hypertrophic breast. Acta Chir Scand 1962; 124:521.
7. Robbins TH. A reduction mammaplasty with the areola nipple based on an inferior dermal pedicle. Plast Reconstr Surg 1977; 59:64.
8. Courtiss EH, Goldwyn RM. Reduction mammaplasty by the inferior pedicle technique. Plast Reconstr Surg 1977; 59:500.
9. Skoog T. A technique of breast reduction. Acta Chir Scand 1963; 126:453.
10. Schwarzmann E. Die Technik der Mammaplastik. Chirurgie 1930; 2:932.
11. Weiner DL, Aiache AE, Silver L, Tittiranonda T. A single dermal pedicle for nipple transposition in subcutaneous mastectomy, reduction mammaplasty or mastopexy. Plast Reconstr Surg 1973; 51:115.
12. Strömbeck JO, Malm M. Priority grouping in a waiting list of patients for reduction mammaplasty. Ann Plast Surg 1986; 17:498.
13. Strömbeck JO. Benign diseases of the female breast. Surgical treatment and cosmetic aspects. Excerpta Medica International Congress Series 412. Proceedings of the VIII International Congress of Gynecology and Obstetrics, Mexico City, 17–22 Oct, 1976. Amsterdam: Excerpta Medica, 1977:184.
14. Strömbeck JO. Reduction mammaplasty: In: Georgiade NG, ed. Aesthetic breast surgery. Baltimore: Williams & Wilkins, 1983:146.
15. Strömbeck JO. Macromastia in women and its surgical treatment. Acta Chir Scand 1964; Suppl 341.
16. Strömbeck JO. Reduction mammaplasty by upper and lower glandular resections. In: Goldwyn RM, ed. Plastic and reconstructive surgery of the breast. Boston: Little, Brown, 1976:195.
17. Strömbeck JO. Late results after reduction mammaplasty. In: Goldwyn RM, ed. Long-term results in plastic and reconstructive surgery. Boston: Little, Brown, 1980:722.
18. Strömbeck JO. Reduction mammaplasty. In: Strömbeck JO, Rosato FE, eds. Surgery of the breast. New York: Georg Thieme Verlag, 1986:277.

CHAPTER 18

Vertical Bipedicle Reduction Mammaplasty

MARCIA A. FITZPATRICK, M.D.

Perhaps no single operation in plastic surgery better illustrates the ingenuity of the surgeon in adjusting and modifying an operative procedure to achieve an optimal aesthetic and reconstructive result than reduction mammaplasty. Many pioneer surgeons were intrigued by the concept of giving maximal reconstruction with relief of symptoms while still being able to preserve aesthetic contour and (progressing even further) function.

In the early twentieth century France and Germany were the sources for most published material on new surgical techniques, including those for reduction mammaplasty. Morestin, a protopioneer in that after 1904 he limited his practice and teaching to plastic and maxillofacial surgery, spoke at many surgical society meetings on breast surgery and included his description of a horizontal repair of an asymmetric breast.[1,2] Erich Lexer, while at Freiburg, published a technique of reduction mammaplasty in which, after circumscribing the areola, he removed skin and subcutaneous tissue as a strip to the site of the new areola, fixating the areola to its new position.[3] This caused the hypertrophic breast tissue to bulge below the nipple. The bulge was then resected as a wedge. The resultant closure approximated an inexact inverted T.

In 1928, Biesenberger described his method of reduction mammaplasty, which he proposed to use uniformly for all patients.[4] He pioneered the concept that a single operation with modification of only a variable, in this case the lateral markings, could be used for most patients. He believed that it was this freehand latitude given to the surgeon to adjust the lateral marks that gave the predictably good aesthetic results. This operation was used by many surgeons in Europe and the United States for more than 20 years. However, as the reported number of patients operated on worldwide steadily increased, avascular necrosis of the nipple was reported as a complication of this technique.

Two other operative procedures for reduction mammaplasty in the surgically creative decade of the 1920s deserve mention because of their influence on later surgeons. First, Thorek in 1922 described an amputation of breast tissue and nipple with survival of the nipple in its new position as a free graft.[5,6] Second, Emil Schwarzmann in 1930[7] was to antedate both Strömbeck and Skoog[8] with his description of a flap that was to carry breast tissue, areola, and nipple as a unit. He also modified the Biesenberger technique to leave a small rim of dermis around the areola to improve its vascularity.

Strömbeck, attempting to address the significant problem (incidence reported as 3 to 15 percent) of avascular necrosis of the nipple and areola, combined the principles of protective dermis and breast pedicle flap. In 1960, he published his hallmark report on a bipedicle flap based horizontally and carrying the nipple-areola complex.[9] Initial results from this operation were excellent, dramatically reducing the incidence of avascular necrosis. It could easily be standardized and taught. However, surgeons soon noted that although the operation increased safety, there were some difficulties with aesthetic appearance. A flat, inferior breast frequently resulted, and in very large-breasted women and older patients the operation assumed more difficulty. In a young, moderately large-breasted woman with a good skin brassiere, the operation remains a good one and in fact still enjoys widespread popularity in Europe.

In the latter part of the 1960s, Paul K. McKissock attempted to solve the problem of inversion of the nipple as it was infolded in the Strömbeck procedure by changing the direction of the dermal pedicle. He also believed correctly that the use of a keyhole pattern that was too wide was the reason for flatness of the breast. He changed the site of breast mass excision to control the width of the breast. McKissock emphasized strict adherence to the operative markings, in contradistinction to Biesenberger's freehand technique.[10] Over the next 10 years this was to become a widely used breast reduction surgery technique in the United States[11] until the advent of the inferior pedicle and central mound techniques.[12]

APPLIED ANATOMY

Predominant arterial blood supply and venous drainage patterns of the female breast were extensively described by Maliniac.[13] He firmly believed as a consequence of his findings that all breast operations should make an attempt to preserve the three main blood vessels to the breast, i.e. the intercostal, the lateral thoracic, and the internal mammary, which supplies the greatest percentage (60 percent). Other authors, including Aufricht[14] and Climo and Alexander,[15] plotting statistical variance of the percentage contribution of these three vessels, raised the question whether attempts should be made to identify at surgery a specific vessel for preservation. They concluded that the breast was so well randomly vascularized that it made absolutely no technical difference to the end result. The preponderance of successful reduction mammaplasty surgical techniques support this concept that blood supply entering the breast from one direction is sufficient to vascularize all contiguous breast tissue.

Although the venous drainage system assumes extreme importance in topics related to carcinoma of the breast, it does not really have any surgical importance in the treatment of mammary hypertrophy. The venous drainage systems consist of a superficial system draining into both internal mammary and superficial cervical veins, and a deep system draining exclusively into the internal mammary venous system.[16]

Innervation of the mammary gland does not usually merit more than a short summation in most anatomy texts. However, it assumes premier importance to the surgeon contemplating performing reduction mammaplasty because of the psychological nuances of breast sensation, especially nipple sensation, to the patient. Sir Ashley Cooper published his text on the anatomy of the breast in 1840.[17] Most of his notations remain accurate. The lateral nerve supply to the breast comes from the anterior rami of the third to sixth intercostal nerves and medially from the second to sixth rami of the intercostal nerves. Hricko was one of the first investigators to point out the large size of these lateral cutaneous nerves, and first commented on the importance of the anterior branch of the fourth lateral cutaneous nerve.[18] He believed that this constituted a major nerve to the nipple, and perhaps the only single nerve that was significant in sensation. Other breast sensation of the areola and skin is derived from the anterior cutaneous branches of the second to sixth intercostal nerves. Courtiss and Goldwyn and others have pointed out that it is this importance of the lateral cutaneous branch of the fourth intercostal nerve that has led to the embracing of techniques that include its course in the vascular pedicle to the nipple and areola.[19] Almost all patients undergoing reduction mammaplasty show some diminution of sensation postoperatively. As would be expected, the more extensive the procedure and the greater amount of breast tissue removed, the more disturbances there are in sensation, with the amputated breast tissue and free nipple graft transfer patients showing the least amount of sensation 2 years postoperatively. Reinnervation seems to proceed from the periphery, and insensibility is not uniform between one breast and the other, or even between areas of the same breast. The reasons for this are unknown.[20]

Subunits of alveolar lobules and ducts compose the approximately 16 lobes of the breast. Hormonal secretions cause a marked individual response in these anatomic units, both during the monthly cycle and also at different stages of the reproductive cycle. Pregnancy causes a marked proliferation of the lobular alveolar units with subsequent milk formation. The normal menstrual cycle progresses from a compact stroma to proliferative change through epithelial secretions and back to a compact stroma phase secondary to hormonal variations. Finally, menopause causes cessation of hormonal simulation, which leads to involution of the breast tissue and replacement by varying amounts of fat. In mammary hypertrophy, genetic factors obviously can potentiate the end-organ response to hormonal stimulation. The overall body habitus also influences breast size.

PATIENT SELECTION

At the initial preoperative consultation, the surgeon must assess the usual preoperative factors such as the patient's previous medical history and medications taken, and the symptomatology that gave the major impetus to seek surgery. All forms of breast surgery introduce potentially deep-seated psychosexual feelings, and this must be carefully assessed. Goin and Goin discussed the psychology of reduction mammaplasty.[21,22] Surgeons must be aware of this and tailor their discussion to these individual differences. In the author's practice it has been unusual for the woman over 50, married and with grown children, to be concerned to a major degree with the scars on the breast caused by reduction mammaplasty. The same is not true, however, in the 20-year-old who is not married, is sexually active, and is concerned about her perceived unattractiveness to her sexual partner if the scars are severe.

In my experience with 363 patients who have

presented for bilateral reduction mammaplasty, and 82 patients who have had unilateral reduction mammaplasty, presenting symptoms may vary with the age of the patient. Table 18-1 lists the symptoms recorded in this group. It is interesting to note how the age of the patient affects the presentation of symptomatology to the surgeon. It is unusual to find a patient over the age of 50 whose major concern is breast appearance. Most older women describe a long-held desire to seek the operation; most younger women (under the age of 25) relate feelings of frustration with verbal sexual harassment and restriction of physical exercise.

Other than the obvious factors of height, weight, and stature, specific attention during the physical examination should be paid to the presence or absence of breast asymmetry and associated problems, such as an inverted nipple.

A measurement is taken of the location of the nipple in relation to the sternal notch, and the length the nipple will have to be moved to its new location. If the initial measurement exceeds 40 cm, this is the limit that McKissock[23] arbitrarily puts on the subsequent use of his operation. It is possible to extend this length another 8 or 10 cm, but this might lead to unnecessary risk to the pedicle, and usually leaves a residual breast mass that is bulky to close because it does not fit the skin brassiere. In these cases, breast amputation with a free nipple-areola graft is the best technique.

The last portion of the preoperative consultation is devoted to an in-depth question and answer session with the patient. It is at this time that it is easiest to judge the psychological suitability of the patient for the proposed surgery. It is also the best time to introduce the concept of autologous blood donation in patients with breasts large enough for significant blood loss of 400 ml or more to be a danger. Patients have proved extremely responsive to the availability of autodonation no matter what their age group.

After completing the preoperative consultation, I select the technique for surgery on the basis of the following criteria:

TABLE 18-1 Symptoms Recorded in 363 Patients

	Age at Operation		
	<25	25-45	>45
Breast discomfort	121	115	76
Neck and shoulder pain	51	31	52
Back pain	38	86	12
Physical activity restriction	80	49	6
Aesthetic appearance	111	91	9
Emotional considerations*	7	0	1
Other physical signs (shoulder grooving, intertrigo)	5	37	44

*Mild depression, social withdrawal

1. The vertical pedicle technique of McKissock is used in (a) the young patient with good skin brassiere and tense bulky breasts; (b) the young patient with either very large, obese breasts or smaller but extremely ptotic breasts, with a sternal notch-to-nipple distance even exceeding 40 cm, but less than 48 cm; and (c) the older patient with hypertrophic breasts and either normal stature or moderate obesity.
2. Breast amputation with free nipple graft is indicated in the older patient who has very ptotic breasts exceeding the proposed nipple distance of 40 cm or who is obese, or in the young patient with true gigantomastia.

One caveat must be mentioned in regard to tailoring the operation to the patient. Most nipple transposition reduction mammaplasty procedures, including the McKissock technique, are not "short scar" procedures, although they may be somewhat modified if the breast has relatively small hypertrophy. If the young patient with moderate breast hypertrophy specifically requests an attempt to shorten the scars and is a suitable candidate for such an operation, a procedure such as that described by Marchac and de Olarte[24] should be used.

OPERATIVE PROCEDURE

Preoperative Markings

With the patient sitting erect, I begin by marking the proposed new position of the nipple on the breast. This is the most critical decision made in the pattern design, because proper placement reduces the possibility of postoperative "high riding" of the breasts, one of the most difficult contour problems to correct. A plumb line is drawn from the midclavicle through the true meridian of the breast (Fig. 18-1). (Common sense dictates that the "wall-eyed" nipple may be somewhat lateral to this meridian and will be somewhat corrected by moving it.) Nipple position is then chosen relative to the inframammary line, which has been drawn and extends medially and laterally as far as necessary to remove excess skin. Laterally, in the truly huge breast, the scar can sometimes be improved by extending the line transversely rather than by following the curvilinear breast shape. The nipple must be located *exactly* at the height of the inframammary line, and this can be done by a variety of techniques. Positioning the nipple several centimeters above, as advocated by early publications, has been shown to cause abnormally high nipples on postoperative examination.

McKissock's original method of placing obstetric forceps at the clavicular and inframammary lines, with the measurement superimposed on the breast, provides a safe, reliable way to mark nipple location. Others use a complicated series of "normal" mea-

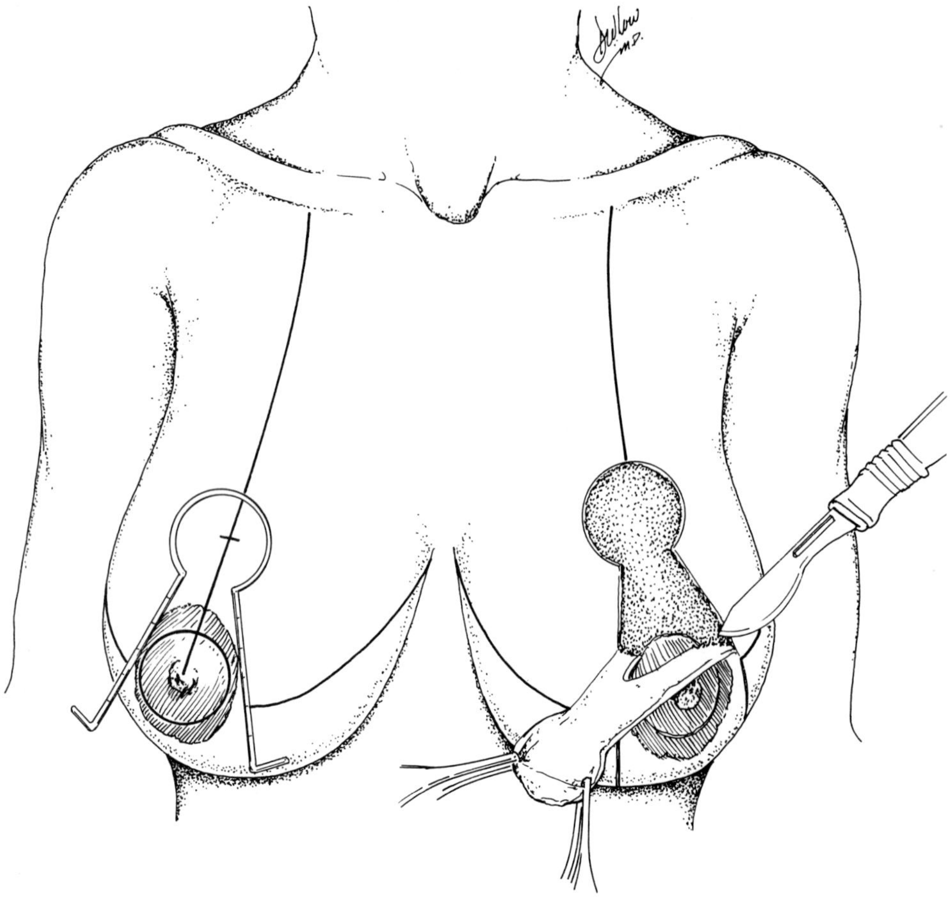

FIGURE 18–1 Preoperative markings for the vertical bipedicle reduction mammaplasty technique are demonstrated on the right breast. The nipple is located at the height of the inframammary line. The McKissock keyhole adjustable pattern is used, and 5-cm vertical limbs are planned. The pedicle is deepithelialized on the left breast, maintaining the integrity of the dermal bridge at the superior aspect of the new areolar site.

surements and intersecting lines. My own preference is a free-hand method with the fingers on the inframammary line and the thumb on the breast skin. By relating the nipple position to the inframammary line *only*, such dictums as "Locate 18 to 22 cm from the sternal notch"[25] become moot. Variation from this nipple location occurs only in mastopexy when, to match a reconstructed breast, a compromise point must be found higher.

Keyhole patterns come in many varieties, which may be used without impeding the vertical vascular pedicle. The commercial McKissock marker is easily adjusted, as the entire keyhole pattern with vertical lines of 5 cm are drawn on the patient (Fig. 18–1). I modify the length of the vertical limb to 6 cm in the very large breast of an obese woman over 50; this helps to avoid closure tension and vascular embarrassment. Nowhere is McKissock's adherence to strict preoperative planning as important as in keeping close the proximity of the vertical limbs to the side of the areola.[26] Although it is common to have to modify the amount of skin centrally at closure, it is safer for the inexperienced surgeon to do this, especially in the case of the "maxi-areola" breast, than to face an almost impossible closure-contour difficulty. Extensions of the vertical limb are then drawn by dotted lines to the inframammary line to note the extent of the deepithelialization.

The breast is gently pulled medially, and the lateral vertical line advances to the meridian point of the submammary line and held. A line is marked along this, superimposed on the inframammary line, representing the amount of skin brassiere to be removed. The medial vertical line is pulled to the meridian point, while the excess of brassiere on the breast medial aspect is marked. The boxlike shape of the breast, which this was believed to prevent, has been found to change with postoperative progression of time.

A line is drawn in the midsternal plane, the measurement of each breast from the sternum to the inframammary line median point is verified, and from here the line to the lateral edge is made the same as the opposite breast. This completes the markings.

Surgical Technique

With the patient asleep in the supine or 30-degree head elevation position, preoperative markings are scored and the patient is prepared and draped. A standard 4.5-cm hardware washer or Freeman "cookie cutter" is then used to mark the areola to fit the keyhole pattern. Some authors have reported injecting a dilute solution of lidocaine (Xylocaine) with epinephrine at this point to assist with hemostasis. It is my preference to request the anesthetist to control the perioperative blood pressure during the actual removal of breast tissue to a level at which the dermis minimally bleeds, approximately 15 to 20 mm Hg below the normal pressure.

Deepithelialization then proceeds with as much attention paid to the integrity of the position of the dermal bridge superior to the areola as to the inferior areola (Fig. 18-1). Although the dermal bridge does not guarantee the success of the operation and nipple inviolability, the superior portion of the dermal bridge, which can be very thin, does add another measure of safety in preservation of the blood supply of the nipple.

After deepithelialization is complete, the electrocautery knife is used to begin to outline the vertical bipedicle. For the neophyte in this technique, and for resident training purposes, it is usually easier to begin by resecting lateral breast tissue. The reason for this is that if too much undermining of the pedicle occurs, it is possible to remove a minimal amount of skin and breast tissue medially to ensure nipple vascular safety. Also, if too much beveling occurs under the medial edge approaching toward the lateral, the entire pedicle may move to an extreme lateral position, with resultant difficulty in closure and contour deformity.

The incision is carried vertically down to the chest wall, starting at the inframammary line and directed superiorly. Beginning at this point provides better control of the evolving vascular pedicle. The upper limit of the incision is within the circular part of the keyhole pattern. In the left breast it ends at 2 o'clock, in the right at 10 o'clock; in the smaller breast it is possible to end this incision lower, at 4 o'clock. This helps preserve a vessel that consistently enters the pedicle between the position of 1 and 3 o'clock.

It should be remembered that the end result of a McKissock reduction mammaplasty leaves a central bipedicle folded on itself superiorly, with small amounts of breast tissue left medially and laterally, sufficient to shape the breast to the desired size.[11,26] Superiorly the breast is removed to accommodate the folded pedicle. To form the lateral pedicle, the assistant holds the main mass of the breast. The surgeon can develop the lateral skin pedicle containing the subcutaneous fat and sufficient breast to give the anticipated size. The residual breast not attached to the skin is then freed from the pectoral fascia. This allows the entire residual lateral mass of breast to be moved as a single unit. In dissecting superiolaterally, it is important to avoid beveling toward the skin, because the skin can be mechanically injured, and laterally the same care must be used to avoid injury to the axillary contents.

In a very large breast, once the lateral pedicle has been formed, it is sometimes easier to start the excision of the residual breast mass inferiorly. This allows control and identification of the vascular and nerve supply.

McKissock, in recent presentations, advocated leaving a layer of breast tissue over the pectoral fascia to diminish further the risk of nerve damage and residual numbness of the nipple.[23] However, there is a low incidence of nipple numbness with this technique, making this an optional maneuver.

The largest amount of breast tissue is removed from this lateral location. Expedience usually dictates rapidity of surgery, with attention only to the larger-bore vessels at the actual time of electrocautery dissection. Meticulous hemostasis is ensured before proceeding to the medial pedicle. My experience with breast reduction procedures performed by means of electrocautery and "modified hypotension" anesthesia is that there is excellent control of blood loss, so that a reduction can be achieved with minimal blood loss, less than 350 ml in 90 percent of patients.

A saline-soaked pack is placed into the lateral operative site, and the electrocautery is again used to carry the dissection on the medial side of the central pedicle, proceeding from the inframammary line in a superior direction to 10 o'clock on the keyhole pattern in the left breast. This is a critical juncture. Extreme care must be taken to bevel the incision *away from the vascular pedicle* proceeding from the chest wall. Prudence must be used here; it is safer to allow a pedicle to be thicker than it would normally be until operative mastery and experience is gained with this technique. Although the pedicle is approximately 5 to 7 cm in width, it is sometimes possible to thin this pedicle to the point at which the vessels can be seen as a gossamer-thin pedicle entering the overlying dermis. Experience with the McKissock operation should be extensive before this extreme dissection is attempted.

With the center pedicle thus preserved at the appropriate width in the lower portion containing the blood vessels, the incision can be rapidly extended down to the chest wall to totally free the medial edge of the pedicle from the medial skin flaps (Fig. 18-2). This dissection must be continued to a more superior level than the actual cessation of the skin markings, in order to allow the appropriate folding after subsequent removal of a central core of breast tissue. Allis clamps or similar tenacula are then used to hold the medial breast mass while the appropriate medial flap is fashioned, again leaving sufficient breast on the skin to achieve proper thickness and shape. Medially, most surgeons leave a somewhat thicker amount of attached breast tissue inferiorly, in an attempt to mimic the medial cleavage of the average female breast.

After formation of the pedicle flap, the residual breast is removed from beneath the skin flaps (Fig.

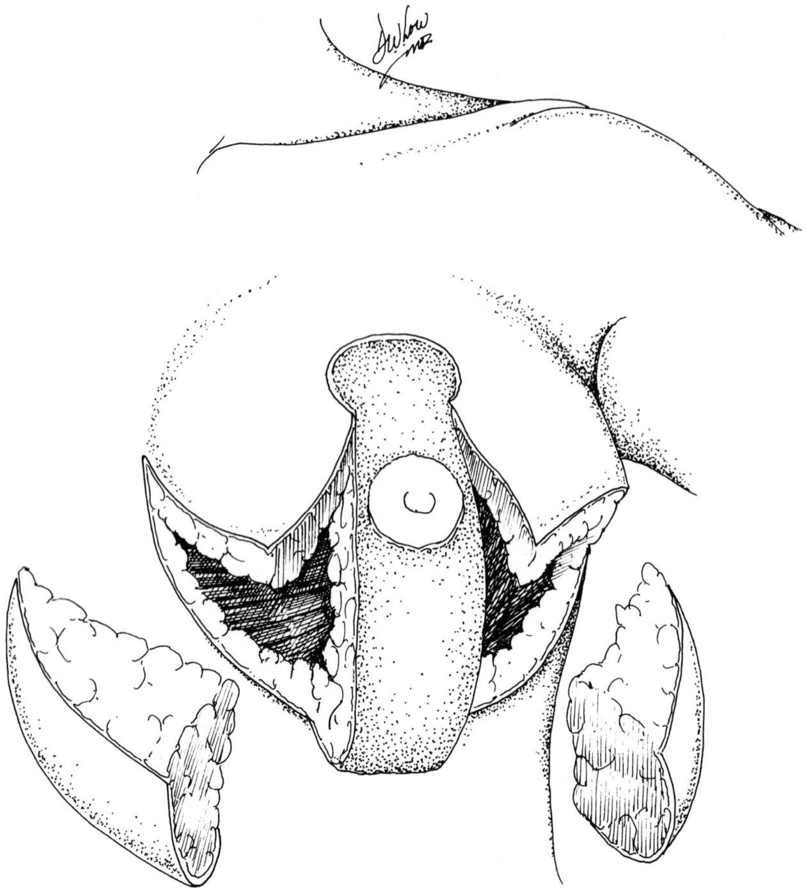

FIGURE 18–2 The base of the pedicle varies between 5 and 7 cm in width. While full thickness of breast tissue is preserved beneath the pedicle, initial incisions are deepened to the fascia of the chest muscles. Medial and lateral wedges of skin and breast tissue are then removed.

18–2). Hemostasis is again achieved in the medial breast. The surgical assistant then gently holds the pedicle from the chest wall, and the surgeon proceeds to remove a circular core of tissue from underneath the superior pedicle, again taking into account the breast size desired. If McKissock's procedure is used as a mastopexy, it is possible that almost no tissue is removed from this location, and the breast is simply folded upon itself.[26] Obviously, in reduction mammaplasty, different weights of breast tissue are removed.

Errors in the McKissock mammaplasty can compromise the aesthetic result or endanger its safety. A common mistake made by a surgeon inexperienced with the technique is inadvertent undermining of the central pedicle: this can destroy its blood supply. Starting the dissection on the lateral side helps prevent this. The second most common mistake is failure to remove the appropriate amount of tissue necessary to achieve easy closure with an excellent contour. In the breast, when an attempt is being made to give the tightest of skin brassieres, i.e. in a young woman's breast, it is desirable to thin the superior portion of the central pedicle to only dermis with a small amount of tissue beneath it. Great care must be taken and the nipple must be closely observed while the surgeon is trimming the amount of tissue; again, with experience it is easier to judge the amount of tissue that can be safely removed. If the surgeon keeps in mind a three-dimensional view of the specimen, it is usually necessary to remove more breast tissue superiorly, underneath the skin marking, than might at first be thought necessary, to allow the pedicle to fold for the appropriate shaping of the breast (Fig. 18–3*A*).

With the operative procedure essentially complete, the specimen is weighed for comparison with the opposite side. The wound is irrigated copiously with either antibiotic solution or sterile saline, and again checked for hemostasis. A point of frequent bleeding that may be overlooked in hemostasis is on the underside of the superior half of the pedicle, which will be infolded. A drain of choice is laid along the chest wall, and the closure begins by approximating the points of the keyhole. At this point in the procedure, it will be obvious whether any subsequent skin removal is needed at the vertical limbs of the inverted-T closure, after it is judged how much "dog-ear" or excess skin there is laterally. The vertical limb length of 5 to 6 cm is again checked. It is my preference at this point to loosely approximate the breast with several towel clips, and judge the ease of

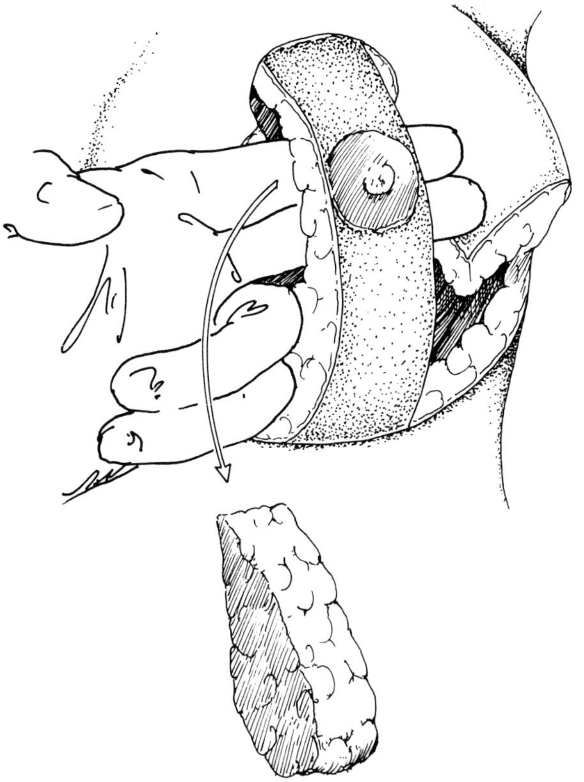
A

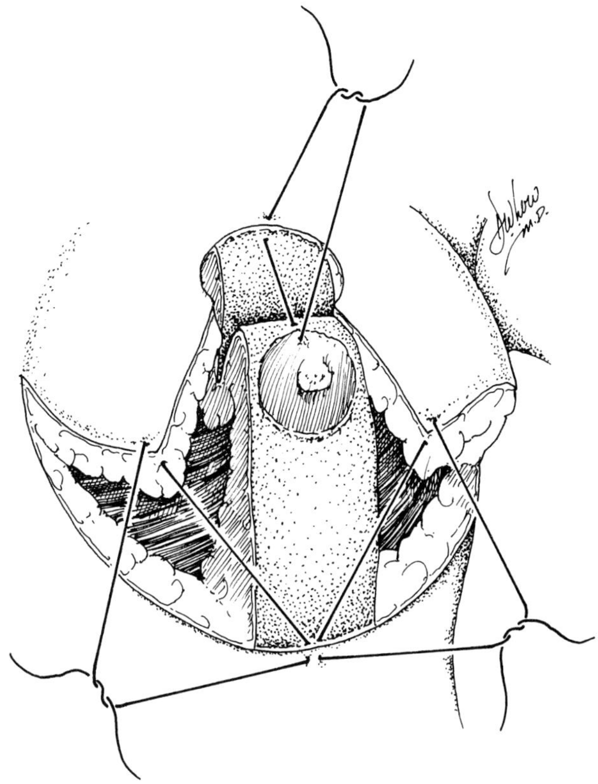
B

FIGURE 18–3 *A*, Breast tissue is removed from beneath the pedicle, more tissue being removed superiorly than at the base of the pedicle. This allows folding of the pedicle for appropriate shaping of the breast. *B*, The vertical lines are approximated to the midline of the base of the pedicle, and the superior suture in the nipple-areola complex is placed in the 12 o'clock position at the deepithelialized part of the superior pedicle. The upper limit of the incision may extend within the keyhole pattern to allow folding of the pedicle. This incision ends at the 2 o'clock position on the left breast and at the 10 o'clock position on the right.

closure and also the approximate size in comparison with the opposite breast.

If the skin flap closure is tight at this point, the tightness will be apparent in the vertical portion of the inverted-T incision. If tightness occurs, the breast *must* be opened and more tissue removed to preserve vascularity. As previously mentioned, the usual site of the excess tissue is superiorly where the pedicle folds, although occasionally more lateral tissue also has to be removed (Fig. 18–4*A*). It is very unusual for it to be necessary to remove any of the medial breast tissue remaining.

Once the surgeon is satisfied with the size and symmetry and satisfied that closure tension is minimal, the actual closure begins. It proceeds medially from the sternum to a point 1 inch or so from the vertical limb, and then resumes from laterally to the same point; a decision is made regarding whether the limbs need to be trimmed for appropriate closure. Although the vertical limb of the inverted T may be skewed either way 15 degrees or so, it is much better technique, especially in the early stages of this operation, to leave the limb totally vertical. The skin closure is made with a subcuticular suture, either absorbable or a nonabsorbable pull-out suture. The vertical limb is then closed in the same two-layer fashion (Fig. 18–3*B*).

The nipple is closed as the last step. If there has been any altering of the limbs of the keyhole where they come together, it is very important at this point to check the aperture with the "cookie cutter" to ascertain that it has maintained its preoperative size and shape. If there is a discrepancy, the appropriate amount of skin is removed to make the circle accurate. The nipple is sutured with several everting sutures at the dermis level, and again it is the surgeon's preference whether to use a subcuticular or a running suture to close the areola (Fig. 18–4*B*). Steri-Strips are used to reinforce the closure, and either an Ace bandage or a pressure tape support dressing over bandages completes the dressing of the wound.

POSTOPERATIVE COURSE

After surgery, the patient remains hospitalized for 24 to 48 hours. The continued use of perioperative antibiotics postoperatively is up to the personal preference of the surgeon. After removal of the

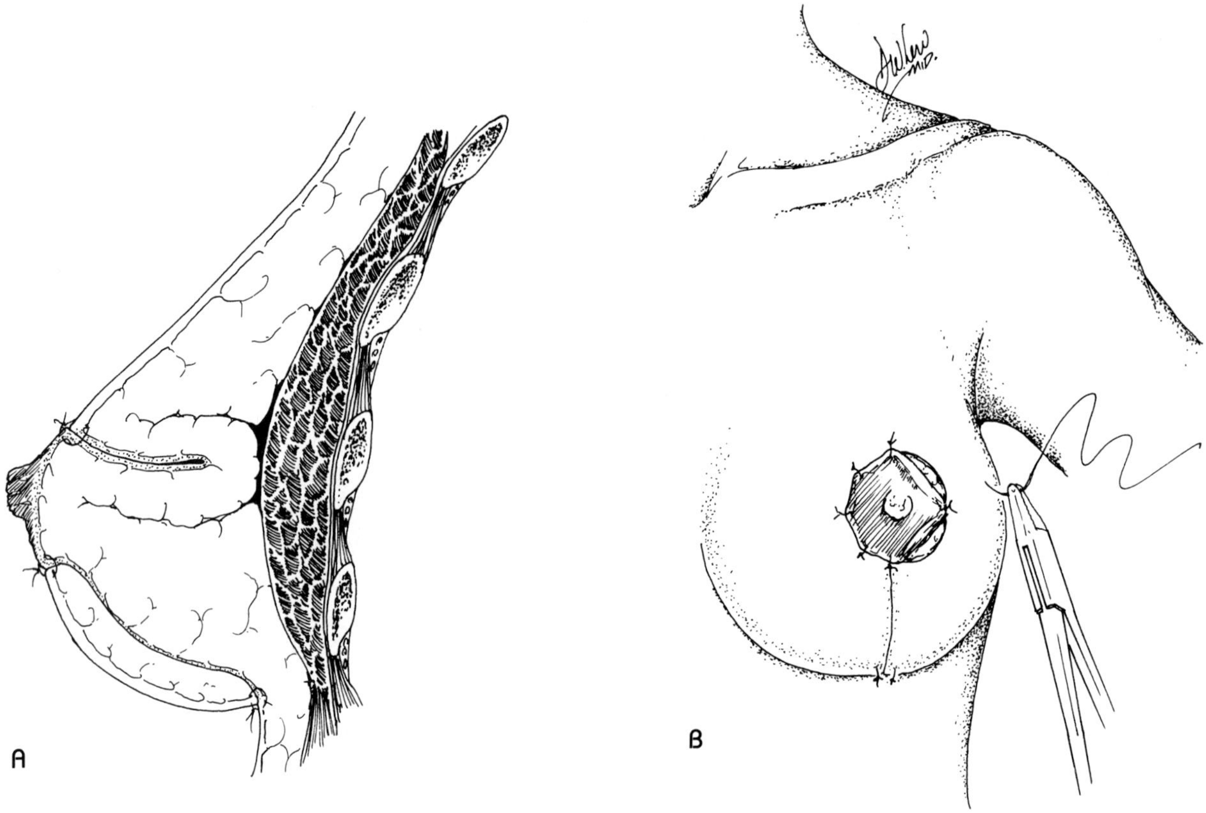

FIGURE 18–4 *A*, Removal of excess breast tissue from beneath the superior part of the pedicle allows folding without tension. Note the relative thickness of the breast tissue behind the superior and inferior parts of the pedicle. *B*, Nipple-areola closure is the final step in the procedure. Adjustments in the skin flap may be necessary during suturing to ensure a circular closure.

drains, the patient is sent home and encouraged to continue gentle support to the breast, with a bra, for the first several weeks postoperatively. Light physical exercise such as walking can begin immediately, but extreme physical activity such as tennis and advanced aerobics are contraindicated until approximately 1 month after surgery. Six months after surgery a routine postoperative mammogram is obtained in all patients over the age of 30 as a baseline, because it has been reported that reduction mammaplasty causes mammographic changes in most women. The patient is followed at intervals for 1 year, in some cases for 18 months, to monitor the progression of the scars, which are notorious for slow resolution. Although women of reproductive age have been counseled that they will be unable to nurse a child after surgery, it has been an interesting postoperative experience, substantiated by other authors, that in this series 60 percent of a small number of patients who attempted to nurse were successful. Other authors have reported a higher incidence of successful nursing after nipple transposition reduction mammaplasty than previously believed.[27]

RESULTS

Reduction mammaplasty provides a high degree of patient satisfaction. In the series of patients surveyed, 93 percent would undergo surgery again. Five percent would change their breast size, most feeling that they would like to be smaller in size. Only 2 percent of the patients would elect not to have the surgery again, either because of chronic pain postoperatively or for aesthetic considerations. Interestingly, the over-45 age group is the most vocal in its praise of the operation for its effect on physical and mental wellbeing.

By the late 1970s Woods and colleagues[28] were reporting that the McKissock procedure gave superior aesthetic results with a good margin of safety in comparison with procedures previously described, such as those by Strömbeck and Skoog. Although later techniques introduced now yield the same good aesthetic results with the same margin of safety, McKissock's procedure remains an excellent operation for the predictability of its results (Figs. 18-5 and 18-6).

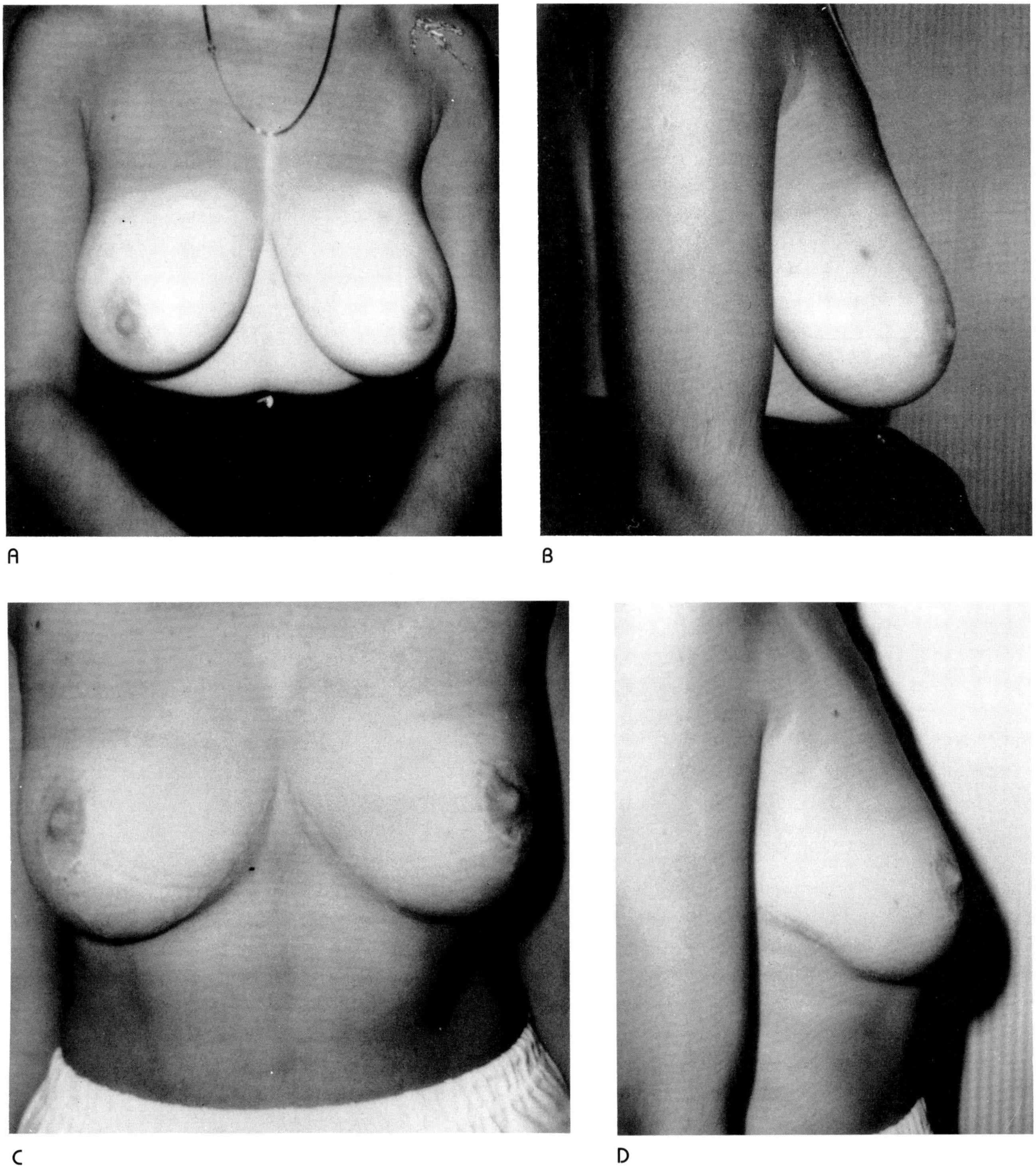

FIGURE 18-5 *A, B,* Preoperative views of a 23-year-old woman before vertical pedicle reduction mammaplasty. *C, D,* Three years after surgery the breast shape is maintained, with good nipple location.

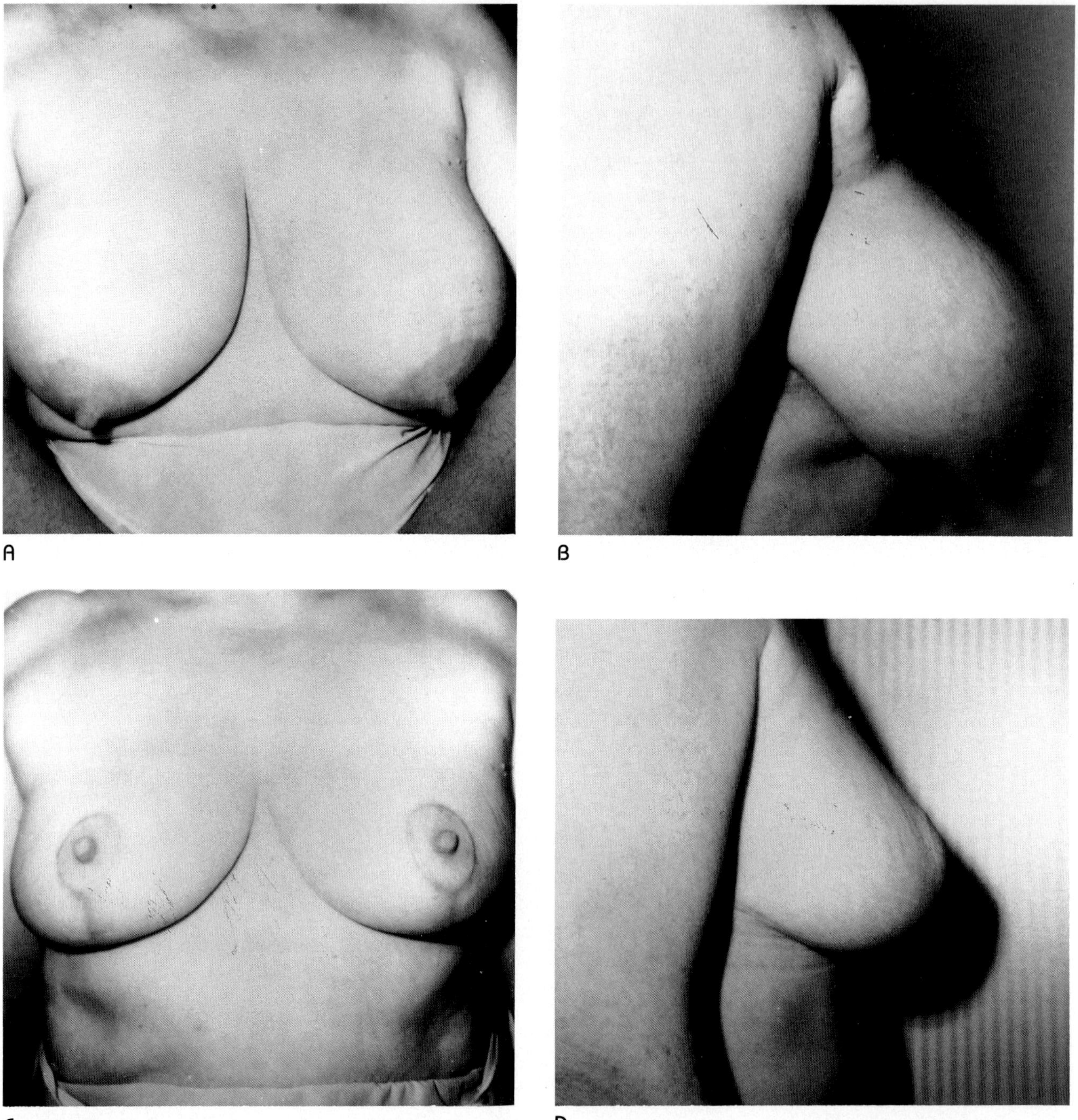

A B C D

FIGURE 18–6 *A, B,* A 39-year-old woman with very large ptotic breasts. The nipple measured 38 cm from the suprasternal notch. The vertical bipedicle technique was used. *C, D,* Seven months after surgery the nipple shape and projection are excellent, with good breast contour.

COMPLICATIONS

Serious complications are infrequent (Table 18–2). They include the following:

Nipple Loss. The one patient in this series with a total loss of the nipple was a 63-year-old obese woman whose nipple had to be moved 40 cm. Retrospectively, she was a poor candidate for the operation and should have had a breast amputation with free nipple graft procedure. She did not require hospitalization for treatment of the complication.

Partial Nipple Loss. Two partial nipple losses have occurred (1) in a 29-year-old black patient with technical factors compromising nipple viability, and

TABLE 18-2 Complications (Reduction Patients Only) (N = 363)

Nipple necrosis	
Total	1
Partial	2
<10%	7
Hemorrhage	2
Fat necrosis	5
Infection	5
Wound slough	
Major	3 (2 Fat necrosis)
Minor (inverted and puncture)	24
Minor wounds (cysts, scars)	40
Nipple malposition (high)	3
Nipple sensory loss (partial)	27

(2) in a 65-year-old white patient who developed significant fat necrosis with infection; she required hospitalization and subsequently lost approximately 20 percent of the nipple.

Hemorrhage. Two patients were readmitted to the hospital within 7 days after reduction mammaplasty for drainage of a hematoma of one breast. In both of these patients the bleeding vessel was found to be in the posterior portion of the pedicle. The results in both were subsequently satisfactory.

Infection. Three patients required hospitalization for infection. One was a woman in her mid-40s with no predisposing factors who had developed a staphylococcal infection that necessitated hospitalization for 5 days. Both of the other two patients were over the age of 60 and were hospitalized for treatment of an infection that followed fat necrosis. Two of the three patients subsequently required resection of a painful calcific mass.

Emotional Factors. One patient with no history of such an event experienced a full-blown psychotic episode regarding body image approximately 3 weeks after reduction mammaplasty. She responded to psychiatric therapy. Two other patients reported severe depressive reactions, which were not treated and were recognized by the patients after surgery as a response to changing body image at the time. Both returned to normal within 3 months.

ADVANTAGES AND DISADVANTAGES

Common features that favor McKissock's operation include safety and predictability. Although initially the breast may look "boxy" and "square" and have a fullness or lumpiness in the superior pole, this rapidly resolves postoperatively, so that by 6 weeks after surgery the breasts appear to have a normal shape and have lost most of their flatness in the inferior pole. It is important to stress this fact to the surgeon when this operation is first undertaken, because to form a sufficiently tight skin brassiere, it is sometimes necessary to have this unnatural-appearing superior pole immediately postoperatively. The patient should be reassured that this will resolve.

The safety of McKissock's procedure, with a superior vascular pedicle bringing a blood supply to the nipple, makes this suitable for use in resident training. By leaving the pedicle a full 5 to 7 cm in width until the end of the procedure, it becomes easier to guide the resident in the early stages of three-dimensional thinking and preservation of blood supply with a fallback margin of safety. Until experience is gained, it is much easier to guide the resident through the vertical parallel cuts of the McKissock procedure than through the nuances of the inferior pedicle and central mound techniques. It also imparts an ultimate appreciation of the amount of tissue needed superiorly to avoid a flat superior pole of the breast. Aesthetic results remain predictably good and are similar to those from other techniques that use a form of vertical pedicle. Although one who uses this procedure frequently would like to postulate that leaving the nipple attached to a superior bridge of tissue produces a more predictable projection and fullness of the superior whole, it is not possible to support this belief with scientific evidence.

The only disadvantage of the McKissock procedure is that for some surgeons it adds several minutes to the operative time. The problem of "bottoming out" of the breasts over a long postoperative period of years remains to be solved.

References

1. Morestin H. Hypertrophic mammaire. Bull Mem Soc Anat Paris 1905:602.
2. Morestin H. La réduction graduelle des difformités tegumentaires. Translation and comments by Converse JM. Plast Reconstr Surg 1968; 42:72.
3. Lexer E. Hypertrophie bei der Mammae. Munch Med Wochenschr 1912; 59:2702.
4. Biesenberger H. Eine neue Methode der Mammaplastik. Zentrablbl Chir 1928; 55:2382.
5. Thorek M. Possibilities in the reconstruction of the human form. NY Med J 1922; 116:572.
6. Thorek M. Histological verification of efficacy of free transplantation of the nipple. Med J Rec 1931; 134:474.
7. Schwarzmann E. Die Technik der Mammaplastik. Chirurgie 1930; 2:932.
8. Skoog T. A technique of breast reduction. Acta Chir Scand 1972; 49:245.
9. Strömbeck JO. Mammaplasty: Report of a new technique based on the two-pedicle procedure. Br J Plast Surg 1960; 13:79.
10. McKissock P. Reduction mammaplasty with a vertical dermal flap. Plast Reconstr Surg 1972; 49:245.
11. McKissock PK. Reduction mammaplasty by the vertical bipedicle flap technique. Clin Plast Surg 1976; 3:309.
12. Courtiss E, Goldwyn RM. Reduction mammaplasty by the inferior pedicle technique. Plast Reconstr Surg 1977; 59:500.

13. Maliniac JW. Arterial blood supply of the breast. Arch Surg 1943; 47:329.
14. Aufricht G. Mammaplasty for pendulous breasts. Empiric and geometric planning. Plast Reconstr Surg 1949; 4:13.
15. Climo MS, Alexander JE. Intercostothelial circulation: Nipple survival in reduction mammaplasty in the absence of a dermal pedicle. Ann Plast Surg 1980; 4:128.
16. Gray L. Anatomy of the human body. Dross CM, ed. Philadelphia: Lea & Febiger, 1959.
17. Cooper A. The anatomy of the breast. London: Longman, 1840.
18. Edwards EA. Surgical anatomy of the breast. In: Goldwyn RM, ed. Plastic and reconstructive surgery of the breast. Boston: Little, Brown, 1976.
19. Courtiss EA, Goldwyn RM. Breast sensation before and after plastic surgery. Plast Reconstr Surg 1976; 58:1.
20. Haagensen CD. Diseases of the breast. Philadelphia: WB Saunders, 1988.
21. Goin JM, Goin MK. Changing the body: Psychological effects of plastic surgery. Baltimore: Williams & Wilkins, 1981.
22. Goin MK, Goin JM, Gianini MH. The psychic consequences of a reduction mammaplasty. Plast Reconstr Surg 1977; 59:530.
23. McKissock PK. Presentation at the 23rd Annual Symposium on Cosmetic Surgery, Miami, FL, Feb., 1989.
24. Marchac D, de Olarte G. Reduction mammaplasty and correction of ptosis with a short inframammary scar. Plast Reconstr Surg 1982; 69:45.
25. McKissock PK. Discussion: Precision in breast reduction. Plast Reconstr Surg 1988; 82:642.
26. McKissock PK. Reduction mammaplasty. Ann Plast Surg 1976; 2:321.
27. Zacher JB. Breast feeding after reduction mammaplasty. Presented at the American Society of Aesthetic Plastic Surgeons, New Orleans, April, 1986.
28. Woods JE, Borkowski JJ, Masson JK, et al. Experience with and comparison of methods of reduction mammaplasty. Mayo Clin Proc 1978; 53:487.

CHAPTER 19

Superior Pedicle Reduction Mammaplasty

DANIEL L. WEINER, M.D.

A successful breast reduction operation requires a combination of the following three basic maneuvers:

1. Movement of the nipple-areola complex as a viable entity to a more desirable superior location that has been preoperatively determined and marked.
2. Resection of adequate amounts of breast tissue to accomplish the reduction, followed by reconstruction of the smaller but well-formed mammary eminence.
3. Finally, resection of the excess skin and closure of the new skin brassiere to facilitate reshaping and contouring of the reduced breast, producing the final aesthetic result.

There are several acceptable surgical options to accomplish each of these three steps, successfully moving the nipple, resecting the breast, and tailoring the skin. Procedure selection is always according to the surgeon's individual preference. All plastic surgeons are ultimately trying to identify the operation that will be applicable in all cases of ptosis and hypertrophy and will produce uniformly excellent results.

In the early 1960s, plastic surgeons focused their attention on the migration of the nipple-areola complex on a pedicle, in order to preserve normal nipple appearance, function, and sensitivity.[1,2] This concept was introduced in preference to the previously employed free nipple grafts. In 1972 we reported a superiorly based dermal pedicle that gave freedom of mobility while preserving the nipple with its cutaneous sensation and circulation intact.[3] We had been obliged to isolate the nipple-areola complex in selected cases of subcutaneous mastectomy and mastopexy, solely on its surrounding dermis. It survived and flourished on only its dermal bed, retaining contractility and sensation. This confirmed and was supported by Schwartzman's original work, which established the cutaneous origins and cutaneous circulation of the nipple.[4] It followed that if the circulation of the nipple was cutaneous (from a random dermal network), the nipple could be isolated and supported on an adequately designed skin or dermal pedicle. Therefore, there was thought to be no need for breast parenchyma to provide circulatory support.[5] This was our finding. Our choice was a pedicle that was superiorly based and would not restrict movement in a superior direction. Subsequently, there have been many variations of our original work on dermis-based pedicles for nipple transposition. This has included "composite pedicles" with breast parenchyma in addition to dermis. We have used this variant in selected patients. Other authors have based the pedicles at different points on the compass rose: i.e., south (inferior) and east and west (lateral pedicles).[6-8] Our preference of origin still remains due north in the direction of the nipple migration. The contributions of others over the past 20 years[9] only further serve to confirm our original premise that the best results in breast reduction relating to form and function are obtained with some type of dermis-based pedicle for nipple-areola complex migration.[10,11]

There are also a number of techniques by which the surgeon may resect the excessive breast tissue, excise excess skin, and reconstruct the new skin brassiere. The plastic surgery literature is filled with a multitude of personal experiences and preferences that include individual approaches to modifying and tailoring the breast and skin to achieve the final result.

TRADITIONAL PROCEDURES

Presurgical marking of the new nipple location as well as the pattern of skin resection is universally accepted. These decisions are often modified during surgery, frequently after intraoperative repositioning of the patient.

The breast resection, shaped as a cone, wedge, or keel, is usually checked by weighing the portions of specimen removed.[12] Thus, breast reduction often becomes an "art form"[13] that depends on the individual surgeon's skill, judgment, and experience with a particular technique. There has yet to evolve a universally accepted standard operation, with consistently reproducible results, to be performed by any trained plastic surgeon. The wide acceptance of so many variations in breast reduction technique attests to the inability of surgeons to identify one procedure applicable to all types of breast hypertrophy and ptosis.

SUPERIOR DERMAL PEDICLE AMPUTATION REDUCTION TECHNIQUE

After 18 years of improving and modifying the superior pedicle technique, we now have developed a complete operation that we feel meets all the criteria for a uniformly successful breast reduction technique.[14] It is a basic two-stage procedure.

1. Isolation of the nipple-areola complex on a true superior dermal pedicle, followed by transposition of the complex to its new predetermined location.
2. A direct, simple, amputative type of mammary resection of the hypertrophied breast and skin en bloc, following presurgical markings. Simple closure is accomplished with no twisting, torsion, or rotation of breast pedicles. There is no undermining of the skin, and no dead space is created. Edge-to-edge closure is accomplished safely and efficiently in a proven simple method.

This basic, uncomplicated amputative breast resection can be most effectively accomplished when combined with the superiorly based dermal pedicle technique.

Initially, the superiorly based pedicle, with its intact nipple-areola complex, is carefully constructed and its circulatory status confirmed. The nipple is folded superiorly on its pedicle out of the operative field and tacked into its new position with a few key sutures. The breast resection, skin reduction, and closure can then be accomplished with the amputative technique, unimpeded and with complete disregard for the nipple-areola complex or its pedicle. The resection is totally within the lower breast quadrants following the preoperative Wise skin brassiere markings. The procedure is completed with this single en bloc simultaneous resection of skin and breast tissue, followed by simple primary closure. There is no undermining, no tailoring, no change of position, and no intraoperative decisions. There is no tension on closure because the breast tissue that was preserved includes all of its normal covering skin. It is important that all incisions for resection of the breast be made at right angles to the chest wall, so as to preclude any undermining of the breast or skin that would create deformities or dead space.

After the breast and skin resection, the reconstruction and primary closure establish good shape and contour. Closure of a basic wedge resection of the breast reduces axillary fullness and ensures a round rather than square breast. The skin is approximated under no tension and closed according to the surgeon's individual preference. The simple amputative resection uses the presurgical markings as a guide for *both* skin and breast excision. There is a constant and normal relationship between the remaining skin and remaining breast, ensuring the adequacy of skin coverage and minimal tension on closure. The surgeon will *never* be faced with the problem of a tight closure that will lead to healing complications or produce a square or abnormally shaped breast (i.e., too much breast and not enough skin to close), necessitating additional resection of breast tissue. The superior pedicle amputative procedure is simple, fast, and applicable to all breast hypertrophies and ptosis. The only intraoperative decision is to consider the use of a composite pedicle instead of the true dermal pedicle.

The superior pedicle procedure gives the surgeon the freedom to complete the breast reduction without interruptions and intraoperative judgments. We have performed a complete bilateral breast reduction, assisted only by the scrub nurse, in under 3 hours.

DETAILS OF TECHNIQUE

Pre-operative Markings

The levels of the new nipples are marked with the patient in the sitting position. The anterior projections of the inframammary creases are used as guides. These two markings must be symmetric. The standard wise pattern is used, to determine and mark the new nipple keyhole and the limits of the new skin brassiere (Fig. 19 – 1).[15] The inframammary fold is marked, including its midline point for guide in closure, and all markings are connected for an en bloc simultaneous resection of skin and breast (the amputative technique). The nipple distances from the clavicle are documented on the operative record.[16]

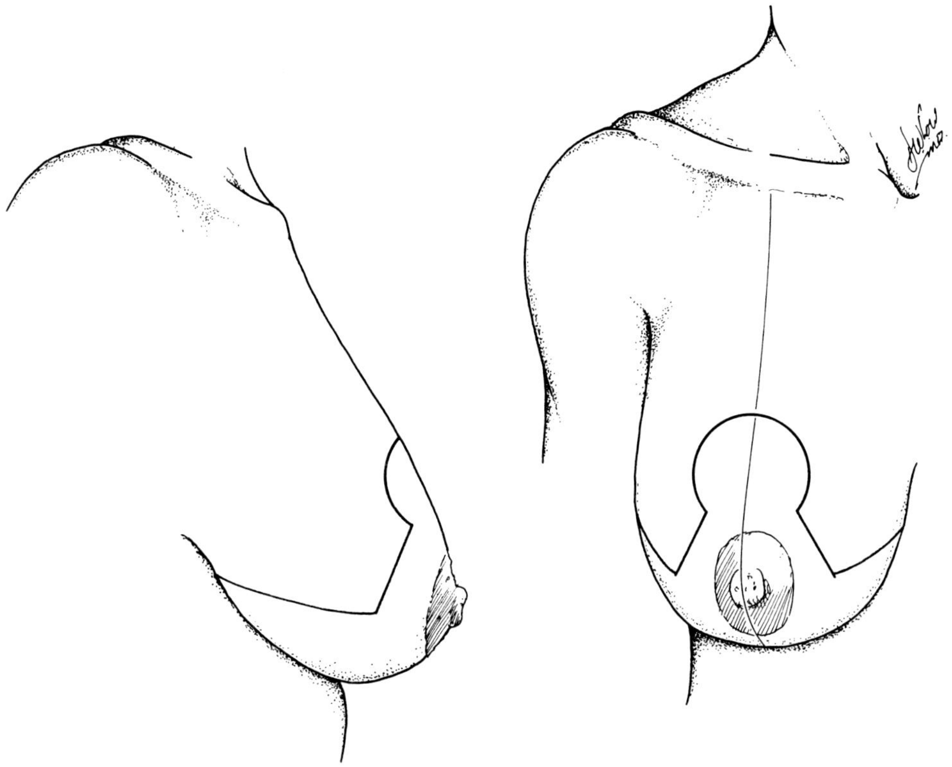

FIGURE 19-1 Preoperative markings are made with the patient sitting. The new nipple location corresponds to the anterior projection of the inframammary fold. The standard Wise keyhole pattern is used as a template for nipple outline and skin incisions.[15]

Operative Procedure

The circular border of the new nipple-areola complex is incised and connected to the keyhole entry points to completely delineate the limits of the superior dermal pedicle. The surgeon must meticulously and carefully de-epithelialize this area, to produce the true dermal pedicle (Figure 19-2). The pedicle must look like a split-thickness skin graft donor site and not like Swiss cheese with fat exposed. This maneuver is best accomplished by compressing the breast to create a distended and fairly rigid working surface, and then using a No. 15 blade to cut to the intradermal plane. The skin that is being removed to be discarded is retracted with a double skin hook, placing maximal tension on the developing intradermal plane. This plane can almost be created by avulsing the epithelial layer skin from its dermal bed. With enough tension, the plane can be developed by barely touching the knifeblade to the separating dermal plane. The technique will preserve an intact dermal bed and create a true dermal pedicle. This is technically the most difficult part of the procedure but is well worth the time and patience required.

The nipple-areola complex is isolated on its superior dermal pedicle by completing a peripheral incision through the dermis. The nipple is elevated with skin hooks, and all its attachments are divided horizontally from the breast at the subdermal level, creating a free nipple on a dermal pedicle. The nipple-areola complex and its pedicle are folded superiorly into its new position, removing it from the operative zone. A few tacking sutures are placed to establish it in its new location.

With the presurgical markings as a guide, the skin and breast are resected simultaneously en bloc to the chest wall, maintaining planes of resection perpendicular to the chest wall (Fig. 19-3). There should be no undercutting of breast or undermining of skin. The breast should be mobilized from the pectoral fascia to facilitate its movement and reshaping. A No. 20 blade or electrocautery facilitates the en bloc breast excision.

Closure of the breast parenchyma is then performed. Resected edge is closed to resected edge, reconstructing the mammary eminence and producing a normal breast projection. We use 4-0 chromic catgut to accomplish this. Suturing of the nipple-areola complex in its new position is then completed. A careful check is made for nipple circulation, torsion of the pedicle, or distortion of the nipple. These can be relieved by back cutting the pedicle or, if necessary, dividing specific attachments (Fig. 19-4). Folding of the pedicle on itself, as it moves superiorly, comprises vascularity, but there normally is still sufficient arterial supply and adequate venous drainage. This can be confirmed clinically by pinching the nip-

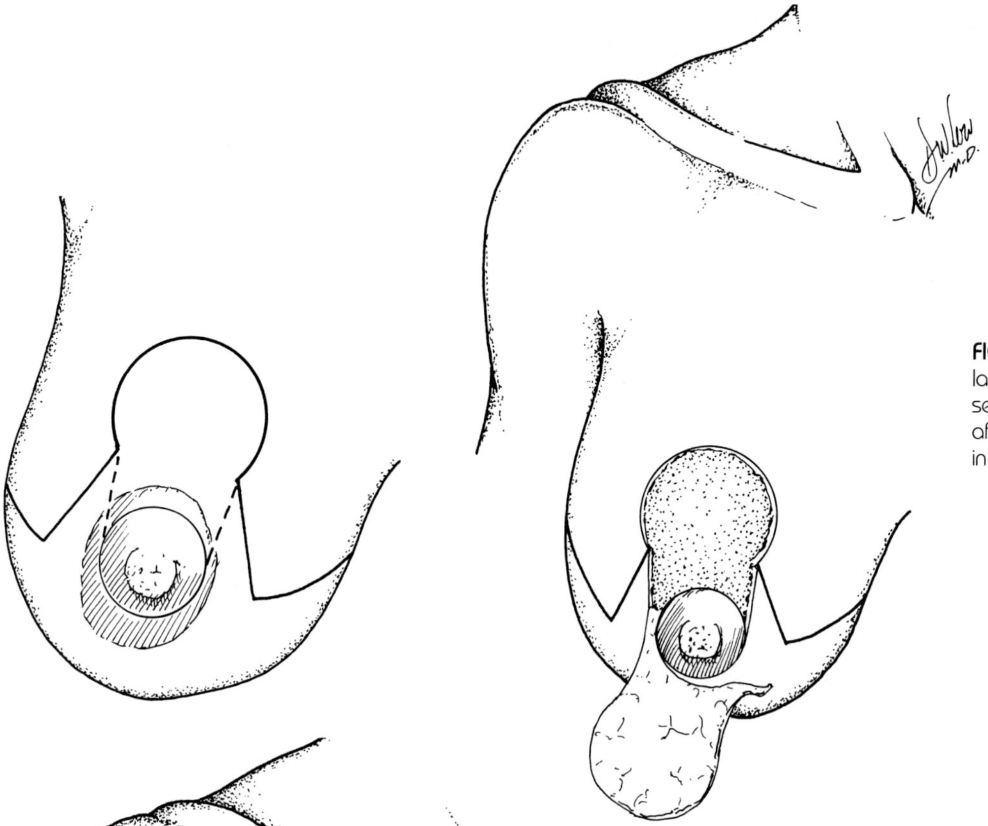

FIGURE 19-2 Cutaneous circulation and sensitivity are preserved on a true dermal pedicle after careful de-epithelialization in an intradermal plane.

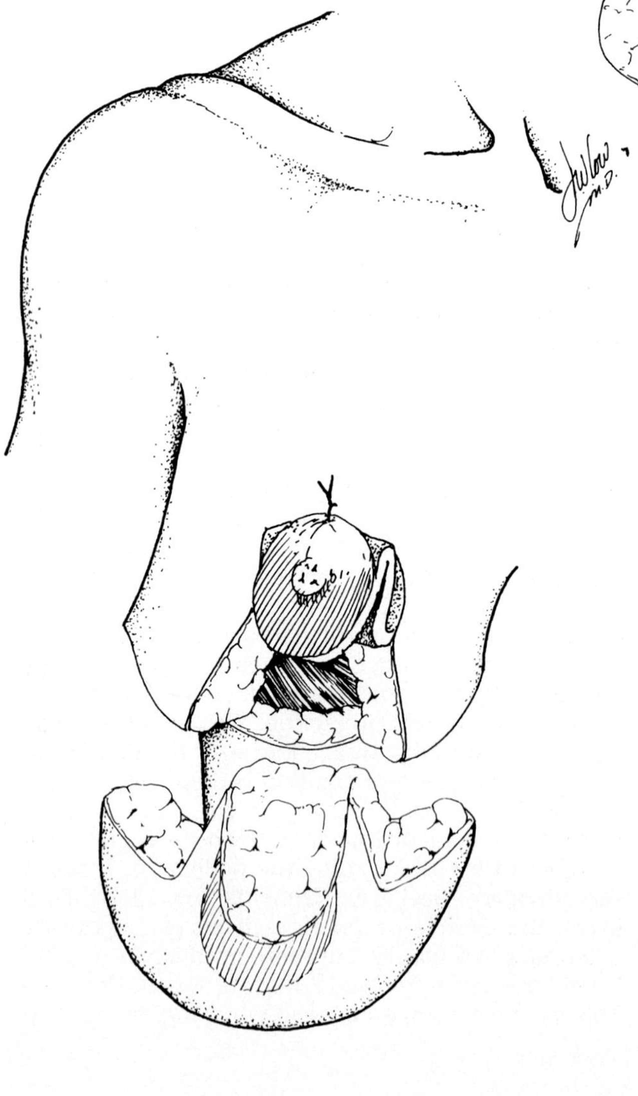

FIGURE 19-3 The nipple-areola complex is removed from the operative zone after folding and attachment to the keyhole in the 12 o'clock position. En bloc resection of skin and breast tissue follows, with incisions perpendicular to the plane of the chest wall.

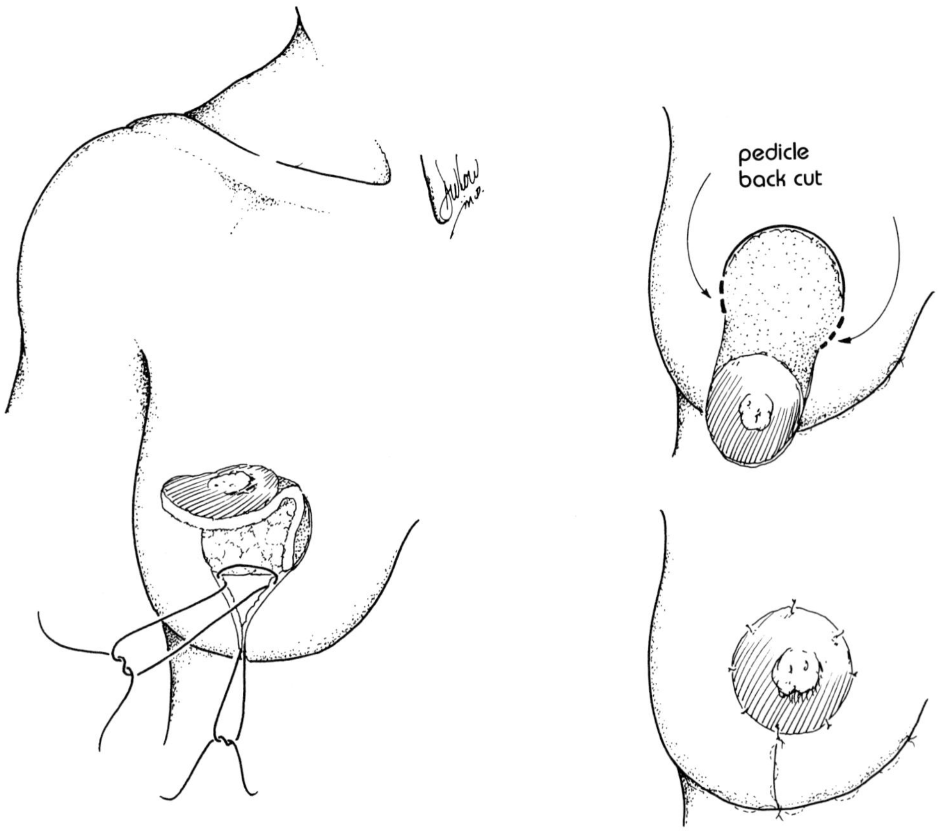

FIGURE 19-4 Breast parenchyma and skin are closed before the nipple-areola complex is inset. Torsion or distortion of the nipple or areola can be avoided with a back cut of the pedicle from the keyhole.

ple with a forceps. Contractility will be maintained if arterial circulation is adequate.

Skin closure is made with 5-0 nylon sutures. A ¼-inch Penrose drain is placed through the lateral incision. Drains are removed on the first postoperative day when the patient is discharged. With the superior pedicle technique, there is no need for operative determinations, positioning, or adjustments. There are no problems with skin flaps, primary closure, or healing. There is no undermining, and therefore no dead space created. Bipolar cautery suffices for all hemostasis, with no need for clamps or suture ligatures.

CHOICE OF DERMAL OR COMPOSITE PEDICLE

We have occasionally isolated a nipple-areola complex on a pedicle up to 15 cm in length. A composite pedicle that includes parenchymal tissue also has adequate (although not necessarily better) circulation, because vascularity is primarily a function of the dermal circulation. Preservation of some parenchyma does not improve sensation in any way. In these patients, major sensation is still a function of the cutaneous branches. Perforating sensory branches from the chest wall are usually sacrificed in traditional composite pedicle techniques, in any case. The only advantage of a composite pedicle is the possible maintenance of some parenchymal connections and an increased potential for lactation (Fig. 19-5). The preservation of some parenchymal tissue usually makes surgeons feel more secure, but as they continue to isolate nipples on dermis alone, they will gain confidence and realize the advantages of the true dermal technique.

The composite pedicle, when used, is often bulky, is more difficult to migrate, and can give a distorted contour and fullness to the nipple-areola complex. It is sometimes necessary to trim excess parenchyma from the composite pedicle to achieve good contour or to relieve too tight a nipple closure.

We now use a composite pedicle only occasionally in younger patients, in whom it is technically easy because of their breast configuration. The simple dermal pedicle, without exception, is flat, more natural in appearance, and better contoured and gives a superior result. It is sometimes necessary to make 0.5-cm back cuts along the pedicle margin at its point of entry to the keyhole to facilitate closure at the 6 o'clock position in the new nipple site (see Fig. 19-4). This is usually when the distance the nipple is to be moved is relatively short. This back cut releases and facilitates nipple movement and skin closure. The larger and the more ptotic the breast,

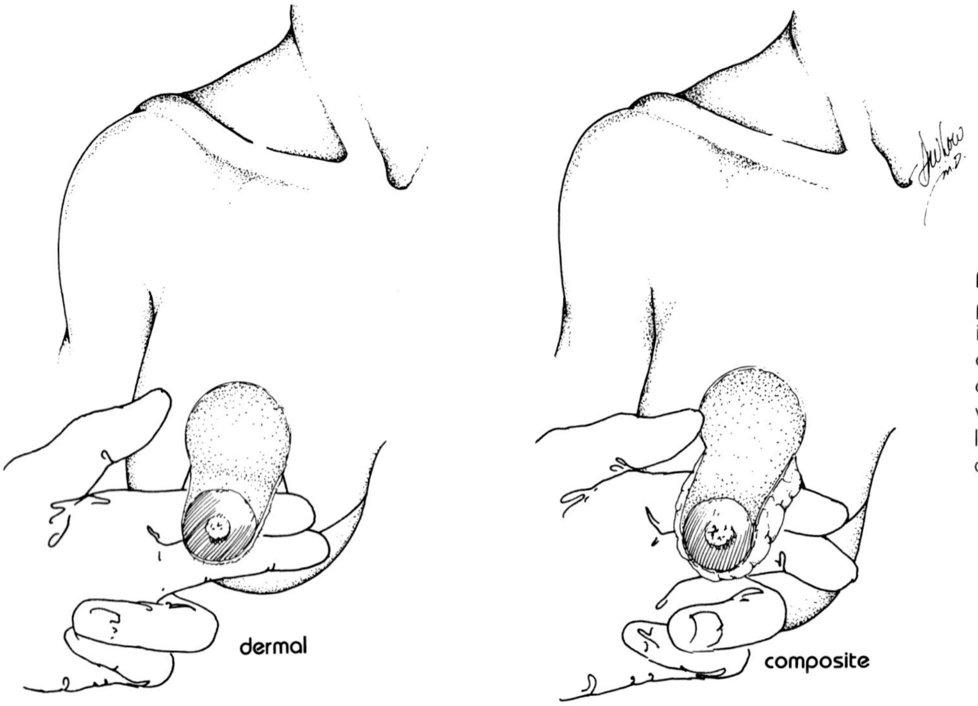

FIGURE 19–5 The author's preference is a dermal pedicle, isolated without breast parenchyma. Inclusion of breast tissue as a composite pedicle may provide an increased potential for lactation and may be appropriate for younger patients.

the easier it is to fold a dermal or composite pedicle into its new position, as more space is available superiorly (Fig. 19–6). In the firm young breast, nipple pedicle migration for short distances is often more difficult to accomplish, but the circulatory demands on the pedicle are also less severe (Figs. 19–7, 19–8).

The pedicle can be initially taken as a composite and then converted to a true isolated dermal pedicle to facilitate nondistorted migration. This adds slightly to operative time.

If the nipple's viability truly appears to be in question and necrosis is a possibility, the nipple should be removed and used as a full-thickness free graft. This is facilitated by previous preparation of the dermal bed. The surgeon can always anticipate some minimal edema and occasional ecchymoses, both of which resolve with time.

LACTATION AND SENSATION

Construction of the dermal pedicle involves division of part if not all of the breast ductal system. Interference with lactation is a sequela but usually not a major concern with most patients. Lactation can be retained if the nipple is left attached to some breast parenchyma with normal ducts. Sensation is always adequate and almost never a source of complaint postoperatively.[17] Revision of hypertrophic scars is not uncommon and may be part of a later tightening of the skin brassiere some 3 to 5 years after surgery.

CONCLUSION

The superior pedicle amputative technique is a single successful procedure, simply described and easily performed, producing uniformly good to excellent results in the hands of any trained plastic surgeon.

The surgeon can have confidence in a superiorly based, adequately prepared dermal pedicle for nipple transposition. The amputative breast reduction that follows is a procedure every plastic surgeon knows, can perform, and trusts. The superiorly based pedicle with its movement to the new site facilitates the simple amputative breast-skin resection, the limits of which were determined preoperatively. There is never a need for pause, hesitation, or major intraoperative determinations, modifications, or anxiety. The two procedures (superior dermal pedicle followed by amputative reduction) combine to give an operation that meets any surgeon's criteria for a successful breast reduction or ptosis procedure. They provide all the advantages of pedicle migration and en bloc resection, including aesthetic appearance, function, primary wound healing with minimal complications, and decreased operative time. This procedure has ended our personal quest for the definitive breast reduction operation. It has had an

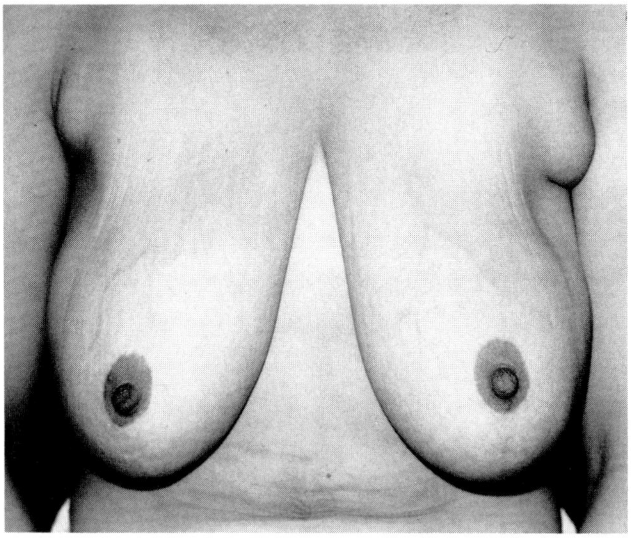

A

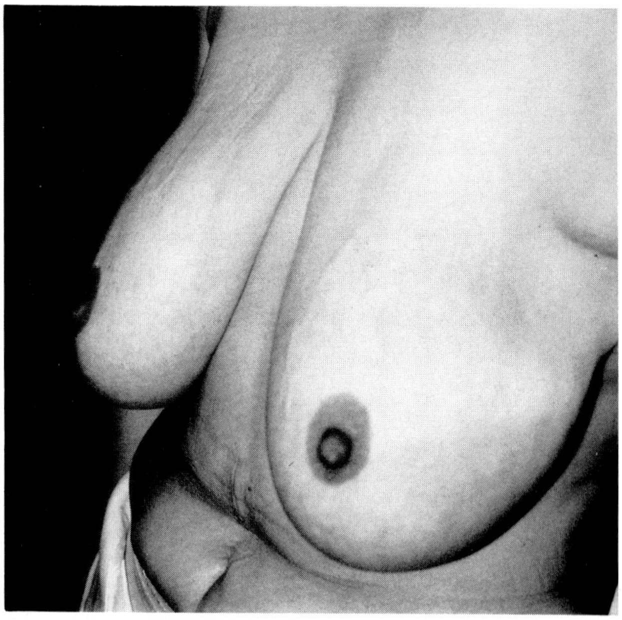

B

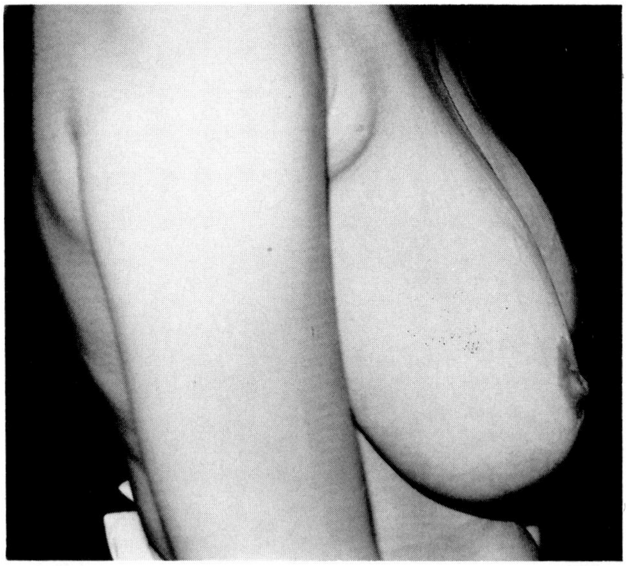

C

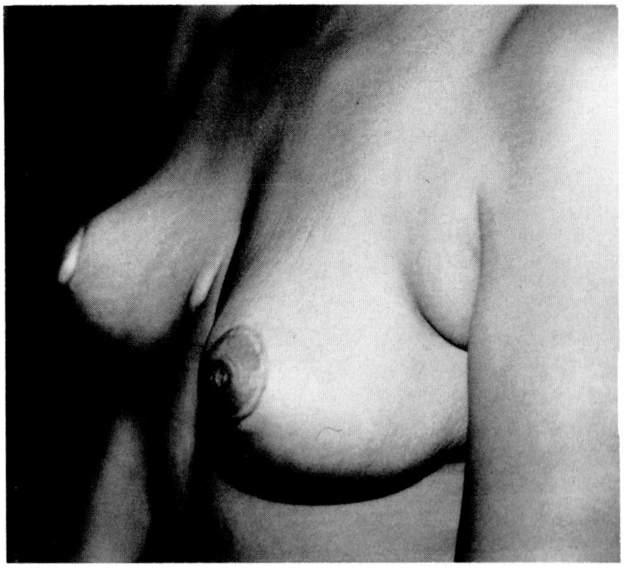

D

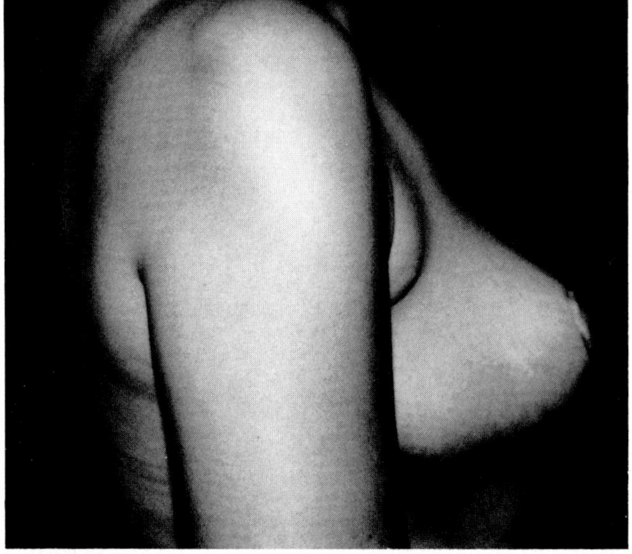

E

FIGURE 19-6 This 38-year-old underwent reduction mammaplasty at age 18. After multiple pregnancies, hypertrophy and ptosis recurred. A repeat reduction mammaplasty-mastopexy procedure elevated the nipple 12.5 cm on a pure dermal pedicle. *A* to *C*, Preoperative frontal, oblique, and lateral views. *D*,*E*, Postoperative oblique and lateral views 1 year after surgery.

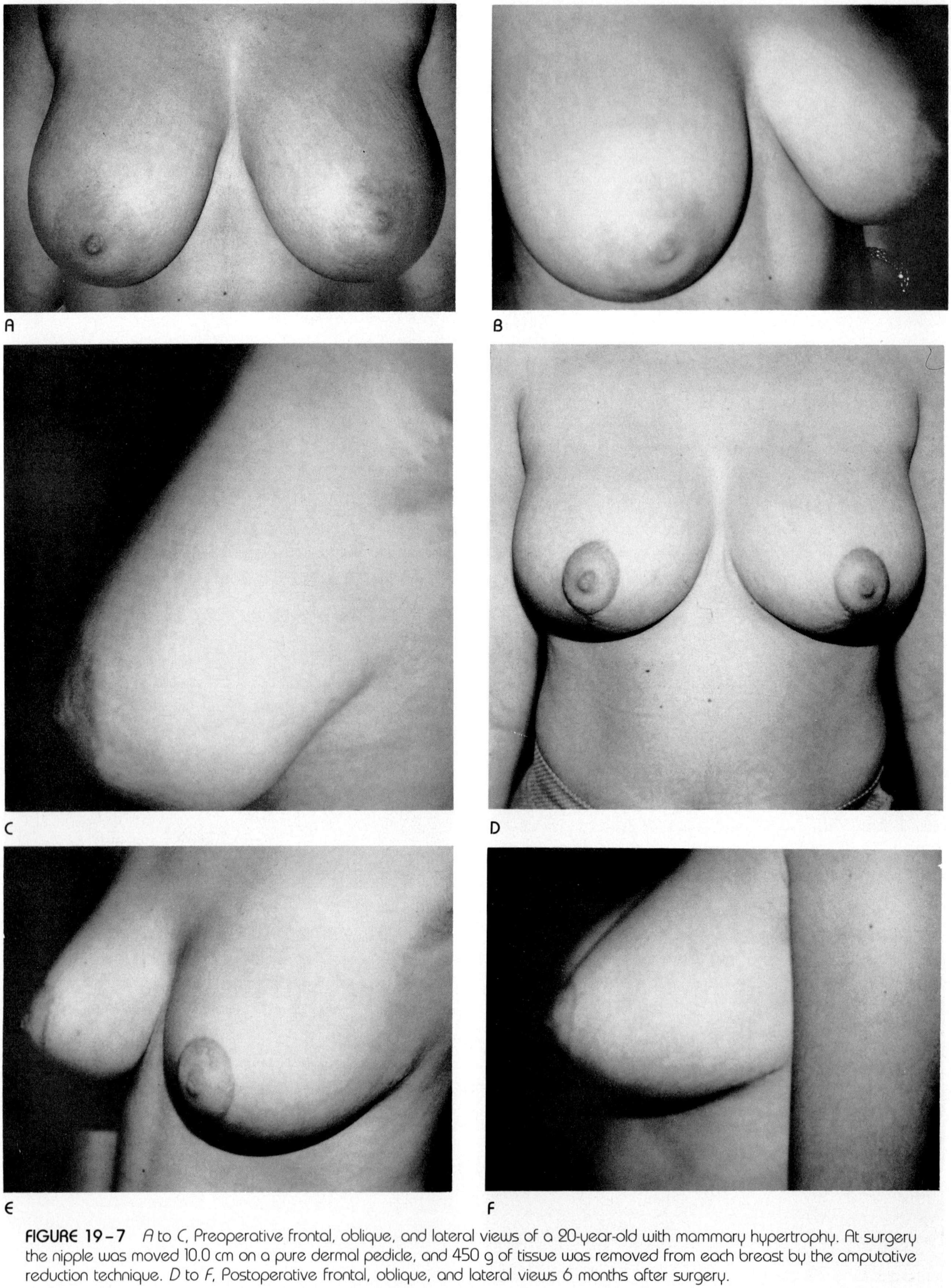

FIGURE 19–7 *A* to *C*, Preoperative frontal, oblique, and lateral views of a 20-year-old with mammary hypertrophy. At surgery the nipple was moved 10.0 cm on a pure dermal pedicle, and 450 g of tissue was removed from each breast by the amputative reduction technique. *D* to *F*, Postoperative frontal, oblique, and lateral views 6 months after surgery.

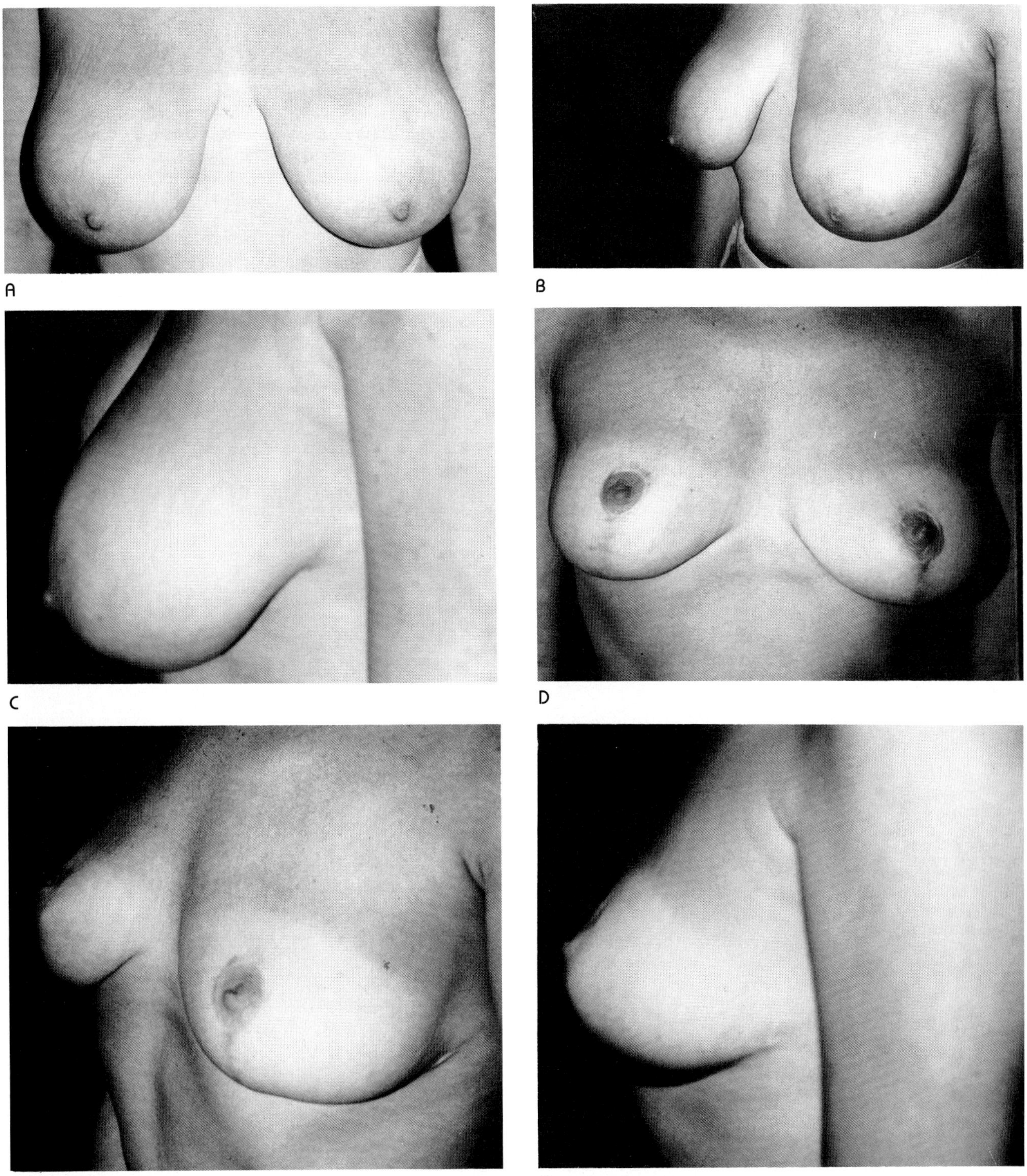

A B C D E F

FIGURE 19-8 *A* to *C*, Preoperative frontal, oblique, and lateral views of a 28-year-old with no history of pregnancy. The amputative reduction mammaplasty technique was used, with 550 g of tissue removed from each breast. The nipple-areola complex was elevated 8.0 cm on a composite pedicle of dermis and breast parenchyma. *D* to *F*, One year postoperative anterior, oblique, and lateral views.

18-year gestation period that offers any competent surgeon the ultimate triad: simplicity, safety, and predictability.

References

1. Strömbeck J. Mammoplasty: Report of a new technique based on the two-pedicle procedure. Br J Plast Surg 1960; 13:79.
2. Skoog T. A technique of breast reduction—transposition of the nipple on a cutaneous vascular pedicle. Acta Chir Scand 1963; 126:453.
3. Weiner D, Aiache AE, Silver L, Tittiranonda T. A single dermal pedicle for nipple transposition in subcutaneous mastectomy, reduction mammoplasty or mastopexy. Plast Reconstr Surg 1973; 51:115.
4. Schwartzman E. Die Technik der Mammaplastik. Chirurgie 1930; 2:932.
5. Maliniac J. Arterial supply of the breast. Arch Surg 1943; 47:329.
6. Cramer LM, Chong JK. Unipedicle cutaneous flap areola nipple transposition on an end-bearing superiorly based flap. In: Georgiade N, ed. Reconstructive breast surgery. St Louis: CV Mosby, 1976:143-156.
7. Hauben DJ. Superior based medial dermal pedicle in reduction mammaplasty. Aesth Plast Surg 1984; 8:189.
8. Conroy WC. Reduction mammaplasty with superior sub-dermal pedicle. Ann Plast Surg 1979; 2:189.
9. Fara M. Reduction mammaplasty with a superior based flap. Acta Chir Plast (Prague) 1983; 16:49.
10. Goulian D. Dermal mastopexy. Plast Reconstr Surg 1971; 47:105.
11. Dufourmentel C, Mouly R. Plastique mammaire par la methode oblique. Ann Chir Plast 1961; 6:45.
12. DeLongis E. Mammaplasty with L-shaped limited scar. Aesthetic Plast Surg 1986; 10:171.
13. Strömbeck JO. Reduction mammoplasty—observations and reflections. Aesth Plast Surg 1983; 7:249.
14. Weiner DL. Reduction mammaplasty using superior pedicle technique. Aesth Plast Surg 1982; 6:7.
15. Wise RJ. A preliminary report on a method of planning the mammoplasty. Plast Reconstr Surg 1956; 17:367.
16. Goldwyn RM. Reduction mammaplasty, Boston: Little, Brown, 1990.
17. Courtiss E, Goldwyn R. Breast sensation before and after plastic surgery. Plast Reconstr Surg 1976; 58:1.

CHAPTER 20

Inferior Segment Reduction Mammaplasty

RICHARD V. DOWDEN, M.D.

BACKGROUND AND HISTORY

General

The inferior segment technique falls into the category of procedures in which the overlying skin flaps are elevated and the breast is refashioned, with an inverted T pattern for the skin and transposition of the nipple. This general approach was suggested by Kraske in 1923, and later elaborated by Axhausen,[2] Lotch,[3] and Biesenberger.[4] The principle of preserving dermis on a pedicle in order to protect blood supply was elaborated by Schwarzmann.[5] Later, Wise described a template pattern for preplanning the skin envelope.[6]

The search continued for a method that would preserve both the sensibility of and the blood supply to the nipple. Several pedicle orientations were tried, and the inferior pedicle methods served this purpose well. In one survey the inferior pedicle techniques were found to have the fewest complications among reduction methods.[7] Techniques employing some type of inferiorly based pedicle make up a spectrum, which has led to unfortunate confusion in the literature. The range varies, from a thin dermal "pedicle" to a full-thickness parenchymal "segment." These must be discussed separately.

Thin Pedicles

In 1967, Kohn and Dalrymple presented a technique that may have anticipated inferior pedicle approaches.[8] Ribeiro reported using for the nipple-areola a very wide inferior dermal pedicle rolled into a cylinder,[9] although at that time he did not use a vertical skin incision. Robbins reported using a wide inferior dermal pedicle technique,[10] and Courtiss and Goldwyn reported a technique with a full-width dermal pedicle base and thickness of 2 cm at the areola and 4 cm at base center.[11] Ariyan described his variation,[12] in which a thin, undermined dermal pedicle was narrowed to 6 cm; Amar and Bosch del Marco presented a similar technique.[13] All of these used a thin pedicle (Fig. 20-1*A*).

The advantages of leaving a greater thickness of breast tissue under the pedicle soon became apparent to many surgeons (Fig. 20-1*B*). Some of Robbins' cases apparently had thicker pedicles.[10] Georgiade and colleagues in 1979 reported using a dermal base 6 to 9 cm wide, 5 cm thick at the areola, and 6 cm thick at the base.[14] Tanski described an inferior dermal-fat pedicle suspended superiorly to serve as an autoimplant for the refashioned skin envelope.[15]

Segments

Next came the true inferior segment techniques (Fig. 20-1*C*). In 1981, Versaci reported his results with increased thickness of the attached flap, leaving full thickness of breast tissue.[16] Labandter and colleagues outlined the technique the following year, using the term "inferior segment" rather than "pedicle" to emphasize that the entire inferior breast is left in continuity with the chest wall.[17] Moufarrege and colleagues reported on this technique,[18] using the term "inferior dermoglandular pedicle" and later "total dermoglandular pedicle."[14] The "maximally vascularized central breast pedicle" as described by Hester and colleagues is the same.[20] The term "inferior segment technique" seems preferable to me.

In a slightly different category are those techniques that also leave a greater bulk of inferior breast tissue but eliminate the dermis entirely. This does

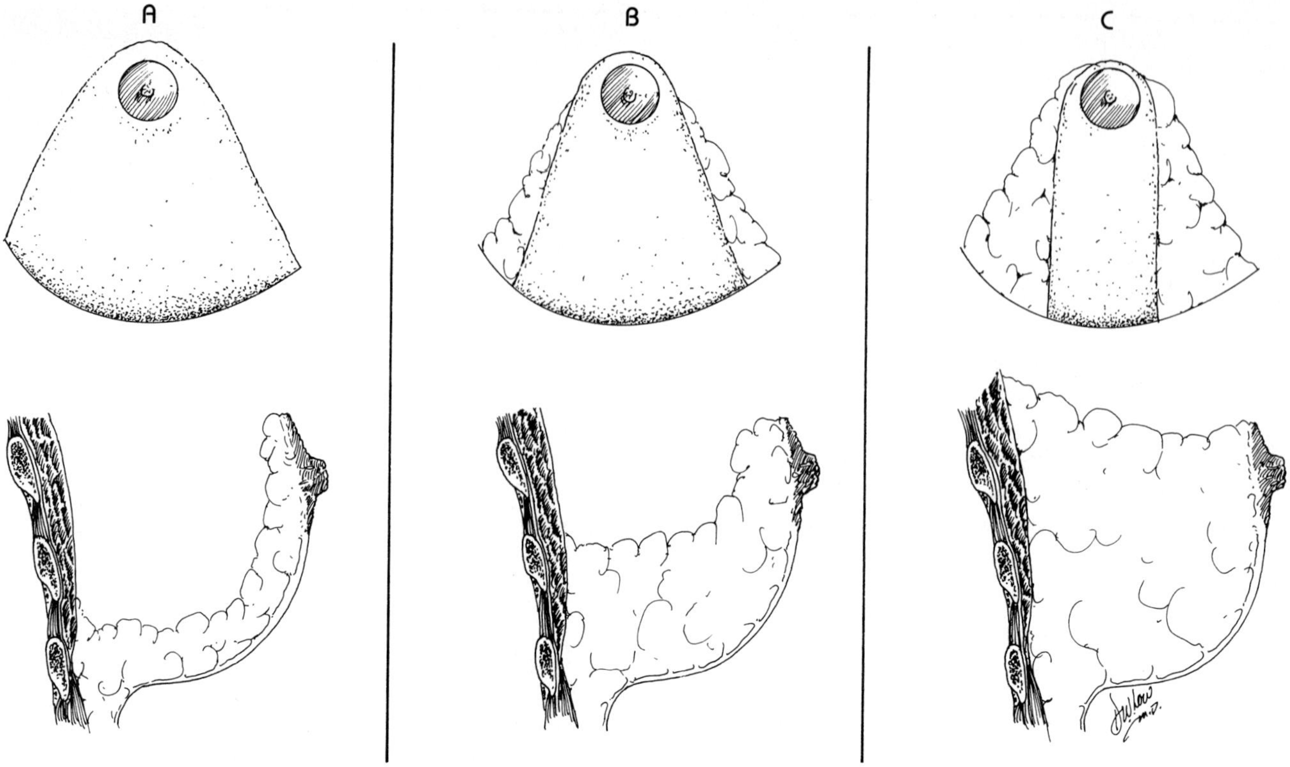

FIGURE 20–1 *A*, Inferior pedicle, thinned to a few centimeters, is designed with a fairly wide base to compensate for the thinness.[9–11] *B*, Inferior pedicle with a thicker base allows narrowing.[10,14,24] *C*, Inferior segment technique features a complete central inferior glandular segment with a narrow strip of dermis.[16–18,20]

not jeopardize the nipple, as clearly demonstrated by others.[21–26]

From this point on I will be discussing only the technique of leaving the nipple on top of a complete parenchymal block of inferior breast tissue extending down to the chest wall, flaring out medially, laterally, and superiorly, and with a roughly rectangular strip of de-epithelialized dermis inferiorly, described in earlier articles as the "inferior segment technique,"[17] "maximally vascularized central breast pedicle,"[20] or "central breast pedicle."[27] I will not be discussing techniques in which the retained dermis is undermined to form a thin pedicle based inferiorly, nor those in which the dermis is removed.

ESSENTIAL ANATOMY

Vascular Supply

The blood supply to the breast is rich and variable. As Maliniac[28] and Aufricht[29] recognized, there is no clearly dominant system that can be predicted to be present because of the multiplicity of sources. As long as a sufficient number of vessels are left to support the remaining breast tissue and nipple, from a vascular point of view the direction from which the blood supply comes does not matter. The breast is supplied by branches from the internal mammary artery, the lateral thoracic artery, some perforating vessels from the thoracoacromial vessels, and significantly from the intercostal vessels inferiorly. In the terminology of Taylor and Palmer,[30] the breast includes portions of the lateral thoracic, internal thoracic, and acromiothoracic "angiosomes." The multitude of breast reduction techniques is testimony to the diversity of blood supply.

The bulk of the breast develops under the deep subcutaneous plexus;[30] as a result, the larger vessels run not far beneath the skin, superficial to the breast tissue. Palmer and Taylor pointed out that because this blood supply comes from the periphery of the breast, the central breast region is supplied only by small vessels.[31] Near the areola, the blood vessels are described as consisting of a superficial and a deep periareolar vascular plexus. The superficial periareolar plexus appears to connect with the veins that lie immediately beneath the dermis of the skin. This in turn means that if the nipple-areola is left on a central breast pedicle in order to protect its nerve supply, it is therefore disconnected from a primary source of blood supply and forced to rely on a secondary system, except for the region of the retained dermis inferiorly. As emphasized in an earlier article,[32] I believe that these inferiorly located veins are an important contribution to the vascular runoff of the nipple-areola. The only *vascular* virtue of retaining the dermis is to protect this subdermal plexus from injury.

Nerve Supply

The anatomic descriptions of the sensory innervation of the breast indicate that it is supplied on its lateral aspect by the anterior rami of the lateral cutaneous branches of the third to the sixth intercostal nerves, and that the medial breast is innervated by the anterior branches of the second to the sixth intercostal nerves.

The precise nerve supply to the nipple remains somewhat mysterious. It seems clear that there is no single nerve whose sole function is to innervate the nipple. Rather, the breast has a rich nerve supply, with overlapping areas of innervation, each capable of reestablishing some degree of sensibility regardless of the technique used. Craig and Sykes described the lateral branch of the third intercostal nerve as the most important,[33] whereas Edwards believed the fourth intercostal to be the most important.[34] The lateral branches of the third and fourth intercostals emerge at the lateral border of the pectoralis muscle where it crosses the interspaces. From there the nerves course medially toward the nipple, entering the breast on its posterolateral aspect 2 cm from its edge.[35] During a reduction mammaplasty, this nerve can be seen and followed for several centimeters, but branching then becomes too extensive to follow.

Courtiss and Goldwyn pointed out that the sensory losses, as well as the interval to return of sensibility, are more likely to reflect the amount of tissue excised than the specific method used.[36] They also found that most patients had considerable sensory loss at the 6-month point, but that only 15 percent of patients still had sensory loss 2 years after surgery. Ariyan theorized that venous congestion of the nipple may lead to decreased sensibility.[12]

Regardless of the reduction technique used, some patients have their sensibility decreased, some stay the same, and for others the perceived sensibility actually increases, the latter being difficult to explain. It has been theorized that the weight of the hypertrophic breast, perhaps through traction on the nerves, renders many of these patients insensate before surgery. No one can say whether postoperative increased sensitivity is due to relief of traction on the nerves, or to increased irritability as a result of removal of inhibition from adjacent nerves. Perhaps the effect is largely psychological because of the increased sensuality that many women feel when they have rid themselves of the excessive size and weight of the breasts. This may account for the fact that good sensibility has been reported after every type of reduction.[33]

Despite the many attempts to quantify the sense of touch around the nipple and areola, finding a way to demonstrate the presence of "normal" sensibility has been elusive. The variability in preoperative status, the lack of truly objective testing, and the psychological overlay all combine to make this difficult to achieve. Nevertheless, the desirable end point is clearly that the patient be pleased with the sensitivity of the nipples after operation. It is the pursuit of this goal that has led to breast reduction techniques that preserve the central and inferior-lateral breast tissue, and thereby the main nerves. Nevertheless, the greater the amount of resected tissue by any technique, the greater is the expected impairment of nipple sensibility.[37]

Nipple Location

According to Pennisi and associates,[38] the nipple should lie over the sixth rib and sixth interspace, approximately 1 to 2 cm lateral to the midclavicular line, in the normal-sized breast. This is a goal for the finished result, but it cannot be used for planning in the hypertrophied breast. Vertical malposition of the nipple is a frequent source of severe patient dissatisfaction;[39] determination of position is discussed later in this chapter.

ADVANTAGES AND DISADVANTAGES

Advantages. The main advantages of the inferior segment technique are its safety and its flexibility. It is safe because the vascularity of the nipple-areola is well protected, and the sensibility is usually good. The technique is flexible because of the independent control one has over the volume of the parenchymal pedicle, the bulk of the overlying flaps, and the position of the nipple. This facilitates a safe progressive approach to reduction and makes this procedure ideally suited for correction of asymmetry.[32]

Disadvantages. One disadvantage of the inferior segment technique is that it may take longer to accomplish, in proportion to how particular one is about achieving symmetry. Another disadvantage stems from its flexibility: the latitude in volume resection of the flaps and of the retained segment can lead to different amounts of resection on the two sides, making a two-team approach unwise.[26] To achieve a truly symmetric result, it is important that the primary surgeon exercise complete control over the resection on both sides, which goal is facilitated by switching sides frequently.

As mentioned earlier, removing the dermis from the inferior segment does not jeopardize the viability of the nipple-areola.[20,24,26] Nevertheless, there are at least two compelling reasons to retain the dermis. First, if necrosis occurs at the T junction, a dermal base is available immediately for either spontaneous re-epithelialization or grafting.[40] Second, if necessary, the nipple-areola can be removed as a split-thickness graft and applied to the dermis of a more vascular caudal part of the inferior segment mobilized upward. Other reasons are that the dermis protects the underlying veins from injury, limits the extent of traction by the assistants, and ensures that the areola does not easily separate off its base. In any event, eliminating this dermis does not result in significant time saving.[41]

I do *not* believe that retention of the de-epithelialized dermis prevents loss of projection with the passage of time, nor that it prevents inferior distention ("dropout") with apparent higher riding of the areola, even if sutured to the pectoral fascia.[42] I am not aware of any maneuver, in any reduction technique, that can prevent this "dropout."

PATIENT SELECTION AND INSURANCE COVERAGE

Motivation

The selection criteria for breast reduction patients have been outlined in Chapter 16, but a few points deserve emphasis. The interference with daily activities caused by breast hypertrophy has long been documented.[43] Studies have clearly shown that most women are driven to seek breast reduction in order to obtain relief of pain and discomfort in the shoulders, neck, and back.[44] The relationship between the symptoms and the hypertrophy of the breasts has been clearly documented, as has the importance of reduction mammaplasty in relieving the symptoms.[45] Explanations have been provided for the observed instances of headache, poor posture, and paresthesia of the hand with breast hypertrophy.[45]

Age

Breast hypertrophy often appears during adolescence, and seldom disappears. It is important for the psychological adjustment of these young women that the operation be performed early, to avoid the psychological trauma inflicted by peers. Postponing of breast reduction may be psychologically detrimental.[46] I believe that the operation should be postponed until growth has stabilized, but have no objections to carrying it out for young women in the 14- to 16-year age range. If the problem is one of rapid continued enlargement, surgery may be needed at a younger age [47] and hormonal manipulation may be necessary.[48]

Body Weight

Many women with breast hypertrophy gain weight in a subconscious attempt to conceal their large breasts, and more easily lose weight after operation than before. Nevertheless, I require obese patients to lose weight before surgery. The larger the size of the breast preoperatively, the less satisfactory is the final result likely to be,[49] and an aesthetically pleasing result is less likely in the obese patient. Strömbeck[50] stated that obesity increases the risk of fat necrosis and areolar necrosis, and cites an incidence of 10 percent in patients more than 16 kg overweight.[39] Pers and colleagues documented increased complications in overweight patients, particularly infection and hematoma, which were five times more frequent in patients more than 5 percent over ideal body weight.[51] Gerner found infection to be ten times more likely, and areolar necrosis four times more likely, in patients more than 5 percent over ideal weight.[52] Furthermore, obesity predisposes to certain postoperative complications, such as deep vein thrombosis, wound infection, and atelectasis.

For all these reasons, I ask my patients to weigh within 5 percent of their ideal body weight. As a rough guide to 5 percent over ideal, I use the following equation: $\text{weight} = \text{height} \times \text{height} \times 0.032$, which is for inches/lbs. For cm/kg I use 0.0023 instead of 0.032 in the equation. Strömbeck and Melm[53] used this formula: ideal weight in $\text{kg} = \frac{2}{3} \times$ height in cm,[50] and Pers and associates[51] presented a graph from life insurance tables.[54] It is clearly undesirable for the patient to lose weight *after* the procedure, because this will contribute to accelerated ptosis.[55] Strömbeck estimated that for each kilogram of body weight lost, the breast loses 20 g of weight.[39] Some patients may not be able to change their eating habits preoperatively, and insistence on weight loss may prevent them from ever having the benefits of the operation;[56] however, this may be preferable to complications.

Pregnancy

Massive breast hypertrophy during pregnancy is rare, estimated at less than one per 100,000 pregnancies, and a paternal etiologic factor has been hypothesized.[57] Once it occurs, it is believed likely to recur with subsequent pregnancies, so consideration should be given to mastectomies as an alternative to reduction for such women considering future pregnancies.[57] The ideal interval between delivery and a reduction operation is not known; planning is easier after involution, but some of the few reported patients underwent the operation within several weeks after delivery.[57]

Insurance

It has been the experience of most plastic surgeons that removal of 200 or more g from each breast is generally sufficient to relieve the musculoskeletal symptoms. Many insurance companies try to use 250 to 300 g as the dividing line between cosmetic mastopexy and corrective breast reduction, and some require greater weights. If the problem is an abnormality outside the normal range for a patient's age, then clearly its correction cannot be considered "cosmetic"; ptosis may be normal, hypertrophy is not. However, an arbitrary weight limit fails to take into account variations in preoperative body habitus and breast size. A patient of small stature could well find that a 200-g reduction relieves her discomfort.[58] The American Society of Plastic and Reconstructive Surgeons states that "weight or amount of breast tissue removed should not be used as the only criterion to determine insurance coverage for reduction mammaplasty." Despite this clear guideline, 250 to 300 g per breast has become entrenched as the cutoff point for health insurance reimbursement. Some health insurers are requesting photographs of the patient's breasts. A specific release should be signed by the patient for this. Unfortunately those who review these photographs often lack the background necessary to realize that photographs cannot illustrate symptoms.

Applicability

All the foregoing considerations apply to any breast reduction technique, and would apply to a free nipple graft reduction as well as an inferior segment reduction. What are the factors that lead to the choice of a segment or pedicle technique over a free graft? The primary advantage over a free graft is the enhanced possibility of preserving nipple sensibility. Although this cannot be guaranteed, it is an objective more likely to be attainable with the inferior segment method than with a free nipple graft, although the literature is replete with attestations of good sensibility after every type of reduction.[33] Therefore, it is the patient whose nipple sensibility is reasonably normal for whom I would choose the inferior segment technique. On the other hand, factors that favor free grafting include impaired nipple sensibility, advanced age, medical problems requiring the shortest possible anesthesia time, and the more massive hypertrophies.[59] Ariyan[12] reported resections up to 3,500 g, and the inferior segment technique has been used successfully by others for even larger reductions. Rather than a weight limit, I use nipple sensibility as the criterion. I have not yet encountered a patient in whom the resection exceeded 2,500 g per side whose sensibility was normal preoperatively.

One of the most important factors in determining whether a patient is a suitable candidate is an assessment of how clearly she understands and accepts the drawbacks and risks of complications and unfavorable results. These are discussed below. If a patient apparently neither understands nor accepts the risk of complications, and the associated possibility of future additional operations, she warrants either repeat counseling or disqualification from the operation.

PREOPERATIVE EVALUATION, COUNSELING, AND INSTRUCTIONS

Counseling

All patients should be made to understand the inherent drawbacks and complications.[37] One drawback is scarring, which may be unsightly and hypertrophic, especially in the parasternal and axillary regions, areas not hidden by the breast. Patients must understand that the appearance of the scars cannot be predicted and that revision may be needed. This is one of the reasons that many surgeons do not show photographs of other patients.[7] Other disadvantages include probable change in nipple sensibility, change of breast shape with time, and probable inability to breast feed, although some patients have been able to lactate to some degree.[19] The main complications of concern relate to tissue necrosis. Most plastic surgery of the breast is based on the assumption that the blood supply is reasonably predictable and dependable,[37] yet variations can be assumed in a small percentage of patients. This will lead to some instances of necrosis of the skin, fat, and nipple-areola even if the surgeon has done everything correctly. Any of these events will likely require subsequent operation.

Weight Loss

For the reasons given above, weight loss is mandatory for the obese candidate. Experience has shown it unwise to preschedule a surgery date for an overweight patient in anticipation of an expected weight loss. My practice now is to have the patient return for another visit after she has attained the desired weight; only then is the operation scheduled. Weight loss can be a reflection of patient motivation.

Transfusion

Transfusion is rarely needed; Bolger and colleagues[26] showed that the use of epinephrine infiltration can reduce the need for transfusion to approximately 1 percent, and electrocautery may eliminate it entirely. Autotransfusion is the ideal way to handle the question of blood replacement for these patients.[60] If the patient lives out of town, her local blood bank can send it on the day of surgery. It is reassuring to the patient that her own blood is on hand should the need arise. However, I am opposed to routinely reinfusing this banked blood, because of the chance of a labeling error, and this is discarded unless a transfusion is absolutely necessary.

Smoking

Because of the detrimental effect of nicotine on the circulation, I ask that patients neither smoke nor use nicotine gum for 3 weeks before surgery. I have not been testing patients' urine for traces of nicotine, although this is certainly a possibility.

I instruct patients to stop taking aspirin or other prostaglandin inhibitors 3 weeks before operation. They are told to return on the preoperative day for further discussion and for measurements, markings, and photographs. They are also instructed in the use of the incentive spirometer and the patient-controlled analgesia apparatus.

Even though the American Cancer Society recommends a first mammogram at age 35, it is my practice to obtain a mammogram before breast reduction in every patient 30 years of age or older. Having had the experience of encountering at operation an invasive carcinoma not visible on mammograms, I now preoperatively discuss that possibility and the treatment options with patients over 30.[61]

PREOPERATIVE MARKINGS

Before operation the patient should be studied carefully, and certain essential guidelines and landmarks established. The more thought given to the design in advance, the greater is the likelihood of an excellent result, especially if there is asymmetry. Even the design-as-you-go method is acceptable only if it is performed with considerable forethought;[62] in practice, one then arrives at precisely the same skin markings. I agree with McKissock[63] that preoperative planning is particularly important if the breast hypertrophy is asymmetric.[32] However, I believe that one should not be inflexibly tied to preplanned markings, because the amount of skin to be removed will depend on the breast volume remaining, and the nipple placement is best determined after skin closure.[3] The surgeon's eye can make the aesthetic adjustments[29] as long as care is taken not to place the nipple too high, and the preoperative markings take care of that.

As advocated by others,[64,65] I design for optimal contour. Some authors[29,66,67] advised against attempting to create a "virginal breast" of uniform radius, but rather recommended creation of a pendulous drooping shape. I disagree with this, believing that no known method is capable of creating a breast that will resist ptosis; time will create sufficient ptosis for every patient.

When. I make the markings on the preoperative day when the patient is in the office for work-up and testing, where she can stand comfortably in a warm room, rather than hurriedly with a sedated patient sitting in a cold operation room.[56] Decisions made with the sedated patient semirecumbent in the operating theater are likely to be fallible,[63] particularly in relation to the vertical position of the nipple.

How. I use a ruler, methylene blue, brilliant green ink, a set of obstetric calipers, two clamps, and a length of silk thread. The markings are initially made in methylene blue, which can be easily erased with alcohol. The final lines are then marked with brilliant green in alcohol,[68] which will persist through preoperative showers and the iodophor prep. I prefer this to silver nitrate or to scratching the skin, which can leave scars if surgery is cancelled. After the marking, photographs are taken, both slides and instant prints. The slides provide a permanent record of the markings for retrospective comparison with the result. The instant print provides the opportunity to review the markings at an unhurried pace the night before operation. Sometimes the prints show apparent small asymmetries that were not noticed in the office, and adjustments can then be decided on.

First, breast meridians are drawn from the midclavicular point down through the desired position of the nipple (Fig. 20–2*A*). In most patients this line will pass through the preexisting nipple position, but not if the nipple is preoperatively too lateral or too medial. On a very large breast, the new nipple location should be slightly medial to the preexisting nipple position. Another guide to the proper position is to use a line 15 degrees medial to a line joining the midclavicular point to the anterosuperior iliac spine.[62]

The most important aspect of the final result is the vertical nipple position. As Dinner and Chait[69] stressed, a nipple that appears high must be avoided. Not only is the nipple position critical in producing an aesthetically pleasing result, but nipple malposition is one of the most common complaints in medicolegal actions after reduction.[70] In particular, a too-high position is difficult to correct.[71] Long-term studies have shown no significant postoperative increase in the distance from the clavicles to the new nipples;[42] when inferior distention does occur, the nipples will appear too high. Such studies also have consistently shown postoperative distention of the breast caudal to the nipple,[42] so care must be taken to keep the nipple low. O'Keeffe put forward the interesting hypothesis that reduction mammaplasty transfers the easily stretchable periareolar skin to a position inferior to the nipple, where it then distends and causes a high-riding nipple.[72]

The upper limit of the nipple position should be

determined in advance. The entire design depends to a great extent on the intended nipple location, so some attempt must be made to establish this. However, the precise nipple location can be adjusted after skin closure,[3] care being taken that the nipple position is not too high. As McKissock said, one takes planning seriously when one considers the too-high nipple to be a virtually uncorrectable deformity.[37]

The midhumeral point is unreliable as a guide to making the vertical position of the new nipple,[66] because after surgery the elasticity of the skin will move the marked point upward after the weight has been removed.[43] Many authors recommend using a fixed measurement from the sternal notch or the midclavicular point,[66] but variations in stature, thoracic cage anatomy, and breast contour do not permit the application of fixed measurements.[43,70] For similar reasons, I do not use prefabricated patterns and strongly advise against their use in asymmetric cases.

To match the nipple position to the patient's anatomy, I use the inframammary fold as the guide to the new nipple position, as recommended by Strömbeck,[73] but rather than relying on my fingers and thumb to transfer this location, I use the obstetric calipers (Fig. 20-2*B,C,D*).[17,63] Using the inframammary crease as the guide is especially reliable in cases of breast asymmetry,[32] because the skin is more stretched on the larger breast than on the smaller breast.[43] If not compensated for, this would result in an excessively high nipple position on the formerly larger side after the weight is removed. The inframammary fold is usually pulled lower a corresponding amount on the larger side.[74] For an average-sized result, the level of the fold is used; for a larger-sized result the nipple should be about 1 cm lower; for a small-sized result, 0.5 cm higher (Fig. 20-3*A*). It is usually preferable to leave younger patients with slightly larger results than older patients.[56,75] Although I predetermine the upper limit of the nipple location, the circular opening is not cut out until the breast has been closed, allowing fine adjustment intraoperatively.[76] I concur with McKissock that large deviations from the preoperative plan are dangerous,[63] particularly if there is a temptation to raise the nipple.

I place the inferior horizontal incision just above the inframammary fold, except at the medial and lateral extremes, where the incision should encroach onto the breast. One must not chase the fold of skin into the axilla, or to the midline. At the medial and lateral margins of a hypertrophied breast, the folds of skin do not truly correspond to the breast tissue, but rather are traction folds of the surrounding skin caused by the weight of the breast; if the breast is supported, these folds disappear. Thus, near the anterior axillary line the correct incision line will depart from the lateral crease and appear to curve upward onto the breast (Fig. 20-3*B*).[16] Therefore, I draw the medial and lateral extremes of this inferior horizontal incision with the patient supine and the breast centralized over the chest.

Care must also be taken to keep the medial end of the incision from encroaching on the midline and from joining with that of the opposite side. This can cause a web of hypertrophied scar that is impossible to eliminate and extremely difficult to camouflage. It is preferable to design the horizontal incision slightly shorter than appears necessary. A small dog-ear is easier to correct than is a too-long scar. Both the medial and lateral extremes of the scars tend to hypertrophy, but the medial ends are more disturbing to the patients, so every effort should be made to minimize the medial extent.

To outline the areola, the patient should be standing and warm so that the nipples are not contracted, otherwise the nipple would be off center. I use a free-hand technique with a ruler, rather than any special marking device.[77] I generally use an areolar diameter of 36 to 42 mm, depending on the desired breast size, but most often about 38 mm. The areola is more vulnerable to necrosis than is the nipple,[37] so it is prudent to keep the areolar diameter as small as aesthetically acceptable.

The length of the vertical limbs depends on the desired size of the result. Too great a length will cause a high-riding nipple; too short can look equally abnormal. If the desired distance from inframammary crease to edge of areola is to be 5 cm,[16] then for an areola of 2-cm radius, the vertical limbs would be 7 cm for an average-sized result, 6 cm for a small final result, and 8 cm for a larger final result (Fig. 20-3*C*). An arc is drawn using the desired length, centered at the estimated new nipple point (Fig. 20-2*E*). Again, it must be stressed that the final position will be determined after closure.

Ramselaar[62] believes that the vertical limbs should be measured only after the skin flaps are developed. His reasoning is that the *medial* vertical line is parallel to Langer's lines and cannot be stretched further, whereas the lateral vertical line cuts across Langer's lines and therefore can be stretched. Maxwell[76] recommended adjusting the nipple-to-inframammary crease length according to the weight of the resected specimen, but I prefer to relate it to the size of the desired result. Clearly, if the sum of the final clavicle-to-nipple distance plus the nipple-to-inframammary crease distance is too small, the breast will be flat and devoid of projection.

The vertical limbs should be kept as close to the areola as practical. I prefer this to methods of pinching the skin to estimate the resection,[78,79] because a tense or flaccid breast makes this method unreliable. Also, I do not use wire keyhole frames, plastic sheet patterns, or the cut-open brassiere method.[80] The amount of divergence of the vertical limbs can be dealt with at the time of closure. If the resection is going to be considerable, a much wider angle of divergence will be used, but this decision can be

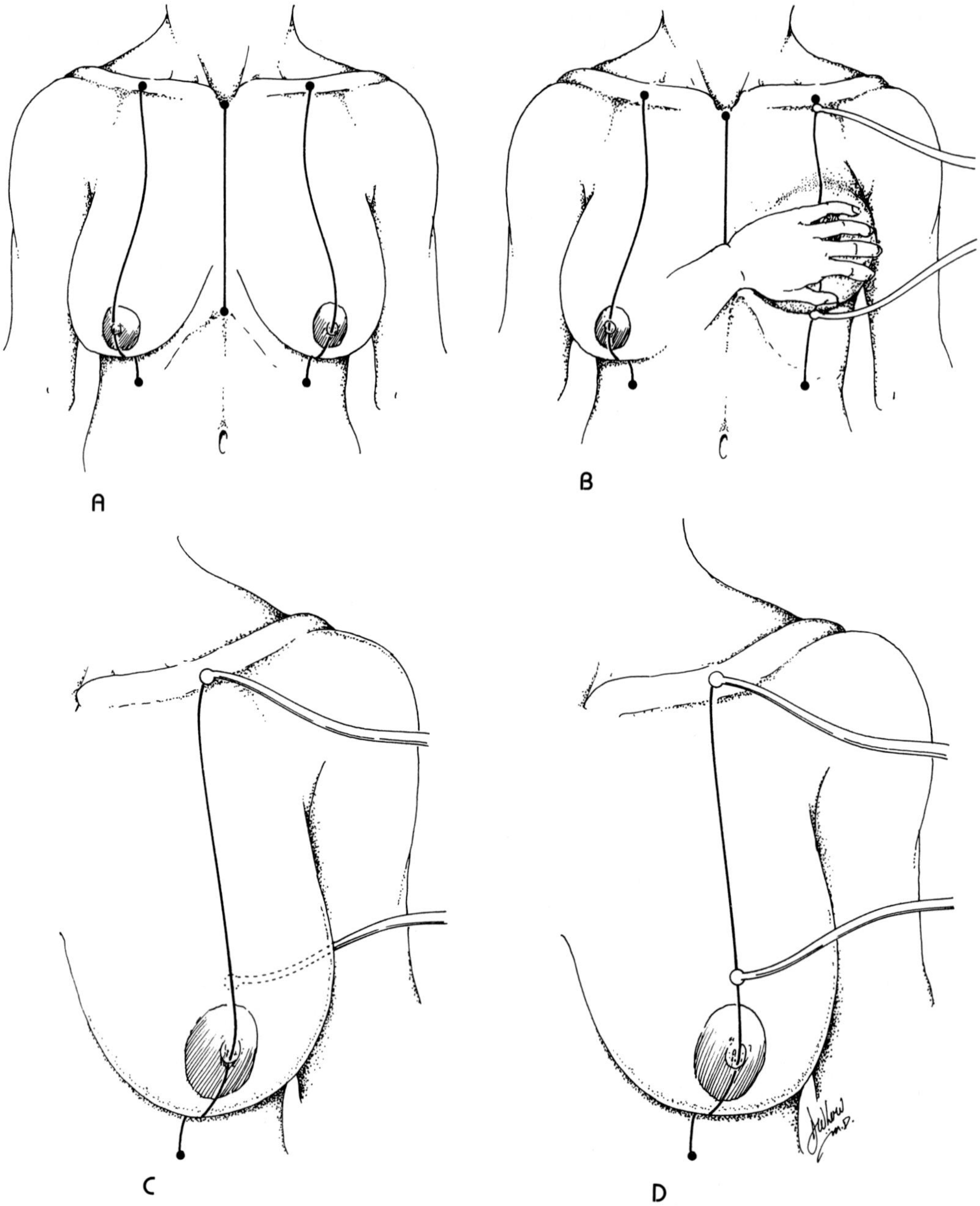

FIGURE 20-2 Preoperative markings are made with the patient in the standing position. *A*, The breast meridians are drawn through the desired nipple locations. *B*, The lower limb of the calipers is placed in the inframammary fold. *C*, The breast is permitted to hang freely and the upper limb of the calipers is adjusted to the clavicles. *D*, Without changing the spacing of the calipers, the lower limb is transferred to the front of the breast for the new nipple height. *E*, The vertical limbs are drawn as in the text, generally diverging only widely enough to skirt the areola. It is not necessary to draw in the new areolar ellipse. *F*, After injection of epinephrine, the epidermis is removed and the incision is made around the deepithelialized area. *G*, After flap elevation the medial and lateral triangles are excised. *H*, The vertical wedge of the keyhole is removed. *I*, The inferior segment is fully delineated as described in the text. *J*, Temporary closure is performed with either staples or sutures, and with the patient upright the position for the nipple is determined.

delayed and the excess removed later, at the end of the procedure. The vertical limbs can curve inward sharply above the areola to meet at the new nipple centers, because any resulting dog-ear at the top will be excised for the areola.[74] If the patient has a breast that is flat in the upper region, she also has relatively little excess skin in a horizontal direction, and all possible skin will likely be needed for closure. In such a patient, the vertical limb angle must be as narrow as possible.[72] This is the reason behind the

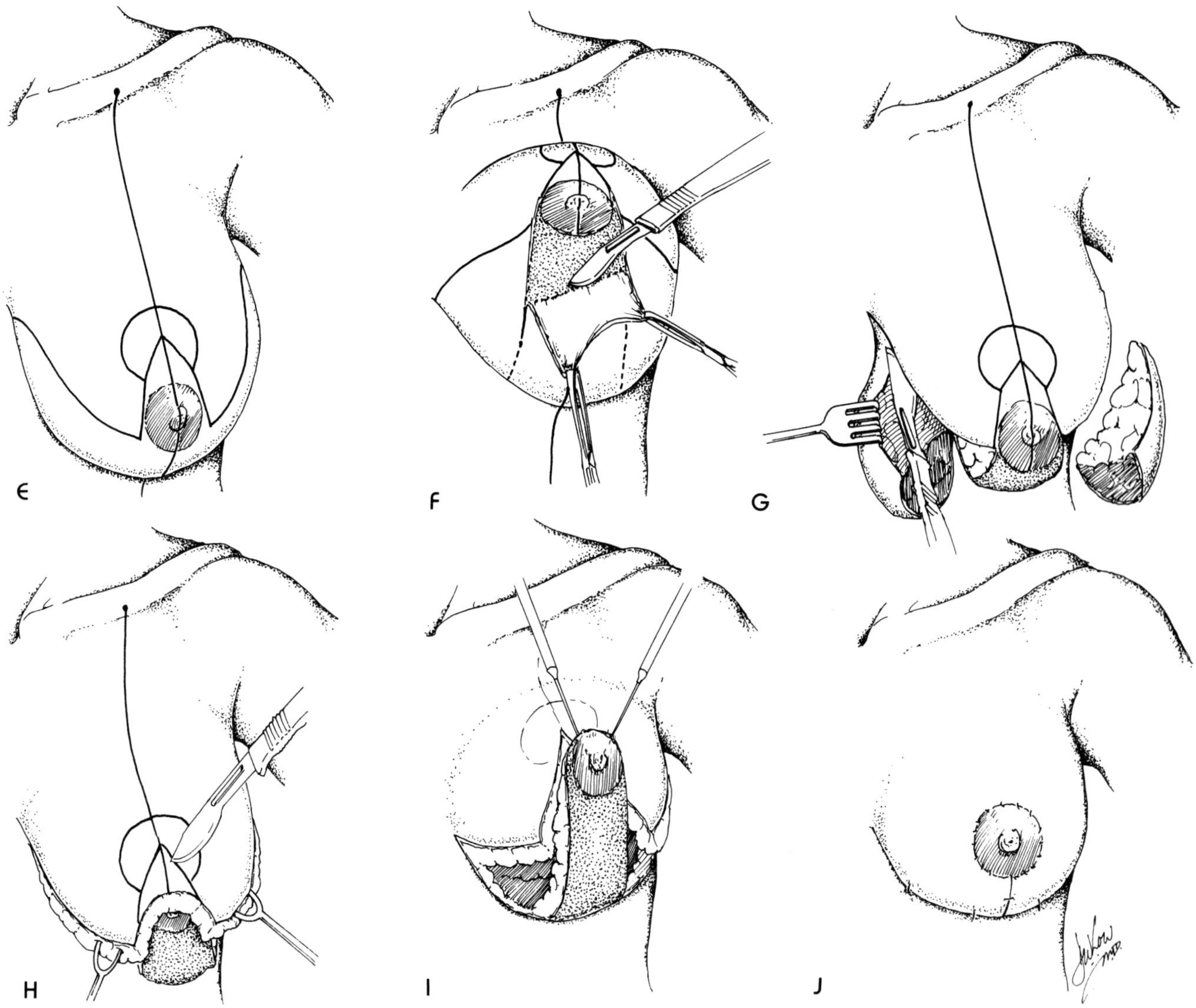

Figure 20-2 *Continued*

admonition of Woods and colleagues[81] that a long breast often requires a narrow angle of the vertical limbs.

To facilitate closure at the T junction, the limbs should diverge no more than needed. One way to ensure this is to premeasure the length of the medial and lateral portions of the inframammary incision, and use these lengths to determine the divergence of the vertical limbs.[82] If it is not possible to design the medial and lateral portions of the upper flap long enough to equal the inframammary incision, one can plan to use a lateral Burow's triangle, or to leave a trapezoid of intact skin on the inferior dermal segment (see Fig. 20-5*C*). Another reason to leave this trapezoid of skin is that if the areola is very large, the vertical limbs will encroach upon it, resulting in pigmented skin being present on the lower breast. Sometimes this cannot be avoided, but the additional scar from leaving a trapezoid of skin inferiorly may be less noticeable than deep pigmentation of the lower breast.

Although I have tried to reduce the length of the horizontal scar without unacceptably lengthening the vertical limb and raising the nipple position, as recommended by Lassus,[83] Marchac and colleagues,[74,84] Peixoto,[85] and Basile,[86] I have not been able to do so consistently, except in smaller hypertrophies in younger patients whose skin elasticity allows it to conform to the decreased volume. Likewise, I do not find myself able to use this technique with the isolated vertical incision method as outlined by Peixoto,[87] Lassus,[88] and Berrimo and colleagues,[89] without leaving the resultant nipple too high, or extending the vertical incision either superior to the nipple or inferior to the breast, except in young girls with modest enlargement. Certainly a horizontal in-

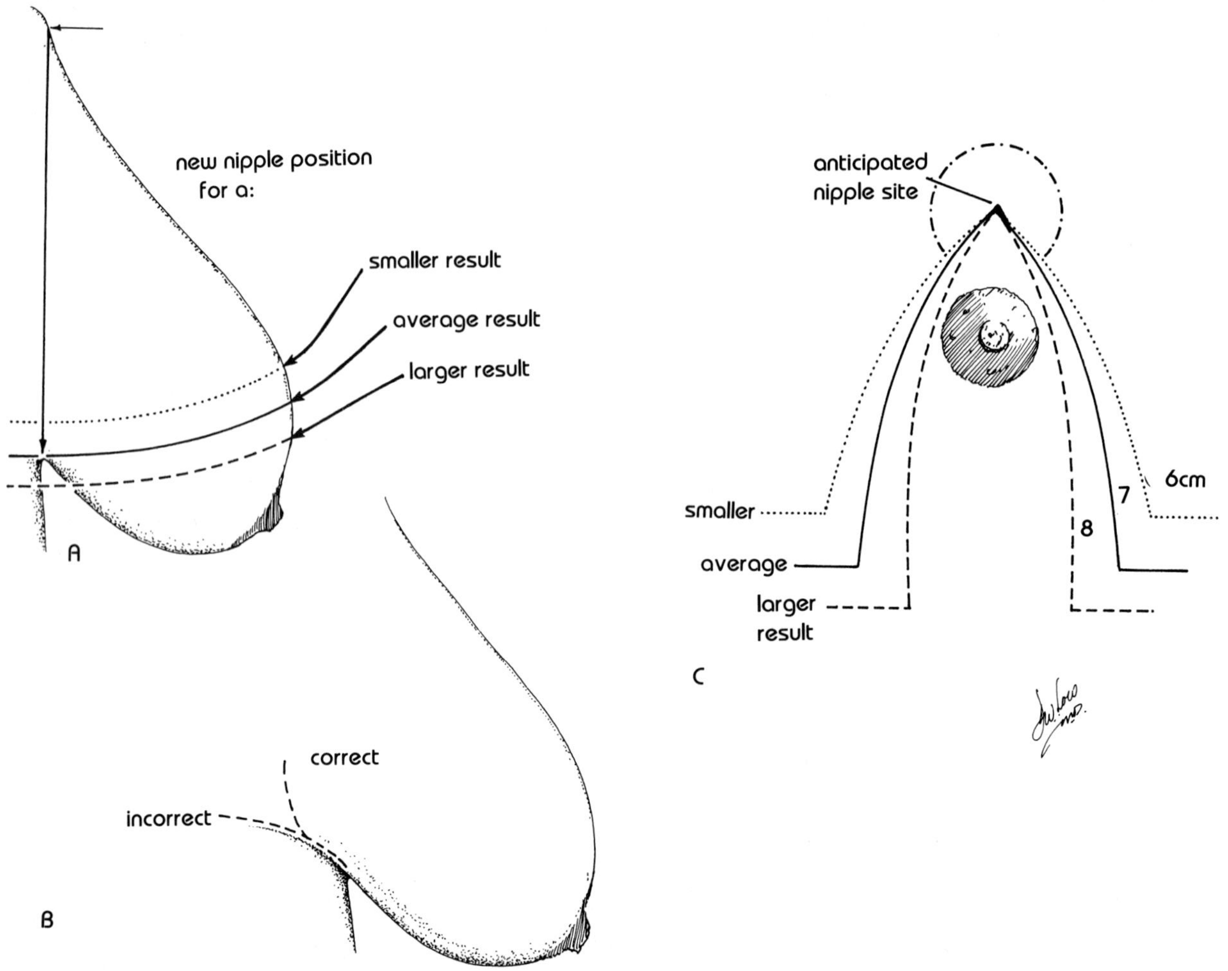

FIGURE 20-3 *A*, The inframammary crease of the hypertrophic breast determines the new nipple position, with 1 cm added for a larger result, and about 0.5 cm subtracted for a smaller result. *B*, Laterally, the line of the inframammary incision should depart from the skin fold and curve upward along the true edge of the breast. The incision may not need to be carried this far, but this is the line to follow if needed. *C*, The vertical limb length also depends on the desired size, and is longer for a large result, shorter for a smaller result.

cision is preferable to an excessively high nipple, or an undesirable shape. This may be an instance in which smaller may not be better.[90]

The superior horizontal incisions are then drawn. At one time, it was recommended that a lazy-S incision be used to gain length for these incisions, but it is not likely that they contribute a significant amount of length.[56] Nevertheless, I do use a very slight S-shape curve laterally in order to tighten the lateral inferior portion of the breast envelope, and to reduce a "boxy" appearance with bulging in that region. An intriguing explanation for "boxiness" put forward by Ramselaar,[62] is that because of the direction of Langer's lines, the skin of the lateral region of the final breast is more distensible than the skin of the medial region. Medially, the incision is a gentle curve when the patient is standing, but is virtually a straight line when she is supine. If the future T-junction site is accurately known in advance, one can make a small inverted Y junction instead of a T, the small peak lessening the stress on the flap corners.[72]

Formerly[17] I predesigned an oval in a horizontal orientation at the time of marking, as recommended by others.[24] However, now that the areola is positioned intraoperatively after closure, it is not necessary to mark this beforehand, although it is an interesting exercise to do so. One sees that a horizontally oriented oval preoperatively is the appropriate configuration, rather than simply a larger circle, as would be needed if the breast skin behaved like a cardboard model.[72]

The de-epithelialized area can be designed at this time. Before discussing the width of the pedicle, the terminology must again be clarified. The literature has not clearly distinguished between thin (dermal) inferior pedicles and thick (parenchymal) inferior glandular segments. As mentioned earlier, this chapter deals with a thick, parenchymal, glandular pyramid, with overlying retained dermis (see Fig.

20–1*C*). If a thin dermal pedicle were to be used, then as Georgiade and associates recommended,[14] the maximal length-to-breadth ratio should be 3:1. However, because the inferior segment technique relies on a thick parenchymal base, this ratio can be exceeded, up to 6:1 in my experience, and as narrow as 6 cm at the base, although I have used 4 cm on occasions. Some patients have large veins visible just under the skin, and sometimes these can be seen clearly on the mammogram. If this is the case, one might expect very few deep veins draining the areolar region. If possible, the significant superficial veins should be included in the area that will become the de-epithelialized dermal pedicle.

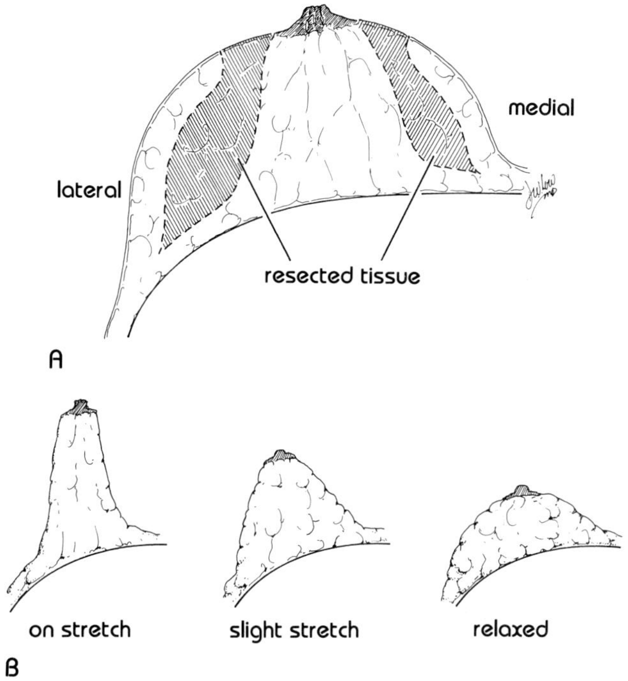

FIGURE 20–4 *A*, The lateral resection is greater than the medial resection. Breast tissue remains on the pectoral muscle, both medially and laterally. *B*, The inferior segment should be elevated during dissection. When relaxed it will collapse into a satisfactory shape if cut as shown. If the tissue is incised when it is in a relaxed state, it is possible to remove too much tissue, undermining the nipple.

OPERATIVE TECHNIQUE

Before Incision

In the operating room, the patient is positioned in such a manner as to permit safe elevation to nearly a sitting position for evaluation at intervals during surgery. Safety measures include a safety belt to prevent shifting, a footboard, and adequate padding to protect prominent points.[91] I prefer the arms abducted and fully supinated, to keep the ulnar nerve away from the supports, although others prefer pro-

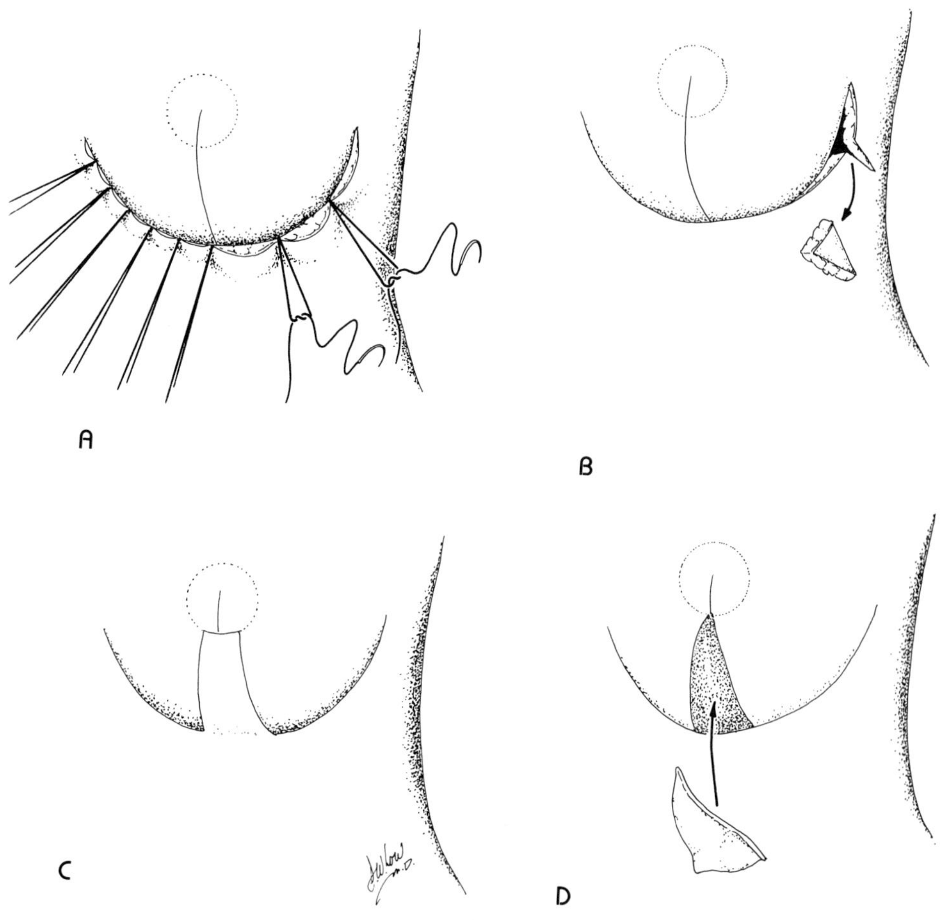

FIGURE 20–5 *A*, One way to deal with the discrepancy of skin in the horizontal incision is to gather the inferior skin in a pleated manner while suturing. *B*, Another method is to remove a Burow's triangle laterally. *C*, If closure difficulty is anticipated in advance, one can defer removal of the epithelium, leaving a trapezoid-shaped area of skin intact. *D*, If the above methods are unsuccessful, the thin skin removed from the deepithelialized area can be replaced as a graft.

nation.[91] I generally use a foam-rubber ring for the head, to prevent pressure alopecia. I use a metal bar securely attached to the table so that the drapes will move with the patient. I generally use pneumatic pump stockings, but elastic bandages would probably suffice. I do not generally use antibiotics, and rarely recommend a urinary catheter. I use either endotracheal general anesthesia or epidural anesthesia; I have not performed this procedure under a local anesthetic. The mammograms and the instant print photograph of the markings are placed where they can be referred to. I use an iodophor prep, which does not remove the brilliant green markings. If the markings are faint, they should be refreshed before the skin preparation.

It has been clearly documented that an epinephrine solution can be injected without untoward reactions,[26,92] although some surgeons prefer not to use it. A considerable proportion of the epinephrine will be sequestered in the excised tissue and removed before it can reach the patient's circulation. Because of this, the older guidelines[93] regarding the maximal amount have been revised: for example, 35 ml of 0.5 percent lidocaine with 1:200,000 epinephrine, repeated after 45 minutes.[26] The use of electrocautery usually keeps blood loss to a minimum, avoiding any need for transfusion, without detriment to the flaps.[26] I do not inject under the areola. Lidocaine cannot be relied on to prevent reflex segmental contracting of the areola, so it is wise to mark the areolar circle in advance, to avoid a noncircular areola.

The Segment

Generally, I begin by de-epithelializing a 1-cm rim around the areola, if the placement of the vertical limbs allows. Any pigmented skin removed can be stored, against the possibility that problems are encountered with the areola. The pedicle is de-epithelialized (Fig. 20-2*F*); this can be done by dermatone,[94-96] but epidermal inclusion cysts may result, especially inferiorly. This may be due in part to the variation in thickness of dermis, increasing from areola to inframammary crease. I also do not use the laser to de-epithelialize,[97] partly because I prefer to save the skin as a graft until after surgery, in case closure of the T junction proves difficult. If preoperative evaluation suggests that closure will be difficult, the epithelium should be retained inferiorly on the pedicle (see Fig. 20-5*C*). Next, the sides of the pedicle/segment are initially cut to a depth of 1.5 to 2 cm, staying close to the de-epithelialized area, except around the areola, where I leave 0.5-cm margin. I agree with Bolger and colleagues[26] that there are no adverse effects from using the electrocautery for the cutting and coagulation. The laser can be used as well, but I find that it has few advantages and is actually more time-consuming.

The medial and lateral flaps are next elevated, using a thickness of 1.5 to 2 cm rather than 3 cm as in our earlier publication.[17] Strömbeck advised minimal undermining,[73] but I find it easier to obtain a good result if the undermining continues superiorly to the top of the breast. The plane between the breast and subcutaneous tissue is often easy to dissect, with very few vessels, and I use this so long as it provides a flap of at least 1.5-cm thickness. The excess medial and lateral skin is removed (Fig. 20-2*G*), and then the vertical wedge is removed (Fig. 20-2*H*). Some surgeons prefer to leave the medial and lateral triangles attached to the superior flap, to be excised later.

The inferior segment is fully delineated, as a pyramid-shaped central mound with gradually sloping sides, leaving a layer of tissue overlying the pectoral fascia medially and laterally (Fig. 20-2*I*).[17] It is important during the resection for the surgeon to change sides at the operating table in order to avoid dissimilar resections, as mentioned by Bolger and colleagues.[26] I do not dissect straight down to the chest musculature, as outlined by Robbins,[40] although he reports no problems from doing so. Very little tissue is resected medially, and the greatest bulk removed superiorly, and laterally to avoid "boxiness" (Fig. 20-4*A*).[11] Laterally the ideal breast ends fairly abruptly in front of the midaxillary line,[37] and tissue is removed to produce this. The shape of the segment depends on the tension under which it is placed during dissection. I prefer to elongate it while cutting in order to avoid undermining or excessive narrowing. When relaxed onto the chest wall, it will generally have a satisfactory contour (Fig. 20-4*B*).

It has long been observed that neither suturing glandular elements to the pectoral fascia[43] nor the use of fascial slings[39] can reduce ptosis, and I have not yet seen any convincing evidence to the contrary. I also do not believe that the dermis of the inferior segment can act to "reinforce" against later ptosis. Furthermore, I believe that extensive folding of the inferior part of the segment can jeopardize the nipple-areola.[59] Occasionally, to accommodate a long de-epithelialized segment, I rotate the nipple about 90 degrees, so that the segment curves medially, then laterally.

Evaluating the Resection

The temporary staple closure (Fig. 20-2*J*) begins at the medial and lateral extremes of the incision, the medial and lateral flaps being advanced toward the T junction, with moderate tension at first, but then minimal tension for the last 3 or 4 cm until the T junction is reached. Any excess skin resulting from the fact that a narrow vertical limb angle was used can be excised at this time. If the skin caudal to the horizontal incision bulges out and looks "overstuffed,"[37] more breast tissue must be resected and staple closure performed again. If closure at the T junction is not easily obtained, there are several actions that can be taken (Fig. 20-5). First, further advancement of the flaps, even to the point of a slight scalloping of the inferior skin, can be performed. Care must be taken to avoid tension in the 3 or 4 cm adjacent to the vertical incision. If this is ineffective, the next consideration is to excise a Burow's triangle from the lateral aspect of the inferior flap (Fig. 20-5*B*). Another approach is to regraft the skin removed from the pedicle (Fig. 20-5*D*). Of course, if this had been anticipated, one could have left a trapezoidal area of skin intact (Fig. 20-5*C*).

The patient is next raised almost to a sitting position. This maneuver must be performed with care to avoid mishaps with equipment, the endotracheal tube, the sphygmomanometer, the monitoring leads, and the patient's extremities. It is well to bear in mind that the breasts must look smaller in the operating room than the desired final size. If additional resection is required, the patient is returned to the supine position, the staples are removed, resection is performed, and restapling carried out. If additional resection is needed but judged likely to impair the nipple circulation, the nipple can be removed, the pedicle advanced and further resected, and the nipple placed as a free graft.[56]

To determine the proper amount of tissue removal, I prefer to rely mainly on varying the desired skin envelope dimensions and then tailoring the contents intraoperatively so that they fit. One can also use the rule of thumb proposed by Regnault and Daniel.[98] As an approximation, if the preoperative chest circumference under the breasts is 32 to 34, 100 g of tissue is removed per desired cup size change; if the measurement is 36 to 38, 200 g; if 40 to 42, 300 g; if 44 to 46, 400 g. I am not accustomed to this method, nor do I measure the volume of the preoperative breast using any of the standard techniques.[53,99] The specimen weights can be compared, but two hypertrophied breasts are rarely the same size, so equal resected weight is not as good a measure of symmetry as is the trained aesthetic eye.

I customarily separate the excised specimens into quadrants so that if histologic examination discloses a carcinoma, its location will be known. Obviously, great care must be taken not to confuse the left and right specimens.[100] The incidence of lobular carcinoma has been reported to be as high as 8 percent;[101] invasive carcinoma is much less likely, but more significant. All patients should have the tissue sectioned serially to look for grossly visible lesions, and it is sometimes helpful to x-ray the slices.[102] Patients over 40 years of age should undergo a more detailed histologic search for microscopic lesions.[101]

Nipple Positioning

At this point, the patient is again brought to a semisitting position for final evaluation of the symmetry and nipple positioning. The principle of final determination of nipple-areola placement being made intraoperatively is an old one[43] that has been frequently rediscovered. If the resection appears to have been adequate and the result symmetric, the exact nipple position can be determined at this time. Again, the nipple must not be located too high; there is even an argument for intentionally placing it 1 cm lower than appears correct, to allow for later inferior expansion.[103]

The diameter of the circular cutout for the areola should be the same as the diameter measured around the areola when the patient was upright. Once this circle is cut, the opening tends to spring into somewhat of a horizontal oval shape. For this reason, I cut the opening slightly narrower in a transverse direction than the predetermined diameter. I do not use a "platform" for the nipple such as one would need to support a thin dermal pedicle.[65] If there is a doubt about poor circulation of the nipple, one can simply de-epithelialize (rather than excise) the circular area, then make a cruciate incision. The resulting four flaps can be folded in to permit retrieval of the nipple and final assessment. If the nipple is healthy, these four de-epithelialized flaps are discarded; if not, the flaps can serve as a base for accepting a free grafted nipple. Final closure can then begin.

Final Closure

The staples within 3 cm of the T junction are removed, any excess skin of the vertical margins is excised, and the vertical incisions are sutured with only moderate tension.[104] For the vertical incision, care should be taken to first suture the deep subcutaneous layer; if this is not done, the deepithelialized tissue can intrude, displacing the subcutaneous tissue and compressing and stretching the vessels to the skin (Fig. 20-6), leading to T-junction necrosis. As all the staples are removed, the incisions can be closed with any type of subcuticular suture. A small dog-ear at each end of the incision will flatten in time, and is preferable to lengthening the scar; this is aided by excising fat from beneath it.[72] The periareolar sutures are best made with suture material placed very close to the incision; this may leave fine marks, but these may actually help blur the otherwise sharp border of the skin-areola transition. I use "untieable" nylon sutures that can be easily untied the next day if there is any areolar compromise, and then subsequently retied without the need for local anesthesia.

I usually use a suction drain on each side, but many surgeons do not. I use no constricting, circumferential, or compression dressings whatsoever, only a light covering of the incisions.[105]

POSTOPERATIVE CARE

If a urinary catheter was inserted, it is removed in the recovery room. Postoperative vasoconstrictors are prohibited. The first night, the patient is kept in a head-elevated position and can get up to

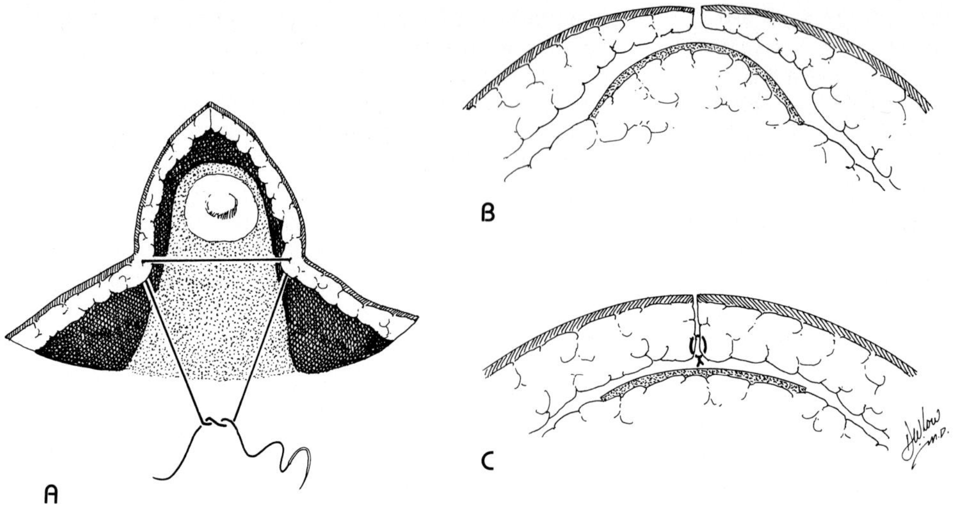

FIGURE 20-6 *A*, The deep subcutaneous layer must be sutured first to prevent displacement of the subcutaneous tissues by the underlying pedicle. *B*, If no effort has been made to approximate the deeper aspects of the subcutaneous tissue, the underlying pedicle will push the tissue aside.

visit the bathroom with assistance. The intermittent pressure stockings are continued overnight. The patient uses the incentive spirometer to prevent atelectasis, and generally has the use of a patient-controlled analgesia pump. Arm motions are unrestricted, except that forceful use is discouraged. When the patient is examined in the evening postoperatively, the nipple-areola is inspected. If this is compromised in any way, the sequence of steps as outlined in Figure 20-7 is begun. The next morning the dressings are changed completely, the drains are possibly removed, and a soft wrap dressing is applied for patient comfort. Ambulation is increased and the patient may eat. The patient is discharged as soon as she can cope at home.

The patient is seen 1 week postoperatively, at which time the sutures are removed. It is acceptable for the patient to begin wearing a bra at this time as long as the waistband is fairly loose and not likely to compress the tissues at the T junction. I permit patients to resume driving after 1 week, although one patient developed a hematoma at the 1-week point while driving vigorously. At 3 weeks, I permit the patient to resume full activity without restriction. After completion of healing and scar maturation, acceptable aesthetic results should be expected. (Figs. 20-8 to 20-12).

The patient should resume breast self-examination within a month after surgery. She will rapidly become acquainted with her own new anatomy and the underlying scar tissue. Any lumps require biopsy.[106]

Six months to 1 year after the reduction, I order a baseline mammogram for patients over 30. The likelihood of an average woman developing a cancer during a 1-year interval has been estimated as between one in 300[107] and one in 600.[108] Any breast reduction produces mammographic changes.[109] After the inferior segment technique, almost all patients have periareolar and inferior pole soft tissue changes as revealed by the mammogram, often asymmetric.[110] Occasionally they may show fat necrosis or calcifications, which usually can be differentiated from cancer.[111] The removal of the large volume of breast tissue may further reduce cancer risk, as suggested by Rees and Coburn[112] and others, and supported by Lund and associates,[113] so this interval appears reasonable.

COMPLICATIONS: AVOIDANCE AND MANAGEMENT

General. The avoidance of complications begins preoperatively with the withdrawal of nicotine and with the mandatory weight loss in overweight patients. The next critical point is the preoperative determination of nipple location and flap design, as mentioned earlier. The perioperative use of pneumatic stockings has also been mentioned.

T Junction. The risk of T-junction necrosis can be reduced by discontinuing nicotine before and after surgery. At the time of closure, T-junction tension should be avoided and care taken to suture the deep layer of the subcutaneous tissue (Fig. 20-6). If necrosis at this site becomes apparent early, the T-junction sutures should be removed, the wound allowed to gape, and secondary closure anticipated. If there is a major skin necrosis of these flaps, one can anticipate fat necrosis and very likely infection.[37] Debridement, wet dressings, and antibiotic coverage are the main treatment.

Hematoma often precedes infection, and both are more common in obese patients, as is fat necrosis. Fat necrosis is signaled by fever, induration, erythema, and drainage. Treatment consists of

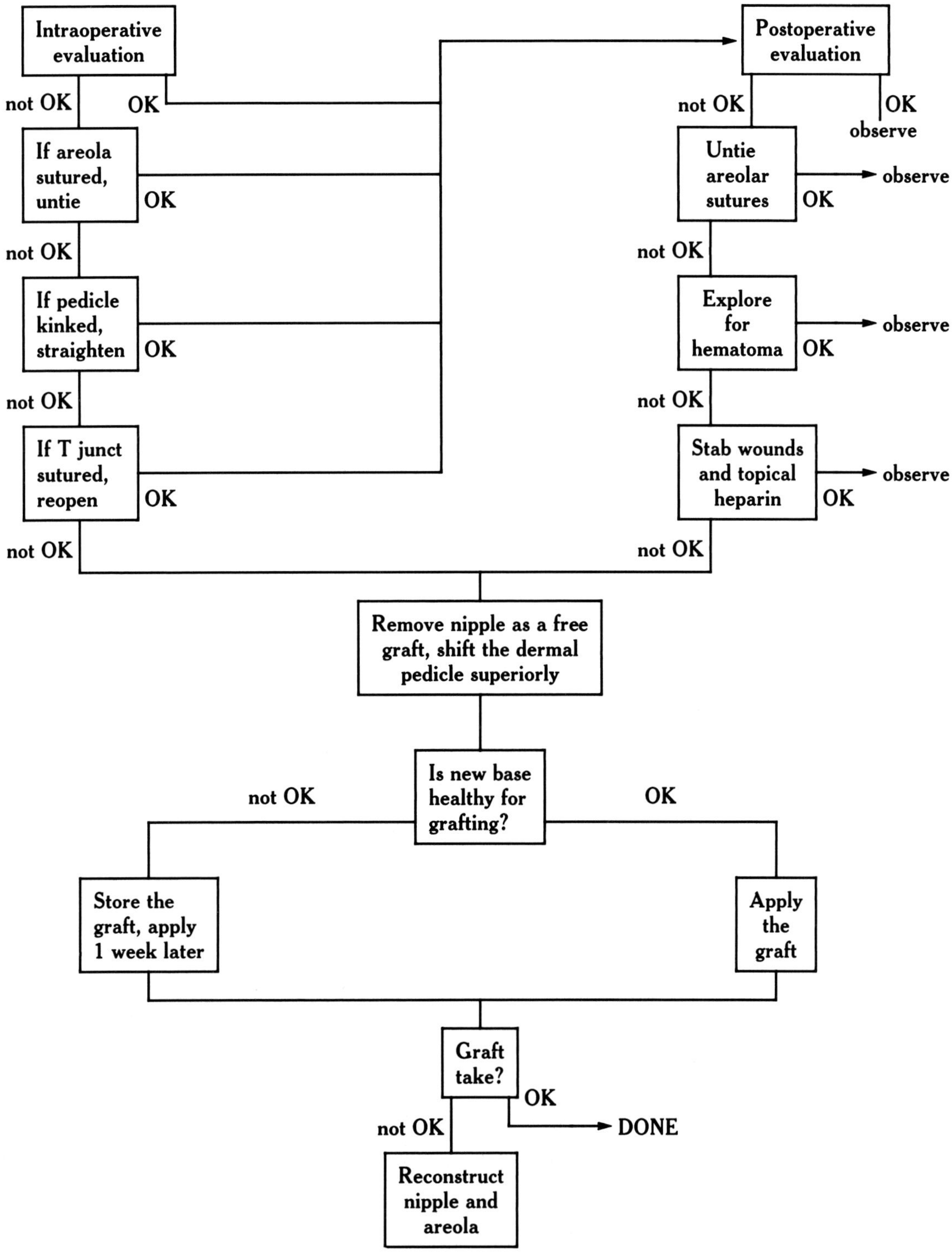

FIGURE 20-7 A typical decision tree for dealing with impairment of nipple-areola ischemia after the inferior segment technique.

drainage, the extent of which is dictated by the degree of the problem. Of course, the patient should not use heating pads on the breasts, which may cause burns.

Nipple-Areola. I avoid injecting the epinephrine solution directly beneath the nipple-areola or into the pedicle itself, and postoperatively I avoid vasopressors. Intraoperatively, one should avoid tension on the breast tissue supplying the nipple-areola, which may avulse small vessels. Undercutting the pedicle is avoided by putting mild, gentle upward traction on the areola to elongate the pedicle

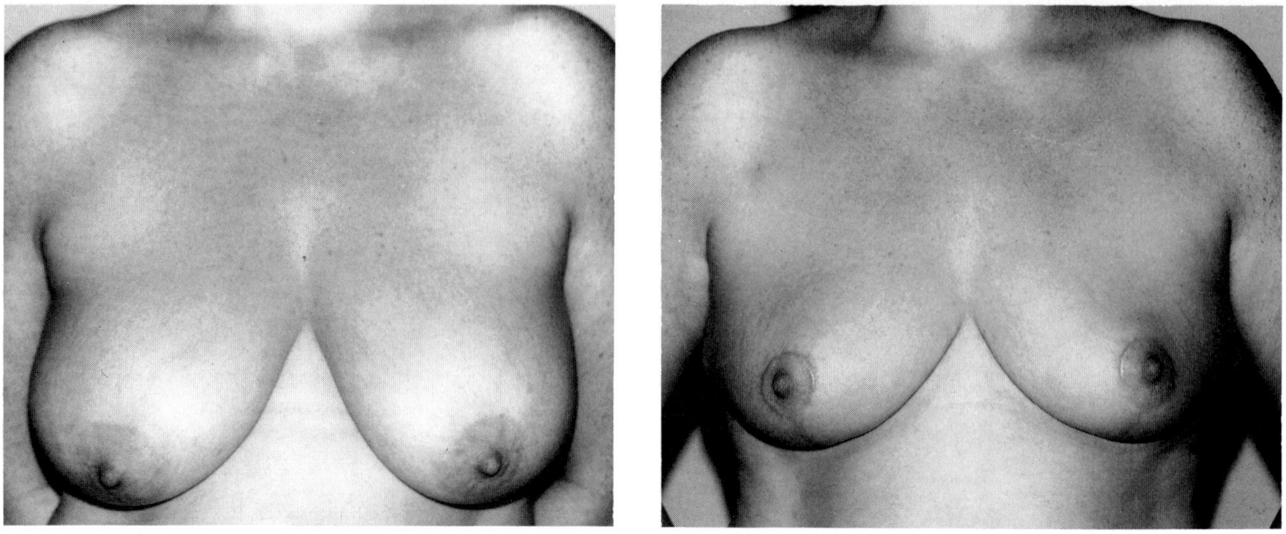

A B

FIGURE 20-8 *A, B,* A 41-year-old woman before and after removal of 520 and 510 g from right and left breasts, respectively.

so that the effect of removing tissue at any one area is clearly seen (Fig. 20-4*B*).

Fluorescein can be used to evaluate nipple perfusion.[114] Nipple-areola circulatory compromise is dealt with as follows (Fig. 20-7). If the nipple appears jeopardized during surgery, I verify that the areola is not under excessive tension, the pedicle not kinked, and the skin closure not excessively tight. If none of these correctable factors is present, the nipple is removed as a free graft. If the circular opening has already been cut for the areola, the de-epithelialized pedicle is shifted upward and the graft applied to its dermal surface.[115] If the circular opening has not been cut, the graft can be applied on the dermis of the breast skin itself.

If the nipple-areola looks well perfused in the operating room, but appears jeopardized that night or the next day, one probable cause is a minute hematoma. I untie the periareolar sutures, evacuate any hematoma present, and, if the nipple still appears in jeopardy, make several stab incisions with a No. 11 blade and begin application of heparin dress-

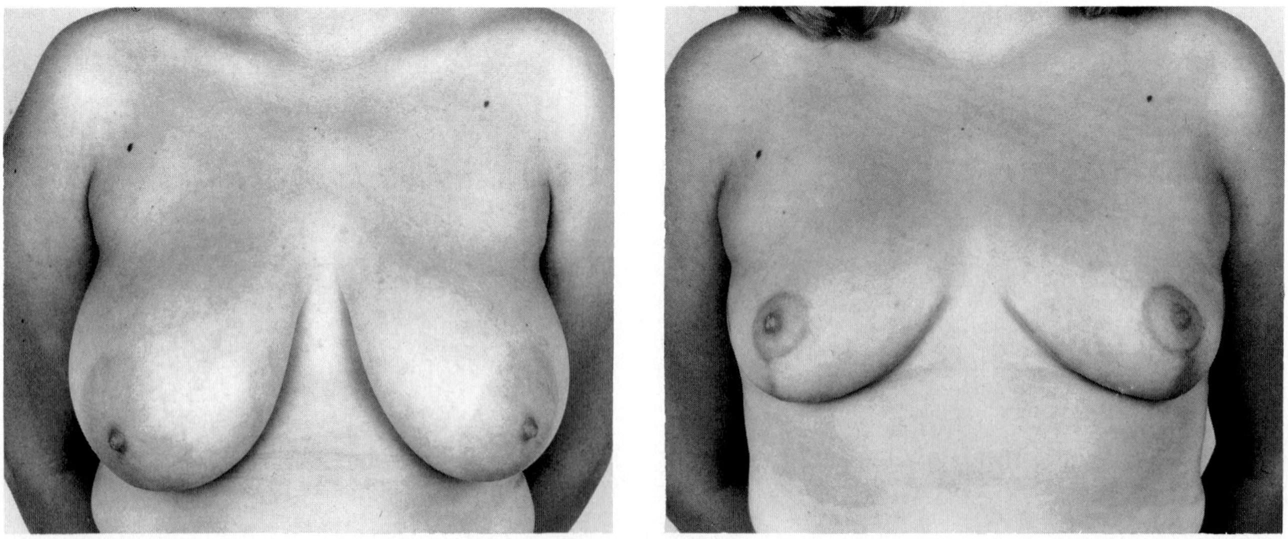

A B

FIGURE 20-9 *A, B,* A 16-year-old woman before and after removal of 475 and 605 g from right and left breasts, respectively. Note the pigmentation below the areola.

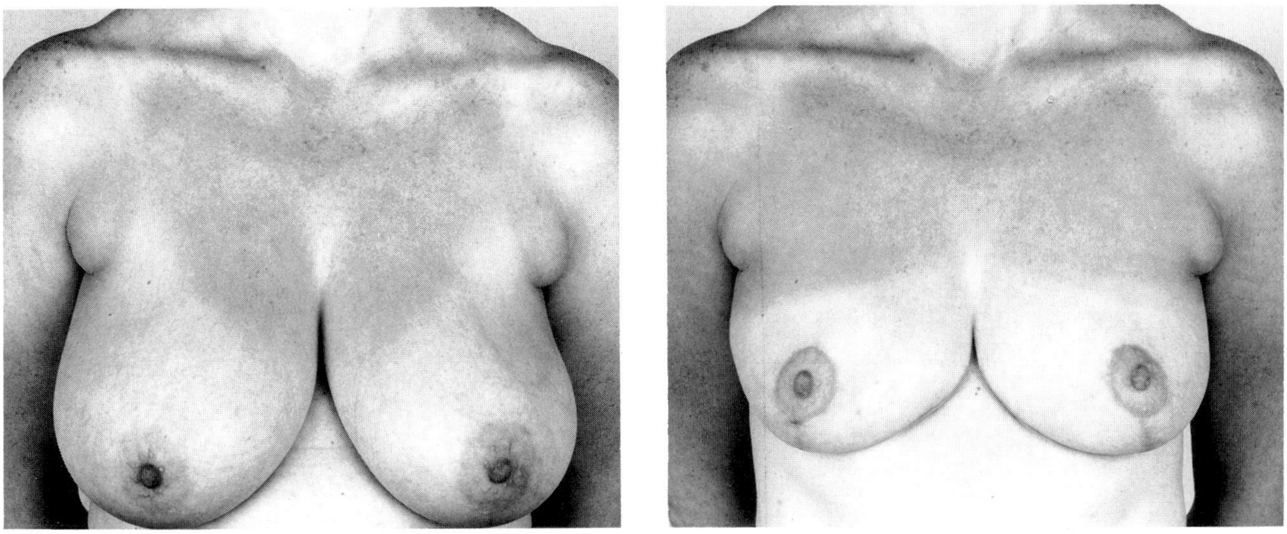

A B

FIGURE 20-10 *A, B,* A 42-year-old woman before and after removal of 615 and 520 g from right and left breasts, respectively.

ings, 10 ml of 1,000 units per ml, changed several times a day. If the nipple improves with this therapy, I continue the heparin for several days. If the nipple does not improve, it is removed as a free graft.

Long Term. Reenlargement of the breasts may occur after weight gain, pregnancy, or continuing growth disorder of the underlying parenchyma.[47,56,57,116] I have not seen a case of galactorrhea after breast reduction, but if this occurs, bromocriptine, 2.5 mg twice daily for 2 weeks, can be given.[117,118] Loss of breast contour without enlargement is usually due to inferior dropout as discussed earlier. Its correction is not complex, merely requiring removal of a horizontal/or vertical wedge of skin.

CONCLUSION

The "inferior segment" technique, not to be confused with "inferior pedicle" techniques, is a safe and reliable method of reducing the hypertrophied breast, an excellent method of correcting asymmetric hypertrophy.

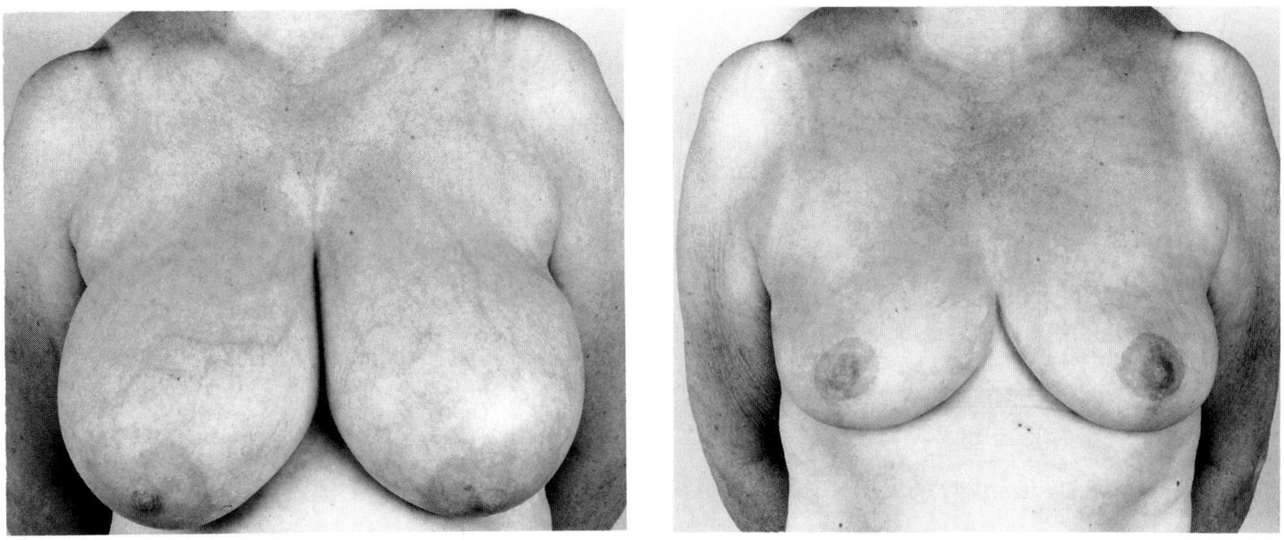

A B

FIGURE 20-11 *A, B,* A 50-year-old woman before and after removal of 942 and 765 g from right and left breasts, respectively.

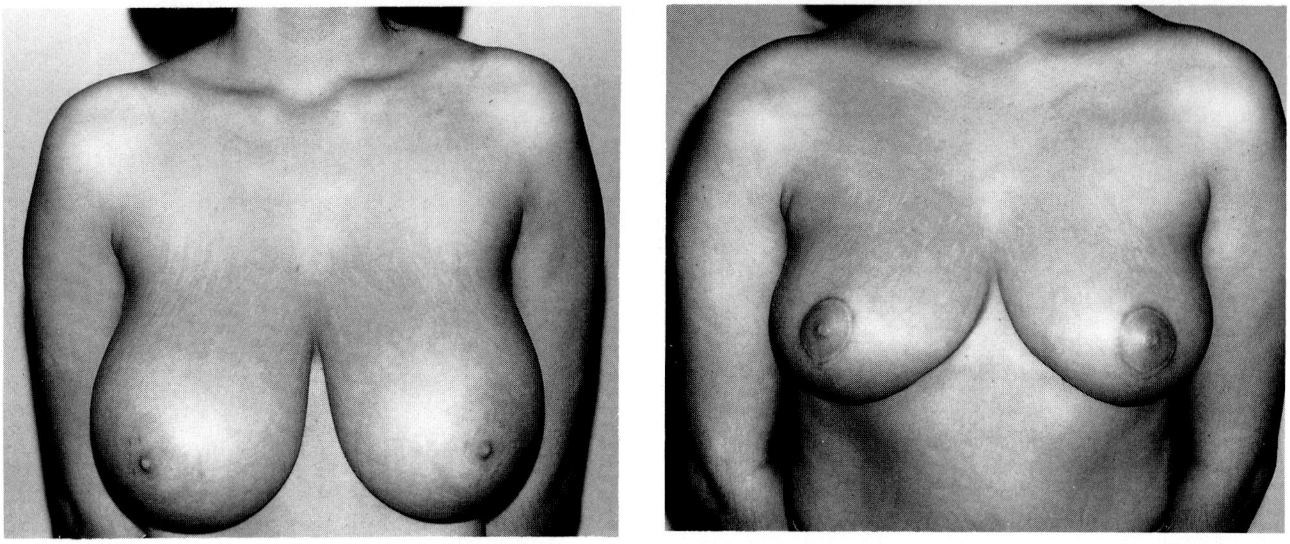

A B

FIGURE 20-12 *A, B,* A 17-year-old woman before and after removal of 950 and 853 g from right and left breasts, respectively.

References

1. Kraske H. Die Operationen der atrophischen und hypertrophischen Hangebrust. Munchen Med Wochen 1923; 70:672.
2. Axhausen G. Plastic surgery of breast. Med Klin 1926; 22:1437.
3. Lotch F. Über Hangebrust plastik. Klin Wochenschr 1928; 7:603.
4. Biesenberger H. Deformitaten und kosmetische Operationen der weiblichen Brust. Vienna: W Maudrich, 1931.
5. Schwarzmann E. Avoidance of nipple necrosis by preservation of corium in one-stage plastic surgery of the breast. Rev Chir Struct 1937:206.
6. Wise RJ. A preliminary report on a method of planning the mammaplasty. Plast Reconstr Surg 1956; 17:367.
7. Hoffman S. Reduction mammaplasty: A medicolegal hazard? Aesthetic Plast Surg 1987; 11:113.
8. Kohn F, Dalrymple J. Plastic reconstruction of the enlarged breast: Report of a new technique. Br J Plast Surg 1967; 20:184.
9. Ribeiro L. A new technique for reduction mammaplasty. Plast Reconstr Surg 1975; 55:330.
10. Robbins TH. A reduction mammaplasty with the areola-nipple based on an inferior dermal pedicle. Plast Reconstr Surg 1977; 59:64.
11. Courtiss EH, Goldwyn RM. Reduction mammaplasty by the inferior pedicle technique. Plast Reconstr Surg 1977; 59:500.
12. Ariyan S. Reduction mammaplasty with the nipple-areola carried on a single narrow inferior pedicle. Ann Plast Surg 1980; 5:167.
13. Amar R, Bosch del Marco G. Reduction mammaplasty using an inferior dermo-glandular pedicle flap. Ann Chir Plast 1981; 26:243.
14. Georgiade NG, Serafin D, Morris R, Georgiade G. Reduction mammaplasty utilizing an inferior pedicle nipple-areolar flap. Ann Plast Surg 1979; 3:211.
15. Tanski EV. A new method for prophylactic mastectomy, reduction mammaplasty, and mastopexy. Plast Reconstr Surg 1980; 65:314.
16. Versaci AD. Reduction mammaplasty for moderate macromastia. Ann Plast Surg 1981; 6:253.
17. Labandter HP, Dowden RV, Dinner MI. The inferior segment technique for breast reduction. Ann Plast Surg 1982; 8:493.
18. Moufarrege R. Plastie mammaire à pedicule dermoglandulaire inférieur. Ann Chir Plast 1982; 27:3.
19. Moufarrege R, Beauregard G, Bosse JP, et al. Reduction mammoplasty by the total dermoglandular pedicle. Aesthetic Plast Surg 1985; 9:227.
20. Hester TR, Bostwick J, Miller L, Cunningham SJ. Breast reduction utilizing the maximally vascularized central breast pedicle. Plast Reconstr Surg 1985; 76:890.
21. Kaplan I. Reduction mammaplasty: Nipple-areolar survival on a single breast quadrant. Plast Reconstr Surg 1978; 61:27.
22. Climo MS, Alexander JE. Intercostothelial circulation: Nipple survival in reduction mammaplasty in absence of a dermal pedicle. Ann Plast Surg 1980; 4:128.
23. Balch CR. The central mound technique for reduction mammaplasty. Plast Reconstr Surg 1981; 67:305.
24. Crepeau R, Klein H. Reduction mammaplasty with inferiorly based glandular pedicle flap. Ann Plast Surg 1982; 9:463.
25. Silversmith PE. re Crepeau, reduction mammaplasty. Ann Plast Surg 1983; 11:266.
26. Bolger WE, Seyfer AE, Jackson SM. Reduction mammaplasty using the inferior glandular "pyramid" pedicle: Experiences with 300 patients. Plast Reconstr Surg 1987; 80:75.
27. Hester TR Jr, Cukic J. Central breast pedicle and "free-hand" technique for alteration of volume and skin envelope of the breast. Clin Plast Surg 1988; 15:613.
28. Maliniac JW. Arterial blood supply of the breast. Arch Surg 1943; 47:329.
29. Aufricht G. Mammaplasty for pendulous breasts. Em-

piric and geometric planning. Plast Reconstr Surg 1949; 4:13.
30. Taylor GE, Palmer JH. The vascular territories (angiosomes) of the body: Experimental study and clinical applications. Br J Plast Surg 1987; 40:113.
31. Palmer JH, Taylor GI. The vascular territories of the anterior chest wall. Br J Plast Surg 1986; 39:287.
32. Dowden RV, Dinner MI, Labandter HP. Breast reduction for asymmetrical hypertrophy. Plast Reconstr Surg 1984; 73:928.
33. Craig RDP, Sykes PA. Nipple sensitivity following reduction mammaplasty. Br J Plast Surg 1970; 23:165.
34. Edwards EA. Surgical anatomy of the breast. In: Goldwyn RM, ed. Plastic and reconstructive surgery of the breast. Boston: Little, Brown, 1976.
35. Farina MA, Newby BG, Alani HM. Innervation of the nipple-areola complex. Plast Reconstr Surg 1980; 66:497.
36. Courtiss EH, Goldwyn RM. Breast sensation before and after plastic surgery. Plast Reconstr Surg 1976; 58:1.
37. McKissock PK. Complications and undesirable results with reduction mammaplasty. In: Goldwyn RM, ed. The unfavorable result in plastic surgery. Boston: Little, Brown, 1984.
38. Pennisi VR, Klabunde EH, Pletsch ME. The location of the nipple in breast reconstruction. Plast Reconstr Surg 1969; 43:612.
39. Strömbeck JO. Reduction mammoplasty: Some observations and reflections. Aesthetic Plast Surg 1983; 7:249.
40. Robbins TH. Reduction mammaplasty by the Robbins technique. Plast Reconstr Surg 1987; 79:308.
41. Kroll SS. A comparison of deepithelialization and deskinning in inferior pedicle breast reduction. Plast Reconstr Surg 1988; 81:913.
42. Reus WF, Mathes SJ. Preservation of projection after reduction mammaplasty: Long-term follow-up of the inferior pedicle technique. Plast Reconstr Surg 1988; 82:644.
43. Schwarzmann E. Die Technik der Mammaplastik. Chirurgie 1930; 2:932.
44. Goin MK, Goin JM, Gianini MH. The psychic consequences of a reduction mammaplasty. Plast Reconstr Surg 1977; 59:530.
45. Letterman G, Shurter M. The effects of mammary hypertrophy on the skeletal system. Ann Plast Surg 1980; 5:425.
46. Wapnir I, Rabinowitz B, Snyderman R. Asymmetrical breasts in an adolescent (letter). Plast Reconstr Surg 1988; 81:813.
47. Hinderer UT, del Rio JL. An unusual case of gigantomasty. Aesthetic Plast Surg 1985; 9:91.
48. Mayl N, Vasconez LO, Jurkiewicz MJ. Treatment of macromastia in the actively enlarging breast. Plast Reconstr Surg 1974; 54:6.
49. Spicer TE. Reduction mammaplasty. In: Selected readings in plastic surgery. Vol 4, No 30, Dec 1987. Dallas, TX: Baylor University Medical Center.
50. Strömbeck JO. Reduction mammaplasty. In: Goldwyn RM, ed. Plastic and reconstructive surgery of the breast. Boston: Little, Brown, 1976.
51. Pers M, Nielsen IM, Gerner N. Results following reduction mammaplasty as evaluated by the patients. Ann Plast Surg 1986; 17:449.
52. Gerner N. The significance of overweight for the occurrence of primary complications after the surgical treatment of breast hypertrophy. Ugeskr Laeger 1985; 147:3578.
53. Strömbeck JO, Malm M. Priority grouping in a waiting list of patients for reduction mammaplasty. Ann Plast Surg 1986; 17:498.
54. Statistic Bulletin Metropolitan Life Insurance Company, Nov 1959.
55. Castro CC. Late results after reduction mammaplasty with curved incisions. Plast Reconstr Surg 1978; 61:862.
56. Goldwyn RM. Comments on Chapter 37 (Reduction mammaplasty). In: Goldwyn RM, ed. The unfavorable result in plastic surgery. Boston: Little, Brown, 1984.
57. Beischer NA, Hueston JH, Pepperell RJ. Massive hypertrophy of the breasts in pregnancy: Report of three cases and review of the literature. Obstet Gynecol Surg 1989; 44:234.
58. Stark RB. A procedure for mammary reduction and mastopexy: Summary of 100 personally performed operations. Aesthetic Plast Surg 1977; 1:145.
59. Hawtoff DB, Levine M, Kapetansky DI, Pieper D. Complications of reduction mammaplasty: Comparison of nipple-areolar graft and pedicle. Ann Plast Surg 1989; 23:3.
60. Mandel MA. Autotransfusion in elective plastic surgical operations. Plast Reconstr Surg 1986; 77:767.
61. Cathcart RS, Hagerty RC. Preoperative and postoperative considerations in elective breast operations. Ann Plast Surg 1989; 22:533.
62. Ramselaar JM. Precision in breast reduction. Plast Reconstr Surg 1988; 82:631.
63. McKissock PK. Reduction mammaplasty. Ann Plast Surg 1979; 2:321.
64. Mathes SJ, Nahai F, Hester JR. Avoiding the flat breast in reduction mammaplasty. Plast Reconstr Surg 1980; 66:63.
65. Schultz RC, Marus NJ. Platform for nipple projection: Modifications of the inferior pedicle technique for breast reduction. Plast Reconstr Surg 1981; 68:208.
66. Penn J. Breast reduction. Br J Plast Surg 1955; 7:357.
67. Berry EP. Geometric planning in reduction mammaplasty. Plast Reconstr Surg 1968; 42:232.
68. Granick MS, Heckler FR, Jones EW. Surgical skin marking techniques. Plast Reconstr Surg 1987; 79:573.
69. Dinner MI, Chait LA. Preventing the high-riding nipple after McKissock breast reductions. Plast Reconstr Surg 1977; 59:330.
70. Pennisi VR. To facilitate the suitable location of the nipple in breast reduction and reconstruction (letter). Plast Reconstr Surg 1987; 80:474.
71. Smith JW, Gillen FJ. Repairing errors of nipple-areolar placement following reduction mammaplasty. Aesthetic Plast Surg 1980; 4:197.
72. O'Keeffe PJ. Draftsmanship for reduction mammaplasty. Ann Plast Surg 1983; 10:465.
73. Strömbeck JO. Mammaplasty: Report of a new technique based on the two-pedicle procedure. Br J Plast Surg 1960; 13:79.
74. Marchac D, Olarte G. Reduction mammaplasty and correction of ptosis with a short inframammary scar. Plast Reconstr Surg 1982; 69:45.
75. Strömbeck JO. Late results after reduction mammaplasty: In: Goldwyn R, ed. Long-term results in plastic and reconstructive surgery. Boston: Little, Brown, 1980.
76. Maxwell GP. Discussion of preservation of projection after reduction mammaplasty: Long-term follow-up of

the inferior pedicle technique, by Reus and Mather. Plast Reconstr Surg 1988; 82:651.
77. Liang MD, Narayanan K. A new disposable breast marker. Ann Plast Surg 1988; 21:85.
78. Pontes R. Reduction mammaplasty—variations I and II. Ann Plast Surg 1981; 6:437.
79. Cardoso de Castro C, Coelho RFS, Cintra HOP. The value of non-prefixed marking in reduction mammaplasty. Aesthetic Plast Surg 1984; 8:237.
80. Gerow FJ, Spira M, Hardy SB. A simplified design of reduction mammaplasty. Plast Reconstr Surg 1974; 53:271.
81. Woods JE, Borowski JJ, Masson JK, Irons GB. Experience with and comparison of methods of reduction mammaplasty. Mayo Clin Proc 1978; 53:487.
82. Gasperoni C, Salgarello M. Preoperative breast marking in reduction mammaplasty. Ann Plast Surg 1987; 19:306.
83. Lassus C. Breast reduction with a vertical scar. Int Surg 1970; 53(I):103.
84. Marchac D, Sagher U. Mammaplasty with a short horizontal scar. Clin Plast Surg 1988; 15:627.
85. Peixoto G. Reduction mammaplasty: A personal technique. Plast Reconstr Surg 1980; 65:217.
86. Basile RD. Mammaplasty: Large reduction with short inframammary scars. Plast Reconstr Surg 1985; 76:130.
87. Peixoto G. The infra-areolar longitudinal incision in reduction mammaplasty. Aesthetic Plast Surg 1985; 9:1.
88. Lassus C. Breast reduction: Evolution of a technique—a single vertical scar. Aesthetic Plast Surg 1987; 11:107.
89. Berrimo P, Galli A, Raimero ML, Santi P. Unilateral reduction mammaplasty: Sculpturing the breast from the undersurface. Plast Reconstr Surg 1988; 82:88.
90. Pitanguy I. Discussion of: Reduction mammaplasty—a personal technique by Peixoto G. Plast Reconstr Surg 1980; 65:226.
91. Letterman G, Schurter M. A sitting position for mammaplasty with general anesthesia. Ann Plast Surg 1988; 20:522.
92. Brantner JN, Peterson HD. The role of vasoconstrictors in control of blood loss in reduction mammaplasty. Plast Reconstr Surg 1985; 75:339.
93. Varejes L. The use of solutions containing adrenaline during halothane anesthesia. Anesthesia 1963; 18:507.
94. Rosenberg L, Tanner B. A fast and simple de-epidermization in corrective mammaplasty. Aesthetic Plast Surg 1984; 8:259.
95. Furnas DW, Turpin IM. Use of the drum dermatome for deepithelialization of pedicles in reduction mammaplasty. Ann Plast Surg 1982; 9:510.
96. DeWet HC. The use of a drum dermatome in reduction mammaplasty. Plast Reconstr Surg 1973; 52:448.
97. Becker DW Jr, Bunn JC. Laser deepithelialization: An adjunct to reduction mammaplasty. Plast Reconstr Surg 1987; 79:754.
98. Regnault P, Daniel RK. Breast reduction. In: Regnault P, Daniel RK, eds. Aesthetic plastic surgery, principles and techniques. Boston: Little, Brown, 1984: 499-538.
99. Ramirez MA. Calculation of the volume of the normal and the hypertrophic breast. Aesthetic Plast Surg 1980; 4:239.
100. Crikelair GF, Malton D. Mammaplasty and occult breast malignancy: Case report. Plast Reconstr Surg 1959; 23:601.
101. Bondeson L, Linell F, Ringberg A. Breast reductions: What to do with all the tissue specimens? Histopathology 1985; 9:281.
102. Kallen R, Broome A, Muhlow A, Forsby N. Reduction mammoplasty: Results of pre-operative mammography and patient inquiry. Scand J Plast Reconstr Surg 1986; 20:303.
103. Carvalho CGS, Baroudi R. Mammaplasties: Surgical refinements of the nipple-areola complex. Ann Plast Surg 1982; 8:458.
104. Pacik PO. The trifurcation headache. Plast Reconstr Surg 1981; 68:975.
105. Ely JF. Guidelines for reduction mammaplasty. Ann Plast Surg 1981; 6:424.
106. Isaacs G, Roznet L, Tudball C. Breast lumps after reduction mammaplasty. Ann Plast Surg 1985; 15:394.
107. Baker LH. Breast cancer detection demonstration project: Five-year summary report. CA 1982; 32:194.
108. Humphrey LJ. Invited comment (to Pennisi and Capozzi). Ann Plast Surg 1984; 12:345.
109. Robertson JLA. Changed appearance of mammograms following breast reduction. Plast Reconstr Surg 1977; 59:347.
110. Brown FE, Sargent SK, Cohen SR, Morain WD. Mammographic changes following reduction mammaplasty. Plast Reconstr Surg 1987; 80:691.
111. Isaacs G, Rozner L, Tudball C. Breast lumps after reduction mammaplasty. Ann Plast Surg 1985; 15:394.
112. Rees TD, Coburn R. Breast reduction: Is it an aid to cancer detection? Br J Plast Surg 1972; 25:144.
113. Lund K, Ewertz M, Schou G. Breast cancer incidence subsequent to surgical reduction of the female breast. Scand J Plast Reconstr Surg 1987; 21:209.
114. Singer R, Krant SM. Intravenous fluorescein for evaluating the dusky nipple-areola during reduction mammaplasty. Plast Reconstr Surg 1981; 67:534.
115. Wray RC, Luce EA. Treatment of impending nipple necrosis following reduction mammaplasty. Plast Reconstr Surg 1981; 68:242.
116. Ryan RF, Pernoll ML. Virginal hypertrophy. Plast Reconstr Surg 1985; 75:737.
117. Bruck JC. Galactorrhea: A rare complication following reduction mammaplasty. Ann Plast Surg 1987; 19:384.
118. Bronson DL. Galactorrhea after reduction mammaplasty. Plast Reconstr Surg 1989; 83:580.

CHAPTER 21

Parenchymal Techniques of Reduction Mammaplasty

JAMES C. GROTTING, M.D.

Parenchymal breast reduction techniques are those methods that leave the nipple-areola complex pedicled on the major remaining portion of the parenchymal mound. Technically speaking, virtually all types of breast reduction that carry the nipple-areola complex on a pedicle are attached in one way or another to the breast parenchyma, but in this chapter only those techniques in which the parenchymal mound is reduced either by tangential surface shaving or radial or undersurface resection with conization are discussed.

In general, these techniques fall into two categories. First, if the surface of the breast parenchyma is to be reduced by tangential shaving, the skin and subcutaneous fat of the breast must be elevated. Very limited or no undermining of the breast parenchyma is done in order to preserve the blood supply. In the second category, the parenchyma is left attached to the overlying skin and subcutaneous tissue, with reduction of the parenchyma by radial wedge excision, and varying degrees of undermining and reduction of the base of the breast from its undersurface. At the risk of oversimplification, for the purposes of this chapter we will refer to the first category as *central mound techniques* and the second as *radial resection and undersurface sculpturing techniques.*

CENTRAL MOUND TECHNIQUES

Background and History

Central mound techniques of breast reduction consist of total free dissection of skin and subcutaneous tissue, surface modification of the gland, and usually some degree of skin envelope reduction. It is difficult to identify a single early author who can be given the credit for this concept. Between 1901 and 1930 almost all the technical methods of breast reduction were attempted, some based on a knowledge of anatomy and others completely ignoring the vascular anatomy of the breast.[1] However, in 1923 Lotsch from Magdeburg, Germany, described a procedure that probably comes closest to the techniques currently in use.[2,3] In 1928 Biesenberger from Vienna, Austria, introduced a variation on the technique in which he completely dissected the skin and followed this with an S-shaped modification of the gland. He then rebuilt the conical shape of the breast, displacing the nipple-areola complex upward and outward. The skin was then redraped and the excess removed in a final inverted T-shaped scar.[4] Biesenberger's operation achieved great popularity even until the 1960s, despite reports of skin necrosis and losses of the nipple-areola complex.

Other modifications of the basic technique were offered by Wise, who proposed tangential excision of glandular parenchyma using a plastic form fit over the anterior surface of the gland, and Festge, who removed surface parenchyma circumferentially around the nipple-areola complex.[5,6] Currently, the most widely used modification of the central mound technique is perhaps that offered by Hester and colleagues.[7,8]

Essential Anatomy

Various modifications of the central pedicle technique have been made in order to maximize the blood supply to both the nipple-areola complex and the skin flaps. The blood supply of the breast is well known. It receives branches from the lateral thoracic artery, intercostal perforators, and pectoralis major perforators and from the internal mammary artery. The arrangement of these vascular arcades has led to the concept of a hypovascular zone beneath the breast itself surrounded by a hypervascular zone at the periphery.[9] Therefore, any resection of the central parenchymal mound should begin at least 2 to 3 cm away from the chest wall circumferentially in order to maximally preserve branches from the major vascular pedicles (Fig. 21-1).[7,8]

The innervation of the nipple-areola complex comes mainly from the anterior and lateral cutaneous nerves of the third, fourth, and fifth intercostal nerves.[10] The fourth lateral cutaneous nerve is the single most important branch supplying sensitivity to the nipple. On the left breast, this nerve enters at approximately the 4 o'clock position, and on the right breast at the 8 o'clock position. Dissection in these regions should be minimal.

Elevation of the skin flaps is safest if the flaps are kept at least 2 cm thick. This often requires that some parenchyma be kept with the skin flaps for maximal viability. The flaps also should not be undermined beyond 2 to 3 cm from the chest wall circumferentially.

Patient Selection

The central mound technique of breast reduction appears to be best suited for patients with a breast shape that is wide based and who require reduction in the 300- to 1,000-g range. It is more difficult to use with predictability in severely ptotic breasts or those with a tubular shape.

Preoperative Evaluation and Markings (Hester Modification)

With the patient in the sitting position, the inframammary fold is marked. The new nipple position is then estimated at 1 to 2 cm above the inframammary fold projected onto the anterior surface of the breast. If the breasts are asymmetric, adjustments may be made medially or laterally so that the end result is a similar shape on both sides. A curved tangent is then drawn down along the nipple-areola complex on both sides to the inframammary fold, resulting in a triangular segment. The amount of skin to be removed in the horizontal direction below the nipple-areola complex can be estimated by pinching the skin between the thumb and index fingers. It is best to be conservative at first, because more can be trimmed later if necessary (Fig. 21-2).

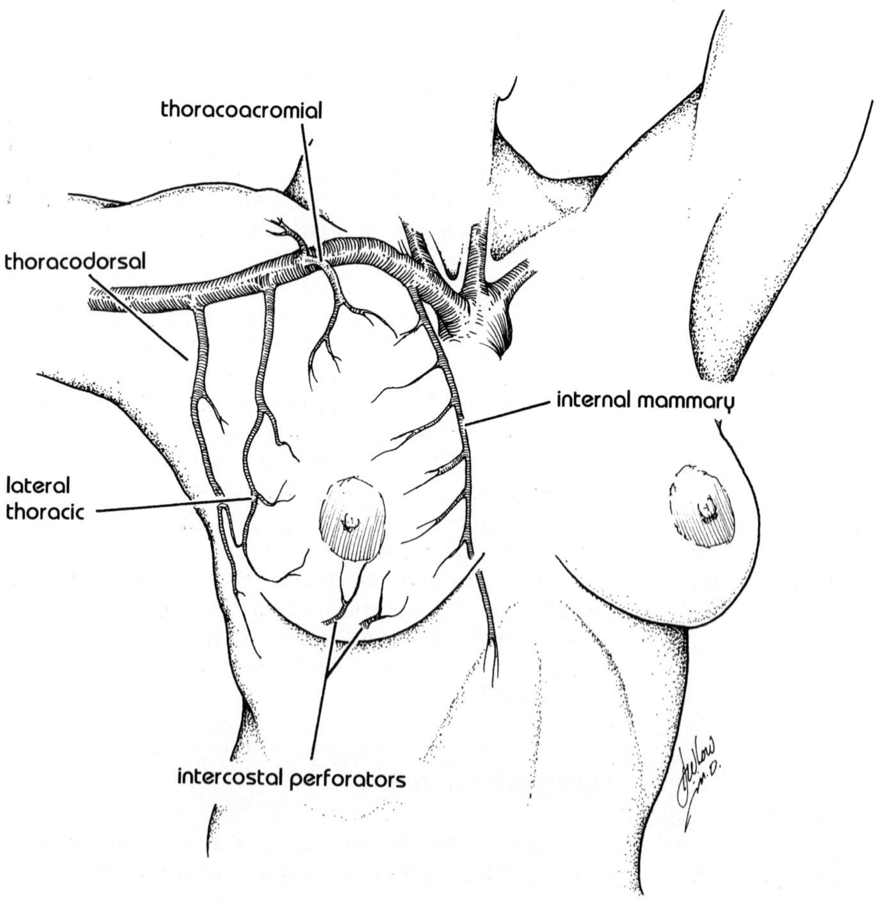

FIGURE 21-1 The major sources of the arterial blood supply to the breast. (Adapted from Hester TR, Bostwick J, Miller L, Cunningham SJ. Breast reduction utilizing the maximally central breast pedicle. Plast Reconstr Surg 1985; 76:890.)

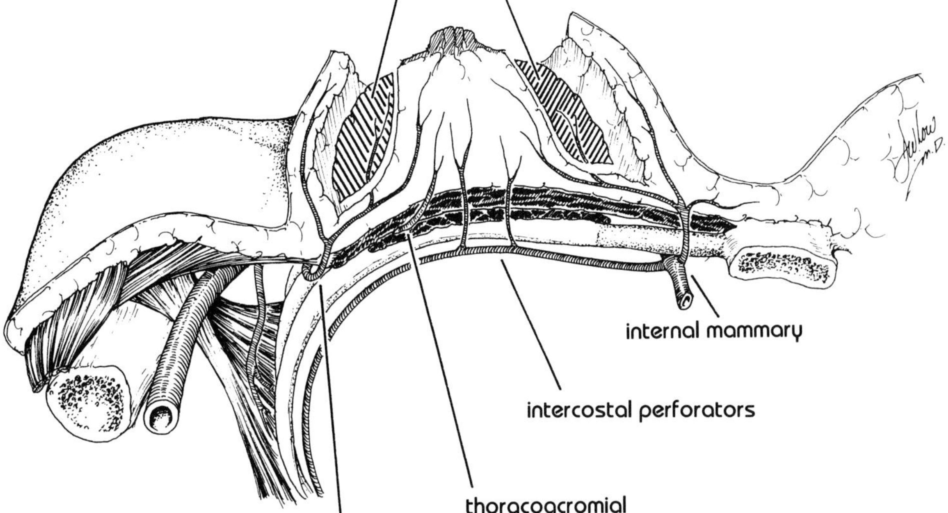

FIGURE 21-2 The anatomic basis for the central pedicle technique of reduction mammaplasty. (Adapted from Hester TR, Bostwick J, Miller L, Cunningham SJ. Breast reduction utilizing the maximally central breast pedicle. Plast Reconstr Surg 1985; 76: 890.)

Details of Surgical Technique

After the breasts have been marked, I prefer to infiltrate in the planes of dissection with a solution of 0.5 percent lidocaine and 1:200,000 epinephrine. This means that transfusion is rarely needed. The triangular segment is de-epithelialized around the areola and inferiorly to the inframammary fold. As mentioned, the skin flaps are kept uniform and at least 2 cm thick. The medial flap is dissected first, followed by the lateral flap and finally the superior flap. The dissection stops at least 2 to 3 cm from the chest wall in order to maximally preserve blood supply to both skin flaps and parenchyma.

The parenchymal mound is then reduced by tangential planing over all segments. Most glandular tissue is usually resected over the lateral surface of the cone; less is resected medially and superiorly. Ramselaar recommended resection in six planes with avoidance of the sensory nerve to the nipple at the 4 o'clock position on the left side and the 8 o'clock position on the right side.[8]

The skin reduction is then accomplished in a "freehand" manner. The gland and nipple-areola complex are pushed superiorly as the skin flaps are drawn caudally, and temporary vertical closure is then accomplished. If further skin must be removed, Allis clamps or mattress sutures with a straight Keith needle help approximate the amount of skin to be resected along the vertical limb of the closure. Large medial and lateral dog-ears are then resected, advancing the skin flaps toward the apex of the T to minimize the length of the horizontal scar. Approximately 30 percent of the total weight of the reduction is accomplished by removal of these dog-ears.[8]

The nipple-areola complex is then exteriorized at the desired point by simply resecting or de-epithelializing an appropriate disc of skin (Fig. 21-3).

Results

Moufarrege reported his experience with over 700 cases of breast reduction using his modification of the central mound technique. Very few complications were reported, with good nipple sensation and normal lactation in 20 patients who became pregnant after the reduction.[11] Hester and colleagues reported 65 patients with reductions ranging between 90 and 1,300 g per breast.[8] Again the technique was shown to produce relatively few major complications, with a slightly increased incidence of postoperative temporary skin induration and small hematomas because of the wide undermining.

Advantages and Disadvantages

The advantages of this method are the preservation of the maximal blood supply to the nipple-areola complex while at the same time allowing maximal movement in the level of the nipple position. From an aesthetic standpoint, treating the breast parenchyma and the skin flaps as separate elements allows reassembly of the components in virtually unrestricted proportions (Fig. 21-4). This flexibility of

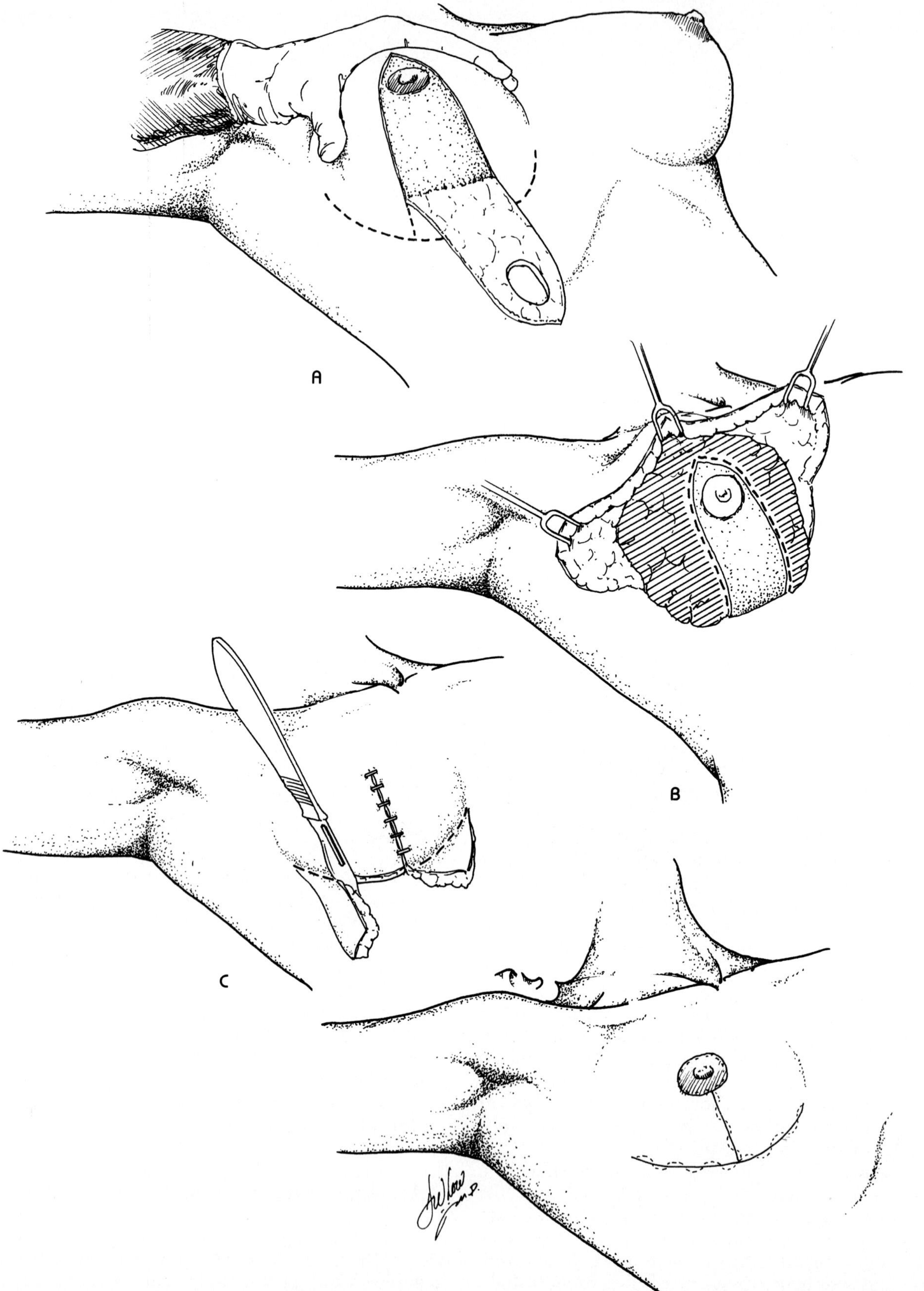

FIGURE 21–3 *A*, Preoperative markings for the central pedicle technique demonstrating the area to be de-epithelialized. *B*, The extent of glandular resection is indicated by horizontal lines. Usually more is resected laterally than either superiorly or medially. *C*, Temporary closure and resection of excess skin medially and laterally. *D*, Final closure.

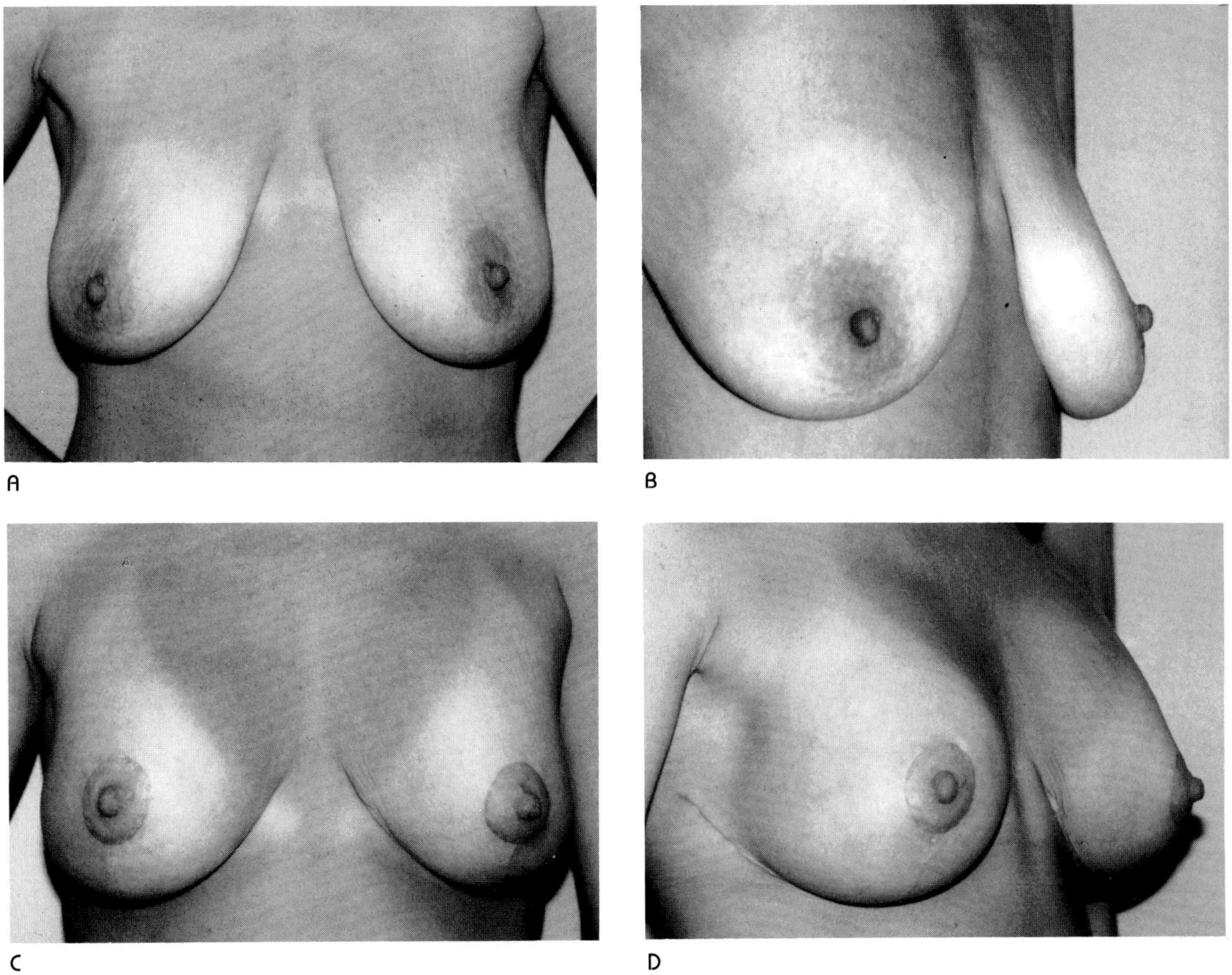

FIGURE 21-4 *A*, A 30-year-old woman with severe ptosis and glandular atrophy: preoperative view. *B*, Oblique preoperative view. *C*, Mastopexy carried out using the central mound technique. A submuscular polyurethane-covered implant was placed at the same time. *D*, Oblique postoperative view.

the central mound technique is of great advantage to a surgeon who likes a freehand sculpturing technique. However, a predetermined pattern can just as easily be used. Theoretically, with the preservation of maximal parenchymal glandular tissue, lactation and breast feeding is possible in the premenopausal woman.

The disadvantages relate to the possible complications that can occur from wide skin undermining. Pitanguy also pointed out the ectodermal origin of the gland from the skin, noting that skin undermining destroys this relationship and possibly the suspension of the gland.[12] However, if one is careful not to dissect too close to the chest wall, skin complications are rare. This technique also requires a certain level of experience and good aesthetic judgment to achieve the best results. Appropriate patient selection, as in every technique of breast reduction, is essential.

RADIAL RESECTION AND UNDERSURFACE SCULPTURING TECHNIQUES

Background and History

The first author to approach the gland from its undersurface appears to have been Thomas in 1882, in an operation designed to remove benign tumors. In the early 20th century, many authors described various techniques of breast reduction involving discoid pattern resections.[13-15] Dissatisfaction with unfavorable results from skin undermining techniques led to a variety of techniques for resecting parenchyma from the undersurface of the gland without skin undermining. In the modern era, Arié developed a technique of breast reduction using an almond-shaped resection below the areola.[16] Pitanguy modified this by beginning the incision above the areola at the point at which the nipple would ultimately be elevated.[17] In Pitanguy's technique (Fig. 21-5), the new nipple position (point A) is determined by placing a hand in the inframammary fold and projecting this level to the anterior surface of the breast in the midclavicular line. The angle of the vertical limbs (points B and C) is determined by pinching the skin on either side to determine the points that can be easily brought together without tension. This determines the amount of skin and breast to be resected in this area. Points D and E essentially demarcate the medial extent of the sulcus and its lateral extent without extending beyond the anterior axillary line. The resection includes virtually the entire inferior portion of the gland as well as a keel-shaped segment beneath the nipple-areola complex. The medial and lateral pillars of parenchymal tissue can then be approximated and the incisions closed in a T-shaped fashion.

Pitanguy's technique stimulated other authors to approach the gland in this fashion, leaving the parenchyma attached to the dermis. Most recently, modifications have sought to shorten the inframammary portion of the scar.

Patient Selection

In all the techniques to follow, the best results seem to be most predictably achieved in cases of

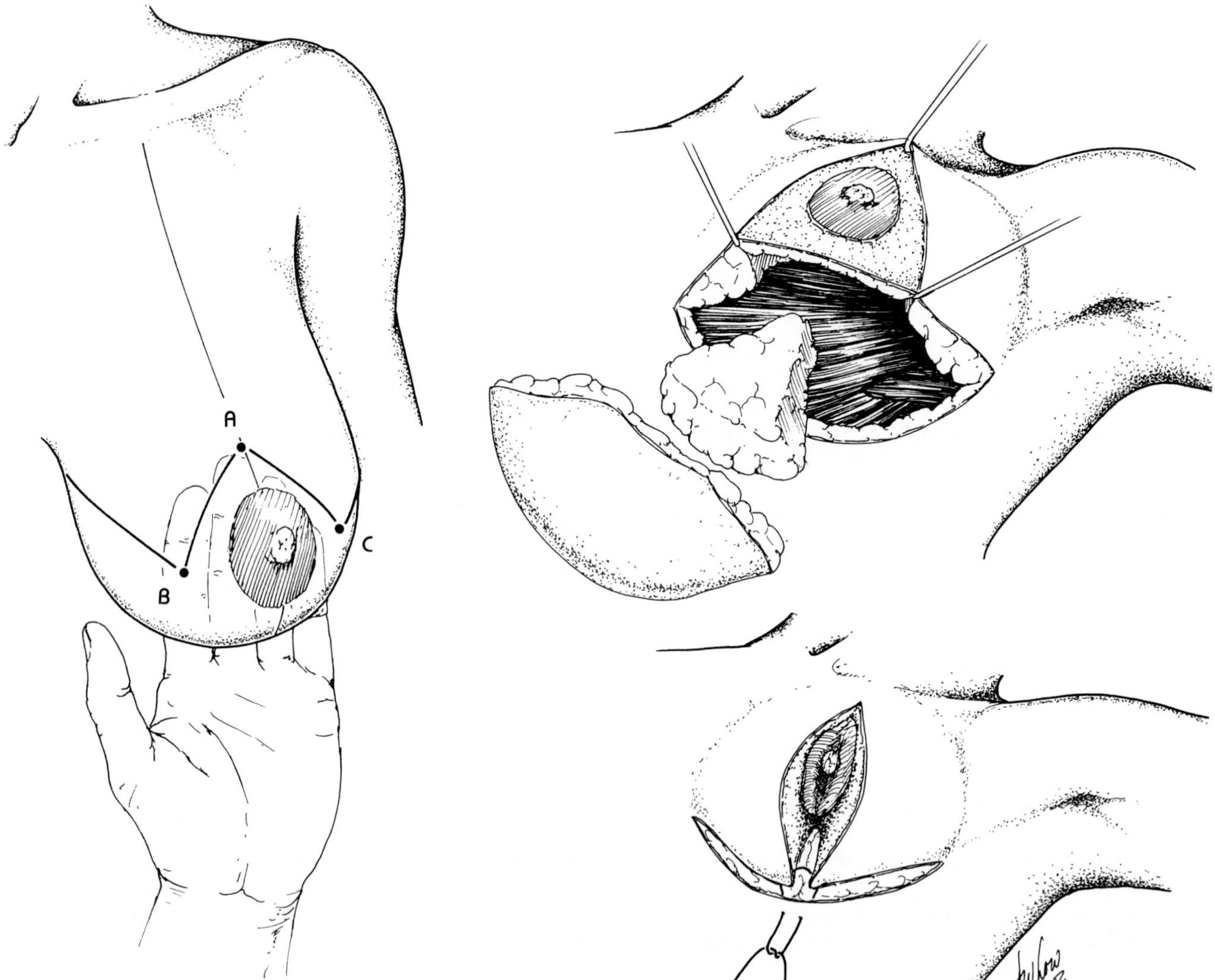

FIGURE 21-5 *Left*, The A point in Pitanguy's method of reduction mammoplasty is determined by the level of the inframammary fold at the midline of the breast reflected onto its anterior surface. Points B and C are varied, depending on the elasticity or redundancy of the skin. *Upper right*, The resection of the gland is carried out primarily in the inferior pole and a radial wedge beneath the nipple and areola. *Lower right*, Initial closure is achieved by bringing points B and C together at the midline of the breast in the inframammary fold.

mild to moderate hypertrophy not exceeding 800 g. In general, the larger the breast, or the greater the ptosis, the more difficult it is to produce an acceptable result with short scars. Therefore, for true gigantomastia, techniques such as the inferior pedicle or free nipple grafting may give more freedom to bring the nipple-areola complex to the desired level without tension. Nevertheless, surgeons who are experienced with undersurface sculpturing techniques are able to achieve predictably good results, even in patients with larger breasts.

Peixoto Technique

Among modern authors, Peixoto has been one of the main proponents of sculpturing the breast from its undersurface through limited incisions. The concept is that of the breast representing a cone whose altitude can be lowered by resecting its base (Fig. 21-6).[18-20] In 1980, Piexoto published his technique for breast reduction and mastopexy. The essential components are as follows. First, the skin resection may vary from none at all to a considerable amount

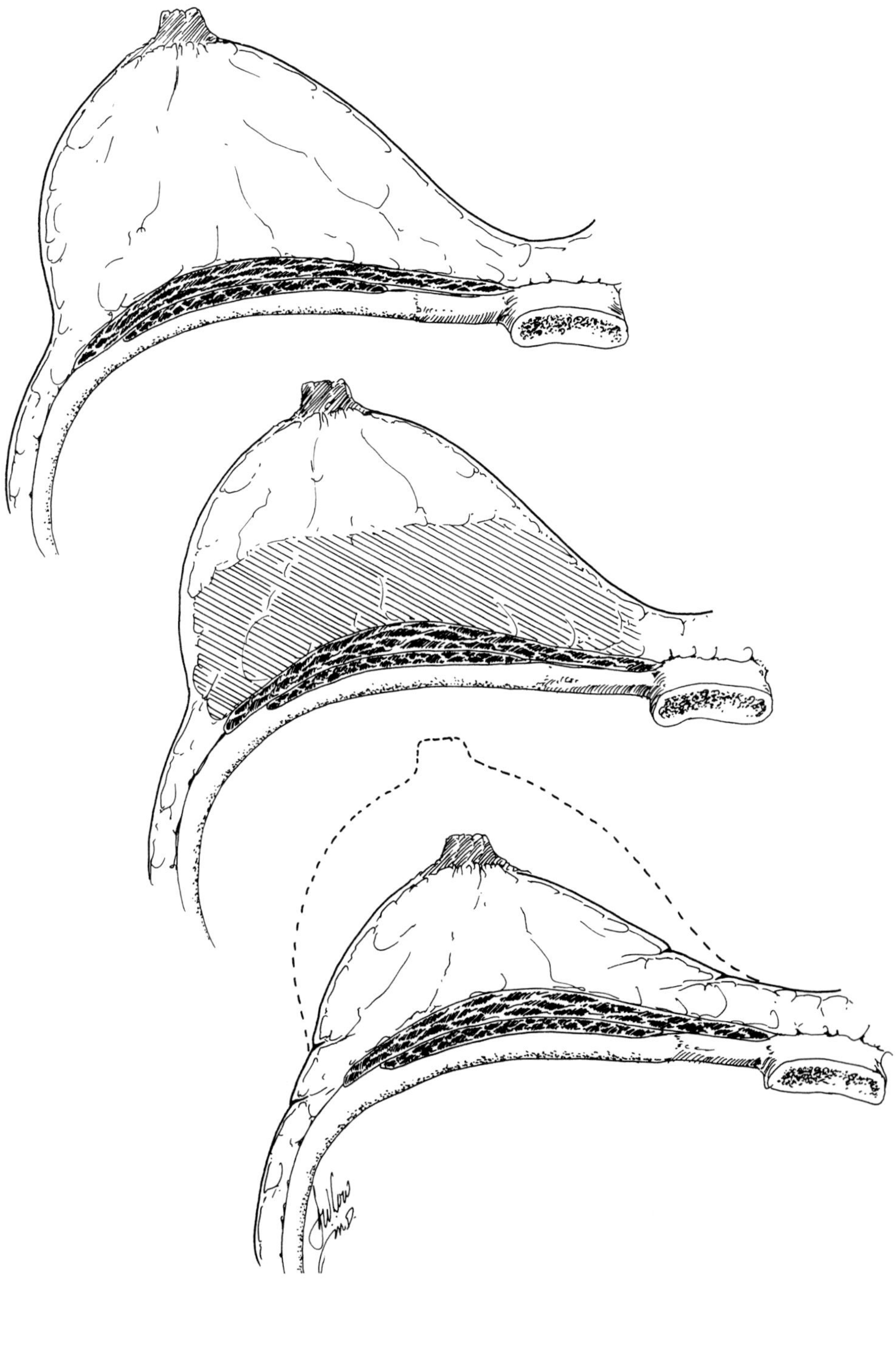

FIGURE 21-6 In Piexoto's view, it is unnecessary to excise a large amount of skin when the skin has normal contractility. By resecting glandular parenchyma at the base, the skin can be expected to contract much as it does after a mastectomy. Of course, with damaged skin and large numbers of striae, the skin cannot be expected to contract as much.

in cases of gigantomastia. The final scar is limited to the periareolar area and a single vertical segment, with occasional need for a short horizontal scar just above the inframammary fold. The gland is completely freed from the pectoralis fascia, and the base of the gland is amputated in an oblique fashion in every case to reduce the height of the cone and conform to the chest wall. The variety of markings is seen in Figure 21-7. The amount of excess skin to be resected is estimated using the bidigital pinch technique, both above the nipple-areola complex and horizontally below. The method also depends on the natural elastic qualities of the skin to shrink to fit the new glandular cone. If the breast is excessively wide, a V-shaped excision is also carried out beneath the nipple complex.

Complications

Peixoto reported very few complications with this technique but stated that the method is more difficult to use in elderly patients with giant hypertrophy. Other authors have pointed out the tendency for widening of the vertical scar and the inability to raise the nipple-areola complex more than 6 cm.[21] Also, if the skin does not shrink to the desired breast shape, secondary revisions may be necessary. This is particularly true in large glandular resections, for which Piexoto occasionally recommends a two-stage technique.

The Marchac Technique

In an effort to combine glandular remodeling from the undersurface with a short horizontal scar, Daniel Marchac combined techniques published by several other authors. He credited Dufourmentel and Mouly with the development of a wedge resection of glandular tissue corresponding to a parenchymal elliptical excision going from areola to axilla. After developing some experience with Pitanguy's method as well as the resection techniques of Arié, Marchac

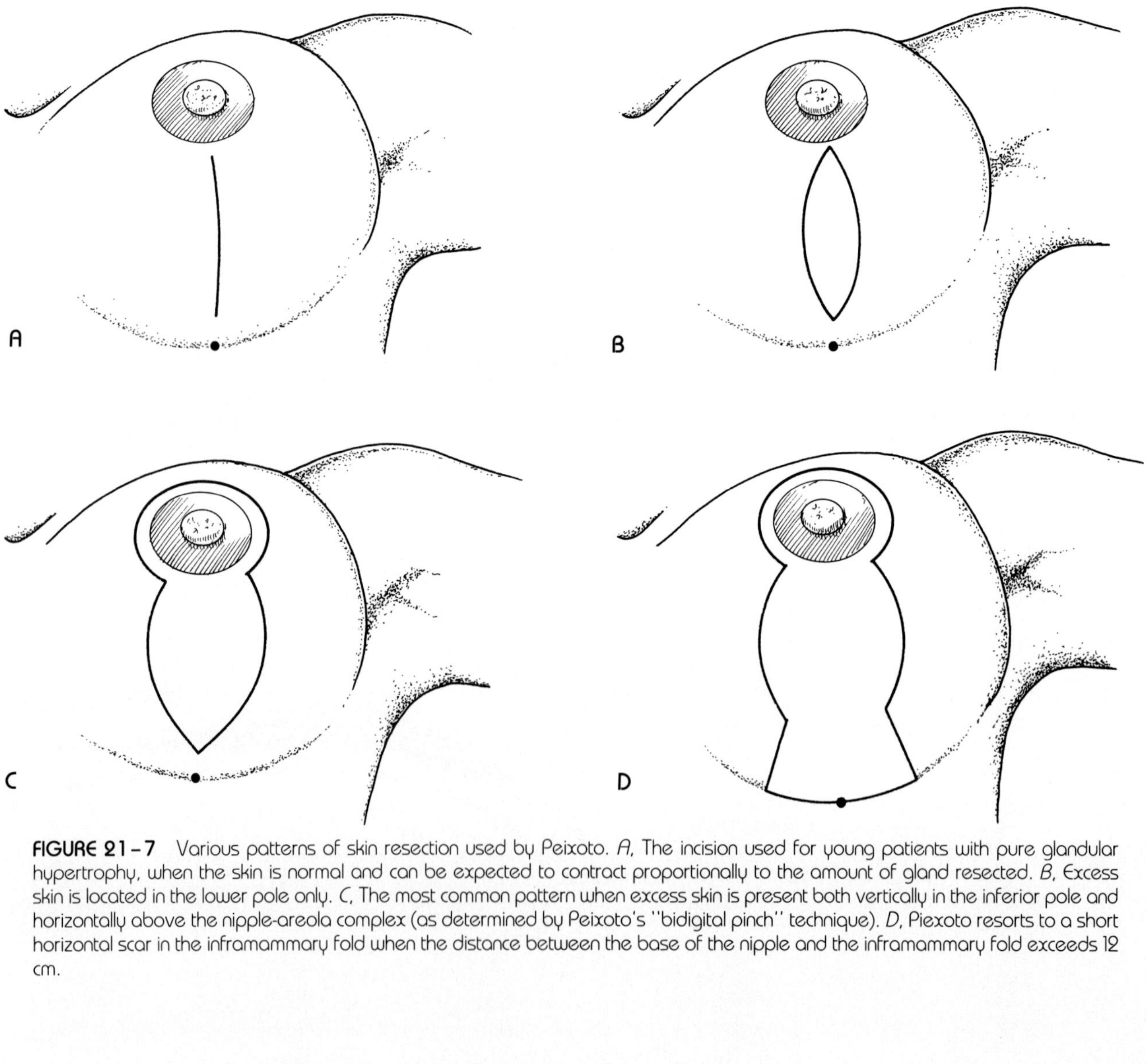

FIGURE 21-7 Various patterns of skin resection used by Peixoto. *A*, The incision used for young patients with pure glandular hypertrophy, when the skin is normal and can be expected to contract proportionally to the amount of gland resected. *B*, Excess skin is located in the lower pole only. *C*, The most common pattern when excess skin is present both vertically in the inferior pole and horizontally above the nipple-areola complex (as determined by Peixoto's "bidigital pinch" technique). *D*, Piexoto resorts to a short horizontal scar in the inframammary fold when the distance between the base of the nipple and the inframammary fold exceeds 12 cm.

blended the three techniques together, adding the idea of stopping the vertical excision above the inframammary fold to convert some of the lower breast skin into abdominal tissue.

The breast can be marked in the operating room with the patient in the semisitting position. The following markings are made (Fig. 21-8):

1. The vertical axis of the breast is marked where the nipple and areola will be relocated. In the average patient, this line is usually 8 to 10 cm from the vertical midline.
2. By moving the breast first laterally and then medially, the medial and lateral sides of the estimated skin excision are marked. These line up with the vertical axis of the breast.
3. The medial and lateral sides of the skin excision are then connected with a curved line parallel with the inframammary fold but approximately 5 cm above it. By pinching the medial and lateral lines together, the markings are checked to make sure there is no excessive tension after the skin resection.
4. Five-cm limbs are then marked upward from the inferior curved line that will represent the vertical closure of the eventual T-shaped scar. From these points a semicircle is drawn above the nipple-areola complex to connect the two sides. A small indentation is made on either side of the upper point of the vertical closure line to ultimately diminish tension on the periareolar closure.

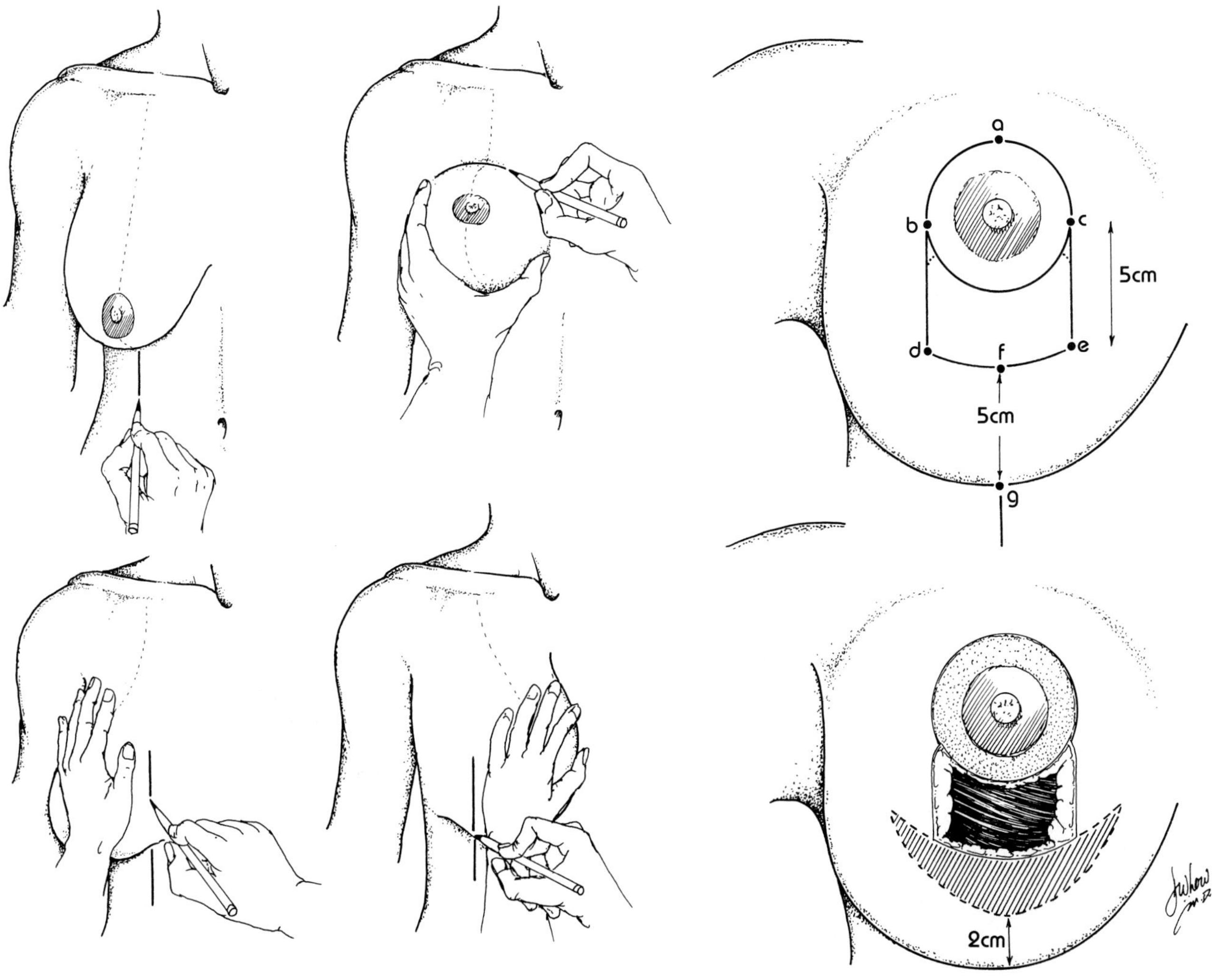

FIGURE 21-8 The markings of the Marchac reduction mammoplasty technique. The midline of the breast (a–f–g) and the upper extent of the parenchyma are marked. The skin resection is determined by gently moving the gland laterally and medially and drawing a line that corresponds with the midline of the breast (b–d, c–e). The skin between these two lines is then pinched to estimate whether this amount of skin can be safely removed. For most reductions the initial horizontal line (d–f–e) is marked at 5 cm and parallel with the inframammary fold. Ultimately the new inframammary fold moves up approximately 2 cm higher than the original fold (g). See text for details. The upper pole of the areola will ultimately end up at point a.

Marchac recommended marking a scale from the midclavicle to the nipple on each side to aid in placing the nipple-areola complexes at the same level after reduction. The key points are then tattooed. The semicircle down to the level of the indentations is de-epithelialized. Below this point the medial and lateral limbs are incised full thickness through the skin. Between the indentations the breast parenchyma is incised to about 2-cm thickness. The inferior breast skin is elevated with some subcutaneous fat down to the inframammary fold. The entire gland is then undermined to the superior extent of the breast tissue.

The resection of the gland is carried out in a vertical wedge beneath the nipple and areola and the base, in a manner similar to Pitanguy's method. The breast is suspended by placing a key suture beneath the nipple-areola complex, anchoring it to the fascia at the superior portion of the undermined gland. As this suture is tied down, a superior fullness is created. The medial and lateral parenchymal pillars are approximated along the 5-cm vertical skin markings. The vertical skin closure should come together with no tension following the parenchymal approximation.

The lower portion of the remaining breast tissue is freed up and trimmed as necessary to empty the area between the old inframammary fold and the new one, which is usually 2 cm higher. This is the unique feature of this type of reduction, which purposefully raises the inframammary fold. The medial and lateral dog-ears are then simply excised through the shortest possible horizontal incision. The details of this technique are presented in several earlier reports by Marchac and colleagues.[22–24]

Postoperative Care

One of the most important factors in the postoperative care of patients who have undergone this type of reduction is the wearing of a brassiere with a relatively wide elastic band to assist in the molding of the new inframammary fold and the flattening out of the breast skin that has been converted to abdominal wall skin.

Results

In Marchac's own series of 176 patients operated on between 1977 and 1986, he achieved a pleasing shape in most cases and a lasting correction that actually improved with time.[23] Fifty percent of the patients had normal sensation; 25 percent reported transient diminution but subsequent recovery; 7 percent experienced permanent attenuation of sensitivity. Compression below the new inframammary fold is essential to prevent sliding of the breast tissue into the space between the old inframammary fold and the new one (Figs. 21–9, 21–10).

Pontes currently has developed his own modification of a similar method, attributing the resection technique to Lexer.[25,26] In Pontes' technique the medial and lateral lines are drawn in an almond shape extending from the estimated point of the nipple position to, and ending approximately 1 to 2 cm above, the inframammary fold. The method then calls for a variable glandular resection, depending on the size and shape of the breast. Usually, a vertical wedge of tissue is resected with some removal of the base. Ribeiro described a similar method of marking the skin, which he referred to as "the lozenge technique."[27] In this method an inferiorly based flap is used to increase projection and fill the superior portion of the breast.

Other Techniques of Skin Reduction

As can be seen, the various techniques discussed in this chapter involve parenchymal reduction and skin resection in an effort to minimize scars. There are several other important techniques of dealing with the skin excess that will be mentioned only briefly here.

L-Shaped Scars

The lateral method of reduction mammaplasty is generally credited to Hollander. In the 1960s, Dufourmentel and Roullete used the oblique technique with a wedge resection of glandular tissue corresponding to the skin excision. Kesselring and Meyer developed a technique for reduction of breast volume across the base of the breast and taking up some of the excess skin in the periareolar area, with the remainder in an L-shaped or curving incision toward the lateral inframammary fold.[28] Bozola from Brazil refined the J or L mammaplasty to keep the scar as short and lateral as possible just above the inframammary fold (Fig. 21–11).[29] In this technique the A point is marked according to the Pitanguy method. The M point is on the midline of the breast and represents the most anteriorly projecting point on the breast. This may or may not correlate with the nipple. Using the A–M distance as a radius, a semicircle is drawn with the M point at its center. The A–M distance is then also used to mark a curving resection of skin at the base of the breast to rotate the scar into a J or L-shaped incision. In both the Kesselring-Meyer and Bozola techniques, if there is a large amount of ptosis, a short medial resection of skin is also made to avoid lengthening the lateral incision past the anterior axillary line. In smaller breasts, Bozola is able to accomplish the reduction through a single vertical incision, as advocated by Peixoto and others.

Maillard described a form of Z-plasty developed from the oblique techniques to keep the scar in the vertical portion of the breast between the areola and the inframammary fold. This is accomplished by re-

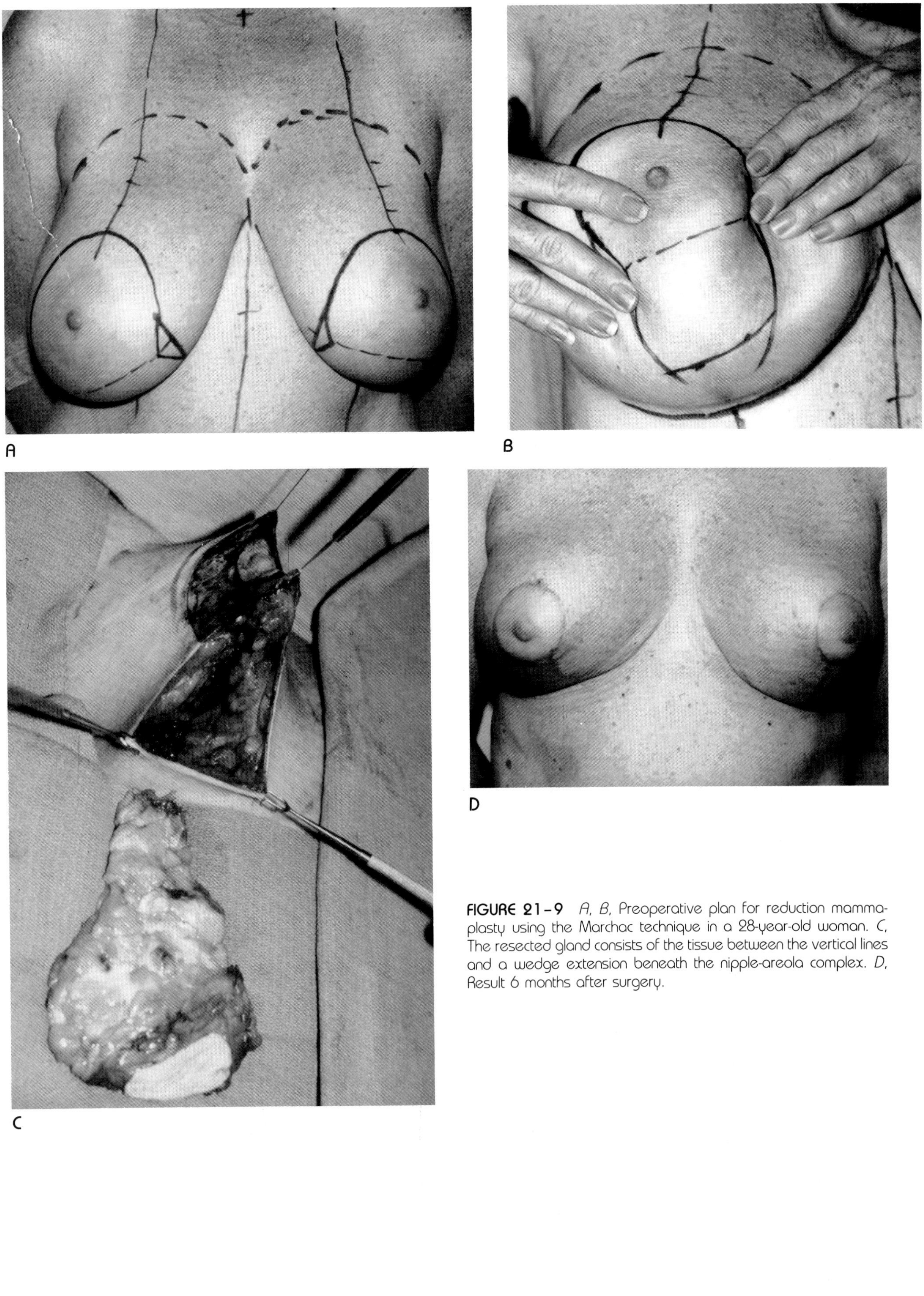

FIGURE 21–9 *A, B,* Preoperative plan for reduction mammaplasty using the Marchac technique in a 28-year-old woman. *C,* The resected gland consists of the tissue between the vertical lines and a wedge extension beneath the nipple-areola complex. *D,* Result 6 months after surgery.

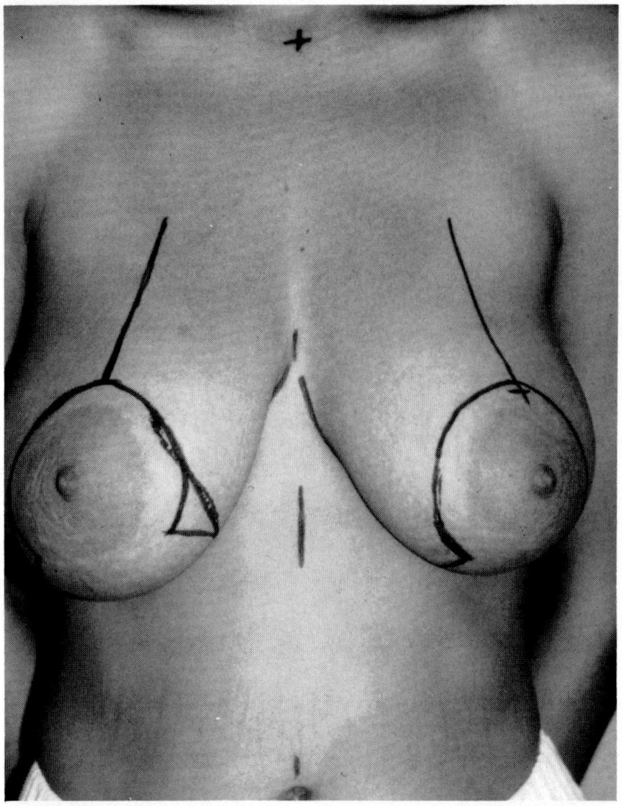

A

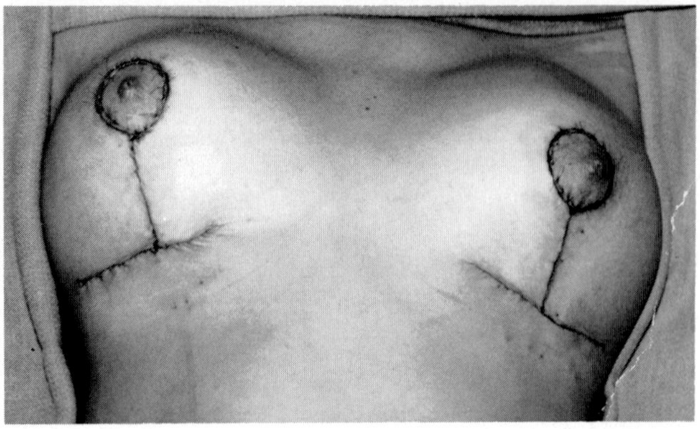

B

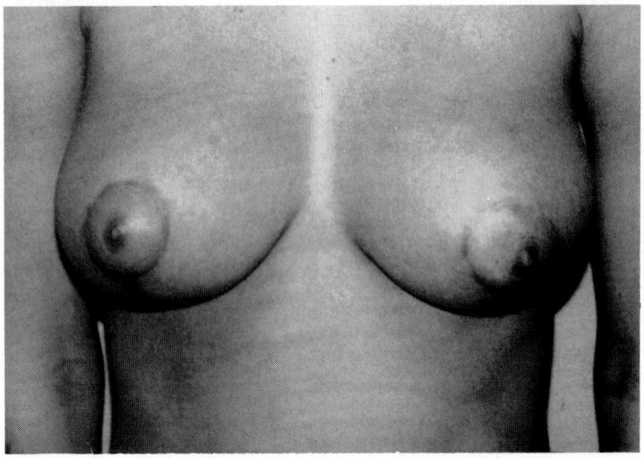

C

FIGURE 21–10 *A*, Marchac reduction preoperative plan for a 26-year-old patient. *B*, After resection and initial closure. *C*, Result 1 year after surgery.

secting the base of the breast through an "arched gateway" type of figure (Fig. 21–12). This creates two triangular-shaped flaps. After the nipple-areola complex has been raised to the appropriate level, the medial flap is drawn around the complex to take up the excess skin, closing much like the diaphragm of a camera. The lateral triangular flap is then brought into the inframammary fold so that the closure is shaped much like a Z-plasty. Maillard produced his best results in younger patients with less than 500 g resected, but also was able to use the technique in patients with up to 900 g resection.

Over the past decade, the trend in reduction mammaplasty has been toward reshaping the parenchymal mound either from its surface or from its base, followed by tailoring of the skin to resect the excess with as short scars as possible. Many of these techniques rely on the expected shrinkage of the skin that seems to occur best in younger patients, but always occurs to some extent, as seen in subcutaneous mastectomy patients. However, the larger the reduction and the greater amount of ptosis present, the more difficult it is to produce a natural shape with short scars. These patients, perhaps, offer the greatest challenge in reconstructive and aesthetic breast surgery.

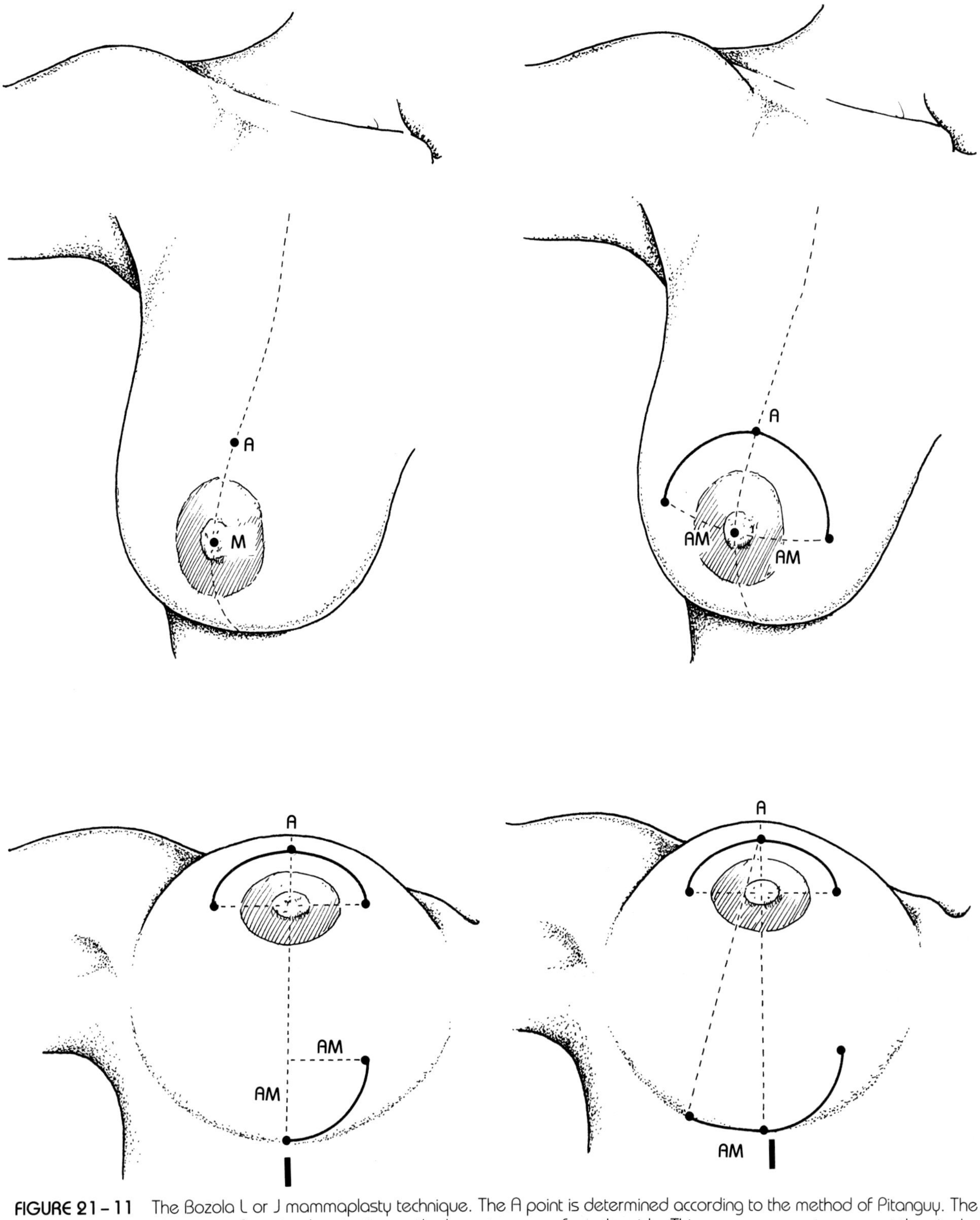

FIGURE 21-11 The Bozola L or J mammaplasty technique. The A point is determined according to the method of Pitanguy. The M point represents the point of maximal projection on the breast as seen from the side. This may or may not represent the nipple. The A–M distance is then used to make all the other markings as shown. A curving resection of skin at the base of the breast allows rotation of the breast closure into a J- or L-shaped scar.

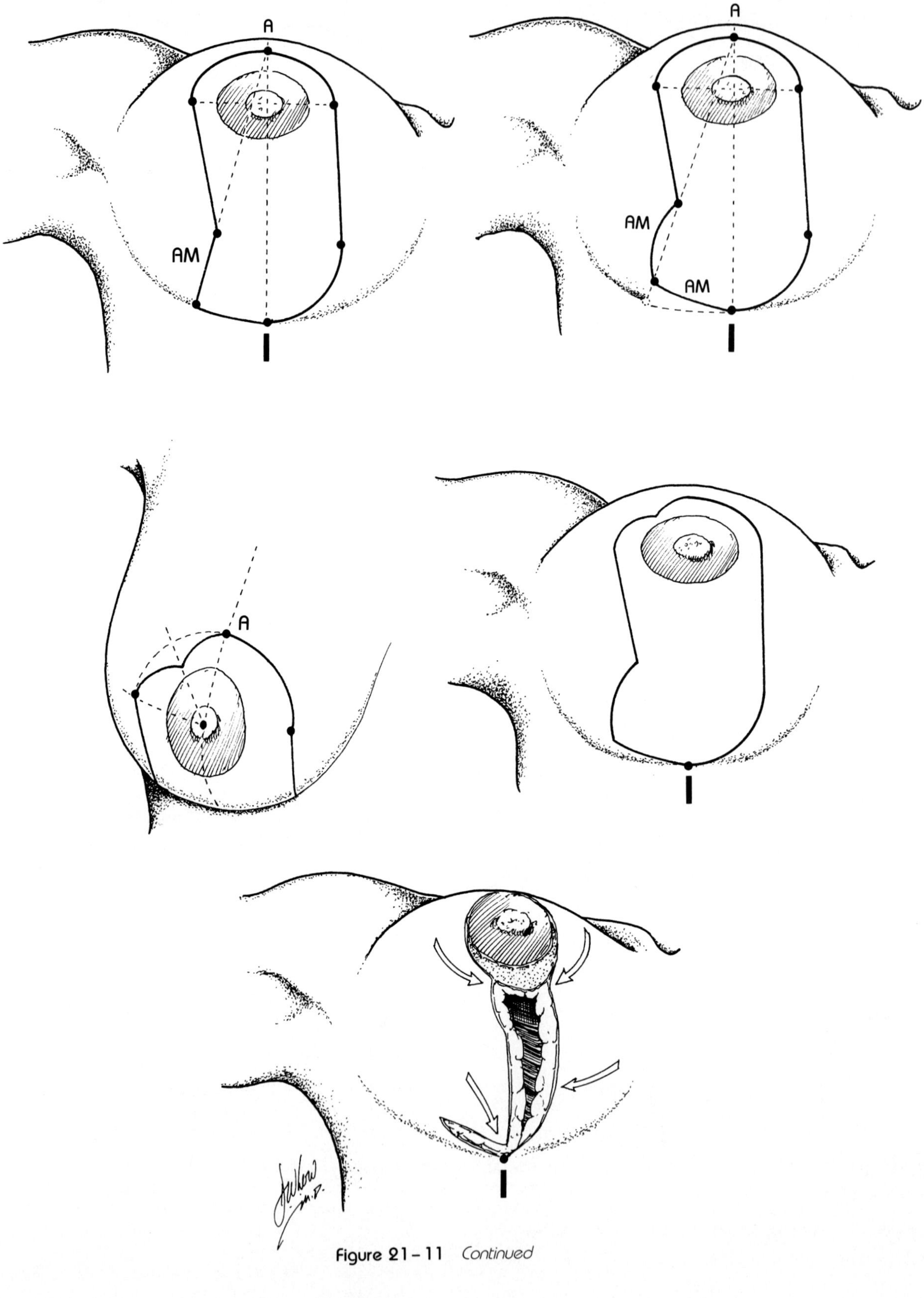

Figure 21–11 *Continued*

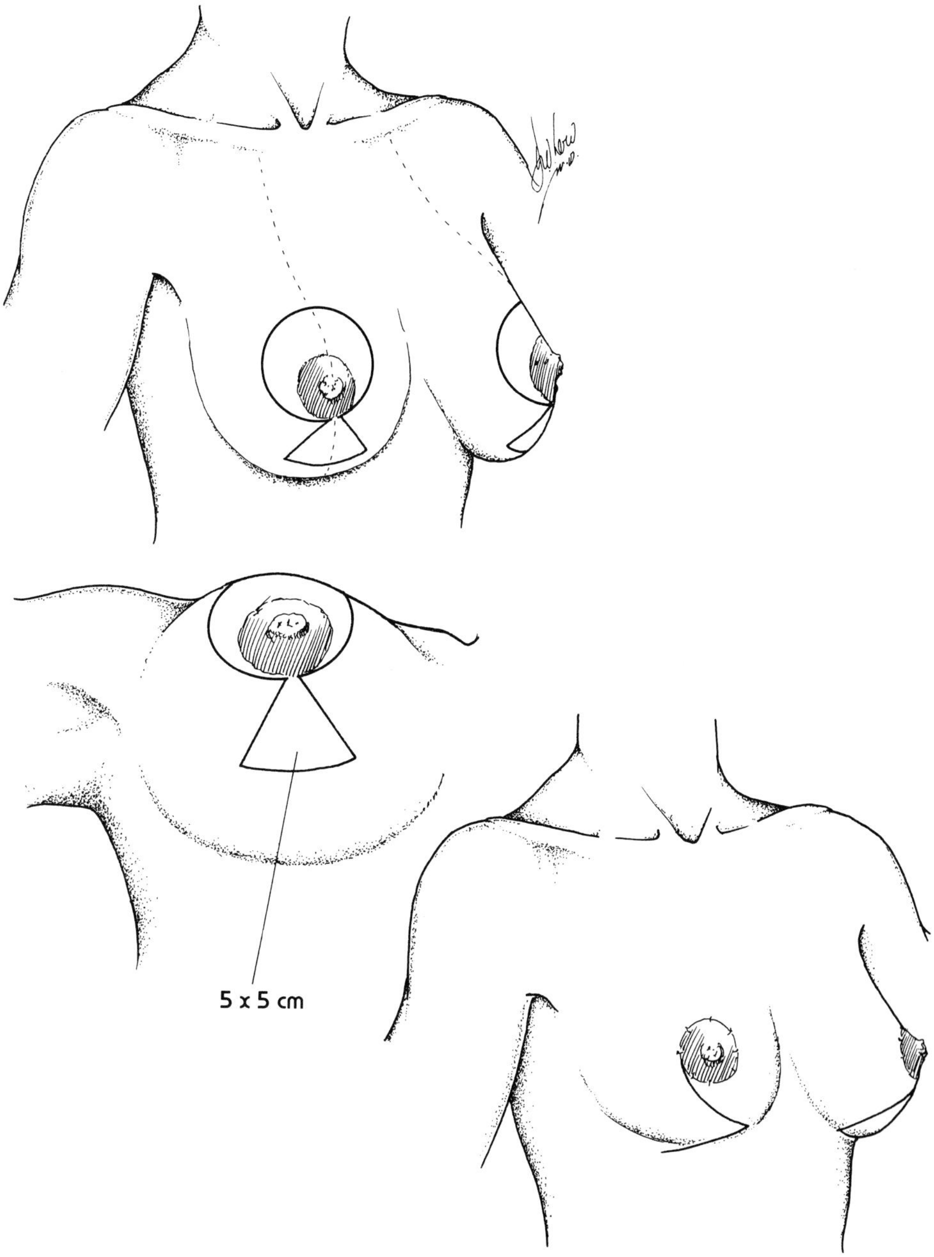

FIGURE 21-12 Maillard's technique is similar to that of Marchac. However, the excess skin below the nipple-areola complex is handled as a Z-plasty that tightens the periareolar skin much like the aperture of a lens.

References

1. Psillakis J, de Oliveira MC. History of reduction mammoplasty. In: Goldwyn RM, ed. Reduction mammoplasty. Boston: Little, Brown 1990:1.
2. Lotsch F. Über Hangebrustplastik. Zentralbl Chir 1923; 50:1241.
3. Lotsch F. Über Hangebrustplastik. Zentralbl Chir 1928; 7:603.
4. Biesenberger H. Eine neue Methode der Mammaplastik. Zentralbl Chir 1928; 55:2382.
5. Wise RJ. Preliminary report on a method of planning the mammoplasty. Plast Reconstr Surg. 1956; 17:367.
6. Festge O. Eine abgewandelte Technik bei der Mammaplastik zur Vermeidung von Mamillen- und Gewebsnekrosen. Zentralbl Chir 1960; 85:2365.
7. Ramselaar JM. Precision in breast reduction. Plast Reconstr Surg 1988; 82:631.
8. Hester TR, Bostwick J, Miller L, Cunningham SJ. Breast reduction utilizing the maxillary vascularized central breast pedicle. Plast Reconstr Surg 1985; 76:890.
9. Palmer JH, Taylor GI. The vascular territories of the anterior chest wall. Br J Plast Surg 1986; 39:287.
10. Craig RDP, Sykes PA. Nipple sensitivity following reduction mammoplasty. Br J Plast Surg 1970; 23:165.
11. Moufarrege R. Reduction mammoplasty by the total dermoglandular pedicle. Aesthetic Plast Surg 1985; 9:227.
12. Pitanguy I. Reduction mammaplasty; a personal odyssey. In: Goldwyn RM, ed. Reduction mammaplasty. Boston: Little, Brown, 1990:95.
13. Warren JC. Plastic resection of the mammary gland. Ann Surg 1907; 45:801.

14. Morestin H. Hypertrophie mammaire traitée par la resection discoide. Bull Chir Paris 1907; 33:649.
15. Guinard R. In discussion by Morestin H. "Hypertrophie mammaire traitée par la resection discoide." Bull Soc Chir Paris 1970; 33:651.
16. Arié G. Una nueva tecnica de mastoplastia. Rev Lat Am Cir Plast 1957; 3:22.
17. Pitanguy I. Mammaplastias estudo de 245 casos consecutivos e apresentacao de tecnica pessoal. Rev Bras Cirurg 1961; 42:201.
18. Peixoto G. Reduction mammoplasty: A personal technique. Plast Reconstr Surg 1980; 65:217.
19. Peixoto G. Reduction mammoplasty. Aesthetic Plast Surg 1984; 8:231.
20. Peixoto G. The infra-areolar longitudinal incision in reduction mammoplasty. Aesthetic Plast Surg 1985; 9:1.
21. Goldwyn RM. Comments on Chapter 23. In: Goldwyn RM, ed. Reduction mammoplasty. Boston: Little, Brown, 1990:362.
22. Marchac D, DeOlarte G. Reduction mammoplasty and correction of ptosis with a short inframammary scar. Plast Reconstr Surg 1982; 69:45.
23. Marchac D, Sagher U. Mammoplasty with a short horizontal scar. Evaluation and results after nine years. Clin Plast Surg 1988; 15:627.
24. Marchac D. Reduction mammoplasty with a short horizontal scar. In: Goldwyn RM, ed. Reduction mammoplasty. Boston: Little, Brown, 1990:317.
25. Lexer H. Zur Operation der Mammahypertrophie und der Hangebrust. Dtsch Med Wochenschr 1925; 51:26.
26. Pontes R. Personal communication, 1990.
27. Ribeiro L. The lozenge technique. In: Goldwyn RM, ed. Reduction mammoplasty. Boston: Little, Brown, 1990:365.
28. Kesselring U, Meyer R. Reduction mammoplasty with the L-shaped suture line. In: Goldwyn RM, ed. Reduction mammoplasty. Boston: Little, Brown, 1990:305.
29. Bozola AR. Reduction mammaplasty; preferred techniques. In: Goldwyn RM, ed. Reduction mammaplasty. Boston: Little, Brown, 1990:407.

CHAPTER 22

Reduction Mammaplasty with Free Nipple Graft

VINCENT R. DIGREGORIO, M.D.

When a plastic surgeon is faced with a patient judged both physically and psychologically suitable for reduction mammaplasty, one of the fundamental decisions concerns the choice of technique. Usually, the technique will include transfer of the nipple and areola on a pedicle, or will require removal of the nipple-areola complex and replacement as a free graft.

Early in my career, I frequently wrestled with this dilemma, attempting to choose from among the multiplicity of techniques available. I have developed certain decision-making principles that I now use when planning reduction mammaplasty.

1. If the operation is primarily a "pexy" procedure and requires elevation of the nipple-areola complex by 3 cm or less, I use a single superior pedicle technique.[1]
2. If the proposed procedure is primarily a reduction mammaplasty with an estimated nipple-areola elevation of 3 cm or more, I use a free nipple graft technique. The technique discussed in this chapter has been developed over a number of years and is one that I have come to think of as a *pyramidal reduction mammaplasty* (PRM).

This chapter concisely describes free nipple graft reduction mammaplasty using the "pyramidal technique." This technique, with minor variations, is similar to other reduction mammaplasty techniques that reconstitute the final breast form using a central wedge excision, but with one critical variation: In the PRM, the ultimate inferiorly-facing plane resulting from the removal of the ptotic inferior hemisphere of the breast (the base of the pyramid) is rotated a full 90 degrees and is ultimately attached high up on the pectoralis fascia as a breast pyramid.

RATIONALE FOR USE OF THE PYRAMIDAL REDUCTION MAMMAPLASTY

Pyramidal reduction mammaplasty is a technique that (1) is relatively easy to perform; (2) produces excellent and consistently reproducible results; (3) is adaptable to a wide variety of breast shapes and body types; (4) is not compromised by technical concerns about the vascularity of the pedicle and subsequent nipple viability; and (5) allows determination of the final nipple placement as the last step in the procedure, giving great latitude to the nipple-areola location. Furthermore, once the final location is established, it is secure and is not subject to the late postoperative dislocation and distortion caused by contraction and distortion of a nipple-areola complex–carrying pedicle.

DISADVANTAGES OF PEDICLE TECHNIQUE

When any of the multiplicity of dermal or parenchymal nipple-areola complex–carrying techniques are used, the shape of the breast and location of the complex may often be compromised by maneuvers designed to ensure the viability of the complex.

There is a greater possibility of total loss of the nipple-areola complex with the pedicle technique. Although it is difficult to determine the extent of slough following reduction mammaplasty by a pedicle technique, some suggestion of this incidence can be made by inference. In an article on the advantages of using intravenous fluorescein for evaluating the ischemic nipple-areola complex during reduction mammaplasty, Singer and Kraut[2] described four instances of duskiness or loss of the complex in 31 patients, an incidence of approximately 13 percent—an unacceptably high complication rate for an elective cosmetic operation. In my personal series of well over 200 pyramidal breast reductions with free nipple graft, there has been no loss of the complex, total or partial.

Late postoperative scar retraction of the complex-carrying pedicles may cause subsequent retraction and distortion of the complex or of the entire breast structure.

It is my impression that nipple-areola–carrying pedicle procedures in general, because of the prolonged dissection and considerations of pedicle viability, produce greater blood loss. I have never had to use a blood transfusion in PRM, and therefore consider preoperative type and cross-matching or autotransfusion preparations unnecessary.

DISADVANTAGES OF FREE NIPPLE GRAFTS

When a free nipple graft is used, the nipple-areola complex may not have as much projection as with pedicle approaches. This may or may not be the case. However, I believe the primary objective of the operation, from the patient's prospective, to be breast shape, not primarily nipple-areola complex appearance and projection. We, as surgeons, may have mistakenly focused on nipple-areola appearance, selecting techniques that compromise breast shape because of pedicle consideration, and thus inadvertently subverting the patient's primary objective.

There is an inability to lactate after the free nipple-areola graft. The ability of a breast reduced by the pedicle technique to lactate is theoretically possible, and isolated patients have been known to lactate and complete a breast-feeding program.

PATIENT SELECTION

As indicated above, if the patient is an acceptable candidate for reduction mammaplasty, the critical decision to be made centers around the extent of nipple-areola complex elevation. If the distance between the present location of the nipple prominence and the new nipple location is less than 3 cm, I use a single superior pedicle technique. If the distance of the new location is greater than 3 cm, I use the technique described below.

PREOPERATIVE EVALUATION

As with any other elective procedure, a complete and thorough litany of operative risks and consequences must be discussed in great detail with all preoperative patients. This discussion must include the possibilities of anesthetic misadventures, hemorrhage, infection, fat necrosis, inability to lactate, and loss of the nipple-areola complex. In addition, any consideration of reduction mammaplasty must include an in-depth discussion of postoperative scarring.

POSTOPERATIVE SCARRING

Patients frequently have the misunderstanding that "plastic surgery" can be performed without scars. This misapprehension must be addressed, especially in discussions of reduction mammaplasty, in which the total length of scar probably exceeds that in any other plastic surgical or reconstructive procedure. In addition, the scars often are not the "hairline" type anticipated by the patient.

Although as a general rule I try not to show preoperative and postoperative photographs to patients, I make an exception in the case of reduction mammaplasty. It is impossible for the patient to visualize the extent and the length of the scars, even with diagrams, without photographs. The latter should show patients with average results, not the best postoperative examples. This is done in order to stress the extent of scarring, not to advertise my best results. Furthermore, I indicate that the objective of the procedure is to substitute one abnormality for another, i.e., trading large, awkward breasts for breasts that have a more acceptable appearance but are obviously surgically scarred. I tell all patients that once they are topless, observers will easily determine that they have had a surgical procedure.

ULTIMATE SIZE OF THE BREASTS

Patients often ask what the ultimate size of their breasts will be. This has always been a difficult question to answer, first because it is difficult to estimate accurately the volume of breast tissue to be removed and correlate this with breast size, and second because brassiere manufacturers' sizing patterns vary. The size of the bra, as can best be determined, is calculated by measuring the chest circumference at the inframammary line and adding an arbitrary number of five. Therefore, a woman with a chest circumference measuring 29 inches at the inframammary line would have a breast size of 34. Cup size is another more arbitrary matter. Research presented in a paper given at the meeting of the New York Regional Society of Plastic and Reconstructive Surgery in 1978 indicated that the average cup size differential was 90 ml among several manufacturers tested.[3] Furthermore, in preparation for this textbook, I conducted personal telephone conversations with several brassiere manufacturers, failing to obtain any objective criteria for determining cup size.

I therefore tell my patients that their postoperative numerical bra size will remain constant, and I attempt to estimate the size of the reduction in terms of cup size: e.g., the change will be from a 34D to a 34B. Again, I stress that this is only an estimate, and that the ultimate size will be determined by surgical circumstances and the judgment of the surgeon during the operative procedure. The patient is reassured that I will try to harmonize her breast size with her body type in accordance with her general preoperative goals, i.e., to be very small or very full.

Because abnormal breast hypertrophy is frequently an affliction of young girls, timing of the operation is critical. My criteria in young girls is that they must have attained a stable breast size and maintained that constant size for at least 6 months. Obviously, operating on girls with actively increasing breast size may necessitate additional future procedures.[4-6] A thorough breast examination is performed on all women before surgery, and a baseline mammogram is obtained in women over 35 years of age.

All the above is discussed with the patient at the initial preoperative visit. At this time, I also provide patients with two Hibiclens sponges to be used in a full torso scrub, neck to pubis, posterior axillary line to posterior axillary line on the night before and the morning of admission. I prefer to perform this surgery in the hospital as a regular admission or same-day surgery admission basis, and not as an ambulatory surgical procedure.

PREOPERATIVE MARKINGS

The patient is seen the evening before surgery for final discussion and preoperative markings. These markings are critical to the ultimate success of the operation. They must be made with the patient standing, not sitting or in the supine position, because this is the position on which the patient and surgeon ultimately make the final assessment as to the postoperative result and satisfaction.

The following are the steps used in breast markings. They usually take no more than 5 minutes to complete.

1. Find the midline of the sternal notch (point S) (Fig. 22-1).
2. Establish the breast axis from the clavicle to below the inframammary fold (Fig. 22-2). The breast axis is used in this context as the roughly vertical line on which the new nipple-areola complex will be centered, approximately halfway between the medial and lateral bases of the breast. Because of breast or nipple asymmetry (Fig. 22-3, and see Fig. 22-10), this is not necessarily the midline of the breast.
3. Establish the central point of the new nipple-areola complex (Fig. 22-4, points A and A′). This is the most subjectively established point in the preoperative marking process, and is es-

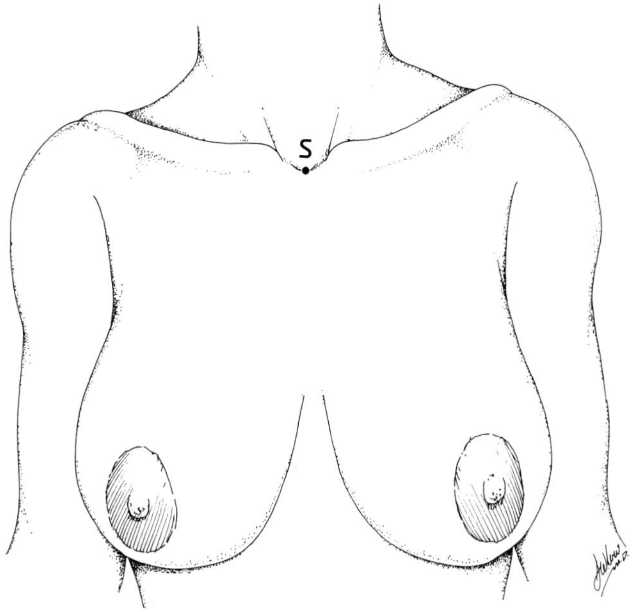

FIGURE 22-1 The first step in marking is to establish the midline at the suprasternal notch.

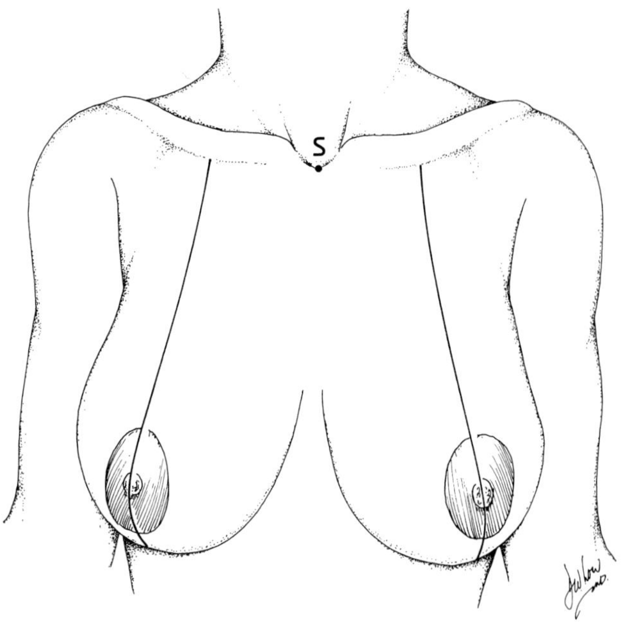

FIGURE 22-2 The breast axis is half the distance from the medial to the lateral base of the breast.

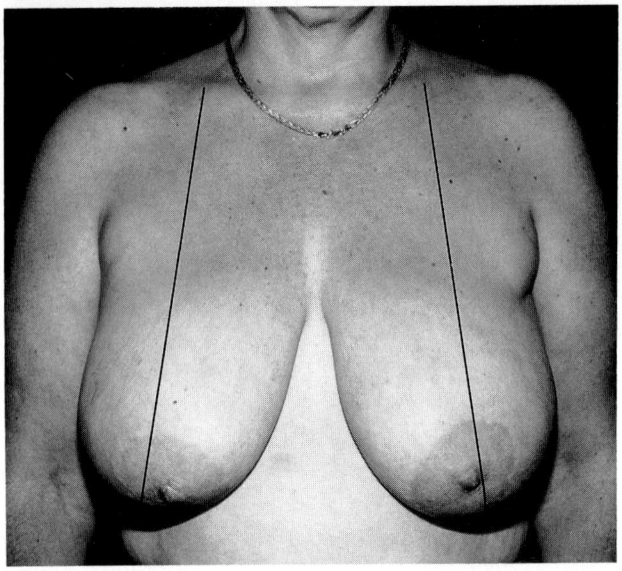

FIGURE 22-3 Breast asymmetry in hypertrophic breasts. Note that the breast axis in this case does not course through the nipple.

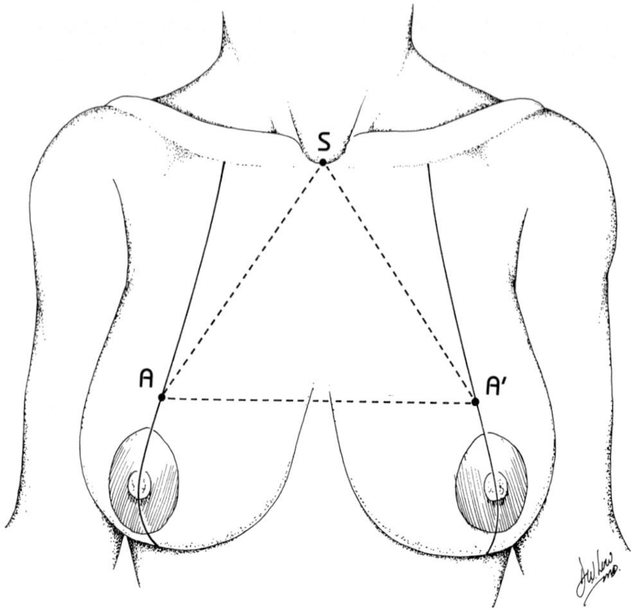

FIGURE 22-5 The equilateral triangle S-A-A′ is established.

tablished at a position 2 to 3 cm above the inframammary line on the breast axis by palpating the inframammary line with one hand and establishing point A with the other. Consideration must be given to the traction forces of gravity on the skin, especially in heavy breasts. Therefore, the breasts should be elevated proportionately during marking to compensate for these forces. Note that point A is the nipple summit and not the 6 or 12 o'clock position of the nipple-areola complex. In addition, point A is established solely in relationship to the preexisting inframammary fold, and not in relationship to distance from the clavicle or to a relative position on the humerus. When points A and A′ have been established, the distances SA, SA′, and AA′ should be equal (Fig. 22-5), thus establishing an equilateral triangle. There may be exceptions in extreme cases of very tall or very short, stout women.

4. Using a pattern (Fig. 22-6), establish the angles of the incision (approximately 97 degrees) and the length of the arms, thereby establishing points B to B′, and C to C′ (Fig. 22-7). In my experience, this pattern can be used in most women, except in the extreme example

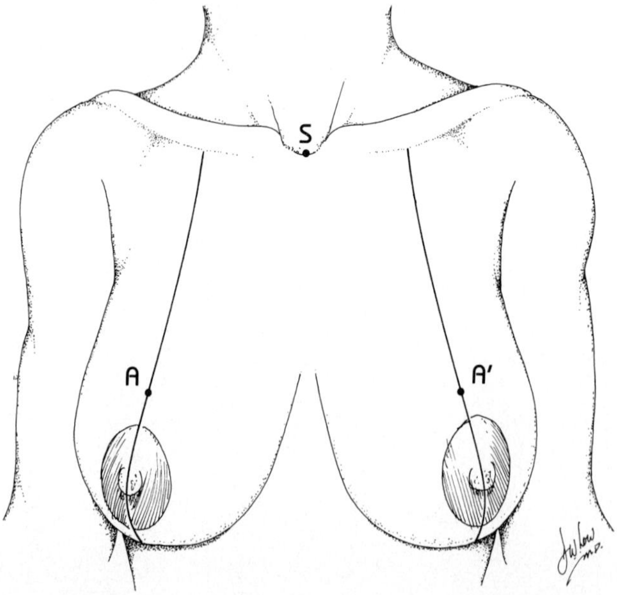

FIGURE 22-4 The central point of the new nipple-areola complex (points A and A′) is determined in relationship to the inframammary fold.

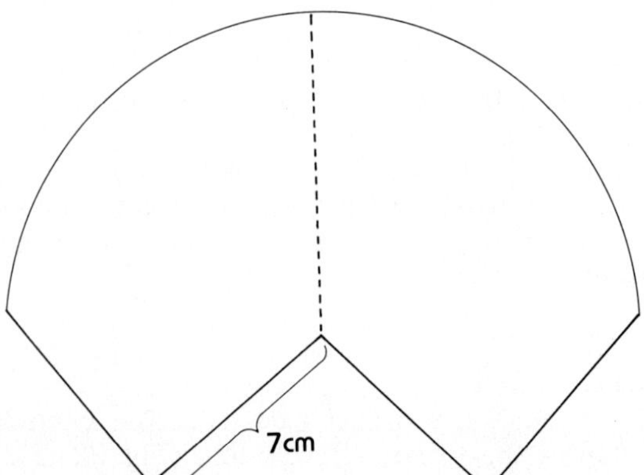

FIGURE 22-6 Pattern used to establish angles C-A-B and C′-A′-B at approximately 97 degrees.

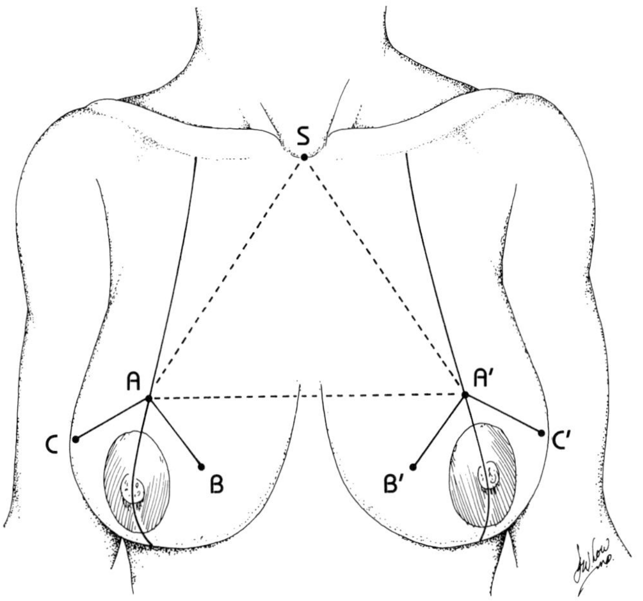

FIGURE 22-7 Points B, C, B′, and C′ are established by using the pattern.

of the very wide breast for which the angles must be proportionately increased. However, this is a rare occurrence, and if the surgeon is in doubt, this accommodation of increased angle can be made during the procedure.

5. Establish the lateral limits of the horizontal incision (Fig. 22-8). Medially these (points D and D′) are obvious. However, when these two medial breast points are very close to one another or meet, or when there is a preexisting web across the sternum, they must be staggered to prevent postoperative cicatricial webbing.
6. Care must be taken when establishing the lateral limits of the horizontal incision (point E). This point is always above the natural lateral extension of the inframammary line and is usually between the anterior axillary and midaxillary line. If point E is located in the natural extension of the inframammary line (point F), it will invariably be too low postoperatively (Fig. 22-9).
7. Establish the horizontal incision by connecting points D and E.
8. The distances B to D and C to E should roughly equal or approximate the distance E to D in order to establish the desired breast shape and projection (Fig. 22-10).

OPERATIVE PROCEDURE

Just as the preoperative breast markings are performed with the patient in the standing position, and for the same reasons, the operative procedure must be carried out with the patient in as much of the vertical position as possible. This is best accomplished in the padded chaise lounge position (Figs. 22-11, 22-12).[11] The elements of this position are (1) table back at 50 degrees plus from horizontal, (2) table break at 20 degrees plus from the horizontal position, (3) leg break at 30 degrees minus from horizontal position, and (4) footboard at 90 degrees plus from the leg position of the table.

Two additional precautions should be taken. First, pneumatic, cycling, antiembolic stockings should be used as a guard against lower-extremity

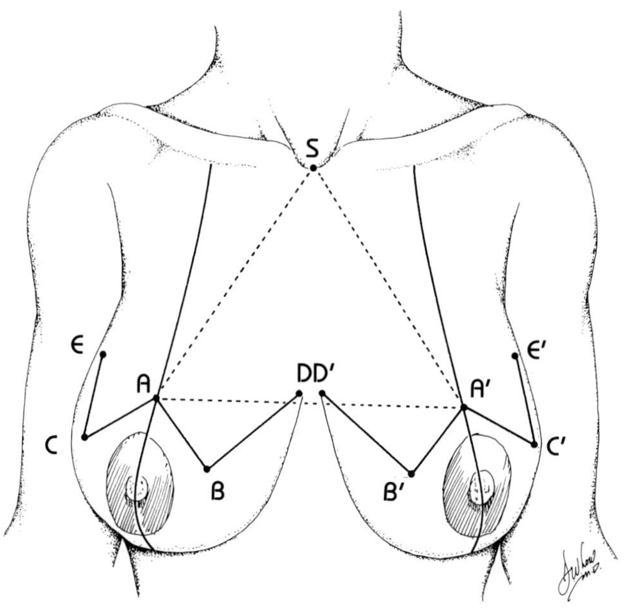

FIGURE 22-8 Points D, E, D′, and E′ are the medial and lateral limits of the horizontal incision.

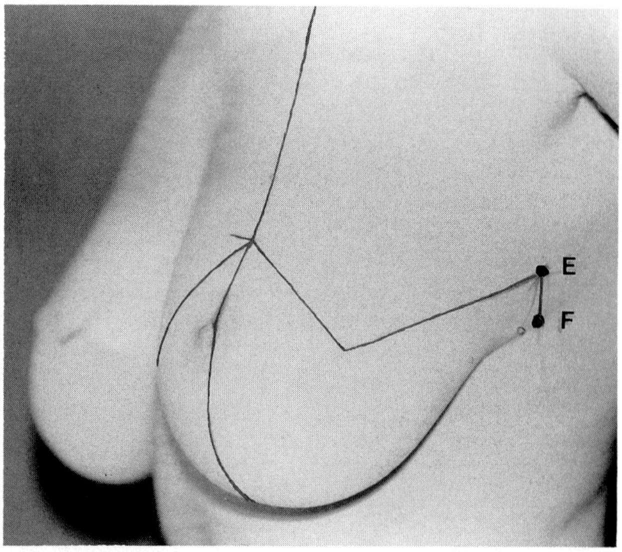

FIGURE 22-9 Point E is always located *above* the natural lateral extension of the inframammary line (F).

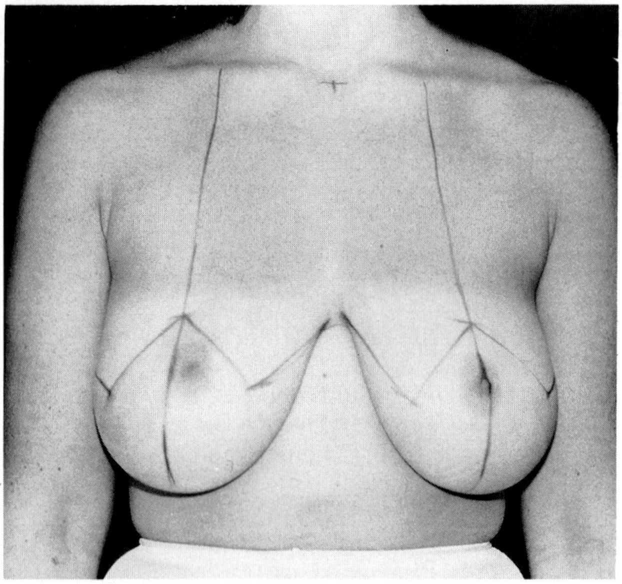

FIGURE 22-10 Patient at completion of preoperative breast markings. Note that the breast axis is lateral to the nipple-areola complex on the right breast. Also note the transsternal breast webbing necessitating staggering of points D and D′.

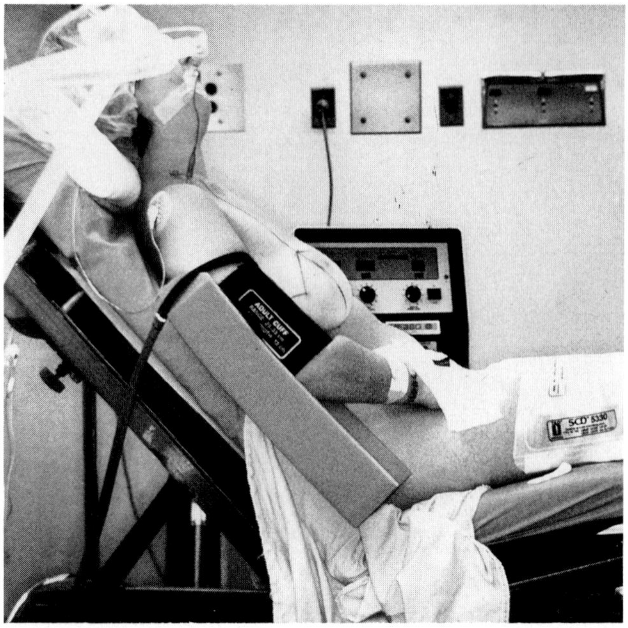

FIGURE 22-12 Lateral view of the padded "chaise lounge" position.

thrombosis and subsequent embolization. Second, the head should be taped in the anatomic position across the forehead to prevent sideway slumping of the head with subsequent shoulder, torso, and breast distortion. The anesthesiologist must be made aware

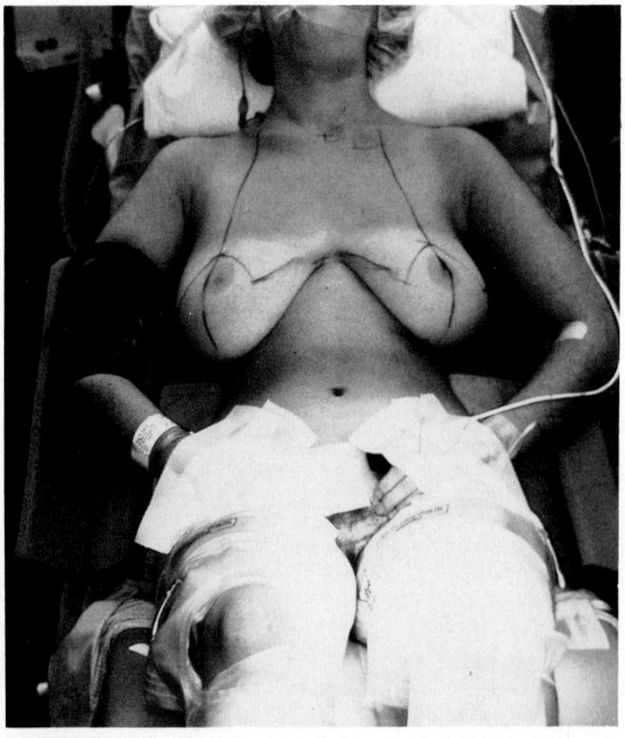

FIGURE 22-11 Frontal view of the padded "chaise lounge" position.

of the importance of maintaining this position during the procedure, because once the patient is draped, the former is in the best position to observe the head and shoulders. The hands are then taped into position in the inguinal area, and the elbows, popliteal surfaces, and plantar surfaces of the feet are padded.

The patient is then prepped and draped in the usual sterile fashion, and great care is taken to allow maximal exposure of the base of the neck, clavicles, lateral chest, and abdomen, in order to maintain proper perspective of the torso and breasts during the procedure.

The surgery is performed one breast at a time. All dissection should be performed by the same surgeon, because as much information is obtained by the sensation of the dominant hand cutting, and the sensation of the nondominant hand palpating and retracting, as by visual clues.

The new nipple-areola complex is marked using a 38-mm circular "cookie cutting" pattern. The complex is next removed as a composite graft, including nipple, areola, and as much smooth muscle as possible. There is an easily defined dissection plane just below the dermis that allows removal of the complex with all the nipple and some of the smooth muscle fibers of the complex intact. The complex is placed aside in a nutritive solution for further use.

At this point, a line is drawn 2 cm distant from and parallel to the lines A to B and A to C (Fig. 22-13). The inverted V thus transcribed is then de-epithelialized to be used to further strengthen the intrinsically weak vertical junction section of the inverted-T incision during final suturing. Skin incisions B to D, C to E, and D to E are made through the skin

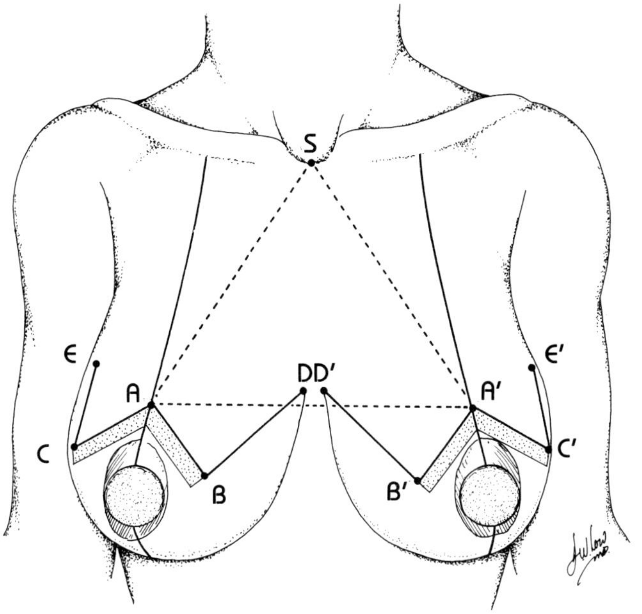

FIGURE 22-13 Central deepithelialized inverted V is used to reinforce the suturing of the intrinsically weak vertical incision.

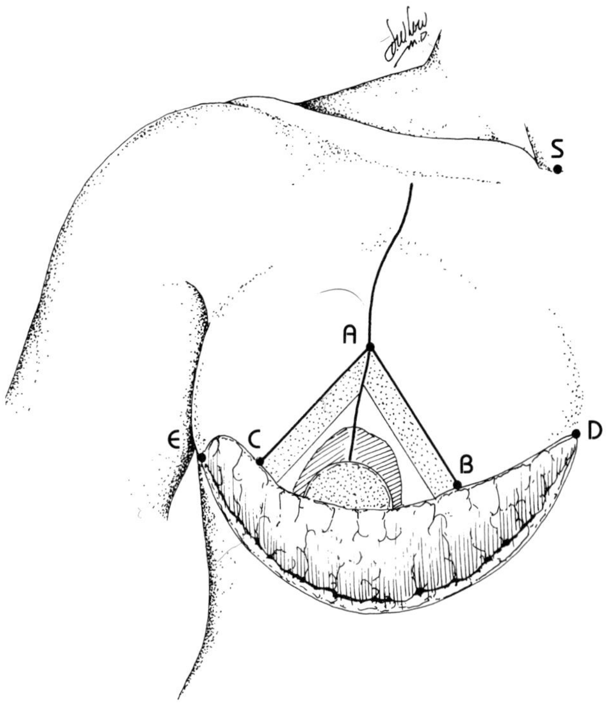

FIGURE 22-14 The inferior planar surface is established after removal of excess inferior breast tissue.

and into the underlying tissue. In an effort to minimize bleeding and conserve time, all dissection after this point is made by electrocautery using the spatulate tip.

The breast is then dissected off the chest wall at the level of the pectoralis major fascia. This dissection is made the entire width of the incision and to a point 5 cm below the clavicles. As discussed below, this cephalic extension of the superior dissection is necessary in order to rotate the base of the breast 90 degrees and suspend it cephalically from the pectoralis fascia, thus establishing the new breast pyramid.

The inferior portion of the breast below the line D to E is then removed, creating a flat, downward surface that we shall call the inferior planar surface (Fig. 22-14). This surface will ultimately become the new base of the pyramid when rotated 90 degrees. Care must be taken to remove adequate amounts of tissue from both the medial and lateral aspects of line D to E to ensure good breast projection and to prevent a flat or square-looking breast.

A keel-shaped section is next removed from the central portion of the breast.

At this point, a stout single skin hook is placed at point A, and the breast is elevated away from the chest wall, thus approximating the ultimate breast shape (Fig. 22-15). This maneuver allows the surgeon to evaluate breast size and shape and to determine the extent of any additional resection. When the resection is judged adequate, the new breast can be finally shaped and secured.

The medial and lateral aspects of the inferior planar surfaces are next approximated, with the resultant reconstituted inferior planar surface rotated 90 degrees onto the chest wall in one step. This is the key concept of the PBR, i.e., the 90-degree rotation and ultimate suspension of the reconstituted inferior planar surface (the pyramidal base) high on the chest wall (Fig. 22-16). The medial and lateral

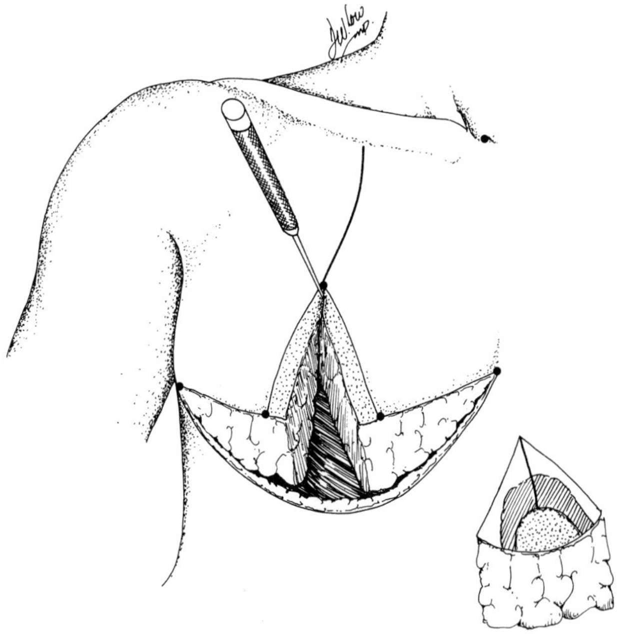

FIGURE 22-15 A central keel-shaped section is removed and the new breast shape is approximated by use of a single skin hook.

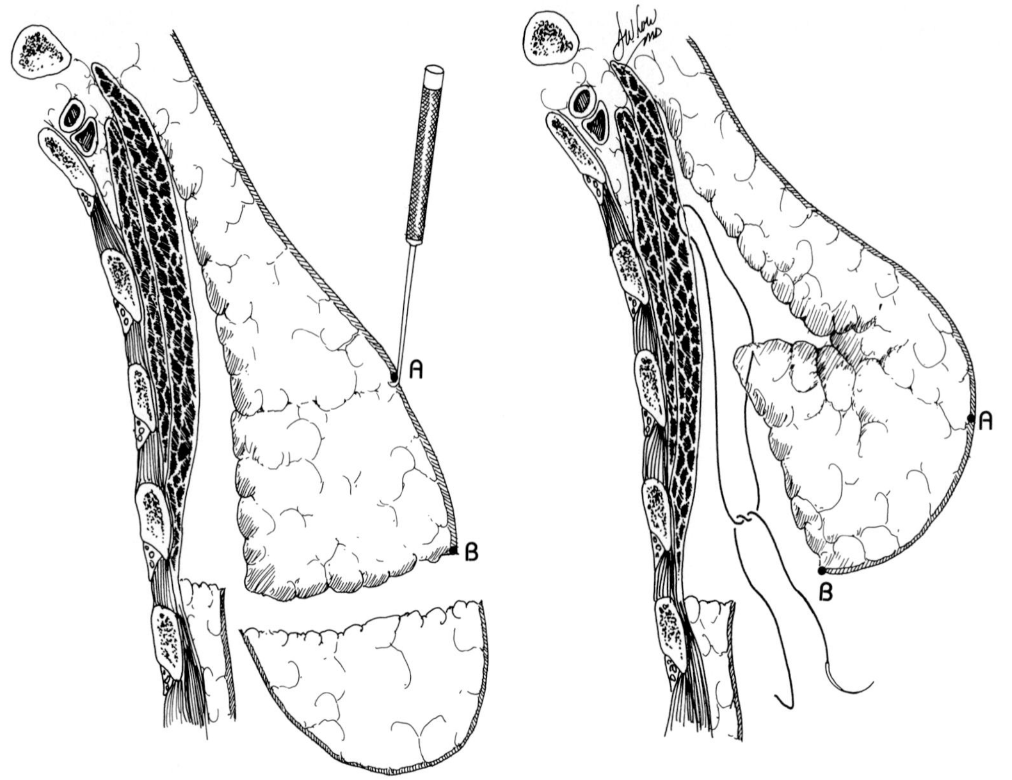

Figure 22–16 The reconstituted inferior planar surface is rotated 90 degrees and attached to the pectoralis fascia high on the chest wall.

aspects of the reconstituted inferior surface are united using a simple suture of 2-0 polyglycolic acid (PGA) suture. However, the suture is not cut but approximated to the pectoralis fascia high on the anterior chest. Continuous suturing procedes inferiorly until the skin points B and C (see Fig. 22–7) meet at the inframammary horizontal line. Thus, the breast has been fashioned into a pyramid and rotated and suspended in one step.

Again, using a single skin hook to approximate breast shape, the vertical and horizontal incisions are temporarily closed with stainless steel staples.

Attention is next turned to the opposite breast and the same procedure is carried out, correcting for any differences in breast volume. Temporarily closing the skin incisions and shaping the breast with stainless steel staples allows the surgeon to ensure that both breasts are equal in size and shape, and that appropriate adjustments are made before permanent sutures, other than the suspensory rotational sutures are placed, (Fig. 22–17). Once the surgeon is satisfied with the breast shape and volume, the incisions are closed in the following fashion: (1) 2-0 PGA to the depths of the breast tissue in the horizontal plane, (2) 4-0 PGA horizontal mattress sutures to the dermis of the horizontal incision and dermal flaps of the vertical incision, and (3) 3-0 monofilament nylon to the horizontal and vertical

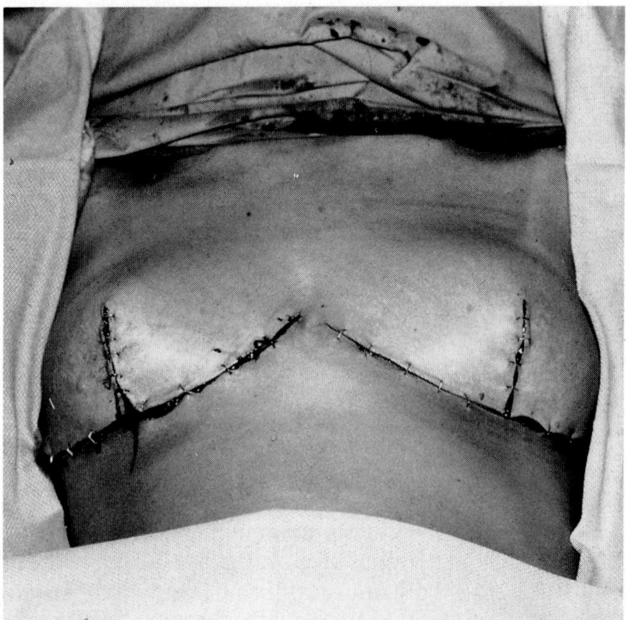

FIGURE 22–17 Points B and C are joined at the horizontal incision. Both breasts are closed temporarily with stainless steel staples.

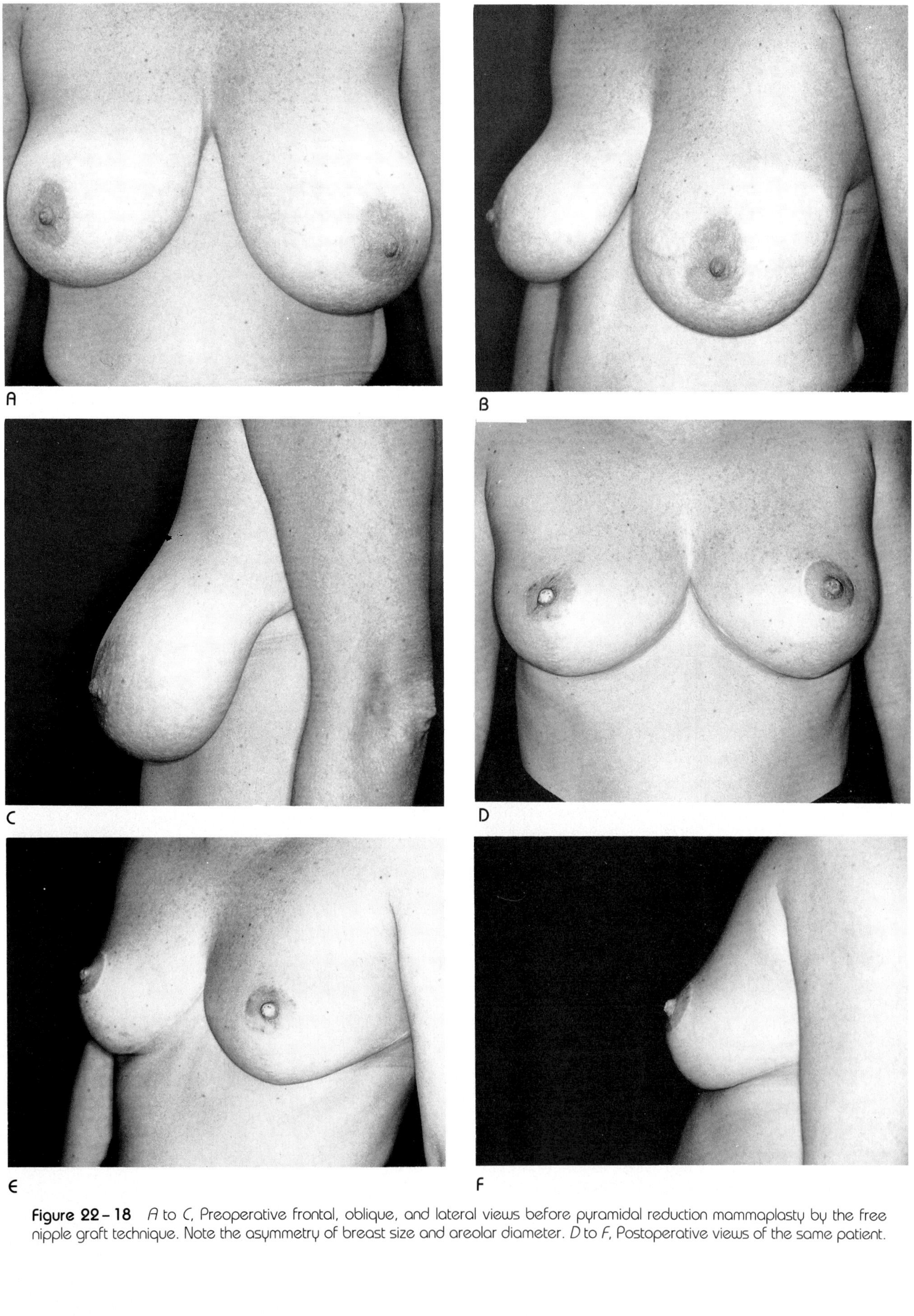

Figure 22-18 *A* to *C*, Preoperative frontal, oblique, and lateral views before pyramidal reduction mammaplasty by the free nipple graft technique. Note the asymmetry of breast size and areolar diameter. *D* to *F*, Postoperative views of the same patient.

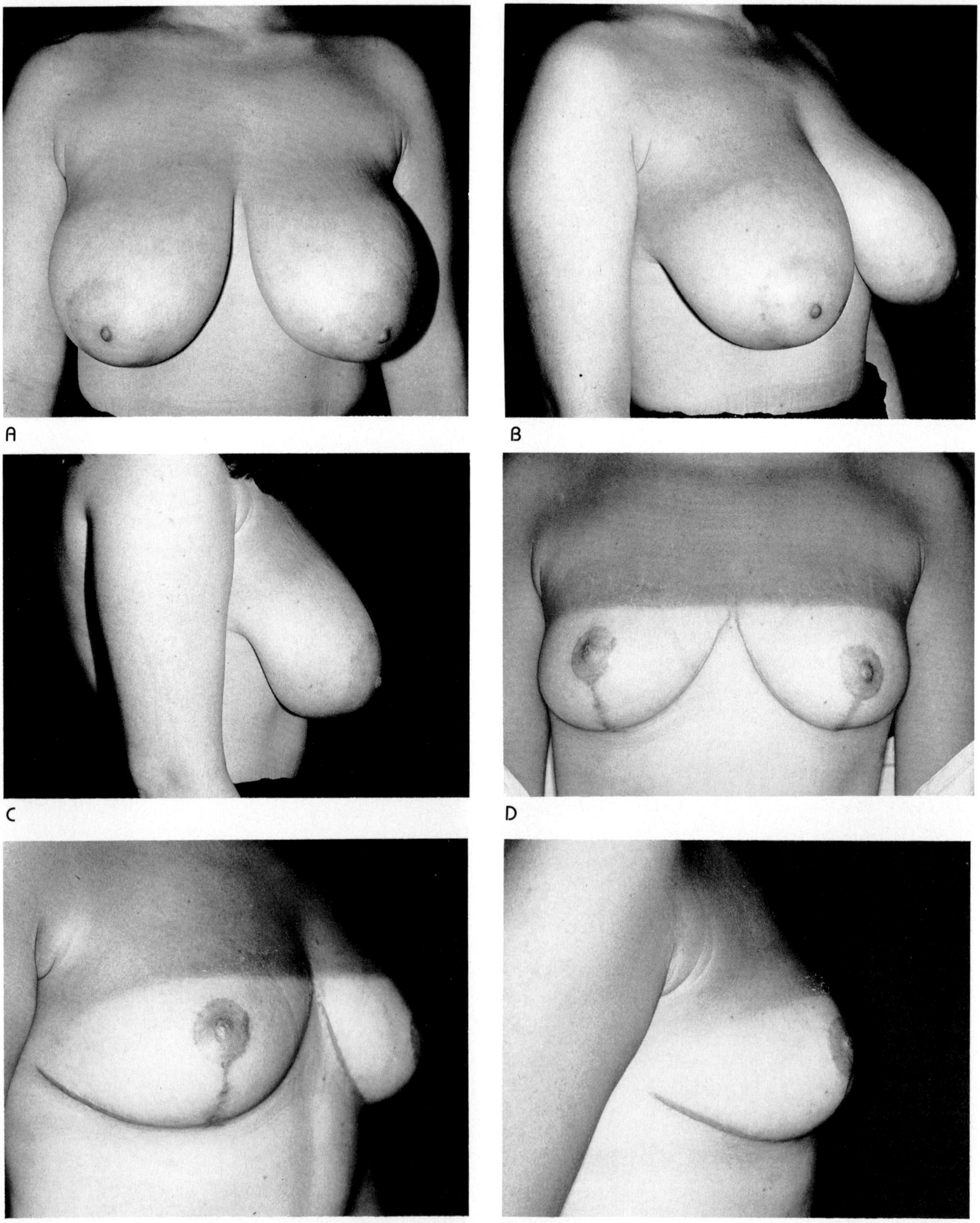

FIGURE 22-19 *A* to *C*, Preoperative frontal, oblique, and lateral views. *D* to *F*, The same views 6 months after reduction mammaplasty by the free nipple graft technique.

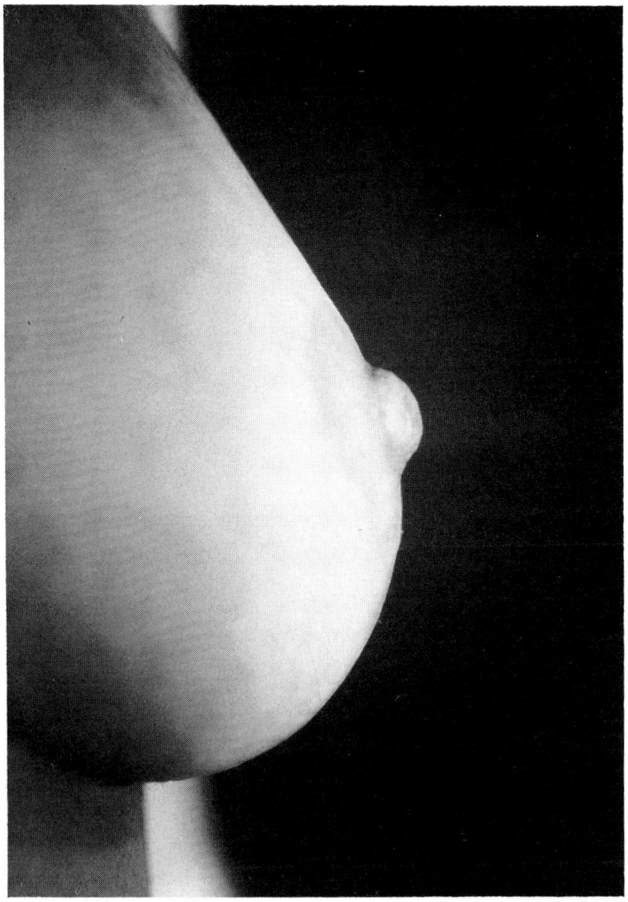

G

Figure 22-19 *Continued*

incisions in an intradermal fashion. Closed suction drainage is used if necessary.

Attention is then turned to the location of the nipple-areola complex, which ideally should be at the previously determined point A. Using the same 38-mm template as a guide, the location is temporarily inked in around point A. The surgeon next steps to the foot of the table to evaluate the location of the symmetry of the complex. This can best be determined from the position at the foot of the table, with the patient in the semisitting, padded "chaise lounge" position.

The flexibility of the free graft technique now becomes apparent, because a minor correction in placement of the complex (even as small as a few millimeters) creates significant improvement in the aesthetic appearance of the breast. The surgeon can feel confident that this position will suffer no postoperative dislocation through late contractions of the pedicle.

Once the final position of the nipple-areola has been determined, the circumscribed area is carefully deepithelialized. Hemostasis by electrocautery is avoided in the deepithelialized area and is obtained by use of dilute epinephrine solution to the donor site for a few minutes. Attention is then turned to the composite nipple-areola graft, which, after removal from the nutritive solution, is sutured into place with 5-0 silk tieover sutures placed at the 1 to 12 o'clock position, and a 5-0 nylon running locking perimeter stitch. Little or no debulking of the graft is carried out before placement. The silk tieover sutures are then tied over cotton moistened with mineral oil. Mineral oil is used to ensure long-term plasticity of the dressing; saline-moistened cotton, when dried, becomes hard and cakelike, and may increase sheer force on the nipple-areola complex with movement.

The final dressing consists of a single layer of gauze dressing over the incisions and nipple-areola, and a snug-fitting, previously autoclaved brassiere, available in most sizes in the operating room.

POSTOPERATIVE CARE

On the first postoperative day, the wounds are examined for postoperative complications. The drains are removed if there has been less than 30 ml of drainage and if the drainage is seen to be decreasing.

Patients are cautioned to avoid strenuous activity and to keep their elbows at their sides in an effort

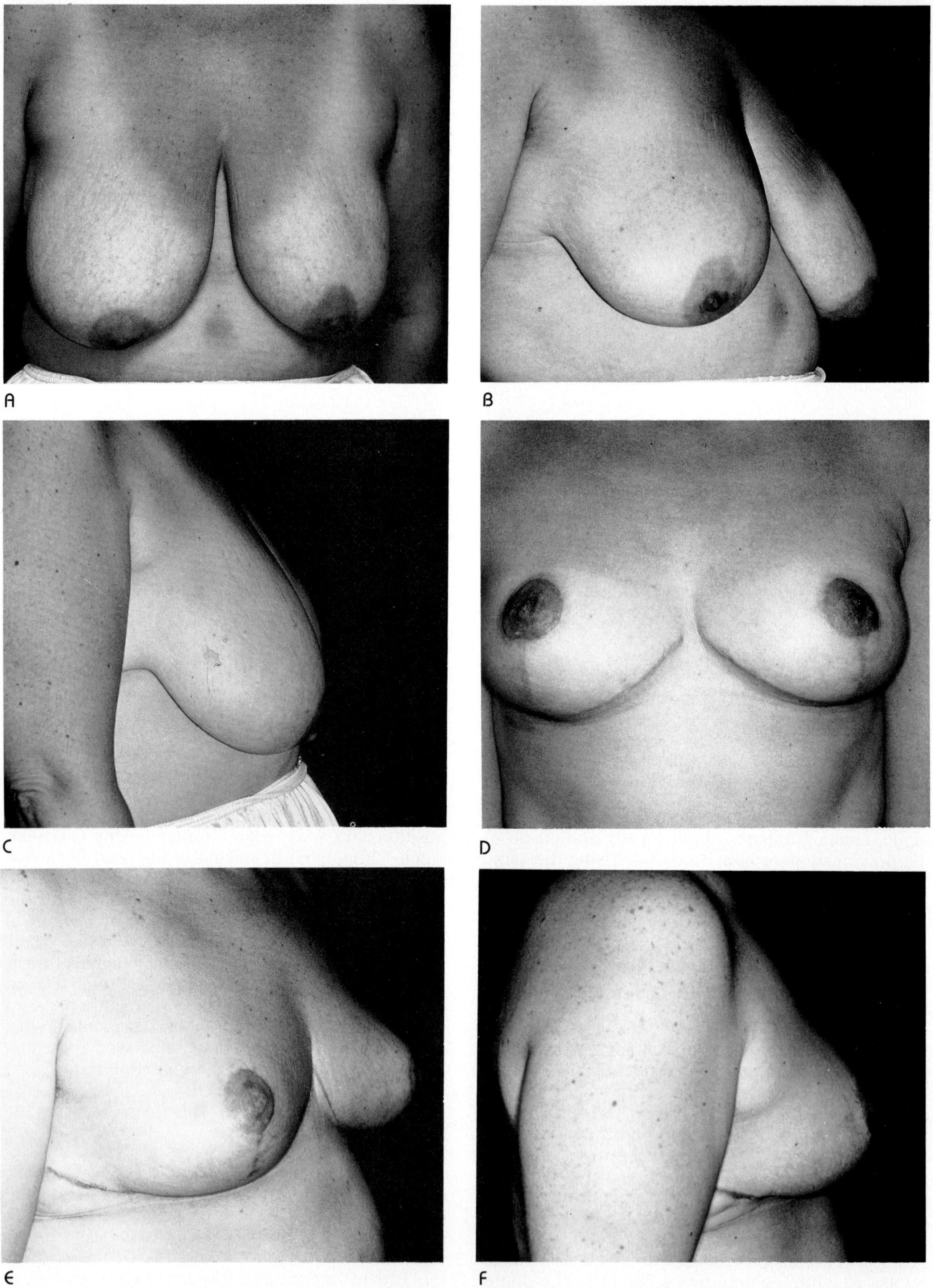

FIGURE 22–20 *A* to *C*, Preoperative views of a patient with hypertrophy and asymmetric ptosis. Note the close approximation of the medial breast points over the midsternum. *D* to *F*, Similar views after surgery. The points D and D′ were staggered during preoperative marking to prevent cicatricial webbing across the sternum.

to minimize breast movement over the underlying pectoralis fascia.

Tieover dressings are removed after 8 to 10 days. It is not unusual to observe a small amount of epidermolysis at the summit of the nipple at this time. This is treated with peroxide cleansing and a mild antibiotic ointment application three times a day. Intracuticular sutures can be removed at 10 to 14 days. Patients may resume full overhead activity after 1 month. A brassiere should be used 24 hours a day for the first month and during strenuous physical activity for the next 3 months. Significant changes in postoperative mammograms have been demonstrated after reduction mammaplasty.[7] Therefore, a postoperative baseline mammogram is obtained 6 months after surgery and shared with the referring physician who will be doing the long-term follow-up breast examination.

RESULTS

My patients and I have been delighted with the consistently excellent, reproducible postoperative results of the pyramidal breast reduction mammaplasty with free nipple graft procedure (Figs. 22-18 to 22-20). In our practice, by design, my associates and I perform a full spectrum of plastic and reconstructive procedures from acute burn management to primarily elective aesthetic procedures. My experience has been that reduction mammaplasty patients, as a group, are the most consistently satisfied and grateful of all our patients.

References

1. Weiner DL, Aiache AE, Silver L, et al. A single dermal pedicle for nipple transposition in subcutaneous mastectomy, reduction mammaplasty, or mastopexy. Plast Reconstr Surg 1973; 51:115.
2. Singer R, Kraut S. Intravenous fluorescein for evaluating the dusky nipple-areola during reduction mammaplasty. Plast Reconstr Surg 1981; 67:534.
3. Sperling R. An attempt to quantify breast cup size by manufacturer. Presented at the New York Regional Society of Plastic and Reconstructive Surgery, New York Academy of Medicine, 1978.
4. Mayl N, Vasconez LO, Jurkiewicz MJ. Treatment of macromastia in the actively enlarging breast. Plast Reconstr Surg 1974; 54:6.
5. Cardoso de Castro C. Subcutaneous mastectomy for gigantomastia in an adolescent girl. Plast Reconstr Surg 1977; 59:575.
6. Goldwyn RM. Voice of polite dissent. Plast Reconstr Surg 1977; 59:746.
7. Robertson JLA. Changed appearance of mammograms following breast reduction. Plast Reconstr Surg 1977; 59:347.

C H A P T E R 23

Non-Hypertrophic Breast Ptosis

ARTHUR G. SHIP, M.D., D.M.D.

Procedures to correct breast ptosis have developed almost as a by-product of the progressively sophisticated surgery for gigantomastia. The Bames[1] and Maliniac[2] pioneering multistage techniques for reducing hypertrophic breasts evolved to one-stage operations. Beisenberger,[3] Aufricht,[4] and Gillies and Marino[5] popularized such techniques. They all employed degloving of the gland, with selective quadrant resection to construct a conical shape, and redraping and tailoring of the skin envelope. Fat and glandular necrosis as well as skin loss led to a high incidence of secondary healing. Many surgeons fixed the reshaped gland to the prepectoral fascia or muscle, although some relied on the skin envelope to retain the contour of the reshaped gland and to prevent ptosis. Occasional reports described dermal grafts sutured to the chest wall to prevent glandular descent. Others suggested that resuspending the gland with fascia lata or dermal strips alone could correct ptosis.

CLASSIFICATION

Breast ptosis is conventionally evaluated by the relationship of the nipple level to the inframammary fold. Regnault[6] classified ptosis by the extent of descent of the nipple:

1. First-degree or minor ptosis. The nipple lies at the level of the submammary fold, above the lower contour of the gland and skin brassiere.
2. Second-degree or moderate ptosis. The nipple lies below the level of the fold but remains above the lower contour of the breast and skin brassiere.
3. Third-degree or major ptosis. The nipple lies below the fold level at the lower contour of the breast and skin brassiere.

Lalardrie and Jouglard[7] recognized two categories of ptosis (Fig. 23-1). Cutaneous ptosis, or descent of the gland accompanied by elongation of the skin of the upper half of the breast, corresponds to Regnault's classification. Glandular ptosis is characterized by the discoid flat breast with the nipple-areola complex at or above the level of the inframammary fold. The skin does not appear to participate in the phenomenon of breast descent, or does so to a minimal extent. Regnault referred to this "dished-out" appearance of the gland that has settled caudally as pseudoptosis. This undesirable configuration is the consequence of many well-intentioned surgical procedures. In such cases the nipple-areola complex has been displaced cephalically and the existing breast tissue has been recontoured in the caudal half of the breast, only to settle out and descend with time.

Descriptions in the literature of the mechanisms producing ptosis remain conjectural at best. Among alleged causes are postpartum or postmenopausal glandular regression, weight loss, the dermochalasis of aging, the stretching caused by pregnancy or monthly enlargement, and a host of even less well documented factors such as gravity or inadequate garment support. There is no consistent attributable cause of any single manifestation of ptosis. Nipple, skin, and gland do not follow the same pattern of descent. Ptosis of the breast must be considered a multifactorial phenomenon.

EVOLUTION OF SURGICAL TECHNIQUES

In 1958 Gillies and Marino[5] published one of the earliest papers to address surgery of the small ptotic breast. They refined Beisenberger's glandular shaping and characterized it as the "periwinkleshell" principle. They were prescient in their criticism of reliance on the skin envelope for the major component of ptosis correction: "The simple cure might appear to lie in forcing the gland into the desired shape and securing this by tightening the skin around it. This maneuver is disappointing because in

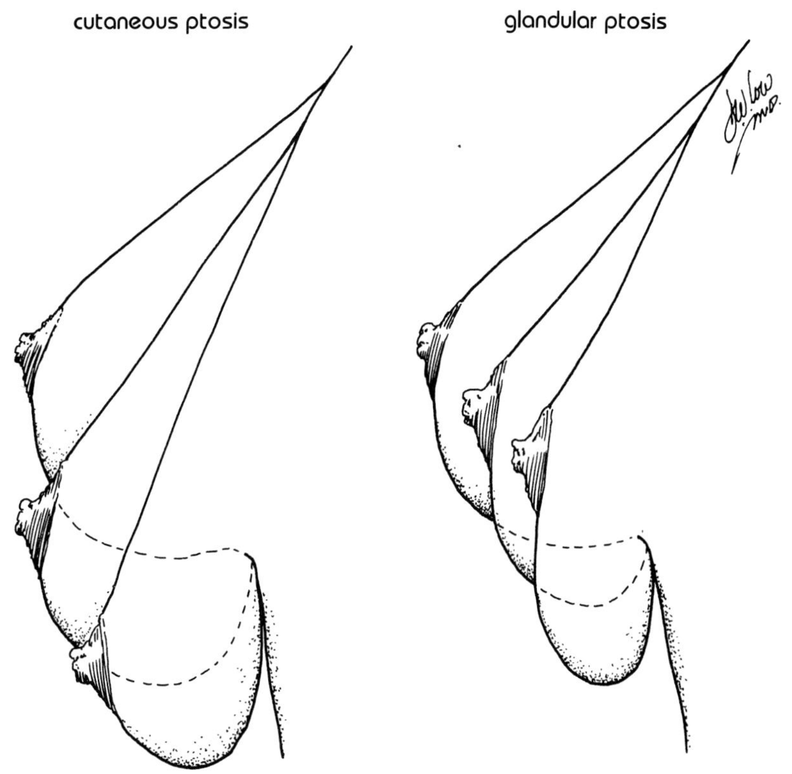

FIGURE 23-1 With cutaneous ptosis, descent of the gland is accompanied by elongation of the skin of the upper half of the breast. Glandular descent with very little skin laxity results in a nipple-areola complex positioned at or above the inframammary fold level, characterizing glandular ptosis.

a short time the skin stretches, permitting the gland to slip back to its former position. As the nipple has been secured in a higher position and remains there, the final deformity is worse than the original." This warning appears to have gone largely unheeded.

Longacre[8] pioneered the use of contiguous pedicled dermis-fat tissue to augment the volume of the reconstructed small breast. The use of contiguous pedicled tissue has found continued favor in the work of many others.[9-17] However, final shape ultimately depends on skin envelope tailoring.

Postoperative descent of parenchyma inevitably followed most forms of breast reconstruction. As early as 1925 Passot described fixation of parenchyma to the muscle "to prevent the breast from sliding down."[18] Maliniac[2] declared that "firm fixation of the breast to the pectoralis muscle is indispensable to a good end result." He utilized both nonabsorbable suture material and dermal loops obtained from deepithelialized redundant skin (Fig. 23-2). Various fixation techniques were incorporated into the breast procedures of Arie,[19] Mir y Mir,[20] and others. Dermal suspension only was advocated by da Silva.[21] Lewis[22] used strips of fascia lata to secure parenchyma to the chest wall at the second rib. Johnson[23] advocated using Marlex mesh, and Piotti[24] advocated using Mersilene mesh. Fixation of parenchyma to the chest wall or muscles has been included in procedures described by Hinderer,[10] Pitanguy,[25] Figallo,[26] and others.

Strömbeck's 1960 report heralded a new era in breast surgery.[27] He shifted the prevailing techniques of wide skin undermining to preservation of the skin-parenchyma interface. This increased the safety factor in breast reduction and ptosis surgery, reducing the incidence of complications. Others soon followed with pedicle techniques that respected the integrity of the skin-gland relationship.[28-30] The "periwinkleshell" principle used to shape the gland was "rediscovered" by Dufourmentel and Mouly,[31] who repositioned caudally displaced parenchyma by spiral rotation to the upper pole, thus converting the flat discoid breast into a new conical shape (Fig. 23-3). The Dufourmentel and Mouly breastplasty, perceived by many as more appropriate for ptosis correction than for reduction, transposed gland without separation of overlying skin and thus without formation of a separate skin brassiere. This procedure over time resulted in derotation of the "periwinkleshell" pedicle and unacceptable medial displacement of the nipple-areola complex.

Operations designed to correct nonhypertrophic ptosis by altering the skin envelope only (without the use of large alloplastic implants) appeared in fairly rapid succession after the 1968 description by Kahn and colleagues[32] using the Strömbeck technique. These authors removed only skin in the lower transverse crescent of the pattern. Goulian further simplified the technique by removing epidermis

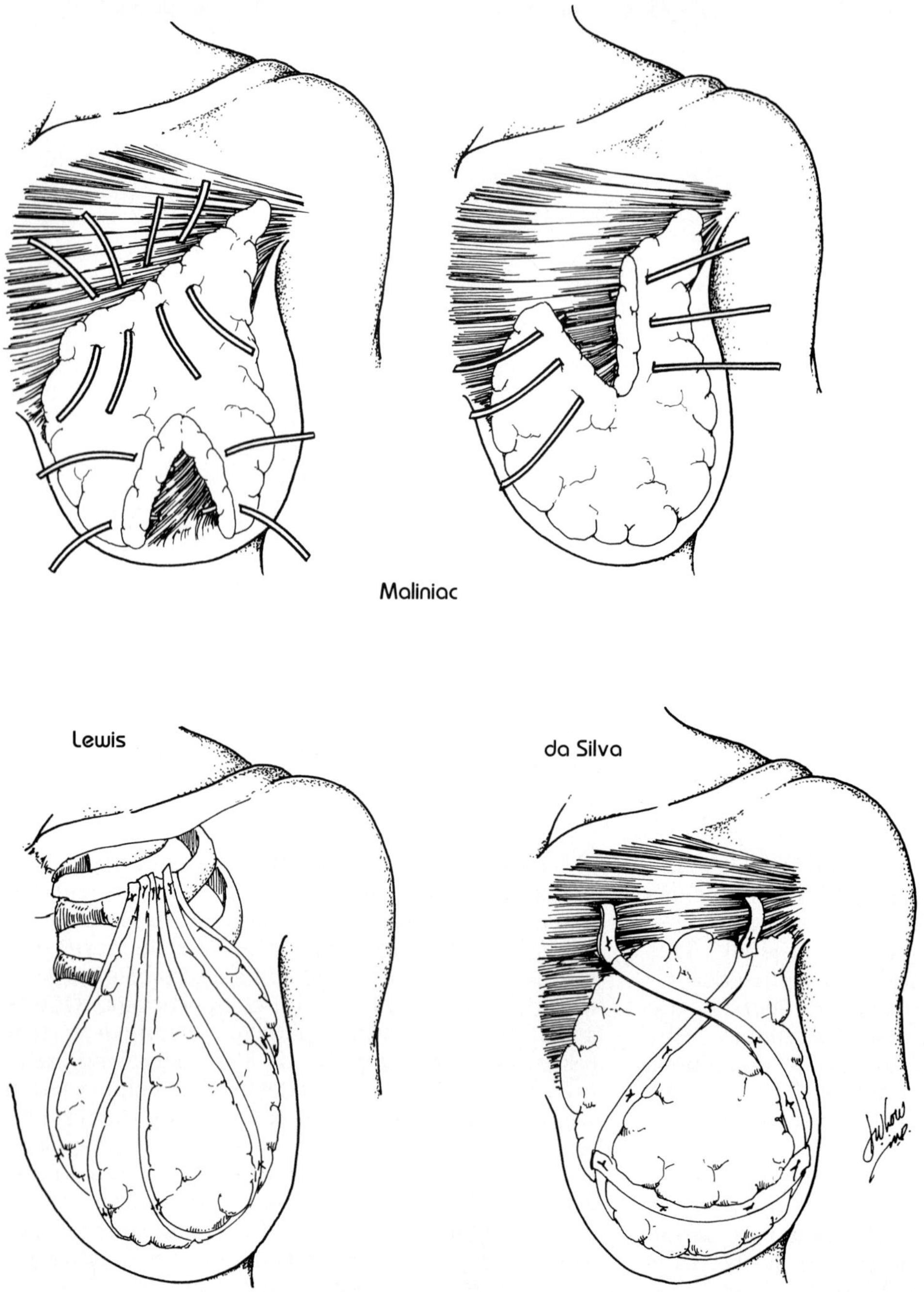

FIGURE 23-2 Various fixation techniques have been incorporated into procedures for ptosis correction. Maliniac used nonabsorbable suture and dermal loops from deepithelialized redundant skin.[2] Lewis advocated fascia lata suspension to the second rib.[22] da Silva fixed the gland to the pectoralis muscle with dermal strips.[21]

within a modified keyhole pattern, inverting breast tissue and relying on the tightened skin envelope for shape and support (Fig. 23-4).[33]

In 1976 Bartels and associates,[34] displeased with the resultant anchor-shaped scars, advocated periareolar skin excision. In 1980 Gruber and Jones,[35] referring to this "donut" mastopexy, noted the unfavorable character of the periareolar scars and, even more important, observed that with time the breast parenchyma exhibited a tendency to resume its previous shape. Also in 1980, Erol and Spira[36] described the correction of nonhypertrophic ptosis by suture invagination of the glandular tissue after degloving via a circumareolar incision. They claimed an improved breast shape and satisfactory scars, but were unable to describe long-term results in their small series of only six patients. Essentially, these procedures "stuff" the residual breast tissue into a tight skin envelope, with the bulk of the parenchyma residing in the caudal half of the reconstructed breast.

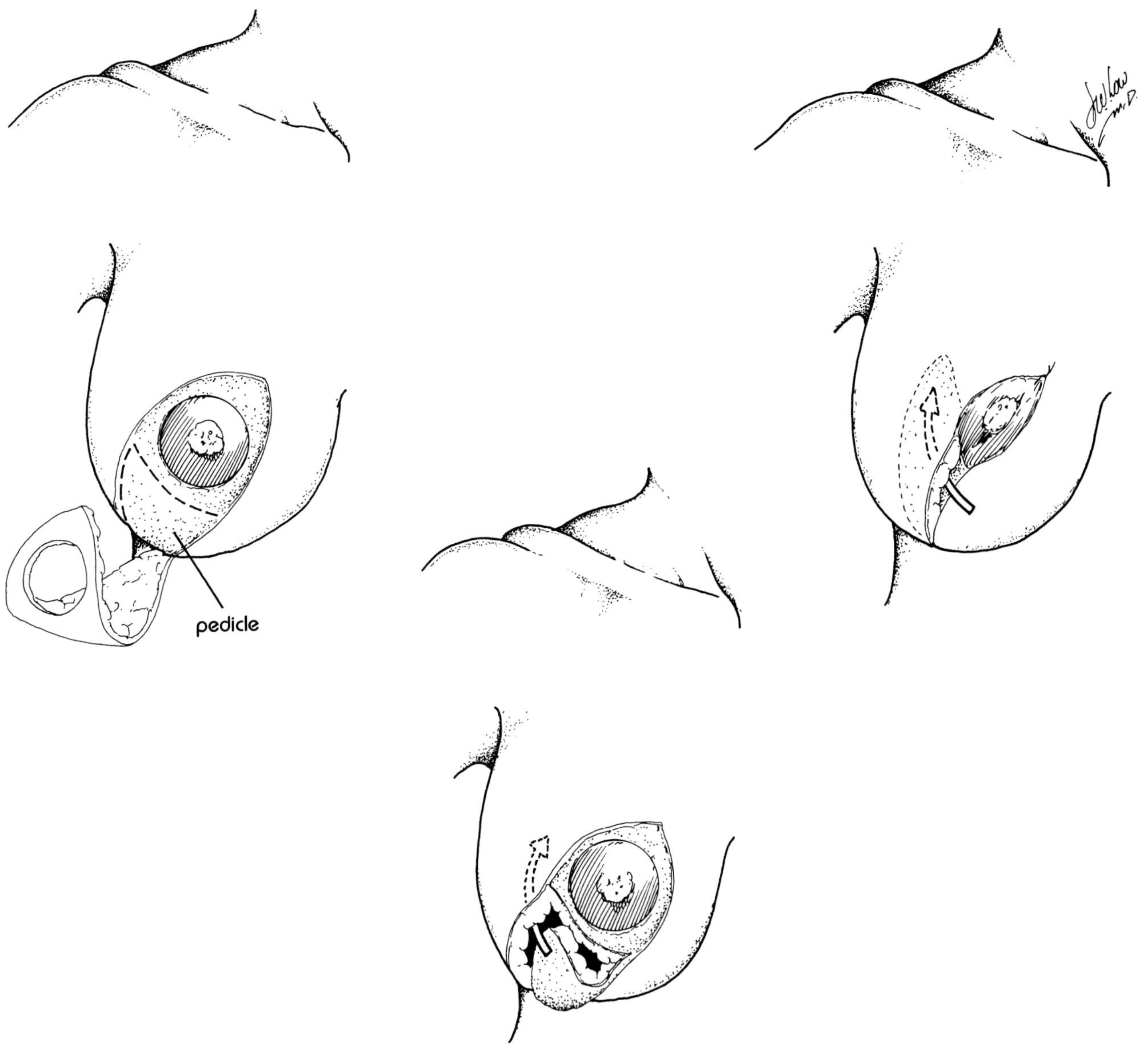

FIGURE 23-3 Spiral rotation of breast parenchyma to the upper pole converts the flat discoid breast into a conical shape with the Dufourmentel-Mouly procedure.[31]

The extensive stretching of the scars, documented by Wray and colleagues,[37] and elongation of the skin result in eventual recurrence of the deformity, i.e., recurrence of ptosis. In 1988 Reus and Mathes[38] reiterated the need for internal support rather than dependence only on a skin brassiere.

Regnault and associates in 1988[39] recognized that a more aggressive approach was required, especially when the breast volume was adequate but located largely in the lower quadrant. In an attempt to produce increased fullness of the upper pole of the breast, they devised the "minus-plus" mastopexy: excision (minus) of lower pole glandular excess and augmentation (plus) of the upper quadrant with a breast implant. McKissock[40] supported this view and stated that ptosis correction requires the placement of an alloplastic implant to provide superior pole fullness.

In 1989 Ship and colleagues[41] described the dual-pedicle dermoparenchymal mastopexy (DPM) for correction of nonhypertrophic ptosis. This procedure incorporates autoaugmentation of the superior pole of the breast, elevation of the nipple-areola complex, and fixation to the chest wall. Redundant caudal breast tissue is deepithelialized, divided into two dermoparenchymal pedicles (Fig. 23-5), crossed, spirally rotated, and fixed to the pectoralis fascia cephalad to the nipple-areola complex. This

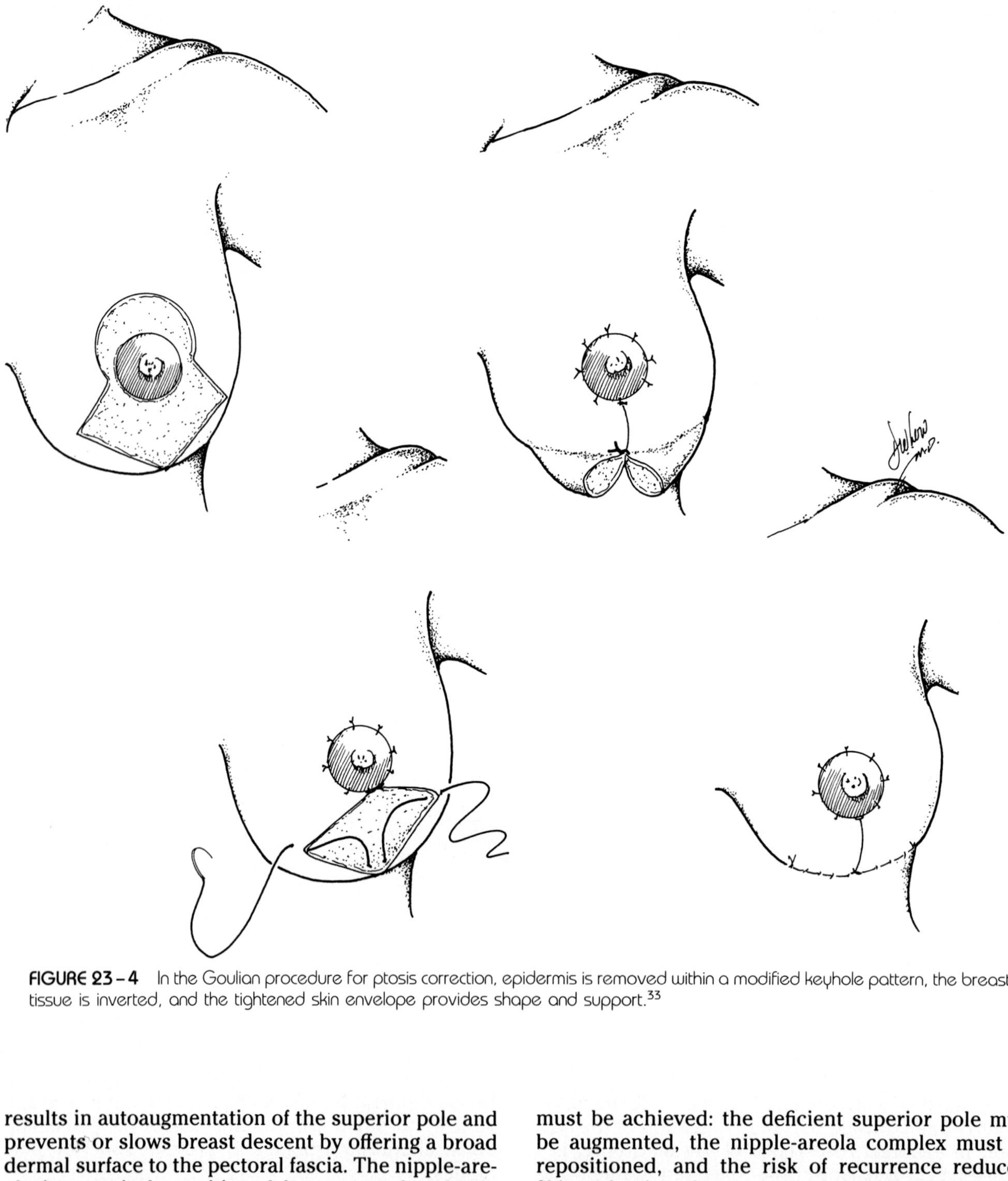

FIGURE 23-4 In the Goulian procedure for ptosis correction, epidermis is removed within a modified keyhole pattern, the breast tissue is inverted, and the tightened skin envelope provides shape and support.[33]

results in autoaugmentation of the superior pole and prevents or slows breast descent by offering a broad dermal surface to the pectoral fascia. The nipple-areola is superiorly positioned by means of a classic "superior pedicle" technique that displaces the bulk of the remaining gland cephalically.

CONCLUSION

It is apparent that there is no single procedure that corrects all forms of breast ptosis. Several goals must be achieved: the deficient superior pole must be augmented, the nipple-areola complex must be repositioned, and the risk of recurrence reduced. Skin reduction alone, or together with glandular imbrication, fails to augment the superior pole and results in early recurrence of ptosis. Placement of an implant superiorly may be followed by glandular descent with a resultant "double-bubble" appearance. The dual-pedicle mastopexy introduced by the author, although limited to ptosis requiring 7 to 8 cm of nipple elevation, addresses the remaining essential elements of ptosis correction.

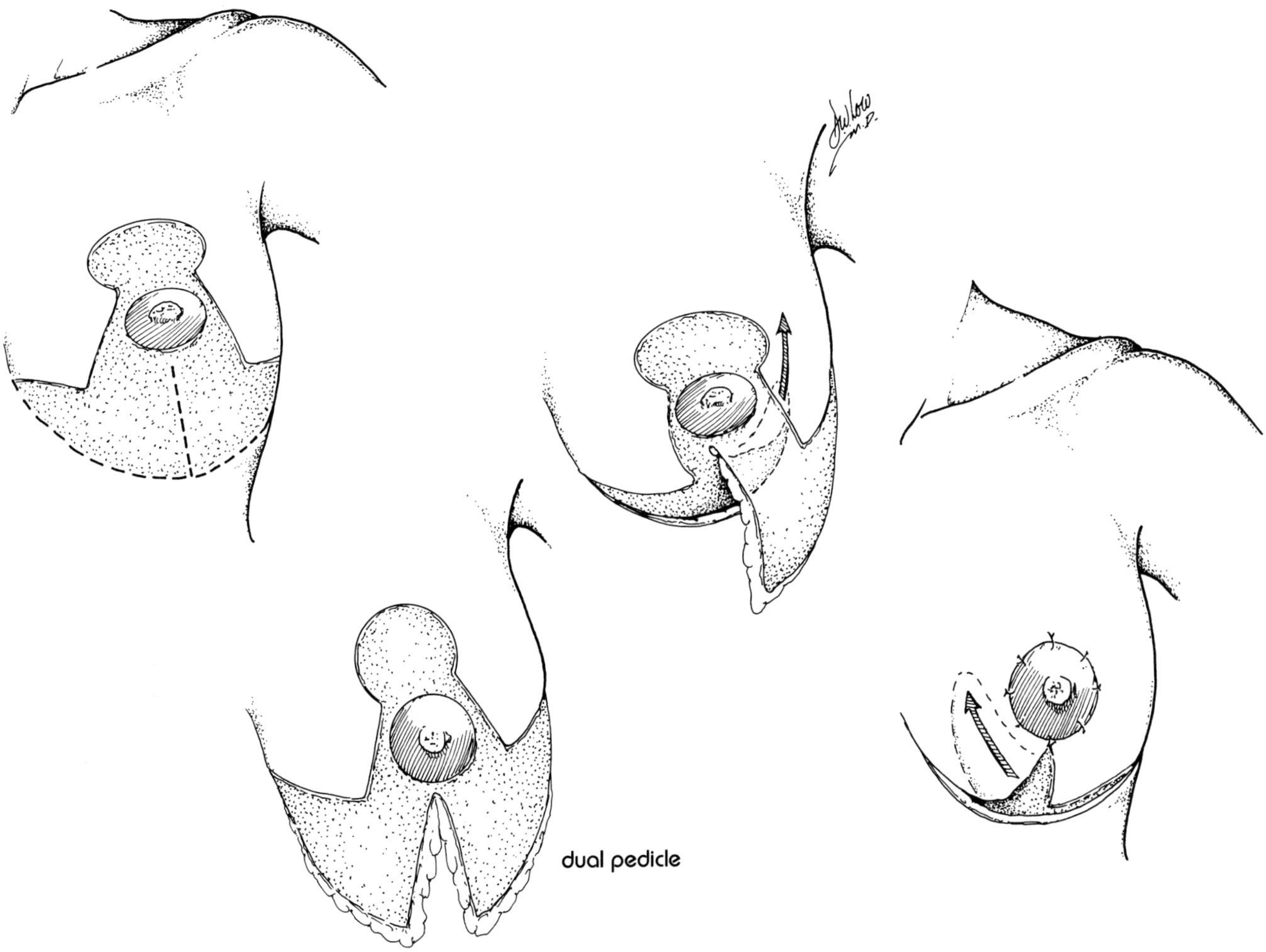

FIGURE 23-5 The author's technique provides auto-augmentation of the superior pole of the breast and fixation to the chest wall. The nipple-areola is positioned cephalically by means of a "superior pedicle technique." The redundant caudal tissue is divided into two dermoparenchymal pedicles that are crossed, spirally rotated, and fixed to the pectoralis fascia.[41]

References

1. Bames HO. Reduction of massive breast hypertrophy. Plast Reconst Surg 1948; 3:560.
2. Maliniac JW. Breast deformities and their repair. Baltimore: Waverly Press, 1950.
3. Biesenberger H. Deformitaten und kosmetische operationen der weiblichen brust. Vienna: Mandrich, 1931.
4. Aufricht G. Mammaplasty for pendulous breasts. Plast Reconstr Surg 1989; 4:13.
5. Gillies Sir H, Marino H. The "periwinkleshell" principle in the treatment of the small ptotic breast. Plast Reconstr Surg 1958; 21:1.
6. Regnault P. Breast ptosis. Clin Plast Surg 1976; 3:139.
7. Lalardrie J-P, Jouglarde J-P. Chirurgie plastique du sein. Paris: Masson & Cie, 1974.
8. Longacre JJ. Surgical reconstruction of the flat discoid breast. Plast Reconstr Surg 1956; 17:358.
9. Baroudi R, Lewis JR Jr. The augmentation-reduction mammaplasty. Clin Plast Surg 1956; 17:358.
10. Hinderer JT. The dermal brassiere mastoplasty. Clin Plast Surg 1976; 3:349.
11. North JF. Mammary hyperinvolution and ptosis. Br J Plast Surg. 1975; 28:310.
12. Figallo E. Surgical treatment of mammary ptosis without hypertrophy. Plast Reconstr Surg 1977; 60:189.
13. Hrivnakova J. A new modification of Bigg's operation for the correction of ptosis with a short inframammary scar. Plast Reconstr Surg 1982; 69:45.
14. Marchac D, de Olarte G. Reduction mammaplasty and correction of ptosis with a short inframammary scar. Plast Reconstr Surg 1982; 69:45.
15. Ely JF. The devil's incision mammaplasty. Aesthetic Plast Surg 1983; 7:159.
16. Ho LCY. The small ptotic breast: Reposition auto-augmentation mammaplasty. Br J Plast Surg 1983; 39:196.

17. Reich J. Mammaplasty with reduction of the lower central breast segment. Br J Plast Surg 1983; 36:196.
18. Passot R. La correction esthetique du prolapsus mammaire par le procède de la transposition du mamelon. Presse Med 1925; 33:317.
19. Arie G. Una nueva tecnica de mastoplastia. Rev Latinoam Cirurg Plast 1957; 3:23.
20. Mir y Mir L. Reduction mammaplasty. Plast Reconstr Surg 1968; 41:352.
21. da Silva G. Mastopexy with dermal ribbon for supporting the breast and keeping it in shape. Plast Reconstr Surg 1964; 34:403.
22. Lewis GK. A method of mastopexy with fascia lata transplants. J Int Coll Surg 1956; 26:346.
23. Johnson GW. Central core reduction mammaplasties and Marlex suspension of breast tissue. Aesthetic Plast Surg 1981; 5:77.
24. Piotti F. Experience with a vertical technique in mammaplasty. Aesthetic Plast Surg 1981; 5:349.
25. Pitanguy I. Mamaplastias. Rev Latinoam Cirurg Plast 1963; 7:139.
26. Figallo E. Surgical treatment of mammary ptosis without hypertrophy. Plast Reconstr Surg 1977; 60:189.
27. Strömbeck JO. Mammaplasty: Report of a new technique based on two-pedicle procedure. Br J Plast Surg 1960; 13:79.
28. Skoog T. A technique of breast reduction. Acta Chir Scand 1963; 126:453.
29. McKissock PK. Reduction mammaplasty by vertical bipedicle flap technique. Clin Plast Surg 1976; 3:309.
30. Weiner DL, Aiache AE, Silver L, Tittiranonda TA. Pedicle flap technique for nipple transposition in subcutaneous mastectomy, reduction mammaplasty or mastopexy. Plast Reconst Surg 1973; 51:115.
31. Dufourmentel C, Mouly R. Modification of the "periwinkleshell operation" for small ptotic breasts. Plast Reconstr Surg 1968; 41:523.
32. Kahn S, Hoffman S, Simon BE. Correction of non-hypertrophic ptosis of the breasts. Plast Reconstr Surg 1968; 41:244.
33. Goulian D. Dermal mastopexy. Plast Reconstr Surg 1988; 82:644.
34. Bartels R, Strickland DM, Douglas WM. A new mastopexy operation for mild or moderate breast ptosis. Plast Reconstr Surg 1976; 57:687.
35. Gruber RP, Jones JR. The "donut" mastopexy: Indications and complications. Plast Reconstr Surg 1980; 65:34.
36. Erol OO, Spira MA. Mastopexy technique for mild to moderate ptosis. Plast Reconstr Surg 1980; 65:603.
37. Wray, RC Jr, Holtman B, Weeks PM. Factors in the production of inconspicuous scars. Plast Reconstr Surg 1975; 56:86.
38. Reus WF, Mathes SJ. Preservation of projection after reduction mammaplasty: Long-term follow-up of the inferior pedicle technique. Plast Reconstr Surg 1988; 82:644.
39. Regnault P, Daniel RK, Tirkanits B. The minus-plus mastopexy. Clin Plast Surg 1988; 15:595.
40. McKissock P. Personal communication.
41. Ship AG, Weiss, PR, Engler AM. Dual pedicle dermoparenchymal mastopexy. Plast Reconstr Surg 1989; 83:281.

CHAPTER 24

Complications of Reduction Mammaplasty

SAUL HOFFMAN, M.D.

According to Goldwyn, the ideal reduction mammaplasty should be safe, simple, speedy, bloodless, and relatively scarless, producing a breast of normal appearance and function.[1] Results continue to improve, but we are still a long way from this ideal. However, the operation can be very gratifying because most patients are happy to be relieved of their symptoms and are pleased with their new appearance. Many are motivated to achieve further improvement by means of diet and exercise.

Unfortunately, complications and poor results do occur. This chapter discusses the complications with particular attention to prevention and management.

AVASCULAR NECROSIS

Avascular necrosis was common with the older methods of reduction mammaplasty such as the one described by Biesenberger, in which the mammary gland is widely dissected from the overlying skin (Fig. 24-1).[2] With modern techniques, major tissue loss is now rare, but small areas of skin necrosis, particularly at the junction of the vertical and horizontal incisions, are not infrequent (Fig. 24-2).

In a personal review of 100 cases performed with the Biesenberger technique before 1963, almost 25 percent had vascular complications with varying degrees of skin and fat necrosis. In 1946 Ragnell gave up the Biesenberger operation because of circulatory disturbances in one third of his patients.[3] In 1952 Conway rated a 27 percent major complication rate with transposition techniques in 110 patients, and satisfactory results in only 54.5 percent.[4] On the other hand, when he performed free composite nipple grafts, his success rate was 95 percent, and the transplanted nipples regained sensation and erectility.

By 1958 McIndoe and Rees were able to decrease the complication rate to 11 percent by using a modified Biesenberger procedure.[5] Their complications included hematoma, loss of nipple (four partially, one totally), infections, wound separation and slough, fat necrosis, cerebral thrombosis or embolism, and pleurisy. It is interesting that the main complication was hematoma, which they were able to control with hypotensive anesthesia. They reduced the incidence of circulatory complications by preserving a "mesentery" of fat-containing branches of the lateral thoracic artery.

By 1976 the complication rate had been reduced even further.[6] Although a few surgeons continue to perform this operation, most have abandoned it in favor of procedures requiring less extensive undermining. In 1988 Hester described an operation in which the skin was also widely undermined.[7] The peripheral portion of the gland was then reduced, the skin envelope draped over it, and the excess skin excised. Despite the wide undermining, the complication rate in 218 patients was low. There was one almost total nipple-areolar loss (0.3 percent) and three minor areolar losses (0.9 percent). There was one infection and a revision rate of 10 percent (usually for scars).

In 1963 Strömbeck presented a procedure with minimal undermining in which the nipple is supported on medial and lateral pedicles.[8] He showed some excellent results, prompting surgeons to adopt and modify his procedure. His postoperative complications rate in a series of 670 patients included hematomas in 2.7 percent, fat necrosis in 2.1 percent, complete areolar necrosis in three patients, and skin necrosis requiring skin grafts in five. Hypertrophic scars, recurrence of hypertrophy, and postoperative sagging occurred infrequently. The result was deemed to be excellent by 67 percent of his patients, good by 20 percent, and poor by 1 percent.

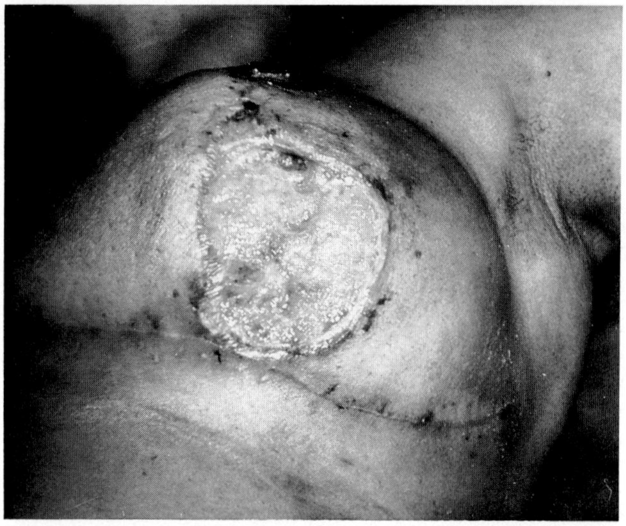

A

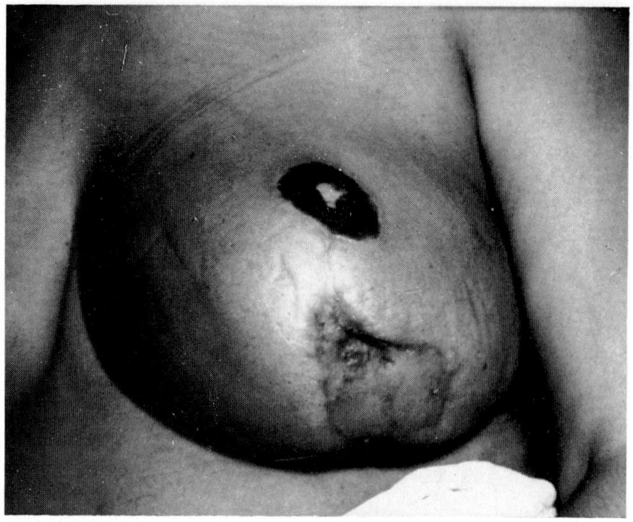

B

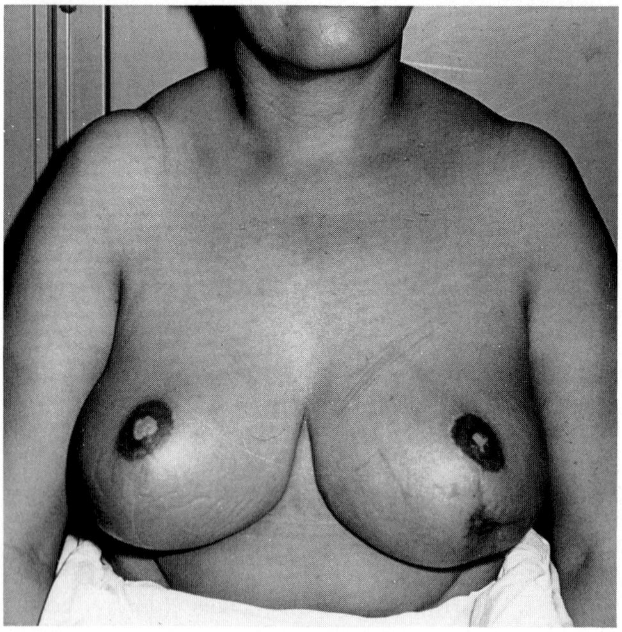

C

FIGURE 24–1 *A*, Major skin loss in a 49-year-old woman after a Biesenberger type of reduction mammaplasty. *B*, After a split-thickness skin graft. *C*, One year postoperatively. Note the depigmentation of the free-grafted nipple.

Since Strömbeck's report, many techniques using a variety of pedicles have been described. Two of the most popular procedures are the vertical dermal flap of McKissock and the inferior pedicle technique.[9–13]

In a review of 100 cases in which the inferior pedicle technique was used between 1984 and 1989, the rate of vascular complications was less than 1 percent. It is difficult to compare an operation popular 25 years ago with procedures performed today, because much has changed in terms of better training, improved instrumentation, electrocautery, and so forth.

Factors responsible for avascular necrosis are described below.

Vascular Disease. A careful history should be taken to rule out diseases that may affect the blood vessels. It is now widely recognized that in heavy smokers there is a higher incidence of vascular complications after surgery.[14,15] Patients with diabetes have small vessel disease, which may affect healing. Care must also be taken when operating on patients who have received corticosteroid therapy for long periods (Fig. 24–3). In general, it is safer to perform an amputative mammaplasty with free nipple grafting in the presence of vascular disease.

Tension. When the skin envelope is too small in relation to the amount of breast tissue, necrosis is likely to occur. Careful preoperative planning reduces this possibility. A small triangle of skin interposed between the medial and lateral flaps at the junction of the vertical and horizontal incisions

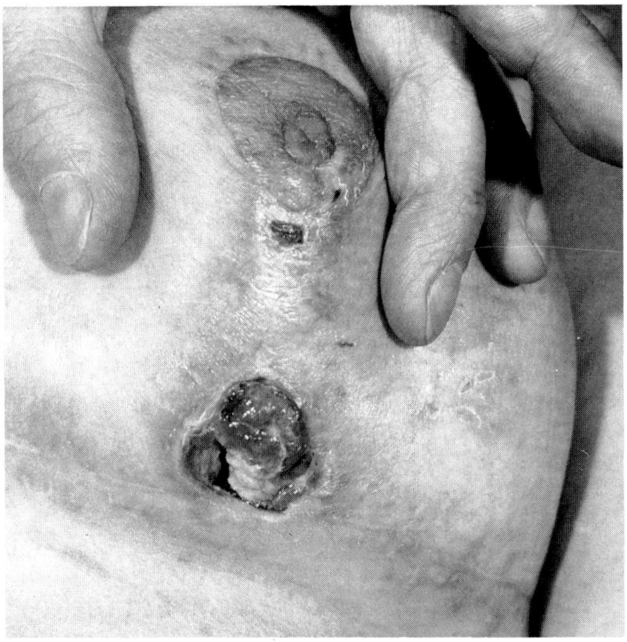

FIGURE 24-2 Tissue loss at the junction of the vertical and inframammary fold incisions.

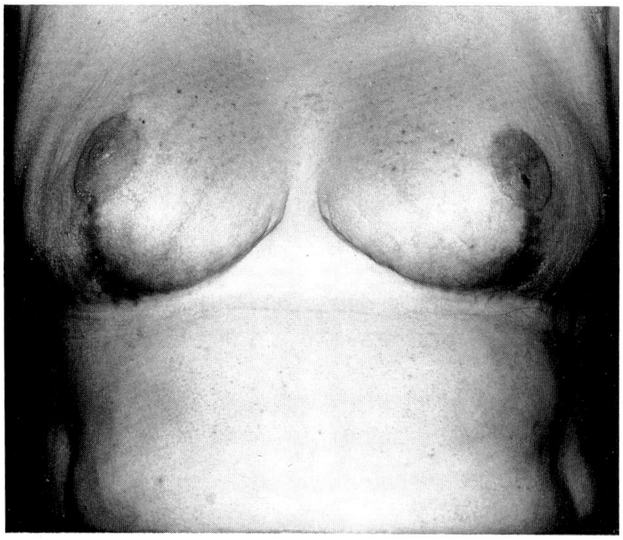

FIGURE 24-3 Postoperative result of an amputative reduction mammaplasty in a 43-year-old woman who had been on high doses of prednisone for several years for chronic eye disease. Wounds healed slowly, with attenuation of the vertical scars. There was atrophy of the dermal layer of the skin.

makes it possible to round off the corners of the flaps, thereby minimizing skin loss at this critical point (Fig. 24-4).

It is important to understand the circulation of the breast in order to minimize vascular complications. For example, in the inferior pedicle operation the width of the pedicle is not critical, but the blood vessels contained in the layer of fat above the pectoralis fascia must be preserved (Fig. 24-5). The blood vessels to the pedicle are easily injured when the pectoralis fascia is widely exposed.

The circulation is assessed intraoperatively, and if the nipple appears compromised, it is safer to transplant it as a free full-thickness graft. Usually, the flaps are sutured before positioning and placement of the nipple. This allows the surgeon to evaluate the nipple circulation and make an adjustment in nipple position before the final stages of the operation.

Ordinarily, a full-thickness circle of skin is removed and the nipples are sutured into position. It is preferable to leave a 1-cm peripheral dermal shelf to support the nipple-areola complex. To convert the

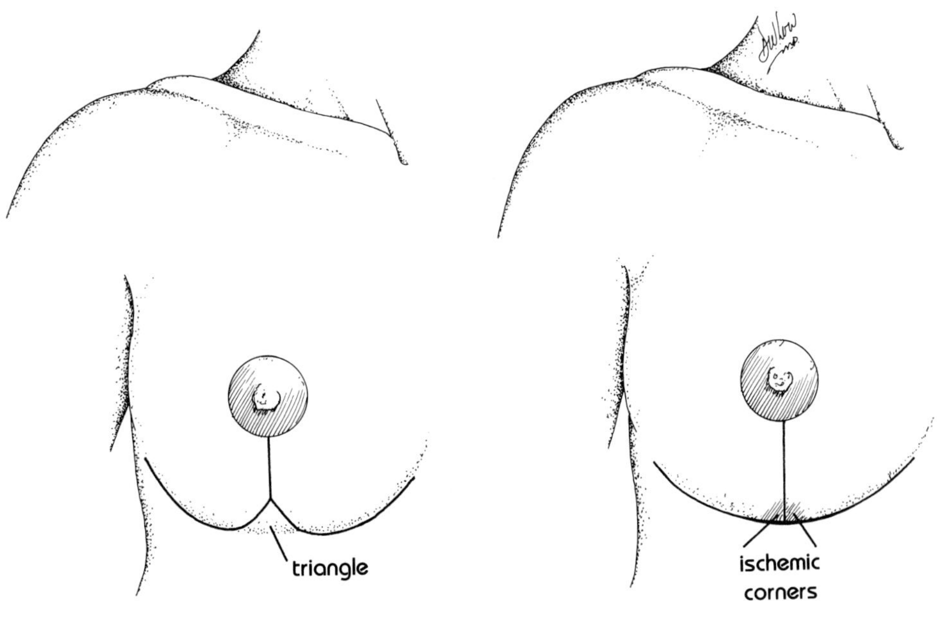

FIGURE 24-4 A triangle of skin interposed between the flaps helps prevent the ischemia commonly seen at the corners of the flaps.

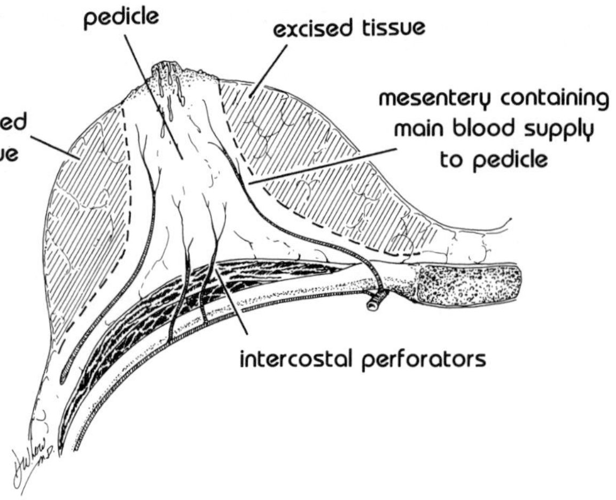

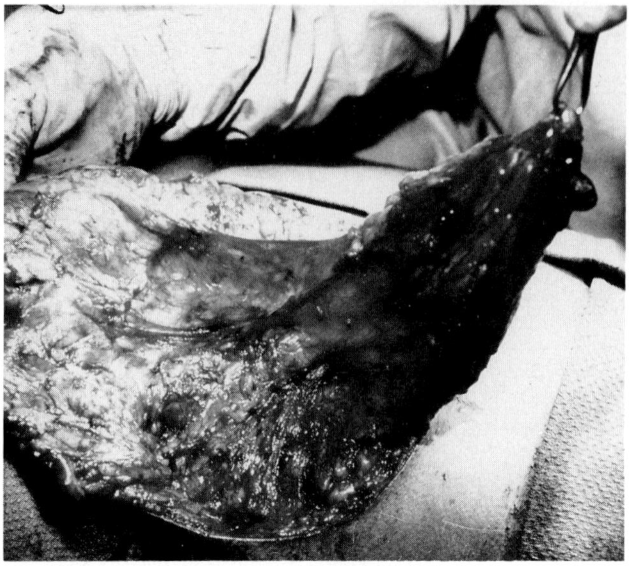

FIGURE 24-5 *A*, Vascular anatomy of the inferior pedicle technique. *B*, Intraoperative view demonstrating the "mesentery" to the inferior pedicle.

operation to a free nipple graft, the recipient site is prepared by removing a partial-thickness circle of skin.

When the nipple appears compromised in the immediate postoperative period, it may be necessary to return the patient to the operating room to explore the pedicle. If the circulation does not improve after exploration of the pedicle, the distal devitalized portion of the pedicle can be excised and the nipple grafted to the dermis on the proximal portion of the pedicle.

If necrosis does occur, it is best to wait for spontaneous demarcation and separation. A superficial loss will heal with minimal deformity, so a conservative approach is best for all but the most major losses, which may require grafting (Fig. 24-6). Loss of the nipple-areola complex is usually accompanied by necrosis of the distal portion of the pedicle. This may lead to a depressed scar that requires major revision and nipple-areolar reconstruction.

In over 100 cases in which the inferior pedicle technique was used, I have seen only one significant loss of the nipple-areola complex.

In a personal series of 50 free nipple grafts there were several superficial losses, mostly in the central nipple area, but none required revision. Gradinger reported loss of a free nipple graft in one of 156 patients.[16] It is interesting that he uses this technique in 20 percent of his reduction mammaplasties. Although this seems high, it is a safer approach than pushing the transposition procedures to their limits and inviting a higher incidence of complications.

Avascular necrosis or infection leads to more extensive scarring, but hypertrophic scars can occur even after uneventful healing. Should hypertrophic or keloidal scarring be considered a complication, since it is to be expected in a certain percentage of cases? In an analysis of 50 cases of reduction mammaplasty involved in litigation, most complaints concerned the scars.[17] For purposes of this discussion, therefore, hypertrophic or severe scarring will be considered a complication.

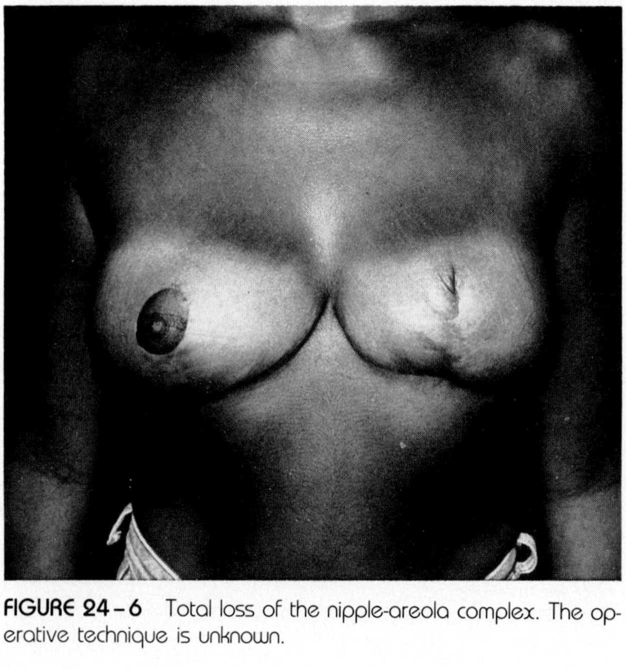

FIGURE 24-6 Total loss of the nipple-areola complex. The operative technique is unknown.

FAT NECROSIS

Fat necrosis is more common in obese patients. It may become manifest in the immediate postoperative period by temperature elevation, tenderness, induration, and sometimes mottling of the overlying skin. When skin loss accompanies fat necrosis the resultant ulceration usually granulates and epithelializes, leaving a depressed scar. Without skin loss, there may be continuing drainage of clear, cloudy, yellowish, fatty fluid, which may continue for several days or weeks. Areas of fat necrosis can remain as hard lumps that may become worrisome but usually disappear after several months. Meticulous attention to detail, careful removal of devascularized particles of fat, and closure without undue tension help to avoid this complication. Overzealous use of electrocautery may contribute to fat necrosis. Adequate drainage for 24 to 48 hours postoperatively is also recommended.

Wound infection after reduction mammaplasty is uncommon. When it does occur, it usually accompanies tissue necrosis and resolves with removal of the necrotic tissue. I have not found prophylactic antibiotics to be necessary.

Because complications are more common in obese women, it is logical for them to lose weight before surgery. Furthermore, the extent of the reduction can more readily be determined in a patient who is at the ideal weight. This should be discussed at the initial consultation and every effort made to lose the necessary weight before surgery.

Significant fat necrosis will result in loss of volume, which may necessitate augmentation of the smaller breast or further reduction of the larger one.

Complications related to the use of electrocautery have also been seen. One must be certain that the equipment is in proper working order and that the patient is carefully grounded. The tip of the cautery should be guarded at all times if burns are to be prevented.

Awareness of possible complications is the first step in their prevention. The patient should be properly positioned and all pressure points padded. Brachial plexus injuries and ulnar nerve palsies have been reported. Temporary loss of occipital scalp hair from prolonged pressure has been seen.

SELECTION OF PATIENTS AND PROCEDURE

Complications can be minimized by proper patient selection and by choice of the appropriate surgical technique. I agree with Gradinger, who believes that free nipple transplantation reduces the complication rate in women with very large breasts.[16] Specifically, his indications for this procedure are (1) postmenopausal women who are very large and have little or no pleasurable nipple sensation; (2) patients with large, tender, painful, lumpy breasts that are difficult to examine; (3) patients with hypertrophy and nipple inversion; (4) the postmastectomy patient whose remaining breast is hypertrophied; and (5) patients with gigantomastia. Of course, the free nipple graft operation would certainly eliminate the possibility of breast feeding and destroy any pleasurable sensation.

Necrosis and infection may lead to irregularities of contour, asymmetry, and excessive scarring. Unsatisfactory results can also occur without complications, but nevertheless are included in this discussion.

HYPERTROPHIC SCARRING

From an aesthetic point of view, the major problem with reduction mammaplasty is the scarring (Fig. 24-7). Although most women with severe breast hypertrophy are willing to accept hypertrophic scars, some are not. Young women with minimal hypertrophy may be very unhappy with the appearance of the scars. I have seen women with average scars after reduction mammaplasty who were extremely angry because they had been told that the scars would be inconspicuous. Some had consulted attorneys. Patients must, therefore, be made aware of the unpredictable nature of scars following this operation. In most cases, a verbal description is not sufficient. McKissock recommended showing *honest* photographs of average results illustrating the appearance of hypertrophic scars on the breast.[18] Goin pointed out that showing photographs to a patient in

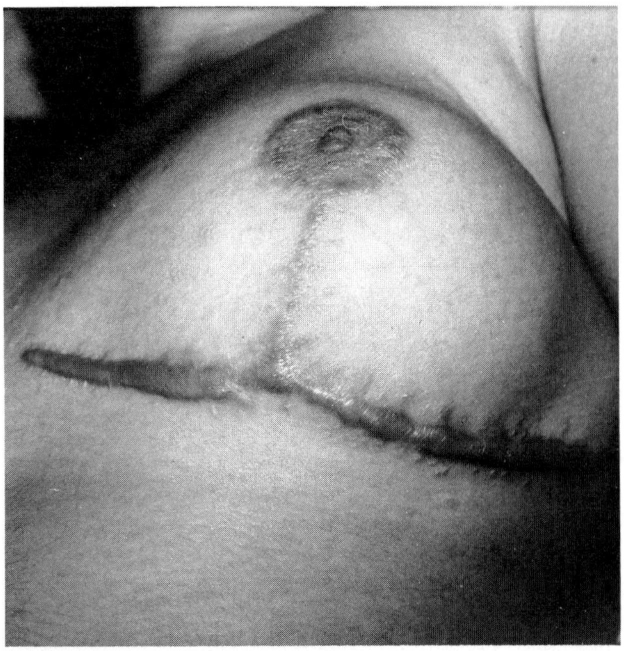

FIGURE 24-7 Severe hypertrophic scars in a 21-year-old woman 1 year after reduction mammaplasty.

a preoperative consultation can be useful to diminish rather than enhance her expectations.[19]

Efforts to modify and reduce the length of the scars have been somewhat successful for the moderately hypertrophic breasts. Regnault has been able to eliminate the medial scar with her "B" technique.[20] Although she demonstrated excellent results from resection with up to 1,300 g in a large number of patients, her method has not been widely accepted.

Peixoto reported good results from a very short inframammary fold incision in 582 patients.[21]

Marchac and DeOlarte also described a method of shortening the transverse limb of the incision, making the scars less conspicuous than with traditional techniques using the Wise pattern.[22] This procedure creates a new, higher inframammary fold and does not appear to work well with large hypertrophies.

Basile was able to reduce large breasts using a similar method.[23] These techniques are promising but have not yet replaced the standard operations with longer incisions.

Benelli has recently described a periareolar mammaplasty in which the only scar is periareolar.[23a]

Scar hypertrophy is usually temporary and may gradually subside over several years. Intralesional steroids can relieve the hypertrophy but often result in a spread, depressed, and depigmented scar.

Scar revision is occasionally effective, perhaps because there is less tension than at the original operation. Compression and massage can help to minimize the extent of the recurrence of the hypertrophy after revision. Silicone gel applied to the scar has been described as a treatment for scar hypertrophy.[24] All these methods may be necessary to minimize recurrence of marked scar hypertrophy.

LOSS OF SENSATION

Other negative results of this operation that should be discussed with the patient are loss of the ability to lactate and loss of nipple sensation, which can vary from slight and temporary to complete and permanent.

Craig and Sykes reported the incidence of permanent loss of sensation to be as high as 20 percent in transposition techniques and 50 percent with free nipple grafting.[25] They noted a considerable discrepancy between subjective and objective findings and stressed the importance of preoperative assessment, because some patients with gross hypertrophy had diminished sensation.

These authors also performed anatomic dissections and determined that the nipples and areolae were supplied by branches of the third, fourth, and fifth intercostal nerves. A knowledge of the anatomy of these nerves helps to prevent interruption of sensation in aesthetic breast surgery.

AESTHETIC COMPLICATIONS

Reduction mammaplasty is often performed to relieve symptoms, but it is nevertheless an aesthetic operation. Although normal breasts can have many different sizes and shapes, aesthetically pleasing breasts must be the right size for the patient, shapely, nonptotic, and symmetric. Aesthetic complications are those in which these criteria are not met. When the result is satisfactory, the patient and doctor usually agree. Occasionally, the patient is unhappy with a good result or pleased when the result falls short of expectations.

Proper patient selection, choice of the appropriate procedure, and careful preoperative planning, as well as meticulous attention to detail in the operating room, will minimize the aesthetic complications discussed below.

Inadequate Reduction. Patients who feel that their breasts are still too large after surgery will be very unhappy (Fig. 24-8). In the preoperative consultation, it is important to discuss expectations regarding size. Once again, photographs can help to provide insight into the patient's wishes. An appropriate procedure is then selected. For example, in order to reduce gross hypertrophy adequately, amputation and free nipple grafting may be indicated.

Photographs should be available in the operating room to remind the surgeon of the preoperative appearance. With experience, one can estimate accurately the amount of tissue to be resected. Weighing

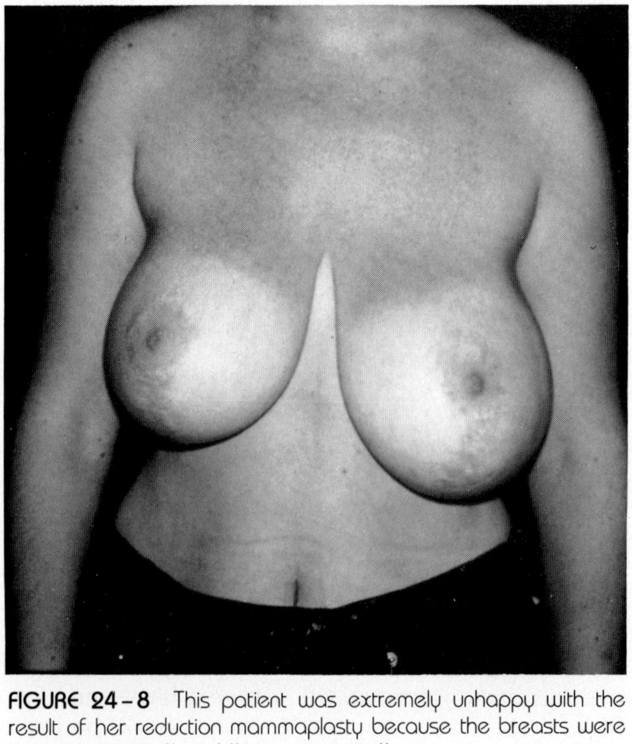

FIGURE 24-8 This patient was extremely unhappy with the result of her reduction mammaplasty because the breasts were "much too large" and "not symmetric."

the specimens in the operating room can be especially helpful in cases of asymmetry. The patient must be made to understand that perfect symmetry is impossible to achieve.

Over-reduction. In older women with marked ptosis, most of the breast tissue may have descended well below the inframammary fold. When an amputative mammaplasty is performed, it may be found that insufficient breast tissue remains (Fig. 24-9). Enough tissue should be left to augment the upper portion of the breast. It is helpful to leave breast tissue based on an inferior pedicle and then trim it to the desired size after assessment with the patient in a sitting position.

Asymmetry. In order to avoid significant asymmetry after reduction mammaplasty, a careful examination should be made preoperatively. Several days before surgery the patient is seen in the office for marking, which is done with a 20 percent solution of silver nitrate and the patient in a standing or sitting position (Fig. 24-10). The marks remain for approximately 10 days and will not wash off. After the specimens have been removed, the patient is again placed in a position sitting up at 90 degrees and reevaluated; it is impossible to assess volume, symmetry, and nipple position accurately in a supine position.[26,27]

Bottoming Out. With time the skin relaxes, allowing the breast to descend so that the nipple position changes (Fig. 24-11). In order to have the nipple properly positioned relative to the mammary gland, the distance to the inframammary fold must be kept short (less than 7 cm). The ideal position is determined with the patient sitting at the end of the procedure and the distance then shortened by 1 to 2 cm to allow for the postoperative change. Moderate

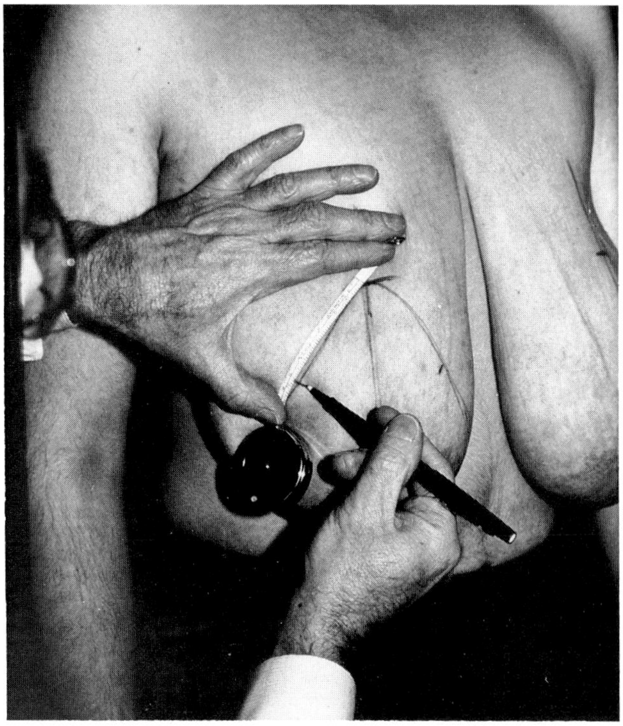

FIGURE 24-10 Preoperative marking with the patient standing.

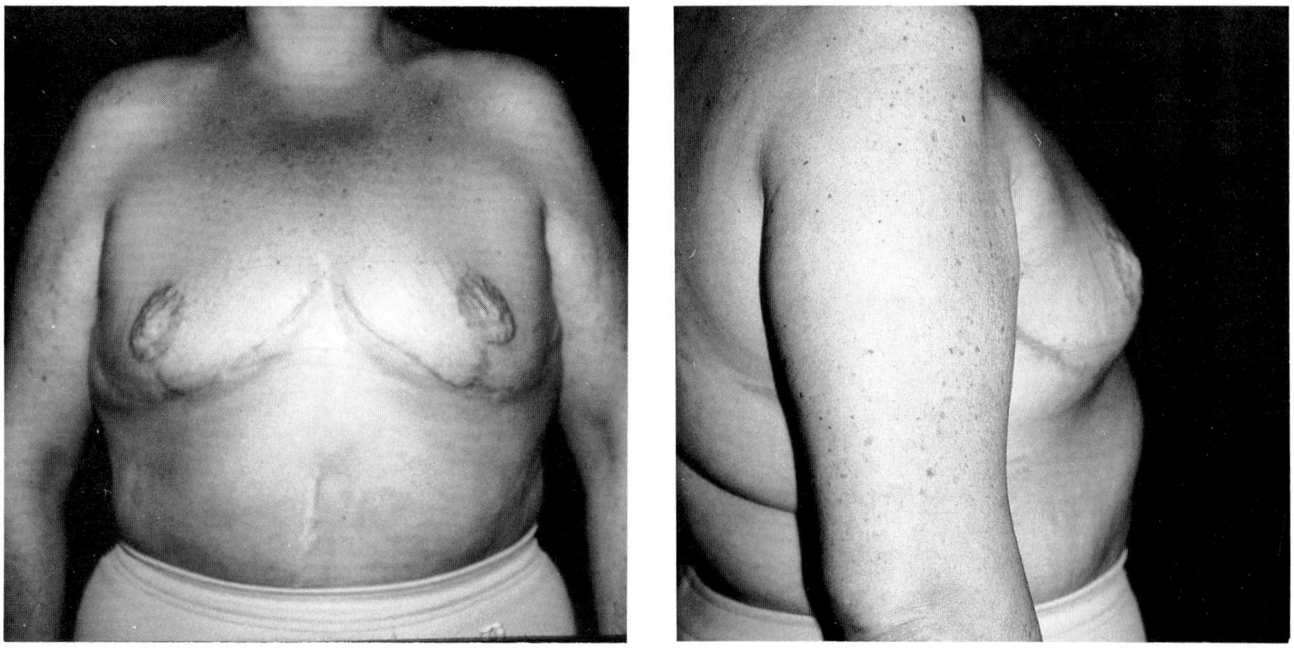

A B

FIGURE 24-9 *A, B,* This woman's breasts were very large and ptotic and she wanted them to be small. She was unprepared for the overreduction, however, and felt as though she had had a mastectomy.

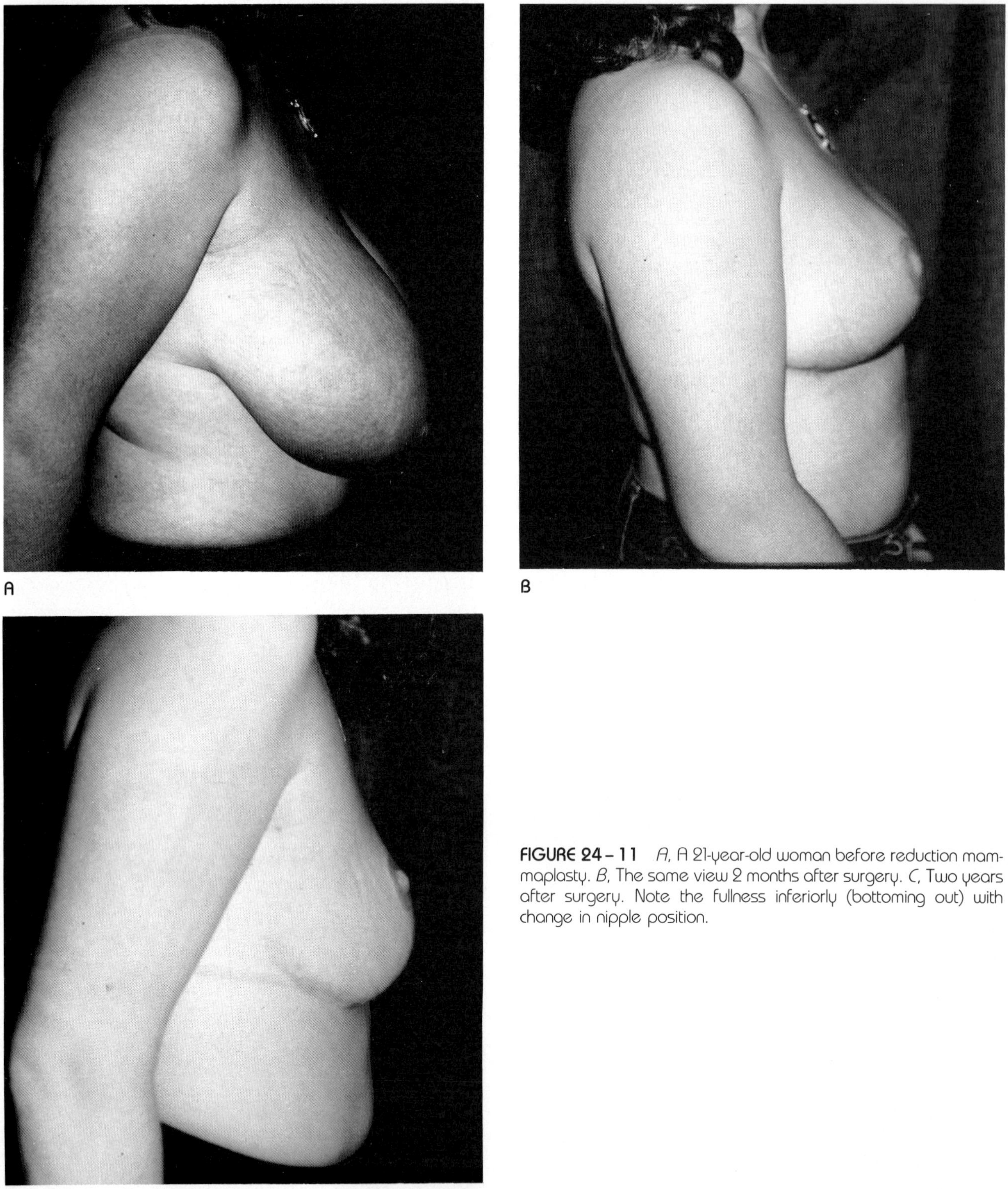

FIGURE 24-11 *A*, A 21-year-old woman before reduction mammaplasty. *B*, The same view 2 months after surgery. *C*, Two years after surgery. Note the fullness inferiorly (bottoming out) with change in nipple position.

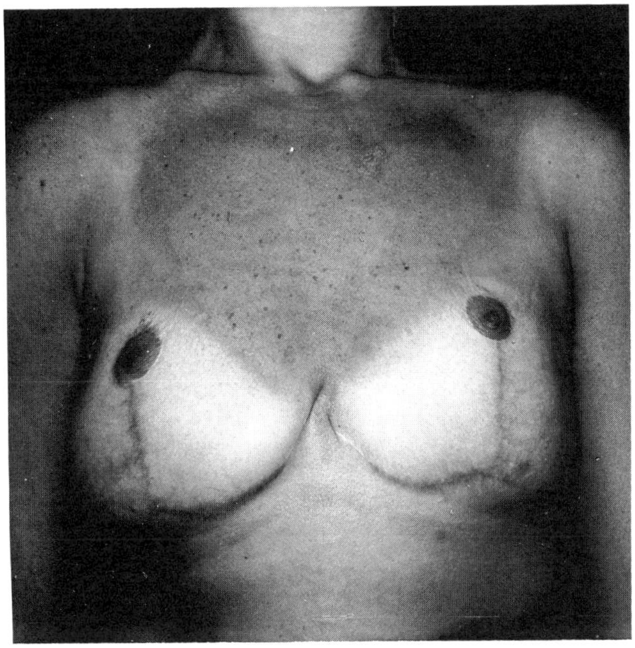

FIGURE 24–12 Postoperative photo showing high nipple position.

degrees of bottoming out can be improved by resecting additional skin. However, when the nipple is situated very high postoperatively, lowering it will result in conspicuous and disfiguring scarring above the nipple (Fig. 24–12).

Complications such as bottoming out may not become apparent in the immediate postoperative period. In order to evaluate results properly, patients should be followed for a minimum of 3 years. In some patients deformities developed after 5 years.[31] Occasional critical reviews of patients allow us to determine the efficacy of a particular procedure. In 1965 Gupta undertook such a review of the contemporary procedures used in breast reduction, concluding that the Biesenberger operation produced some good results but that there was a tendency to bottom out with time.[32] He stated that the Strömbeck procedure resulted in less postoperative sagging but produced a tendency toward inverted nipples. From these observations, modifications developed.

It is difficult to obtain adequate follow-up in this group of patients, and the many variables make comparison of results invalid.

Vilain reported on his long-term results but could not determine whether they were better or worse than those from other methods; he also could make no conclusion about nipple sensation.[6]

MEDICOLEGAL IMPLICATIONS

Most women who undergo reduction mammaplasty are happy with the results. However, a considerable number of malpractice actions result from this procedure.[17] Eleven percent of plastic surgeons who responded to a questionnaire stated that they had been sued at least once by an unhappy patient after a reduction mammaplasty. It is imperative, therefore, to inform the patient properly about the risks, complications, and expected results.[30] The best defense against malpractice action is to proper documentation of the informed consent procedure. This can consist of a note in the patient's record stating that all the risks have been explained to her, or a consent form that lists all the risks and possible complications. The use of audio and even video tapes to record the interview has been recommended.

MANAGEMENT OF CARCINOMA FOUND DURING REDUCTION MAMMAPLASTY

In addition to a careful physical examination, preoperative mammograms are indicated in patients aged 35 to 40 years, or earlier if they are in a high-risk category, e.g., a strong family history of breast cancer.

If a suspicious tumor is found during a reduction mammaplasty, a frozen section plus a wide excision (lumpectomy) should be performed and the reduction mammaplasty completed. Definitive treatment might then consist of radiotherapy or mastectomy. Mastectomy following a reduction mammaplasty can be performed through the original incision (inverted-T).[33] Primary reconstruction in these patients often requires a tissue expander, because the skin flaps will be tight.

SECONDARY SURGERY

Patients should be informed about the common complications and told that revisional surgery is occasionally needed. Those who are well informed are able to cope much better when problems do occur. For example, since it is usual to keep the scars short, dog-ears are common and often require secondary removal. Women forewarned of this accept it readily.

A frank discussion of fees should also cover the costs of secondary surgery. It is not unusual for a mastopexy to be required several years after a reduction, because ptosis does occur with time. Excision of the previous scars and excess skin without moving the nipple is usually all that is needed.

Major corrective surgery can be difficult. A knowledge of all the principles of aesthetic and reconstructive breast surgery is essential (Fig. 24–13).

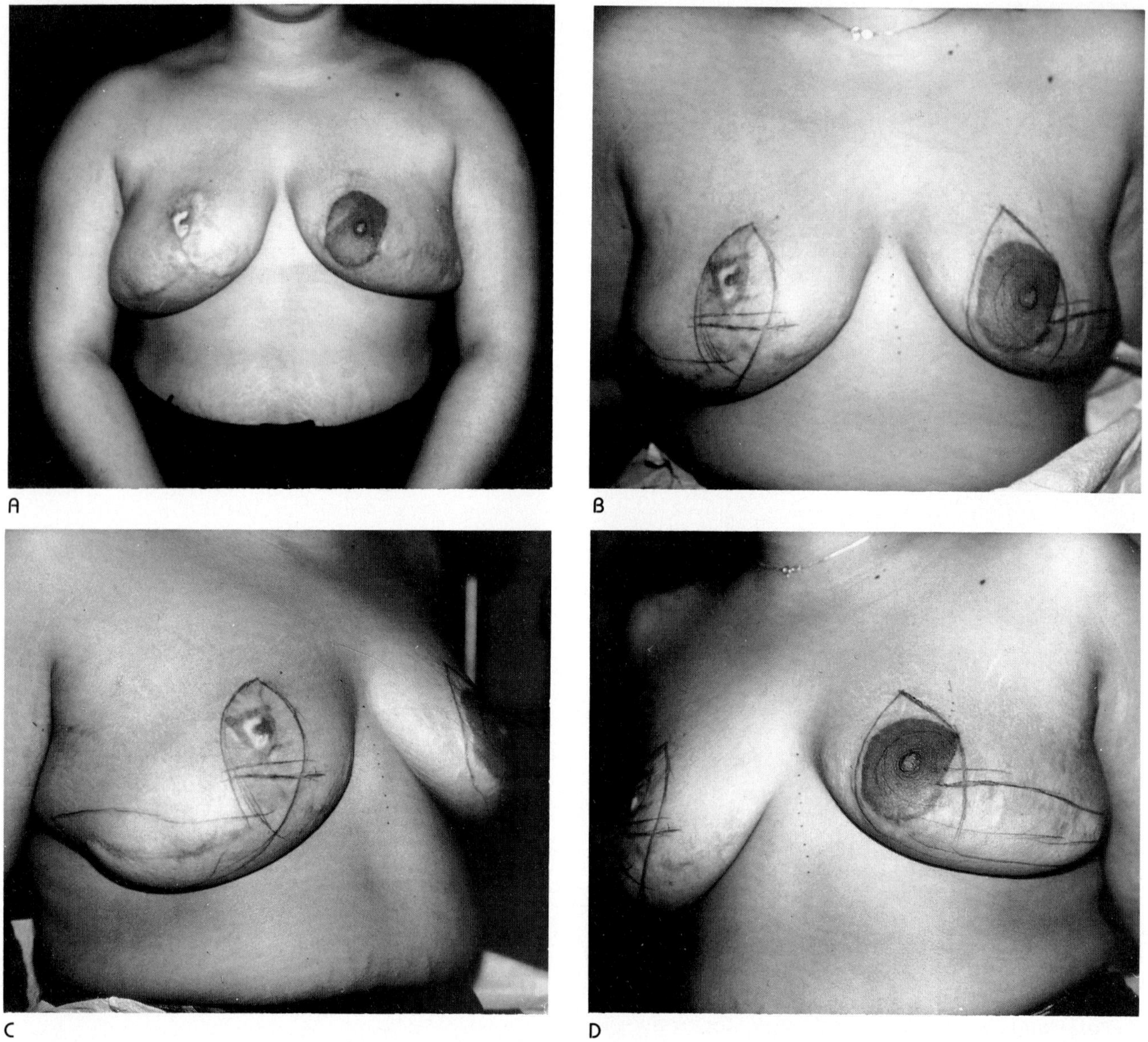

FIGURE 24 – 13 *A*, This unfortunate 35-year-old woman underwent reduction mammaplasty performed by an untrained surgeon. Note the loss of the right nipple and areola. Note the medial placement of nipples and the wide malpositioned scars. *B*, The plan of revision included excision of the scars and the remaining left nipple. The breasts were recontoured and the nipples repositioned. The right nipple was reconstructed by sharing the left side, and both were replaced as full-thickness grafts. *C*, Oblique view before revision. *D*, Oblique view. *E*, Six months after surgery, good symmetry of breasts and nipples is seen. Scars above the nipple could not be avoided. *F*, Oblique view 6 months after surgery.

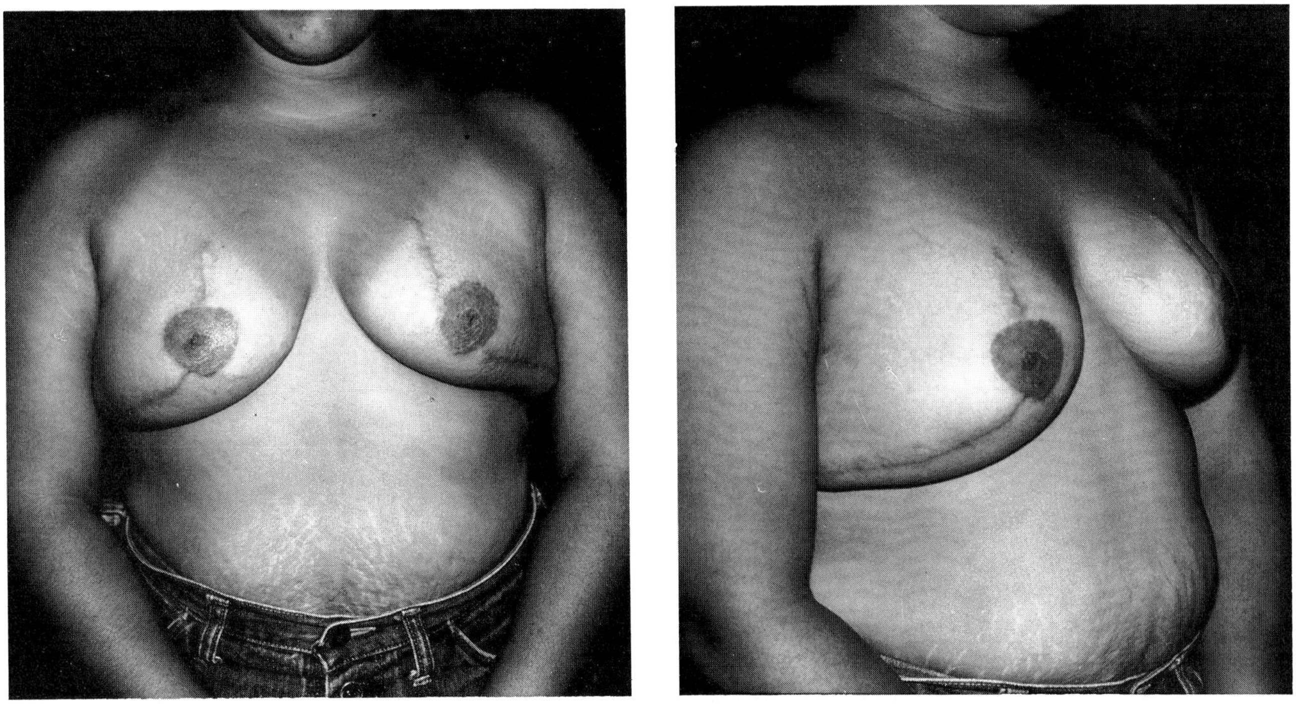

E F

Figure 24-13 *Continued*

References

1. Goldwyn RM. Remarks on reduction mammaplasty. In: Goldwyn RM, ed. Plastic and reconstructive surgery of the breast. Boston: Little, Brown, 1976:147.
2. Biesenberger H. Eine neue Methode der Mammaplastik. Zentralbl Chir 1928; 55:2382.
3. Ragnell A. Operative correction of hypertrophy and ptosis of the female breast. Acta Chir Scand (Suppl) 1946; 113:13.
4. Conway H. Mammaplasty analysis of 110 consecutive cases with end results. Plast Reconstr Surg 1952; 10:303.
5. McIndoe AM, Rees TD. Mammaplasty: Indications, technique, and complications. Br J Plast Surg 1958; 10:307.
6. Vilain R. Modification of the Biesenberger procedure. In: Goldwyn RM, ed. Plastic and reconstructive surgery of the breast. Boston: Little, Brown, 1976:155.
7. Hester TR, Cukic J. Central breast pedicle and "free hand" technique for alteration of volume and skin envelope of the breast. Clin Plast Surg 1988; 15:613.
8. Strömbeck JO. Reduction mammaplasty in upper and lower glandular resections. In: Goldwyn RM, ed. Plastic and reconstructive surgery of the breast. Boston: Little, Brown, 1976:195.
9. McKissock PK. Reduction mammaplasty with a vertical dermal flap. Plast Reconstr Surg 1972; 49:245.
10. Ribeiro LA. A new technique for reduction mammaplasty. Plast Reconstr Surg 1975; 55:330.
11. Robbins TH. A reduction mammaplasty with the areola-nipple based on an inferior dermal pedicle. Plast Reconstr Surg 1977; 59:64.
12. Courtiss E, Goldwyn RM. Reduction mammaplasty by the inferior pedicle technique. Plast Reconstr Surg 1977; 59:500.
13. Georgiade NG, Serafin D, Morris R, Georgiade G. Reduction mammaplasty utilizing an inferior pedicle nipple-areolar flap. Ann Plast Surg 1979; 3:211.
14. Rees TD, Liverett DM, Guy CL. The effects of cigarette smoking on skin-flap survival in the face lift patient. Plast Reconstr Surg 1984; 73:911.
15. Nolan J, Jenkins RA, Kunihiro K, Schultz RC. The acute effects of cigarette smoke exposure on experimental skin flaps. Plast Reconstr Surg 1985; 75:544.
16. Gradinger GP. Reduction mammaplasty utilizing nipple-areola transplantation. Clin Plast Surg 1988; 15:641.
17. Hoffman S. Reduction mammaplasty: A medical legal hazard? Aesthetic Plast Surg 1987; 11:113.
18. McKissock PK. The unfavorable result in plastic surgery. In: Goldwyn R, ed. Plastic and reconstructive surgery of the breast. Boston: Little, Brown, 1984:745.
19. Goin JM. On showing photographs preoperatively to patients (letter). Plast Reconstr Surg 1974; 54:90.
20. Regnault P. Reduction mammaplasty by the "B" technique. Plast Reconstr Surg 1974; 53:19.
21. Peixoto G. Reduction mammaplasty: A personal technique. Plast Reconstr Surg 1980; 65:217.
22. Marchac D, De Olarte G. Reduction mammaplasty and correction of ptosis with a short inframammary scar. Plast Reconstr Surg 1982; 69:45.
23. Basile RD. Mammaplasty: Large reduction with short inframammary scars. Plast Reconstr Surg 1985; 76:130.

23a. Benelli L. A new periareolar mammaplasty: The "round block" technique. Aesth Plast Surg 1990; 14:93.

24. Mercer NSG. Silicone gel in the treatment of keloid scars. Br J Plast Surg 1989; 42:83.
25. Craig RDP, Sykes PA. Nipple sensitivity following reduction mammaplasty. Br J Plast Surg 1970; 23:165.
26. Smoot EC, Ross D, Silverberg B, Ruttle M, Newman LM. The sit-up position for breast reconstruction. Plast Reconstr Surg 1986; 77:60.
27. Letterman G, Schurter M. A sitting position for mammaplasty with general anesthesia. Ann Plast Surg 1988; 20:522.
28. Herman S, Hoffman S, Kahn S. Revisional surgery after reduction mammaplasty. Plast Reconstr Surg 1975; 55:422.
29. Hoffman S, Schiavetti A. A reduction mammaplasty with legal implications. Ann Plast Surg 1982; 9:506.
30. Hoffman S. Medicolegal aspects of reduction mammaplasty. In: Goldwyn R, ed. Reduction mammaplasty. Boston: Little, Brown, 1989:60.
31. Hoffman S. Recurrent deformities following reduction mammaplasty and correction of breast asymmetry. Plast Reconstr Surg 1986; 78:55.
32. Gupta SC. A critical review of contemporary procedures for mammary reduction. Br J Plast Surg 1965; 18:328.
33. Hoffman S. Mastectomy with a T-shaped incision. Breast Dis 1988; 1:135.

SECTION 5

BREAST RECONSTRUCTION

CHAPTER 25

Surgical Treatment of Breast Cancer

THOMAS G. FRAZIER, M.D.

Probably no other single aspect of medicine in the 20th century has undergone such significant evolution as the primary treatment of breast cancer. Aided largely by the prospective randomized trials of the National Surgical Adjuvant Breast Project (NSABP), surgical scientists have been confronted with irrefutable data concerning the natural history of breast cancer and the impact of various local and regional treatments on outcome.

The subsequent disproving and rejection of the halstedian hypothesis has opened new avenues for breast cancer research. The concept of breast cancer as a systemic disease, almost from its inception, has more logically taken its place in the overall scheme of our knowledge about this disease. Clearly, two major factors are paramount in any treatment of cancer, but particularly that of breast cancer: (1) survival and (2) local control of the tumor.

Of perhaps equal importance in present society is the preservation of quality of life by optimizing cosmesis as part of the therapeutic approach.

To see the future, one must examine the past. Therefore, a working knowledge of the historical landmarks in breast cancer surgery should be part of every surgeon's background. The modern era of breast cancer really dates to the late 19th century when Halsted at Johns Hopkins[1] and Willy-Meyer in Great Britain described what has become known as the "classic" radical mastectomy. This really was not a new operation per se, but simply a compendium of the thoughts of their various surgical colleagues and the state of knowledge regarding breast cancer at that time. The belief that breast cancer was a predictable disease that spread from the breast through the lymph nodes into the lung, liver, and finally bone in a rather orderly fashion was the essential element in the development of the radical mastectomy. The radical extirpation of the breast, fascia, muscles, and nodes that drained the breast, if done promptly, could interrupt this progression and cure the patient! Perhaps as a tribute to Halsted's surgical fame and reputation, this theory went largely unchallenged until the 1950s, when Haagenson and Stout[2] first described their criteria against radical mastectomy. Clearly the reevaluation of the use of radical local and regional therapy for local tumors with grave signs of systemic spread was a logical step that incredibly took almost 50 years to be expressed. Refinements to the radical mastectomy, such as the addition of radiation therapy to the other lymphatic drainage from the breast, or the surgical removal of such nodes (the so-called "superradical" of Urban and Baker,[3]) only served as a clear indication that our knowledge of the metastatic patterns of breast cancer was still in its infancy. Not until Protocol B-04 of the NSABP, published in 1974, did we begin to challenge the halstedian concepts of our surgical forefathers. That study evaluated radical mastectomy and total mastectomy with and without radiation in a randomized clinical fashion. The primary aim was to ascertain whether radical mastectomy and total mastectomy with radiation were equivalent procedures, particularly in patients with clinically positive lymph nodes. The subsequent conclusions of this trial demonstrated that after 10 years, treatment of the clinically involved axillary nodes by either radical mastectomy or radiotherapy leads to equal survival patterns.[4] It was of particular interest that for patients with clinically negative nodes, total mastectomy plus nodal radiation, or even total mastectomy and observation of the axillary nodes with subsequent surgical dissection only for the 20 percent of patients who went on to develop clinical evidence of disease, also led to equal survival results. Because this was a randomized study, one would expect that 40 percent of the patients who were under observation only should have had positive axillary nodes, yet these eventually became clinically positive only half the time. This study was certainly among the first to show that survival in breast cancer is not dependent on local and regional therapy, and paved the way for what is probably the greatest single clinical trial in the history of surgery: Protocol B-06, the initial results of which were published in 1985.[5]

In the interim between 1974 and 1985, the changes to modified mastectomy had begun in full force, using different approaches from a number of investigators, each of whose names are now connected with variations on the theme of total mastectomy and axillary dissection. The Patey or Handley procedure[6] is a variation of total mastectomy and axillary dissection, which includes the removal en bloc of the pectoralis minor muscle. This does provide a slightly greater access to the axillary nodes for dissection, and therefore is still in favor with many surgeons who believe that en bloc resection is essential to total extirpation of the tumor. The Auchincloss mastectomy[7] divides the pectoralis minor while leaving it in place, allowing again for slightly better visualization and easier removal of the nodes. The Madden approach,[8] on the other hand, leaves both the minor and major intact, relying on retraction and the capability of the individual surgeon to remove all the nodes without cutting either muscle. The benefits of these approaches are discussed later in this chapter.

When Protocol B-06 was conceived and eligible patients began to accrue in April, 1976, the overall aims were to compare segmental mastectomy and axillary dissection, with and without radiation to the breast, with total mastectomy and axillary dissection. Eligible patients who had tumors 4 cm or less in diameter, with or without clinical axillary node involvement, were randomized to one of the three groups, (1) to test whether segmental and axillary dissection with or without radiation of the breast would be equivalent to total mastectomy and axillary dissection, and (2) to determine whether cosmetically acceptable preservation of the breast could be achieved without unfavorably influencing treatment failure and mortality rates, as well as morbidity. Obviously a third aim was to evaluate the clinical significance of microscopic multifocal breast tumor in the group who had neither radiation or total mastectomy. Two of these areas can now be addressed.

DEFINITION OF NATURAL HISTORY

Of patients who underwent lumpectomy alone, 28 percent had recurrence in the breast as a "second event" at 5 years, and that number increased to almost 40 percent at 8 years. This group of patients needs a better predictive treatment, if possible; i.e., one that allows knowledge of which patients are likely to experience recurrence if they are treated by segmental resection alone. This is discussed later in the chapter. It is critical to decide whether multifocal disease will ever become clinically important, or whether breast cancer may in some ways mimic some of the studies on multifocal disease of the thyroid in which other areas of malignancy may be present, but may never become clinically important.

VALUE OF RADIATION

Radiation in Protocol B-06 was given to the breast only, not to other node groups, i.e., the supraclavicular, internal mammary, or axillary nodes. Only 8 percent recurred as an "event" in the breast at 5 years, and that number was essentially the same at 8 years. The value of radiation for local control in the breast has thus been established. Clearly at 5 years, however, 100 patients receive radiotherapy to obtain control in the 20 percent who actually benefit from the radiation. It is hoped that not so much time will be needed for radiation therapists to move away from "radical radiation therapy" (the inclusion of supraclavicular and internal mammary nodes in the radiated fields, as well as the area of axillary dissection) as was required for surgeons to understand the patterns of disease spread.

STATUS OF AXILLARY DISSECTION

From both B-04 and B-06 protocols, it has become obvious that the axillary dissection really serves as a prognostic indicator, and very rarely is therapeutic. The status of the nodes was thought for many years to be an indicator of the aggressiveness of the tumor, and as such the hallmark for adjuvant systemic therapy. Clearly, the single most important factor in the prediction of recurrence is the presence of positive nodes. To evaluate node-negative patients who even in the Stage I and II trials would have at least a 25 to 30 percent chance of having recurrence, Protocols B-13 and B-14[9] were initiated and activated in August, 1981. The early data from these studies suggested that most patients should undergo systemic therapy regardless of nodal status, and although there has been no impact on survival this early in the trials, the impact on recurrence suggests that some form of adjuvant therapy may be of value for almost every patient, and that the value of axillary dissection itself may be in a state of flux.

All these changes, however, cannot obscure the primary goals of therapy—local control and survival—and although mastectomy clearly remains the best choice for local control, the key question that must eventually be answered is whether long-term survival in patients who have failed radiation therapy and undergone salvage mastectomy is affected by the delay in performing mastectomy. Unfortunately, or perhaps fortunately, too few recurrences have been described after radiation for a definitive statement regarding this to be made. "Salvage mastectomy" may in fact eventually prove to be as therapeutic as initial mastectomy, but this cannot be confirmed with certainty at this time. Therefore, the standard by which all treatments must be judged is mastectomy. The various surgical approaches currently employed are discussed below.

RADICAL MASTECTOMY

In my opinion, this procedure should be mentioned for historical purposes only. Even for tumors that are adherent to the muscle, my current approach is to widely excise the muscle at the point of adherence, with at least a 1-cm margin (the so-called saucerizing technique), and follow with either local radiation therapy or systemic adjuvant therapy, almost irrespective of nodal analysis. The morbidity rates related to arm edema, delay or loss of shoulder function, and chest wall deformity clearly outweigh any theoretical advantages of radical mastectomy. The plastic surgeon will continue, however, to be confronted with this procedure on occasion, particularly in patients who in the course of having a modified radical mastectomy have had the pectoralis major muscle denervated and, with subsequent atrophy, have a sunken defect requiring excessive skin and probably muscle coverage.

MODIFIED RADICAL MASTECTOMY

The appropriate technique for this procedure is to use a transverse or oblique incision that removes the nipple and as much of the breast parenchyma as possible, by cutting flaps that approximate the thickness of the patient's subcutaneous fat in other areas of the thorax (Fig. 25-1*A*). Usually this dissection occurs in the superficial layer of the superficial fascia, and should include any parenchymal breast tissue that extends into the axilla. Although this is sometimes a difficult plane of dissection, care with this technique should remove over 98 percent of the breast tissue. On the chest wall the deep layer of the superficial fascia should be removed with the breast, and usually an attempt should be made to preserve the very thin layer of deep fascia that overlies the pectoralis major and the serratus muscle (Fig. 25-1*B*). The key question in approaching the axilla is again to define the purpose of the axillary dissection. Most surgeons agree that the goal is to stage patients adequately, and although many patients are not upstaged by taking the level III, or highest, nodes (the so-called apical segment), I still prefer to remove that segment, particularly in premenopausal patients for whom upstaging could be particularly important with regard to adjuvant chemotherapy. Using a Richardson retractor, adequate exposure can be obtained by retraction only, without sacrifice or division of

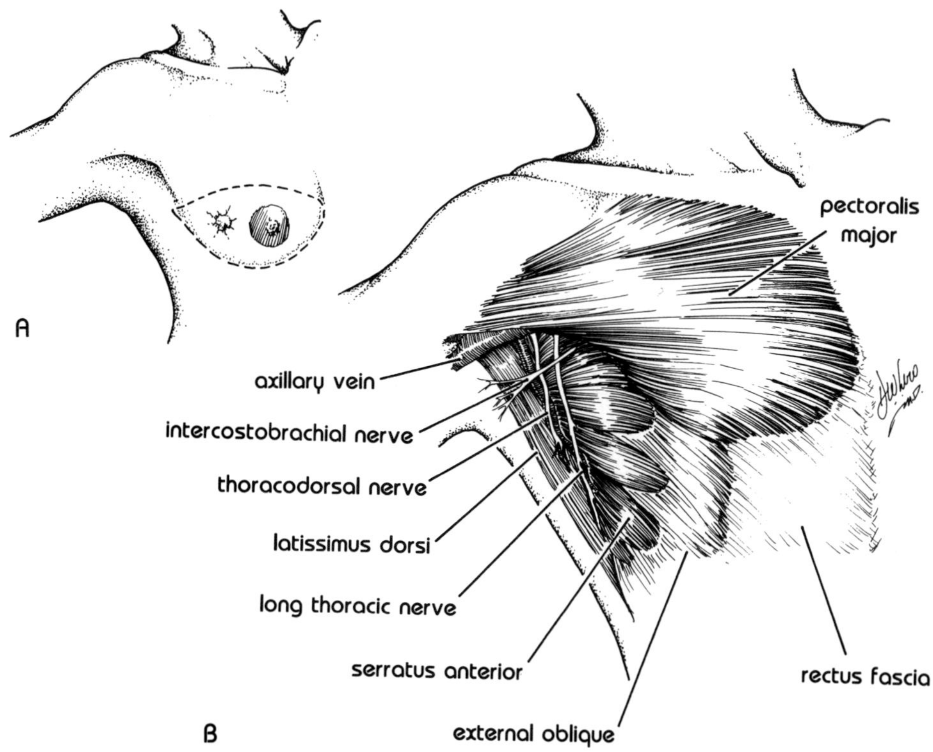

FIGURE 25-1 *A*, A transverse or oblique incision is standard for exposure to perform a modified radical mastectomy. The nipple-areola complex should be included within the incision. A margin of at least 1 cm from all palpable borders of the tumor is essential. *B*, The axillary vein is the upper limit of the axillary dissection, and the anterior border of the latissimus dorsi muscle is the lateral limit. The long thoracic and thoracodorsal nerves are preserved, in addition to at least one or two branches of the intercostobrachial nerve. If immediate reconstruction is planned, it is important to preserve the junctions of the pectoralis major and external oblique muscles with the rectus fascia.

the pectoralis minor muscle. My own preference is to avoid injury to both the lateral and medial branches of the nerves to the pectoralis major, thereby minimizing any risk of atrophy of the major muscle. Some surgeons believe that the removal of Rotter's nodes (the inter- and intrapectoral nodes) can be accomplished only by removal of the pectoralis minor. Although this may be true, such an approach will almost always sacrifice both innervations to the pectoralis major, and the subsequent atrophy of the major is an unacceptable price to pay, in my opinion, for the theoretical advantage of removing Rotter's nodes. The cosmetic defect that plastic surgeons face after this is generally one that can be easily reconstructed via the established submuscular approach.

AXILLARY DISSECTION

The limits of the axillary dissection should not go above the axillary vein, nor is dissection extended laterally beyond the anterior border of the latissimus dorsi muscle. Such an approach has not altered our lymph node counts (mean 25.9 nodes), and I make every effort to preserve not only the long thoracic and thoracodorsal neurovascular bundle but also at least one or two branches of the intercostobrachial nerve (Fig. 25–1*B*). Preservation of these last structures has made a profound difference in patient mobility and comfort, and requires only a few extra minutes of dissection.

There usually is a palpable node or two laterally at the level where the thoracodorsal nerve dips into the muscle, and this generally is also taken as a separate lateralmost level II node segment (Fig. 25–1). As mentioned, I take care not to injure any component of the thoracodorsal neurovascular bundle, because preservation of this is important if the patient ever requires reconstruction with a latissimus dorsi muscle flap.

BIOPSY

Although most patients, on the basis of the data from the NSABP Protocol B-06, would be logical candidates for breast conservation surgery, only 40 percent of our patients have chosen this option. This compares with 25 to 30 percent in the NSABP trials and 15 percent nationwide. However, it is still preferable to plan the biopsy with future therapy in mind. Many of our current patients are diagnosed with fine needle cytology, and present for definitive surgical treatment without any encumbrance from a previous biopsy scar, we have continued to use innovative incisions at the time of mastectomy to improve the cosmetic result and save additional skin for the immediate or subsequent reconstruction. The best result from biopsy itself requires meticulous hemostasis to encourage seroma and prevent hematoma. The biopsy should be done as a segmental resection with a portion of normal surrounding tissue taken, thereby making reexcision of the biopsy site unnecessary and providing a better cosmetic result, although our own studies have shown that there may still be as many as 25 percent of patients who have residual tumor, despite pathologically clear margins.[10] I never reconstruct the breast tissue itself, and always close the biopsy without a drain, using a subcuticular closure and $\frac{1}{4}$-inch Steri-Strips.

ADDITIONAL TECHNICAL POINTS

Use of Fluorescein

Since our first immediate reconstruction in 1977, I have used fluorescein injection for every patient, using 10 cc. of 100 mg per cc as the dose, evaluated the skin with a Wood's lamp, and trimmed the skin flaps as necessary. This is particularly important in patients who smoke, but the routine use of fluorescein to assess flap viability has virtually eliminated flap necrosis in patients undergoing mastectomy, either with or without immediate reconstruction.

Incisions

Clearly the transverse or Stewart incision is cosmetically preferable and is our goal for all mastectomy patients. As previously stated, lateral-based incisions can be used for lower outer quadrant radial biopsies, and other innovative incisions may also be used. It is essential to plan the incisions with the plastic surgeon before initiating the mastectomy itself, in order to obtain the best cosmetic result. The question of the optimal amount of skin to be excised remains to be answered. Our current approach is to make the incision at least 1 cm from the previous biopsy or palpable margin of the tumor (Fig. 25–1*A*). Although I always remove the nipple-areola complex as part of the incision, on occasion we have approached certain preinvasive lesions by coring the nipple from the skin flap and removing it with the breast, preserving the patient's own areola.[11] Use of a 1-cm margin has *not* changed our local recurrence rate.

Drains

We use two drains routinely, one to the anterior chest wall and one to the axilla. Currently I prefer the closed Jackson-Pratt system, bringing both out through separate incisions hidden by the brassiere. It is better not to bring the drains out through the axillary hair, because the scarring occasionally makes eventual shaving of the axilla difficult. The drains are removed when drainage is below 30 ml for

24 hours, or 10 ml for the last 8-hour shift. It is clear that increased or persistent drainage is a function of nodal involvement[12] and is not related to early mobilization of the arm. Consequently, I encourage immediate mobilization and use of the arm beginning on the day of surgery.

AXILLARY DISSECTION ALONE

It is important to remember in patients undergoing breast conservation surgery with axillary dissection and primary radiation therapy that cosmesis is a primary goal. I therefore make a vertical incision in the axilla, just anterior to the hair-bearing line. This not only gives a superior cosmetic result but also avoids the hair-bearing area and makes future shaving and personal hygiene easier. Again, a single closed system drain is used through a separate stab wound hidden beneath the brassiere or swimsuit line.

CHOICE OF CORRECT PROCEDURE

Clearly, we are practicing in an era of options for the treatment of primary breast cancer. It is essential, however, that treatment not be dictated by the mass media, but rather that the patient have a full understanding of the rationale behind the various choices. Each patient's tumor is as individual as the patient herself. Certain tumors and situations are not amenable to breast conservation, and these must be treated by modified radical mastectomy, with or without immediate reconstruction. These are summarized briefly in Table 25-1. It is important for the surgeon to remember that any breast conservation procedure that does not provide a good aesthetic result is really a less than adequate operation. Therefore, all patients need to be counseled on the basis of tumor factors, treatment factors, and patient factors.

TABLE 25-1 Considerations in Evaluation of Breast Conservation Therapy versus Modified Radical Mastectomy

General Factors	Histologic and Tumor Factors
Patient preference	Presence and extent of microscopic involvement of tumor margins
Age	Histologic features of tumor
Pregnancy	Tumor size in relation to breast size
Other medical conditions	Nipple discharge
connective tissue disorders	Multiple lesions revealed by palpation or mammography
heart disease	Evidence of diffuse or multicentric disease
	Location of primary tumor

Tumor Factors

Tumor factors involve the cancer itself, its aggressiveness under the microscope, multifocality, associated lobular neoplasia (or lobular carcinoma in situ), and several other considerations. It is particularly important to note that although most invasive cancers can be treated by segmental resection and axillary dissection, many ductal carcinomas in situ (DCIS) involve the breast so diffusely that they cannot be excised by partial mastectomy, and many women who have these prognostically favorable tumors require total mastectomy, with or without immediate reconstruction or delayed reconstruction. In selecting patients, two major criteria are important: (1) the potential for recurrence in the breast, especially in comparison with the local regional failure of modified radical mastectomy; and (2) the overall appearance of the breast after resection—the avoidance of a major cosmetic deformity. The latter may be determined by the size of the primary tumor, the size of the breast, the location of the tumor, and the extent of surgical margin necessary. Mammography plays an extremely important role in analysis of the breast, both preoperatively and occasionally after a segmental resection for suspicious calcifications has been carried out. Patients with two nonadjacent malignant lesions in the same breast, revealed either by palpation or by mammography, are very poor candidates for breast conservation therapy. The main reason is that the cosmetic results from multiple wide local excision and radiation boosts are satisfactory. Second, these patients may have large concentrations of tumor cells left within the breast, which are unlikely to be totally eradicated by radiation therapy. A good general rule in any therapy for breast cancer is that the greater the tumor burden, the higher is the probability of local failure, and for that matter, of distant failure also. In most series, increasing tumor size has been associated with a higher risk of local failure. Similarly, the greater the number of axillary lymph nodes involved, the greater is the risk of local failure. This is equally true of local regional failure after mastectomy. The mammogram is probably most important in showing extensive malignant microcalcification. Fifty percent of patients who have extensive microcalcifications are found to have more than one quadrant of the breast involved pathologically when mastectomy is performed.[13]

The location of the tumor is also a consideration in selection of treatment. Patients who presented with nipple discharge and a subareolar lesion were found to have a high failure rate when treated with conservative breast surgery and x-ray therapy if the nipple and areola were preserved.[14] In fact, subareolar tumors, regardless of size, were actually excluded from treatment in the original Protocol B-06. It is also important that subclinical involvement of the nipple and/or areola may occur in 50 percent of invasive tumors within 4 cm of the nipple-areola complex, even without associated nipple discharge.[15]

Thus, it appears that recurrence is clearly more common in patients who do not undergo a complete gross excision of the primary tumor. A controversy then arises concerning the maximum size of the primary tumor acceptable for treatment. In the Protocol B-06 trial, local recurrence was 6.5 percent in patients with T1 tumors and 9.6 percent in those with T2 tumors who received segmental resection, axillary dissection, and radiation therapy. On a more practical basis, it is extremely difficult to achieve a good aesthetic result when tumors larger than 5 cm must be removed, unless the patient has very large breasts. As previously mentioned, in our own studies, despite pathologically clear margins, as many as 25 percent of patients have residual tumor in the mastectomy specimen. This creates an important controversy over grossly clear versus microscopically clear margins, partly because assessing the margins is a technically difficult problem for the pathologist. It is essential that the pathologist ink or otherwise identify the margins of resection, by cutting the specimen so that they can be clearly identified on the microscopic examination. This is further complicated when a sample of the tumor is taken for estrogen and progesterone receptor analysis, as well as for DNA histography and cathepsin D analysis. Thus, the actual decision regarding the margins becomes more and more difficult for the pathologist. The histologic evaluation of tumors in Protocol B-06 so far has not found any significant histologic factors that influence failure rate, but a study by the Joint Center for Radiation Therapy in Boston has shown at least two factors to be important in the subsequent risk of local recurrence.[16]

Many factors, such as dosage to the primary site, nuclear grading, the size of the primary tumor, clinical axillary status, lymphatic vessel invasion, and blood vessel invasion were examined in this study. On multivariant analysis, the only factors that had a statistically significant impact on the local recurrence rate were the presence of extensive intraductal component (EIC) and very young patient age (less than 35 years). The group with extensive intraductal involvement had a 24 percent risk of breast cancer recurrence at 5 years and 32 percent at 10 years, compared with only 6 percent at 5 years and 14 percent at 10 years for patients without an EIC. Patients categorized as being in the EIC category were those in whom two features were simultaneously present: (1) intraductal carcinoma as a prominent portion of the primary mass and (2) intraductal carcinoma that clearly extended beyond the infiltrating margin of the tumor (predominantly noninvasive tumors with only focal areas of invasion were also included in this category). Why patients with an EIC were at such a high risk of local recurrence is not entirely clear. It is likely that these patients have a greater residual tumor burden after gross excision than do other patients. It may be that because negative margins were required for inclusion in Protocol B-06, many patients in this category did not have negative microscopic margins, and therefore underwent mastectomy in that randomized study. Thus, if the margins are involved and the patient can cosmetically undergo a reexcision of the scar and previous segmental resection site, it should be done before conservative therapy is considered. Our own practice is to reexcise; if on reexcision the margins are still positive, the patient is informed that she is at high risk for local recurrence and should be treated by mastectomy as the optimal therapy. When reexcision is not technically possible or cannot be done without causing severe breast deformity, mastectomy is clearly more desirable.

Some other important histologic features may be those associated with infiltrating lobular carcinomas. A number of authors have reported that patients with infiltrating lobular carcinoma may have slightly higher recurrence rates than those with infiltrating ductal histology.[17]

Our own experience is that lobular carcinomas tend to produce very little reaction on physical examination, and the tumor often extends widely throughout the breast. Associated microcalcifications may or may not be seen radiologically, making these extremely difficult to diagnose both on physical examination and mammography. Thus, we tend to look very carefully at patients with lobular carcinoma for multifocality, and pay particularly close attention to them at follow-up.

The effect of age is a controversial subject. The study from the Joint Center for Radiation Therapy showed that patients under the age of 35 had an increased frequency of recurrence, and also a higher frequency of EIC. We have found that our younger patients often are from very high-risk families, and they therefore may be a genetic variant as a potential cause of tumor. Whether this is related to hormone analysis or general aggressiveness of the tumor in these young patients must be a matter for speculation at the present time. However, we tend to favor mastectomy for younger patients, not only because of the histologic and frequently genetic factors, but also because most are estrogen and progesterone receptor negative, and therefore are offered chemotherapy as an adjuvant. Some authors have already reported that the combination of radiation therapy and chemotherapy produces a less desirable cosmetic result, and since the goal for younger patients is not only survival but good aesthetics, we have tended to obtain our best cosmetic results from mastectomy and immediate reconstruction.

Treatment Factors

Treatment factors involve the availability of radiation therapy in the patient's locale and the ability to handle 5 weeks of therapy, 5 days a week. In addition, the patient's medical or cardiac history rarely may be so precarious as to exclude the option of mastectomy.

Patient Factors

Patient factors are an essential part of the decision process, and it is here that the art of medicine plays a major role. Some patients do not want their breast removed under any circumstance; others do not want to be concerned about the possibility of additional surgery in the future, even if that chance is only 8 percent or lower. The philosophy of life as a glass of water—half empty or half full—is of paramount importance in the patient's mental well-being, and attitudinal factors become extremely important.

Clearly, the goal of every oncologic surgeon must be to individualize an appropriate therapy for each patient. The triumvirate of survival, local control, and cosmetic result, or quality of life, must be the guiding principles of the decision-making process. Keeping in mind that there is no right answer for every given patient, but only a right answer for any given patient, this goal can be successfully achieved.

References

1. Halsted WJ. The results of operations for the cure of cancer of the breast performed at the Johns Hopkins Hospital from June 1889 to January 1894. Johns Hopk Hosp Bull 1894-1895; 4:297.
2. Haagenson CD. Disease of the breast, 3rd ed. Philadelphia: WB Saunders, 1986.
3. Urban JA, Baker HW. Radical mastectomy in continuity with en bloc resection of the internal mammary lymph node chain. Cancer 1952; 5:992.
4. Fisher B, Redmond C, Fisher ER, et al. Ten year results of a randomized clinical trial comparing radical mastectomy and total mastectomy with or without radiation. N Engl J Med 1985; 312:674.
5. Fisher B, Bauer M, Margolese R, et al. Five year results of a randomized clinical trial comparing total mastectomy and segmental mastectomy with or without radiation in the treatment of breast cancer. N Engl J Med 1985; 312:665-673.
6. Handley R, Thackray A. Conservative radical mastectomy (Patey's operation). Ann Surg 1969; 170:880.
7. Auchincloss H. Significance of location and number of axillary metastasis in carcinoma of the breast: A justification for a conservative operation. Ann Surg 1963; 153:37.
8. Madden JL, Kandalaft S, Bourque R. Modified radical mastectomy. Ann Surg 1972; 175:624.
9. Fisher B, Constantino J, Redmond C, et al. A randomized trial evaluating tamoxifen in the treatment of patients with node negative breast cancer who have estrogen receptor positive tumors. N Engl J Med 1989; 320:479.
10. Frazier TG, Wong WY, Rose D. Implications of accurate pathologic margins in the treatment of primary breast cancer. Arch Surg 1989; 124:37.
11. Bland KI, O'Neal B, Weiner LJ, Tobin CR. One stage simple mastectomy with immediate reconstruction for high risk patients. An improved technique: The biologic basis for ductal glandular mastectomy. Arch Surg 1986; 121:221.
12. Petrek JA, Rogato A, Knauer C, et al. Axillary lymphadenopathy: A prospective randomized trial of thirteen factors influencing drainage, including early or delayed arm mobilization. Presented at the Annual Meeting of the Society of Surgical Oncology, San Francisco, 1989.
13. Danoff B, Goodman RL. Identification of a subgroup of patients with breast cancer in whom conservation surgery and radiation is contraindicated (abstract). Int J. Radiat Oncol Biol Phys 1985; 11 (Suppl 1):104.
14. Recht A, Danoff BS, Solin LJ, et al. Intraductal carcinoma of the breast: Results of treatment with excisional biopsy and irradiation. J. Clin Oncol 1985; 3:1339.
15. Suehiro S-I, Inai K, Tokuoka S, et al. Involvement of the nipple in early carcinoma of the breast. Surg Gynecol Obstet 1989; 168:244.
16. Osteen RT, Connolly JL, Recht A, Silver B, Schnitt SJ, Harris JR. Identification of patients at high risk for local recurrence after conservative surgery and radiation therapy for stage I or II breast cancer. Arch Surg 1987; 122:1248.
17. Schnitt SJ, Connolly JL, Silver B, Recht A, Rose MA, Harris JR. Infiltrating lobular carcinoma of the breast: Results of treatment with conservative surgery (S) and radiotherapy (RT) (abstract). Int J Radiat Oncol Biol Phys 1988; 15 (Supp 1).

CHAPTER 26

Partial Mastectomy and Radiation Therapy

W. EARLE MATORY, JR., M.D.

The potential multicentric nature of breast cancer increases the difficulty the surgeon faces in establishing the amount of breast resection necessary to achieve tumor control. There is no question that microscopic foci are left behind after both conservative and radical cancer management. Subserial histologic sections after modified radical mastectomy indicate the presence of remote foci of tumor in 40 to 50 percent of specimens.[1-4] Residual cancer was noted in 63 percent of 203 simulated partial mastectomies by Rosen and colleagues.[5] Persistent tumor was observed in 26 percent of patients after partial mastectomy for lesions less than 2 cm in diameter, and in 38 percent after resection of lesions greater than 2 cm in diameter. Conservative management is based on the premise that limited resection of tumor will remove gross cancer involvement and that radiation will eliminate residual microscopic carcinoma. Prospective randomized trials indicate no difference in disease-free, distant disease-free, and long-term survival for total mastectomy versus partial mastectomy and radiation at 5, 8, and 10 years, respectively.[6-8] Patients in whom solitary recurrence develops may be addressed with salvage mastectomy without known change in survival.[9-12]

The National Surgical Adjuvant Breast Protocol suggests that individuals with Stages I or II breast cancers (tumors smaller than 4 cm in diameter) are most amenable to partial mastectomy.[3] Ideally, all gross tumor must be resected. Contraindications are less well defined but include pregnancy. A large resection in a small breast is relative contraindication. A multifocal or poorly defined primary tumor that is not amenable to complete resection is a poor candidate for conservative cancer management. A very large breast may be a contraindication to adequate radiation therapy.

Although partial mastectomy with radiation therapy now serves as a viable option in the management of primary operable breast cancer, a vast diversity of techniques has been described. These range from the quadrantectomy of Veronesi and colleagues[13] and Crile and associates[14] to the limited lumpectomy of Fisher and colleagues.[3] The rapid evolution of lumpectomy has preceded a consensus among surgeons as to standard operative technique. The goals of breast conservation cancer management are local tumor control and cosmesis. The aesthetic results, however, are often disparate from one surgeon to another and from one patient to the next. In many instances the procedure is that of individualized art form, without discrete anatomic boundaries. The following summarizes a critical review of several hundred partial mastectomies, their cosmetic outcome, and what I consider to be a more consistently aesthetic approach to conservative cancer management.[15]

RATIONALE AND PLANNING

Objective aesthetic outcome is influenced primarily by surgical technique, and then the effects of radiation. The primary factors contributing to surgical defects include size of resection relative to breast size, location of tumor, orientation of skin and parenchymal resections, and parenchymal closure (Table 26-1). The latter two factors are most easily influenced by the surgeon, who must be familiar with lines of resting skin tension within the breast (Fig. 26-1). The ideal operative design must include adequate resection of tumor, maintenance of nipple position, and preservation of conical shape in each region of the breast (Fig. 26-2).

The most important surgical contribution to failure of local tumor control is inadequate resection. According to Westbrook and Gallager,[16] early intraductal cancer growth is confined to the ductolobular

TABLE 26-1 Factors Contributing to Surgical Defects After Partial Mastectomy

Size of breast relative to size of resection
Location of tumor
Orientation of resections
Parenchymal closure

system. On the basis of the orientation of the ductal system, a transverse ellipse may not completely excise the tumor (Fig. 26-3). However, radial excision of the ductal system may potentially increase the adequacy of resection. Further support for radial resection of skin or parenchyma is illustrated in Figure 26-4.

Skin incisions should be oriented along lines of resting skin tension.[13] Langer's lines, represented by concentric circles around the nipple, are inappropriate for skin incisions.

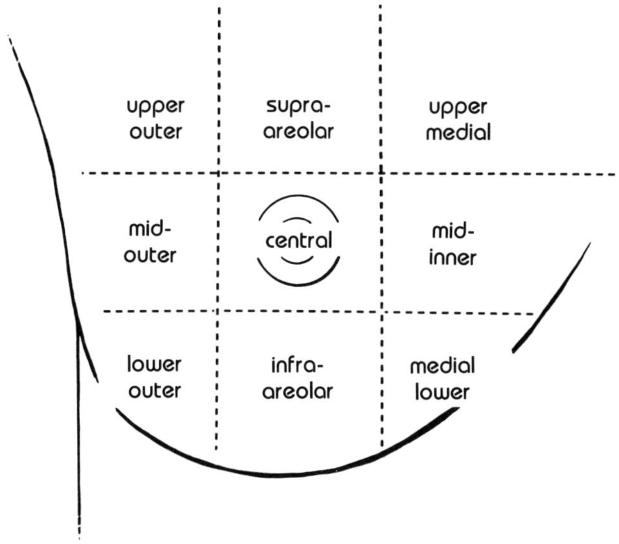

FIGURE 26-2 Resections within various regions have different effects on breast contour.

OPERATIVE TECHNIQUE

Both breasts should be prepared within the operative field, to permit a comparison with the contralateral breast. If desired, the contralateral breast can be isolated with sterile transparent drapes. The tumor is identified and the skin incision outlined along resting skin tension lines. The incision rarely needs to be longer than 5 cm. Local anesthesia of choice is injected. It is important during the initial incision to carry the skin incision down to the level of intended resection. Once this is completed, the scalpel is used to elevate skin and fat above this plane to allow for radial parenchymal resection. This allows for independent closure of the skin and fat, which helps to camouflage underlying volume loss or breast distortion. The tumor is removed with a 1- to 2-cm margin of normal tissue.

After resection, the specimen is placed on a towel and sutures are placed in it to orient the pathologist. Metal clips can be placed along the resection margin for subsequent identification by the radiation oncologist; this is particularly helpful for identifying any residual tumor.

Parenchymal approximation is necessary after resections in the upper breast and when larger resections have been performed. Interrupted 3-0 absorbable sutures are placed in fibrous parenchyma, minimizing the amount of fat incorporated into the suture. The patient's trunk may be elevated at this point to allow comparison of gravitational forces on each area of the breast. If distortion has resulted after suture ligation, sutures may be removed. The overlying skin and fat flaps are approximated with dermal closure and tape strip applied to the skin.

Axillary Dissection

A radial incision devised for both the partial mastectomy and axillary dissection may initially preserve cosmesis. However, separate incisions

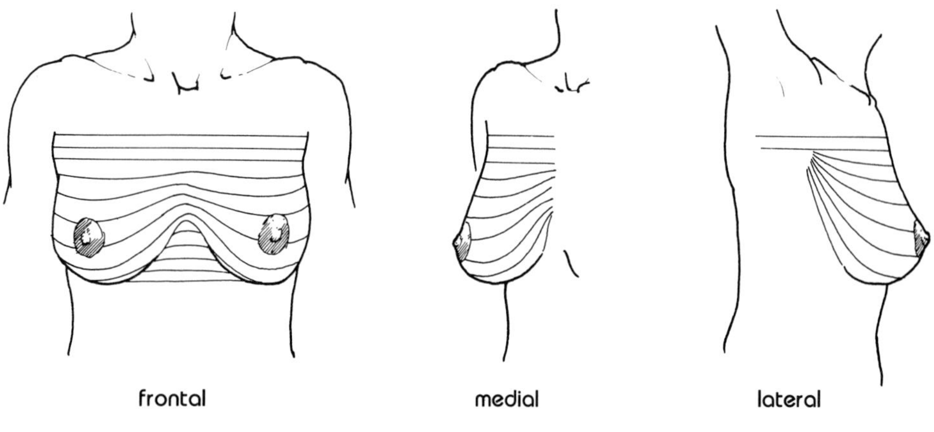

FIGURE 26-1 Lines of resting skin tension in the breast should be used as guides in planning skin incisions for partial mastectomy.

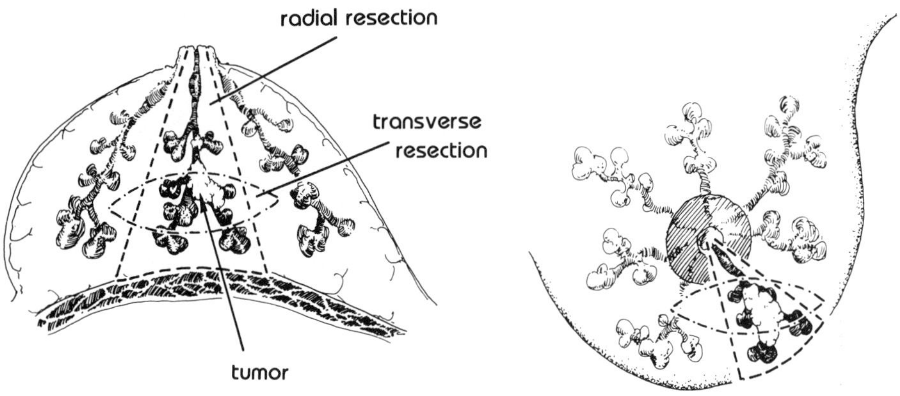

FIGURE 26-3 Rationale for radial parenchyma resection.

should be used unless the tumor is within 5 cm of the axilla. After radiotherapy, upward and outward retraction of breast tissue will occur. The incision is limited anteriorly and posteriorly by the lateral pectoral and latissimus borders. Transverse orientation further minimizes abnormal scarring. A length of 6 to 8 cm provides adequate exposure to complete the axillary dissection, with preservation of the axillary vein and artery, the long thoracic nerve, and the intercostobrachiocutaneous nerve. Transection of the latter may lead to troublesome paresthesias and dysesthesias of the inner arm. A level I and II dissection provides adequate node sampling with minimal resultant arm and breast edema.

COSMETIC IMPROVEMENT BY INCISION DESIGN

Conservative management may lead to the same complications noted with other forms of diagnostic and therapeutic breast cancer management. Particular pitfalls from partial mastectomy are discussed later.

When inadequate resection of gross tumor involvement is noted by the pathology department, reexcision is usually required. Radiation therapy provides some tumor control for gross involvement, but local recurrence rates are far lower after complete resection of all gross tumor.

Using the techniques described above, loss of cosmesis is usually referable to orientation of skin resections or contour deformity caused by parenchymal approximation. The initial biopsy usually determines the orientation of the subsequent partial mastectomy skin incision. A transverse resection in the supraareolar area for the initial biopsy will necessitate a similar incision for the partial mastectomy. If the biopsy incision is excised, there will be resultant upward nipple retraction. The same applies to the infra-areolar areas of the breast. If supra-areolar or infra-areolar cancer is suspected, a radial skin incision can be outlined. Subsequent skin resection can be performed with minimal deformity. It is preferable that the initial biopsy be performed by the surgeon who is to administer definitive cancer management.

The decision to use parenchymal approximation should not be finalized until the gravitational forces on the breast have been assessed. The patient must be placed in a sitting position and the contour compared with the contralateral breast.

The location of the tumor within the breast is the primary determinant of the type of incision to be made. Representative incision designs for various tumor locations are described below.

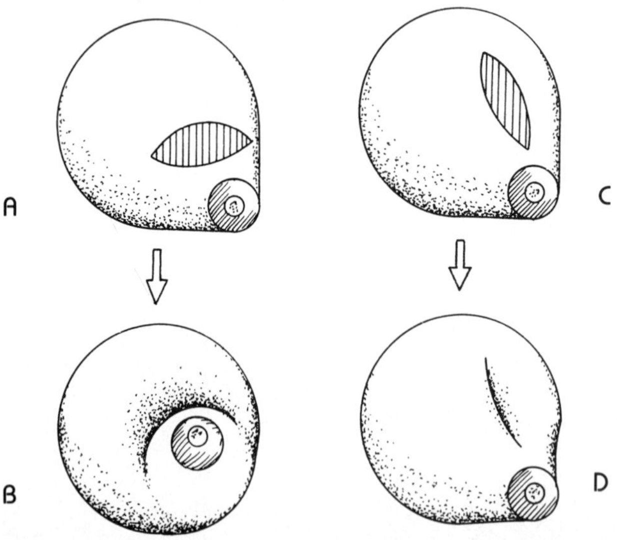

FIGURE 26-4 *A, B,* A transverse resection of skin or parenchyma will cause a shortening of one side of the cone with resultant breast distortion and nipple displacement. *C, D,* Preservation of the conical shape requires radial resection of skin, often followed by reapproximation of parenchyma.

Right Upper Outer Transverse

In the patient who has had an upper outer quadrant excisional biopsy, loss of fullness may develop in the upper breast. This may be further exaggerated by the biopsy. The orientation of previous resection necessitates a parallel elliptical resection of parenchyma with a 1-cm wide skin resection. In the absence of precise details of the original dissection or when there is postbiopsy induration, it is difficult to determine the amount of tissue to resect. Adding a 1- to 2-cm margin of grossly normal tissue can lead to a sizable resection for a relatively small tumor. Once removed, the specimen margin is sutured and oriented for the pathologist. Representative biopsies of the walls of the defect are sent for frozen section as necessary. The resultant 5- × 8-cm defect extends to the pectoralis fascia. When the tumor is adjacent to the pectoral fascia, fascia can be excised if desired. If the parenchyma is approximated, significant breast and nipple retraction will result. Interrupted absorbable sutures are placed in the deep dermis. Skin is approximated with a running absorbable dermal suture and tape strips are applied. The noted distortion and volume loss are exaggerated in the sitting position (Fig. 26-5).

Supra-areolar Transverse

The supra-areolar area is perhaps the most difficult in which to achieve optimal cosmesis. This region is the most visible within the breast. It is also the thinnest, so that any resection results in visible contour deformity. A 5-cm transverse skin incision placed directly over the tumor is adequate for exposure. Skin and fat are elevated from the parenchyma in the plane superficial to the level of planned resection (Fig. 26-6).

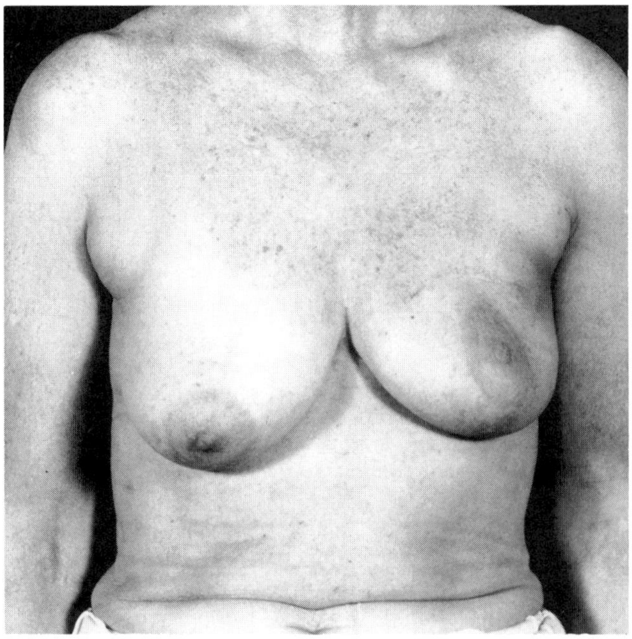

FIGURE 26-5 When a supra-areolar skin resection is needed, even a 1-cm wide skin resection leads to upward nipple and breast displacement, as demonstrated in the left breast above.

Supra-areolar Radial

A radial skin incision yields comparable exposure. A 5-cm incision is usually adequate, but may be extended along with circumareolar margin if desired. A subcutaneous plane is developed to identify the tumor. The cancer is resected, the breast undermined, and a layered closure performed. There is minimal visible change in breast volume or nipple position. The radial incision is more highly visible.

Centric Circumareolar

When the tumor lies within 2 cm of the areola, a circumareolar incision can be performed. Dissection greater than 2 cm from the areola will lead to nipple retraction due to radiation fibrosis. Up to 180° of the circumference can be used without resultant areolar distortion or ischemia (Fig. 26-7). Deep dermal sutures align the circumareolar incision, which is followed by a continuous dermal suture. Minimal deformity is noted in both the supine and sitting positions.

Centric-Nipple Resection

The incidence of synchronous microscopic nipple cancer associated with carcinoma of the breast may be as high as 30 percent.[17] Significant likelihood of microscopic nipple involvement is noted most commonly with proximity to the nipple. After resection of the primary tumor, any remaining microscopic cancer is treated with radiation. Current primary indications for a nipple resection include gross nipple involvement or tumor location within 1 to 2 cm of the nipple. The ellipse is transversely oriented. Incisions are carried directly to the pectoralis fascia, which may be resected if tumor proximity dictates. The width of resection is adjusted to achieve adequate tumor margin. Undermining in a suprafascial plane is accomplished inferiorly and superiorly to the resection. The parenchyma is closed (Fig. 26-8). Centric resection is one of the most aesthetic procedures after conservative cancer management because breast contour is preserved. Nipple-areolar reconstruction can be performed by a plastic surgeon if desired.

Infra-areolar

A transverse skin or parenchymal resection in the infra-areolar area will result in downward nipple displacement (Fig. 26-9). Conversely, a radial skin incision in the lower breast at the time of biopsy allows subsequent elliptical or wedge resection with minimal breast distortion (Fig. 26-10). The wedge is outlined and resected, carrying the incision to the

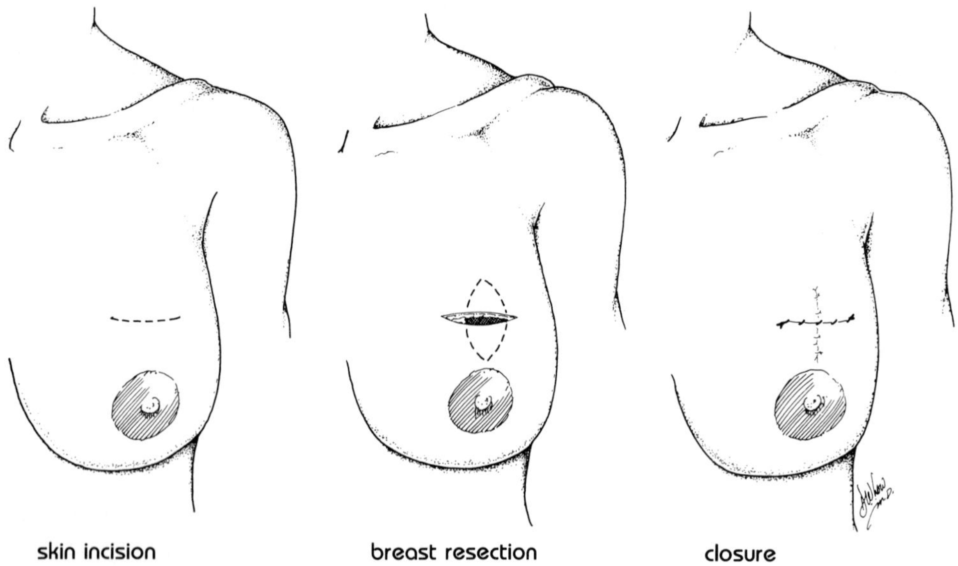

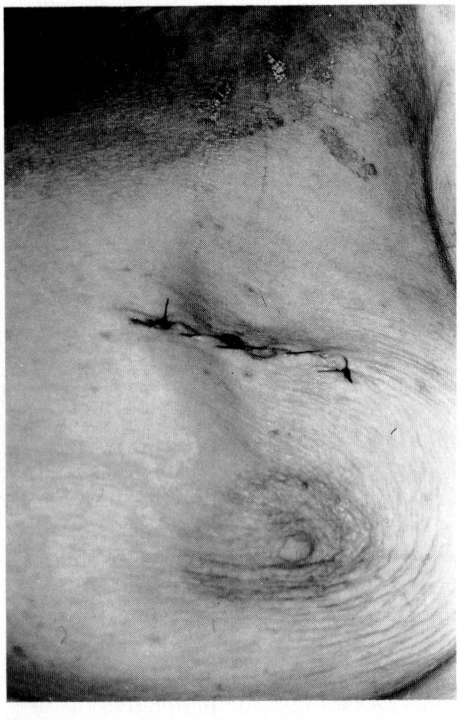

FIGURE 26-6 *A, Left,* For tumors in the supra-areolar location, a transverse skin incision is made. *Center,* A radially oriented wedge of breast tissue is resected. The gravitational pull of the lower breast will tend to separate the depths of this wound. To minimize this effort, the breast is undermined in a suprafascial plane. *Right,* Parenchyma and fascia are approximated before skin closure. *B,* After closure, the skin wound is in the direction of the lines of resting skin tension.

level of the fascia. The breast is undermined and dermis is closed. Closure of the parenchyma and skin can be facilitated by extending the incision into the inframammary fold.

The above examples show that some degree of creativity is required for conservative tumor resection in each respective breast. Using the principles stated above, one can design a resection and closure of the breast that maintains an optimal cosmetic appearance.

RADIATION FACTORS CONTRIBUTING TO LACK OF COSMESIS

Distortion of the breast by radiation has four primary causes. These causes are (1) the total dose; (2) the use of supplemental radiation; (3) overlapping of radiation fields; and (4) concurrent chemotherapy. The negative effect of total radiation dose has been greatly reduced by time-dose fractionation and by the improved administration of supplemental

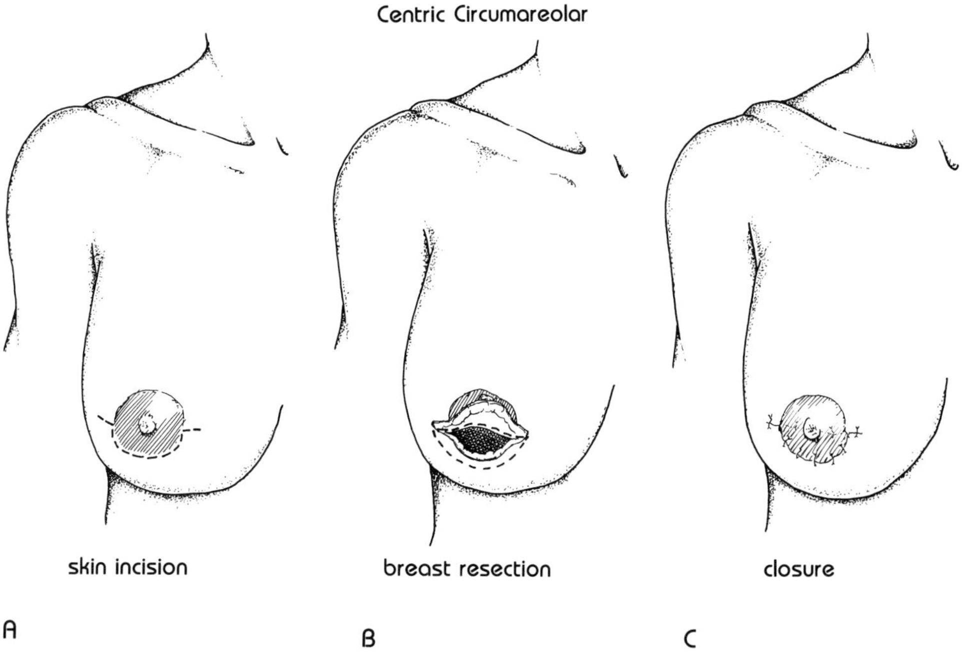

FIGURE 26-7 *A*, A 5-cm long circumareolar incision is optimal for exposure of lesions within 2 cm of the nipple. *B*, A radially oriented ellipse is outlined with close to a 3:1 width-to-length ratio to prevent dog ears. Tumor is resected. *C*, Parenchyma is approximated with absorbable suture, and skin closure is completed.

irradiation. By utilizing time-dose fractionation (giving multiple small doses of radiation over an extended period), the marked tissue destruction not uncommonly noted 10 years ago has not been seen in studies of the author's patients.[15]

Supplemental radiation augments the dose administered to those patients with positive resection margins and to those patients with invasive intraductal carcinoma. Interstitial implants and electron beam represent the two forms of supplemental therapy commonly used. The advent of electron beam has brought forth distinct advantages. The beam applies a concentrated blast of radiation, thus enhancing tumor kill. There is minimal destruction of normal tissue, making this technique particularly useful in the small breast.

After assessment of the relative contributions of surgery and radiation with and without boosts (Table 26-2), we found that over two-thirds of our patients had significant breast retraction and fibrosis prior to any radiation treatments. Retraction was slightly enhanced following tangential field expo-

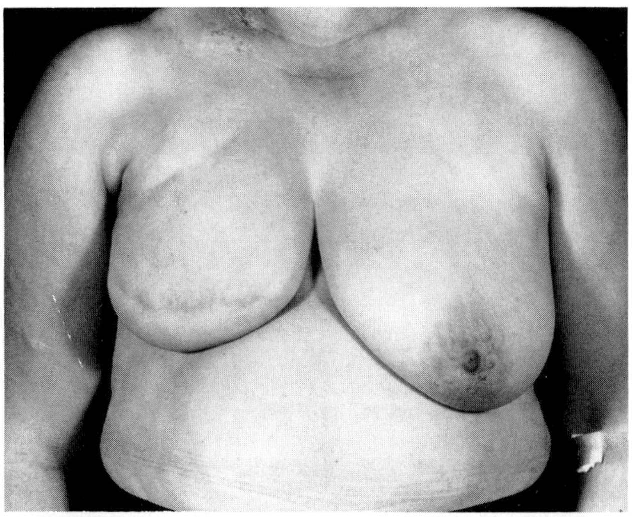

FIGURE 26-8 A 35-year-old patient 25 months after centric-nipple resection and radiation. Note the preservation of conical breast contour. Nipple reconstruction can be performed after healing and scar maturation.

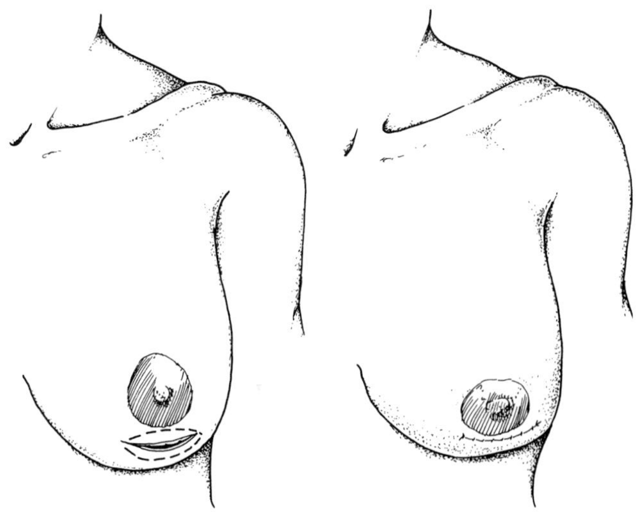

FIGURE 26-9 A transverse skin or parenchymal resection in the infra-areolar area will result in downward breast displacement. This occurs despite undermining of parenchyma to the inframammary fold.

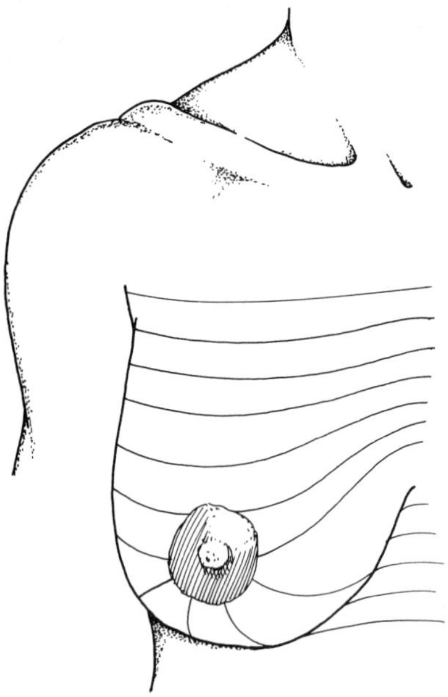

FIGURE 26-10 Proposed skin incisions for partial mastectomy, using lines of resting skin tension.

TABLE 26-3 Functional and Cosmetic Deformities Following Conservative Surgery and Radiotherapy in 57 Patients

Arm		Breast	
Edema	1	Edema	57
Supraclavicular fibrosis	0	Asymmetry	46
Shoulder resection	0	Fibrosis	36
Matchline effect	0	Telangiectasia	24
		Tenderness	15
		Hyperpigmentation	12
		Loss of sensation	11
		Fat necrosis	8

(From Matory WE Jr, Wertheimer M, Fitzgerald TJ, et al. Aesthetic results following partial mastectomy and radiation therapy. Plast Reconstr Surg 1990; 85:739.)

sure, but was markedly increased following supplemental boost. Telangiectasia was significantly augmented by supplemental radiation.

Of 12 patients who received adjunctive chemotherapy during radiation treatments, 10 noted significant fibrosis and retraction. These findings were more than expected based on surgical determinants of cosmesis.

All patients we have studied received tangential field radiation. Areas of overlap result in exaggeration of the desired tissue destruction. This causes a scorching of tissues, i.e., a matchline effect. The use of lead blocks minimizes overlapping and the resultant tissue burn. By optimizing tissue dose homogeneity, breast retraction, telangiectasia, and fibrosis can be minimized.

The physiologic changes are numerous following partial mastectomy and radiation (Table 26-3). Significant symptomatology in the ipsilateral upper extremity was rare. Breast edema was seen in all patients studied, but usually receded by 24 months. Asymmetry caused by fibrosis and retraction was seen in over 80 percent of our patients. Fat necrosis occurred in eight patients, six of whom were large breasted. In five of these patients, necrosis followed chemotherapy. These individuals were not evaluated prior to radiation, therefore we cannot assess the surgical contribution to fat necrosis.

TABLE 26-2 Boost Effect

	Postoperative	Unboosted	Boosted
Significant breast retraction	16/24(66.6%)	2/24(8.3%)	6/24(25%)
Telangiectasia	0	3/15(20%)	12/15(80%)

(From Matory WE Jr, Wertheimer M, Fitzgerald TJ, et al. Aesthetic results following partial mastectomy and radiation therapy. Plast Reconstr Surg 1990; 85:739.)

CONCLUSION

The initial biopsy should be performed by the surgeon responsible for definitive cancer management. By adjusting the orientation of skin and parenchymal resections, the aesthetic appearance can be optimized. Skin incisions in the upper breast may be placed parallel to resting skin tension lines. Parenchymal resections are best when radially oriented. If skin resections are anticipated, a radial orientation is preferable, particularly in the lower breast. Supra-areolar radial skin resections are more aesthetically satisfactory.

Parenchymal approximation is necessary after resections in the upper breast and when large resections have been performed. An associated skin resection may minimize breast distortion. Consultation with a plastic surgeon for operative planning may be of benefit to achieve the desired aesthetic result.

References

1. Qualheim RE, Gall EA. Breast carcinomas with multiple sites of origin. Cancer 1957; 10:460.
2. Gallager HS, Martin JE. The study of mammary carcinoma by mammography and a whole organ sectioning —early observations. Cancer 1984; 53:623.
3. Fisher B, Bauer M, Margolese R, et al. Five-year results of a randomized clinical trial comparing total mastectomy and segmental mastectomy with or without radiation in the treatment of breast cancer. N Engl J Med 1985; 312:665.
4. Tinnemans JGM, Wobbes T, van der Sluis RF, et al.

Multicentricity in nonpalpable breast carcinomas and its implications for treatment. Am J Surg 1986; 151:334.
5. Rosen PP, Fracchia AA, Urban JA, et al. "Residual" mammary carcinoma following simulated partial mastectomy. Cancer 1975; 35:739.
6. Veronesi U, Zucali R, Del Vecchio M. Conservative treatment of breast cancer with the QUART technique. World J Surg 1985; 9:676.
7. Fisher B, Redmond C, Poisson R, et al. Eight-year results of a randomized clinical trial comparing total mastectomy and lumpectomy with or without irradiation in the treatment of breast cancer. N Engl J Med 1989; 320:822.
8. Sarrazin D, Le M, Rouesse J, et al. Conservative treatment versus mastectomy in breast cancer tumors of microscopic diameter of 20 millimeters or less. The experience of the Institut Gustave-Roussy. Cancer 1984; 44:209.
9. Clarke DH, Le M, Sarrazin D, et al. Analysis of local-regional relapses in patients with early breast cancers treated by excision and radiotherapy: Experience of the Institut Gustave-Roussy. Int J Radiat Oncol Biol Phys 1985; 11:137.
10. Vilcoq JR, Calle R, Stacey P, et al. The outcome of treatment by tumorectomy and radiotherapy of patients with operable breast cancer. Int J Radiat Oncol Biol Phys 1981; 7:1327.
11. Kurtz MJ, Spitalier MJ, Amalric R. Results of salvage surgery for local failure following conservative therapy of operable breast cancer. Front Radiat Ther Oncol 1983; 17:84.
12. Harris JR, Recht A, Amalric R, et al. Time onset and prognosis of local recurrence following primary radiation therapy for early breast cancer. J Clin Oncol 1984; 2:37.
13. Veronesi U, Saccori R, Del Vecchio M, et al. Comparing radical mastectomy with quadrantectomy, axillary dissection, and radiotherapy in patients with small cancers of the breast. N Engl J Med 1981; 305:6.
14. Crile G, Cooperman A, Esselstyn CB, Hermann RE. Results of partial mastectomy in 1973 patients followed from five to ten years. Surg Gynecol Obstet 1980; 150:563.
15. Matory WE Jr, Wertheimer M, Fitzgerald TJ, et al. Aesthetic results following partial mastectomy and radiation therapy. Plast Reconstr Surg 1990; 85:739.
16. Westbrook KG, Gallager HS. Intraductal carcinoma in the breast. A comparative study. Am J Surg 1975; 130:667.
17. Largos M, Gates B, Westdahl PR, Richards V, Alpert B. A guide to the frequency of nipple involvement in breast cancer. Am J Surg 1979; 138:135.

CHAPTER 27

Prophylactic Mastectomy with Reconstruction

JOHN R. JARRETT, M.D.

Subcutaneous mastectomy, although first reported before 1920, was an uncommon procedure before the development of silicone bag-gel mammary prostheses for use in reconstruction in the early 1960s. Although these prostheses produced satisfactory results in routine augmentation mammaplasty, their placement in the subcutaneous space after subcutaneous mastectomy was associated with a very high rate of complications. These included severe fibrocapsular contracture (Fig. 27-1) and implant exposure, with resultant loss if even a small area of skin developed ischemic necrosis.

To combat this problem, some surgeons performed very incomplete adenomammectomies by leaving a thick layer of subcutaneous fat and tissue, which improved skin viability but not the softness. This combination of poor aesthetic results with inadequate and thus ineffective mastectomies resulted in many unhappy patients, and the procedure fell into disfavor with most oncologic and reconstructive surgeons. The introduction of submuscular reconstruction immediately after subcutaneous mastectomy[1,2] resulted in significantly fewer objections from both patients and surgeons to the original procedure. The compressive force of the dynamic muscle tissue covering the implant flattens it significantly in the early postoperative period, producing a capsule with a broad base. Therefore, after muscle stretching allows the implant to drop and project, the diameter of the capsule is great enough to allow the implant to expand when compressed, which is the hallmark of a soft reconstruction (Fig. 27-2). The early flattening of the implant also enhances skin vascularity by removing all implant pressure from the skin. In addition, with the implant totally covered by muscle, small areas of ischemic skin necrosis can be treated conservatively without endangering the implant, thus allowing surgeons to perform a much more complete glandular resection with skin flaps as thin as those in mastectomies for cancer. This last fact has enabled surgeons to readily convert prophylactic mastectomies into the therapeutic mastectomy of choice if carcinoma is found during the prophylactic mastectomy.

PATIENT SELECTION

Risk Assessment

According to the 1988 figures of the American Cancer Society, the projected lifetime risk of occurrence of breast cancer in American women was 10 percent, and 140,000 new cases were expected to be diagnosed in 1989. Despite improved diagnostic techniques and education of the public regarding self-examination and mammography, breast carcinoma remains the leading cause of cancer deaths among women. The American Cancer Society figures indicate that 25 percent of new breast cancer patients had identifiable factors placing them at increased risk before their diagnosis of carcinoma, suggesting that 36,000 of the anticipated new breast cancer patients in 1988 have been candidates for prophylactic surgery. Surgeons recommending and performing any type of prophylactic mastectomy are doing so in the belief that removal of 95 to 98 percent of breast tissue will significantly reduce or eliminate the risk of the patient's developing carcinoma.

The ideal patient for prophylactic mastectomy therefore is one who: (1) is at proven high risk for carcinoma; (2) shows significant mastopathy on physical examination and mammography; and (3) is unwilling to continue with nonsurgical surveillance and management.

The only factors that produce significant increased risk are (1) biopsy-proven high-risk tissue;

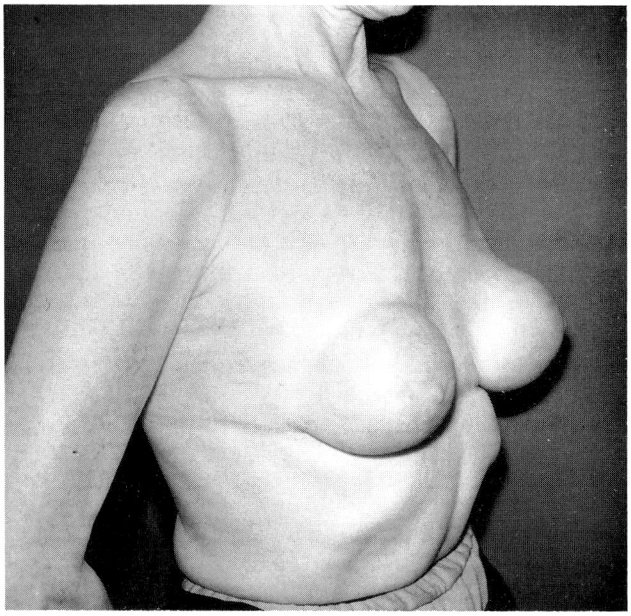

FIGURE 27-1 Severe fibrocapsular contractures in a patient with subcutaneous placement of implants after subcutaneous mastectomies. (From Riley W. Plastic Surgery Educational Foundation Instructional Courses. Vol 1. St. Louis, MO: CV Mosby, 1988.)

(2) a strong family history of breast carcinoma; and (3) contralateral breast carcinoma.

In reference to biopsy-proven risk, the College of American Pathologists in 1986, in conjunction with numerous surgeons and oncologists, issued a consensus statement[3] listing the relative risk associated with pathologic entities found in breast biopsies. The statement identified pathology findings that are not associated with an increased risk of cancer, including adenosis, apocrine metaplasia, gross cystic disease, fibroadenoma, duct ectasia, and mild hyperplasia. The report listed moderate or florid hyperplasia and papilloma with fibrovascular core as producing a cancer risk of 1.5 to two times normal, whereas atypical ductal or lobular hyperplasia was considered to involve a five times normal risk.

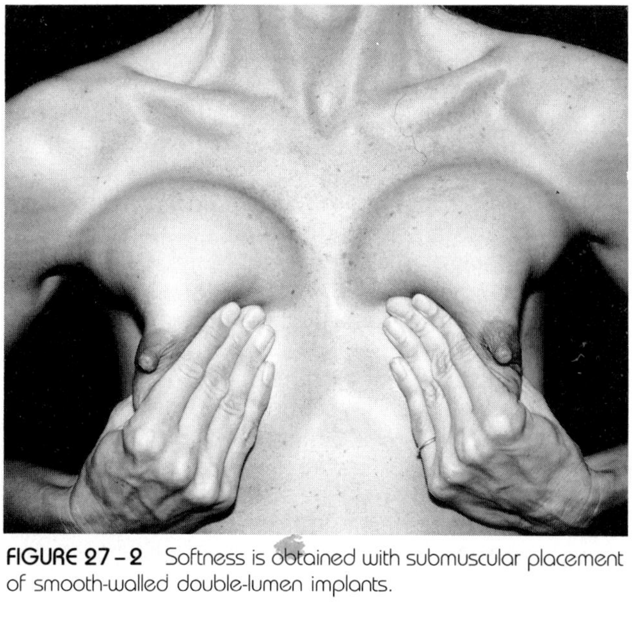

FIGURE 27-2 Softness is obtained with submuscular placement of smooth-walled double-lumen implants.

Family history is the second major factor to be considered in risk assessment. Familial breast cancer is defined as the presence of premenopausal breast cancer in two or more first-degree relatives, and it carries a risk of five to six times normal.[4,5] In addition, patients with familial carcinoma are 15 to 20 years younger at diagnosis[6] than those with sporadically occurring disease, and have a risk of bilaterality at least three times greater than normal.[7]

Premenopausal breast cancer occurring in one first-degree relative imparts a 2.5 to three times normal lifetime risk, which is doubled if that relative had bilateral carcinoma. Postmenopausal carcinoma in a sister or mother produces only a slight risk elevation, possibly up to 1.5 times normal.[7] Pre- or postmenopausal carcinoma in second-degree relatives carries little, if any, proved increased risk according to current genetic information, although carcinoma in several second- or third-degree relatives often results in increased anxiety about carcinoma. Nulliparity, early menses, and late onset of menopause are also considered very slight risk-elevating factors.

The third major factor capable of increasing the risk of breast carcinoma is the presence of carcinoma in the contralateral breast. Leis[8,9] pointed out that because many patients do not live long enough after developing breast carcinoma to have much chance of developing contralateral disease, the observed rate is much higher if only patients under 50 years of age with stage 0 or 1 disease are evaluated. Following such patients, Leis has confirmed that the risk of contralateral diagnosis becomes significant, increasing approximately 1 percent per year of survival.

Patients with invasive lobular or multifocal ductal carcinoma are also considered to be at particular risk for contralateral disease.

Indications for Surgery

A proved increased risk in conjunction with significant fibrocystic mastopathy in a patient who is unwilling to continue with conservative management is a primary reason to consider a surgical alternative. Taking into account the factors discussed above, a patient's actual risk can be fairly accurately assessed. I recommend consideration of prophylactic mastectomy for patients with a documented risk of 2.5 times normal or greater when routine surveillance is made difficult and inaccurate by significant fibrocystic mastopathy on physical examination and mammography.

From the earlier discussions of risk assessment,

the following situations place a patient in a projected lifetime risk of five times normal:

1. Two or more first-degree relatives with premenopausal breast carcinoma.
2. One first-degree relative with bilateral premenopausal breast carcinoma.
3. Biopsy-proven atypical ductal or lobular hyperplasia.
4. Biopsy-proven ductal or lobular carcinoma in situ.
5. Contralateral carcinoma plus a. One or more first-degree relatives with premenopausal breast carcinoma, or b. A biopsy finding of florid hyperplasia.
6. Contralateral carcinoma when the pathology is lobular or multifocal.

There is a lifetime risk of 2.5 to 3 times normal in one of the following situations:

1. A single first-degree relative with premenopausal breast carcinoma.
2. Contralateral carcinoma of favorable prognosis in a patient under 50 years of age.
3. A biopsy of florid hyperplasia or papilloma with fibrovascular core.

Patients without a proved risk of 2.5 times normal and significant fibrocystic mastopathy may be considered for prophylactic mastectomy when the breast examination is regarded as inaccurate and worrisome, and if this condition is accompanied by mammograms that are interpreted as inaccurate because of dysplasia and/or microcalcifications dense enough to cover a small malignancy. Many such patients have a history of recurrent cysts and masses treated by aspirations or biopsies. Such individuals, although at no proven increased risk, may have legitimate anxiety or actual cancerphobia, and thus be worthy of consideration for prophylactic mastectomy. They obviously must be informed that any such surgery is intended primarily to remove tissue of concern, relieve their anxiety, and (it may be hoped) improve the quality of their lives. The decision for surgery in these patients should have the support of an oncologic surgeon.

Severe silicone mastopathy and legitimately incapacitating mastodynia may be reasons to consider mastectomies that would be regarded as therapeutic rather than prophylactic. I prefer, however, that such surgery be considered only for a patient who has failed to obtain relief from conservative therapy, and when the procedure is recommended by a general surgeon who has evaluated that patient.

PREOPERATIVE EVALUATION AND CARE

Informed Consent

Because of the popularity of, and widespread dissemination of information regarding, purely aesthetic breast surgical procedures, it is very easy for patients contemplating prophylactic mastectomy with reconstruction to assume that the operation will enhance their appearance. This confusion is more prevalent in this operation than it is for either delayed or immediate reconstruction following mastectomy for carcinoma, when the patient is obviously aware of the severity of the deformity without reconstruction. Failure to provide a thorough basis for informed consent may result in the surgeon being satisfied with the treatment but the patient, because of unrealistic expectations, being displeased with her appearance.

My patients are therefore told, verbally and in writing, that although every effort will be made to produce a result that will enable them to maintain a satisfactory self-image, this is not an "aesthetic" procedure and they should not undergo the operation unless they are willing to accept an appearance that is less attractive than their current one.

In order that there can be no confusion regarding expectations, I provide a written description of each of the complications that could happen (plus disclaimers regarding other problems that could arise), along with information about the incidence of each complication within my practice. This is signed by the patient after a personal review with me. The list of complications includes sensory loss, hematoma, wound infection, implant problems, fibrocapsular contracture, and skin necrosis. I also show photographs of average results, including various incisions, plus other views depicting problems such as early postoperative deformity with implant asymmetry and complications such as skin necrosis. I warn the patient that a history of smoking, especially within a month of surgery (preoperatively or postoperatively), is associated with a high incidence of skin or nipple-areolar necrosis, which may result in additional surgery and even removal of the prosthesis if it becomes exposed.

Preoperative Preparation

Surgery is usually scheduled for 1 month or more from the time of initial consultation to allow time for patients to donate two units of autologous blood (unless designated donor blood is available), to eliminate salicylates and other anti-inflammatory drugs that might interfere with blood coagulation, and for smoking patients to discontinue tobacco use. Time-released iron capsules, which are tolerated better than iron tablets, are started 1 or 2 weeks before the first unit of autologous blood is donated. All patients are seen a second time in the office for the purpose of reviewing the procedure and providing informed consent, because it is very unlikely that any patient can absorb the intricate details of this surgery and risks in one office visit. A second visit allows the patient an opportunity to ask questions after having thoroughly studied the information provided at the first consultation.

SURGICAL TECHNIQUE

Anesthesia

Moderate hypotensive anesthesia, usually produced by sodium nitroprusside, has been helpful in minimizing blood loss. Complete muscle paralysis is essential for creation of the submuscular pocket and for obtaining complete muscle closure over the implants. Intravenous narcotics, administered both before completion of surgery and in the recovery room, are of great benefit in allowing the patient to have a slow, smooth emergence with a minimum of significant pectoral muscle contractions that could threaten to disrupt the integrity of the muscle closure.

Incision Choices

Before choosing incisions, all surgeons must determine whether they feel it appropriate to leave the nipple-areola complex attached to the skin. Those who prefer the "total mastectomy" concept obviously have to use an incision allowing nipple-areola removal. I believe there are no concrete data indicating any therapeutic value in nipple-areola removal for benign breast disease. Whereas carcinoma has been reported in nipple grafts used in reconstruction when the nipples were removed from breasts containing malignancies, it has not been reported after mastectomies for benign disease. Removal of all fibrous tissue under the areola leaves nothing more than the ductal tissue within the nipple-papilla. Most surgical oncologists agree that the remaining papilla is at extremely low risk for carcinoma and also can be very easily evaluated. Because even modified radical mastectomies leave microscopic breast tissue under the skin flaps, indicating less than 100 percent removal, and because prophylactic mastectomy flaps can be created equally as thin (Fig. 27-3), the ductal tissue within the nipple papilla should be the only difference between completeness of glandular resection between prophylactic mastectomies performed through inframammary incisions and incisions that remove the nipple. Consideration of these factors has led me to continue to choose the prophylactic mastectomy incision that will produce the best aesthetic result for the individual patient. Because an inframammary incision is inconspicuous (Fig. 27-4), I use it whenever it is anatomically possible (Fig. 27-5).

A review of my series reveals that the breasts of one third of my patients are large or ptotic enough to require a surgical reduction of the skin brassiere, whereas the inframammary incision has been used in the remaining two thirds. Owing to early postoperative flattening of the implants from muscle compression, most patients who receive inframammary incisions require skin suspension with tape in the early postoperative period to allow skin muscle adhesion to occur with the nipple in the proper position.[2] Four-inch wide Conform tape* is applied on the

*Kendall Hospital Products, Boston, MA 02110.

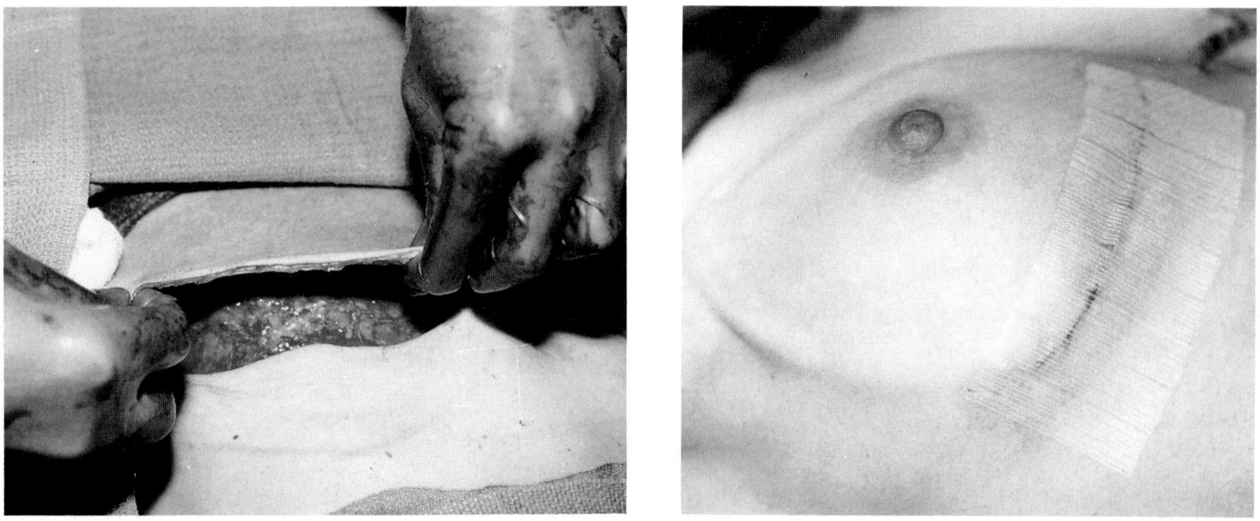

A B

FIGURE 27-3 *A*, A skeletonized skin flap, easily as thin as a flap resulting from a modified mastectomy for cancer. *B*, A 5-mm round suction catheter prominently visible between skin and muscle emphasizes the thin nature of the entire skin flap. (From Gant TD, Vasconez LO. Post-mastectomy reconstruction, 2nd ed. Baltimore: Williams & Wilkins, 1988.)

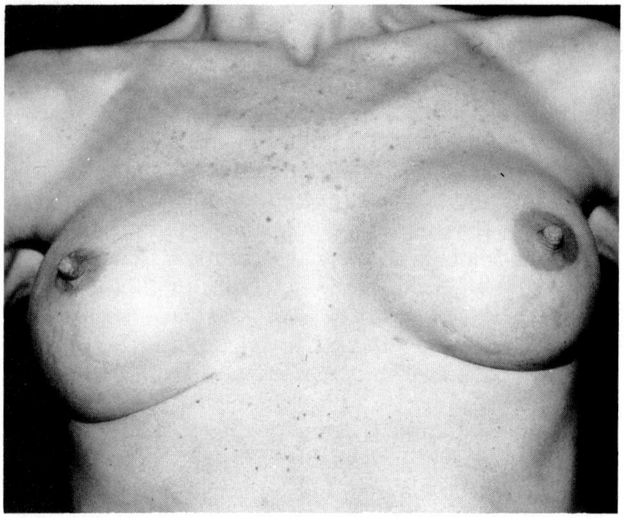

FIGURE 27-4 Inconspicuous 10-cm inframammary scars after subcutaneous mastectomies. (From Riley W. Plastic Surgery Educational Foundation Instructional Courses. Vol 1. St Louis, MO: CV Mosby, 1988.)

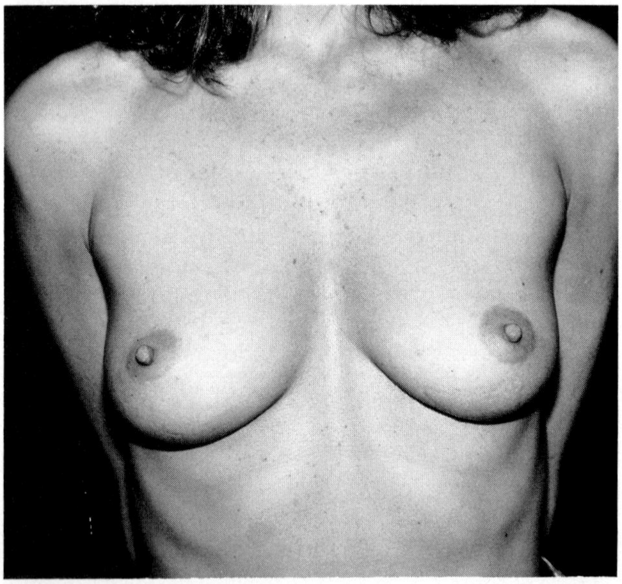

A

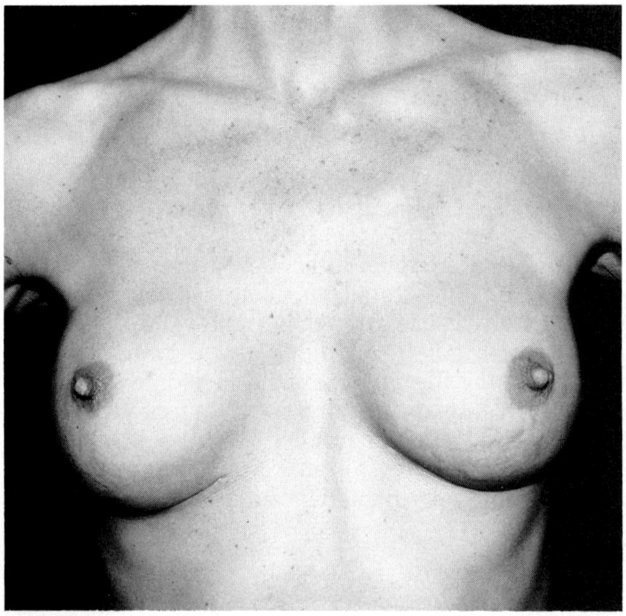

B

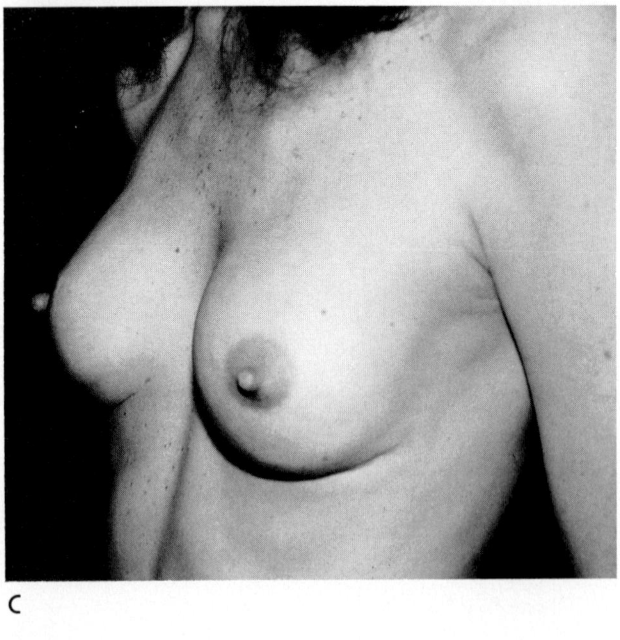

C

FIGURE 27-5 *A*, Preoperative view of a candidate for subcutaneous mastectomy with small breasts. *B*, *C*, Postoperative views showing the aesthetic result obtained with 10-cm inframammary incisions. (From Gant TD, Vasconez LO. Post-mastectomy reconstruction, 2nd ed. Baltimore: Williams & Wilkins, 1988.)

operating room table (Fig. 27-6*A, B*) and changed as necessary with the patient standing 1 or 2 days after surgery to position the nipple properly. The tape is again changed on a weekly basis for up to 6 weeks; it produces very little skin reaction or maceration because of its hypoallergenic and porous nature.

This taping technique has been used successfully in patients with moderate ptosis in whom the skin shows signs of good elasticity. To date, 3 cm is the greatest nipple elevation achieved by taping, and for ptosis requiring more than 3 cm of correction there should be surgical reduction of the skin envelope (Fig. 27-6*C, D*).

Patients requiring this surgical reduction should have the nipple-areola transferred as a free graft rather than on a dermal pedicle, if it is to be used in the reconstruction. Nipples transferred on pedicles, in association with proper thinning of flaps, suffer avascular necrosis in a significant number of patients,[10] even without a history of smoking. When nipple-areola complexes are transferred as grafts, there uniformly is good take of the areolae and vary-

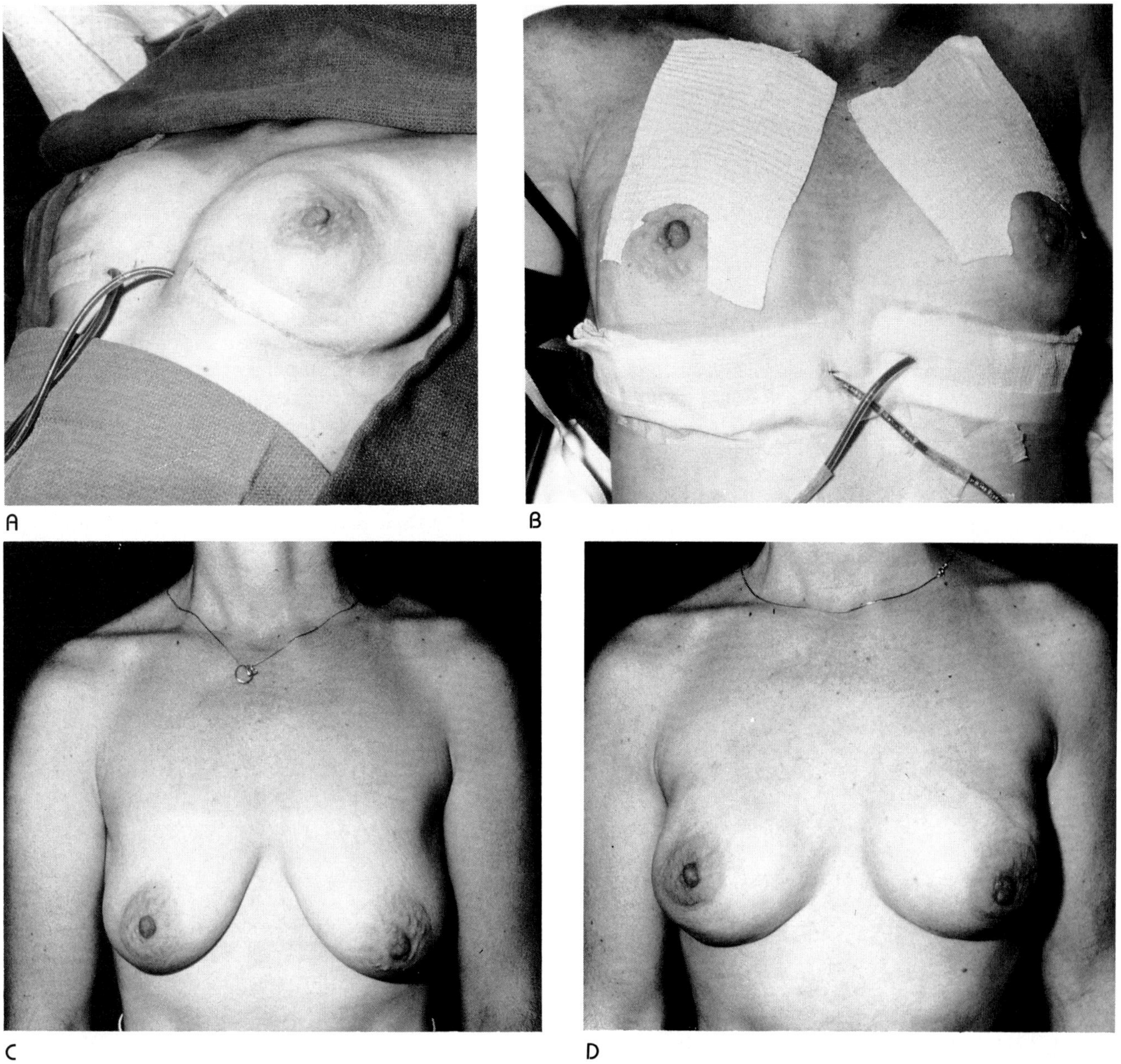

FIGURE 27-6 *A*, Loose skin at the end of subcutaneous mastectomy with reconstruction. *B*, Conform tape is applied with the patient in the supine position. *C*, Preoperative view of same patient. *D*, Postoperative view showing a nipple position 3 cm higher than preoperative measurements, demonstrating the effectiveness of the nonsurgical mastopexies with skin taping. (From Gant TD, Vasconez LO. Post-mastectomy reconstruction, 2nd ed. Baltimore: Williams & Wilkins, 1988.)

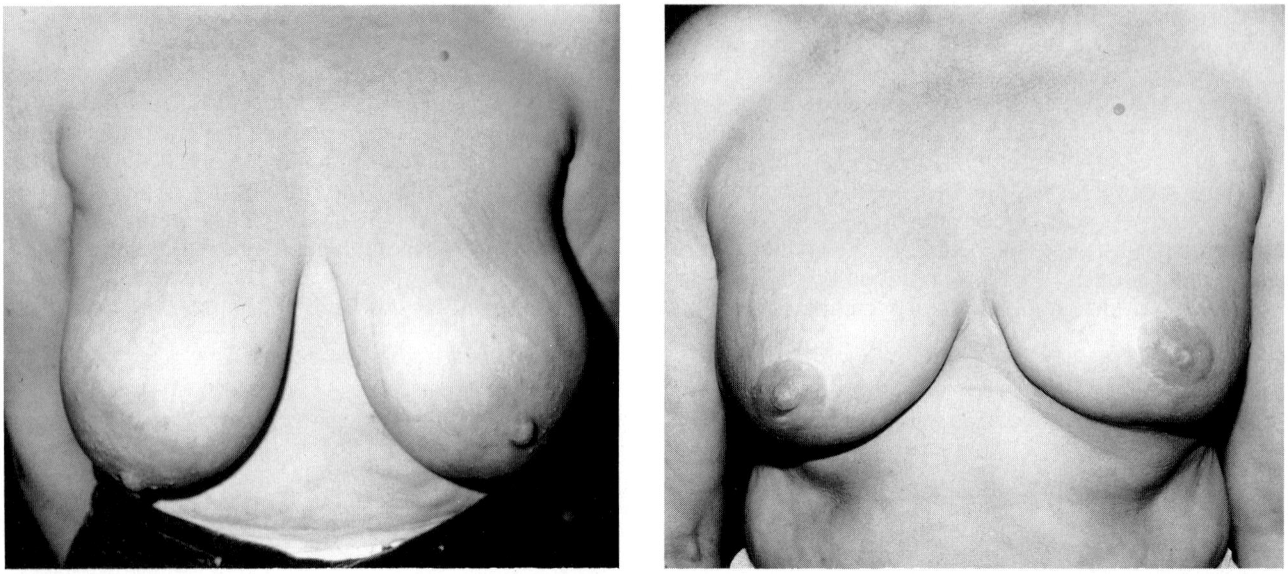

A B

FIGURE 27-7 *A*, Preoperative and *B*, 12-year postoperative views of a patient who received subcutaneous mastectomies with inverted-T skin reduction incisions and nipple grafting. (From Riley W. Plastic Surgery Educational Foundation Instructional Courses. Vol 1. St. Louis, MO: CV Mosby, 1988.)

ing degrees of nipple papillary survival in nonsmoking patients.

I have used only two types of skin resection incisions, the inverted-T (Fig. 27-7) or the elliptical (Fig. 27-8) (transverse or oblique), transferring nipples as grafts. The inverted-T incision, however, should be used only in nonsmokers if skin necrosis is to be avoided in the skin adjacent to the vertical closure line between the nipple and inframammary line. This incision also is not recommended for narrow or tubular breasts or those with extremely large areolae that make up 50 percent or more of the transverse width of the lower part of the breast, where removal of the skin containing the areola would result in an excessively tight vertical closure. In such patients, an elliptical skin excision will remove skin only in one dimension, resulting in better skin flap vascularity than with the inverted-T incision.

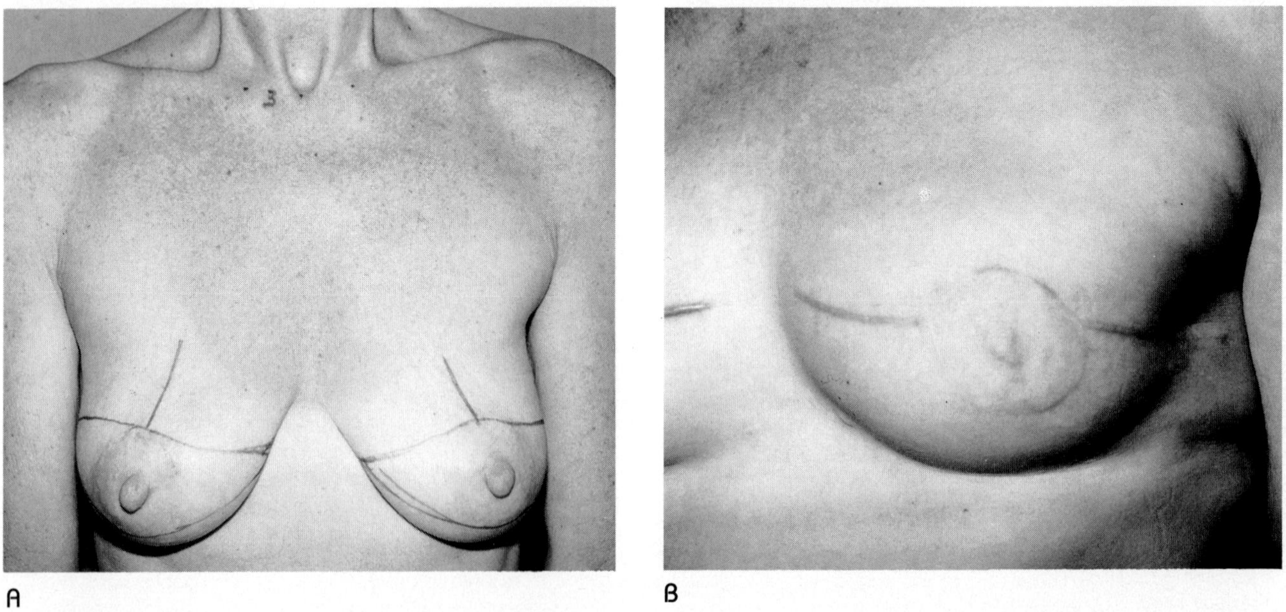

A B

FIGURE 27-8 Subcutaneous mastectomies with elliptical incisions and free nipple graft. *A*, Preoperative markings. *B*, Typical final appearance. (From Riley W. Plastic Surgery Educational Foundation Instructional Courses. Vol 1. St Louis, MO: CV Mosby, 1988.)

A breast-halving incision with or without skin resection may even be preferable to the inframammary if it is necessary to operate on a patient who smokes, because skin on both sides of the incision will require a shorter span of subdermal vascular bridging than the skin between the inframammary incision and the areola.

Through the incision of choice, glandular resection is performed aided by hypotensive anesthesia to decrease blood loss. I prefer to begin with the deep dissection, preserving pectoralis and serratus muscle fascia, before the subcutaneous dissection, in order to be able to remove the breast tissue as soon as possible after completing the more vascular subcutaneous dissection. The specimens are weighed (to assist in implant size selection) before sending them to the pathology department for gross examination and frozen section, if indicated. Skin flaps should be thinned by scissor dissection of all protruding fat globules and fibrous tissue, while preserving the subdermal plexus of vessels. All subareolar fibrous tissue can be safely removed in nonsmokers, leaving the ductal tissue in the papilla as the only gross remnant of ductal tissue. If preferred, the nipple papilla can be removed like an apple core and the areolar tissue "pursestringed" without affecting the vascularity of the skin around the areola.

The pathologist is asked to evaluate the tissue while hemostasis is being obtained. Submuscular reconstruction is begun upon receipt of a negative pathology report. Because of eventual implant protection by total muscle cover, the skin flaps of any incision used for prophylactic mastectomy should be thinned to leave no more subcutaneous tissue than would be left in a mastectomy performed for cancer, other than for the ductal tissue within the nipple papilla (see Fig. 27-3).

Submuscular Reconstruction

After complete glandular removal, submuscular reconstruction is begun by making a 7- or 8-cm incision through the serratus anterior muscle and a portion of the rectus abdominis muscle down to the sixth rib (Fig. 27-9), or whatever portions of ribs are in line with the inframammary incision. This incision is placed over the anterior surface of the chest, with the medial end usually 3 or 4 cm from the edge of the sternum, in order to work through an area of relatively thick muscle tissue, as opposed to the very thin muscle found more laterally deep to the serratus fascia. These muscles are then sharply dissected from the intercostals of the fourth and fifth interspaces until the subpectoral plane is entered, where blunt dissection is often adequate, other than for removal of the origins of the pectoralis from the fourth and fifth ribs. Care is taken to preserve all sternal attachments of the pectoralis major muscle and to stay on top of the pectoralis minor muscle in order to avoid high-riding implants.

The most difficult part of the dissection, however, is laterally, where serratus muscle fibers must be dissected from the ribs and left attached to the overlying serratus fascia, while maintaining continuity with the pectoralis fascia. Scissor dissection is very useful to free the muscle tissue up from the fourth, fifth, and sixth ribs lateral to the end of the incision through the serratus anterior fibers on the sixth rib. Laterally, dissection is rarely carried as far as the midaxillary line in order to keep the implant well centered. Any tears in the muscle during this dissection can be repaired before implantation. Sizer implants are then used bilaterally to help check for pocket size and symmetry, after which final adjustments in the pocket can be performed.

Inferiorly, the serratus and rectus are dissected off the inferior border of the sixth rib and usually down onto the surface of the sixth interspace, or a distance of 1 to 2 cm inferior to the desired inframammary line. Final implant size is determined by the size of the submuscular pocket that can be produced. Barring any severe rib cage abnormality, 300- to 400-ml implants are commonly used.

Whereas some surgeons prefer to create the submuscular pocket by splitting the fibers of the pectoralis and then bluntly dissecting inferiorly and laterally under the serratus anterior, I have not abandoned the direct approach on the sixth rib, as originally described in 1978. Using this approach, I have not had implants extrude, and I am better able to create good inframammary definition.

Lower Thoracic Turnover Flap

The inframammary line approach to submuscular reconstruction also allows one to use a lower thoracic turnover muscle flap to ensure complete muscle enclosure in cases in which the serratus anterior or the lower pectoralis is excessively tight, deficient, atrophied, or damaged during dissection. I originally used this flap to salvage breast reconstruction patients with inferiorly displaced implants following capsulotomies. Successful use of this flap in several such cases led to its employment in primary submuscular reconstruction after either prophylactic mastectomy or modified radical mastectomy when the lower pectoralis and serratus fascia were removed during the mastectomy (for oncologic reasons), or when the lower muscle was too thin, friable, or excessively tight to allow adequate muscle closure.

The technique involves dissection of the skin and subcutaneous tissue from the muscle fascia from the inframammary incision inferiorly to the costal margins. This is followed by the development of either a U- or a crescent-shaped incision (Fig. 27-10), depending on the length of muscle flap required,

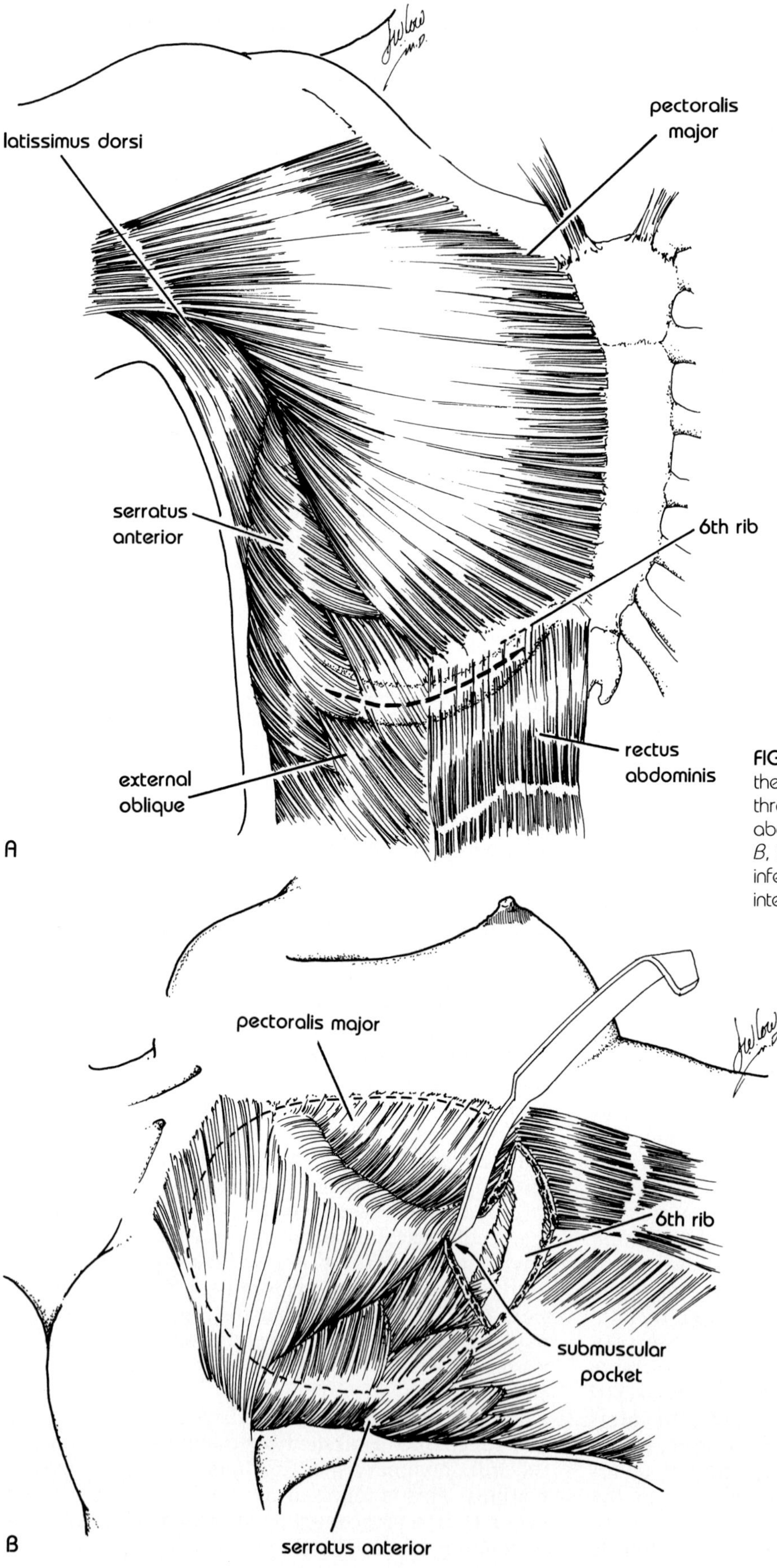

FIGURE 27–9 *A*, The preferred approach to the submuscular pocket begins with an incision through the serratus anterior and rectus abdominis muscles at the inframammary line. *B*, Sharp dissection is needed to develop the inferior pocket over the fourth and fifth interspaces.

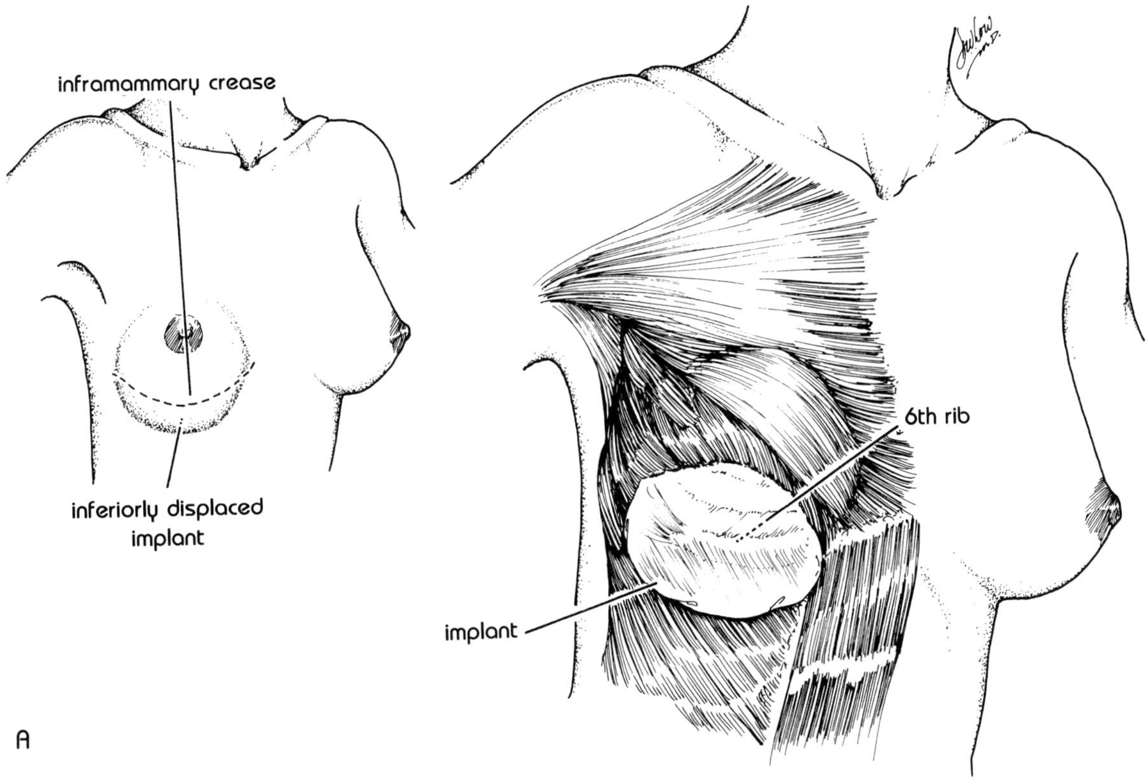

A

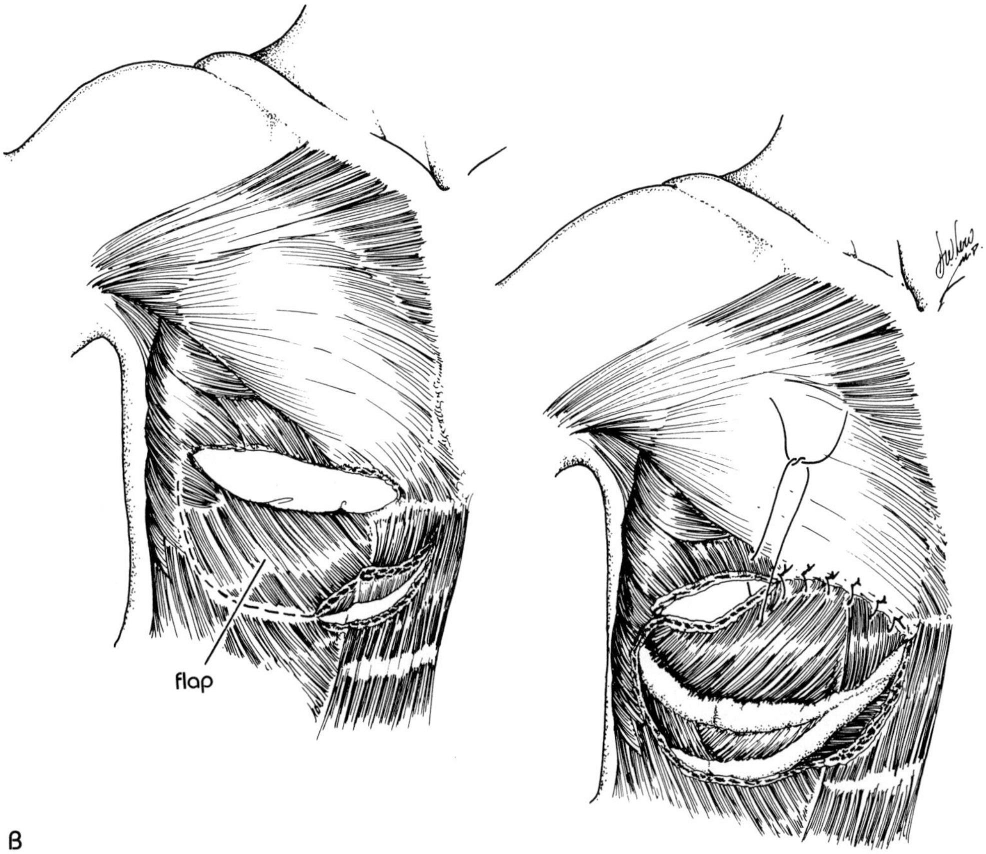

B

FIGURE 27 – 10 *A*. When muscle cover is deficient, inferior displacement or exposure of the implant in the subcutaneous position can be prevented with a muscle turnover flap. *B*, The lower thoracic muscle turnover flap is based on the sixth rib and sixth interspace. The location of the flap incision through the rectus abdominis and external oblique muscles depends on the length of flap required.

through the rectus abdominis and external oblique muscles, leaving them attached to the sixth rib and sixth interspace for neurovascular supply, and dissection of the flap retrograde to allow the flap to "turnover" the lower part of the implant. This turnover muscle flap is then attached to the pectoralis and serratus muscle tissue covering the superior portion of the implant. This not only provides excellent muscle cover, but also allows the implant to rest on this sling, or shelf, of muscle projecting straight out from the rib cage, providing a very precise inframammary crease.

Hypotensive anesthesia is discontinued as soon as the primary muscle dissection is accomplished on the second breast, so that normotensive pressures, and thus accurate hemostasis, can be obtained before implant placement and final closure.

Implants

Single-walled silicone bag gel prostheses were primarily used in the mid-1970s until gel bleed was described and found often to be associated with capsular contractures. I switched to Heyer-Schulte inflatable implants around 1978, but changed to double-lumen implants in 1981 after experiencing deflations in nearly 50 percent of the inflatables. At the present time, the newest generation of low-bleed, round, double-lumen implants are used with great satisfaction. My specific preference is for a free-floating inner bag with both bags constructed of low-bleed silicone. I prefer a saline volume equal to 10 percent of the silicone volume in the outer lumen along with 15 mg of Solu-Medrol. Using these doses and with complete muscle cover over the implant, I have not experienced any evidence of cortisone atrophy. Because of the flattening effect of the muscle cover, however, low-profile implants are not recommended. This policy eliminates some of the double-lumen prostheses currently produced. Some of these lower-profile double-lumen implants may be used successfully in augmentation mammaplasty; my attempts to use them in complete submuscular reconstruction have produced an unsatisfactory appearance on the operating table, necessitating immediate exchange for the better shape produced by the round double-lumen implants, which have a smaller diameter but greater projection.

I have not had a positive experience with tissue expanders in these cases, and prefer to use serial expansion with regular implants if the first implants are not deemed large enough. After complete muscle stretching, and if the pocket is truly large enough, it is not difficult to place a larger implant through a short inframammary incision under local anesthesia, because no capsulotomy or other dissection is required. In such cases, however, I do not add Solu-Medrol into the outer lumen of the second implant.

I have no experience with either polyurethane-covered or textured silicone implants, primarily because of continued satisfaction with current implants and a very low rate of capsular contracture with the techniques described in this chapter. In all patients reoperated on because of fibrocapsular contracture, I have obtained a satisfactory result using double-lumen replacement implants with Solu-Medrol in the outer lumen.

Conversion to Cancer Surgery

It is not difficult to convert prophylactic mastectomies performed through any one of the above-described incisions into a cancer ablative procedure if malignancy is found during the pathologic evaluation that forms part of the procedure. Any form of skin reduction incision pattern has been found to produce excellent exposure for a low axillary lymphadenectomy, and this dissection has also been performed adequately after extending an inframammary incision several centimeters into the axilla. Pectoralis fascia removal does not jeopardize implant cover in patients in whom the tumor is found close to the deep dissection level, although interruption of fascial continuity between the serratus anterior and pectoralis major muscles may threaten the integrity of the muscle cover unless a lower thoracic turnover flap is used.

The nipple papilla can easily be removed with pursestring closure of the areola when the inframammary incision has been used. Recipient nipple sites in skin reduction patterns should not be de-epithelialized until a negative pathology report has been obtained in order to include the nipple-areola complex with the specimen if cancer is found.

POSTOPERATIVE CARE

In the immediate postoperative period, arm motion and activity is kept to an absolute minimum in order to not stimulate postoperative bleeding and to protect the muscle repair. In addition, compressive dressings are avoided to preserve skin vascularity. Most patients are hospitalized for 2 or 3 postoperative days or until they are able to get in and out of bed without pushing or pulling themselves with their arms. Drains are left in place draining both subcutaneous and submuscular pockets until no more than 1 ml per hour per breast of serous fluid is produced over a 12-hour period; this usually takes 3 to 5 days. Gentle stretching exercises and isometric contractions of the pectoral muscles are combined with gentle implant massage the day after drains are removed. Patients are encouraged to increase the amplitude of the stretching exercises and the force of their massage within the limits of comfort. They should perform these activities four times daily for at least 3 months and then once a day for the rest of their lives.

Patients are asked to wear a camisole instead of a brassiere for a minimum of 3 months to avoid possible obliteration of the inferior aspect of the subserratus pocket, which would result in superior displacement of the implant. Many patients become extremely comfortable with their internal muscle support and never return to wearing a bra. Even after 3 months, a snug bra may produce pain from pressure on the ribs where the muscle dissection was carried out.

Strenuous physical activities are discouraged for 4 to 6 weeks after surgery, although many patients are able to return to office-type work 3 or 4 weeks postoperatively. They are encouraged to resume normal aids to daily living upon discharge from the hospital, and are usually allowed to drive a car about 10 days later. Sleeping on the back is preferred during the first 2 postoperative weeks, after which any comfortable position may be used.

RESULTS

As of January 1990, my personal series includes slightly more than 1,000 breasts in over 600 patients followed for up to 14 years with a mean follow-up of 6 years. Numerous patients operated on in the early part of the series would not meet the more stringent requirements for surgery at the present time. Records indicate that many of these patients were not at any proven increased risk for carcinoma, but were operated on because of the presence of fibrocystic disease with recurrent nodules requiring aspirations and/or biopsies and mammograms showing dense dysplasia, which raised fears of carcinoma in patients and their primary physicians. This series has now been restructured so that a separate follow-up is being conducted of patients who have a proved risk of at least 2.5 times normal; this includes those with a family history of premenopausal breast cancer in one or more first-degree relatives, those who have contralateral carcinoma, and those in whom there are biopsy findings of atypical hyperplasia or severe hyperplasia. Slightly more than 50 percent of the 600+ patients fit into this category, and none of these high-risk individuals have developed carcinoma postoperatively. Only one patient in my entire series has developed a small subcutaneous malignant nodule in the upper outer quadrant, which was discovered 11 years after subcutaneous mastectomies performed for relief of incapacitating mastodynia. The initial surgery, performed in 1978 purely for pain relief, left more subcutaneous tissue than current procedures used for cancer prophylaxis.

These numbers are obviously too small to provide any conclusive opinions about the prophylactic nature of this operation, but I believe the numbers indicate a trend. At least these patients are uniformly easy to examine, especially in comparison with their extremely inaccurate and difficult preoperative status as a result of the nodular nature of the breast tissue. There are no failures of reconstruction in the entire series, although approximately 12 percent of the entire series of patients required secondary surgery.

COMPLICATIONS

The earliest postoperative problem seen is hemorrhage with hematoma formation, which usually is evident in the postoperative recovery room but occasionally develops after the patient returns to the surgical ward. The incidence of this complication has been significantly reduced (1) by the elimination of all salicylates and anti-inflammatory drugs preoperatively, (2) by discontinuing hypotensive anesthesia and returning the patient to a normotensive state before final hemostasis is obtained (usually including transfusing autologous blood before wound closure rather than in the recovery room after the blood pressure drops), (3) by keeping the patient suitably sedated in the recovery room, and on the ward by prompt administration of intravenous analgesics, (4) by restricting arm motion to limit the pectoralis function, and (5) by forbidding smoking before surgery to reduce postoperative coughing.

A round Jackson-Pratt drain left between the skin and the muscle tissue covering the implant can be a useful guide for the nurses to check for signs of early subcutaneous hematoma. A hematoma is not present if the tube can be easily palpated, assuming that the entire breast skin is available for inspection and not covered by dressings.

Skin ischemia is common in the early postoperative period, particularly if the patient is improperly warmed and is hypothermic upon arrival in the recovery room. Rapid warming usually produces prompt improvement in such cases. However, these situations can easily be prevented by keeping warming pads on the operating table, warming inhalation anesthetics and intravenous fluids, and by wrapping the head with towels to reduce heat loss.

Pharmacologic agents can also be used to improve skin flap viability in the early postoperative period. Ten- or 20-mg nitroglycerine skin patches can be readily applied in the immediate postoperative period and have been found effective in improving ischemic skin flaps and nipple-areola complexes. Although these patches are reported to have a 24-hour life span, I have found that their effectiveness diminishes after 12 hours. I therefore adopted a routine of applying a 10-mg nitroglycerin patch in the recovery room, adding a second one 12 hours later, and changing each at 24-hour intervals, so that one of the patches is always fresh each 12 hours.

Woods and Meland[10] also reported clinical success with use of intravenous steroids to improve ischemic skin flap viability, a program supported by laboratory experiments of Zarem and colleagues,[11] in which dramatic improvement was produced in ischemic skin flaps by the use of intravenous steroids.

Ischemia leading to full-thickness necrosis, which is most commonly found in patients who smoke, can usually be successfully treated in a very conservative manner without exposure or loss of the implant, as long as the implant has been completely enclosed by muscle. Regular wound management of a dry eschar is carried out by covering the eschar with either Betadine or Silvadene dressings, allowing them to separate spontaneously, or by debridement and skin grafting as indicated. Implant displacement or herniation, especially into the axilla, has been reported only in conjunction with entry into the submuscular space through the pectoralis major or the pectoralis-serratus junction at the lateral border of the pectoralis. This problem has never occurred in the more than 1,000 breast procedures in my series using the direct approach on the sixth rib to enter the submuscular space. However, I have found in several patients an implant projecting 1 to 2 cm too far inferiorly owing either to excessive subserratus dissection or, in one case, to an unrecognized submuscular hematoma beneath the pectoralis forcing the implant too far inferiorly. Minor degrees of this problem can easily be corrected by having the patient wear a brassiere with an elastic lower portion that maintains pressure over the serratus, allowing it to readhere to the intercostal muscle tissue. In three patients I performed a capsullorrhaphy with success.

Although the incidence of fibrocapsular contracture has been greatly reduced with total muscle cover of the implants, these conditions still occur. However, they are relatively infrequent and usually of a less severe nature than those resulting from implants that are not covered by muscle tissue. An accurate analysis of the first 483 patients in my series, representing 821 breasts and with follow-up ranging from 1 to 12 years, showed Baker Class II or III contractures occurring in 13.3 percent of breasts, with no Baker Class IV contractures. Most of these Class II or III contractures were not reported by the patients but were merely described as part of a follow-up examination. Fewer than half of these patients required surgical capsulotomies. Because a significant number of these contractures occurred in patients who had single-lumen bag gel prostheses during the early part of the series, and who were found to have gel bleed when the capsulotomy was performed, a second analysis was made of 495 breast reconstructions with double-lumen implants followed for 1 to 5 years. This second series showed an 8 percent incidence of Baker Class II or III contractures, and again, fewer than half were symptomatic and required treatment. By using the current generation of double-lumen implants in which both lumens are constructed of low-bleed silicone, I believe it is realistic to anticipate less than a 10 percent patient incidence of symptomatic capsular contracture.

CONCLUSION

Surgeons recommending and performing prophylactic mastectomy must do so in the belief that removal of approximately 95 percent of the breast tissue will have a significant effect on reducing or eliminating a high-risk patient's chances of developing breast carcinoma. This philosophy of treating benign breast disease should be considered consistent with current forms of treatment for malignant breast tissue, which admittedly include leaving microscopic elements of breast tissue attached to skin flaps of modified radical mastectomies, and leave the vast majority of breast tissue when cancer is treated by lumpectomy and radiation. Surgeons performing this procedure are encouraged to follow up as many of their high-risk patients as possible, so that meaningful data can be obtained about the true effectiveness of prophylactic mastectomy in preventing breast carcinoma.

The techniques described in this chapter have allowed me to perform thorough mastectomies and immediate reconstruction with a low morbidity rate and very satisfactory final aesthetic results that are well accepted by most patients.

References

1. Jarrett JR, Cutler RG, Teal DF. Subcutaneous mastectomy in small, large or ptotic breasts with immediate submuscular placement of implants. Plast Reconstr Surg 1978; 62:702.
2. Jarrett JR, Cutler RG, Teal DF. Aesthetic refinements in prophylactic subcutaneous mastectomy with submuscular reconstruction. Plast Reconstr Surg 1982; 69:624.
3. Cancer Committee of the College of American Pathologists. Is fibrocystic disease of the breast precancerous? Arch Pathol Lab Med 1986; 110:171.
4. Lynch HT, Harris RH, Organ TH, et al. Management of familial breast cancer. Arch Surg 1978; 113:1053.
5. Lynch HT, Algano WA, Lynch JF. Genetic counseling, familial breast cancer and surgeon's responsibility. Plast Reconstr Surg 1980; 66:303.
6. Lynch HT, Guirgis H, Brodkey F, et al. Early age of onset in familial breast cancer. Arch Surg 1976; 111:126.
7. Anderson DE. A genetic study of human breast cancer. J Natl Cancer Inst 1972; 48:1029.
8. Leis HP. Bilateral breast cancer. Breast Dis Breast 1981; 7:13.
9. Leis HP. Managing the remaining breast. Cancer 1980; 46:1026.
10. Woods JE, Meland NB. Conservative management in full thickness nipple-areolar necrosis after subcutaneous mastectomy. Plast Reconstr Surg 1989; 84:258.
11. Zarem HA, Hayden B, Soderberg R, et al. Effect of corticosteroid administration in ischemia-ischemic injury. Plast Reconstr Surg 1988; 82:865.

CHAPTER 28

Psychosocial Factors in Mastectomy and Reconstruction

WENDY S. SCHAIN, Ed.D.

BREAST CANCER AS A BIOPSYCHOSOCIAL DISEASE

Mastectomy has been referred to as the surgery women fear most, and breast reconstruction as the operation they never dreamed possible or believed available only to the rich and famous. The history of the technology of breast reconstruction is almost 100 years old and dates back to the early operation performed by Czerny in 1895,[1] but accounts of psychosocial sequelae attendant on this reparative procedure do not appear in the literature until around the mid-1970s. The reporting of the emotional consequences of reconstructive mammaplasty parallels a time period. This phase, characterized by the use of silicone implants to restore the shape of the missing breast after mastectomy, was described by Snyderman as the "modern era" in breast reconstruction.[2]

For the purposes of this chapter, the author encourages readers to consider breast cancer and breast reconstruction as a biopsychosocial phenomenon consisting of an outcome predicated on the interaction of a multiplicity of factors. Contributing variables interact in a unique configuration in any individual woman to produce the manifest response. Nevertheless, a general combination of factors appears both with considerable frequency and to a predictable magnitude for one to make some broad, sweeping statements about coexistence, if not cause and effect.

According to Meyerowitz,[3] there are three major categories of variables that influence the intensity and duration of psychosocial adaptation to breast cancer (Table 28-1).

Of the list of contributing factors acknowledged, some of the most critical are possibly age or life stage, quality of marital sexual relationship, and availability of support persons (the last two factors often overlap). To comprehend the ultimate psychological response to this crisis demands an understanding of the life stage cycle the woman has reached when she develops breast cancer. What are the important goals and tasks in her life stage that she fears will be interrupted, delayed, or permanently eliminated by the cancer and related treatments? For a nulliparous 37-year-old, the prospect of becoming sterile because of cytotoxic chemotherapy threatens psychological adjustment in ways qualitatively different from a 62-year-old widow's response to systemic antiestrogen medication.

A pervasive theme for breast cancer patients is the threat to body image and the meaning and investment a woman has attributed to her breasts as indicative of who she is, how sexually attractive she feels, and how essential her breasts are to her overall self-esteem. It has been suggested that women who are multifaceted as women (i.e., have strong identities) see themselves as resourceful and able to adapt more easily to mastectomies than women who are more traditional and strongly invested in their physical appearance as primary determinants of their self-esteem.[4] Because many women today have a choice of treatment alternatives, one must take into account personality characteristics and coping strategies in recommending primary therapy. Ideally, recommendations for treatment should be a collaborative effort based on an understanding of the biology of the disease, the psychology of the individual

TABLE 28–1 Summary of Variables Examined in the Psychological Literature on Breast Cancer and its Treatment

Psychosocial Impacts of Breast Cancer and its Treatment

- Psychological discomfort
  - Depression
  - Anxiety
  - Hostility
- Changes in life patterns
  - Physical discomfort
  - Marital sexual upset
  - Reduced activity level
- Fears and Concerns
  - Mastectomy mutilation
  - Cancer death

Variables That Influence Intensity and Duration of Psychosocial Impact

- Premorbid variables
  - Patient characteristics
    - Importance of physical appearance of breasts to patient
    - Age
    - Preoperative expectations
  - Environmental characteristics
    - Preoperative preparation by surgeon
    - Quality of sexual relationship with partner
- Postmastectomy Variables
  - Coping
    - Denial and related defenses (intensity and selectivity)
    - Search for causes (self-blame and projection of blame)
  - Environmental variables
    - Time elapsed since surgery
    - Availability of support (physician/surgeon, spouse and family, other patients)
    - Additional medical therapies (radiotherapy and chemotherapy)

(From Meyerowitz BE: Psychosocial correlates of breast cancer and its treatments. Psychol Bull 1980; 87:108. Copyright 1980 by the American Psychological Association.)

woman (including her self-esteem and coping strategies), and the way in which she imagines that a particular treatment will affect her quality of life.

Over the last 20 years as a psychotherapist who has counseled women with breast cancer, trying to help them make decisions about treatment and to facilitate their postoperative adjustment, I have uncovered certain predispositional profiles that seem to indicate which women will fare better emotionally with one treatment or the other. Whenever medically feasible, the recommendation for a particular surgery should (1) correspond to the woman's belief about what she needs to maintain her quality of life and (2) reinforce her existing coping strategies and support her belief about the efficacy of that treatment.

Specifically, will a 6-week course of radiation therapy help her feeling that she is in a sense buying an insurance plan against her breast cancer, or will such daily treatments undermine her usual coping strategy of denial? If this defense is threatened, the woman may confront certain issues that reduce her functioning effectively and interfere with her routine or career. Such a change in adaptation could jeopardize her self-esteem and feeling of autonomy.

CULTURAL CONTEXT AND CONTRIBUTION

No woman faces the prospect of breast cancer surgery and possible removal of that socially prized organ de novo. She comes to the operating room with a profusion of images and feelings about the importance and value of her breast and with attitudes about the curability or fatality of the disease.

Anthropologists may someday label this time in our cultural heritage as the "mammocentric era," an interval in history when enormous amounts of psychic energy and capital resources went into glamorizing, idealizing, and sensationalizing the female breast. For centuries, artists and poets have exalted the female form and highlighted its aesthetic and symbolic meaning. Human breasts may sometimes be referred to as end organs and be described as only mammary glands, but they are rarely viewed dispassionately. This part of the anatomy elicits a strong mixture of lustful, nurturant, and dependency reactions. A woman's breasts are often (1) equated with her ability to attract a member of the opposite sex, (2) reflective of her capacity to reproduce and nourish her offspring, (3) revealing of her level of libidinal desire, and (4) viewed as synonymous with her self-confidence, self-esteem, and sense of sexual desirability.

How this critical and convoluted connection between breasts and feminine identification comes into being, and what the factors are that undermine or reinforce its development, are not altogether clear. However, the dynamics operating are sufficiently strong and predictable to force us to consider certain questions related to the psychosocial outcome of breast cancer in order to try and minimize resulting morbidity.

1. What happens to the woman and her significant other when she develops breast cancer and is faced with the need either to remove or alter such a value-laden organ?
2. What are the ramifications for her body image, her quality of life, and her sense of overall effectiveness?
3. How can we identify women at high risk for emotional distress and intervene early enough to avert or minimize long-term morbidity?
4. What role does breast reconstruction play in restoring or reestablishing this special connection if mastectomy is the elected treatment, and when is the optimal timing for this operation?

The anthropologist Susan Brownmiller[5] helps us to understand this strong and powerful connection between gender role identity, preoccupation with breasts, and self-esteem. She asked:

". . . where does this whole issue of femininity and sexuality start? At what age does a girl begin to view her assets and count her deficient parts? When does she close the bedroom door and begin to gaze privately into the mirror—pull in her stomach, throw out her chest and pose again in search for the most flattering angle? At what age does the process begin? This obsessive concentration on the minutiae of her physical being . . . (a preoccupation that) will occupy some portion of her waking hours . . . quite possibly for the rest of her life."

Although the exact nature of this occurrence is elusive, it must be borne in mind that a breast cancer diagnosis and subsequent treatment tend to intensify this obsession about breasts or their absence (in the case of mastectomy), and may contribute to mild or marked emotional distress for a brief or a very protracted period. Clarification of why this is so, and identification of precipitating and remedial factors contributing to the psychosocial consequences for breast cancer reconstruction patients, is a major theme throughout this chapter.

PSYCHOLOGICAL REACTIONS TO MASTECTOMY

Breast conservation therapy is rapidly becoming an acceptable alternative to mastectomy,[6] but surgical removal of the diseased breast still remains the standard of care in most regions of the United States. The psychosocial literature reports a range in type and magnitude of emotional distress after mastectomy and attributes the morbidity to a variety of factors. The earliest discussion of emotional factors in breast carcinoma dates back to 1952 in an article by a well-known group of psychoanalytically oriented psychotherapists, who described a list of behavioral characteristics in 40 women who had the disease.[7] These psychological precipitators, as they were viewed, included (1) a masochistic character structure, (2) inhibited sexuality, (3) inhibited motherhood, (4) a facade of pleasantness covering an inability to discharge or deal appropriately with hostility or aggressiveness, (5) unresolved conflict with the mother handled through denial and unrealistic sacrifices, (6) a delay in securing treatment, and (7) a frequent picture of chronic depression with vague feelings of anxiety, guilt, strong self-criticism, and self-condemnation.

The original research for a causal link between personality type and subsequent breast cancer has been a recurring theme in the literature and has alternately emerged into prominence and been eclipsed into obscurity for almost 40 years. The early papers were reports based on data secured from the psychoanalytic psychotherapies of women with confirmed diagnoses of breast cancer. These were clinical interpretations and speculation of personality structure that was alleged to predate diagnosis and was reflective of an ongoing depressive component. There was no attempt to conduct scientific studies with control of critical variables or to use a comparison group of matched women without this disease.

The first generation of substantive research in this area did not emerge until the late 1970s when investigators attempted to document the psychological and sexual consequences of breast cancer treatment rather than describe its possible precipitators.

There remain today, however, recurrent themes of a connection between the development of cancer and diminished host resistance, again correlating depression or loss and changes in immunocompetence. The most recent wave of interest in this topic has spawned a group of scientists committed to the study of psychoneuroimmunology and investigating ways in which the mind-body connection may play a role in cancer incidence and outcome.[8-10] An update of findings describing possible correlations between psychological factors, endocrine or neural pathways, and immune functions that may influence tumor progression or regression is contained in a book by Norman Cousins, *Headfirst: The Biology of Hope.*[11]

Herberman and Ortaldo presented preliminary data that suggests a connection between breast cancer and natural killer cells. Their research demonstrated that behavioral interventions can affect these naturally occurring cytotoxic agents,[12] a finding that may have significant implications for future treatment planning. More defensible conclusions in this area may expand our repertoire of therapeutic agents in the battle against breast cancer, as well as identify noninvasive strategies that may alter the outcome of the disease. Schain and colleagues are currently developing a pilot project to measure whether life style modification and cognitive therapy can influence the immune responses of daughters of breast cancer patients.[13]

For the most part, for the last 20 years, discussions of psychological factors and breast cancer have focused primarily on adaptation to surgery with the intention of finding ways to minimize the identified morbidity, not alter the course of the disease. Maguire and colleagues[14] and Morris and associates[15] reported a significant degree of depression and anxiety in their study populations. They concluded that approximately 27 to 32 percent, respectively, of the mastectomy patients acknowledged depression and sexual difficulties after surgery. Jamison and colleagues,[16] in their first study of the mastectomy patient, found that 23 percent of their study sample were emotionally distressed and also reported sexual dysfunctions. A moderate number also reported depression, sleep disturbances, and occasional suicidal ideation. A later study conducted by Wellisch and associates[17] on the partners of these mastectomy patients concluded that more than one third of the men rated the impact of the mastectomy as negative, and that approximately 17 percent of these male partners admitted that they had not looked at their wife naked during the first year after the mastectomy operation.

SEXUAL ADAPTATION AFTER MASTECTOMY

The focus in the literature on male-female interaction after mastectomy is rather sparse, and only a few studies to date have either examined the interpersonal interaction of couples subsequent to breast cancer surgery or made more detailed inquiries about their sexual and intimate responses. In 1978 Frank and associates[18] reported that about one third of the mastectomy patients they investigated had not resumed intercourse for 6 months, and that nudity and self-display become an issue for a significant proportion of women. Silberfarb and colleagues[19] found that 22 to 31 percent of their mastectomy patients reported reduced frequency of intercourse and other sexual disturbances. A specific description of these other sexual disturbances has been difficult because most of the research studies restricted their review of sexual dysfunction to include only change in frequency or satisfaction with intercourse.

In a small retrospective study of women volunteers, Abt[20] asked mastectomy patients to describe the changes they were experiencing in a wide variety of sexually related behaviors that could impact on sexual satisfaction. Her results revealed that half of the women surveyed admitted to experiencing between three and six changes in their sexual relations in the direction of decreased frequency, decreased satisfaction, or both. The behaviors documented were kissing, undressing, sleeping nude, acting seductively with one's partner, initiating sex, and having sexual fantasies. Clearly there is a much broader range of activities in addition to intercourse that influence an individual's or a couple's reporting of sexual satisfaction. Sophisticated research in this area must tap the broad spectrum of behaviors that may be affected by cancer surgery and related treatments. Changes in these behaviors can affect both genital sexual responses and interpersonal interaction and affectionate behaviors, thereby diminishing the quality of life.

BODY IMAGE DISTORTION AND RELATED RESPONSES

Grinker[21] added much-needed insight into and sensitivity to this matter by describing some additional problems that may occur:

> *"The dread of exposing one's self to one's spouse as crippled, damaged, incomplete or dying may cause sexual inhibition or abstinence. Intimacy in sexual body functions may be affected by shame and embarrassment. Mutilation (viz. mastectomy) may make exposure and nudity extremely painful. Self disgust may be displaced and projected on to the partner . . . there may be an increase in the outrage that the partner displays any interest in sex. In fact, normal interest may be seen as an invasion of the rights of the "damaged person." . . . Lack of self-esteem and a relative feeling of emotional poverty in survivors may prevent the resumption of their previous relationship."*

The nuances of the disturbance in sexual functioning after mastectomy, and the complexity of the intrapsychic variables affecting the onset and duration of this problem, are best explained by the results of some early research in this area. Clifford and associates[22] conducted two studies to learn more about the nature of the relationship between sexual responses and marital satisfaction after the loss of a woman's breast. They concluded that the impact on the marital relationship was directly in proportion to the degree of upset experienced by the woman. Specifically, if the mastectomy patient could restrict her upset to a small part of her self-evaluation (namely, her breast area per se) and not let it spill over and spoil her self-esteem or sense of sexual desirability, the consequences for the couple would be less devastating than if the woman felt totally diminished by the surgical alteration.

This latter possibility occurs with some frequency and is clearly depicted by an excerpt from a book by a well-known journalist who has had a mastectomy. She portrayed the insult she felt in her sexual self-esteem.[23]

> *"I did not worry that my husband would no longer find me attractive. He found me attractive. He wanted me. The crazy thing was I did not want him. He still found me attractive, all right, but I did not. I no longer found me attractive. I was damaged goods and I knew it . . . I was mutilated, a deformed person. If you feel deformed, it's hard to feel sexy."*

Perhaps it is in this aspect of postmastectomy anguish, the area of feeling deformed and so unlike one's former self or other women of similar age, that breast reconstruction may have its most benefit. If, as Clifford and associates intimated, mastectomy does not create a major subtractive effect (but remains an isolated wound), the woman may not feel that her overall value and attractiveness would be significantly improved by breast reconstruction. Her motivation for such an operation may therefore be negligible. On the other hand, if she feels terribly diminished by the missing breast and can compartmentalize the feeling of defectiveness, repair of that area may have a significant salutary impact and elevate her overall sense of self-esteem.

POSSIBLE INTERVENTION STRATEGIES

Kolodny and associates[24] stated that the male superior intercourse position may become preferable for women who have undergone mastectomy because they feel that their partners will not be subjected to such an obvious and visible confrontation with their missing organ. When the woman is in the female superior posture, it is more likely that the male partner is looking directly at the missing area, and both individuals may be more aware of what that loss means, in terms of erotic value and also threat to life. Other positions such as the lateral scissors (or side by side) allow for more flexibility in maneuvering, and also support a less stark confrontation of the loss following breast cancer surgery.

In an effort to address sexual rehabilitation with mastectomy patients and their partners, Wabrek[25] strongly encouraged physicians to inquire about the sexual and interpersonal relationship that existed before the onset of disease and its treatment. This is an important prerequisite before one can comfortably recommend remedial strategies. This is because if the couple were at risk because of poor communication skills or lack of sexual satisfaction before the diagnosis, the added burden of coping with cancer and its vicissitudes may be overwhelming. Under such circumstances a specially trained mental health professional or sex therapist should be contacted so that early attention to possible sexual morbidity may avert the magnitude of dysfunction that could ensue. Considerable psychological anguish is caused by unmet needs in sexual rehabilitation, and as Kolodny and associates succinctly stated:[24]

> *"It is both comfortable and convenient for the physician to forget that oncology patients continue to have sexual feelings (and to assume) . . . that such patients are no longer interested in sex."*

The psychosexual implications of cancer and related treatments can best be understood by asking some relatively simple questions relating to the impact of the surgery on the patient emotionally and physiologically, and how these changes influence the ways in which she relates to her partner. Specifically, one might ask:

1. In what ways has your mastectomy affected your psychological well-being and moods?
2. In what ways has your surgery (or treatment) affected your feelings about yourself as a woman and as a sexual partner?
3. In what ways do you feel your mastectomy has affected your spouse (or lover)?

There is a need to be explicit in gathering this information and not to be too polite by asking banal questions such as "How are things in the bedroom since your operation?" One needs to inquire rather specifically about nudity, comfort in sleeping in bed with one's partner, feelings about having one's breast or incisional area fondled, and simply the sensation of being hugged and whether this response precipitates discomfort and self-consciousness? Not all physicians wish to or should take a history of sexual problems, but they should acknowledge the fact that breast cancer surgery may indeed create some changes in feelings about one's self and one's sexuality. Sensitive inquiry into the sexual responses of the woman often permit the patient to feel she is viewed as a whole person and not some treatment statistic. Several references for those interested in more in-depth evaluation and intervention in this area are to be found in *Sexuality and Chronic Illness* by Schover and Jensen[26] and in an article by Schain describing the fact that "a sexual interview is a sexual intervention."[27]

In summary, it is vital to be alert to several major variables that can affect sexual adaptation after cancer surgery: (1) psychological factors that include moods such as depression or anxiety, (2) feelings about one's self and body image, (3) physiologic sensations that may have to do with pain or sensitivity in the actual area of treatment, (4) lubrication difficulties that may be associated with hormonal depletion after systemic chemotherapy or antiestrogen medication, (5) relationship factors such as lack of openness about sharing feelings related to each other or the mastectomy experience, and (6) premorbid sexual inhibitions.

INTERPERSONAL SUPPORT AFTER MASTECTOMY

For more than 20 years the exclusive focus in psychosocial adaptation to breast cancer has been the female patient and her reaction to medical intervention. Postmastectomy adaptation, however, is a multifactorial response and must include assessment of both intrapersonal and interpersonal variables.

The quality of social support has been receiving increased press coverage both as a factor in adjustment to the disease and as a possible predictor of the onset and progression of breast cancer.[28-30] It may appear self-evident that husbands of mastectomy patients have an important role in the emotional recovery of women with breast cancer, but the nature of that support is often ill defined and poorly researched.

There are now a number of seminal articles on partners of mastectomy patients. However, the reports are largely anecdotal and clinical and almost exclusively refer to partners being male. This is neither accurate nor realistic. However, the discussion of sexual sequelae of breast cancer in a lesbian relationship is a separate treatise with some problems shared with the heterosexual couple, but also a host of problems unique to a homosexual pair. This chapter focuses on the male partner's reaction to breast cancer and reconstructive surgery. Mildred Hope Witkin[31] is perhaps the first health professional to address this issue. In her article "Sex Therapy and Mastectomy" she clearly states that the husbands of these women must not only deal with their wife's trauma and fears about her life and her body alterations, but also face their own fears relating to death and mutilation. How to accomplish this goal emotionally is not well indicated in this article, but specific steps to take regarding desensitization of sexual avoidance are outlined. For some couples, the logical starting point to improve communication is the verbal exchange of feelings; for others, recreating a loving and gratifying sexual interchange can open up the other area of sharing feelings that increase a sense of intimacy.

THE MAN'S RESPONSE AFTER MASTECTOMY

Until recently the focus in discussion of psychosocial sequelae of breast cancer was the individual patient and her symptoms, with minimal or no discussion of the couple interaction and how that relationship might facilitate or undermine the woman's psychological adaptation. The emotional reactions of the partner of a breast cancer patient, and his ability to help nurture his wife and at the same time quell his own anxieties about this crisis, are poorly understood and significantly underinvestigated. There are, however, a sporadic number of articles that say how critical the male partner is in facilitating his partner's emotional recovery from breast cancer.

An interesting discussion by Gates[32] may help explain much of the distress experienced by the postmastectomy couple. He asserts that many of the husbands of breast cancer patients he has counseled complain of very angry and aggressive reactions from their wives. These men admit they do not know how to handle this problem, because the woman is also seen as fragile and somewhat vulnerable. They repeatedly ask why would a woman who is so distressed and in need of help strike out against the person on whom she is likely to be most dependent? The author's explanation is to compare that interaction with the drowning person who strikes out in desperation at the swimmer trying to save her. Sometimes feelings of helplessness and fear are translated into hostility and attack. This may be the result of an unconscious need to create, in the other person, the level of pain and anxiety experienced by the wounded woman herself. The advice given by Gates under this circumstance is to provide understanding of the woman's pain and to give reassurance and support in an active and assertive fashion, but with very clear limits about what kinds of angry expression are tolerable. These kinds of firm, but loving behaviors are needed from the husband to dissipate the wife's distress, neutralize her victimizing behavior, and reduce his own negative feelings about the whole trauma.

Another critical issue is how to define or interpret support. It must be understood that it is the perception of support that is critical to adjustment, and not just the illusion of support or a specific behavior per se. Baider and De-Nour[33] studied the psychosocial adjustment of 35 women with lumpectomies and their spouses, and compared them with a well-matched group of 27 mastectomy patients and their partners. The series of self-report questionnaires revealed no significant differences between the psychological adjustment of women undergoing the two different treatment regimens or that of their partners. There was, however, moderate congruence between the distress of the woman patient and that of her husband. Bader concluded from this study of breast cancer patients and their partners in Israel that "the most common reaction to breast cancer is depression, but the incidence and severity reported varies considerably." Bader goes on to conclude that breast cancer is a "family affair" and that couples who have an open communication about how the experience affects them show less psychological morbidity individually and collectively.

Because it appears that the spouse or lover is critical to the adjustment of the breast cancer patient, the following discussion concentrates on the role he is expected to play in this drama. In addition, there will be references to research and clinical interpretations that allow us to understand this seriously neglected support person and his unique trials and tribulations. The male partner is expected to be the major support person for the married woman, but one should ask who is to support the support person? Where is this font of strength supposed to spring from and how can one help maximize the nuturance and endurance so necessary in this ordeal?

Being a marriage partner has been shown to be a predictor of adjustment to health problems in general and to mastectomy in particular. However, simply having support available does not in and of itself represent *feeling support.* In fact, as Bloom and colleagues acknowledged, some relationships can have a deleterious effect on a person's adjustment.[34] It is not merely the presence of a partner that is potentially therapeutic, but the nature of the interaction between the partners. Some men are so narcissistic that they cannot distance themselves from their own needs long enough to be emotionally available to their wives during their convalescence. Usually many men do not know how to be emotionally available and intimate in the interpersonal sense. Most women want support in terms of affectionate responses, communication about feelings, and verbal expression of caring from their partners. They are more likely to be appreciative of an honest exchange of concerns about how the mastectomy is going to affect their husband than of a ride to run errands that he might be willing to provide.

Sabo and associates[35] provided an in-depth understanding of the other person in this relationship and explained the man's reaction and adjustment to mastectomy. Instead of merely supplying prescriptions for helping husbands, the authors offered an architectural blueprint of the male psyche in our culture. Their interpretations are gleaned from a study of 24 men over many months. They used clinical interviews, observations from a multisession support group for men whose partners had breast cancer, and a battery of self-report questionnaires. They concluded that society dictates behaviors that reinforce denial, especially in men who are directed not to be disclosing of feelings or too emotionally expressive. "The traditional 'husband-provider' role may encourage men to mask or deny inner emotions . . . because in our society marital role functions usually revolve around instrumental functions for husbands and expressive functions for wives." Men generally show their support of women by some kind of caretaking responses, but most women want them to be more communicative and verbally expressive of thoughts and feelings. However, it is possible that under the threat of the breast cancer crisis, most men retreat into the traditional stoic role and away from the intimacy that their wives desperately crave.

This defensive and solitary posture combined with years of social training in keeping a "stiff upper lip" compels most men to move through their wife's cancer experience alone and unsupported. This for them is often a painful and agonizing journey. In recognition of this common situation, Sabo and associates strongly encouraged the need for and endorsed the value of a support group for men going through this experience. They acknowledged that such an opportunity for sharing is valuable in two important ways. First, groups of this type cut through the psychological and social barriers and encourage introspection and self-disclosure for the man. Second, practicing emotional expression of this type, in a protected setting, can carry over to the husband-wife interaction at home. Usually, when men reported back to the group that this is indeed what they did, they said that their wives perceived this response as genuine support and that the sharing of feelings had a tendency to enrich rather than complicate the marital relationship (as they may have erroneously believed). Most wives complain of a lack of sharing of feelings rather than the absence of tangible support, so increasing this type of communication is likely to be experienced positively. Most individuals, however, need specific assistance in this area. Fortunately, current professional and lay literature contains written documents, both substantive reports and personal accounts, that offer a wide range of help for the woman who has breast cancer and for the important people in her life on whom she relies to soften the blow of this ordeal (i.e., her spouse or lover).

A popular book that bears testimony to these issues consists of a detailed description of the emotional struggles of two men when the women they love receive cancer diagnoses.[36] It is written by a former Chicago policeman and a San Antonio newspaper reporter. Both men said they were paralyzed with panic when they learned their wives had breast cancer. More important, however, both these men reinforced the notion of how critical social support was for their own psychological adjustment and secondarily for assisting their wives' emotional recovery.

Social support is an essential and necessary condition for optimal adjustment, but it may not be sufficient. Some other factors required for successful adaptation to mastectomy are reflected in a profile proposed by Cobliner in 1977:[37]

1. A high self-image and an absence of irrational ideas about cancer.
2. A positive image of femininity that suffers little alteration, if any, as a result of the disease or its treatments.
3. Strong faith in the doctors.
4. A high degree of trust in the clinic or hospital where the patient is treated.
5. A belief in the efficacy of the particular treatment.
6. An opportunity for patients to confide their worries and intimate concerns to another person, usually of the same sex.
7. Involvement in an activity or occupation that provides satisfaction.
8. Good relationships with husband, sexual partner, or close friends that change slightly or not at all after the onset of illness or treatment.
9. Concordance between life expectations and degree of attainment.
10. The nature and success of any previously attempted resolutions of a life crisis.

Successful adaptation appears to reflect past and present coping strategies that permit integration of the mastectomy experience with a gratifying life style. Until about 5 years ago, the conclusions about psychosocial adaptation of breast cancer patients were postulated solely on women who had undergone surgical removal of the diseased breast (i.e., mastectomy). Whether the same criteria for healthy resolution and adjustment apply to women whose breast is spared is the subject of an ongoing debate. Less than radical surgery for breast carcinoma was not popular or readily available in the United States until the 1980s, so a more broad-based investigation of psychosocial sequelae to breast cancer surgeries is a fairly recent event.[38–41] The important issues to be explored under these circumstances are:

1. Does elimination or amputation of the breast categorically erase negative psychological trauma or is there a universal distress that transcends the type of treatment?
2. If given a choice of surgery that does not compromise survival, would all women opt to preserve this cherished part of their anatomy?

If the answer to this last question is "no," and preliminary research findings indicate that this is the case, it becomes imperative to determine who these women are who will fare better psychologically with breast conservation or mastectomy, and to disseminate that information among the health professionals ministering to their care.

Treatment recommendations based on a more rational understanding of the psychological dynamics of the woman who must receive the therapy could significantly reduce psychological morbidity, enhance feelings of well-being and effectiveness, and optimize the quality of life.

PSYCHOSOCIAL SEQUELAE OF BREAST RECONSTRUCTION: INTRAPERSONAL AND INTERPERSONAL

It is not clearly determined how many of the approximately 130,000[42] breast cancers diagnosed annually are treated by mastectomy or, of the proportion who undergo radical surgery, what percentage elect breast reconstruction. "An estimated 98,000 breast reconstructions were performed in 1984 in the United States compared with 20,000 in 1981."[43] What the total numbers of these operations are at present and how many of them require breast implants is not clearly established. Data collected by the American Society of Plastic and Reconstructive Surgeons suggest that these numbers are changing rather rapidly. At a recent FDA meeting held in Washington, DC to discuss the risks and benefits of silicone breast implants, the number of implants used for reconstruction was estimated to be approximately 25 percent.[44] Conservatively, then, one can speculate that 13,000 to 20,000 breast reconstructions are performed each year. Some of these reconstructions do not require the use of an internal breast implant, a factor that is relevant to an evaluation of the cosmetic or psychological outcome.

CHANGING TIMES: CHANGING TRENDS

The reasons for the marked increase in the number of breast reconstructions performed are varied and heterogeneous and involve technical improvement, societal endorsement for the procedure, and sophisticated consumerism. Specifically, there has been a growing trend for less radical procedures that leave more available tissue to build a reconstructed breast contour. Second, the technology of reconstructive surgery has advanced markedly to allow multiple options in the selection of a procedure best suited to an individual woman and one that is likely to give her a more acceptable "breastlike" outcome with fewer complications than in the past. Third, there is enhanced appreciation for quality of life issues and psychological well-being following breast cancer surgery. Fourth, women consumers are more sophisticated and active and are demanding a more participatory role in their medical care and in the decisions about their treatment.

Although there is a tidal wave of information regarding women's health issues and extensive opportunities for exposure to information about breast reconstruction, a sizeable population of women remain mildly or moderately unfamiliar with this option. Research conducted in 1982 by the National Cancer Institute on attitudes about breast cancer revealed that almost 40 percent of the women surveyed indicated that they would be interested in breast reconstruction, but that approximately 30 percent were unaware that such an operation existed.[45] The variation in knowledge and awareness of breast reconstruction is both situational and psychological. Some women do not want to have to face this issue until it is something that they personally have to deal with. Others who may have had a breast cancer operation are either uneducated about this topic or too passive to confront their physician about alternatives to mastectomy and living their life with one or both breasts missing. There is still lingering ambivalence and marked geographical variations in practices of providing women with information about treatment options, and encouraging them to seek out individuals who have had this experience and are willing to disclose the risks and benefits as they experienced them. Rural regions and European countries have very different methods of popularizing this concept than large metropolitan cities such as New York or Atlanta. An Italian study remarked how less than 53 percent of the mastectomy patients surveyed even knew that breast reconstruction was a rehabilitation option.[46]

As publicity about the possible hazards of breast implants mounts and popular reports sensationalize the potential dangers of this device, more women will be informed (albeit misinformed).[47] Certain recently published texts and public accounts have managed to present more balanced and comprehensive discussions of the advantages and disadvantages. One of the most accessible is that of Berger and Bostwick.[48] There is an ever-increasing need to transfer the knowledge about breast reconstruction in general and breast implants specifically to the public so that they know where to obtain accurate information, know how to identify and report complications, and are in a better position if necessary to make a rationally directed choice about this operation.

Numerous reports[3,17,18,49] have documented the fact that a significant proportion of the emotional morbidity associated with mastectomy is due to the loss of the breast and the resulting negative impact on body image. If this is the rule rather than the exception, one must wonder why all women who have to sacrifice their breast in the treatment of this disease do not elect to reconstruct the missing body part. Specifically, one must inquire which women seek out breast reconstruction to restore their lost body part and which women choose not to do so. Slightly more than a decade ago it was believed that only those women who could not adjust to the physical defect treated by mastectomy would consider breast reconstruction. It was assumed that these women were less able to cope with their altered body image and so would go in search of replacing their missing breast. Allegedly, the other group of women who did not seek out reconstruction were thought to be better adjusted and could accept their disfigurement with appropriate resignation and learn to live with their amputation. In the last 10 to 15 years, various researchers have not only challenged this assumption, but presented clinical case material and empirical finding to refute it. Clifford[50] was probably the first social scientist to investigate this problem and study women who had undergone delayed reconstruction at some time after their mastectomy. He concluded that women who sought "restitution" for their surgically altered body were exhibiting evidence of positive coping and assertive, effective problem-solving behavior, not neurotic compensation. The desire for and active effort to change an undesirable physical defect, which is indeed correctable today, is more likely the outgrowth of adaptive coping responses than of a maladapted defensiveness.

Another research team exploring motives underlying the choice for breast reconstruction evaluated a cohort of women after their mastectomy. The study populations of 83 women who sought reconstruction were compared with 50 of their mastectomy counterparts who did not want this operation.[51] The results of this study further supported Clifford's conclusions of the adaptive value in seeking breast reconstruction. The women who sought reconstruction were seen as well adjusted, devoid of any clinically significant psychopathology, and able to maintain a high level of psychosocial functioning. The antiquated notion that only discontented women who cannot accept their defect or adjust to the harsh blow that life has dealt them go in search of restitution has been laid to rest.

MOTIVES FOR BREAST RECONSTRUCTION

Women's motives for seeking reconstruction after mastectomy can be classified in different ways. One of the most useful distinctions was derived from a research study investigating two groups of women matched for age and time interval since mastectomy.[52] The first group seeking reconstruction was interviewed preoperatively and 2 months after surgery. The other group, women not seeking reconstruction, was also interviewed twice within a 2-month period. From her analysis, Daniels found that the two groups did not appear significantly different on a number of psychological variables, suggesting that reconstruction patients, as a whole, did not exhibit greater problems in all areas of functioning after mastectomy.

Specifically, the reconstructed patients in comparison with their mastectomy controls did not show significant differences in the following feelings or conditions: (1) major threat of cancer, (2) minor threat of cancer, (3) threat of mastectomy, (4) sense of control, (5) satisfaction in love relations, (6) satisfaction in sexual relations, (7) social acceptability, (8) health status, (9) life satisfaction, (10) morale, (11) depression, (12) anxiety, (13) hostility, (14) satisfaction with their prosthesis, and (15) overall body satisfaction.

On the other hand, the list of significant differences between the two groups studied is very illuminating and reveals that reconstructed patients reported a higher dissatisfaction with their breasts, expressed more negative concerns regarding their femininity and sexual attractiveness, and admitted more self-consciousness about wearing an external prosthesis, both in public and in private. The last has been repeatedly supported in other publications, which suggest that women who find their external prosthesis cumbersome, contributory to self-consciousness, or restrictive in clothing are more motivated to seek breast reconstruction surgery.[53] In addition to explaining some of the variance in seeking breast reconstruction, the issue of comfort with a prosthesis adds to a very central theme in distinguishing between women who elect to have this restorative surgery and those who do not; the latter group is seen as not having as intimate a connection between their body image and their self-esteem.

From Daniels' research it was also concluded that women who sought breast reconstruction scored higher in the test for self-esteem. Although this appears contradictory, it is possible that a higher general self-esteem contributes to a woman's feeling worthwhile enough to want to do something to reduce her discomfort and correct the physical defect, rather than passively ignore such underlying needs. A high level of self-esteem and initiative will foster a woman's pursuit of her goals in spite of certain obstacles encountered.

Significant differences found between the women seeking reconstruction and those electing not to have that surgery were in the following areas: (1) impact of the mastectomy, (2) dissatisfaction with breasts, (3) negative concerns with regard to femininity, (4) negative concerns with regard to sexual attractiveness, (5) public self-consciousness, (6) private self-consciousness, (7) somatic symptoms higher in the reconstructed population, (8) social support perceived lower in the reconstructed population, and (9) self-esteem higher in the reconstructed population.

The correspondence between body image and overall sense of self-worth has been alluded to in numerous reports,[19,21] as has the well-researched notion that loss of a breast significantly diminishes body image.[3,49,54] Given the assumption that for most women a negative body image follows mastectomy, one must look for more complex contributions to the fact that all women who lose a breast do not experience the same degree of insult or negative aftereffect. As suggested by Teimourian and Adham,[55] reconstruction may be experienced by many women as a "reverse mastectomy": a procedure that can create a neutralizing of the destructive effect of the loss of such a significant body part. A better understanding of the role that body image plays in a woman's sense of efficacy and worth has significant implications for counseling patients regarding breast reconstruction and predicting satisfaction with outcome.

A PRIVATE BODY IDEAL VERSUS A PUBLIC BODY IMAGE

Again Daniels helps us with this critical concept. In her work, she hypothesized that the difference between women seeking reconstruction and women not seeking reconstruction could be explained by the ways in which they prioritized two basic organizing principles: (1) their *body ideal* and (2) their *public body image concept.* Women who favor a body ideal generally are more concerned about how their body should look than about how it actually does appear. Conversely, those who favor a public body concept are more concerned about how their body appears to others and what those other important people's reactions are going to be in terms of possible rejection or acceptance.

Some women experience mastectomy as an assault on their idealized body image, not because they fear other people's depreciation or rejection, but because they see it as markedly deviant from how they had looked previously or how they want to look now. Reconstruction is therefore viewed as an opportunity to achieve their idealized view of how they want their body to be. If indeed the results are congruent with the woman's expectations (which does not mean perfection, but does mean that they correspond to the notion she has of what she wants in terms of private or public impact), then she is likely to be pleased and psychologically rewarded. For example, a woman who is driven to pursue restitution to recapture her idealized body image might make the following comment: "I really do think my partner is as responsive and interested in my body as he ever was, but I can't stand to look at it (my mastectomy scar) myself or even think of him caressing my breast area. I am the one who cannot accept what has happened to me."[52] This notion of viewing acceptance or rejection from a solely individual vantage point reflects the "inner-directed" rather than "other-directed" sources of dissatisfaction or satisfaction. The woman who is motivated to achieve her idealized body image through her reconstruction is propelled into action by self-determined needs and may be minimally influenced by the reactions of her significant other.

This organizing principle of ideal versus public body image orientation has significant implications for the choice of and satisfaction from breast reconstruction. One can speculate that women primarily motivated by a public body image orientation will be strongly influenced by how they imagine their partners or other important people to perceive them after their mastectomy. If they experience or fantasize that their partners find them less physically or sexually attractive, and if this perception contributes to a reduced satisfaction with their quality of life, they may indeed seek reconstruction. If, however, the outcome of the reconstructive surgery does not result in improved relationships with these people, or does not appear to offer enhanced opportunity for positive reinforcement from others in the near future, such women may be disappointed or depressed after their operation. In addition, women who underwent immediate breast reconstruction at the time of the mastectomy might experience a cumulative impact of negative emotions subsequent to the operation. In summary, it might be assumed that women who have enjoyed a life experience characterized by a positive, fairly confident physical self-image can endure the temporary disfigurement of mastectomy. This is particularly true if they intellectually or in fantasy get themselves through the disfiguring phase and project their image into the period after the restorative operation. Conversely, for women who have endured negative feelings about their physical appearance for a long time and have been particularly dissatisfied with their breasts, the mastectomy experience (or an unacceptable breast reconstruction outcome) may exacerbate their sense of unacceptability. This latter outcome is known as the "medical confirmation of a defect" and may explain why some women are so distraught after mastectomy and reconstruction. Alterations or mutilation to the part of their body that was consciously or unconsciously viewed as inadequate unfortunately serves to confirm their feeling of being "defective" and unacceptable. Sensitive inquiry before mastectomy, and certainly before reconstructive surgery, can help to illuminate a woman's characteristic perception of her physical self and its relation to her overall sense of self-esteem.

Two other important insights to add to the body ideal versus public body concept distinction are (1) an understanding of how limited or widespread the woman's feeling of being "defective" or altered is and (2) how short term or enduring is the dissatisfaction with her body. If a woman has enjoyed her breasts and felt them to be attractive and is confident about her body image appeal, a sudden and marked alteration of that feeling is likely to be extremely painful, but transient. For this type of woman, reconstructive surgery that restores her general sense of body balance and attractiveness is likely to be extremely therapeutic, with an obvious and almost immediate improvement in psychological adaptation.

Another group of women, however, may be characterized as having been self-conscious about their breast size or shape since puberty. For women with long-term and chronic dissatisfaction about their breasts, reconstruction may be only mildly beneficial. If, in addition to feeling diminished in terms of their breast attractiveness, these women have had negative feelings about a variety of other physical characteristics over a long period (or experience a generalized sense of inadequacy), another insult in the form of mastectomy may be experienced as overwhelming and seriously undermine their psychological equanimity and self-esteem. It is probable that for this subset of mastectomy patients, breast reconstruction alone (without corrective or reeducative psychotherapy) may not be sufficient to reduce the emotional morbidity unleashed by the surgical removal of the breast.

TIMING OF BREAST RECONSTRUCTION

Both popular and professional wisdom today support the notion that breast reconstruction in general has a salutary effect on a mastectomy patient's psychological adaptation, especially in the areas of feeling physically intact, whole, and more similar to her premorbid body image. The issue is no longer whether to reconstruct a woman who requests this operation, but when in the course of the treatment is the most propitious time to recommend the reconstruction. Earlier views about the timing of breast reconstruction were rooted in the belief that a patient could better appreciate the result of a reconstructed breast only after she had lived with the defect of mastectomy and truly mourned the loss of her natural breast.[56] A number of surgical oncologists and breast reconstruction surgeons[57] proposed that that mastectomy patient would most likely value the cosmetic appearance of her new breast when she had experienced the discomfort of an external prosthesis and/or the sadness and inconvenience of living without a part of her body. In addition to the belief about patient satisfaction being predicated on first living with an unsatisfactory body condition, there were serious caveats about possible medical hazards associated with early breast reconstruction.[58]

Dowden and colleagues[59] helped allay these concerns about immediate breast reconstruction from a biologic perspective. They appealed to the profession to recognize that a sizeable population of breast cancer patients would benefit from immediate restoration, and that such a reparative procedure would not adversely affect the group of women who might experience a recurrence of their cancer. More recent information about the relationship between immediate breast reconstruction and cancer detection or promotion has not refuted these authors' claim. A study conducted to evaluate recurrence of carcinoma in 118 patients who underwent mastectomy and immediate breast reconstruction revealed that 14 women (12 percent) suffered a recurrence of cancer and 10 (9 percent) died of cancer within a median follow-up of 2.3 years.[60] As postulated, an adverse outcome in the morbidity of this group was associated with the well-known prognostic factors for breast cancer and not with the presence of an internal breast prosthesis. Disease-free survival and overall survival was comparable with previously reported findings in mastectomy patients who did not undergo breast reconstruction. The authors stated, with supporting evidence, that immediate breast reconstruction should be offered routinely for breast reconstruction patients, because outcome depends on the biology of the tumor and not the presence of a prosthesis. In the absence of any obvious negative impact on patient survival and the fact that insertion of an internal implant seems to pose no threat to tumor status, decisions about timing of breast reconstruction need to be predicated on the woman's psychological state and the benefits alleged to accrue from immediate restoration.

Noone and associates,[61] in an early research study, investigated this issue and concluded that there was no less satisfaction in the immediate reconstruction patients than in those women who delayed this surgery. Teimourian and Adham,[55] in a survey of patients who had delayed reconstruction, found that approximately 90 percent reported being quite satisfied with their outcome. Noone and associates concluded that 92 percent of the immediate group were satisfied with the results. Such a high level of satisfaction in the immediate reconstruction group would tend to disprove the older notion that living with the deformity was a necessary requisite to patient satisfaction of the reconstruction. The research of Dean and colleagues[62] in the the United Kingdom also supported the psychological advantage of immediate breast reconstruction in reducing psychiatric morbidity after mastectomy, especially in women whose marital relationships were compromised. Schain and associates concluded that "the sooner the better" was a reasonable recommendation for many mastectomy patients to undergo reconstruction. In a study of 60 patients, they found that the women who had undergone immediate reconstruction were less anxious, less depressed, and less hostile to their doctors than the study group who delayed their reconstruction.[63]

Interestingly, in the U.K. study, the mastectomy patients were randomized to immediate versus delayed reconstruction, and only a very few of the latter group elected to have reconstruction at a later date. The authors concluded that although reconstruction does seem to benefit a sizeable population of mastectomy patients, those who are interested in undergoing this procedure will select themselves fairly early in the postoperative period. Information discussed earlier in this chapter regarding idealized versus public body image orientation may help to explain this selection process. Other contributing factors to the ultimate decision may be:

1. The presentation of information about breast reconstruction at the time of the cancer diagnosis.
2. Financial constraints of individual women when reconstruction is not carried out as part of the health care system of that country or underwritten by third-party carriers.
3. Changes in a woman's life that might affect how she prioritizes her private versus her public body image (e.g., divorce or career change that necessitates more flexibility in the wardrobe).

Another study conducted in the Netherlands also confirmed that immediate breast reconstruction was a much appreciated operation that resulted in a high level of patient satisfaction.[64] Interestingly, this study added more precise information about possible interaction between timing of the reconstruction, type of operative procedure, and ultimate degree of satisfaction. From a sample of 122 patients operated on between 1980 and 1984 who underwent three different types of breast reconstruction surgery, 95 women were assessed for follow-up at least 1 year after reconstruction. No significant differences in psychological satisfaction were found for the three different types of operations, but there were marked differences in satisfaction with cosmetic results. Simple insertion of a prosthesis in the subpectoral region without a flap produced the least satisfactory aesthetic results. The transverse rectus abdominis myocutaneous flap (TRAM) and latissimus dorsi flap procedures produced a higher level of expressed satisfaction, but the rectus abdominis flaps resulted in higher complication rates.

Another interesting study comparing two different methods of breast reconstruction disclosed opposite findings favoring the TRAM operation.[65] The TRAM procedure provided a more satisfactory reconstruction with few major complications, a higher degree of patient satisfaction, and less patient dissatisfaction (a factor not often assessed and distinguished from satisfaction). It is possible that this particular study was conducted by a group of surgeons especially expert in the TRAM flap procedure, and that those patients therefore suffered fewer complications. The psychological reports on the patients in this study must be interpreted with caution, as they were not assigned their operation, but were free to choose their type of reconstruction surgery. Perhaps only the most motivated chose the more complicated TRAM procedure. Nevertheless, reports of patient satisfaction are very revealing and may be used to help recommend the operation most likely to provide satisfactory results with the individual patient. The TRAM flap patients usually perceived their reconstruction to be of higher quality, and expressed significant relief in the definitive and time-limited nature of the procedure. Patients who underwent tissue expander implant (TEI) surgery remained apprehensive and suspicious that they would eventually experience problems with the implant.

TISSUE EXPANDER IMPLANT SURGERY

Irrespective of the final decision over which type of reconstruction provides a more satisfactory outcome and for whom, there is little doubt today that the tissue expander implant (TEI) procedure is one often used. The medical complications and cosmetic results compared with other types of reconstruction are still unclear, as is the psychological impact of a breast implant that requires repeated inflation over a "reasonable" period of time. It is important to inquire whether repeated intrusions to expand the prosthesis, which can cause excessive focus on the treated breast, are more beneficial or more of a burden to the patient. A report by Goin and Goin[66] evaluated in depth, by clinical interview, the psychological experiences of ten women undergoing this type of reconstruction. The women revealed a wide range of reactions to TEI, the most constant of which was a willingness to talk about their experience in the hope of helping others. They said they chose this type of reconstruction because they did not want a "big" operation and were hoping to avoid additional scars. Allegedly, all patients stated that they remembered being told the procedure would take 4 to 6 months. They wanted completion as quickly as possible but were willing to tolerate what was necessary to avoid additional visible tell-tale marks. General findings from this study revealed that most of the patients admitted feeling pleasure immediately after the implant was in place. Several women stated that weekly visits to the office for injection of fluid into the expander was a routine event for them that did not cause any serious distress or disruption of activities. In fact, some admitted that the experience was positive to the extent that they could share this information with friends and co-workers even though they had been secretive about their mastectomy. About half of the study group described the steady inflation and enlargement as painful; one woman described the sensation as a feeling that the object was changing from "a friend to a foreign thing." Another woman was so negatively affected by the growing size and changing shape that she said, "It feels like a thing, like a growing tumor, not a breast." The others experienced the gradual change more positively. Another patient undergoing the expansion phase expressed how she felt it was a type of rebirth and simulated what she remembered as she developed during her adolescent period. Gradual expansion of the breast region represented for some of these women an opportunity to adjust slowly to the reappearance of their femininity and body integrity. In general, most of whatever negative feelings may have been unleashed during the expander experience disappeared as soon as the expander was replaced by the permanent implant.

There appears to be considerable heterogeneity in women's reaction to the TEI method of breast reconstruction. Some of this variability may be rooted in body image experiences of many years earlier. Interestingly, another possible contributory factor associated with negative reactions to the expansion process is a sensation of being "stretched" and the feeling of being "off balance" during most of the phase. In addition to adjusting to the inflation process and whatever physical discomfort may be related, there is an ongoing need to make accommodations (albeit small) in one's body image and style of dress. At the point when the reconstructed breast is hyperinflated, a major adjustment must occur to camouflage the enlarged implanted breast and to modify the contralateral breast to achieve symmetry. Additional patient education about these possible psychological sequelae might minimize the morbidity that has been described. However, such acknowledged discomfort does not appear to eliminate the desire for this type of operation.

Considerable variation in reaction to the expander experience does exist and needs to be researched more thoroughly. More detailed inquiry of prospective candidates for this procedure should include such questions as:

1. What was adolescence like for you as your breasts began to develop?
2. How did you experience other changes in your breast size or shape during pregnancy or weight loss or gain?
3. What coping strategies do you have to distract yourself when you feel upset about your breast cancer and body image?
4. Are you familiar with ways to camouflage the difference in your breast symmetry (e.g., patterned blouses, a short-term prosthesis)?

Attention to such issues might help prepare candidates for this procedure and help select those women who might fare better psychologically with a flap operation, and one that is more definitive and provides more rapidly achieved symmetry. As suggested in Oncology Nursing Forum,[67] the nurse's role in assisting women during this phase of breast cancer rehabilitation can be very helpful. Specifically the nurse can provide concrete information about possible problems and complications to be monitored and reported. She can also be particularly helpful in assisting patients to handle anxiety about the finished product and the time it may take. She may also offer practical hints and suggestions necessary to accommodate the asymmetrical breast projection inherent in the expansion phase.

IMPACT OF PARTNER

Most women claim that the wish for reconstruction is strictly personal and has nothing to do with their husband. However, the research by Daniels[52] has added to our understanding of women whose primary incentive for reconstruction is predicated on achieving an idealized body concept as opposed to those who wish to achieve a more acceptable public body image (perhaps to please a mate). However, it is evident that the reactions of the partner from the time of the mastectomy affect the patient's view of herself, and therefore her interest in the reconstruction effort. Information on husbands' reactions to reconstruction and the effects, negative or positive, that it may have on their interpersonal or sexual interaction with their wives is seriously lacking, and this has not been studied in any systematic manner. However, one study by researchers from Memorial Sloan Kettering investigating anecdotal comments made by husbands of mastectomy patients, revealed that approximately one-third of these men were slightly or moderately opposed to their wives' breast reconstruction.[51] The specific reasons for their reactions were not disclosed. This study concluded that many women were so strongly motivated to seek this operation that they pursued the option over serious objections from family, friends, and physicians. Again, the woman who is motivated to achieve her idealized body image may persist in reaching her goal through rather assertive behaviors, ones more likely to be tolerated in the 1990s by medical professionals and significant others. Interestingly, the same study reported that 13 percent of all patients thought no one had been supportive of their decision; 39 percent of the married women said that their spouses had not reinforced their desire for this operation.

The largest group of husbands studied voiced their own ambivalence about reconstruction, and varied in their ability to understand their wives' need or motives for this operation, but did say they wanted them to do what would make them happy. The patient with this type of spouse feels fairly free, albeit somewhat alone, in her decision to go ahead with this surgery because the needed feedback from her partner is so ambiguous.

Another group of male partners are too involved in their own reactions and fears to really listen to their partner and instead vocalize their own distress. Some women view this upset as concern for their well-being and respond with reassurance for their partners. However, they find it more difficult to accept the surgery because they traditionally have to take care of their husband's physical and emotional well-being rather than concentrate on their own recovery. "You don't have to do this for me" is another message not infrequently voiced by a spouse. Although this type of comment may sound selfless, it does not really support or encourage the woman to explore her needs and to act in her own best interest. Passive endorsement is not equivalent to active support.

In general, couples are often unwilling to disclose their fears, anxieties, disappointments, and honest reactions toward issues such as cancer and loss of a significant body part (Dakoff and colleagues).[68] There is often a need to protect the other person and to preserve the notion that the man is a nice person who would not say something hurtful about how awful it might look for his "woman" to have one or both breasts missing. An open exchange of feelings and needs often is delayed or eliminated in some cases. Not infrequently, however, these unspoken feelings are converted to nonverbal reactions that may be detrimental to the relationship and experienced as hostility or passive obstructionistic behavior. It is important when the patient is married or in a committed relationship to invite the partner to come in and discuss his or her possible fears and concerns about the intended reconstruction.

Another reaction often communicated is the partner's sincere concern for the patient's well-being and the wish for her not to have to undergo any more surgery or trauma. If the woman can communicate the feeling that reconstruction is perceived as an additive and not a subtractive or traumatic experience, the partner may be less fearful of the outcome and more able to empathize with the desired results.

SEXUAL RESPONSIVENESS AND RECONSTRUCTION

Another critical factor is the view that the breast cancer patient has about her sexuality and how critical a role her breasts play in her sense of physical attractiveness and sexual desirability. Breast reconstruction has been found to increase sexual responsiveness,[54,55] but the source of this outcome is not clear and clinical examination of this issue has been sorely lacking. This may be because the relationship between body integrity and sexuality is assumed to be uncomplicated. More likely, the paucity of research is due to the delicate subject matter and the difficulty in establishing and executing scientific methodology. However, an interesting laboratory investigation conducted several years ago by Gerard[69] added considerable insight into this complex phenomenon. Gerard compared the sexual arousal of mastectomy patients with that of women who had also undergone reconstruction. This was accomplished by the use of a photoplethysmograph to document vaginal blood flow as an index of sexual excitement while the women were listening to romantic and erotic tapes. Her findings revealed that women who had been reconstructed were more easily sexually aroused than their mastectomy counterparts. The clinical interpretation of this finding appears to be related to the anxiety that mastectomy patients often feel about their altered body and the increase in self-consciousness experienced as a result of being different from the way they were previously, and also from the way they perceive other women to be. They are often obsessed with their body disfigurement and this distracts them from being able to concentrate their energies on the lovemaking experience. Instead of being able to tune into the pleasurable aspects of the sexual stimulation and related good feeling that could be unleashed, the mastectomy patients were more likely to be focused on their body's differentness: feelings that make it difficult to relax and abandon one's self to more positive experiences. The women who were reconstructed, it appeared, could distance themselves from concentrating on the physical aspects of their altered breast (or self-perceived defect) and enter into the fantasy or real sexual experience. There was a notable difference between the two study groups in regard to the lag time between the stimulus and reaction, and also in terms of the magnitude of the sexual arousal measured. The mastectomy patients had more difficulty getting "turned on."

The above findings have serious implications for health professionals in terms of understanding the connection between women's sexual reactions and their interest in breast reconstruction. Although some breast reconstruction patients say they do not have erotic sensations in the reconstructed breast, the link between body parts and sexual responsiveness is much more complex than the presence or absence of specific sexual organs. Breast reconstruction facilitates a reintegration of body image and contributes to feeling whole again (Berger and Bostwick).[48] This finding is clarified by Nathan and Johanning,[70] who reported that the closer a woman can remain to her presurgical state physically, the less distress she may feel generally and the less disrupted she may be specifically in regard to her sexual responsiveness.

In an effort to add further understanding to the relationship between intact breast image and sexuality, Wellisch and colleagues[71] constructed a study to evaluate the difference in the psychosexual outcome of women who had undergone breast reconstruction and who subsequently elected either to have or not to have nipple-areola reconstruction. The nipple-added group (n = 33) compared with the non-nipple-added group (n = 26) reported significantly greater contentment with breast reconstruction in regard to (1) overall satisfaction, (2) satisfaction with nude appearance, (3) satisfaction with size, (4) satisfaction with breast softness, and (5) satisfaction with the sexual sensitivity of the reconstructed breast.

Findings from this study are noteworthy, even though the researchers did not specify the different types of breast or nipple reconstruction performed. In summary, the nipple-added group expressed increased satisfaction with the sexual responsiveness in their reconstructed breast. The addition of the nipple-areola complex to the reconstructed breast mound could not itself increase erotic response. This reported reaction must have to do with somatosensory reactions rather than anatomic or physical connections. The identified outcome is therefore likely to depend on a complex set of psychological variables, the most important of which is the "sense of completeness" and the visual appeal of an intact breast and nipple contour experienced by the woman and responded to by her partner. Adding the nipple-areola not only makes the breast look more natural to the patient and her partner, but also makes it appear more familiar and more like the way it was. A major clue to understanding this response lies in the fact that the more a woman is likely to experience herself as unchanged or undamaged, the more she is likely to forget (although not deny in a pathologic sense) that she was surgically altered. This speculation has implications for understanding both the psychological adaptation of mastectomy patients, and the alleged improved body image and sexual responses of breast cancer patients who are treated with conservative surgery. The population of conservatively treated breast cancer patients most often achieves a postoperative physical appearance closest to the presurgical body image.

CONCLUSION

For almost a century, mastectomy has been the standard of care for the breast cancer patient. Women, their partners, and their doctors all had to accept with varying degrees of resignation or rage the physical mutilation and psychological morbidity suffered with the amputation of such a prized part of the anatomy. Today, mastectomy is only one option in the clinical armamentarium of breast cancer surgery. There are a variety of alternatives for primary and adjuvant treatments. This process of choice is both a blessing and a burden for the patient and her physicians in evaluating the relative risks and benefits of various procedures.

Irrespective of primary surgery, breast reconstruction remains a central theme in treatment and rehabilitation. It may be chosen at the time a mastectomy is performed as primary surgery, or it may become a necessary option if a woman has had breast conservation therapy, relapses, and needs a subsequent salvage mastectomy. This latter group of breast cancer patients has not been studied in any detail, but should be evaluated so that health professionals can communicate more candidly with them about the anticipated psychosocial consequences of their therapy.

Almost all women today are likely to be candidates either for breast preservation or for reconstruction if mastectomy is the elected or required surgery. The painful and distressing image of a woman with a Halsted radical mastectomy, an obvious concavity, and a "washboard" chest is almost an obsolete phenomenon. Even though the treatment outcome for this disease has changed only marginally in the last 10 years, the prospect of permanent disfigurement and social and sexual isolation is rapidly becoming an anachronism. Neither breast conservation surgery nor breast reconstruction is a procedure without complications, but the benefits tend to be impressive, especially when carefully considered and matched with patient selection variables. One study in the Netherlands[72] found that only one of 100 patients who had been reconstructed regretted her choice. The others were extremely satisfied, and of those 96 happy patients, 14 revealed that the reconstructive procedure was "absolutely psychologically vital." Numbers like this represent an impressive endorsement for the therapeutic value breast reconstruction can provide.

Age and stage of disease no longer seem to be major contraindications for this procedure. Patient motivation and physician concordance are the determining factors. What remains essential is to distinguish more clearly the psychological variables likely to predict patient satisfaction, and those that suggest possible dissatisfaction and/or resulting psychological morbidity. Critical questions are:

1. In what ways will my quality of life be better if I have breast reconstruction and how will the different procedures affect my style of life and routine activities?
2. Are the results likely to be congruent and match my major motivation for this procedure (i.e., I want to be closer to an idealized body image *or* I want to have breasts that look good in different clothes because I want to continue my modeling career).
3. I feel pretty good about my body image in general, but the change in my breast area causes me considerable distress. Is this likely to go away with reconstruction?

In general, if the woman can imagine that her psychological state will be improved by the reconstruction and that it will allow her to maintain her social, sexual, and leisure time pursuits with little alteration, she is likely to be grateful and pleased with the outcome. However, if the type of procedure or the use of an implant exacerbates her preoccupation with her body and intensifies her fears about an underlying cancer, the outcome might be problematic.

Because the human condition is so variable and unique, overgeneralizations do not serve this issue well. What is primal is to spend time with the woman considering this procedure, to inquire about her imagined reaction to the various questions posed, and to share with her how likely it is that her expectations can be met by the operation agreed on. The need for continued health vigilance and for monitoring psychological changes in one's life that might alter the satisfaction with the breast reconstruction should be reinforced.

References

1. Czerny V. Plasticher Ersatz der Brustdruse durch ein Lipom. Zentrabl Chir 1895; 27:72.
2. Snyderman RK. Symposium on neoplastic and reconstruction problems of the female breast. St Louis: CV Mosby, 1973.
3. Meyerowitz BE. Psychosocial correlates of breast cancer and its treatments. Psychol Bull 1980; 87: 108-131.
4. Scott DW, Eisendrath SJ. Dynamics of the recovery process following initial diagnosis of breast cancer. Psychosocial Oncol 1985-1986; 3:53-66.
5. Brownmiller S. Femininity. New York: Simon & Schuster, 1984:25.
6. Harris JR, Hellman S, Silen W. Conservative management of breast cancer: New surgical and radiotherapeutic techniques. Philadelphia: JB Lippincott, 1983.
7. Bacon CR, Renneker R, Cutler M. A psychosomatic survey of cancer of the breast. Psychosom Med 1952; 14:453.
8. Levy S, Schain WS. Psychological response to breast cancer: Direct and indirect contributors to treatment outcome. In: Lippman M, Lichter A, Danforth D, eds. Diagnosis and management of breast cancer. Philadelphia: WB Saunders, 1988:439-456.
9. Pettingale KW, Morris T, Greer S, Haybittle JL. Mental attitudes to cancer: An additional prognostic factor. Lancet 1985; 8431:750.
10. Levy S, Herberman R, Malush A, et al. Prognostic risk assessment in primary cancer by behavioral and immunological parameters. Health Psychol 1985; 4:99.
11. Cousins N. Headfirst: The biology of hope. New York: EP Hutton, 1989.
12. Herberman R, Ortaldo J. Natural killer cells: Their role in defense against disease. Science 1981; 214:24-30.
13. Schain W, Levy S, Herberman R. Familial breast cancer: A life enhancement intervention. Grant proposal, 1990.
14. Maguire GP, Lee EG, Bevington EJ, et al. Psychiatric problems in the first year after mastectomy. Breast Med J 1978; 963-965.
15. Morris T, Greer HS, White P. Psychosocial and social adjustment to mastectomy: A two year follow-up. Cancer. 1977; 40:2381-2387.
16. Jamison KR, Wellisch DK, Pasnau RO. Psychosocial aspects of mastectomy: The woman's perspective. Am J Psychiatry 1978; 235:432-436.
17. Wellisch DK, Jamison KR, Pasnau RO. Psychosocial aspects of mastectomy: The man's perspective. Am J Psychiatry 1978; 135:543-546.
18. Frank D, Dornbruch R, Webster S, et al. Mastectomy and sexual behavior: A pilot study. Sexuality Disability 1978; 1:16.
19. Silberfarb P, Maurer LH, Crouthamel C. Psychosocial aspects of neoplastic disease: I. Functional status of breast cancer patients during different treatment regimens. Am J Psychiatry 1980; 137:450-455.
20. Abt V. The impact of mastectomy on sexual self-image, attitudes and sexuality. J Sex Education Ther 1978; 4:43-46.
21. Grinker RR. Sex and cancer. Med Aspects Hum Sex 1976; 10:130-139.
22. Clifford E, Clifford M, Georgiade NC. Breast reconstruction following mastectomy. II. Marital characteristics of patients seeking this procedure. Ann Plast Surg 1980; 5:343-346.
23. Rollin B, First you cry. New York: New American Library, 1977:58.
24. Kolodny RC, Masters WH, Johnson VE. Textbook of sexual medicine. Boston: Little, Brown, 1979:274.
25. Wabrek AJ. Rehabilitative intervention: Intervention with couples. Proceedings of the Workshop on Psychosexual and Reproductive Issues Affecting Patients with Cancer. San Antonio, TX: American Cancer Society, 1987.

25a. Wabrek AJ, Wabrek CJ, Burchell RC. Marital and sexual counseling after mastectomy. In: Green R, ed. Human sexuality: A health practitioner's text, 2nd ed. Baltimore: Williams & Wilkins, 1979:215-225.

26. Schover LR, Jensen SB. Sexuality and chronic illness: Comprehensive assessment and treatment. New York; Guilford Press, 1989.
27. Schain WS. A sexual interview is a sexual intervention. Innovations in oncology nursing. Meniscus, PA 1988; 4:2.
28. Wortman CB, Dunkel-Schetter C. Interpersonal relationships and cancer: A theoretical analysis. J Social Issues 1979; 35:120-151.
29. Peters-Golden H. Breast cancer: Varied perceptions of social support in the illness experience. Soc Sci Med 1982; 15:483-492.
30. Bloom J. Social support, accommodation to stress and adjustment to breast cancer. Social Sci Med 1982; 16:1329-1338.
31. Witkin M. Sex therapy and mastectomy. J Sex Marital Ther 1975; 1:290-302.
32. Gates C. Husbands of mastectomy patients. Patient Counseling and Health Information: 1980:38-41.
33. Baider L, De-Nour AT. Breast cancer—a family affair. In: Cooper CL, ed. Stress and breast cancer. Baltimore: John Wiley, 1988:155.
34. Bloom JR, Ross RD, Burnell E. The effect of social support on patient adjustment after breast surgery. Patient Counseling and Health Education 1978; 1:1-9.
35. Sabo D, Brown J, Smith C. The male role and mastectomy support group and men's adjustment. J Psychosocial Oncol 1986; 14:19-31.
36. Murcia A, Stewart B. Man to man: When the woman you love has breast cancer. New York: St Martin's Press, 1989.

37. Cobliner G. Psychosocial factors in gynecological or breast malignancies. Hosp Physician: 1977; 10:38.
38. Schain WS, Edwards BK. Gorell CR, et al. Psychosocial and physical outcomes of primary breast cancer therapy: Mastectomy vs excisional biopsy and irradiation. Breast Cancer Res Treat 1983; 3:377-382.
39. Lasry JC, Margolese RG, Poisson R, et al. Depression and body image following mastectomy and lumpectomy. J Chronic Dis 1987; 40:529-534.
40. Steinberg MD, Juliano NA, Wise L, et al. Psychological outcome of lumpectomy vs mastectomy in the treatment of breast cancer. Am J Psychiatry 1985; 142:32-39.
41. Kemeny M, Wellisch DK, Schain WS. Psychosocial outcome in a randomized surgical trial for treatment of primary breast cancer. Cancer. 1988; 62:1231-1237.
42. Cancer facts and figures. New York: American Cancer Society, 1988.
43. Plastic surgery experiences healthy increases. News release of the American Society of Plastic and Reconstructive Surgeons, Chicago, May 16, 1985.
44. FDA General Surgical and Plastic Surgery Devices Subcommittee Meeting on Risks and Benefits of Silicone Implants, Washington, DC, January 1989.
45. National Cancer Institute Survey on Knowledge about Breast Cancer, 1982.
46. Sorrentino P, Baccaglini U, Ruffatto MT, et al. Mastectomized woman's acquired knowledge about and attitude towards breast reconstruction. A prospective survey on 100 cases. Ital J Surg Sci 1988; 18:17-23.
47. Sperling D. The risk of breast implants. USA Today, November 11, 1988.
48. Berger K, Bostwick J. A woman's decision: Breast care, treatment and reconstruction. St Louis: CV Mosby, 1984.
49. Polivy J. Psychological effects of mastectomy on a woman's feminine self concept. J Nerv Ment Dis 1977; 164:77-87.
50. Clifford E. The reconstruction experience. The search for restitution. In: Georgiade NG, ed. Breast reconstruction following mastectomy. St Louis: CV Mosby, 1979:22-35.
51. Holland JC, Rowland JH. Patient rehabilitation and support: Psychosocial reactions to breast cancer and its treatment. In: Harris J, Helliman S, Henderson C, et al, eds. Breast diseases. Philadelphia: JB Lippincott, 1987:632-645.
52. Daniels E. Breast reconstruction post mastectomy: A psychosocial study. Doctoral dissertation. University of California San Francisco, 1984:46.
53. Vah Dam FS, Bergman RB. Psychosocial and surgical aspects of breast reconstruction. Eur J Surg Oncol 1988; 14:141-149.
54. Schain WS, Jacobs E, Wellisch DK. Psychosocial issues in breast reconstruction: Intrapsychic, interpersonal and practical concerns. Clinical Plast Surg 1984; 11:237-251.
55. Teimourian B, Adham MN. Survey of patients: Responses to breast reconstruction. Ann Plast Surg 1982; 9:321-325.
56. Holland JC, Rowland JH. Psychological care of the patient with cancer. Handbook of psycho-oncology. New York: Oxford University Press, 1989:188-208.
57. Lester LJ. A critical viewpoint by a general surgeon toward reconstructive surgery after mastectomy. Clinical Plast Surg 1979; 16:15.
58. Silva Neto JB, Fontelles JA, Assis P, et al. Results of radical mastectomy for stage I and II breast cancer: Implications for breast reconstruction. Breast 1983; 9:2022.
59. Dowden RV, Blanchard JM, Greenstreet RL. Breast reconstruction, timing and local recurrence. Ann Plast Surg 1983; 10:265-269.
60. Johnson C, Van Heerden JA, Donohue JH. Oncological aspects of immediate breast reconstruction following mastectomy for malignancy. Arch Surg 1989; 124: 819-823.
61. Noone RB, Frazier TG, Hayward CA, et al. Patient acceptance of immediate reconstruction following mastectomy. Plast Reconstr Surg 1982; 69:632-638.
62. Dean C, Chety U, Forrest AR. Effects of immediate breast reconstruction on psychological morbidity after mastectomy. Lancet 1983; 26:459-462.
63. Schain WS, Wellisch DK, Pasnau RO, et al. The sooner the better: A study of psychological factors in women undergoing immediate versus delayed breast reconstruction. Am J Psychiatry. 1985; 142:40-46.
64. Mansel RE, Horgan K, Webster DJ, et al. Cosmetic results of immediate breast reconstruction post mastectomy: A follow-up. Breast J Surg 1986; 73:813-816.
65. McGraw JB, Horton CE, Grossman JA, et al. An early appraisal of the methods of tissue expansion and the transverse rectus abdominis musculocutaneous flap in the reconstruction of the breast following mastectomy. Ann Plast Surg 1987; 18:93-113.
66. Goin M, Goin J. Growing pains: The psychological experience of breast reconstruction with tissue expansion. Ann Plast Surg 1988; 21:217-222.
67. d'Angelo TM, Gorrell CR. Breast reconstruction using tissue expanders. Oncol Nursing Forum 1989; 16: 23-27.
68. Dakoff GA, Taylor SE, Collins RL. Family support and the cancer patient. Paper presented at American Psychological Association Convention, New York, August 1987.
69. Gerard D. Sexual functioning after mastectomy: Life vs Lab. J Sex Marital Ther 1982; 8:305-315.
70. Nathan EP, Joanning HH. Enhancing marital sexuality: An evaluation of a program for the sexual enrichment of normal couples. J Sex Marital Ther 1985; 11:157-164.
71. Wellisch DK, Schain WS, Little Jr JW, and Noone RB. The psychological contribution of nipple addition in breast reconstruction. Plast Reconstr Surg. November 1987:69-704.
72. Asplund O, Korlof B. Late results following mastectomy for cancer and breast reconstruction. Scand J Plast Reconstr 1984; 18:221-225.

CHAPTER 29

Immediate Reconstruction After Mastectomy

R. BARRETT NOONE, M.D.

As techniques for breast reconstruction after mastectomy have improved, reconstructive surgeons have turned their attention to determining the appropriate timing. Traditionally, reconstruction gained acceptance as an important factor in the rehabilitation of the breast cancer patient when it was performed some time after the mastectomy. Waiting for the mastectomy wound to heal and mature, assessing the complete histologic nature of the tumor and therefore the patient's prognosis, allowing for completion of postoperative adjuvant radiation therapy or chemotherapy, and giving the patient adequate time after the mastectomy to reflect on her choices have been helpful in promoting acceptance of reconstruction.

However, this traditional concept of delayed reconstruction has not been ideal for many women. Accordingly, searches for alternatives have included a concerted effort toward breast conservation treatment, such as lumpectomy and radiation therapy, in addition to a desire to achieve earlier, if not immediate, reconstruction. The growth in acceptance of immediate reconstruction after mastectomy has paralleled the development of an improvement in the techniques of breast reconstruction.

Immediate reconstruction gained acceptance slowly in the United States, but was introduced by Hueston and McKenzie in Australia in 1970.[1] This was approximately the same time that early attempts at delayed reconstruction began in the United States. The slow acceptance of immediate reconstruction appears to have its basis in a number of issues. General surgeons were concerned that the addition of reconstruction at the time of mastectomy would compromise their ability to provide the most complete surgical procedure possible, and might increase the surgical complication rate following mastectomy. Psychiatrists expressed their concern that emotional sequelae would occur if the patient did not go through the loss and bereavement process associated with a mastectomy before entering the reconstructive phase. Some oncologists were worried that immediate reconstruction would limit their ability to provide necessary adjuvant therapy after the mastectomy, and would possibly delay or inhibit the detection of local or regional occurrences of the tumor during follow-up. Plastic surgeons, in addition to the above considerations, were concerned that the aesthetic quality of the reconstruction would not be as good as with delayed reconstruction. They also thought that the patient would not appreciate the reconstruction so much as if she were encouraged to "live with" the deformity for a time.

Armed with the conviction that the advantages of immediate reconstruction would outweigh the expressed disadvantages, we began to address some of the above concerns at our institution in 1977.[2-5] Other centers studying the principles and techniques of immediate reconstruction added to the knowledge and acceptance of this mode of timing.[6-11] On the basis of this experience, there has been a growing acceptance of immediate reconstruction by the physicians involved with the care of the breast cancer patient. The late 1980s saw a distinct trend toward increases in the number of immediate mastectomy reconstructions.[12]

ADVANTAGES OF IMMEDIATE RECONSTRUCTION

The advantages of breast reconstruction at the time of mastectomy can be considered in the following categories: (1) economy; (2) psychology; (3) availability; (4) total breast cancer care; (5) relations with the general surgeon; and (6) aesthetic considerations.

Economy

The advantage of *economy* has been demonstrated in other forms of immediate reconstruction after cancer ablation therapy, such as head and neck reconstruction. Applied to breast cancer, the various forms of economies in performing breast reconstruction immediately after mastectomy are obvious. They include *economy of finances,* in limiting the extirpative and reconstructive procedures to a single, general anesthetic with a single hospital admission. The hospital stay after mastectomy with immediate submuscular reconstruction is comparable with that of mastectomy without reconstruction. At the Bryn Mawr Hospital, a sample patient population between January 1985 and January 1987 was evaluated for length of stay. During that 2-year period, 62 patients received a modified radical mastectomy without immediate reconstruction; the average length of stay was 6.27 days. In the same period, 94 patients underwent modified radical mastectomy with immediate breast reconstruction; the average length of stay was 6.77 days. The hospital stay of one-half day longer for patients undergoing reconstruction certainly appears to be justified when compared with the length of stay that would be needed for a second hospital admission if reconstruction were to be started on a delayed basis with another operative procedure. This length of stay also compares favorably with the average length of stay of 8.9 days for patients younger than 70 years of age who underwent mastectomy for cancer without reconstruction, and who formed the basis of the statistic in the Federal Register, which governs rules and regulations for implementation of fiscal reimbursements to hospitals under the DRG Program.[13]

Although two or more subsequent operations may be required to complete the reconstructive project, including the nipple-areola complex reconstruction and secondary revisions of the immediate procedures, these are usually performed on an outpatient basis with less cost of hospitalization. In a review of 185 immediate reconstructive procedures at our institution, 113 patients received secondary operations, yielding a total of 1.61 operations per patient. If this same group of patients were to have initiated reconstruction on a delayed basis, the total number of operations per patient would likely be much higher, in the range of 2.6. In this study of secondary procedures, 26 percent were for nipple-areola complex reconstruction; 12 percent for capsulotomy, capsulorrhaphy, or adjustment of the implant; and the balance for procedures on the opposite breast. The opposite breast procedures were usually done at the same time as the secondary surgery on the operated breast.

Economy of time is equally important. As more and more women are pursuing careers in the workplace, and because incomes depend on their contributions, the clear advantage of one major hospitalization and recovery period rather than two is obvious. Time away from families and small children can essentially be halved with the immediate approach to reconstruction. A major concern of many patients facing mastectomy is the general anesthetic with its attendant risks. Limiting the need for general anesthesia to slightly more than one procedure is regarded by many women as a major advantage. Also, the postoperative morbidity of both procedures, particularly the expected discomfort, can be combined in a single recovery period.

Psychology

As illustrated later in this chapter, initial concerns that a negative psychological impact may be seen in a patient who has an immediate reconstruction have been shown to be largely unjustified. These studies actually support an easier recovery and rehabilitation for women who have the immediate procedure. It may even be appropriate to suggest that a psychological boost at the time of facing the major life crisis of breast cancer may have a positive overall effect, not only on surgical treatment, but also on tumor-host relationship. If psychological influences affect the course of any malignant condition, they may be likely to do so in such a chronic malignancy as breast cancer.

Availability

An immediate reconstruction program essentially offers reconstruction to almost any woman who desires it. Many women, if not given the immediate option, would not return for reconstruction on a delayed basis. Within the entire population of women facing mastectomy, there is a subgroup who are by nature unassertive. For them, an elective decision to re-enter the hospital to initiate a course of breast reconstruction with additional major surgery and recovery is not likely to be made. These women seemingly regard this second procedure as a selfish act, whereas they would be willing to undergo the placement of an implant reconstruction at the time of mastectomy. Perhaps this lack of assertion is one reason why the reported incidences of nipple-areolar reconstruction in reconstructive patients as a whole is less than one third. The availability of reconstruction to all women at the time of mastectomy also provides them with an alternative to lumpectomy and radiation therapy. Many women, fearful of the drastic change in femininity associated with mastectomy, opt for the less drastic procedure of partial mastectomy followed by radiation. Immediate reconstruction offers these patients the alternative of avoiding irradiation if they so desire.

Total Breast Cancer Care

Before the introduction of breast reconstruction for mastectomy, approaches to the breast cancer patient were generally made by the general surgeon and oncologist and perhaps the radiation therapist. The introduction of the concept of reconstruction to the patient as a part of her total breast cancer care is now well accepted in most major centers and is the course generally followed when the patient undergoes mastectomy. If the reconstruction is done on an immediate basis, this total care concept of providing emotional support and reinforcement to the patient can begin immediately. Close cooperation with the general surgeon, resulting in a two-team approach to mastectomy and reconstruction, still gives the general surgeon the opportunity to ensure the completeness of mastectomy that otherwise would be present in the absence of reconstruction. Although the skin incisions are planned on a team basis preoperatively, the general surgeon retains the firm decision regarding the margins to be used surrounding the biopsy site of the primary tumor and the extent of skin to be resected, as well as the thickness of the skin flaps and removal of fascia or muscle if indicated. In the latter instances, immediate reconstruction can still be performed by the use of either local muscle flaps (described below) or distant myocutaneous flap reconstruction.

In the past, concerns were expressed that the placement of a silicone prosthesis might have a detrimental effect on the immune response in the host and adversely affect the ability of the body to inhibit recurrent or metastatic disease. To date, there has been no clinical or experimental evidence to indicate an impairment in the immunologic response because of the presence of silicone prostheses. Experimental data on mammary implants in the rat laboratory model indicated no adverse immunologic effects.[14,15]

In our experience with immediate reconstruction in clinical Stage I patients, there has been tumor involvement in axillary lymph nodes in approximately one third of the patients.[4] These patients, and a growing number who are clinically node negative but who have negative hormonal receptors, are offered systemic adjuvant chemotherapy after mastectomy. If reconstruction is performed on a delayed basis, the reconstructive effort should be delayed until completion of the adjuvant chemotherapy course, which in most centers is approximately 6 months. However, if reconstruction is done on an immediate basis, the chemotherapy program may begin at the completion of the mastectomy wound healing, and the patient is not forced to wait an artificially long time until chemotherapy is completed. This gives a significant positive reinforcement to the patient receiving chemotherapy. In our experience, no alteration in either the initiation or duration of treatment of adjuvant chemotherapy occurred because of immediate reconstruction, and no complications of reconstruction were attributed directly to adjuvant therapy. I believe there is no justification for delay in beginning treatment, even if the prosthesis seems to be at risk. Initial concerns that the presence of an implant or flap used in immediate reconstruction may delay or inhibit the detection of local recurrences have not been substantiated.

Relations with General Surgeon

One distinct advantage of an immediate reconstruction program is that it provides harmonious communication between the general surgery and plastic surgery services. When two teams work closely together, mutual benefit and education can be noted. For example, cooperative incision design with the general surgeon allows the performance of a more aesthetically pleasing mastectomy. The general surgeon may even report more attention to technical detail when working on the same operative field as the plastic surgeon. The availability of immediate reconstruction to surgeons providing primary oncologic care allows them to suggest immediate reconstruction to the patient as an alternative to lumpectomy and irradiation, if she so desires. If immediate reconstruction were not available to the general surgeon, perhaps more women would opt for lumpectomy and irradiation. Communication regarding reconstructive patients also leads to greater communication in other areas of mutual interest between general surgery and plastic surgery, such as improvement in the care of the trauma patient.

Aesthetic Considerations

There are many elements necessary for an ideal reconstructive result after mastectomy. These include the achievement of symmetry with the opposite breast, a natural breast fullness, a certain amount of ptosis (which may depend on the age of the patient and the general laxity of body tissues), and appropriate location of the nipple-areola complex. The timing of the reconstruction appears to be less important than some of the other factors in achieving the ideal aesthetic result. However, immediate reconstruction does offer certain aesthetic advantages. Working in unscarred tissues and with muscles that have not atrophied because of denervation, the plastic surgeon can control muscle expansion more freely at the time of dissection. This allows for more ease in the control of the submuscular pocket. Of equal importance are the benefits derived from collaboration with the general surgeon in both the planning of the skin incision and the extent of the mastectomy deformity itself. Preoperative incision design by both plastic surgeon and general surgeon can greatly enhance aesthetic results by placing incisions in areas that can be concealed by most clothing. It is well known that hypertrophic scars after mastectomy most commonly occur in the medial mastectomy in the parasternal area. This is the anatomic area most commonly seen when V-neck clothing and bathing apparel is worn. With the exception of rare upper, inner quadrant primary lesions, incisions in the parasternal area can be avoided altogether with proper preoperative cooperation. One of the reasons some of these scars have existed with the traditional mastectomy is because of excision of the dog-ear deformity at the medial aspect of the mastectomy scar. This excision can be avoided with immediate reconstruction, because much of the expendable skin and subcutaneous tissue is incorporated into the reconstruction.

Early objections to immediate reconstruction were that the aesthetic results would not be as good as those with delayed reconstruction. I do not share this view. Given the ability to coordinate planning and proper incisions with the general surgeon and given the opportunity to work with unscarred, fresh muscle and skin, I believe that the immediate results of prosthetic reconstruction should essentially be the same as, if not better than, delayed reconstruction. There appears to be no difference in aesthetic results between patients who have a temporary tissue expander at the time of the immediate procedure and those who receive a flap reconstruction if it is needed, when these techniques are compared with similar procedures in delayed reconstruction. Although some consider that the patient in the immediate situation may expect less from the procedure and be pleased with it regardless of the aesthetic result, there is no reason that the reconstructive surgeon should expect a less than desirable result if reconstruction is performed at the time of mastectomy.

PSYCHOLOGY OF IMMEDIATE BREAST RECONSTRUCTION

As noted above, one of the major advantages of immediate reconstruction is the significant psychological boost given the patient facing a cancer diagnosis. It has been known that the impact of mastectomy, added to the fear of recurrence of cancer, produces an alteration of mood, body image, sexuality, femininity, and social and occupational functioning.[16] Psychological theories related to loss and bereavement provided a major area of resistance to immediate breast reconstruction,[17] suggesting that a woman must mourn the loss of her breast by experiencing its absence before being able to adapt in the other aspects of her life.[18] The mourning process includes a sequence of denial, anger, depression, despair, and (it is hoped) eventual acceptance. In the past, those treating breast cancer believed that women who sought reconstruction were having difficulty in completing the mourning process by not adapting to and eventually accepting the loss of the breast.[14]

The theories of reaction to loss and the necessity for bereavement have been challenged in recent years. The psychiatric literature began to support the view that reconstruction is the only solution to the real disfigurement caused by mastectomy.[20] Plastic surgeons suggested that even planning the reconstruction with the patient before her mastectomy, in an effort to allow her to look forward to the reconstruction after healing from the surgery, reduced the negative consequences of the mastectomy.[21] These psychological benefits of reconstruction were found to be even more important when the reconstruction was performed at the time of mastectomy. Clifford evaluated signs of depression and stress in postmastectomy patients and found that the expected signs were not present in those who had undergone immediate reconstruction.[22] Stevens and associates compared patient groups with respect to the timing of reconstruction and found that those undergoing immediate reconstruction expressed less change in feelings of attractiveness and femininity than patients who underwent delayed reconstruction, as well as a noticeable absence of the sense of mutilation.[23] These authors suggested that immediate reconstruction does alter the mourning process, because mourning for the breast begins in both groups even before the mastectomy with the anticipation of the breast loss. They also noted that patients seem to be satisfied with the cosmetic result, regardless of the time of mastectomy. However, the reconstructed breasts are better integrated into the body image when immediate reconstruction is performed, being experienced as a "restoration" for the removed breast rather than a "replacement." Goin and Goin evaluated the psychological impact of immediate reconstruction on patients who had undergone previous mastectomies and delayed reconstructions on the opposite breast, and concluded that no psychological benefit was present in a delayed environment.[24] These authors also reported that many of their patients expressed a wish that reconstruction could have been done at the time of mastectomy. Dean and colleagues also emphasized the salutary psychological effects of immediate reconstruction, showing that less psychiatric morbidity was present in patients undergoing immediate intraoperative repair than in those who delayed the reconstruction.[25]

Our group challenged the concept that patients should experience the deformity of a mastectomy in order to be satisfied with the results following reconstruction. Our study of a consecutive series of patients undergoing immediate reconstruction demonstrated a high degree of patient acceptance, and emphasized the importance of proper preoperative education of the patient in order for her to accept the reconstruction as a breast substitute without having "lived" with the deformity.[2] We also evaluated the psychosocial correlates of immediate versus delayed reconstruction in a combined patient series.[26,27] In studying these patients, a psychological evaluation was performed of nine major areas of functioning: somatization, obsessive-compulsive reactions, interpersonal sensitivity, depression, anxiety, hostility, phobic anxiety, paranoid ideation, and psychoticism. These were determined in groups of patients who underwent either delayed or immediate reconstruction. Results of this study questioned a number of previous assumptions about breast reconstruction, especially about the timing of reconstruction. Contrary to an earlier prejudice that women who seek breast reconstruction are maladapted and "unable to accept their defect,"[19] both groups of patients studied were normal on psychological testing and very similar to a normative group of adult women of comparable age. When timing of reconstruction was compared with sociodemographic data, requests for immediate reconstructive procedures came from a group entirely comparable with those opting for conventional delayed reconstruction. Therefore, it was not only the younger, unmarried, or more highly educated woman who sought immediate reconstruction. Such requests for reconstruction on an immediate basis, then, depend on the knowledge of availability as presented to the patient by the general surgeon or physician initially concerned with cancer care. Another assumption challenged by our findings is that the patient benefits from "living with her deformity" and that her satisfaction is "enhanced by such exposure."[28] There was no significant difference between our immediate and delayed groups; 96 percent of the former and 89 percent of the latter reported satisfaction with the breast reconstruction procedure.[26,27] There is, in fact, clinical evidence that a woman who undergoes immediate reconstruction is more likely to incorporate the new breast into her body image and thereby achieve a higher level of comfort and satisfaction from the onset.[23]

Reduction in the psychological distress caused by mastectomy appears to be a major benefit of immediate reconstruction. Although patients who undergo either immediate or delayed reconstruction both experience a cancer diagnosis and a major body alteration, it appears that those who have immediate reconstruction do not experience the magnitude or duration of psychological symptoms and seem to experience an earlier return to former psychological equilibrium than women who live for a time with the deformity of mastectomy. When asked to recall the emotional distress relating to the cancer surgery experience, the women in our immediate study group reported significantly less distress than those who underwent delayed reconstruction. It appears that maintenance of a breast contour in the postoperative period after mastectomy may lessen the trauma of the ablative experience and may influence subsequent adjustment in a positive manner. Perhaps the end point of reconstruction may be the same for women in both the immediate and delayed groups, with a facilitated return to normal psychological function. However, the presence of a breast contour created at the time of mastectomy may ease the type or magnitude of the burdens carried by the patient in the journey toward this end point.

PREOPERATIVE CONSIDERATIONS

The Immediate Reconstruction Team

A successful program of immediate reconstruction must be based on a concept of essential cooperation between the general surgeon performing the mastectomy and the plastic surgeon responsible for reconstruction. Although a medical oncologist is included in the care of many patients, the essential personnel in every case are the general surgeon and the plastic surgeon. For the ultimate benefit of the patient, from the standpoints of tumor care and reconstructive results, it is absolutely necessary that clear lines of responsibility be established between these surgical specialists. The general surgeon must have complete control over surgical decisions regarding tumor treatment. Although modifications in approach, such as incision design, can be suggested by the plastic surgeon, the responsibility rests with the general surgeon to provide optimal care for the patient and the tumor. The general surgeon is also in the unique position of controlling the candidacy of patients for immediate reconstruction. The primary care physician, lay literature, former patients, family, and friends may all stimulate the concept of immediate reconstruction for the breast cancer patient, but it is the general surgeon who must have confidence in the efficacy of the procedure and must suggest it to the patient. This surgical specialist has been shown to be the stimulating influence in the great majority of women who receive reconstruction immediately.[2] Unless the plastic surgeon is prepared to manage the diagnosis and treatment of the complete range of breast disease, benign and malignant, and maintain a proficiency in all aspects of breast cancer, he or she should not perform the extirpative procedure of mastectomy. Likewise, the general surgeon should direct all aspects of the reconstructive procedure to the plastic surgeon.

Implicit in any team approach are potential difficulties in the arrangement of preoperative consultations as well as intraoperative scheduling for a combined procedure. Time considerations and constraints between the general and plastic surgeon may be awkward at the beginning of a reconstructive program, but such concerns are generally well resolved with experience. Because the two-step biopsy is now the standard of care in the treatment of breast cancer, multiple preoperative consultations and frequent second opinions are common for the patient attempting to arrive at a decision regarding treatment. A 2- or 3-week interval may frequently elapse between the time of diagnosis and the actual surgical treatment. In this interval, there is ample opportunity for the patient to be seen as an outpatient in the plastic surgeon's office for the purpose of discussing potential immediate reconstruction. The patient may also be seeking consultation with a medical oncologist and a radiation therapist as well as the general surgeon. The plastic surgeon should be prepared to evaluate the patient in a preoperative consultation setting within a short period after being requested to by the general surgeon. The patient is often in need of emotional support and the plastic surgeon can be helpful by accommodating the patient on brief notice. Intraoperative cooperation is also essential, but is not difficult for practiced teams. If the combined procedure is scheduled as the last operation on the day's surgical agenda, the general surgeon may then, at the completion of the mastectomy, address the family and leave the operating suite or hospital. The general surgeon finds that the time required for postoperative and hospital visits is also reduced, because wound care is provided by the plastic surgeon. The plastic surgeon may schedule his or her portion of the immediate reconstruction procedure between cases in the schedule or during completion of ongoing work in another operating room, especially if residents or surgical assistants are available to assist with closure and dressings. We have discovered that, rather than constricting our operative schedule, the immediate reconstruction program has actually increased the case load on any given operative day.

Diagnosis and Decision for Mastectomy

After suspicion of breast carcinoma has been raised by noninvasive techniques such as breast self-examination, mammography, ultrasonography, or thermography, a two-step approach is made to the ultimate tissue diagnosis of the breast cancer. The first step consists of either fine-needle aspiration cytology or open surgical biopsy. At our institution, an accuracy of 97.5 percent in 1,000 consecutive cases of fine-needle aspiration cytology was reported.[29,30] A positive cytologic result for malignancy is considered conclusive. If the cytologist is in doubt, the patient undergoes open biopsy, usually as an outpatient under local anesthesia. If she is thought to be a candidate for mastectomy with immediate reconstruction, the biopsy incision should be planned with the reconstruction in view. For most biopsies, incisions outlined in the National Surgical Adjuvant Breast Project (NSABP) protocol are used.[31] These include radial incisions for tumors located below the transverse line of the nipple, and circumferential areolar incisions for tumors near the nipple. These incisions usually allow for creative planning of skin flaps to include resection of the biopsy site and nipple-areola complex in order to perform a complete mastectomy and prepare for immediate reconstruction.

In addition to the tumor diagnosis, factors concerning the general health of the patient are evaluated. Age is not considered a deterrent to immediate reconstruction if the patient's general health is sufficient for her to undergo the anesthetic and operative trauma dictated by a mastectomy. Chronic tobacco smoking is an important preoperative indicator. Because of potential skin flap ischemia and necrosis in women who are heavy smokers, these patients are asked to discontinue smoking 2 weeks before surgery and to continue this abstinence in the 2 weeks immediately afterward. If implant reconstruction is planned, the mastectomy skin flaps are carefully evaluated in this group of patients during surgery; if there is any question of marginal viability, either immediate reconstruction is not performed, or a limited soft tissue expansion procedure is used, with very careful and slow expansion in the postoperative period.

Plastic Surgery Consultation

If one of the options for treatment of the tumor is mastectomy with immediate reconstruction, preadmission consultation with a plastic surgeon should be held within 1 week of the positive biopsy diagnosis. Before this consultation, the patient may already have predetermined expectations of the possible results from reconstruction. These ideas may have been discovered in her own readings or in discussion with friends or cancer groups, or may have been placed by her cancer surgeon. Inherent in these are biases and sometimes unrealistic expectations that the plastic surgeon must assess at the time of the patient's initial office visit. The consultation must be unhurried and must be scheduled in the plastic surgeon's office before admission to the hospital, in an effort to give the patient sufficient time to reflect on the consultation and arrive at a thoughtful decision about reconstruction. It is difficult for both the patient and the plastic surgeon to conduct this consultation and arrive at a proper decision if the evaluation is made after admission to the hospital, such as the night before or the morning of surgery. Approximately 30 minutes should be planned for a proper preoperative consultation.

At the consultation, the patient is given full information about breast reconstruction, including both immediate and delayed procedures. Many patients opt to have a reconstruction on a delayed basis for one of a number of reasons, and this option should be available.

A family member or other supportive person is encouraged to be present at the consultation. Details of technical options are reviewed, including the limitations of the specific procedures. This is done by showing photographs of unreconstructed mastectomy defects and average results following the reconstruction, both immediate and delayed procedures. Most patients have known at least one person who has had a mastectomy, but few have seen the deformity.[2] Despite a lengthy and detailed review by her general surgeon, the patient frequently has no concept of what a mastectomy scar will look like or where it will be placed. Reviewing photographs of the unreconstructed deformity is essential for the patient who has never seen a mastectomy defect. This simple demonstration seems to provide a substitute for the experience of living with a mastectomy deformity.[2] Results demonstrating patients with and without a brassiere are shown. Typical results of nipple-areola reconstruction and mastopexy or reduction mammaplasty procedures of the opposite breast are shown, it being emphasized that these are usually performed as secondary procedures. It is made clear that immediate reconstruction is frequently a two-stage procedure, with adjustments to the prosthesis or myocutaneous flap reserved for a later date, often 3 to 6 months after the mastectomy. It is helpful to reassure the anxious patient by showing her a photograph of a typical patient after reconstruction wearing the same bra on discharge from the hospital that she wore before mastectomy. This simple demonstration emphasizes the concept of immediate reconstruction and reinforces the idea of an immediate return to societal activities.

One of the more time-consuming aspects of the preoperative consultation is the choice of technique to be used in the reconstruction. As discussed later, all currently available techniques may be applied on an immediate basis. A combined decision is made by the patient and plastic surgeon, based on many factors. A compromise should not be made in selection of the proper or ideal technique in an effort to proceed on an immediate basis. For example, if both the patient and plastic surgeon agree that the transverse rectus abdominis myocutaneous (TRAM) flap procedure is most ideal for her, and if the patient is unable to devote the time necessary for recuperation from this procedure, it should be performed on a delayed basis. On occasion, this type of patient may opt for temporary submuscular implant reconstruction at the time of mastectomy in order to provide the emotional support for a less than ideal result, with a plan to return at a later date for the more extensive myocutaneous flap procedure. Multiple factors are used to assess the appropriateness and type of technique to be used. The patient's height, the chest wall appearance, the general body habitus, the presence of obesity, the degree of ptosis of the opposite breast, the location of the biopsy site, and any history of tobacco use are all important criteria. Most patients undergo either submuscular silicone reconstruction or soft tissue expansion. Both the silicone implant and the tissue expander should be demonstrated during the consultation, allowing the patient to actually feel the material. Even though a submuscular implant may be the preferred and planned choice, technical factors at the time of surgery may indicate a need for slower skin flap expansion. Therefore, it is best to prepare the patient for either a silicone prosthesis or a soft tissue expander, reviewing the timing of expansion and the potential need for a second procedure if a temporary expander is used.

The possible complications of the surgical procedure are then described. The possibility of scar capsule contracture is outlined, and reassurance is given that future capsulotomy may be an option for the patient. This is frequently done at the time of nipple-areola reconstruction. Photographs are taken before the patient leaves the examining area. Because emphasis is placed on future patient education, the patient is rarely reluctant to be photographed. She is reassured that she will be seen again by the plastic surgeon in the hospital immediately before surgery, at which time preoperative incision planning will be made in cooperation with the general surgeon. The patient is encouraged to contact the plastic surgeon at any time before the surgical procedure if additional questions or difficulties arise.

COOPERATIVE INCISION DESIGN

Before surgery, the general surgeon and plastic surgeon cooperate in designing an incision to provide exposure for effective tumor surgery by mastectomy and axillary dissection, as well as the best aesthetic result (Fig. 29-1). Incision design is planned to minimize postoperative scarring in the parasternal area, especially in that region of the anterior chest above the plane of the nipple-areola complex. The mastectomy should include all pigmented skin in the complex as well as the biopsy or needle aspiration site. The width of the excision around the biopsy site is determined by the general surgeon, who must provide an adequate excision of the tumor with safe surgical margins. We prefer at least a 1-cm margin around the biopsy site. A simple extension of the incision in the superolateral direction toward the low axilla should give sufficient exposure for axillary lymph node dissection. It is not necessary to excise skin toward the anterior axillary area as a part of the initial mastectomy incision. Unnecessary skin excision in this area may lead to postoperative axillary scar contractures, or at the least tightening of the skin in that area, which may be uncomfortable in the early postoperative period. The plastic surgeon may decide to incorporate some of the redundant skin into local flap shifts at the time of closure, and will manage medial dog-ear redundancy, also at the time of wound closure.

Suggested incisions for varied locations of the primary tumor are presented in Figure 29-1. The usual oblique type of incision is most commonly used, having application for both upper outer quadrant and lower inner quadrant lesions. Variable

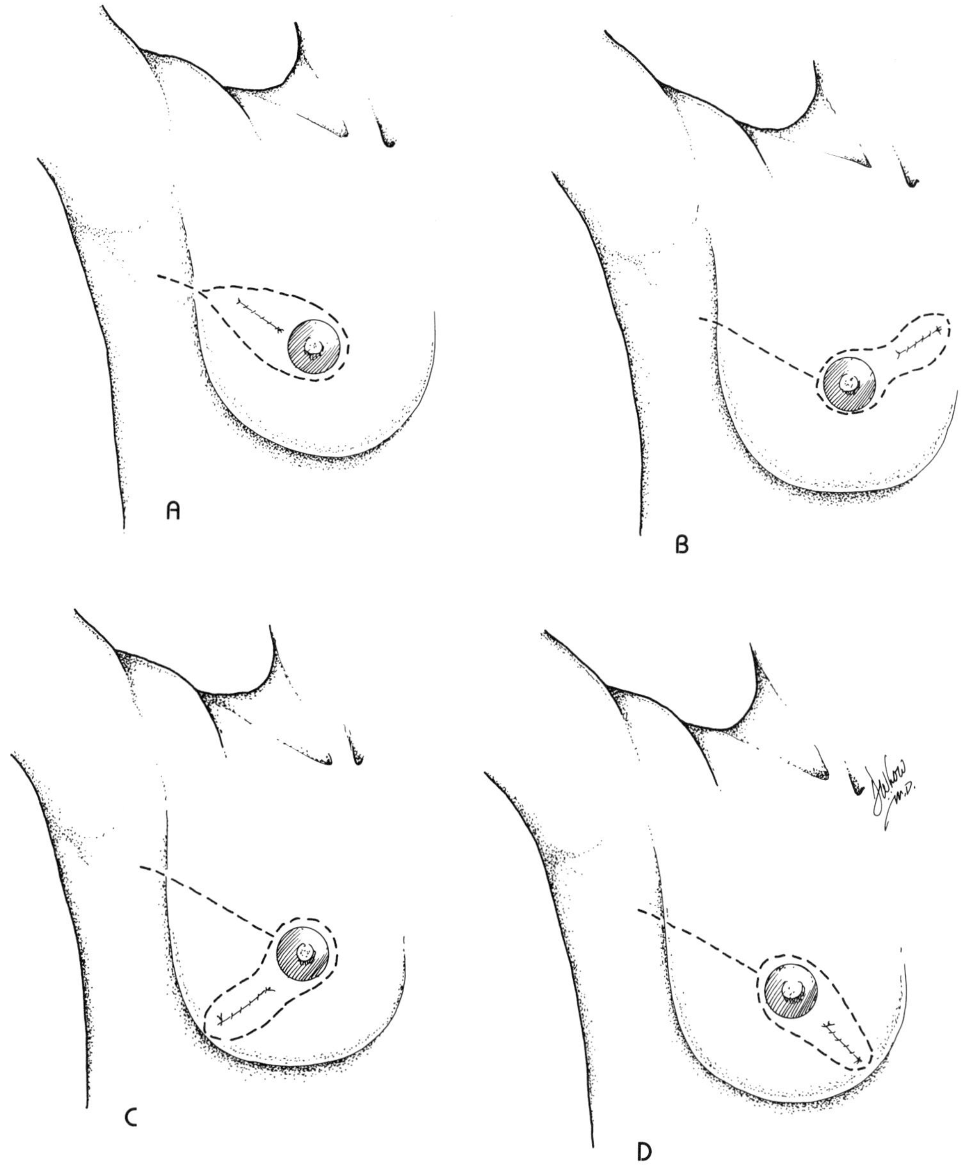

FIGURE 29-1 Incisions for mastectomy with immediate reconstruction should be planned to avoid scars in the parasternal area if possible. They can be designed to give exposure for axillary dissection while incorporating the biopsy site and nipple-areola complex. Suggested incisions for specific tumor location include *A*, upper outer quadrant, *B*, upper-inner quadrant, *C*, lower outer quadrant, and *D*, lower inner quadrant.

amounts of skin are resected, depending on the location of the lesion, with a generous amount of skin preservation along the sternal border with upper outer quadrant lesions. A laterally based triangular flap has been very useful for lesions in the lower outer quadrant, because it provides generous exposure for both the mastectomy and axillary dissection and results in a scar that is entirely lateral to the vertical plane of the nipple-areola complex (Fig. 29-2). Scars resulting from upper inner quadrant lesion resection are unavoidable in the parasternal area, but can be extended in imaginative designs to include the nipple-areola complex and provide axillary exposure, while at the same time leaving sufficient skin for rotation in an effort to minimize tension along the sternal border and therefore reduce the tendency toward hypertrophic scarring (Fig. 29-3). The inframammary fold is marked on both sides for a guide during surgery and reconstruction. Incisions are marked with standard surgical marking pencils designed to withstand surgical preparation solutions.

At the time of incision design, the questions and concerns of the patient are addressed for the final time. She is reminded that for approximately 48 hours after surgery she will notice an orange tint to the skin and urine because of the use of intravenous fluorescein during surgery to assess the viability of skin flap margins.

The plastic surgeon should encourage general surgical colleagues to avoid excising the pectoralis minor muscle or dividing the pectoral nerves, the thoracodorsal neurovascular bundle, and, preferably, the intercostobrachial nerve. The goals of imme-

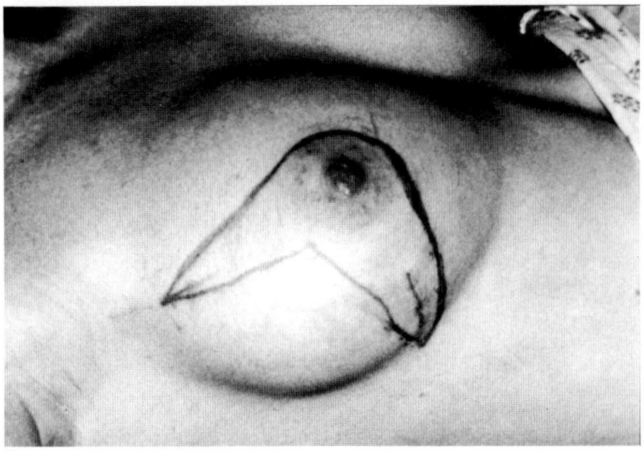

A

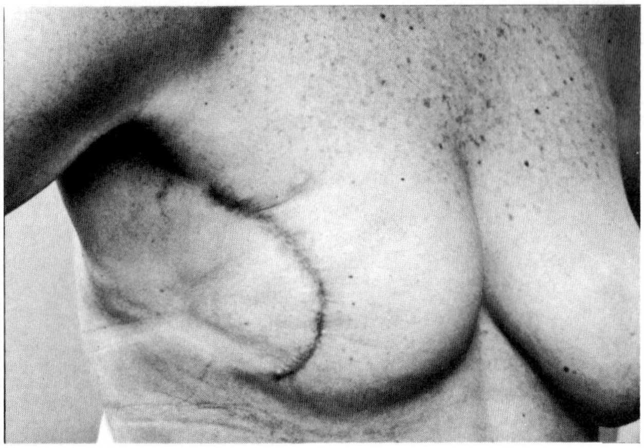

B

FIGURE 29-2 *A*, Incision designed at surgery for mastectomy with the lesion near the inframammary fold in the lower outer quadrant results in a laterally based "triangular" flap closure. *B*, Six weeks after surgery the resultant scar avoids the central and medial reconstructed breast and is easily covered with clothing.

diate reconstruction cannot be fulfilled ideally if subsequent muscular wasting and infraclavicular depression reverses what was originally an encouraging early result. The general surgeon must also be asked to make a particular effort to leave intact the fascia overlying the musculature in the inferomedial quadrant of the breast. Intact fascia in this region makes it technically easier to elevate the pectoralis major muscle in continuity with the medial aspect of the rectus abdominis fascia. This request becomes inappropriate only when the lesion itself is in this quadrant, fortunately one of the less common locations within the breast. A rapid elevation of the breast from the inferomedial quadrant without strict attention to preservation of all fibrous connective tissue covering the muscle in this area can present the plastic surgeon avoidable incumbrances to a straightforward and satisfactory result.[32]

TECHNIQUES FOR IMMEDIATE RECONSTRUCTION

Selection of Appropriate Technique

The goal of the surgical team is eradication of the tumor and reconstruction of the breast using the procedure or series of procedures that give the best aesthetic result and the least morbidity.

The basic techniques used in immediate recon-

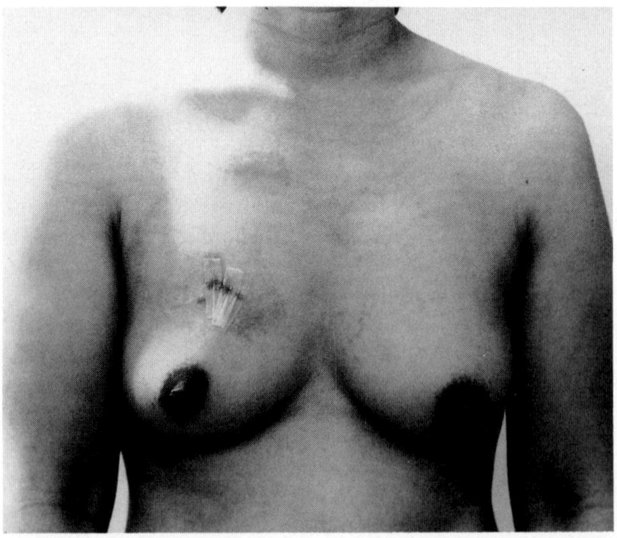

A

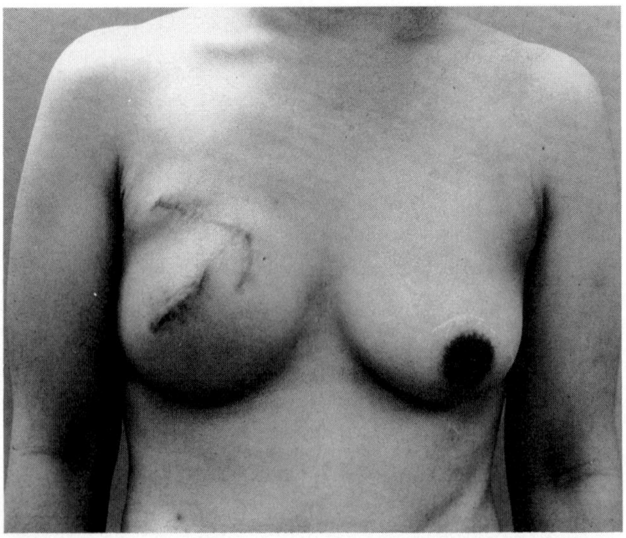

B

FIGURE 29-3 *A*, An upper quadrant biopsy site and nipple-areola complex are included in the same incision with a lateral extension for axillary dissection. *B*, The resultant "inverted anchor" scar avoids the superior and medial sternal areas as much as is possible in this location.

struction include (1) submuscular silicone implant reconstruction; (2) soft tissue expansion, with placement of either a temporary or permanent expander at the time of mastectomy; (3) the TRAM flap; and (4) latissimus dorsi musculocutaneous flap reconstruction. Less common procedures, such as the various free tissue transfer techniques described in a later chapter, may also be used on an immediate basis. The choice of technique is determined by a number of factors including age; breast size; body habitus; tumor location, size, and pathology; size, configuration, and future surgical plans for the opposite breast; ancillary health indicators such as a history of heavy cigarette smoking; and socioeconomic and life style considerations. The technique is almost always chosen during the preoperative consultation with the plastic surgeon, although some alterations may be necessary at the time of surgery, depending on local tissue factors. Therefore, if a submuscular implant reconstruction is planned, the possibility of tissue expansion should be introduced during the preoperative consultation. Of course, deviation from the preoperative planning of either the latissimus dorsi or rectus abdominis flap should be a very rare occurrence.

Surgical Considerations Common to All Techniques

Preoperatively, all patients are given intravenous cephalosporin as antiobiotic prophylaxis. The additional use of corticosteroids and nifedipine for patients undergoing TRAM flap reconstruction is discussed below. General anesthesia is induced and supplemental muscle relaxation drugs are used. The initial position and preparation of the patient are planned in concert with the general surgeon. The entire thorax is prepared, including the opposite breast, with povidone-iodine solution. The ipsilateral arm is prepared and draped freely within the operative field so that it may be mobilized throughout the procedure by both the general surgeon and plastic surgeon. If the TRAM flap is to be used, the preparation extends to the upper thighs bilaterally and to the bed line at both lateral aspects. For the latissimus dorsi flap, the patient is placed in a lateral decubitus position for initial skin preparation, sterile drapes are stapled to the skin at the thoracic spine in the midline, and the patient is returned to the recumbent attitude for the mastectomy.

The mastectomy is then performed by the general surgical team. After delivery of the specimen, the operative field is thoroughly irrigated with sterile water. The general surgeon makes the final decision regarding the appropriate reconstruction. He may wish to consult with the pathologist regarding aspects of the primary tumor site or axillary contents before making his decision. In our experience, it has been very rare to abort the reconstructive phase of the procedure. Any significant frequency of such an occurrence would be an indication of poor patient selection or poor interspecialty cooperation, and it would inflict considerable psychological trauma on both patient and family. Even the most sincere postoperative explanations may not deter the patient from the conviction that hers is a hopeless situation when reconstruction is delayed at this point.[32]

As in any two-team cancer procedure, gloves, gowns, and instruments are changed when the plastic surgical team enters the operative field. The surgical drapes are covered with clean, sterile drapes for the reconstructive procedure. The surgical specimen is weighed in order to give a rough approximation of the volume to be replaced. The viability of the skin flaps is evaluated by clinical means and by the use of intravenous fluorescein dye, followed by visualization with the Woods' lamp.[33] Nonstaining areas should be excised before skin closure. When implant or tissue expansion reconstruction is to be used, further undermining of the inferior skin flap from the muscle of the thorax and even the upper abdomen may compensate for the loss of tissue after excision of nonstaining areas. Technical considerations regarding treatment of the chest wall musculature vary according to the method of reconstruction selected and are addressed in each of the following sections. After completion of the specific technique, subcutaneous and submuscular drains of the silicone, closed-suction variety are used.

Submuscular Implant Reconstruction

Patient Selection. In most patients, submuscular reconstruction is performed with the conventional silicone implant alone. This is the ideal procedure for the patient with small to moderate-sized breasts and is the most efficient and most economical procedure. When the general surgeon and plastic surgeon plan the extirpation and reconstruction together, consistently good results are achieved by this technique, with a low rate of complications (Figs. 29-4 to 29-6). The basic submuscular implant can also act as a soft tissue expander, and the size of the implant changed at the second-stage procedure if necessary (Fig. 29-7). The submuscular reconstructive technique is performed expeditiously at the completion of the mastectomy, rarely extending operative time for more than 1 hour with practiced teams. Masking of early local recurrence is virtually eliminated by this approach, and this assurance can be offered to the general surgeon and medical oncologist.

Technical Considerations. A complete discussion of the technique for submuscular reconstruction with implants is included in Chapter 30, which provides a solid basis for submuscular implant reconstruction on both a delayed and immedi-

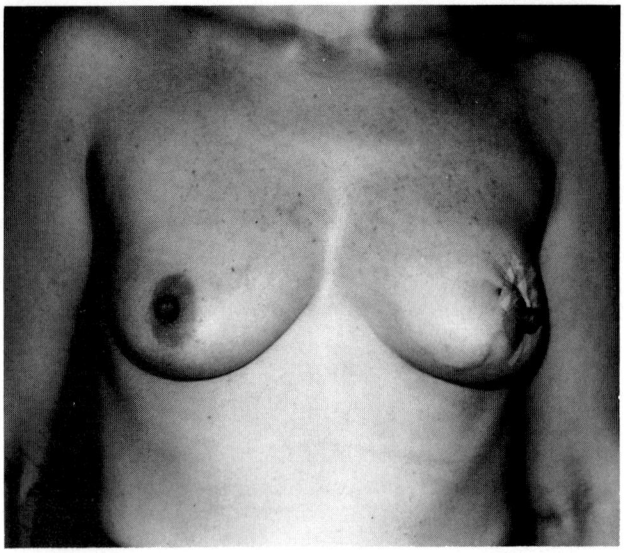

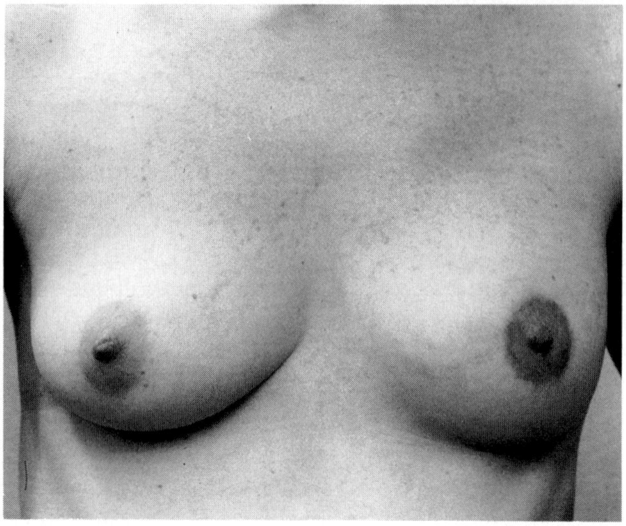

A B

FIGURE 29-4 *A*, This 42-year-old woman with a subareolar tumor location in the left breast was an ideal candidate for submuscular implant reconstruction to achieve symmetry with the small, nonptotic contralateral breast. *B*, One year after immediate reconstruction and 4 months after nipple-areolar reconstruction, symmetry is maintained.

ate basis. The essential element of this reconstruction is the development of a "muscle bra"[32,34] with the ultimate composition of pectoralis major, pectoralis minor, serratus anterior, obliquus externus abdominis, and rectus abdominis muscles. The implant position in the pocket enveloped by the foregoing muscles is essential for providing the best aesthetic result, as well as preventing implant loss. My preference for dissecting the muscle bra is to enter the submuscular pocket by a division of the serratopectoral fascia in a small area, usually over the fourth rib. The dissection is performed with scissors dissection, with a lighted fiberoptic retractor and the assistance of a suction cautery device. The muscle fibers are sharply elevated immediately over the periosteal surface of the nearest rib in both an anterior and a posterior direction. Blunt finger dissection can be used superiorly along the sternal border and in the area of the upper thorax, sweeping the finger underneath the pectoralis minor muscle (Fig. 29-8). Dissection beneath the pectoralis major muscle is usually the easiest part of the operation. The most difficult is at the fourth, fifth, and sixth interspaces and ribs. Especially in the medial aspect of the dissection, sharp dissection is needed to keep the pectoralis major muscle relationships with the rectus abdominis muscle intact (Fig. 29-9). The lower origins of the pectoralis major muscle do not arise from rib but actually from the intervening rectus abdominis muscle, which itself has bony origins superior to the lower pectoralis major. Therefore, dissection of the medial inferior corner of the pocket should involve both a superior and inferior dissection, approaching this juncture mainly from the inferior side in order to prevent a superficial plane between the pectoralis major and underlying rectus abdominis muscles. If the surgeon's finger is inserted beneath the upper edge of the rectus abdominis muscle and this is elevated abruptly toward the juncture with the pectoralis major, sharp dissection along the periosteal attachments of the pectoralis major muscle and the upper rectus abdominis muscle in combination generally frees the inferomedial pocket. With regard to the lateroinferior portion of the pocket, sharp dissection of the serratus muscle from the rib cage is necessary to a position between the anterior and midaxillary lines. The use of the suction cautery is helpful in achieving hemostasis beneath the serratus muscle flap. If the serratus muscle is reflected from superiorly to inferiorly, sharp dissection can then proceed beneath the external oblique muscle in the inferolateral corner of the pocket. This dissection will then be contiguous with the lateral attachments of the anterior rectus fascia, which must be divided in order to complete this portion of the pocket (Fig. 29-9). The lateral rectus abdominis fibers are then elevated from the rib with blunt and sharp dissection, keeping the muscle and fascia superior to it in continuity with the external oblique and serratus anterior muscles. The intent is to elevate all muscles from the periosteum and perichondrium of the underlying ribs and intercostal fascia. After surgery, a temporary periosteal reaction may be noted on bone scan. The follow-up scan after regrowth of periosteum will be normal (Fig. 29-10).

It is my preference to irrigate the submuscular pocket with a cephalosporin solution and to pack the pocket with sponges saturated with a dilute solution of epinephrine. The pocket dissection, when completed and inspected, should extend from a level

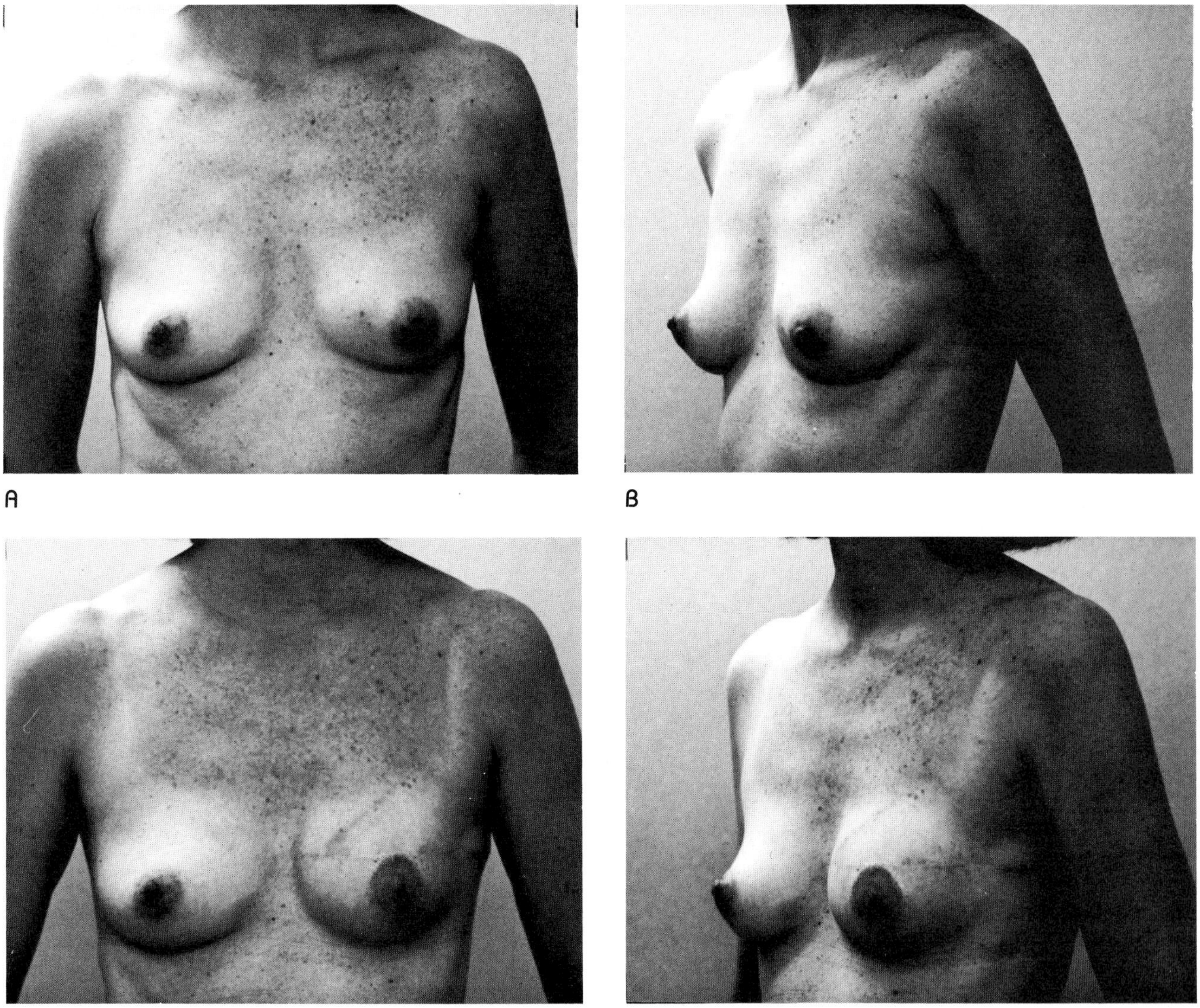

FIGURE 29-5 A 43-year-old woman with infiltrating duct carcinoma of the left breast has a small, nonptotic right breast. *A, B,* Preoperative anterior and left oblique views. *C, D,* Postoperative views 8 months after mastectomy with immediate submuscular reconstruction with a 175-ml implant and 3 months after nipple-areolar reconstruction with an inner thigh graft and the "skate" flap technique.

slightly below the inframammary fold, most often at the sixth interspace, to the clavicle, and from the border of the sternum to between the anterior and midaxillary lines laterally. Care must be taken in evaluating the inframammary fold area. If the pocket is too high, the implant will appear to be high and there will be much less capacity for acceptance of an appropriate-sized implant. Conversely, dissection below the desired inframammary line may provide an implant that is correspondingly low and in need of correction by capsulorrhaphy at a later time. The technique for capsulorrhaphy is described by Spear in Chapter 30.

When a submuscular implant is used, a decision about appropriate volume may be approximated by comparing the weight of the specimen with the size of the proposed implant. This is helpful in the lower ranges of weight but is not appropriate for breast sizes over 500 or 600 g. For the typical patient selected for this technique, our implants usually range between 200 and 400 ml in size (average 330 ml).[4] (For larger women, with large chest-wall diameters and broad shoulders, submuscular implant reconstruction may be insufficient and either temporary or permanent tissue expanders may be needed.) I prefer to use a double-lumen design implant, the outer lumen being adjusted with saline. Some surgeons choose also to use intraluminal corticosteroids or antibiotics. Soft-suction catheters are placed beneath the muscle pocket and beneath the skin flaps before closure. Care is taken in muscle closure to approximate the lateral edge of the serratus ante-

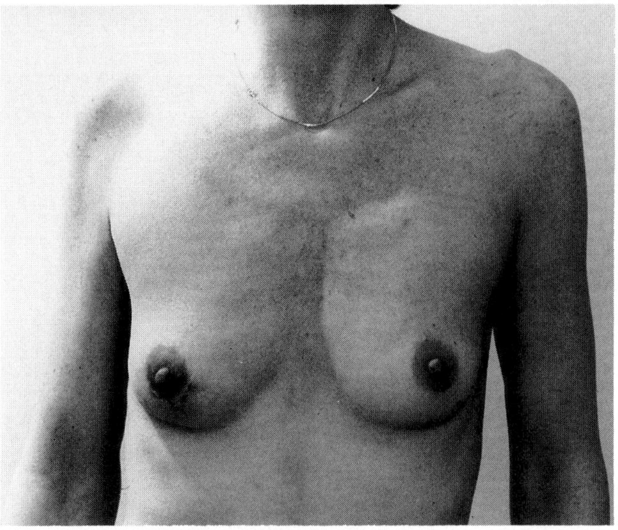

A

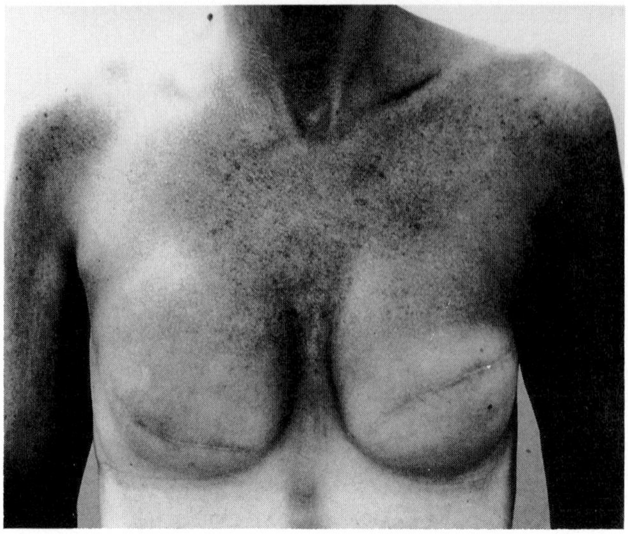

B

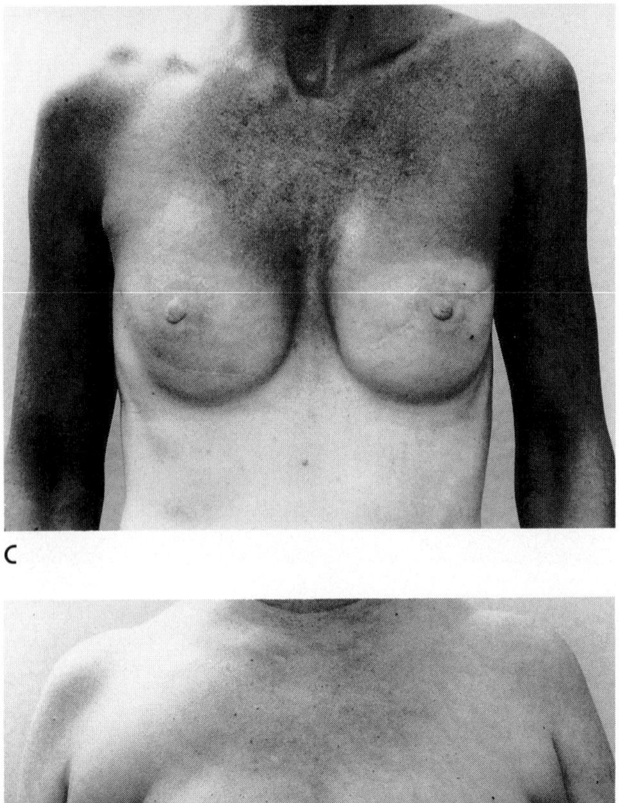

C

FIGURE 29–6 The candidate for bilateral mastectomy is ideal for submuscular implant reconstruction of similar size to achieve symmetry. *A*, A 47-year-old woman with lobular carcinoma in the right breast and high-risk mammographic changes in the left breast desired larger breasts after surgery. *B*, Three months after bilateral mastectomies and submuscular reconstruction with 425-ml gel-inflatable mammary implants. *C*, After skin graft areolar reconstruction and quadrapod flap nipple reconstruction. (From Noone RB, Frazier TG, Murphy JB, et al. Immediate reconstruction after mastectomy for cancer. Adv Plast Reconstr Surg 1987; 4:51–94.)

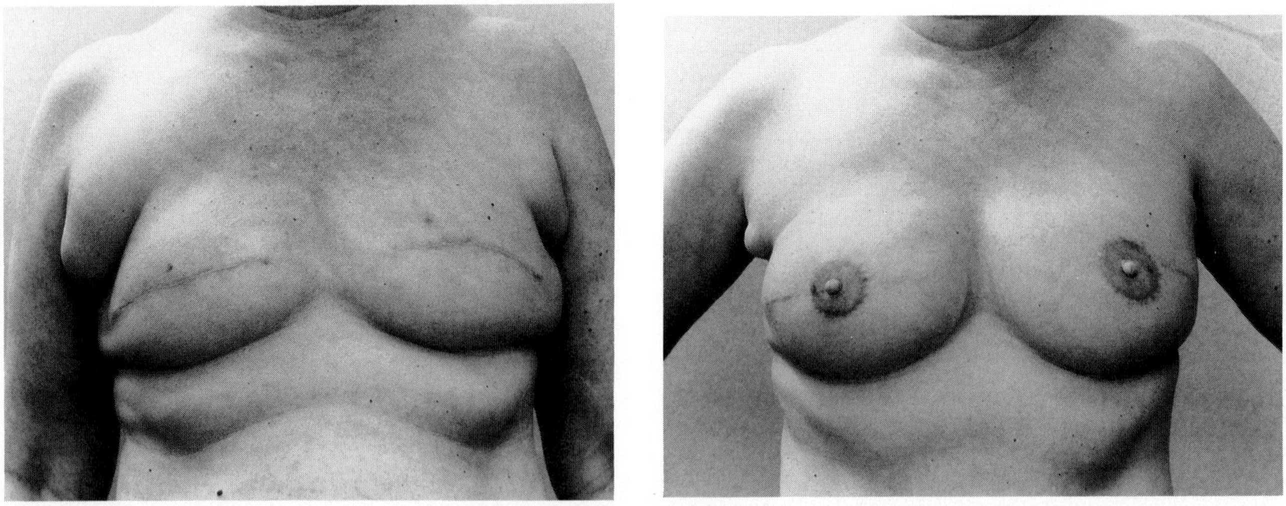

A B

FIGURE 29–7 Submuscular silicone implants may serve as temporary soft tissue expanders, followed by replacement with larger implants at a second operation. *A*, This 54-year-old patient was referred for evaluation after immediate reconstruction with 300-ml implants that provided insufficient volume. *B*, Secondary surgery included replacement with 650-ml gel-inflatable implants, suction lipectomy of the abdomen and axilla, and nipple-areolar reconstruction.

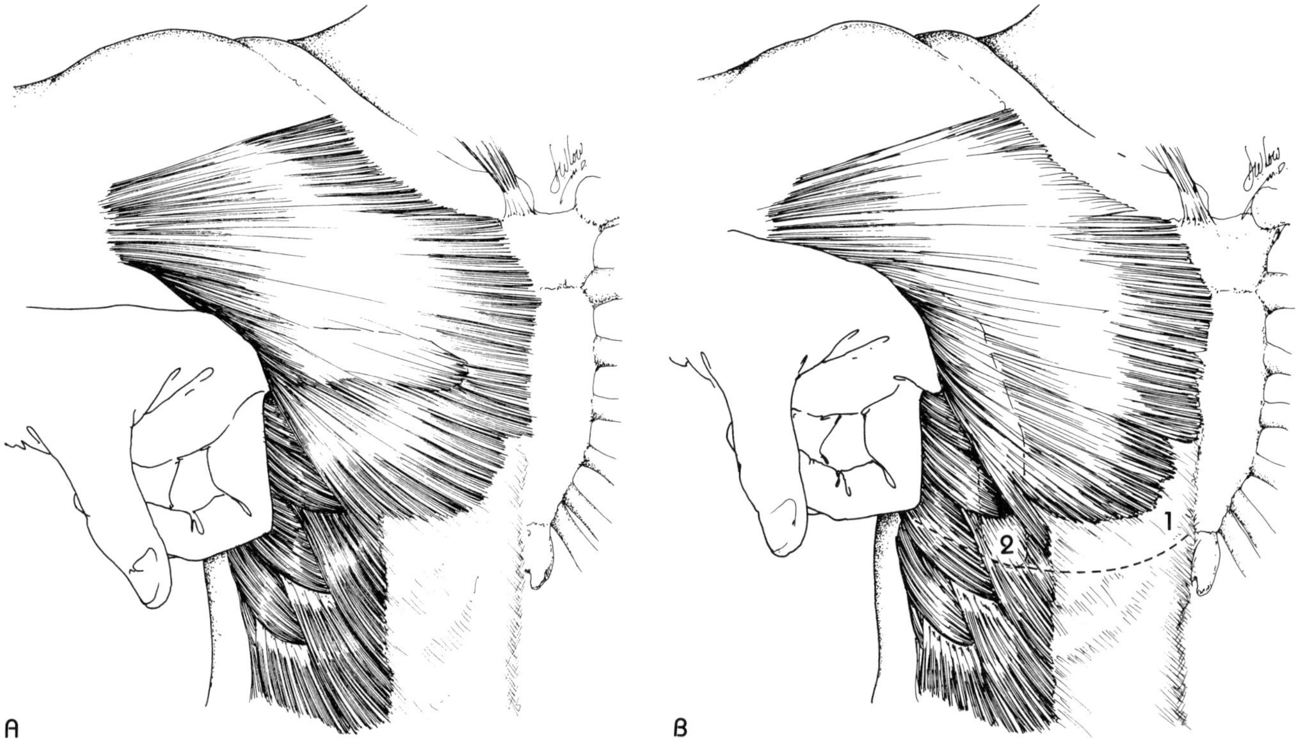

FIGURE 29 – 8 *A*, After the subpectoral plane is entered with sharp dissection, blunt digital dissection can be used superiorly along the sternal border and in the upper thorax. *B*, When resistance to digital dissection is felt at the (1) inferomedial and (2) inferolateral attachments of the pectoralis major, finger dissection must be replaced by dissection with sharp scissors to avoid rupture of the musculofascial juncture.

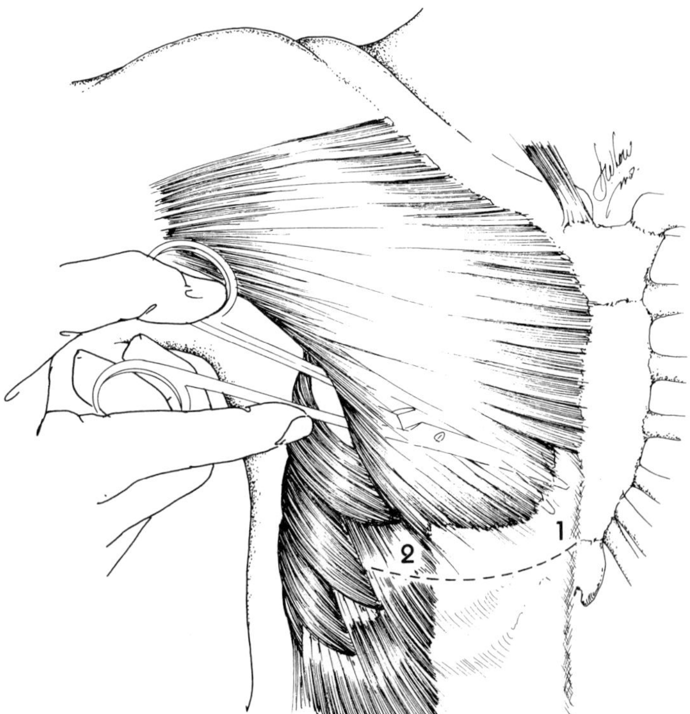

FIGURE 29 – 9 Sharp dissection in the inferior musculofascial pocket is mandatory. Medially, the rectus abdominis fascia is released from costosternal attachments (1). Laterally, the rectus fascia, pectoralis major muscle, external oblique muscle, and serratus anterior muscle are elevated as a unit with sharp dissection to form the lower-outer pocket (2).

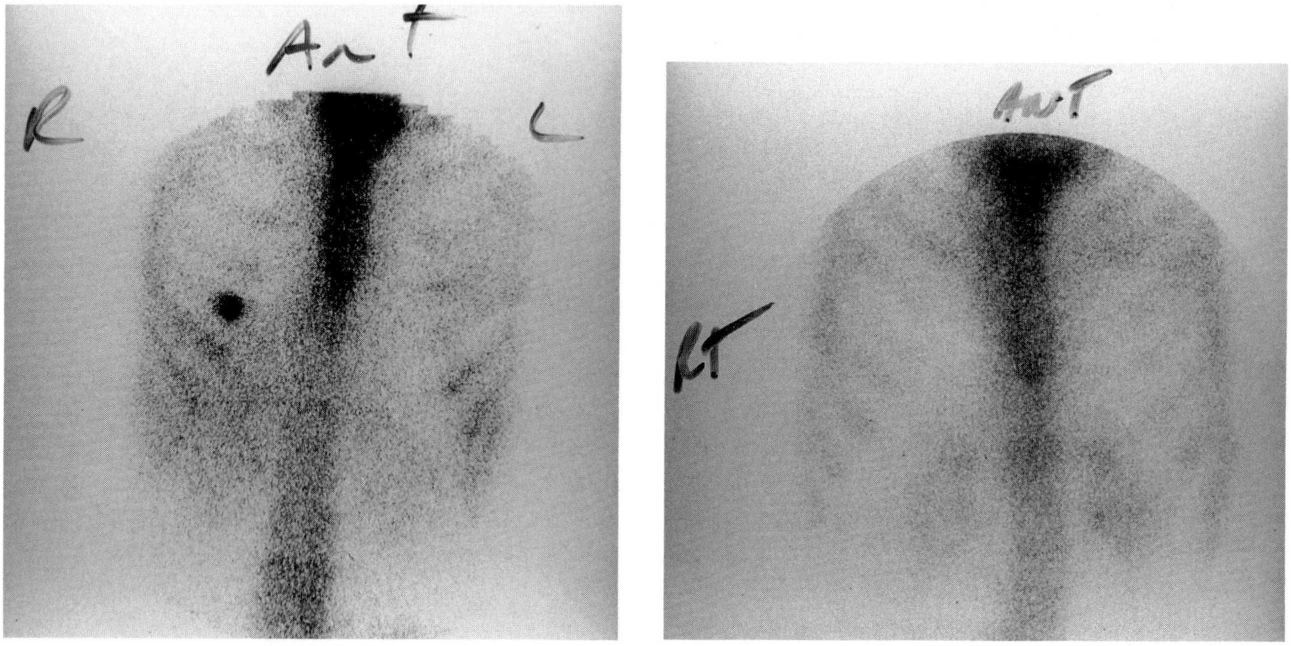

A B

FIGURE 29-10 *A*, Elevation of muscle from the rib periosteum during immediate reconstruction may result in a "false-positive" bone scan because of periosteal reaction after surgery. *B*, After regrowth of the periosteum, the repeat bone scan is normal.

rior and external oblique in achieving closure of the serratopectoral myotomy. I prefer 2-0 Vicryl suture material, because it does not appear to cut through thin muscle tissue as much as its 3-0 counterpart. Before skin closure, intravenous fluorescein dye is used to assess the viability of the skin edges. All areas of questionable viability are excised. Redundant skin (dog-ears) may accumulate medial to the nipple-areola site, and these are excised in a tailored fashion downward and inward, sparing the exposed V-neck area. Careful two-layer closure with intracuticular suture completes the procedure. A bulky dressing is placed in the axilla alone and secured with an elastic wrap that passes over the chest superior to the prominence to the new breast shape.

If disrupture occurs, defying suture repair during dissection of the muscle bra, muscle or muscle-fascia flaps may be introduced to patch the defect.[32, 34] These procedures involve additional surgery and time but are much preferable to leaving significant portions of the implant in contact with the subcutaneous space, inviting contamination and exposure. Coverage of disruptions in the low inferomedial portion can be performed with a broad U-shaped flap of rectus abdominis and external oblique fascia, developed in a turnover fashion. For larger disruptions that may involve a detachment of the pectoralis muscle along the entire inferolateral border from the lower shredded serratus and external oblique muscles, as well as the rectus abdominis, the more significant anterior border strap flap of latissimus dorsi muscle can be transposed. Both flaps have been described by Little and colleagues[34] and modified by Jarrett, as illustrated in Chapter 27. They can be performed without a change in patient position and without extension of the extirpative incisions. Although total muscle cover of the implant is preferable, others have advocated suturing the disrupted portion of pectoralis major border to the undersurface of the inferior skin flap, and then proceeding with slow muscle and skin expansion using the soft tissue expansion techniques.[35-37] Observations on this technique are made below.

Soft Tissue Expansion

Patient Selection. Because the use of soft tissue expanders in breast reconstruction increases patient inconvenience and may lead to a higher incidence of complications, I prefer to use conventional silicone implant reconstruction whenever possible during nonautogenous immediate reconstruction. However, there are specific instances when either a temporary tissue expander or a permanent expander is desirable (Fig. 29-11). These include elderly patients who may have questionable skin flap viability, heavy smokers, patients in whom inadequate muscle cover for the implant cannot be corrected with local muscle flaps, those with a moderate to large contra-

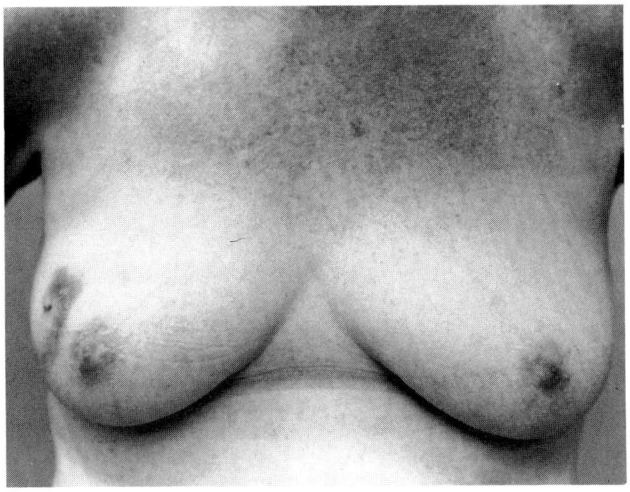

A

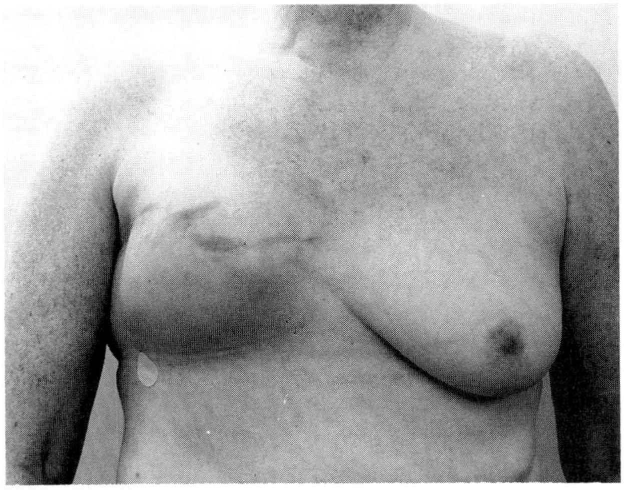

B

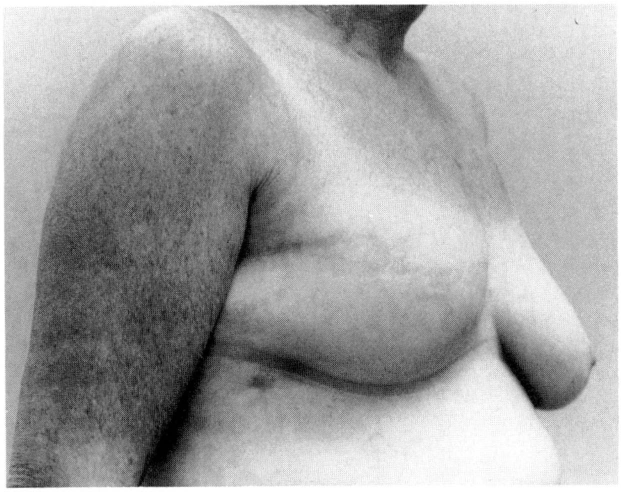

C

FIGURE 29-11 *A*, Soft tissue expansion was selected for this 61-year-old woman with a history of chronic tobacco use. Ischemic skin edges at surgery prompted submuscular placement of a noninflated temporary expander. *B*, After wound healing by epithelialization following separation of marginal skin necrosis, slow expansion was started. *C*, Two months after completion of expansion, the temporary expander was replaced by a permanent mammary implant.

lateral breast in whom contralateral surgery is not desired or is contraindicated, obese patients with a large thorax, and patients with a small breast in whom a large tumor has dictated the need for generous skin excision.

Technical Considerations. The exact details of submuscular pocket dissection and skin flap management, as described above for permanent implant reconstruction, are my preference for surgical wound preparation for tissue expansion. With the permanent expander, I prefer to use a distant fill port placed in a subcutaneous tunnel, usually over the anterolateral rib cage inferior to the location of the bra at the inframammary fold. This places the filling valve at a distance of 6 to 7 cm from the prosthesis, allowing easy palpation for filling after surgery, without concern for perforating the expander as it encroaches on the territory of the filling valve. If the temporary expander is to be used, I select a textured expander with an incorporated "Magnasite" filling port.

Although my preference has been to provide complete coverage of the expander by means of the living muscle bra concept, an increasing number of surgeons are advocating a subcutaneous position for the expander in the caudal portion of the wound. This attitude developed in parallel with attempts to create inframammary fold appearance and ptosis, both of which are difficult with total submuscular cover. Suturing muscle and fascia to the undersurface of the inferior skin flap at a distance from the potential areas of ischemia along the free margin of the flap has been advocated by Paul, Dowden, and Hyland.[35-37] Dowden recommended that the rectus abdominis fascia be left intact, thus leaving the lower portion of the expander or the implant in contact with the subcutaneous tissue of the lower mastectomy flap. He reported a remarkably low exposure of only one implant in over 260 reconstruction patients during a 6-year period.[35]

When placing the expander in a total submuscular position, my preference for inframammary fold creation is to use scar capsule manipulation in a secondary procedure. This is done either at the time of replacement of the temporary expander with a permanent implant, or during a partial capsulectomy if a permanent expander has been used and ptosis is not sufficient. The caudal half of the anterior hemisphere of the capsule is resected during a capsulectomy. This allows lower anterior fullness to develop, creating a ptotic effect (Fig. 29-11*C*). I leave the capsule intact at the superoanterior hemisphere, over the rib cage itself. However, when a temporary expander is replaced with a polyurethane implant, total capsule excision is advocated. When the caudal aspect of the original pocket is created 1 or 2 cm below the inframammary fold, an additional 1 or 2 cm can be added with tissue expansion, allowing for a more definitive inframammary fold at the secondary procedure when the capsule is excised and the dermal skin flap is approximated to the periosteum of the rib at the inframammary fold (Fig. 29-12).

Autogenous Tissue Reconstruction

Patient Selection. Although it represents an added investment in operative time, autogenous tissue reconstruction at the time of mastectomy, especially the use of the TRAM flap, may be the ideal procedure for a young, nonsmoking woman with a generous abdomen (Fig. 29-13). It is particularly suited to patients in whom symmetry with a contralateral breast is desired without the need for surgery on the contralateral breast (Fig. 29-14), patients with moderate contralateral ptosis, or those with a wide chest and a large transverse breast diameter. This technique is also indicated when a generous skin excision is required, either because of the size of the tumor or because of its location relative to the nipple (Fig. 29-15). It is used when the patient is reluctant to undergo reconstruction with silicone implants. It is the procedure of choice for reconstruction following salvage mastectomy for recurrence

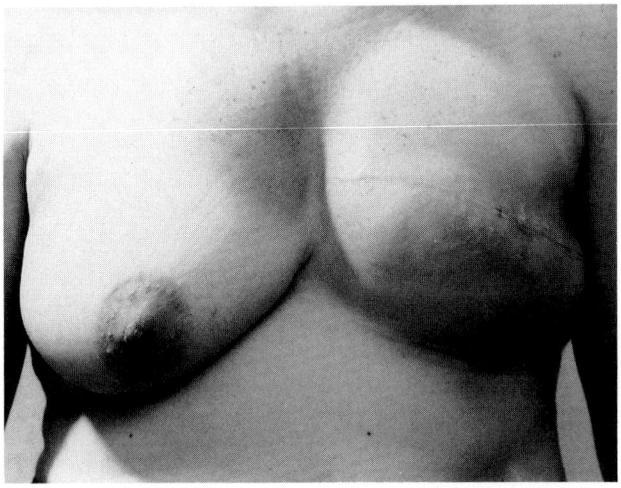

A

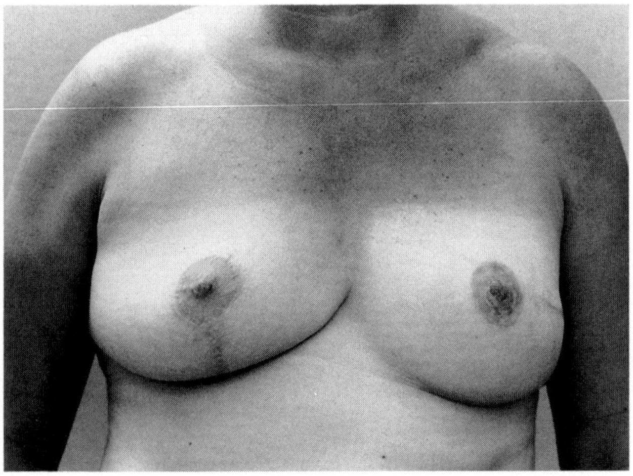

B

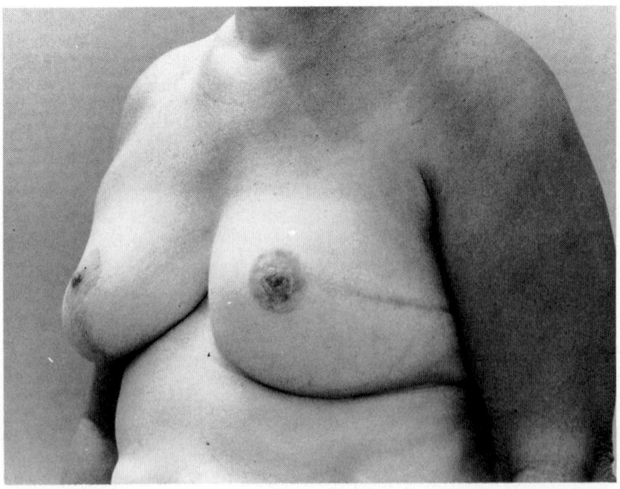

C

FIGURE 29-12 *A*, An additional 1 to 2 cm of caudal displacement of the inframammary fold can be expected after full tissue expansion. *B*, *C*, The position of the inframammary fold remains constant, but ptosis is achieved by resection of the caudal half of the anterior hemisphere of the capsule. (From Noone RB, Frazier TG, Murphy JB, et al. Immediate reconstruction after mastectomy for cancer. Adv Plast Reconstr Surg 1987; 4:51-94.)

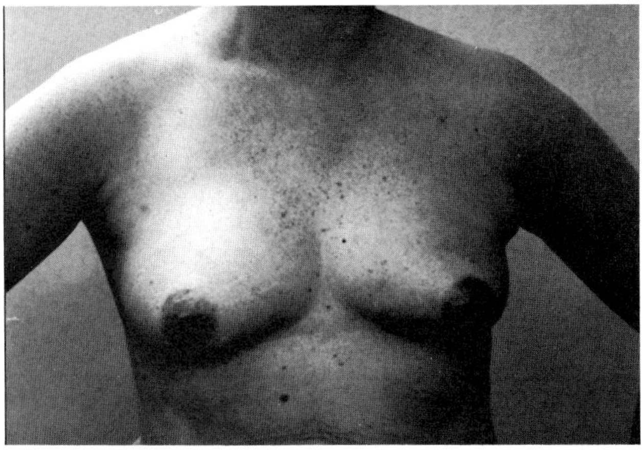

A

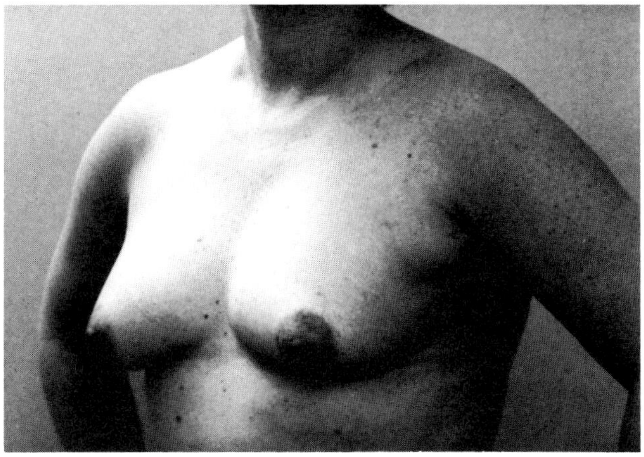

B

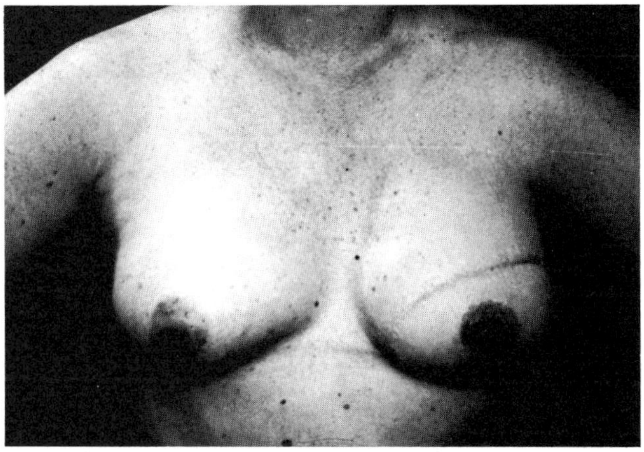

C

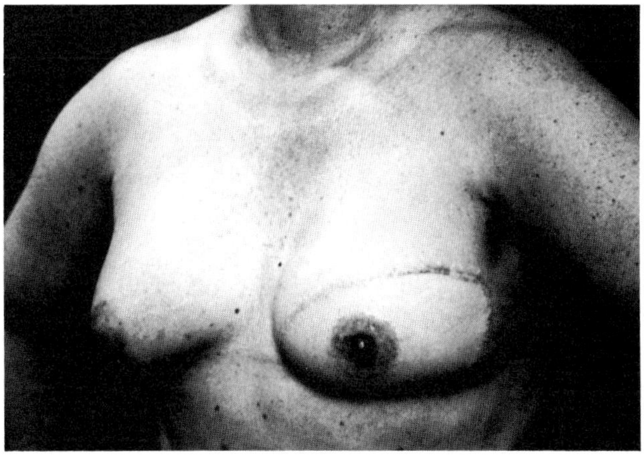

D

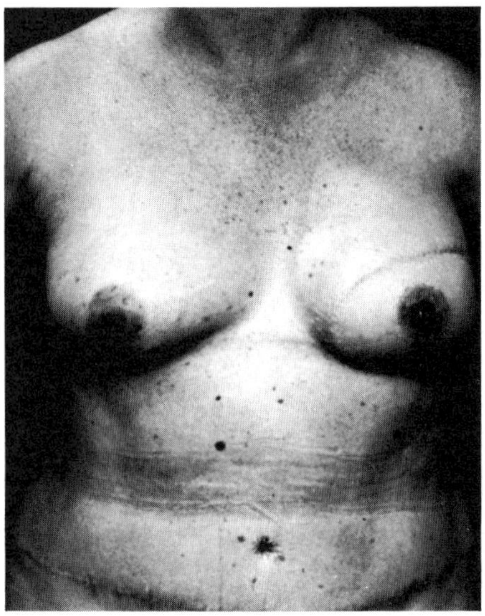

E

FIGURE 29-13 This 42-year-old nonsmoker with moderate glandular and nipple ptosis presented with an intraductal carcinoma of the left breast. The transverse rectus abdominis myocutaneous flap was selected as the procedure that could best match the right breast without the need for contralateral surgery. *A*, Preoperative anterior view. *B*, Preoperative oblique view. *C*, Postoperative anterior view. *D*, Postoperative oblique view. *E*, Postoperative result demonstrating a scar in the middle lower abdomen.

after irradiation failure,[38,39] or for treatment of undesirable results after irradiation (Fig. 29-16).

The relative contraindications include heavy smoking, significant obesity with abdominal wall laxity, and previous abdominal surgical procedures in the flap area. Hartrampf questioned whether a woman who has recently learned of a breast cancer diagnosis can be adequately informed and make a measured decision regarding both ablative breast surgery and a major reconstructive procedure at the

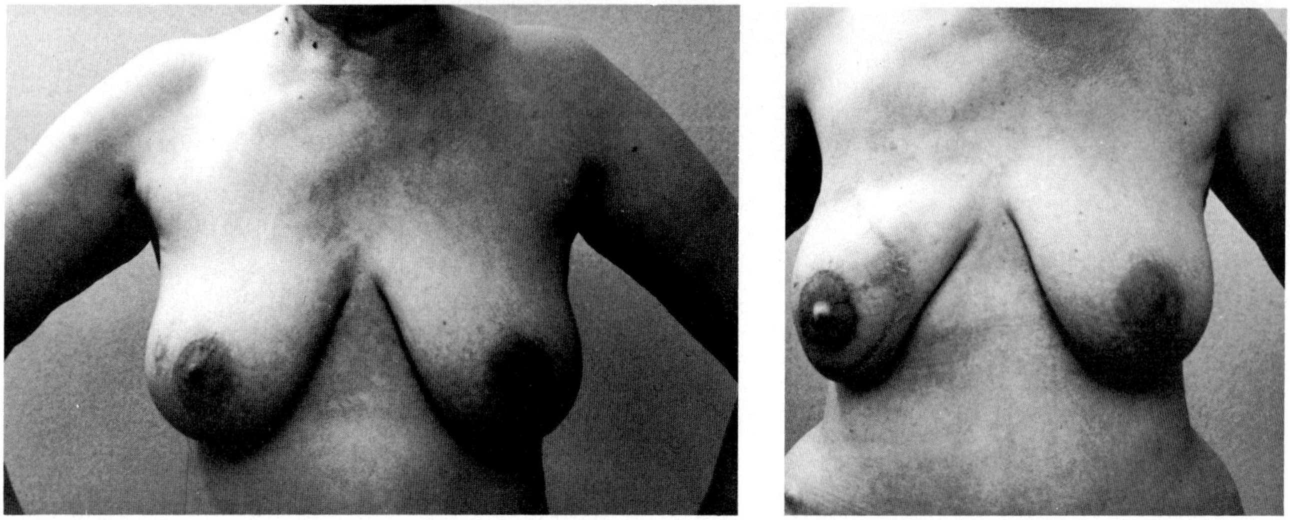

A B

FIGURE 29-14 *A*, Although significant ptosis was present, this 59-year-old woman and her general surgeon requested that no contralateral surgery should be planned for the left breast after a right immediate reconstruction. *B*, When performed as an immediate procedure, the TRAM flap can be sculpted to fill the skin envelope remaining after mastectomy, leading to the desired degree of ptosis.

same time.[40] This may be a relative contraindication to this technique for some women and an absolute contraindication for others. However, the carefully selected patient can realize a significant benefit from the TRAM flap procedure on an immediate basis. Other concerns Hartrampf raised about the TRAM flap included potential contamination of the abdominal area with tumor cells, the unknown histologic margins of the tumor specimen, the potential need for surgery in the contralateral breast, and the difficulty of obtaining autologous blood transfusions in the brief period between diagnosis and surgery. These are all issues that the general surgeon, patient, and reconstructive surgeon must address before the decision to use the immediate TRAM flap is made.

Technical Considerations. Because most patients who are having immediate breast reconstruction undergo surgery within 1 week of consultation, realistic preparation of the abdominal wall by exercise or cessation of smoking is difficult. The patient is prepared for what amounts to a lengthy operative procedure and an extended postoperative course. The initial plan of skin extirpation is modified in the case of autogenous reconstruction alone to drop the lower limb closer to the inframammary fold, so that more abdominal skin can be used and the inferior line of repair will remain hidden in the shadow of the breast. The skin island is planned to be of similar shape but slightly increased overall surface area to the planned extirpation site. Of course, no submuscular dissection is performed in this instance. The caudal edge of the superior skin flap is brought over the de-epithelialized dermis, which is adjusted to allow the skin island to "hang" appropriately for the desired amount of ptosis. The previous inframammary location on the caudal skin flap remains intact and is not undermined. The procedure otherwise is identical to that performed as a secondary procedure in delayed breast reconstruction (see Chapter 34).[41,42]

Conventional transfer of the TRAM island flap as either a single or double pedicle based on the superior epigastric arterial supply is the technique I prefer. Grotting and colleagues compared the use of the abdominal island flap transferred as a free flap based on the deep inferior epigastric pedicle with flap transfer with the conventional technique.[43] Although it requires an excellent level of microsurgical technical expertise, the free TRAM flap appears to be as safe as the conventional technique, and offers the advantages of more limited rectus muscle harvest and an improvement in the medial contour of the breast because of a lack of subcutaneous tunneling. This study found that in the hands of excellent microsurgeons, complications, operating time, estimated blood loss, period of hospitalization, and the return to functional baseline were comparable in both groups. Since there may be an improved vascular supply to the flap with a wider area of tissue perfusion because the lower abdomen is the primary territory of the inferior epigastric vessels, and since less dissection is required with free tissue transfer, especially in the upper abdomen, this technique may continue to gain popularity in the future. However, the decision for its use must be balanced with the experience of the microsurgical team and the operating room facilities available to the surgeon performing immediate reconstruction. Grotting's technique

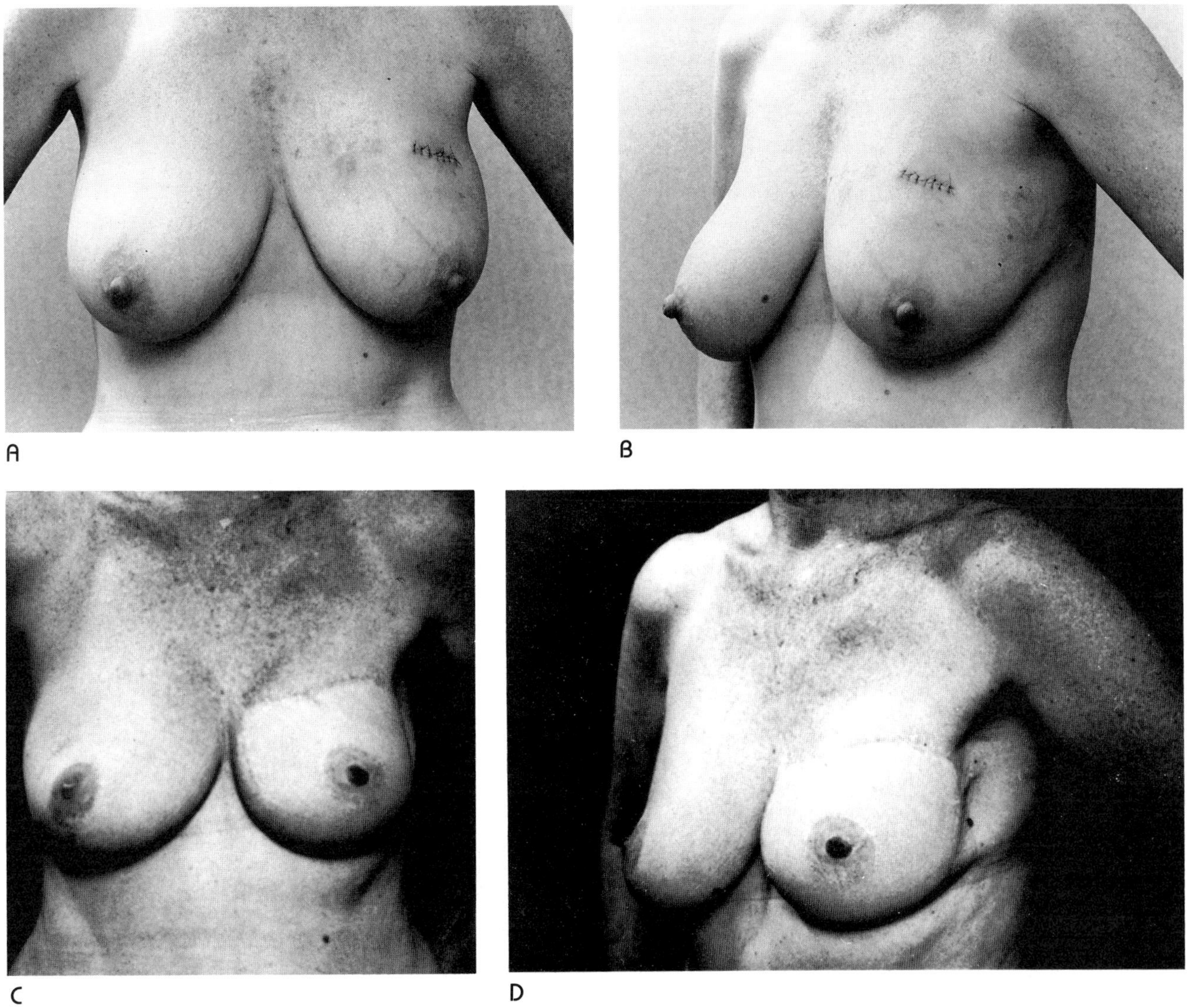

FIGURE 29-15 The size of the breast tumor and its location relative to glandular and nipple-areolar excision at mastectomy may dictate the choice of flap reconstruction. *A, B,* A 49-year-old woman with intraductal carcinoma in a superior location. A generous skin excision was required by the surgeon performing the mastectomy, extending the wound to the sternal border. *C, D,* Postoperative anterior and oblique views. Right reduction mammaplasty 5 months after immediate reconstruction provided excess nipple and areola for shared reconstruction.

utilizes the thoracodorsal vessels, which are usually skeletonized after the axillary dissection. He advocates preserving the serratus branch of the thoracodorsal artery in case a latissimus dorsi myocutaneous flap is needed in the future.

When immediate TRAM flap reconstruction is contemplated, dissection of the abdominal flap can be done by the reconstructive team at the same time that the mastectomy is performed by the ablative team of general surgeons. This requires two sets of surgical instruments, which should be kept separate throughout the course of the procedure. With practiced teams, this combined approach may be expeditious. However, I prefer to allow the general surgeon to complete the mastectomy and then cover the drapes from the ablative portion with clean sterile draping, and then change the instruments entirely before the plastic surgical team enter. This leads to an operating time approximately 1 hour longer than if simultaneous dissection is done, but it enables the reconstructive team to control the operating environment during tedious dissection of the flap and provides greater assurance that the abdominal area is not contaminated from the mastectomy dissection. This method also allows the general surgical team to perform their part of the operation without the proximity of and pressures from the reconstructive team.

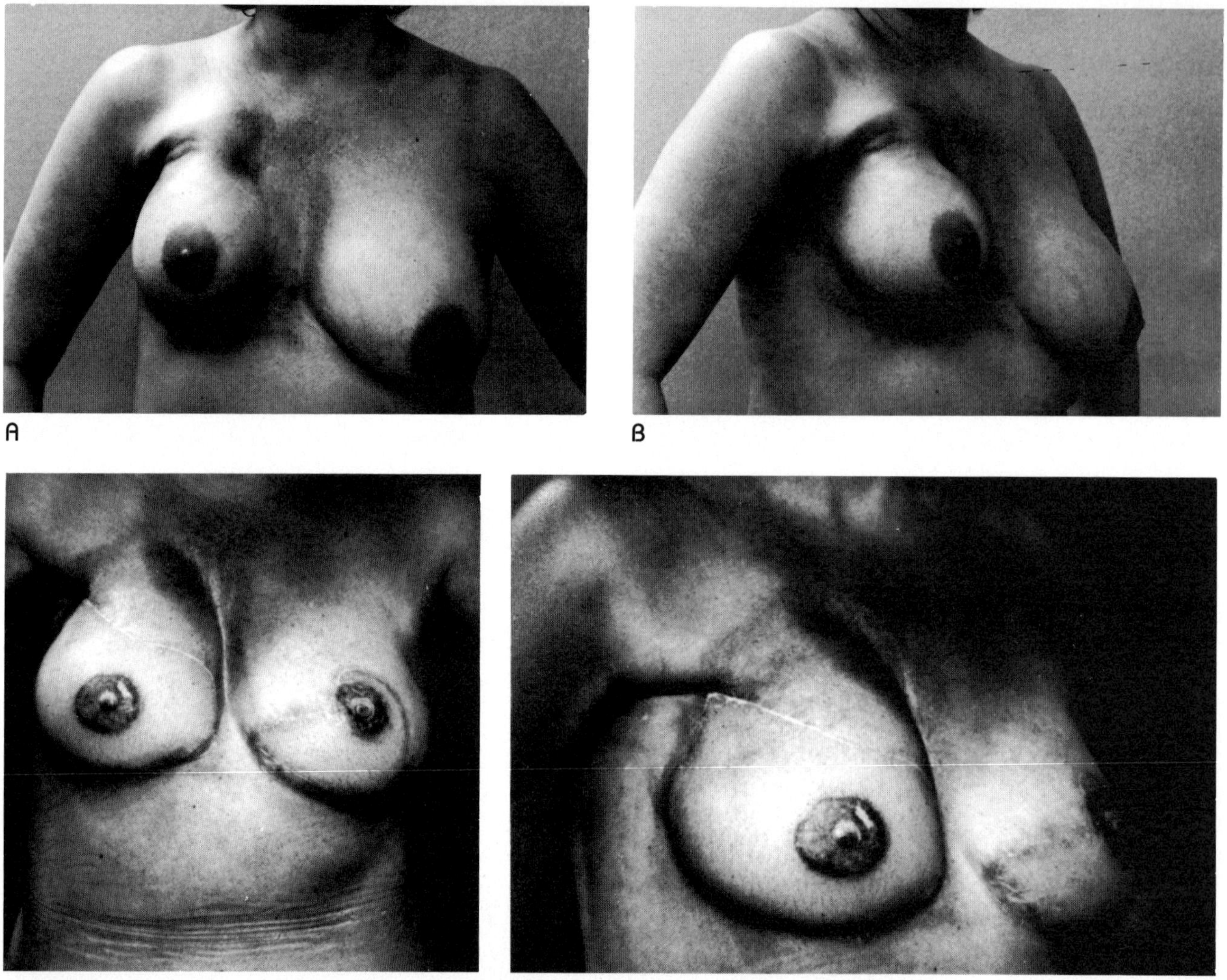

FIGURE 29-16 This 50-year-old woman with a history of both bilateral liquid silicone mammary injections and submammary augmentation mammaplasty developed carcinoma of the right breast. This was treated by lumpectomy, axillary dissection, and radiation therapy with preservation of the implant. She was referred for treatment of painful scar capsule contracture and radiation changes of the thoracic skin. *A, B,* Anterior and right oblique views at initial consultation. The mammogram demonstrated florid silicone mastopathy of the left breast, and a left mastectomy was advised. *C, D,* Bilateral TRAM flap reconstruction was performed at the same procedure with bilateral mastectomies, implant removal, and resection of irradiated skin. The postoperative result is seen 1 year after the mastectomies and 3 months after nipple-areolar reconstruction.

Latissimus Dorsi Flap Reconstruction

Patient Selection. The chief indication for use of the latissimus dorsi flap for an immediate procedure is the resection of a large amount of skin and/or muscle prohibiting implant reconstruction or soft tissue expansion in a patient who does not have sufficient abdominal tissue to provide for TRAM flap reconstruction. The desire to provide ptosis and contralateral symmetry when the abdominal flap is not indicated is also a good indication for the latissimus dorsi procedure. In essence, all the indications listed above for autogenous tissue reconstruction are appropriate for the latissimus dorsi flap when there are abdominal contraindications to the TRAM flap.

Technical Considerations. It is usually known in advance if the latissimus dorsi flap is needed. Therefore, an outline of the flap can be developed on the posterior thorax, corresponding to the elliptic skin excision needed for mastectomy. It is my preference to prepare both breasts and the ipsilateral posterior thorax before the mastectomy, incorporating the ipsilateral arm in a large sterile stockinette. The posterior thorax is kept sterile by stapling sheets and towels to the thoracic spine area and placing the posterior thorax on sterile sheets before the performance of the mastectomy. With experience, the general surgical team can carry out the preparation and draping to the satisfaction of the plastic surgeon. When the mastectomy is completed, the patient can be turned to the lateral decubitus position and the hips appropriately secured to the operating table. A prearranged "bean bag" can then be inflated and the patient's position secured. The ellipse of skin is oriented in a transverse fashion, slightly larger in total surface area than the pattern of extirpation, but similar in surface design to the pattern of extirpation. The plastic surgeon usually has no choice regarding the position or orientation of the flap, because it must be placed exactly into the defect as a patch replica of the extirpation. If there has been muscle disruption during the mastectomy, an extension of the latissimus muscle past the island of skin is helpful in repairing the muscle or fascia tears. The reader is referred to Chapter 33 by Bostwick for a review of the technical considerations involved in flap insertion and implant placement. When performed on an immediate basis, the latissimus muscle flap can be used to augment the existing "living bra" of the pectoralis muscle and its cohorts. Therefore, a large dissection of latissimus muscle is not necessary on an immediate basis, as would be indicated with delayed reconstruction when the implant is placed beneath the latissimus dorsi muscle only.

Compared with TRAM flap reconstruction, the latissimus dorsi offers a shorter operating time, usually a more rapid recovery, and less soft tissue camouflage of the tumor field. These advantages are offset by the patch effect generated by the dorsal skin, the need to change patient positions, the continued potential for scar capsule contracture because an implant is needed, and the visible donor scar and muscle defect in the back.

POSTOPERATIVE CARE AFTER IMMEDIATE RECONSTRUCTION

The patient is admitted to the hospital under the care of the general surgeon. At the completion of the combined procedure, all postoperative care is the responsibility of the plastic surgeon, except that directed toward specific tumor work-up and treatment.

With implant or expander reconstruction, early ambulation is encouraged immediately after surgery in order to minimize the risks of venous complications in the lower extremity. Drains are placed to suction and careful output of drainage is recorded. A circumferential dressing is removed on the second postoperative day and a bra is used to secure wound dressings, usually reinforced with a superiorly placed elastic wrap to keep the prosthesis in a lower position in the pocket. While the drains are in place, the patient is encouraged to use her arms for normal activity, such as hair combing, washing, and eating. The drain that is in contact with the submuscular implant is removed within 3 to 4 days, depending on drainage volumes. The subcutaneous drain is left for a longer time until drainage is less than 30 ml per day, and often is not removed until the first office visit. A complicating factor in immediate reconstruction remains the development of lymphorrhea from the divided axillary lymphatics. This accumulates in the subcutaneous space in the area of the inframammary fold or lateral gutter. If neglected, this lymph-rich fluid will encourage fibrous changes in the overlying skin that will be detrimental to the final result. With implant reconstruction, on the second or third postoperative day, implant massage is begun twice a day in the hospital. Manual manipulation of the implant is carried out, elevating it superiorly in the pocket as far as possible. This occasions the patient considerable discomfort, and analgesics are given at appropriate intervals before such manipulation. By the time of discharge from the hospital, the patient can perform this massage herself. Direct compression massage is continued for 6 months after surgery.

Showering is allowed after the drains have been removed. On occasion the patient may be discharged from the hospital with a drain in place and is instructed to empty and record the drainage at home. Discharge apparel includes an elastic bra without underwire, with or without the addition of the elastic wrap. The patient views and generally accepts the reconstructed result before discharge and welcomes leaving the hospital wearing her premastectomy bra. She is usually followed on an outpatient basis for approximately 1 week after discharge, at which time the surgical wounds are evaluated and massage instructions are reinforced. The intracuticular sutures are removed 2 to 3 weeks after surgery. Follow-up by the plastic surgeon is provided at 4-week, 3-month, 6-month, and yearly intervals unless this routine is interrupted by complications or intervening surgery. Postmastectomy arm and shoulder exercises are allowed as soon as possible after surgery. All regular activity is encouraged 1 month after the operation.

Tissue expansion adds additional consideration to the postoperative routine. The expander is generally expanded to the maximal safe volume at the end of the operative procedure when wound closure is completed. Two or 3 days after surgery the skin flaps are sufficiently relaxed to permit further inflation before the patient is discharged. Postoperative inflation on an outpatient basis at 7- to 14-day intervals is the general routine until the desired size is achieved. At that time, approximately 30 percent overinflation is added, again at intervals dictated by the condition of the wound and the patient's comfort level. This overinflation is maintained for at least 3 months before the volume is reduced and either the full tube is removed in the case of a permanent expander, or the temporary expander is replaced with a permanent implant. It is imperative to perform the outpatient inflation procedures under strict sterile technique. In patients receiving chemotherapy, timing of inflation must avoid the postchemotherapy nadir period.

When TRAM flap reconstruction is used, I prefer to cover the flap with Tegaderm to combine sterile cover with ease of flap inspection. No compression dressings are used over the flap, and only a loose dressing is placed over the abdomen. Abdominal suction drains and the drains used beneath the flap reconstruction in the axilla are removed according to the usual routine, when drainage amounts to less than 30 ml per day. Sequential-pressure antiembolism stockings are continued until the patient is ambulatory, after which standard static stockings are used. Bra placement is delayed until approximately 2 weeks after surgery. No significant abdominal exercises are allowed until 6 weeks after surgery. In general, postoperative management following immediate reconstruction with the TRAM flap is similar to that advocated after delayed reconstruction.

Because simultaneous elevation of the pectoralis major muscle and the latissimus dorsi is added to the extensive dissection of the axilla for lymph node removal, early postoperative shoulder exercises are especially important after immediate latissimus dorsi flap reconstruction. These should be instituted despite the high incidence of seroma formation, which may occur in the caudal end of the posterior thorax. Although it is important to remove the silicone drain in contact with the prosthesis as soon as possible after surgery, generally not later than the fifth day, the drain in the posterior thorax should be left until scant drainage is noted, and then should be removed with care. Frequent development of seroma in the posterior thorax may require aspiration on an outpatient basis.

COMPLICATIONS AFTER IMMEDIATE RECONSTRUCTION

The well-described complications of skin necrosis, seroma, infection and hematoma, may occur after any mastectomy with or without the addition of immediate reconstruction. With an implant in place, these problems can lead to loss of the implant and the accompanying surgical and psychological trauma of an operation for its removal. Therefore, preoperative and intraoperative goals are directed toward preventing the occasion for complications. Preoperative instruction against ingesting blood-coagulation inhibitors, such as aspirin, is given in a standardized list of these medications. During surgery, total muscle cover of the prosthesis, as described above, is the single most important factor in prevention of the implant loss.

After submuscular implant or expander reconstruction, the experience with 244 consecutive immediate breast reconstructions performed at our institution was reported by Castiglione and associates.[44] *Marginal skin necrosis* was the most common complication seen: an incidence of 9.1 percent (21 patients). This usually involved a small amount of skin loss along the wound closure, and occurred despite the routine intraoperative use of fluorescein to assess skin flap viability. Occasionally, larger areas of skin loss may develop. If the condition is recognized early in the postoperative period, nitroglycerin paste is used on the wound in an attempt to salvage questionable areas. Once the limits of necrosis are defined, the patient can be treated conservatively on an outpatient basis, using topical antibacterial ointment along the wound. Necrotic tissue is debrided during office visits and the wound is allowed to heal by contraction and epithelialization. If total muscle cover of the implant was achieved during surgery, the implant usually is not threatened and complete wound healing occurs (Fig. 29–17).

Seroma or fluid collections were noted in 12 patients (5.2 percent) despite the routine use of suction catheter drains as described above. These usually occur in the axilla, lateral gutter, or inframammary fold and may require repeated aspiration. There is little risk to the implant with adequate cover if an intracatheter type of needle is used. It is important to remove all fluid, because even small collections under the skin flaps can lead to fibrosis of the overlying skin and thereby detract from the final aesthetic result.

Infection was noted in 10 patients (4.3 percent) and usually involved a superficial cellulitis, although one case of significant sepsis with hypotension was seen. Cellulitis is usually limited to the skin and responds rapidly to appropriate antibiotic therapy. In the absence of skin necrosis or hematoma, cellulitis itself has not resulted in implant loss.

Hematomas were rare, occurring in four patients (1.7 percent). These are best avoided by meticulous attention to hemostasis and the placement of suction catheters at the time of surgery. A hematoma occurring immediately after surgery is usually heralded by an undue amount of pain in the recognizable firm, tense mass beneath the subcutaneous flap. When recognized, it should be drained immediately in the operating room under sterile conditions because of the threatened exposure of the implant. Given early recognition, drainage, and liberal irrigation, the recognized hematoma should not lead to implant loss (Fig. 29–17).

In our experience, *symptomatic capsule contracture* occurred in 25 patients (10.7 percent), a rate similar to that noted in our delayed reconstructions. This possible outcome is explained to the patient in the preoperative discussion as a common sequelae of the surgery, and the patient is prepared for a two-stage reconstruction. Capsule management by capsulotomy, capsulectomy, or capsulorrhaphy is done at the second procedure, which also includes nipple-areolar reconstruction and management of the contralateral breast. Scar capsule contracture is

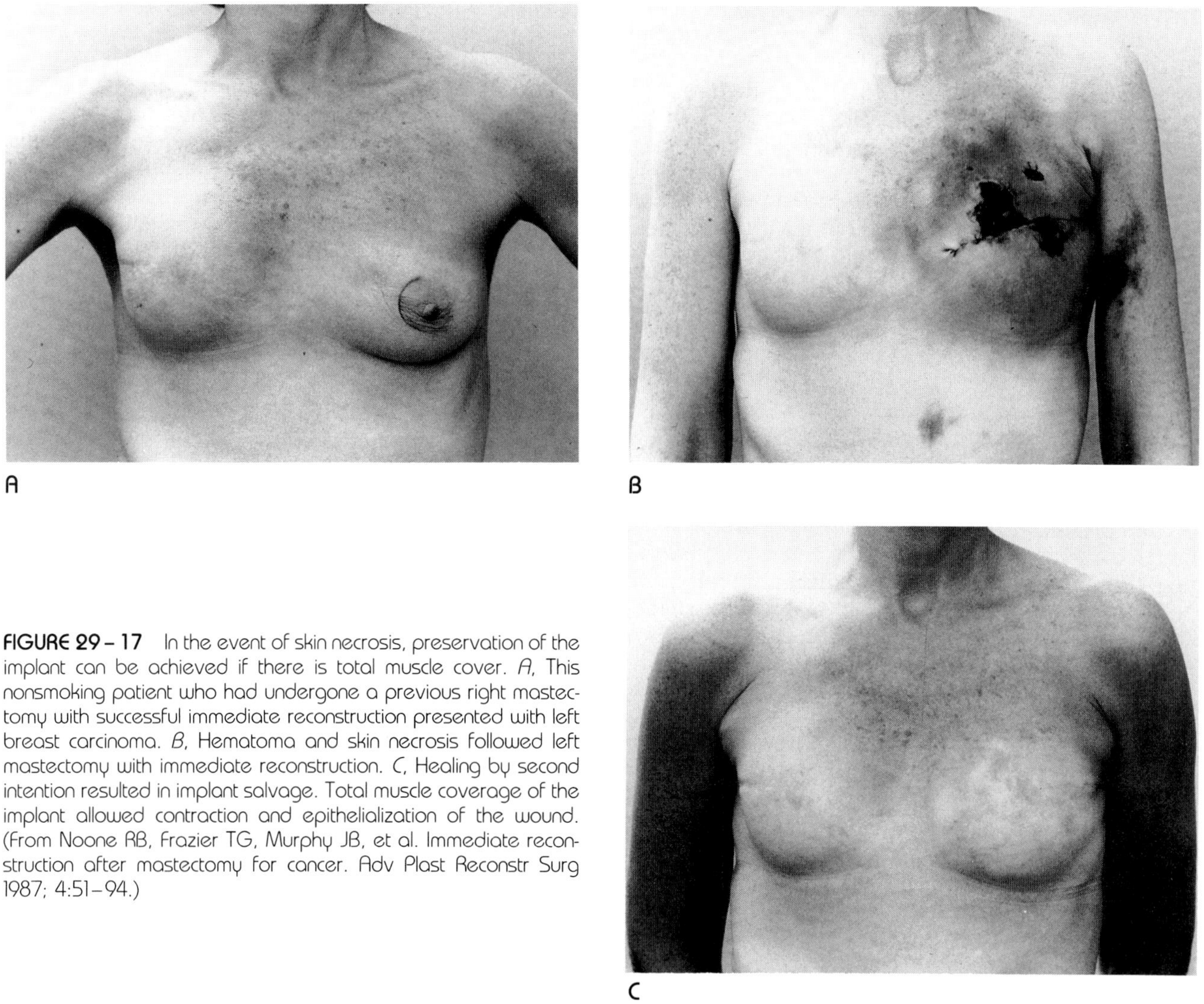

FIGURE 29-17 In the event of skin necrosis, preservation of the implant can be achieved if there is total muscle cover. *A*, This nonsmoking patient who had undergone a previous right mastectomy with successful immediate reconstruction presented with left breast carcinoma. *B*, Hematoma and skin necrosis followed left mastectomy with immediate reconstruction. *C*, Healing by second intention resulted in implant salvage. Total muscle coverage of the implant allowed contraction and epithelialization of the wound. (From Noone RB, Frazier TG, Murphy JB, et al. Immediate reconstruction after mastectomy for cancer. Adv Plast Reconstr Surg 1987; 4:51–94.)

therefore a management problem separate from the other complications described.

Of course, the most devastating complication is that of *implant loss*, not only because of the physical trauma associated with an operation for its removal, but also because of the severe psychological trauma associated with the loss of the restored breast. Preoperative and intraoperative goals are directed toward the prevention of this complication. Fortunately, it is a rare event, occurring in only eight patients in the above series (3.4 percent). It can follow skin necrosis, seroma, infection, and hematoma. Three of the 21 patients with skin necrosis, one of 12 with seroma, one of nine with cellulitis, two of four with hematoma, and the single patient with sepsis suffered loss of the implant. A careful review of the records and operative notes of the patients with implant loss led to a clear understanding of the cause of the loss. In the two patients with hematoma, secondary infection led to implant exposure and loss. For the four patients who lost an implant secondary to skin necrosis or seroma, the common denominator was inadequate muscle cover of the implant so that it was not protected when the infection ensued. Finally, two implant losses occurred in women who had undergone the insertion of tissue expanders. Despite the use of sterile technique with expander inflation, one infection occurred during the course of expansion, and the other presented in septic shock one day after expansion was performed while the patient was probably at the nadir of chemotherapy. Because of this experience, we caution against performing expansion at that stage of chemotherapy. Once it is determined that the implant is exposed or infected, it must be removed and the wound drained adequately. The wound is left to heal by second intention and no further attempt at reconstruction is made until at least 4 to 6 months after implant removal. Many of these patients need autogenous tissue reconstruction.

The above series makes clear that immediate breast reconstruction with implants can be performed with a low complication rate. Prevention of complications involves close collaboration between the general surgeon and the plastic surgeon as well as meticulous surgical technique during the creation of the muscle bra.[32,34] With increased surgical experience, the complication rate should become lower. When complications do occur, they are usually easily managed. Implants can be salvaged in the face of most complications, provided that adequate muscle cover has been achieved at the time of surgery.

SECONDARY PROCEDURES

During the initial consultation, all patients are informed that breast reconstruction, whether immediate or delayed, potentially involves at least a two-stage investment. It is further explained that the goal of the first operation is to produce a soft and relatively normal breast mound, whether the technique be by implant, expander, or autogenous reconstruction. Although symmetry is attempted initially, the details of symmetry with regard to volume, shape, and position are secondary in comparison with a natural appearing breast reconstruction. Patients are informed that achievement of further symmetry must await a second operation 3 to 6 months after the primary reconstruction, almost always as a short-stay procedure on an outpatient basis. At the second operation, "fine tuning" of the reconstructed breast is done and nipple-areolar reconstruction and alteration of the opposite breast are also performed.

If scar capsular contracture has occurred after the initial surgery, this issue is addressed through an open capsulotomy during the second procedure. Secondary procedures on the reconstructed breast usually involve one of five different procedures: (1) open capsulotomy, performed for capsular contracture as well as for implant malposition; (2) capsulorrhaphy, performed for inferior, medial, or lateral malpositioning; (3) soft tissue revision, such as revision of medial dog-ears, excision of subaxillary soft tissue redundancy that follows any mastectomy, or revision of unfavorable portions of the mastectomy scar; (4) exchange of prostheses, either replacing an initial expander or changing the initial implant for reasons of volume or symmetry; and (5) revision of autogenous tissue reconstruction for improvement of the breast mound or for revision of abdominal scars.

The most common of the above procedures is an open capsulotomy or capsulectomy. Any breast mound that does not allow upward elevation of the mammary implant during the external massage maneuver is appropriate for either capsulotomy or limited capsulectomy. The degree of encapsulation may range from the Baker II to the Baker IV classification.[45] Capsulotomy technique involves an incision in a small portion of the mastectomy scar, most often immediately lateral to the pectoralis muscle, followed by a myotomy of the muscle cover and cautery incision of the capsule. After removal of the implant, the capsulotomy may be performed by means of an incision around the total perimeter of the capsule at its juncture with the chest wall, and by radial incisions on the anterior hemisphere of the capsule. An alternative to capsulotomy, capsulectomy, is direct excision of that portion of the capsule that is not adherent to the chest wall. Occasionally, an excision of the inferior portion of the anterior hemisphere of the capsule is all that is necessary. Usually, a new implant is introduced. Suction catheters are used for all capsulotomy or capsulectomy procedures, and drains are left in place for 4 to 8 days after surgery. Immediate massage can be performed with greater vigor than at the primary operation because the extent of dissection, and therefore the level of discomfort, is limited compared with that of the initial procedure.

If the initial level of the implant is too low or if it is displaced in a less than ideal medial or lateral position, these undesirable extensions of the pocket may be obliterated by direct suture, in the procedure called capsulorrhaphy. The anterior capsule of the superfluous pocket is sutured to the posterior capsule. This technique has been effective in correcting ectopic positions in the inferior, medial, and lateral directions. Postoperatively, patients are placed in a supportive brassiere for 3 weeks and instructed to continue the implant massage in an upward direction only.

Nipple-areolar reconstruction is offered to the patient during the second stage as a desirable adjunct to reconstruction of the breast mound. The psychological benefits of nipple reconstruction far outweigh the smaller inconvenience and morbidity of the procedure.[46] Most nipple procedures are done at the second stage, but if significant disparity exists between the two breasts in terms of size, shape, and level, the timing of nipple-areolar reconstruction is delayed to yet a third stage, performed in the office under local anesthesia.

My preference is to use the "skate" flap technique,[47] as described by Little in Chapter 38. The skin graft used to close the nipple donor site for the flap reconstruction will constitute the areola. Differences in color can be adjusted at a later time in the office setting by the use of intradermal tattoo. When the opposite areola is reduced during a concomitant reduction mammaplasty or mastopexy, the discarded excess remains the ideal tissue to use for the ipsilateral areolar reconstruction.

At the secondary procedure, adjustments in the opposite breast are also recommended (Fig. 29–18). These may include (1) reduction mammaplasty, (2) mastopexy, (3) augmentation mammaplasty, or (4) contralateral prophylactic mastectomy with implant reconstruction. The indications for contralateral mastectomy for premalignant disease are discussed elsewhere in this text. In many instances, contralateral mastectomy with reconstruction may be the best

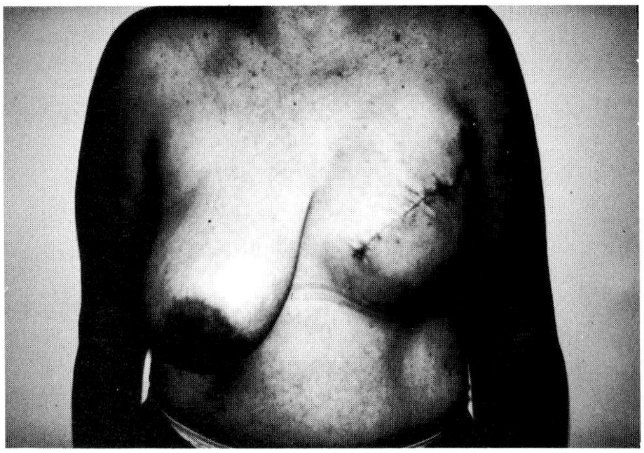

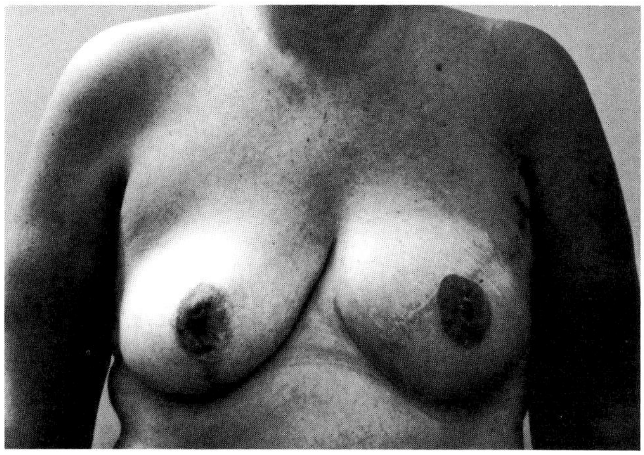

A B

FIGURE 29-18 *A*, This 45-year-old woman received left immediate reconstruction with a 500-ml mammary implant. *B*, Six months after the first operation, right reduction mammaplasty and shared nipple-areolar reconstruction completed the procedure.

choice in providing an optimal aesthetic result on the basis of symmetry, and in decreasing the risk of carcinoma development in the contralateral breast.

ONCOLOGIC CONSIDERATIONS

With the development of submuscular implant techniques, acceptance of immediate reconstruction after subcutaneous mastectomy or other forms of prophylactic mastectomy was almost universal. This acceptance was based on the fact that concerns about compromising the proper treatment of the tumor were not an issue when the mastectomy was done for benign or premalignant disease. However, some of the delays in accepting reconstruction immediately following modified radical mastectomy for cancer were because of concerns expressed by general surgeons, oncologists, and plastic surgeons. These related to potential or theoretically possible limitations on cancer cure, adjuvant treatment, and detection and treatment of recurrent tumor. It remained for these concerns to be answered directly before widespread acceptance of immediate reconstruction could be expected. Specifically, the following areas needed attention.

Completeness of Mastectomy

The two-team approach to mastectomy and reconstruction still gives the general surgeon the opportunity to perform the complete mastectomy that would be performed otherwise in the absence of reconstruction. Although the skin incisions are planned as a team preoperatively, the general surgeon makes the firm decision regarding the margin to be used surrounding the biopsy site of the primary tumor and the extent of the skin to be resected. The nipple-areola complex is considered part of the breast tissue and is always removed with the breast. The immediate reconstruction allows ample exposure of the axilla for complete axillary dissection, the extent of which is determined by the general surgeon. The pectoralis fascia is removed if desired. Deep tumors that invade the pectoralis fascia may require muscle resection. In these instances, reconstruction with local muscle flap techniques, as described above, or by distant musculocutaneous flaps allow for extensive ablative surgery if needed.

Host-Tumor Immunologic Response

Concerns have been expressed that the placement of a silicone implant could have a detrimental effect on the immune response in the host and adversely affect the ability of the body to inhibit recurrent or metastatic disease. There is no evidence to date to indicate an impairment of the immunologic response because of the presence of a silicone prosthesis. Experimental data on mammary implants performed in the rat laboratory model indicate no adverse immunologic effects.[14,15]

Adjuvant Treatment

Our experience with immediate reconstruction in clinical Stage I patients revealed involvement of axillary lymph nodes in approximately one third.[4] This group of patients and some who were node negative with negative estrogen receptors or with large primary tumors were offered systemic adjuvant chemotherapy after wound healing. No change in either the initiation or duration of treatment occurred because of the immediate reconstruction, and no complications of the reconstruction were attributable to the adjuvant therapy. Oncologists generally agree that the most important time to administer adjuvant drugs is in the early course of therapy. I believe there is no justification for delay in beginning chemotherapy even if the prosthesis might seem at risk.

Detection of Recurrences

Concern has been expressed that placement of the silicone prosthesis in the submuscular space may either introduce tumor cells into a new plane of dissection or inhibit detection of recurrences in the local chest wall tissues. In patients who have not undergone reconstruction, it is known that local chest wall recurrences, if they occur, are found in the skin or subcutaneous tissue superficial to the pectoralis major muscle.[48] Detection of such recurrences, therefore, should not be inhibited by the location of an implant behind the pectoralis muscle. The incidence of such local recurrences does not appear to be increased by the submuscular implant immediate reconstructive procedure.[4,49]

CONCLUSION

Experience with immediate breast reconstruction after mastectomy for cancer has led to acceptance of the psychological benefits of this approach and to a refinement in techniques sufficient to produce aesthetic results comparable with those of delayed reconstruction. This experience has diminished concerns about the safety and efficacy of immediate reconstruction. In the rapidly changing field of breast cancer treatment, the woman desiring preservation of feminine form has the clear additional alternative of immediate reconstruction if mastectomy is selected for her treatment.

References

1. Hueston JT, McKenzie G. Breast reconstruction after radical mastectomy. Aust NZ J Surg 1970; 39:367.
2. Noone RB, Frazier TG, Hayward CZ, et al. Patient acceptance of immediate reconstruction following mastectomy. Plast Reconstr Surg 1981; 69:632.
3. Frazier TG, Noone RB. Immediate reconstruction in the treatment of primary carcinoma of the breast. Surg Gynecol Obstet 1983; 157:413.
4. Noone RB, Murphy JB, Spear SL, et al. A six-year experience with immediate reconstruction after mastectomy for cancer. Plast Reconstr Surg 1985; 76:258.
5. Frazier TG, Noone RB. An objective analysis of immediate simultaneous reconstruction in the treatment of primary carcinoma of the breast. Cancer 1985; 55:1202.
6. Rosato FE, Fink PJ, Horten CE, et al. Immediate post mastectomy reconstruction. J Surg Oncol 1976; 8:277.
7. Georgiade GS, Georgiade NG, McCarty KS Jr, et al. Modified radical mastectomy with immediate reconstruction for carcinoma of the breast. Ann Surg 1981; 193:565.
8. Georgiade GS, Georgiade NG, McCarty KS Jr, et al. Rationale for immediate reconstruction of the breast following modified radical mastectomy. Ann Plast Surg 1982; 8:20.
9. Wilkinson LH, Peloso OA, Dail WG Jr. Modified radical mastectomy with immediate breast reconstruction. Arch Surg 1982; 117:579.
10. Webster DJT, Mansel RE, Hughes LE. Immediate reconstruction of the breast after mastectomy: Is it safe? Cancer 1984; 53:1416.
11. Georgiade GS, Riefkohl R, Cox E, et al. Long-term clinical outcome of immediate reconstruction after mastectomy. Plast Reconstr Surg 1985; 76:415.
12. Media Survey. American Society of Plastic and Reconstructive Surgeons, Chicago, 1988.
13. Rules and Regulations, Dept of Health and Human Services, Health Care Financing Administration. Federal Register September 1983:39881.
14. Harris HI. Surgery of breast implants from the point of view of carcinogenesis. Plast Reconstr Surg 1961; 28:81.
15. Schuler FA, Rosato FE, Horton CE. Silicone prosthesis and anti-tumor immunity. Plast Reconstr Surg 1978; 61:762.
16. Renneker R, Cutler M. Psychological problems of adjustment to cancer of the breast. JAMA 1952; 148:833.
17. Parkes MC. Bereavement studies of grief in adult life. London, Pelican Books, 1972.
18. Klein R. A crisis to grow on. Cancer 1971; 28:1660.
19. Goldsmith HS, Alday ES. Role of the surgeon and the rehabilitation of the breast cancer patient. Cancer 1971; 28:1672.
20. Asken MJ. Psychoemotional aspects of mastectomy: A review of recent literature. Am J Psychiatry 1975; 132:56.
21. Snyderman RK, Guthrie RH. Reconstruction of the female breast following radical mastectomy. Plast Reconstr Surg 1971; 47:565.
22. Clifford E. The reconstruction experience: The search for restitution. In: Georgiade NG, ed. Breast reconstruction following mastectomy. St Louis: CV Mosby, 1979:22.
23. Stevens LA, McGrath MH, Drus RG, et al. The psychological impact of immediate breast reconstruction for women with early breast cancer. Plast Reconstr Surg 1984; 73:619.
24. Goin MK, Goin JM. Psychological reactions to prophylactic mastectomy synchronous with contralateral breast reconstruction. Plast Reconstr Surg 1982; 70:355.
25. Dean C, Chetty U, Forrest AP. Effects of immediate breast reconstruction on psychosocial morbidity after mastectomy. Lancet 1983; 26:459.
26. Wellisch DK, Schain WS, Noone RB, et al. Psychosocial correlates of immediate versus delayed reconstruction of the breast. Plast Reconstr Surg 1985; 76:713.
27. Schain WS, Wellisch DK, Pasner RO, et al. The sooner the better: A study of psychological factors in women undergoing immediate versus delayed breast reconstruction. Am J Psychiatry 1985; 142:40.
28. Luce EA. Breast reconstruction after mastectomy. South Med J 1983; 76:190.

29. Frazier TG, Rowland CW, Wollery CT, et al. Cooperative value of aspiration cytology and the diagnostic evaluation of breast masses. J Surg Oncol 1979; 8:353.
30. Frazier TG, Rowland CW, Murphy JT, et al. Value of aspiration cytology in the evaluation of dysplastic breasts. Cancer 1980; 46:2878.
31. Fisher B, Bauer M, Margolese R, et al. Five-year results of a randomized clinical trial comparing total mastectomy and segmental mastectomy with or without radiation in the treatment of breast cancer. N Engl J Med 1985; 312:665.
32. Noone RB, Frazier TG, Murphy JB, Little JW. Immediate reconstruction after mastectomy for cancer. Adv Plast Reconstr Surg 1988; 4:51.
33. Singer R, Lewis CM, Franklin JD, et al. Fluorescein test for prediction of flap viability during breast reconstructions. Plast Reconstr Surg 1978; 6:371.
34. Little JW III, Golembe EV, Fisher JB. The "Living Bra" in immediate and delayed reconstruction of the breast following mastectomy for malignant and nonmalignant disease. Plast Reconstr Surg 1981; 68:392.
35. Dowden RV. Achieving a natural inframammary fold and ptotic effect in the reconstructed breast. Ann Plast Surg 1987; 19:524.
36. Paul MD. Primary breast reconstruction with a subpectoral silicone tissue expander. Ann Plast Surg 1985; 15:404.
37. Hyland WT. Immediate breast reconstruction using the skin expander: A modification in technique. Ann Plast Surg 1988; 21:101.
38. Bostwick J, Stephenson TR, Nahai F, et al. Radiation to the breast: Complications amenable to surgical treatment. Ann Surg 1984; 200:543.
39. Slavin SA, Goldwyn RM. The midabdominal rectus abdominis myocutaneous flap: Review of 236 flaps. Plast Reconstr Surg 1988; 81:189.
40. Hartrampf CR. Discussion: Conventional TRAM flap versus free microsurgical TRAM flap for immediate breast reconstruction. Plast Reconstr Surg 1989; 5:842.
41. Dinner MI, Labandter HP, Dowden RV. The role of the rectus abdominis myocutaneous flap in breast reconstruction. Plast Reconstr Surg 1982; 69:209.
42. Hartrampf CR, Scheflan M, Black PW. Breast reconstruction with a transverse abdominal island flap. Plast Reconstr Surg 1982; 69:216.
43. Grotting JC, Urist MM, Maddox WA, Vasconez LO. Conventional TRAM flap versus free microsurgical TRAM flap for immediate breast reconstruction. Plast Reconstr Surg 1989; 5:828.
44. Castiglione CL, Noone RB, Murphy JB, Little JW III. Complications after immediate breast reconstruction and their management. Plast Surg Forum 1987; 10:221.
45. Baker J. Augmentation mammaplasty. In: Owsley JQ, Peterson RA, eds. Symposium on aesthetic surgery of the breast. St Louis: CV Mosby, 1978.
46. Wellisch DK, Schain WS, Noone RB, Little JW. The psychological contribution of nipple addition in breast reconstruction. Plast Reconstr Surg 1987; 80:699.
47. Little JW III. Nipple-areolar reconstruction. Adv Plast Reconstr Surg 1986; 3:43.
48. Gilliland MD, Larsen DL, Copeland EM. Appropriate timing for breast reconstruction. Plast Reconstr Surg 1983; 72:335.
49. Johnson CH, VanHeerden JA, Donohue JH, et al. Oncological aspects of immediate breast reconstruction following mastectomy for malignancy. Arch Surg 1989; 124:819.

C H A P T E R 30

Reconstruction with Implants

SCOTT L. SPEAR, M.D.

Prosthetic breast reconstruction remains the standard and paradigm by which all other methods of breast reconstruction must be measured. This is true for reconstruction in the case of congenital deformity and after mastectomy. The meteoric growth in the numbers of postmastectomy reconstructive procedures during the late 1970s and the 1980s parallels the development of improved implant materials, better techniques, and the arrival of a less aggressive modified radical mastectomy that often allows reconstruction with an implant alone. Whereas breast reconstruction previously required a prodigious investment by patient and surgeon alike, reconstruction with only an implant, either immediate or delayed, represents an opportunity for a restorative procedure much less forbidding than its predecessors.[1] Some of the earliest strides in simple implant breast reconstruction were reported first by Freeman in 1962 and then by Snyderman and Guthrie in 1971, who described a subcutaneous implant placed after mastectomy.[2-4] Further experience in the same decade was reported by Horton and colleagues in 1974 and Jarrett and colleagues in 1978.[5,6] By 1981 Gruber and associates could report with confidence that submuscular breast reconstruction significantly lowered the risk of capsular contracture compared with subcutaneous breast reconstruction.[7] During the same period, submuscular implant placement proved valuable in lowering the rate of implant exposure from 20 percent or more to 1.5 percent.[8]

At present, immediate reconstruction with an implant at the time of mastectomy still offers the greatest economy to both patient and physician.[9-16] It is the fastest operation to perform and the simplest, it requires minimal blood loss, and it usually does not require a commitment to a second procedure. The typical implant reconstruction, immediate or otherwise, requires about 1 hour and typically results in a blood loss of 100 ml or less. My experience with implant reconstruction patients demonstrates that 40 percent choose not to have a second procedure of any kind, and 55 percent do not need or choose to specifically adjust their implant reconstruction. A particularly popular aspect of implant reconstruction with both patients and physicians is its theoretical and proved transparency in terms of examination for recurrent cancer at the site of the mastectomy. In the same context, within the broader medical community, implant reconstruction has slowly earned a certain respectability as a relatively noninvasive, nonmeddlesome procedure that typically avoids significant sidetracking of other oncologic therapeutic processes such as adjuvant chemotherapy or local radiation.

Tissue expansion has probably seen its greatest application in breast reconstruction, yet I and my colleagues at my institution rarely use it.[17-22] Why? To begin with, as mentioned previously, a significant number of our patients with implant reconstructions never have a second implant procedure. They do not require inflation, deflation, capsulotomy, capsulorrhaphy, fold procedure, filler valve removal, or implant exchange. Any type of expander procedure commits these same patients to a second procedure of some kind, as well as the inconvenience and discomfort of both serial expansion and temporary overexpansion. Work is in progress to develop a true permanent expander, but in the meantime the Becker expander and some other long-term expanders go only partway toward solving some of these problems.[23-25] Tissue expanders also have often produced disappointing results. In our experience with expanders we have found the results often no better than those from simple implant reconstructions, and the complication rate higher. Many of the reports of immediate expander reconstructions describe a significantly higher rate of infection and extrusion than was our experience in 1983.[13] Part of the problem results from the philosophy and timing of expansion. If one expands early, in the first 7 to 10 postoperative days, the advantage of a quick start is obtained, with much of the dissected pocket stretched open early. However, all the components of the wound and the overlying incision are also exposed to this same stress long before sturdy wound healing has taken place. On the other hand, if one waits a minimum of 2 or 3 weeks for substantial healing, the process may be safer, but the opportunity of influencing the wound surrounding the implant at the most opportune time has been lost.

By its very nature, the underinflated tissue expander fails to conform to the implant pocket until it is expanded. Again, the Becker implant with its outer lumen of silicone gel performs best in this regard, because it tends to fill the circumference of the base of the submuscular space reasonably well even when underexpanded. Experience with silicone implants shows that an implant that is mobile and moves freely within a larger space is an implant that can look natural, feel comfortable, and, most important, be soft. Smooth implants, whether silicone, saline, or double lumen, perform best in this regard; textured implants and inflatable expanders, especially those with distant injection sites, clearly perform less well. Thus, although inflatable implants may ultimately expand some of the original implant pocket, they often do so at the expense of allowing other portions of that same pocket to contract prematurely. Our approach of early prosthetic displacement exercises (3 to 4 days postoperatively) has proved very successful in keeping the implant space open and also gradually expanding it.

Although interesting work is in progress with textured nonmobile implants and expanders, the long-term results from these alternative methods are not yet available. The one clear advantage of the tissue expander in breast reconstruction remains the option not to expand or even to deflate an implant when the wound is precarious or exhibits necrosis at the skin level. However, a similar advantage can be obtained by using fluorescein or other tissue perfusion markers to define skin viability accurately at the time of wound closure. We recommend that nonviable skin be excised at the time of closure or soon after if it demarcates postoperatively. Previously we often allowed substantial areas of skin necrosis to heal spontaneously in the presence of a secure muscle closure, but we have now abandoned this earlier approach because of its prolonged healing time, the higher risk of infection, the greater chance of implant exposure, and the negative psychological impact upon patients and others. In practice, most areas of significant skin necrosis (more than 1 cm or so), if missed in the operating room, are excised in the office or at the bedside within a few days of surgery.

In the context of total or near-total implant muscle coverage without overlying skin necrosis, a standard silicone implant of average proportions (200 to 300 ml) should be at low risk for extrusion or infection. Although our average implant size at the time of immediate reconstruction remains about 350 ml, we frequently use 500 ml and occasionally 650 ml or more. In our experience, it fortunately is exceedingly rare in properly selected patients that so little skin is left after both the initial mastectomy and subsequent skin trimming that primary wound closure and healing is prevented. In that unusual scenario with inadequate soft tissue cover, a tissue expander may fare no better than an implant. In practice, in most patients, at the time of reconstruction, we are able to replace the breast with a silicone implant matched milliliter for gram of the mastectomy specimen, up to a weight of 500 g or so. Exceptions include the very large breast (more than 600 g) and the precarious wound environment of both poor muscle coverage and extensive skin loss. In these cases, a smaller implant may be chosen with the intention of replacing it with a larger one at a later date. In this last situation, we have learned that in the breast without capsular contracture (approximately 85 percent of our patients) implants typically perform as gradual expanders quite effectively. They allow, for example, the easy placement of a 600-ml implant in the same space in which a 300-ml implant was placed perhaps with some difficulty at the time of mastectomy 6 months previously. When the local wound environment is particularly unfavorable, one may resort to a complementary flap, a tissue expander (underinflated), or may abandon the immediate reconstruction until a later date.

Much of what is negative about tissue expanders is particularly so in the context of immediate breast reconstruction. The problems of skin necrosis, infection, and implant extrusion are significantly reduced with delayed breast reconstruction, and at the same time the apparent need for skin (i.e., expansion) seems greatest in patients in whom the combination of unrestrained previous excision, contraction, and fibrosis often paints a bleak reconstructive picture. Thus, although we generally favor implants over expanders, this is certainly less so in the delayed situation, especially in a woman with one remaining large breast who has a shortage of skin at the mastectomy site and who is not interested in substantially reducing the normal side. In that situation, a tissue expander, despite its other limitations, is a reasonable option in a patient who prefers a prosthetic reconstruction to one with autologous tissue.

PATIENT SELECTION

Now that there are so many more options in breast reconstruction, the results have improved and many of the methods have become easier, but the selection of techniques ironically has grown more complex. Implant reconstruction must be seen and presented to the patient in the context of expanders, latissimus dorsi myocutaneous flaps, transverse rectus abdominis myocutaneous (TRAM) flaps, and free flaps. In that context, I do not recommend an implant for every situation and actually perform implant reconstructions in only 50 percent of patients, using autologous tissue for most of the remaining 40 percent and tissue expanders only rarely. The selection process is somewhat different in the delayed situation than in the immediate situation, but in both cases some patients for personal reasons reject my advice. Although I may not favor the patient's choice, I comply so long as there is a reasonable chance of success and the patient understands the limitations of the chosen technique and my reservations about it.

Patient examination includes breast size, breast ptosis, previous scars, tumor site and size, recent biopsy scars, axillary lymph nodes, and signs of previous irradiation. The abdomen is also assessed for previous scars, excess skin and fat, and abdominal wall strength. When appropriate, the gluteal and latissimus regions are also surveyed as possible donor sites.

The patient is asked about any family history of breast disease, previous biopsies and mammograms, other significant medical problems, any history of cigarette smoking, and (most important) her underlying goals or fantasies about reconstruction, no matter how optimistic. In many ways, a discussion of the patient's preconceptions is both a good starting point for and an important determinant of the breast reconstruction to be selected. Therefore, early in the consultation, I often ask, "What sort of ideas do you have about your breast reconstruction?" or "Have you spoken with anyone who has undergone a reconstruction?" I try to find out whether the patient has an unspoken agenda regarding the remaining breast or the abdomen. I look for indications for a contralateral mastectomy or contraindications to operating on the other breast. Overall, I try to sense how motivated the patient is, how energetic, and how able to weather the rigors of further surgery and the risk of setbacks. No matter what the physical findings, the data derived from these questions often chart the course of the reconstruction and occasionally require abandoning the plan altogether. Assuming a reasonably informed, realistic, and motivated patient, a good case for prosthetic breast reconstruction is a woman whose opposite breast is small (A or B cup), who is minimally ptotic, and who either has or is anticipated to have, after mastectomy, some laxity of skin at the mastectomy site with intact muscle. If the opposite breast is larger or more ptotic, a prosthetic reconstruction may still be reasonable if the patient is either willing to undergo or, preferably, enthusiastic about contralateral reduction or mastopexy. Very tight skin at the mastectomy site, either apparent or anticipated, substantial muscle deficit, and local radiation is each a fairly strong contraindication to simple prosthetic reconstruction, especially in the face of a large pendulous opposite breast that is not slated for aggressive reduction or mastopexy. When the opposite breast becomes large (C cup) or more ptotic, autogenous reconstruction begins to appear as a significant consideration, and if the breast is very large (D cup or greater), autogenous reconstruction is clearly advantageous. Prosthetic reconstruction in the last situation requires radical reduction or mastopexy to achieve even a reasonable aesthetic solution.

In balancing alternatives, the status of the lower abdomen is often pivotal. A tight and lean abdomen offers little encouragement for autogenous reconstruction and is chosen only when other factors preclude successful prosthetic reconstruction (e.g., previous irradiation or severe skin deficiency). A generous lower abdomen or one with unattractive scars may offer the opportunity of secondary gain in that region by enhancing the donor site while reconstituting the breast. Special caution is advised before the abdominal donor site is chosen in women who are heavy smokers, are poorly motivated, or have a protuberant abdomen by virtue of poor muscle tone rather than generous amounts of superficial fat.

Although advocates of immediate breast reconstruction, we find that patient selection in this situation is often more difficult because the defect is still unknown and must be inferred from the physical findings and history before mastectomy. A large tumor or an awkward upper quadrant biopsy scar can be expected to complicate the planning and increase the required skin resection, thus weighing against facile prosthetic reconstruction. Multiple breast scars from biopsies or previous cosmetic surgery again complicate the planning and increase the likelihood of greater skin loss, either from deliberate resection or from necrosis. The pendulous breast, either large or atrophic, may seem to offer abundant skin left over for the reconstruction, but these patients are particularly prone to extensive skin necrosis because of the sheer length of the flaps often required to complete the mastectomy. Finally, in immediate reconstruction, previous experience with the participating general surgeon often makes it possible to predict whether implant reconstruction is feasible in terms of adequate amounts of viable muscle and skin at the completion of the mastectomy.

PREOPERATIVE PLANNING

After the initial assessment of the patient, it is time to discuss the primary plan and its alternatives. This discussion is relatively simple in a woman with a small breast and a favorable local tissue environment. A simple implant should work well with a reasonable possibility of avoiding a second implant procedure (Figs. 30-1, 30-2). If this patient has already undergone mastectomy, we attempt to retrieve the weight of the breast from the previous operative and pathology records. If it is an immediate reconstruction, we weigh the specimen and match it with an appropriate implant. With encouragement, at this point a significant number of women with small breasts will confess a desire for a reconstruction larger than the original, with an augmentation on the

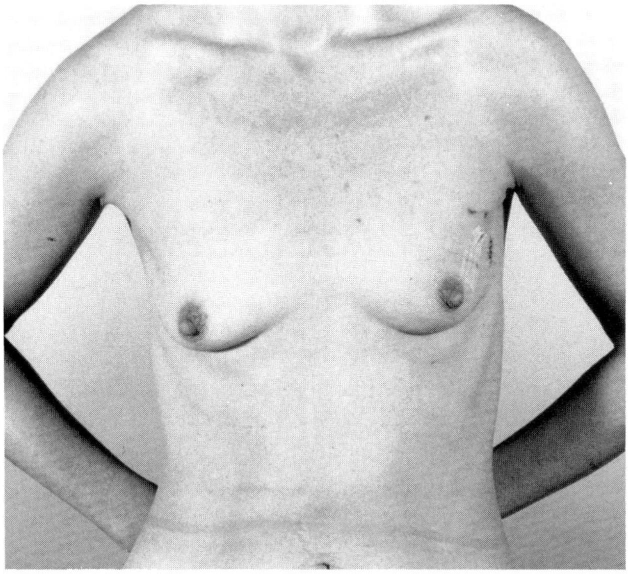

A

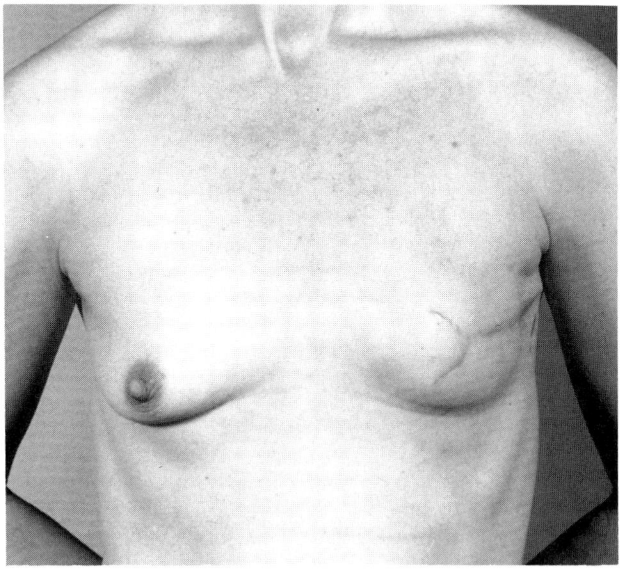

B

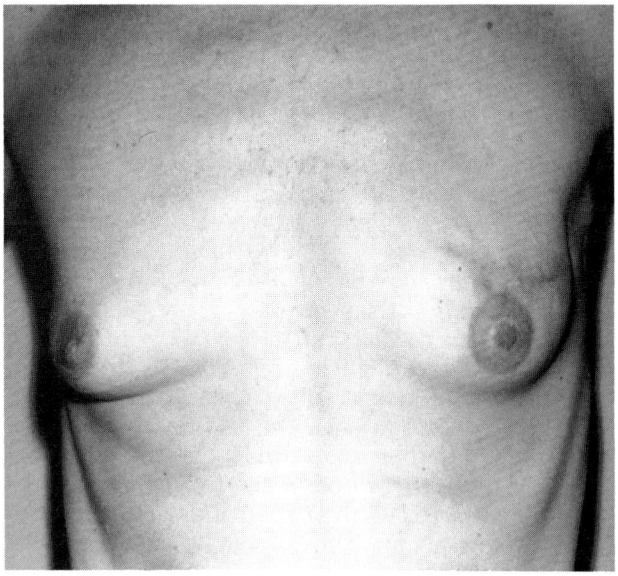

C

FIGURE 30-1 *A*, A 40-year-old woman with a very small breast before immediate breast reconstruction. *B*, After left breast reconstruction with a 120-ml implant. *C*, Completed result after nipple reconstruction and tattoo.

opposite side. In the delayed situation, this is often possible, increasing the reconstruction size typically by 240 ml or so over the mastectomy specimen size and simultaneously augmenting the contralateral breast by the same amount. In the immediate setting, it may be wiser to wait, rather than expose the acute mastectomy wound to the greater stress (Figs. 30-3, 30-4).

In the woman with an ample breast (full B or C cup) and some ptosis, the consultation becomes more complex. Implant reconstruction in this setting is a rough approximation of the normal and nearly always requires at least one adjustment of the implant as well as manipulation of the opposite breast to achieve a reasonable aesthetic outcome (Fig. 30-5). Despite this, many of these patients, especially those less motivated, never have a second procedure. Instead, after the rigors of mastectomy, reconstruction, and chemotherapy, they choose to accept the disappointing compromise of an implant reconstruction that somewhat matches their normal breast only when they wear a brassiere. For a more acceptable outcome in these patients, the initial implant must be thought of as a preliminary expander, with a second larger and permanent implant replacing it approximately 6 months later. It is in this same situation, when a patient is appropriately motivated for both expansion and a second procedure, that an expander makes the most sense. The more difficult part of this consultation relates to the opposite breast, and the most important issue is the risk of disease there. Certain risk factors such as family history,

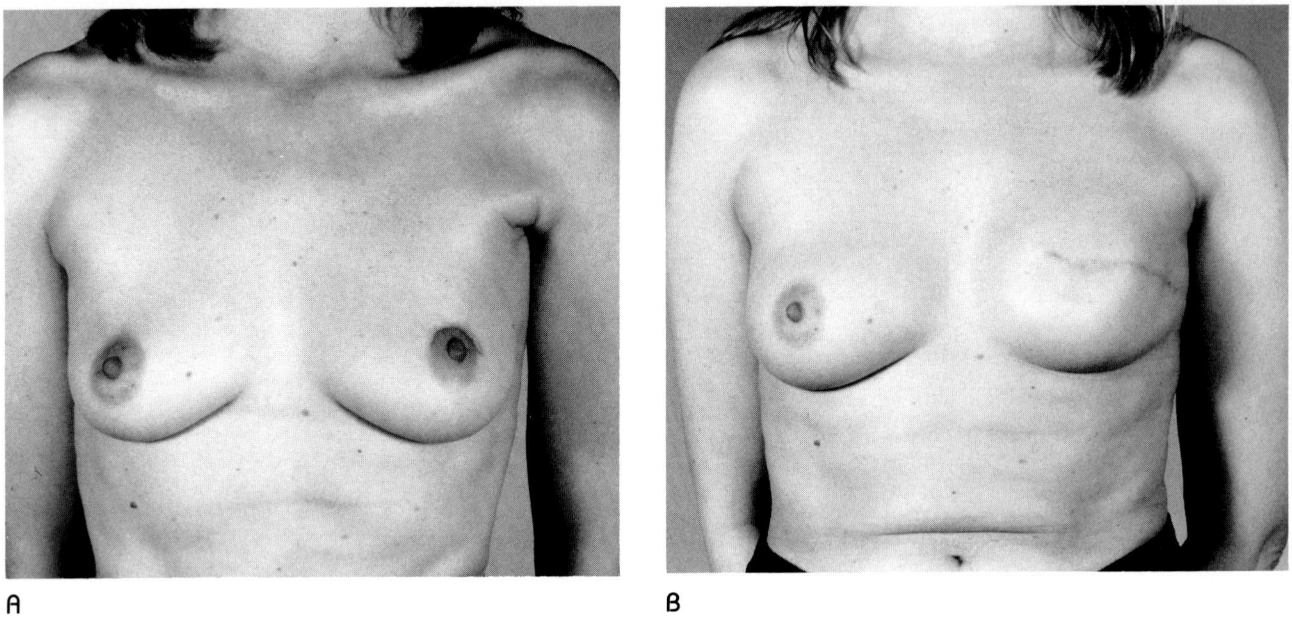

FIGURE 30–2 *A*, A 42-year-old woman with a small but ample breast before immediate breast reconstruction. *B*, After left breast reconstruction with a 200-ml implant. At a later procedure, the patient is scheduled for a minor inferior capsulotomy and nipple-areola reconstruction to be followed by tattoo.

abnormal mammography, lobular carcinoma, multiple previous biopsies, and intraductal disease make contralateral mastectomy a logical option. This is especially so when a reduction is contemplated as the other alternative. When advising a contralateral reduction mammaplasty as part of the plan, therefore, we always review these factors with the oncologist and general surgeon to be certain that we are not interfering with the surveillance of a breast at particularly high risk. Although the same issues pertain somewhat to a contralateral mastopexy, we do not consider that a mastopexy significantly interferes with the follow-up of the patient's normal breast. If contralateral subcutaneous or simple mastectomy is chosen, the reconstruction plan obviously is altered to match an opposite reconstruction rather than the original. When contralateral mastectomy is not appropriate, reduction mammaplasty or mastopexy is most appealing in a patient whose original breast is, for whatever reason, unattractive. For a patient with an attractive large or pendulous breast, adjustment to match the reconstruction is sometimes difficult for the patient to accept. We try to make it clear to these patients that an autogenous breast reconstruction may actually achieve a suitable match more easily than a prosthetic one, even though the initial operation is significantly more complex.

PERIOPERATIVE PROCEDURES

Before surgery, photographs are taken as a baseline and may prove helpful in the operating room. The normal breast is marked to define both its inframammary fold and the shadow of its ptosis in the upper abdomen or lower thorax. If neither mastopexy nor reduction is planned later, the full amount of ptosis is noted. If some later lift is anticipated, a third line is also marked in between the fold and the ptosis shadow line. In delayed reconstruction the previous mastectomy scar is always used, excising it if it is narrow, but incising it only in part if it is fairly spread. The extent of proposed dissection is marked in reference to the marks on the opposite side. Thus for a contralateral small, nonptotic breast, the fold alone is duplicated. Ptosis, when present on the opposite side, is mimicked with an additional curved line drawn to match the ptosis shadow mark on the opposite side. When contralateral adjustment is planned, a third curved line may be drawn midway between the other two. For immediate reconstruction, in addition to the above lines, the extent of skin resection is mapped out to include the nipple-areola, the biopsy site, the tumor surface area, and axillary access. Clearly, one of the major advantages of immediate reconstruction is both controlling and understanding the cutaneous defect from the mastectomy. In small and moderate-sized breasts, skin patterns oriented transversely from the nipple laterally do best. In larger or more ptotic breasts, vertical patterns may work as well so long as the vertical resection does not extend too far superiorly beyond the level of where the nipple would be marked were this a reduction mammaplasty. Superior quadrant tumors, especially medial ones, result in the most awkward excisions, the most postoperative flattening

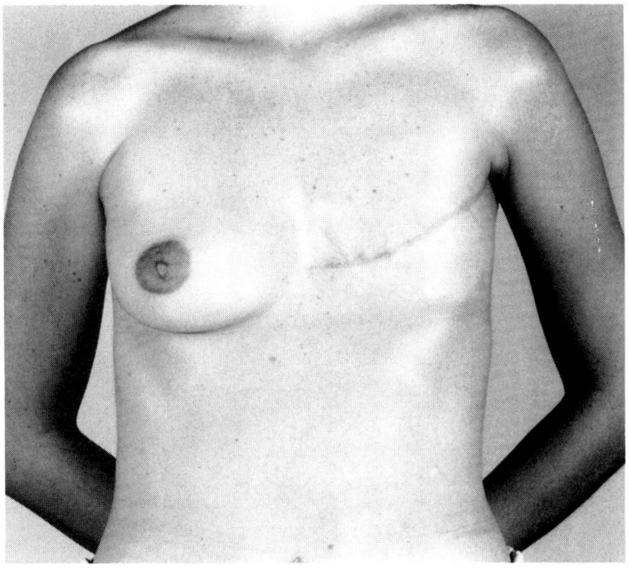

A

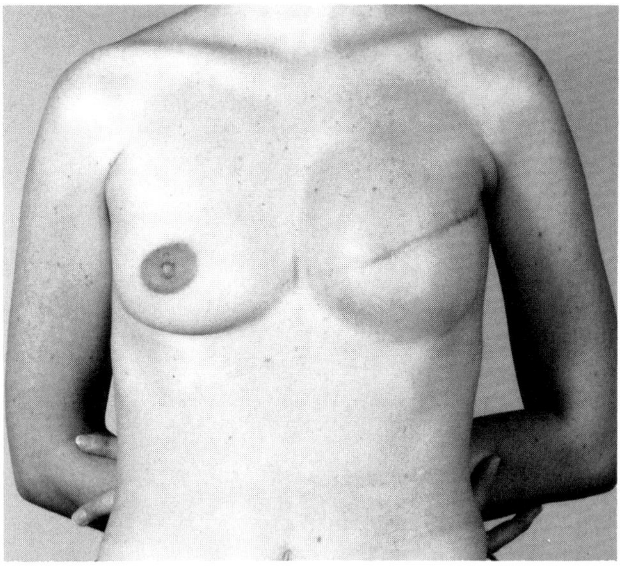

B

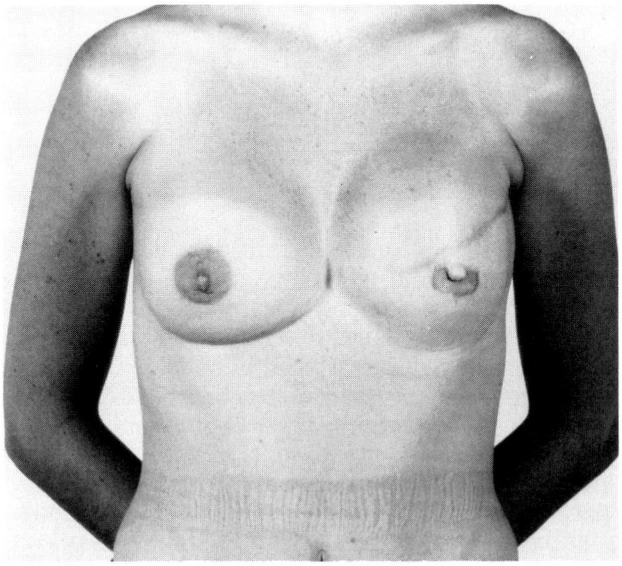

C

FIGURE 30-3 *A*, A 38-year-old woman after left modified radical mastectomy. *B*, After reconstruction with a 365-ml implant. *C*, Four months later after right augmentation with a 200-ml implant, an increase on the left to 420 ml, and partial nipple-areola reconstruction to be followed by tattoo.

of the breast and the most visible and unattractive scars. Inframammary scars from previous augmentation mammaplasty, as well as other breast scars from previous biopsies, increase the likelihood of flap necrosis.

SURGERY

Prosthetic breast reconstruction, immediate or delayed, is virtually always done under general anesthesia. A submuscular dissection is performed using fiberoptic lighting, electrocautery, and blunt dissection. The initial myotomy is created where the individual local circumstances dictate: underlying the mastectomy scar or somewhere between the fourth and fifth intercostal spaces, wherever the fascia seems sturdiest and the eventual skin cover is judged to be most reliable. The muscle is opened to the level of the underlying rib or intercostal fascia. The area of submuscular undermining is enlarged first where the going is easiest, medially near the sternal border and superiorly just inferior to the clavicle. Inferior and lateral dissection proceeds one rib at a time, elevating pectoralis major, rectus abdominis, and serratus anterior muscle fibers from their rib origins under direct vision. Fascia attachments are severed safely after appropriated tunnels have been created overlying the ribs. Submuscular dissection extends to the marked inframammary fold and almost to the midax-

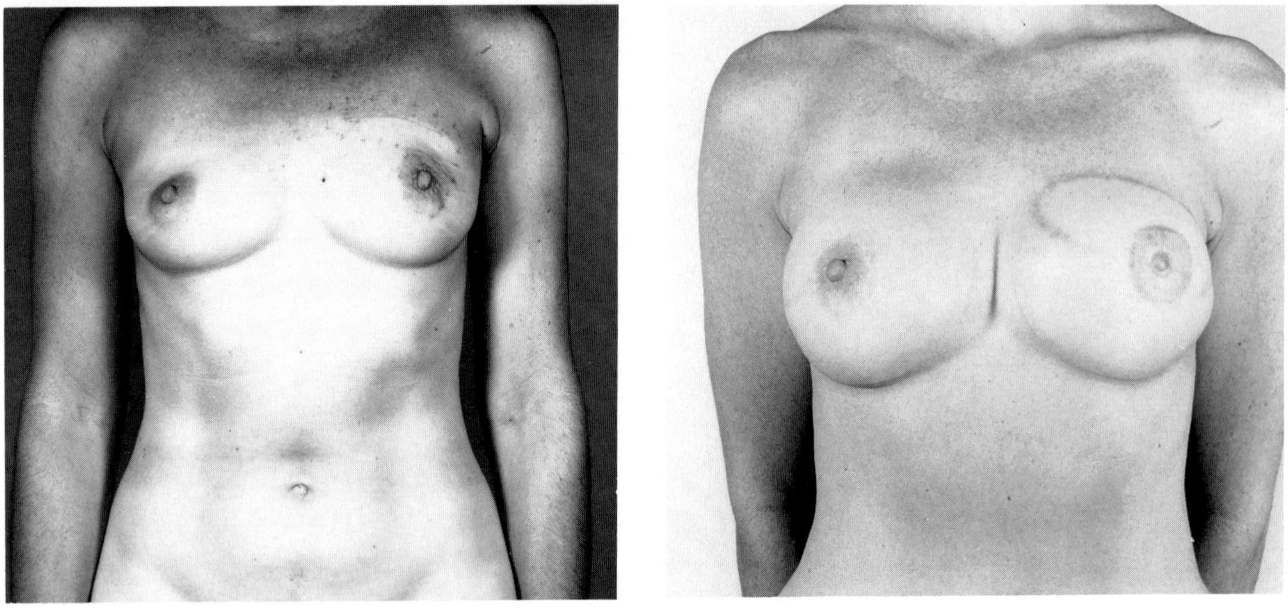

A B

FIGURE 30-4 *A*, A 38-year-old woman before modified radical mastectomy; she was interested in enlargement as well as reconstruction. *B*, The left breast was reconstructed with a 200-ml implant combined with a transverse rectus abdominis myocutaneous (TRAM) flap to replace the large skin excision. The right breast was simultaneously augmented with a 180-ml submuscular implant. Later, a right subcutaneous mastectomy for in situ disease was performed, and the right submuscular implant was increased to 485 ml and the left to 360 ml. Nipple reconstruction and tattoo completed the treatment.

illary line. Blunt and sharp dissection beyond the inframammary fold may be continued to or toward the level of contralateral breast ptosis when judged appropriate. In practice, this may be anywhere from 1 to as much as 6 cm of additional undermining, which need not be (and preferably should not be) rigorously submuscular as was the dissection superior to the fold. Just how far beyond the fold to dissect is a matter of judgment, which in any case can be revised later. A big pocket with a dissection well past the inframammary fold to the level of contralateral ptosis will accept a larger implant. It also tends to minimize early postoperative superior fullness, but can create discomfort where the prosthesis rides below the brassiere, and clearly requires a second operation to create a fold. As a practical compromise, I prefer to limit the inferior pocket extension to 1 or 2 cm below the fold, typically about half the distance between the fold line and the ptosis line. This produces a more commodious implant space, yet minimizes the awkwardness associated with folds of different heights. A fold 1 or 2 cm lower than its opposite need not necessarily be elevated at a later date.

Every effort is made to create an intact muscular brassiere with the original surgical myotomy as its only defect, but it is not unusual for some additional tears to develop in the overlying muscle. In the delayed environment, this is not of particular concern and usually goes unnoticed. In the immediate situation, even small tears are obvious, and larger ones can threaten the success of the entire procedure (Fig. 30-6). In practice, we repair weak areas of muscle with multiple rows of absorbable material. Areas of torn fascia or injured muscle are often repaired before the submuscular dissection to avoid expanding potentially small tears into larger ones. Rarely, the muscle cover may shred to such a degree that is cannot be directly sutured. Three options remain at this point. One may choose to postpone the reconstruction, especially when the skin flaps are also tenuous, the disease is advanced, or the muscle tear is a result of direct excision for locally invasive disease. A second option is to narrow the muscle defect as much as possible and place a smaller implant or expander just to get through this difficult moment. This is appealing in a patient with healthy skin flaps and modest-sized breasts (200 to 400 g). The third option, and my least favorite, is the transposition of a local muscle or fascial flap, either latissimus dorsi or rectus abdominis. The rectus fascia flap is rarely used in my practice because it requires quite a low and difficult dissection to obtain a patch of fascia for a lower medial defect, when in fact these defects are well tolerated even when unrepaired because the overlying skin in that location is usually healthy. The latissimus dorsi muscle flap is used more frequently and can provide an ample muscle strap even when dissected with the patient supine. However, with the patient in this position this is a bloody and difficult dissection, and one that adds substantially to the morbidity of the procedure

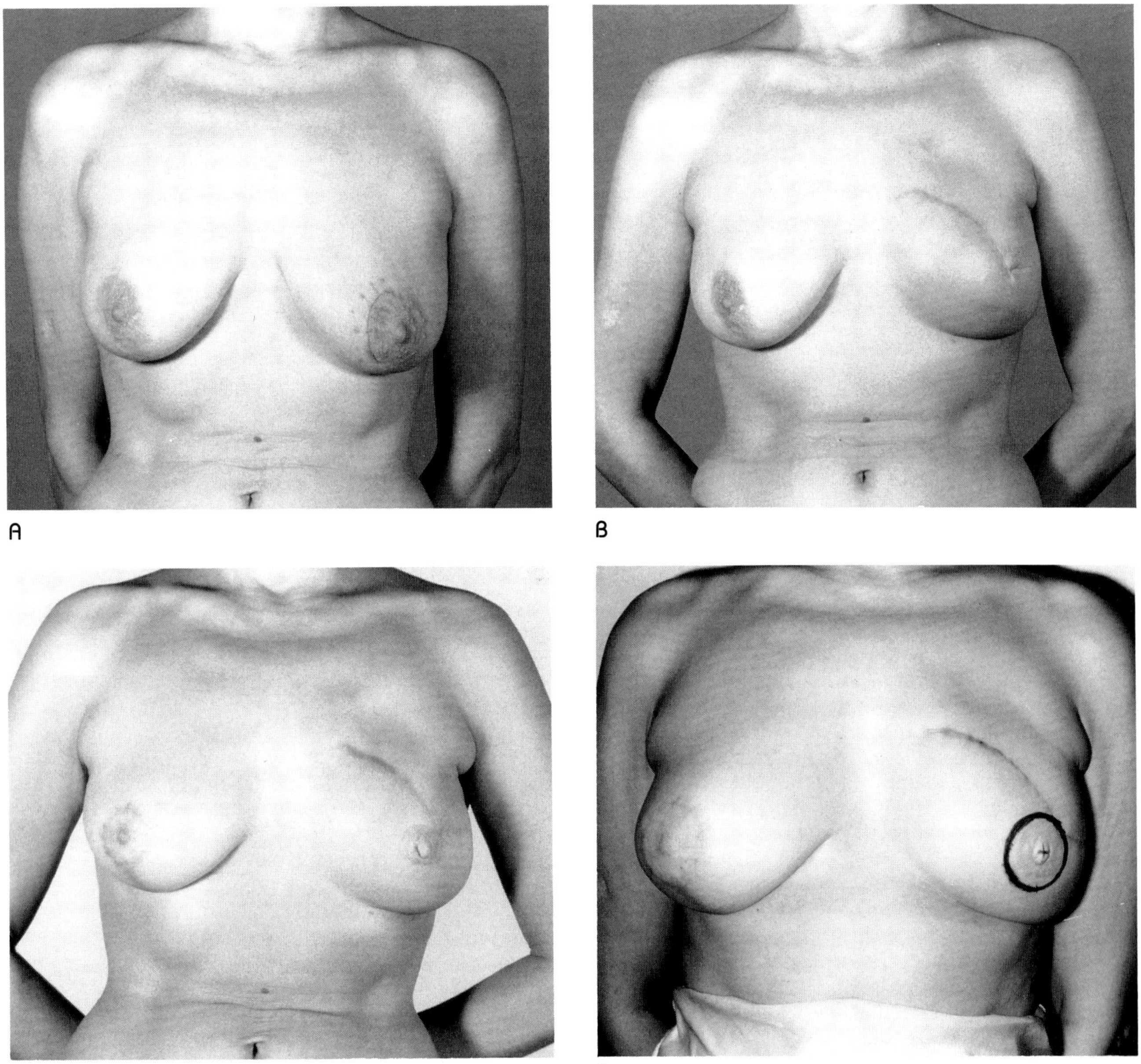

A B C D

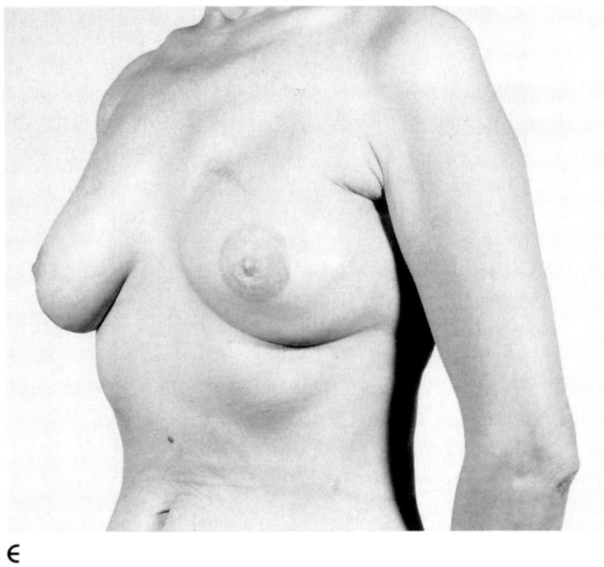

E

FIGURE 30–5 *A*, A 45-year-old woman with C-cup breast before left mastectomy. *B*, After left immediate reconstruction with a 460-ml implant. *C*, After right mastopexy and initial left nipple-areola reconstruction. *D*, Before tattoo. *E*, Finished reconstruction.

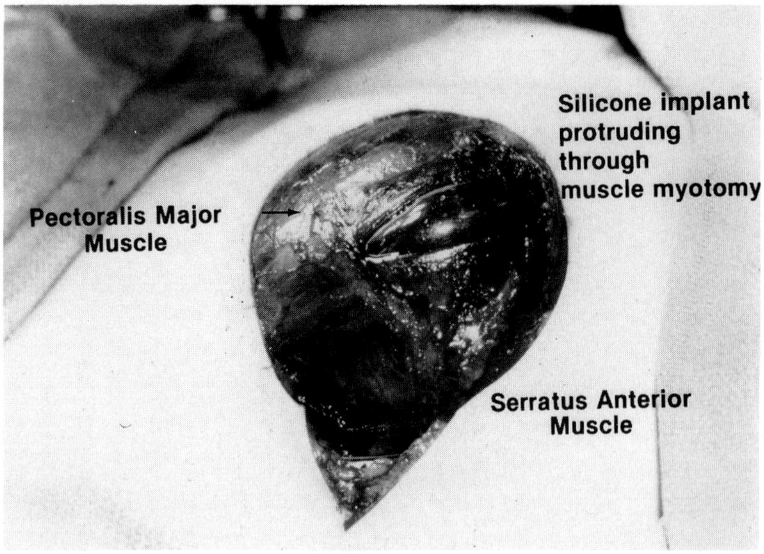

FIGURE 30-6 Typical appearance after modified radical mastectomy and placement of a submuscular implant. The submuscular space usually accommodates implants up to 500 ml and occasionally larger. This allows replacement of the breast on a millimeter of implant per gram of breast basis up to 500 g of breast tissue. Larger breasts require expanders, serial implants, a TRAM flap, or a contralateral reduction mammaplasty.

in terms of bleeding, serous drainage, and discomfort.

After completion of the submuscular dissection, suction drains are placed in the submuscular and, in the case of immediate reconstruction, the subcutaneous space and brought out through the axilla. For convenience, muscle-approximating sutures may be placed at the site of the muscle myotomy before the implant is inserted. In delayed reconstruction, implant sizers may be helpful to select the final implant size, although the previous mastectomy specimen weight is also a helpful guide. With the patient flexed somewhat in a sitting position, the sizer may also help define areas for reshaping the pocket dissection. In the submuscular space, it is much easier to enlarge the space at this stage rather than try to close off an area previously enthusiastically dissected a little too far. In immediate reconstructions, sizers are of little value, but the readily available specimen weight is the ideal size predictor.

Our current preference is a smooth-walled, double-lumen silicone gel and saline implant with a small outer compartment, which is filled typically with 40 ml of physiologic saline to which we add 40 mg percent (16-mg total dose) of methylprednisolone. In these same circumstances, one might also use a saline implant, a simple gel implant, a smooth or textured expander, a textured silicone implant, a reverse double-lumen (Becker-type) silicone-saline expander, or a polyurethane-coated silicone implant. Each of the above approaches may work very well, but we continue to prefer the double-lumen implant with Solu-Medrol added because of its proved reliability during 10 years in over 500 cases of breast reconstruction both immediate and delayed. If other implants, either currently available or to be developed, prove superior, clearly we will upgrade our implant selection.

Before the implant is inserted, the lower panel of the muscular bra is checked for any tight bands that can be partially transected or weakened from within in order to help the implant settle to the most dependent areas of the pocket. With the implant placed beneath the muscle, the myotomy is closed with interrupted 3-0 synthetic absorbable sutures. At this point, in immediate reconstruction, if there is any question regarding skin flap viability, especially in the face of doubtful muscle integrity, intravenous fluorescein is given to evaluate skin capillary perfusion. After preliminary skin approximation, nonfluorescent areas are excised. In order to reduce tension at the site of skin closure, the inframammary region and fold are often undermined by the creation of multiple tunnels directed inferiorly, much as if suction lipectomy of the upper abdomen were being performed. The skin is then closed in layers with key 3-0 absorbable sutures to the deep dermis. Additional intradermal 4-0 synthetic absorbable sutures are used as well as superficial intradermal monofilament pullout sutures or skin staples. Every effort is made to keep the ultimate mastectomy scar as short as possible, and away from the upper or medial aspects of the breast. If skin staples are used, they are removed on the third or fourth postoperative day and replaced with Steri-Strips. At surgery, a light greasy dressing of Xeroform or Vaseline gauze is applied over the skin flaps, with a thin layer of gauze on top of that.

With delayed reconstruction, patients usually return home 1 or 2 days after surgery. Immediate reconstruction necessitates 4 or 5 days of hospitalization. In the delayed group, follow-up occurs 3 to 5 days after surgery when implant displacement exercise instructions are begun. When drainage is minimal (less than 30 ml per day) the submuscular drain is removed. Systemic antibiotic coverage with a cephalosporin is continued until the drain is removed. Careful follow-up is continued at least once weekly for 3 weeks to ensure implant mobility and to monitor for infection or fluid accumulation. After 3 weeks the implant should be somewhat mobile but can be expected still to sit too high, one of the drawbacks of this strategy. The patient is asked to continue displacement exercises four times daily until her next visit in 3 months' time. During this interval, typically about 6 or 8 weeks after surgery, the implant, if mobile, will drop substantially.

Follow-up of the immediate implant reconstruction patient is more complex. During the first 3 or 4 days, careful note is made of any areas of impending skin necrosis. Nearly always, areas of necrosis are excised under sterile conditions at the bedside or in the office within 10 days of operation. The wound is resutured without undermining. Truly large areas of skin necrosis in our experience are exceedingly rare and may require a return trip to the operating room to allow rearrangement of skin flaps for closure. Careful observation and the liberal use of intravenous fluorescein at the initial operation should virtually eliminate this situation. As in delayed reconstruction, displacement exercises begin on the third or fourth postoperative day, but they are done more delicately, especially when the muscle is known to be attenuated. Displacement in these precarious circumstances at this point is limited either to only superior migration or even to none at all. Ten or 14 days later, in the absence of any local wound complications, these exercises can be performed with more vigor, essentially just as in the delayed reconstruction. As in the delayed context, drains are removed as the effluent diminishes, and antibiotics are continued up to that point. Subsequent subcutaneous seromas are carefully aspirated until the skin is adherent to the muscle. After 3 or 4 weeks, when the wound is well healed and the implant mobile, the patient is discharged from observation for 3 months and instructed to continue implant displacement exercises four times daily. This interlude from repeat office visits is welcomed by the immediate reconstruction patient, who is typically in the midst of 6 months of adjuvant chemotherapy at that time.

SUBSEQUENT PROCEDURES

As mentioned, a significant percentage of implant reconstruction patients choose not to undergo a second procedure. This is especially so in the immediate reconstruction group, of whom 50 percent do not undergo any second procedure whatsoever. Submuscular breast reconstruction with a double-lumen implant containing intraluminal corticosteroids represents a method of slow but steady tissue expansion with a mobile implant instead of an expander. Eighty-five percent of these patients can be expected to have a loose pocket with a thin capsule and appropriately stretched out skin within 3 months of the reconstruction. Although capsulotomy would be appropriate in the 15 percent of patients with firm initial results, 85 percent do not require aggressive capsulotomy as part of the second-stage procedure. Forty percent instead have their implants repositioned by selective open capsulotomy, capsulorrhaphy, or both in different areas of the pocket. Patients with a well-developed inframammary fold on the opposite side may benefit from the re-creation of that fold on the reconstructed side, performed as either an internal or external fold procedure. The internal technique described by Pennisi[26] is performed through the original mastectomy scar and obviates the need for additional incisions. Although technically more difficult, it is the procedure I prefer. The external technique of Ryan [27,28] requires a second incision in the inframammary fold (Figs. 30-7 to 30-12). Some patients have only a change of implant size or scar revision. Thirty percent of patients undergo a nipple-areola reconstruction, 35 percent of the immediate reconstructions, and less than 10 percent of the delayed reconstructions. Twenty-five percent of patients have the nipple reconstruction without any other procedure on the reconstructed breast. Capsulotomy performed for capsular contracture requires re-creation of a submuscular space throughout the proposed pocket. The same is true for lowering the fold or shifting the implant medially or laterally. Capsulotomy performed to encourage greater projection or to allow the creation of ptosis requires a different approach. Here the overlying muscle is transected to allow the implant to come into contact with unscarred, distensible subcutaneous fat. To correct the severe flattening often seen on the inferior pole of a breast reconstructed with an implant, serial radial cuts are made transecting overlying capsule, muscle, and fascia in an effort to create a billowing of these lower pole tissues. Capsulotomy to recreate ptosis requires a bivalving type transection of the inferior capsule circumference, followed by centripetal subcutaneous undermining as far as necessary to recruit the necessary skin up onto the lower breast. The inframammary fold is recreated by serial rows of running sutures between the advanced overlying dermis and the posterior capsular tissues, including capsule, periosteum, and intercostal muscles.

Nipple-areola reconstruction can be combined with modest breast adjustments, but should be avoided when major adjustments such as implant lowering or elevating may make the nipple site selection problematic. Likewise, major shifts of the contralateral breast such as in mastopexy, reduction, or mastectomy discourage simultaneous opposite nipple reconstruction because of the increased uncertainty about creating symmetry. Improving standards of breast reconstruction overall demand that the nipple reconstruction phase be postponed until the site can be chosen with greater confidence.

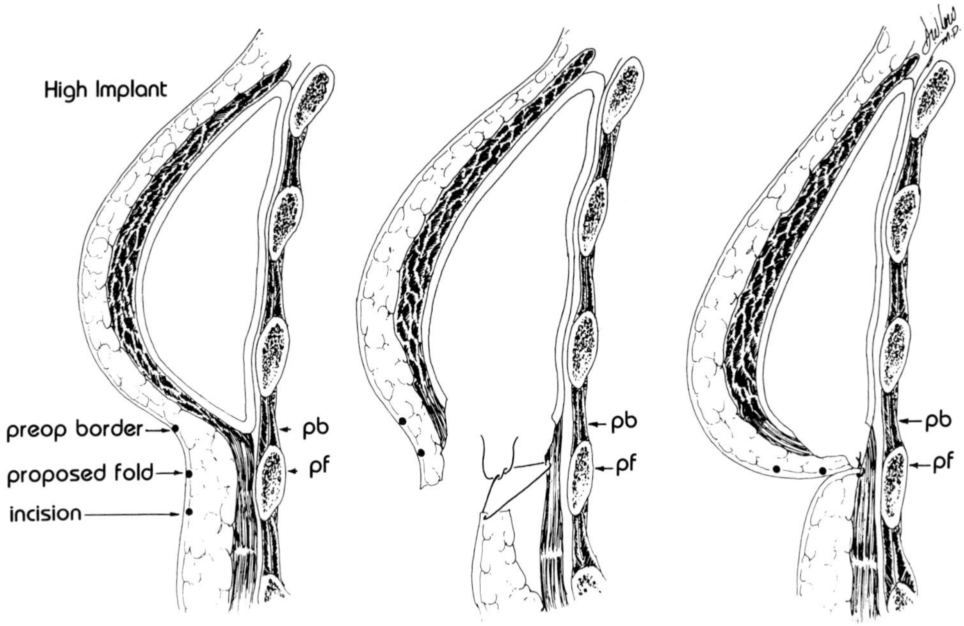

FIGURE 30-7 An open capsulotomy to lower the implant. The capsulorrhaphy is performed at a lower level to help create an inframammary fold. The capsulotomy-capsulorrhaphy can also be performed as a closed technique through the mastectomy scar.

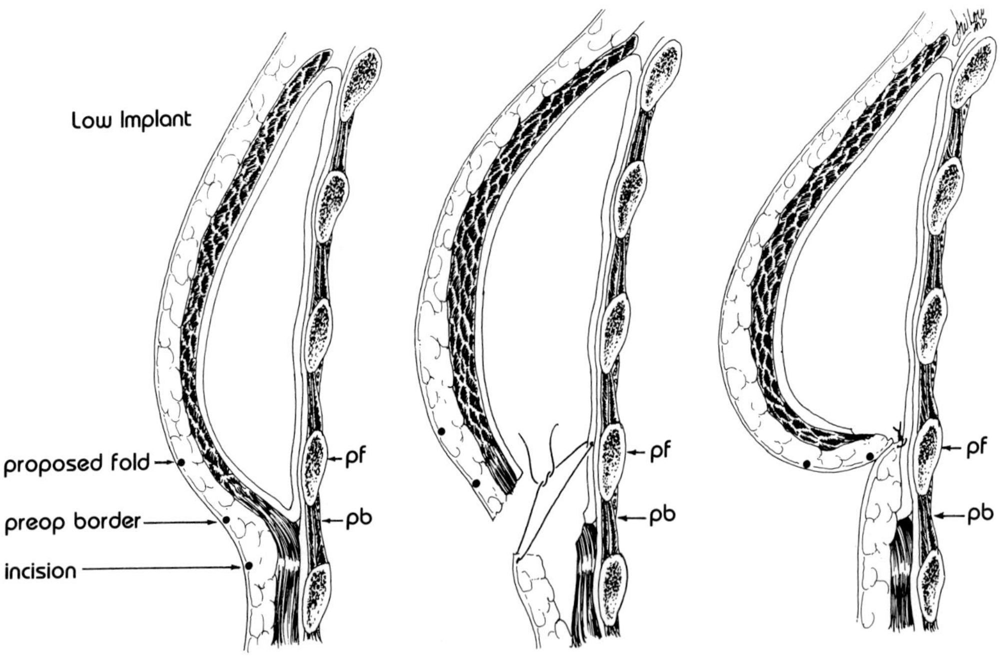

FIGURE 30-8 Raising of an implant with simultaneous inframammary fold formation may be performed through an inframammary incision as illustrated, or by a closed technique.

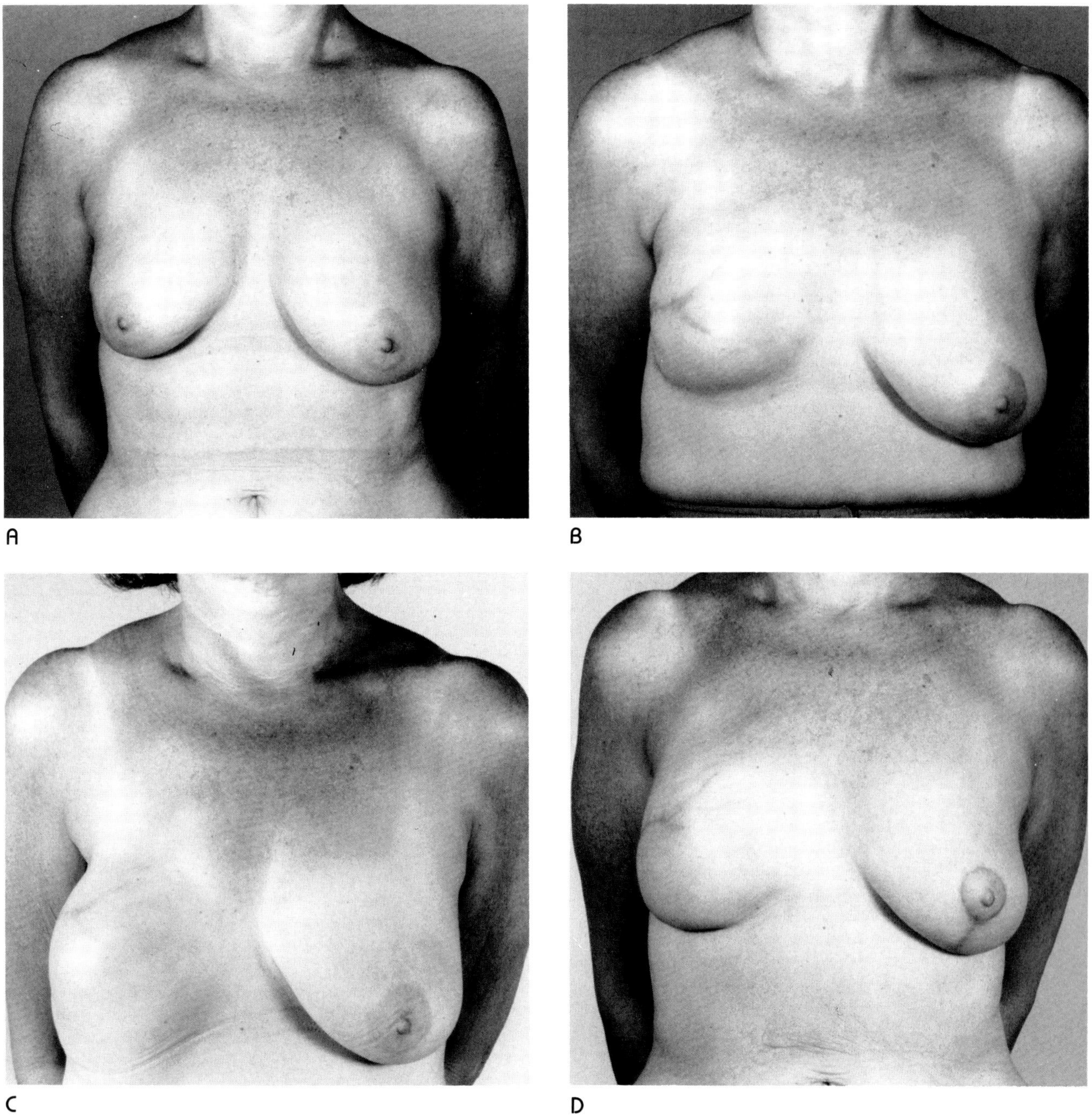

FIGURE 30–9 *A*, A 52-year-old woman before modified radical mastectomy. *B*, After right immediate reconstruction with a 500-ml implant, which produced a breast that was too high and yet smaller than the contralateral. *C*, A capsulotomy to lower the implant and an increase in size has left a different type of asymmetry. *D*, The right breast has been lifted and a new fold developed by capsulorrhaphy while the implant is reduced to 550 ml and the left breast lifted with a mastopexy.

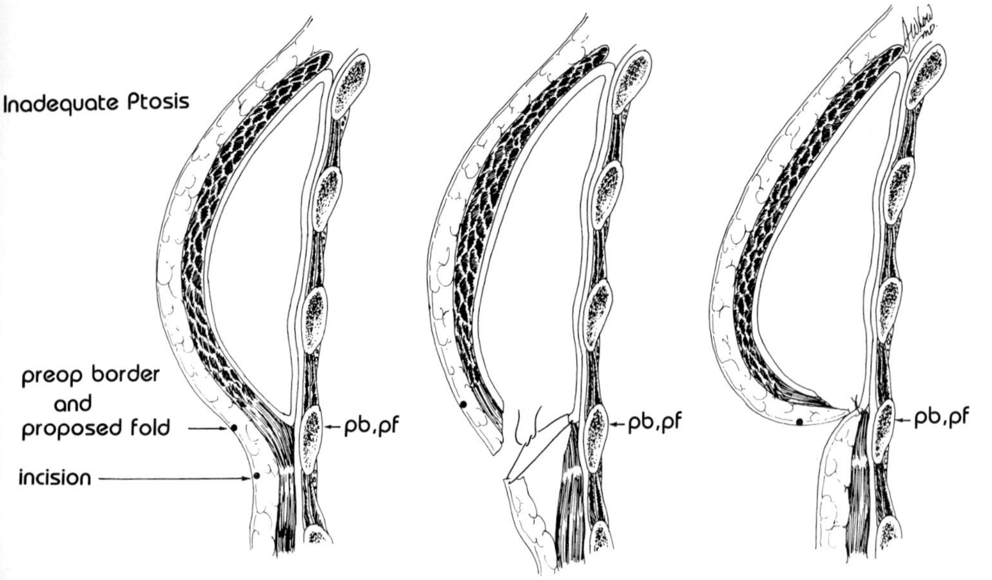

FIGURE 30 – 10 Technique for improved fold definition without significantly elevating or lowering the implant. This may also be performed as a closed capsulorrhaphy.

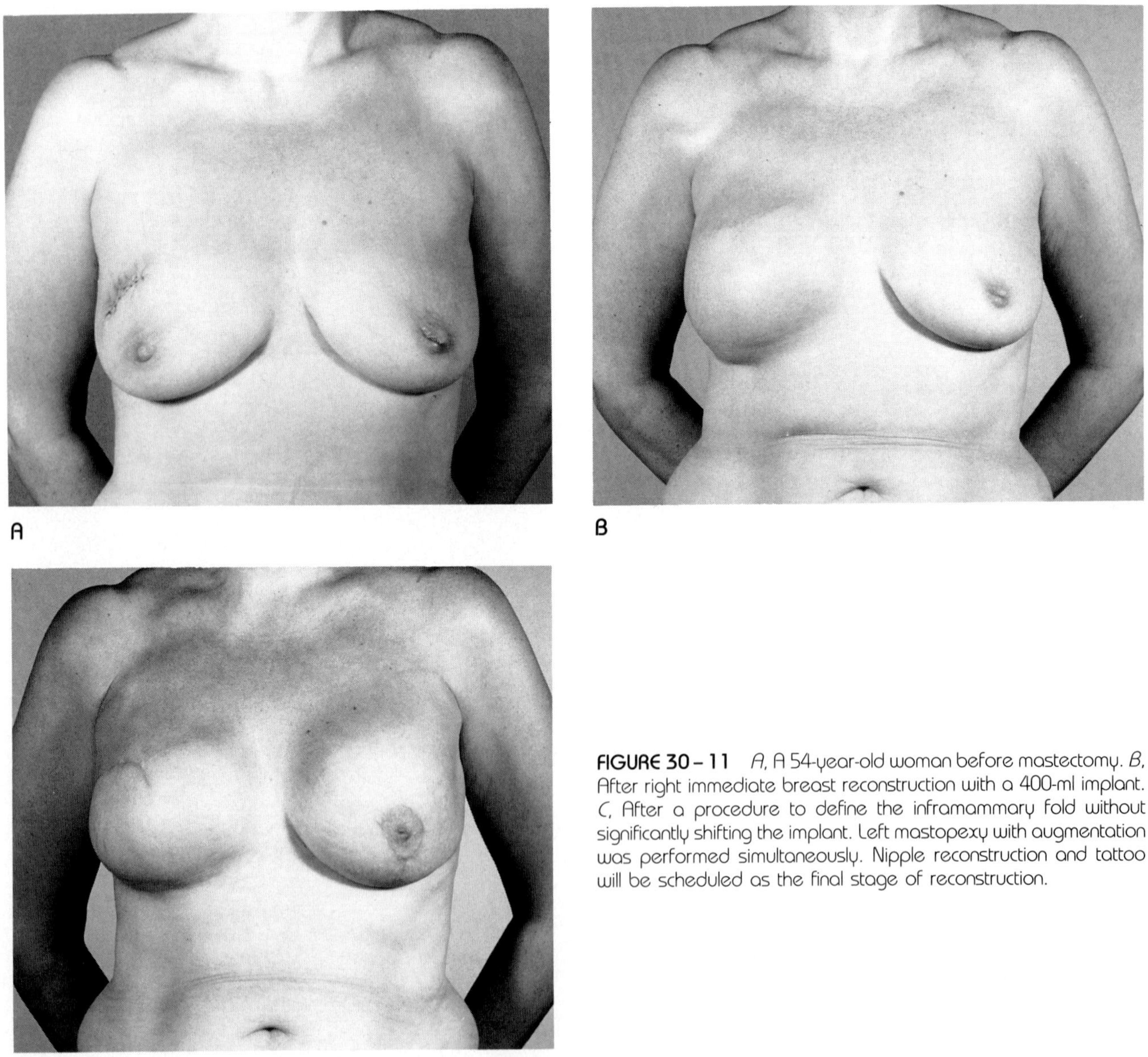

A

B

C

FIGURE 30 – 11 *A*, A 54-year-old woman before mastectomy. *B*, After right immediate breast reconstruction with a 400-ml implant. *C*, After a procedure to define the inframammary fold without significantly shifting the implant. Left mastopexy with augmentation was performed simultaneously. Nipple reconstruction and tattoo will be scheduled as the final stage of reconstruction.

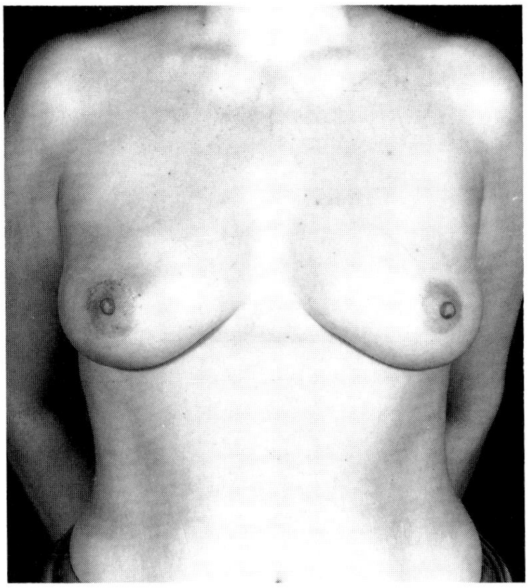

A

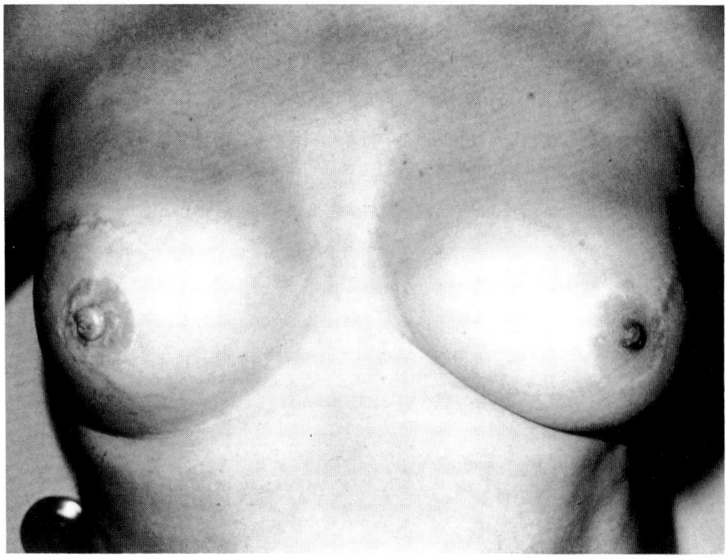

B

FIGURE 30-12 A, A 45-year-old woman before right modified radical mastectomy. B, After right immediate reconstruction with a 500-ml implant, concentric mastopexy on the left breast, a fold definition procedure on the right, an increase in implant size to 600 ml, and nipple reconstruction with tattoo.

CONCLUSION

A reliable scheme of breast reconstruction is proposed that centers on simple initial reconstruction with an implant. Secondary procedures, although not required, are similar to those after expander reconstruction and include capsulotomy, capsulorrhaphy, recreation of the inframammary fold, position adjustments, size adjustments, nipple-areola reconstruction, and matching procedures to the contralateral breast. This economical method has proved both effective and safe over a 10-year period, with few disadvantages. Tissue expanders may be substituted for implants in this regimen, with the clear disadvantage of requiring a second procedure, but with the lure of a more expeditious, controllable, and productive expansion of the remaining breast skin.

References

1. Millard DR. Breast reconstruction after a radical mastectomy. Plast Reconstr Surg 1976; 58:283.
2. Freeman BS. Subcutaneous mastectomy for benign breast lesions with immediate or delayed prosthetic replacement. Plast Reconstr Surg 1962; 30:676.
3. Freeman BS. Technique of subcutaneous mastectomy with replacement; immediate and delayed. Br J Plast Surg 1969; 22:161.
4. Snyderman RK, Guthrie RH. Reconstruction of the female breast following radical mastectomy. Plast Reconstr Surg 1971; 47:565.
5. Horton CE, Adamson JE, Mladick RA, et al. Simple mastectomy with immediate reconstruction. Plast Reconstr Surg 1974; 53:42.
6. Jarrett JR, Cutler RG, Teal DF. Subcutaneous mastectomy in small, large, or ptotic breasts with immediate submuscular placement of implants. Plast Reconstr Surg 1978; 62:702.
7. Gruber RP, Kahn RA, Lash H, et al. Breast reconstruction following mastectomy: A comparison of submuscular and subcutaneous techniques. Plast Reconstr Surg 1981; 67:312.
8. Albo RJ, Gruber RP, Kahn R. Immediate breast reconstruction after modified mastectomy for carcinoma of the breast. Am J Surg 1980; 140:131.
9. Georgiade GS, Georgiade NG, McCarty KS Jr, et al. Modified radical mastectomy with immediate reconstruction for carcinoma of the breast. Ann Surg 1981; 193:565.
10. Jarrett JR, Cutler RG, Teal DF. Aesthetic refinements in prophylactic subcutaneous mastectomy with submuscular reconstruction. Plast Reconstr Surg 1982; 69:624.
11. Georgiade NG, Serafin D, Georgiade G, et al. Subcutaneous mastectomy: An evolution of concept and technique. Ann Plast Surg 1982; 8:8.
12. Georgiade GS, Georgiade NG, McCarty KS, et al. Rationale for immediate reconstruction of the breast following modified radical mastectomy. Ann Plast Surg 1982; 8:20.
13. Noone RB, Murphy JB, Spear SL, Little JW. A 6-year experience with immediate reconstruction after mastectomy for cancer. Plast Reconstr Surg 1985; 76:258.
14. Frazier TG, Noone RB. An objective analysis of immediate simultaneous reconstruction in the treatment of primary carcinoma of the breast. Cancer 1985; 55:1202.
15. Georgiade GS, Riefkohl R, Cox E, et al. Long-term clini-

cal outcome of immediate reconstruction after mastectomy. Plast Reconstr Surg 1985; 76:415.
16. Woods JE. Detailed technique of subcutaneous mastectomy with and without mastopexy. Ann Plast Surg 1987; 18:51.
17. Radovan C. Breast reconstruction after mastectomy using the temporary expander. Plast Reconstr Surg 1982; 69:195.
18. Argenta LC, Marks MW, Grabb WC. Selective use of serial expansion in breast reconstruction. Ann Plast Surg 1983; 11:188.
19. Versaci AD. Reconstruction of a pendulous breast utilizing a tissue expander. Clin Plast Surg 1987; 14:499.
20. Cohen IK, Turner D. Immediate breast reconstruction with tissue expanders. Clin Plast Surg 1987; 14:491.
21. Gibney J. The long-term results of tissue expansion for breast reconstruction. Clin Plast Surg 1987; 14:509.
22. May JW Jr, Attwood J, Bartlett S. Staged use of soft-tissue expansion and lower thoracic advancement flap in breast reconstruction. Plast Reconstr Surg 1987; 79:272.
23. Becker H. Breast reconstruction using an inflatable breast implant with detachable reservoir. Plast Reconstr Surg 1984; 73:678.
24. Becker H. The permanent tissue expander. Clin Plast Surg 1987; 14:519.
25. Becker H, Maraist F. Immediate breast reconstruction after mastectomy using a permanent tissue expander. South Med J 1987; 80:154.
26. Pennisi VR. Making a definite inframammary fold under a reconstructed breast. Plast Reconstr Surg 1977; 60:523.
27. Ryan JJ. A lower thoracic advancement flap in breast reconstruction after mastectomy. Plast Reconstr Surg 1982; 70:153.
28. Ryan JJ. The lower thoracic advancement technique in breast reconstruction. Clin Plast Surg 1984; 11:277.

CHAPTER 31

Reconstruction by Tissue Expansion

LOUIS C. ARGENTA, M.D.

Over the past 15 years, multiple changes have occurred in ablative surgery for breast carcinoma. Concomitant with those changes has been the development of multiple procedures for reconstruction of the breast. The surgeon who undertakes breast reconstruction today faces a large variety of anatomic defects, depending on the size and habitus of the patient preoperatively, the location of the disease, the aggressiveness of the mastectomy, and the individual experience of the ablative surgeon. The reconstructive surgeon should therefore be able to perform all the available procedures for breast reconstruction, ranging from large autologous tissue transfers to the placement of a simple submuscular implant. Surgeons who use the same procedure to repair all defects do themselves and their patients a disservice.

Tissue expansion in which a silicone implant is placed beneath the mastectomy site, is a procedure devised by the late Chedomir E. Radovan.[1] The implant is gradually inflated as local tissues tolerate the reconstruction of a breast mound. Radovan's procedure placed the implant in the subcutaneous space. The vast majority of these reconstructions resulted in significant capsular contracture and subsequent distortion of the reconstructed breast. In the late 1970s it was found that placement of these implants in the submuscular space resulted in safer expansion and a lower incidence of capsular contracture.

Breast reconstruction by tissue expansion is a relatively simple and straightforward procedure.[2,3] There may occasionally be shortcomings, but the overall results are highly acceptable. In 1989, approximately 70 percent of the breast reconstructions performed in the United States involved the use of this technique.

INDICATIONS

The patient who has qualitatively good tissue on the chest wall, but who lacks sufficient tissue for the placement of an implant of sufficient size to achieve symmetry with the opposite side, is the ideal candidate for tissue expansion. The opposite side must be carefully evaluated, because the primary goal of breast reconstruction is to achieve symmetry. If the opposite breast is extremely large and pendulous, the patient must be warned that the tissue expansion will create a rounded, more pubescent breast with limited projection. It is therefore necessary in a patient with a large or pendulous opposite breast to perform a mastopexy or reduction mammaplasty. If the patient objects to this, the transfer of a large flap, either with a latissimus dorsi flap and implant or a transverse rectus abdominis (TRAM) flap is indicated. Patients who are at high risk for contralateral disease or who are candidates for prophylactic mastectomy for other reasons are best reconstructed bilaterally with the use of tissue expanders. It is advisable to employ the same procedure for reconstruction of both sides, if a bilateral mastectomy is contemplated. The combination of an autologous transfer such as the TRAM flap on the mastectomy side and a tissue expander on the prophylactic side does not result in optimal postoperative results.

ADVANTAGES

The advantages of this procedure are numerous and significant. The expander can be placed through the original mastectomy site in secondary reconstruction or even at the time of mastectomy in selected patients. This avoids any new scars. The tissue generated in tissue expansion has characteristics identical to those of the tissue on the chest wall. No new tissue is brought carrying the abnormal color, skin texture, and hair-bearing qualities frequently seen with the TRAM or latissimus dorsi flaps. The size of breast that can be reconstructed varies considerably in most patients. With judicious expansion, breasts of 800 to 1,000 ml can be reconstructed. It is significant that once the basic procedure of tissue expansion is learned, advanced surgical expertise is not required. Both the procedure of expander placement and in some cases a secondary procedure of placing a permanent implant and correcting an inframammary fold are relatively standard techniques that are usually performed in less than 1 hour of anesthetic time. Most of these procedures require minimal hospitalization. Patients tolerate them extremely well with no prolonged period of debility. Most women can return to jobs outside the home or to their work at home within 3 to 5 days. Complications, when they occur, are relatively easy to handle. Infection and extrusion are dealt with by removing the implant and returning to repeat the procedure several months later. There is rarely significant tissue loss, even when implants become infected or are extruded. Major complications such as those encountered with total or partial necrosis of a TRAM flap do not occur.

CONTRAINDICATIONS

Tissues that have undergone extensive radiation as an adjuvant treatment for breast carcinoma are less pliable and have less vascularity than normal tissue. Although a breast mound can be created by expansion, the thinned, firm, irradiated tissue does not result in as pleasing a breast as can be achieved by other techniques involving the transfer of distant tissue. Patients who have undergone classic radical mastectomy do not have sufficient overlying tissue for tissue expansion to achieve adequate results. The transfer of significant amounts of tissue to fill the infraclavicular area can be accomplished only with flaps. Patients who have had primary radiation treatment in the range of 5,000 to 6,000 rads that has failed should not be reconstructed by expansion. It may be technically feasible, but there is an extremely high rate of extrusion and local tissue compromise. Mastectomy and secondary reconstruction with distant flaps or primary reconstruction with distant flaps is the procedure of choice for patients who have recurrences after primary radiation therapy of the breast.

CHOICE OF IMPLANTS

Multiple expanders are available from a wide variety of manufacturers for breast reconstruction. Basically a round expander is used with either an incorporated or a distant valve. The author prefers a distant valve because it may occasionally be difficult to find an incorporated valve in a heavy patient or a patient who develops a significant capsule during expansion. Some manufacturers have tried to develop directional expanders in an attempt to produce a more ptotic breast without mobilization of flaps in a secondary procedure. Unfortunately, all these implants involve the application of directional forces so that maximal force is applied to the area that is going to produce the apex of the breast. This results in significant thinning of this area, which may make reconstruction of the nipple more difficult. Attempts have been made to wrap the cephalad portion of the implant with a more resistant silicone sheet, or to use expanders of multiple thicknesses that preferentially expand in one direction. Recently, breast expanders with textured polyurethane covers have been devised. Although the scientific basis for use of these devices remains nebulous at this time, some physicians feel they are easier to expand and may offer superior results.

The most significant advance in breast reconstruction by tissue expansion has been the development of the permanent expander. Two such devices are available at present, the Becker[4,5] and the Gibney implant (Fig. 31-1).[6] Both of these involve a device with an outer silicone-containing shell and an inner lumen into which the saline is placed. The purpose of these implants is to avoid a secondary procedure to place a permanent implant. Early Becker expanders carried a significant rate of deflation; over the past several years, however, this rate has fallen dramatically with the development of a new valve. With proper patient selection and correct placement of the prosthesis, a significant number of women (in the author's experience, 60 percent) do not require a second procedure to place a permanent implant. Both of these implants have distant reservoirs.

PROCEDURE

The goal of breast reconstruction is to develop a symmetric breast mound that will match the opposite side as closely as possible in base diameter, projection, and contour. It is critical, therefore, not only that the correct size implant be selected, but that the expander be positioned appropriately. The

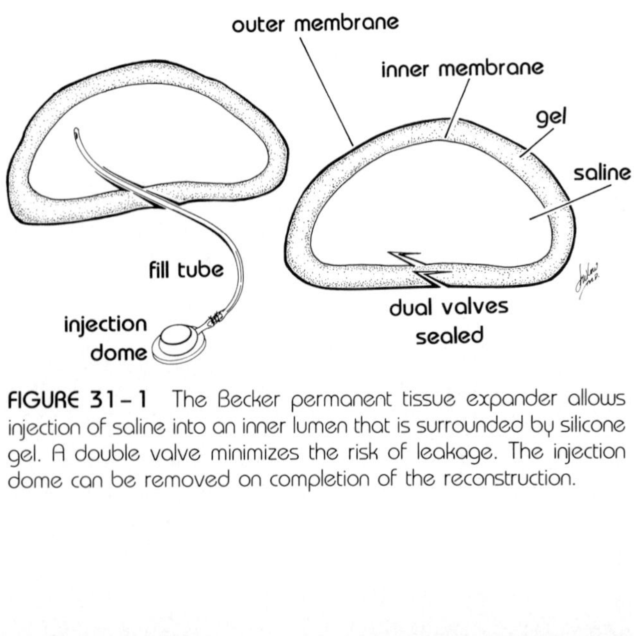

FIGURE 31-1 The Becker permanent tissue expander allows injection of saline into an inner lumen that is surrounded by silicone gel. A double valve minimizes the risk of leakage. The injection dome can be removed on completion of the reconstruction.

size of the implant depends on the size of the breast to be reconstructed. Volumes assigned by manufacturers to expanders are relatively unimportant. The most important feature is the diameter of the base of the implant, which should be slightly larger than the diameter of the base of the remaining breast. An 800- to 1,000-ml implant is usually ideal for the average-sized woman; in a smaller woman, a smaller implant may be indicated.

With the patient standing preoperatively, the location of the remaining breast should be determined and marked appropriately. The apex of the remaining breast should be marked so that the apex of the reconstructed breast will match it. If a ptosis procedure or reduction is to be performed on the remaining breast, the proposed position of the apex of the mound for the remaining breast must be determined so that the reconstructed apex will match it. This apex should correspond to slightly below the center of the implant when conventional expanders are used. When directional expanders are used, experience in determining the maximal excursion of the directional implant is mandatory. Optimizing the apex of the breast mound may require positioning of the inframammary fold of the new breast below the opposite side. Provided that this distance is less than 2 cm, it is well tolerated by the patient.

The general contour of the base of the remaining breast is marked and a slightly larger contralateral pattern drawn. This is used simply to determine the position of the implant placement, but dissection should proceed beyond this implant, especially superiorly and laterally. If the general surgeon has left an inframammary fold intact, that fold is marked and used as the inframammary fold of the new breast.

The patient is placed with both arms taped to the iliac crests in a 15- to 20-degree sitting position on the operating table. The ulnar nerve is protected with appropriate elbow padding. This procedure can be performed under general or local anesthesia, but general anesthesia is usually preferred because dissection in the submuscular plane may be uncomfortable. Epidural spinal anesthesia is useful in some patients and can make this dissection quite simple.

I generally prefer to use the lateral one half or one third of the original mastectomy incision for placement of the prosthesis. If the scar is particularly unsightly or widened, the entire scar can be excised and closed with appropriate subcuticular sutures at the termination of the procedure. Dissection is carried down sharply to the pectoralis muscle medially, and the serratus muscle laterally. The pectoralis major muscle is opened in the direction of its fibers, approximately 2 to 3 cm from its lateral border. This allows preservation of the muscle and makes closure of the wound easier. Once the pectoralis has been entered, dissection is carried both medially and superiorly beneath the pectoralis muscle as necessary. Laterally, the dissection is carried beneath the serratus muscle. In a secondary reconstruction in which there is adequate soft tissue, it usually is unnecessary to bury the entire implant beneath muscle. Once healing has occurred with scarring of the overlying skin to the chest wall, there usually is adequate bulk so that only the medial two thirds of the implant need be covered with muscle. The inferior medial aspect of the pectoralis muscle must be removed from the ribs to allow correct positioning of the implant inferiorly. If the inframammary fold remains from the initial procedure, dissection is carried only 1 or 2 cm below this fold (Figs. 31-2, 31-3). Meticulous hemostasis is mandatory to allow placement of the expander without the need for drains, which may result in contamination of the expander. Seroma is very unusual in secondary reconstruction.

The implant is then placed in the space that has been dissected and should fit loosely without folding. It is important that the entire base of the implant rest comfortably on the anterior chest wall. If an implant with an integrated valve is used, the valve is situated anteriorly. If a distant reservoir is used, as the author prefers, the filling tube is brought out through the lateral margin of the pectoralis or serratus muscle. The filling reservoir is placed in the subcutaneous space, either on the anterior axillary line or below the brassiere line on the anterior chest wall. Most of the reservoirs provided with standard prostheses are of excessive size, and with some experience the smaller pediatric-type reservoir can be used, providing greater patient comfort.

The pectoralis muscle is then closed with 2-0 or 3-0 absorbable PDS or Vicryl sutures. The skin and subcutaneous tissue area are approximated and the skin is closed with subcuticular 2-0 or 3-0 Prolene. The wound is dressed with Steri-Strips, which should be worn as long as possible during the process of inflation. Enough saline is placed into the implant to allow closure of the dead space. No significant tension should be placed on the chest wall, particularly in immediate breast reconstruction.

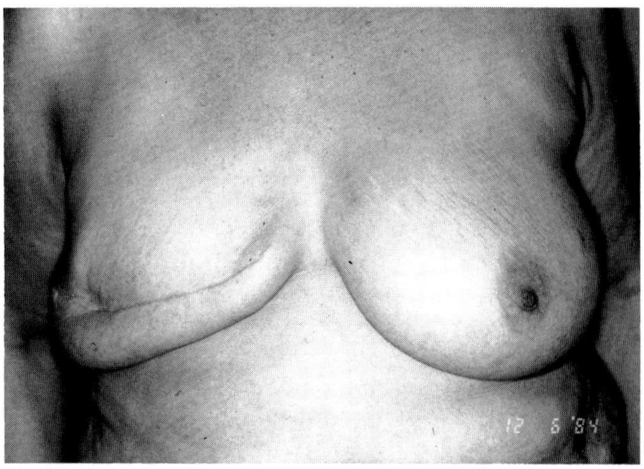

FIGURE 31-2 An ideal candidate for reconstruction by tissue expansion in whom the surgeon has preserved the inframammary fold.

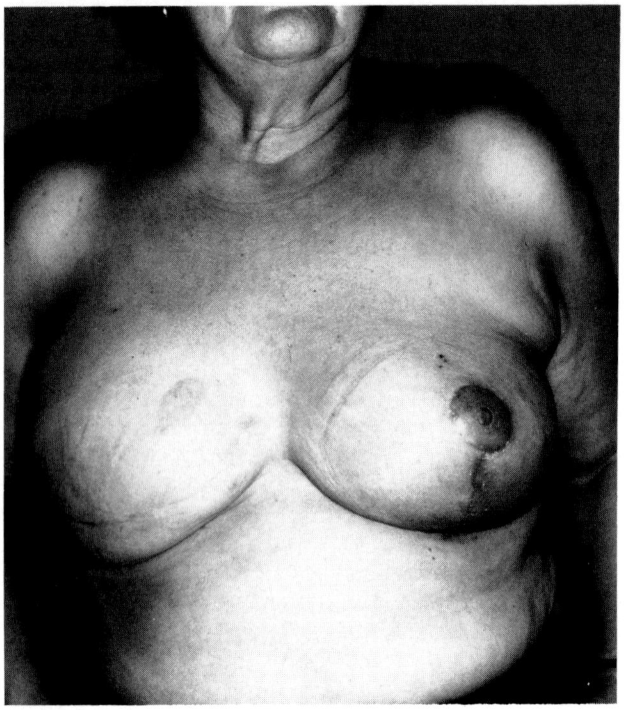

FIGURE 31-3 The patient in Fig. 31-2 after overexpansion and partial deflation. Preservation of the original inframammary fold usually ensures acceptable ptosis of the reconstructed breast. A ptosis procedure on the left was performed without reduction of volume.

INFLATION OF THE EXPANDER

Approximately 10 days to 2 weeks after placement of the implant, the wound achieves enough strength to allow fluid placement for expansion. There are wide variations in the rate at which the expander can be safely inflated. There should therefore be no set schedule for placing a specific amount into the implant at each interval. Enough saline is placed at the time of each inflation so that the tissue overlying the implant becomes tense without being compromised.

I prefer to use a 23-gauge butterfly needle connected with a small tubing to a syringe. This allows some movement of the patient without laceration of the implant reservoir. Injectable saline without preservatives is used. Reports in the literature have mentioned the placement of antibiotics, local anesthetics, and anticontractile drugs in the implant, but I prefer to use saline only. The expander is inflated until tenseness develops in the overlying skin. If the patient complains of discomfort, some saline can be removed. If the overlying skin becomes blanched, saline should be removed until circulation is reestablished.

Valves that are integrated into the implant may be more difficult to palpate, particularly early in the course of expansion. One company has made a magnetic finder for the valve, which facilitates its location.

The patient returns to the office at weekly or biweekly intervals, depending on how the tissue responds to inflation. Usually between five and eight inflations are necessary to achieve an adequate volume for breast reconstruction. Later in the course of expansion, the overlying tissues soften and more saline can be placed with each inflation.

Once volume symmetry has been achieved with the opposite side, the expander should be overinflated. I usually recommend 300 to 400 ml of overinflation, depending on the degree of ptosis I wish to create later. The implant is overinflated and left overinflated for approximately 4 months. My laboratory work has demonstrated that capsules during this interval mature considerably. If the capsule is biopsied upon completion of tissue expansion, a significant number of cellular elements may be found. Several months after overexpansion, the capsule matures and the number of cellular elements decreases significantly. This may contribute to the low incidence of significant capsular contracture after expansion (Fig. 31-4). It has been my impression that if a permanent implant is placed without overexpanding or without allowing the capsule to mature, the rate of capsular contracture increases significantly.

SECOND PROCEDURE

If a standard expansion implant has been employed, it should be replaced with a permanent pros-

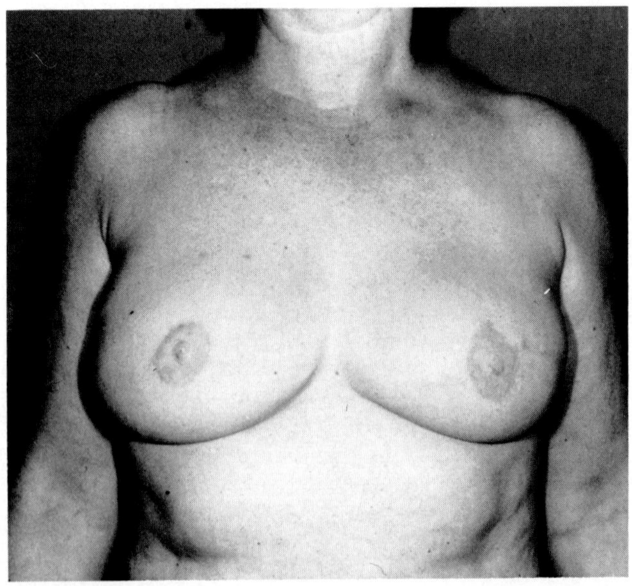

FIGURE 31-4 This patient underwent a two-stage reconstruction of bilateral modified radical mastectomies by tissue expansion. The 520-ml submuscular prostheses have remained soft and present a natural appearance 10 years postoperatively.

thesis. I prefer gel or gel-inflatable combinations for the permanent reconstruction, although textured implants have recently become popular. It has been my experience that if saline-containing prostheses are used, over time they leak and some decrease in size of the implant can be expected.

At this point, creation of a more defined repositioning of the inframammary fold can be accomplished to create ptosis. The amount of ptosis that can be created with this procedure is not as great as that accomplished with a TRAM or latissimus dorsi flap, however. I prefer to mark the apex of the nonoperated breast, either as it stands without surgery or, if a ptosis correction is performed, at the location of the new nipple-areola complex. This position is then marked on the expanded breast mound. If sufficient overexpansion has occurred, there will be excess skin between the site of the new nipple-areola complex and the projected new inframammary fold. It is sometimes helpful to use a heavy-gauge wire, bent according to the contour of the normal inframammary fold, and transpose this in a mirror-image fashion to the opposite side. This wire is then moved up and down on the chest wall to determine the best position for the inframammary fold.

An incision is made at the point that will allow invagination of sufficient tissue to create the desired inframammary fold. The original incision is used or a new one made at the new inframammary fold. I prefer a second inframammary incision that allows direct visualization and localization of the new fold (Fig. 31-5). If a new scar is not desired, creation of an inframammary fold can be accomplished with more difficulty through the original incision.[7] Dissection is carried down to the chest wall and then superiorly until the capsule is entered. The expansion implant is removed, as is the reservoir. The expanded skin on the chest wall and its capsule is then moved superiorly or inferiorly on the anterior chest wall until an appropriate position is reached. Sizers are used to determine the volume of saline to be removed to approximate the opposite breast. If the operator has a difficult time visualizing this preoperatively, the expander can be deflated on the morning of surgery until volume symmetry is obtained. The volume of saline in the implant can then be measured and an implant of appropriate size selected.

The capsule of the expanded tissue anteriorly is sutured directly to the incised capsule posteriorly on the chest wall (Fig. 31-6). This capsule is usually relatively dense and firm and allows the placement of multiple large sutures. I prefer not to suture into the rib bed, because this is usually painful and offers no added strength to suturing to the capsule wall. Permanent 2-0 and 3-0 Prolene sutures are preferred.

The patient is then placed into a sitting position on the table and the apex of each breast mound visualized. It is more important that the apex of the breast mound be on an equal plane than that the inframammary fold be exactly symmetric. Having an inframammary fold 1 or 2 cm below the normal side is well tolerated and may help achieve good symmetry (Fig. 31-7). A fold below 2 cm poses some difficulty with the patient wearing a brassiere and should be avoided if at all possible.

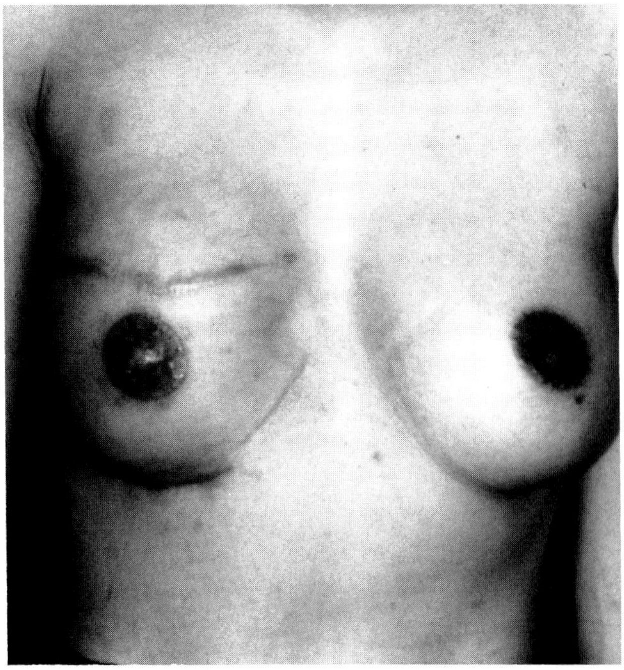

FIGURE 31-5 This patient underwent a two-stage breast reconstruction with tissue expansion. At the second procedure, an inframammary incision was used to define an inframammary fold, as described in the text.

The capsule remaining on the anterior chest wall is then excised, and the skin of the lower chest and abdomen undermined and mobilized superiorly. This is also sutured to a small rim of capsule remaining on the posterior chest wall. The skin is closed with appropriate Prolene sutures.

Positioning of the implant is best accomplished with tape. I prefer foam tape to constricting dressings. This allows mobilization of the overlying skin to appropriate positions.

Gentle movement of the prosthesis is encouraged the day after surgery. Vigorous massage of the prosthesis begins 2 weeks after placement of the permanent implant.

IMMEDIATE BREAST RECONSTRUCTION

Some patients with small, localized breast carcinomas may be candidates for immediate breast reconstruction. Because radiation therapy is infrequently used for control of the local site in the immediate postoperative period, the placement of expanders is an accepted procedure. If metastatic

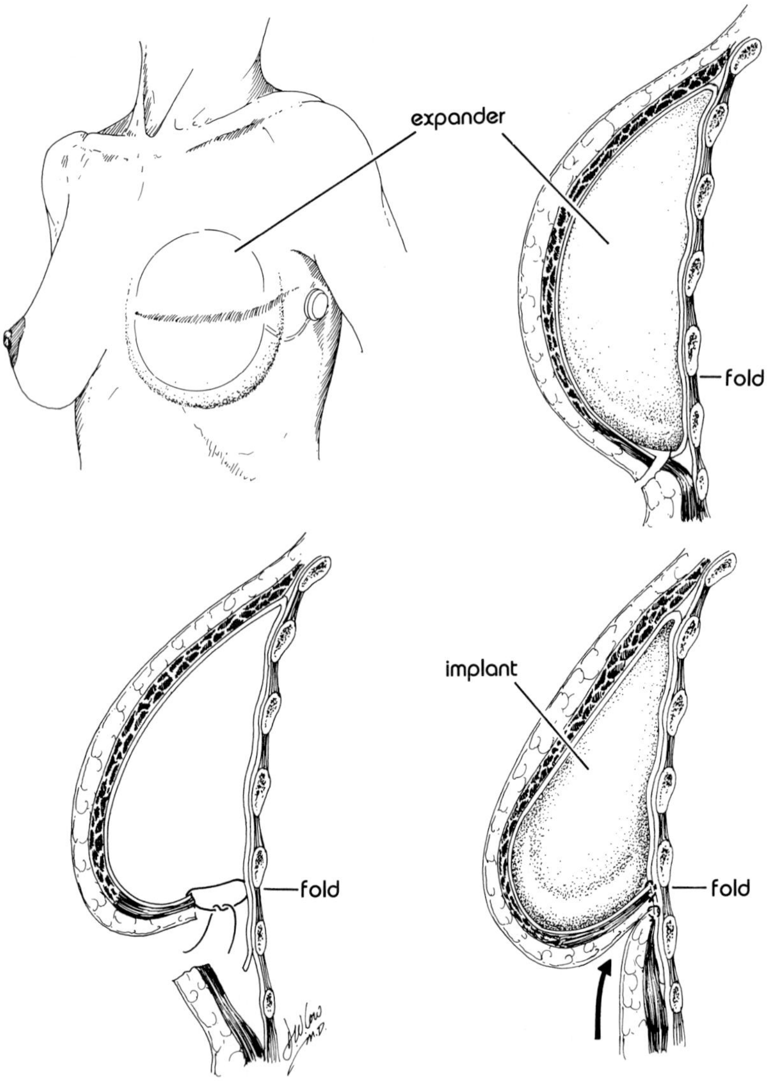

FIGURE 31–6 The technique of creating an appearance of ptosis by secondary adjustment of the inframammary fold begins with overinflation of the expander. The position of the desired fold is determined on the chest wall. Through an inframammary incision the expander is removed and the skin and capsule are moved cephalad, suturing them to the predetermined point. The abdominal skin is undermined and advanced into the inframammary defect.

disease is found after the mastectomy and implant have been placed, the patient can be treated with adjuvant chemotherapy or radiotherapy without significantly compromising the expansion procedure.

Careful preoperative planning is necessary in these patients. The location of the projected breast mound should be marked on the patient preoperatively while she is in the standing position. Both breasts should be prepped into the operative site so that symmetry can be ensured at the time of the procedure. When marking the patient, it is important to take into consideration the amount of skin the general surgeon is going to remove. If an aggressive removal of skin is considered necessary, the plastic surgeon must assess if there is adequate tissue on the chest wall to close the defect or prepare for a flap procedure.

The extent and actual performance of the mastectomy are determined and carried out by the general surgeon with no interference from the plastic surgeon. I feel strongly that the primary objective in this procedure is removal of the carcinoma and that no compromise in its removal should be made for the purpose of reconstruction. Once the surgeon has completed the dissection, the plastic surgeon creates a space beneath the pectoralis muscle. Again, I prefer to split this muscle in the direction of its fibers about 2 cm from its lateral border. Dissection is then carried down to the chest wall and the space developed beneath the muscle. The origin of the pectoralis muscle must be taken down from the ribs; this is easily accomplished with the electrocautery. In some patients, it is necessary to dissect down to the fascia of the rectus abdominis muscle to achieve an adequate pocket. Laterally, the dissection is extended beneath the serratus anterior muscle. If the general surgeon has accomplished an extensive dissection of Rotter's nodes, there may be a disruption in the continuity of the lateral margin of the pectoralis muscle and the serratus and pectoralis minor. Careful dissection is mandatory so that a complete muscle envelope can be developed to prevent migration

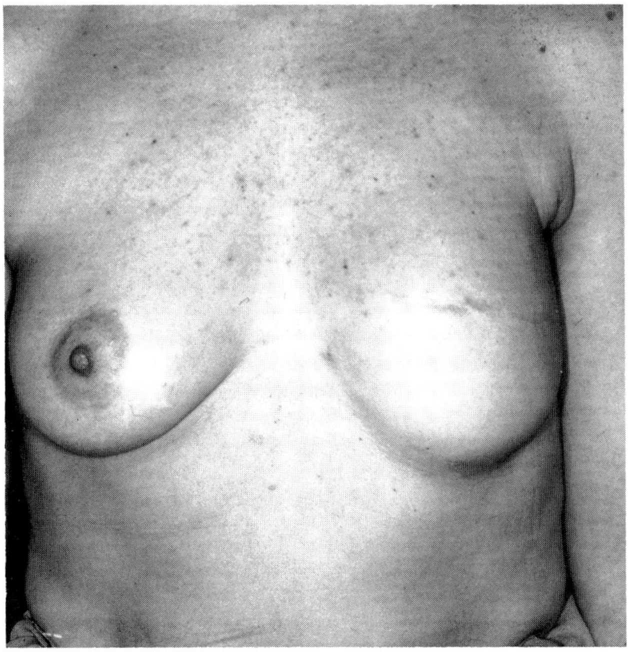

FIGURE 31-7 To create symmetry of the apexes of the breast mounds, the inframammary fold in the reconstructed breast has been moved down almost 2 cm. Displacements of more than this distance can be uncomfortable in a brassiere.

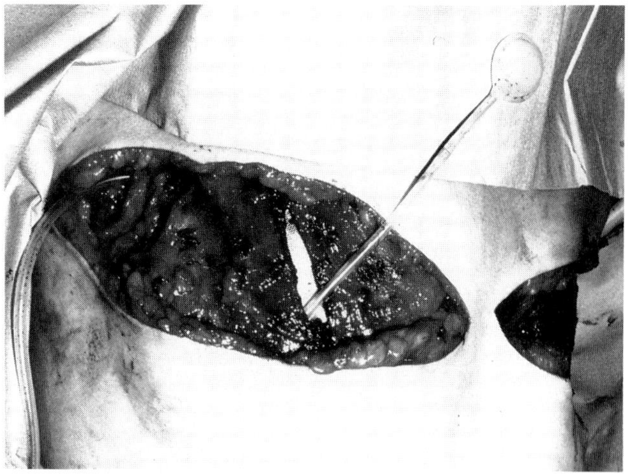

FIGURE 31-8 A bilateral immediate breast reconstruction. In these cases, it is important to completely cover the prosthesis with a muscle envelope extending under the pectoralis and serratus anterior muscles. The reservoir is situated subcutaneously where minimal displacement will occur.

of the prosthesis into the axilla. When more tissue is needed, the pectoralis minor can be taken down from its origin and mobilized laterally on its insertion. It is then sutured to the lateral aspects of the pectoralis muscle. Usually, this is not necessary. As large a dissection is made as is required to accommodate an implant of appropriate size. The implant is then placed in the space and the muscle closed appropriately (Fig. 31-8). If a distant reservoir prosthesis is used, it is important to place the reservoir in a position so that it will not migrate and can be easily found. If an aggressive axillary dissection has been performed, this may result in some difficulty in securing the inflation reservoir in the axilla. Some of these patients are better served by placing the reservoir inferiorly on the anterior chest wall in the subcutaneous space in an area not previously dissected.

Appropriate drains are placed in the submuscular space and into the axilla. It is important that the patient be kept on antibiotics during the mastectomy and for approximately 10 days postoperatively. Until all drainage from the axillary drain has ceased, there is a risk of infection and secondary capsular contracture. The drain, if placed in the submuscular space, should be removed as soon as possible.

Inflation of implants placed at the time of mastectomy can actually be accomplished faster than secondary reconstructions. Once would healing has occurred, usually 2 weeks postoperatively, inflation is begun and proceeds rapidly (Fig. 31-9).

TISSUE EXPANSION WITH TOTAL AND SUBCUTANEOUS MASTECTOMY

Frequently, in conjunction with breast reconstruction, a subcutaneous or total mastectomy is performed on the opposite side. The technique of subcutaneous mastectomy has developed a dubious

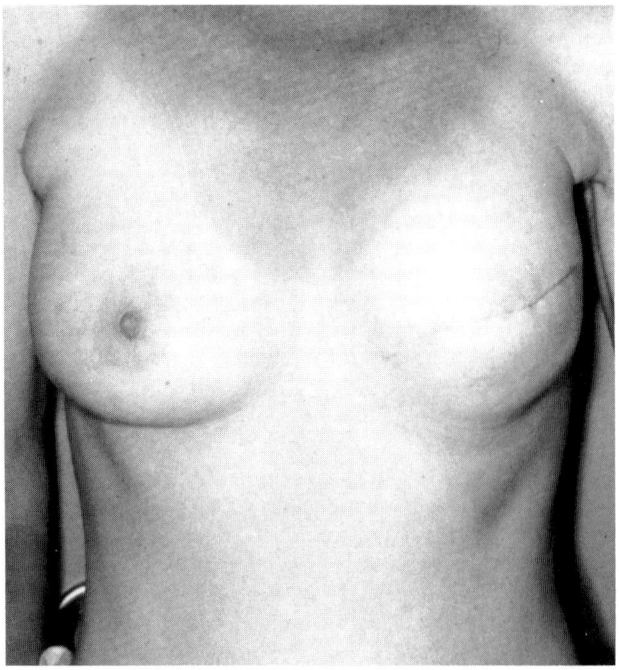

FIGURE 31-9 Immediate breast reconstruction with a Becker permanent expander. This patient has achieved excellent symmetry 4 months after mastectomy with no additional procedures.

reputation in plastic and reconstructive surgery in the past 20 years, although recent studies have demonstrated a probable lower risk of breast carcinoma in these patients. Because of difficulties with significant capsular contractures, skin necrosis, and failure to achieve symmetry, this procedure has been questioned. The use of submuscular tissue expanders allows considerable safety, lower contracture rates, variation in size, and overall improvement of results.

The indications for subcutaneous or total mastectomy vary considerably among surgeons. Subcutaneous or total mastectomy may be performed when there is significant risk of the development of breast carcinoma in the uninvolved side. Particularly in cases of lobular carcinoma and multifocal breast carcinoma, total mastectomy, including removal of the nipple-areola complex, seems desirable. In cases of severe fibrocystic disease, the inability to examine a breast adequately by palpation or radiography, and the inability to achieve symmetry with the opposite breast are lesser indications for prophylactic mastectomy. I prefer a total mastectomy to a subcutaneous mastectomy in most cases because I feel that a more thorough ablative procedure can be performed by removing the nipple-areola complex. Today's techniques of nipple-areola reconstruction have allowed satisfactory reconstruction to replace the resected nipple and areola.

If a subcutaneous or total mastectomy is to be performed on one side in combination with reconstruction of the opposite side, I believe that a breast tissue expander should be placed bilaterally. This allows great latitude in size and shape of the breast so that symmetry can be more easily achieved. Once the total mastectomy has been performed, with or without axillary sampling, a tissue expander is placed by means of the same technique as that for immediate breast reconstruction. It is important to achieve total muscular coverage, because the prepectoral plane has been widely dissected and migration of the implant can be expected, if it is not held in place. The implant is selected on the basis of its base diameter, rather than its volume. Because of the blood and lymphatic oozing that occurs in these patients, it is important that a drain be placed in the prepectoral space and that the patient be kept on antibiotics as long as any serous or lymphatic drainage continues.

After wound healing has occurred, the implants are expanded to maintain symmetry. The expander on the total or subcutaneous mastectomy side often expands much more readily than on the modified radical mastectomy side. It is important not to expand the subcutaneous mastectomy side aggressively, or it may result in an excess that may be difficult to match with the modified radical mastectomy side. It is best to let the latter set the rate for expansion of the subcutaneous mastectomy side.

COMPLICATIONS

Capsular Contracture

The rate of capsular contracture after tissue expansion is less than that seen with placement of simple prostheses. It has been my experience that overexpansion is critical to minimizing the rate of secondary capsular contracture. The expander should be overexpanded by approximately 30 to 40 percent and this implant left in place for at least 4 months. The longer an overexpanded implant is left in place, the better are the results relating to ptosis and softness of the breast after partial deflation. The need for overexpansion wth textured implants has not been clearly defined but there seems to be little lost in overexpanding these implants and deflating them. A prospective study on this question is needed.

In a few patients, capsular contracture develops so rapidly that it is difficult to expand the implant to an appropriate volume. This occurs in about 2 percent of the implants placed. Frequently, these are patients who have had previous implants placed at the time of mastectomy and have developed severe capsular contracture. When this occurs, it is best to return them to the operating room and perform a wide capsulotomy without attempting to remove excessive amounts of the capsule. The implant is then inflated as much as possible in the operating room and rapidly expanded to overcome the rate of capsular contracture. These patients have a higher rate of secondary capsular contracture, and I prefer to place a textured implant in the space when removing the expander. In the future, textured expanders may obviate this problem.

Infection

Like all foreign bodies, tissue expanders may become infected. It has been my impression that expanders placed at the time of mastectomy carry a higher rate of infection than when these implants are placed for secondary reconstruction. This may well be caused by the excessive lymphatic drainage that occurs after the axillary dissection. This lymphatic fluid forms an ideal medium for infection, which may be introduced either during surgery or at the time of inflation. For this reason, patients who have expanders placed at the time of the mastectomy are kept on antibiotics until all drains have been removed and the serum collection in the axilla has subsided.

There have been reports of implants being salvaged after being infected, but these cases are in the minority. Once an implant has become infected, the chance of its successful replacement is small. In some patients the secondary implant has become almost immediately infected with the same bacteria that infected the primary implant, even though it was placed 3 to 4 months after the infected expander was removed. For this reason, if a breast expander does become infected, I recommend that it be removed and 6 to 8 months allowed to pass before reinsertion.

Asymmetry

Ideal symmetry may be one of the most difficult objectives to achieve in any bilateral procedure. If similar ablative procedures have been performed on each side, or particularly if the inframammary fold has been preserved on both sides, symmetry will be better. When standard expanders are used, some degree of repositioning and capsulectomy may allow achievement of a better symmetry when the second implant is placed. With the use of the Becker implant and the permanent textured implants, there may be a tradeoff between the need for a second procedure and the goal of better symmetry. Only careful consultation with the patient will reveal if she is willing to undergo a secondary procedure to achieve a minor, but sometimes significant, degree of improvement in symmetry. The vast majority of patients who undergo this secondary procedure appear to be satisfied. I have recently used high thoracic epidural for these procedures and have been extremely pleased with the degree of patient comfort. This procedure minimizes the complications of general anesthesia and eliminates the discomfort of local infiltrative anesthesia.

THE FUTURE OF BREAST RECONSTRUCTION BY EXPANSION

Although a significant majority of breast reconstructions are performed with tissue expanders, there is still great need for improvement of this technique. The placement of tissue expanders has become such a relatively simple and accepted procedure that many breast reconstructions today are performed by non-plastic surgeons. Rather than attempting to disparage the efforts of others, this author feels strongly that plastic surgeons should seek to consolidate their position by performing a better aesthetic and functional reconstruction. Judicious management of the implant and the overlying tissue, as well as artistry in refining breast reconstructions, is critical. The patient of the 1990s is no longer happy with the simple mound. The development of appropriate ptosis with a minimum of surgery on the contralateral breast should be the objective.

Breast reconstruction should be performed as expeditiously as possible so that the patient who has suffered breast cancer can resume her life with as little interference and loss of time as possible. The reconstructive surgeon should always remember that despite the advances made in breast cancer over the past 20 years, the long-term survival of these patients has not significantly changed. The amount of time that many patients invest in undergoing a breast reconstruction therefore represents time taken away from her family and her life.

References

1. Radovan C. Breast reconstruction after mastectomy using the temporary expander. Plast Reconstr Surg 1982; 69:195.
2. Argenta LC, Marks MW, Grabb WC. Selective use of serial expansion in breast reconstruction. Ann Plast Surg 1983; 11:188.
3. Argenta LC. Reconstruction of the breast by tissue expansion. Clin Plast Surg 1984; 11:257.
4. Becker H. Breast reconstruction using inflatable breast implant with detachable reservoir. Plast Reconstr Surg 1984; 73:678.
5. Becker H. The permanent tissue expander. Clin Plast Surg 1987; 14:519.
6. Gibney J. Use of a permanent tissue expander for breast reconstruction. Plast Reconstr Surg 1989; 84:607.
7. Versaci A. Reconstruction of a pendulous breast utilizing a tissue expander. Clin Plast Surg 1987; 14:499.

CHAPTER 32

Local Flaps in Breast Reconstruction

JAMES J. RYAN, M.D.

Breast reconstruction in the postmastectomy state can be conceived simplistically as the restoration of three basic elements removed by the ablative surgery: a glandular-fat mass of adequate volume, a skin envelope to cover and shape the mass, and the nipple-areola complex. Local tissues are almost always too inadequate to be considered for volume restoration, and therefore are usually involved in supplementing the skin coverage of an implant that provides the volume restoration. Historically, local tissues have been used simply to provide adequate wound closure after mastectomy. The context in which they are addressed here concerns their principal current use as a supplement to the skin envelope in implant reconstruction.

"Local" in this chapter means the use of tissue that has some direct contact with a portion of the mastectomy defect. This may be the skin and subcutaneous element or a deeper muscular layer exposed by surgery. It does not include procedures that have involved the other breast, i.e., "breast sharing."

If one considers the possible options as they present after the most common mastectomy procedure, the modified radical, the mastectomy wound or scar divides the anterior thorax into a more superomedial portion and an inferolateral zone (see Fig. 32-4). Because successful use of flaps involves a zone of excess, an adequate blood supply, and reasonable donor site deformity, consideration of the postmastectomy anterior thoracic situation readily suggests that the superomedial zone offers minimal excess and would be the site of rather conspicuous donor deformity if used as a donor site for local flaps. Thus, virtually all local flaps used in breast reconstruction are planned and taken from the tissues inferior and lateral to the mastectomy defect. This defect is commonly defined by the slightly oblique or transverse mastectomy scar or wound. In a review of the numerous flaps proposed, some are of only passing historic interest. Those that are presently used in common clinical situations will be discussed in more detail.

HISTORY

The first local flap commonly used in the postmastectomy situation appears to be the original latissimus dorsi myocutaneous flap described by Tansini.[1,2] This was based on the posterior axillary fold and included the underlying muscle. In a modified Z-plasty fashion, the tissue composite was moved to provide better closure of the mastectomy defect and some restoration of volume and coverage to the thorax. Indeed, in a patient with a very modest breast volume, an approximation of volume symmetry might be achieved. This technique fell out of favor as the dominant focus of adequacy of ablation in the presence of malignancy cast a shadow across any attempts at reconstruction. Also, in the absence of the ability to restore adequate volume, this most often simply provided a more adequate mastectomy closure and did not approach adequate reconstruction.

A number of local dermal-fat flaps were subsequently introduced. These were almost all based inferiorly and medially and were often large variations of a Z-plasty. They were used more often in the context of restoration for partial breast ablation where a limited volume needed to be restored and local autogenous tissue could be of assistance.[3–6]

As discussed earlier, local tissues usually cannot provide significant volume restoration. Therefore, the development of the silicone implant as a solution to volume deficiency[7] allowed local tissues to be considered for a task more feasible: that of supplementing the skin coverage over the implant.[8] Initially, the local tissues were often simply elevated and again advanced when an implant was placed through the mastectomy incision for a delayed reconstruction. Again, the inferolateral area with its relative zone of excess in some patients proved useful. Advancement of the inferolateral tissues through the mastectomy scar, with attempts to stabilize an inframammary fold, were advocated, notably by Lewis.[9]

A major new flap consideration was the elongated thoracoepigastric flap to both cover and shape delayed implant reconstruction, as proposed by Cronin and associates.[10] Because this was a variation on a very large Z-plasty, the flap required delay and the tip had a precarious blood supply. At the same time, however, a whole new basic concept in flap development was being introduced. The musculocutaneous flap was to give a major thrust to postmastectomy reconstruction, and the latissimus dorsi flap would again take center stage.

The pioneering work of McCraw and colleagues in defining the principle of independent myocutaneous vascular territories was a monumental thrust forward for flap techniques in tissue transposition.[11] One of the major contributions was to define the latissimus dorsi muscle and its overlying skin territory. This provided, in the hands of many, a major step forward in using this muscle for postmastectomy breast reconstruction.[12,13] This would qualify as a local flap in that the latissimus dorsi or a portion of it is almost always in the axillary portion of a mastectomy wound. Very commonly, the skin portion of the musculocutaneous unit is taken as a dorsal skin island. A modification resembling more closely the original description by Tansini was developed to avoid some of the problems with the contrasting pigmentation and texture occasionally seen between dorsal and ventral body skin.[14] By basing the cutaneous paddle along the anterior edge of the muscle, the muscle and skin units really are moved as a large Z-plasty, allowing good definition of an inframammary fold, and supplementation of the breast skin coverage, particularly inferolaterally, over implant reconstruction (Fig. 32-1). Good skin color match can also be achieved (Fig. 32-2) (see Chap. 33). Although a most useful and pioneering flap, the use of the latissimus dorsi decreased as lesser mastectomy deformities were created by more conservative ablative procedures.

In searching for a simpler alternative that might confine the surgery to the ventral body surface, the author was attracted by two considerations: that of the inferolateral zone of relative excess and the importance of the inframammary fold in defining breast shape. With these considerations, the technique of lower thoracic advancement in postmastectomy reconstruction was developed.[15]

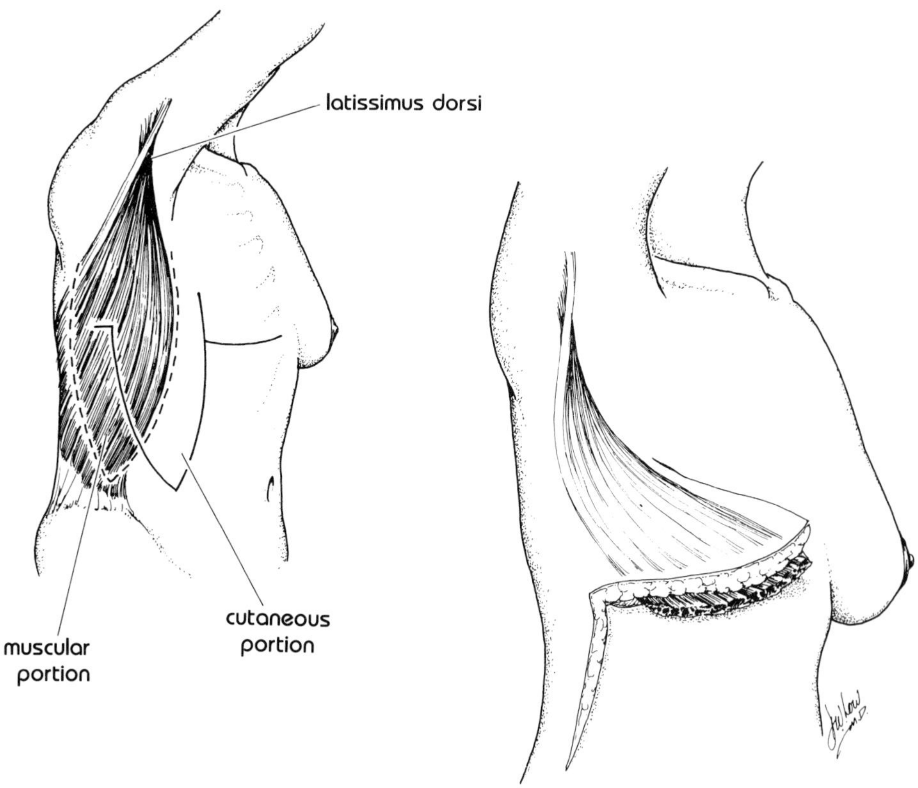

FIGURE 32-1 Modified latissimus dorsi musculocutaneous breast reconstruction in which the cutaneous portion overlies the anterior edge of latissimus muscle with an extended random cutaneous portion. The skin texture and pigmentation closely match the ventral body skin, and the cutaneous donor site lies in the midaxillary line, where it is often easily hidden by clothing and less prone to hypertrophy than scars on donor sites on the back. The inset of the inferior aspect of the cutaneous flap allows for stable definition of the inframammary fold.

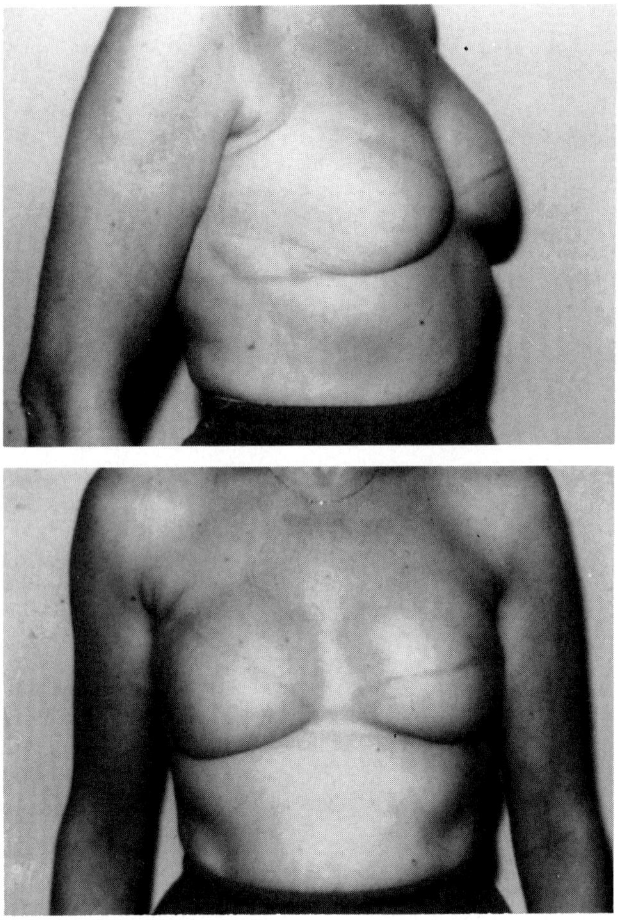

FIGURE 32–2 This patient underwent a bilateral delayed breast reconstruction with modified latissimus dorsi flaps and implants. Note the lateral thoracic donor site of the cutaneous portion and the well-defined inframammary fold. The local skin has a very good texture and pigmentary match to the anterior thoracic skin.

LOWER THORACIC ADVANCEMENT IN POSTMASTECTOMY RECONSTRUCTION

Essential Anatomy

As with most operative procedures, the modified radical mastectomy is interpreted and performed with variations in technique. The following considerations are particularly important to reconstruction: (1) the alignment of the skin resection, whether transverse or vertical; (2) the magnitude of skin resection, and thus the tension of the skin and subcutaneous closure; (3) the uniformity with which the subcutaneous flap dissection is made, contributing importantly to contour irregularities if the fat layer is not dissected uniformly; and (4) denervation of the pectoralis major with subsequent muscle atrophy.

The procedure of lower thoracic advancement works best when there is a well-innervated muscle with good function. The pectoralis major is a tripartate muscle embryologically. Not infrequently, the lower third, and on occasion the lower two thirds, is denervated in removing tissues between the major and minor muscles. This variable innervation and possible denervation and atrophy make the subpectoral implant placement less effective. Contour irregularities can then develop, a depression in the upper or middle thorax after reconstruction, and also less predictable soft tissue expansion over the implant between the pectoralis muscle and the fixed inframammary fold (Fig. 32–3).

At the time of a delayed reconstruction, the chest wall soft tissue presentation can be conceptualized as a delayed myocutaneous unit. After completion of the mastectomy, the chest flaps are sutured into place, where they then adhere to the pectoralis major, a small portion of the pectoralis minor, the serratus anterior, and the remaining chest wall tissues inferiorly. In planning the lower thoracic advancement, the skin and subcutaneous tissues are freed from the chest wall inferiorly, but then superiorly are raised on the pectoralis major muscle. The breast skin cover is then a delayed pectoralis major myocutaneous unit with a random portion inferolaterally beyond the edge of the major pectoral muscle (see Fig. 32–8). This appears to contribute to the increasing safety with which the random portion below the edge of the muscle, and frequently a part

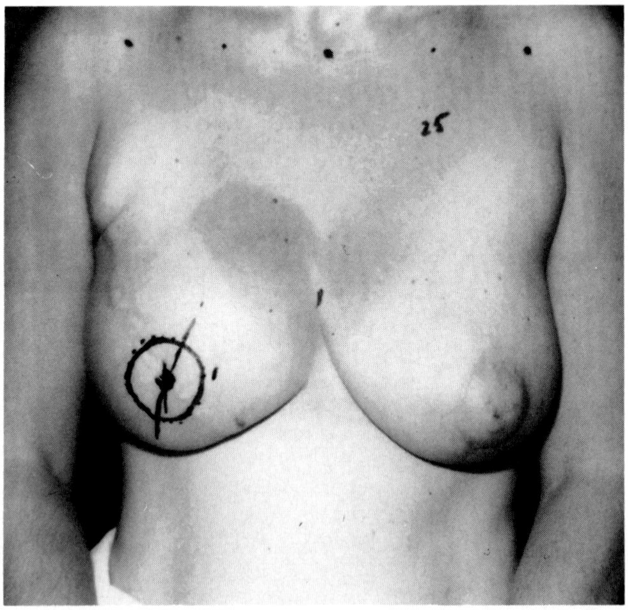

FIGURE 32–3 This patient, who underwent first-stage right breast reconstruction with lower thoracic advancement and subpectoral implant placement, is marked for second-stage planned implant expansion and nipple-areola reconstruction. Note the persisting parasternal and midchest contour deformity produced by a marked atrophy of the middle and lower portions of the pectoralis major muscle.

of the inferior mastectomy flap, can be raised without serious vascular impairment when a period of 4 or more months has intervened. However, vascular problems have arisen and have been reported to the author when the procedure has been attempted within a matter of weeks of the mastectomy. Likewise, subcutaneous fat necrosis is more common when the procedure is performed early in obese patients. Thus, the technique of lower thoracic advancement lends itself to consideration only for delayed postmastectomy reconstruction.

Patient Selection

The technique is very useful in delayed breast reconstruction. It is preferable that it be performed 4 or more months after the mastectomy, and that the latter be well healed with satisfactory mobility of the chest wall soft tissues. If there is marked induration and lack of mobility, an interval of massage is undertaken until tissue mobility is adequate. Also important are the general thoracic configuration of the patient, good pectoralis muscle volume and function, and the direction of the mastectomy scar. Patients with a square or vertically short thorax with good mobility of chest wall tissues, modest but not excessive subcutaneous fat, and a modestly sized remaining breast in the B- to C-cup range (200 to 400 ml) are good candidates. Circumstances that make the procedure more difficult include a very long thoracic configuration, particularly in long, narrow, tight-skinned patients with a flaring lower costal margin, minimal skin mobility, and marked loss of the pectoralis major muscle in its middle or inferior thirds. A low-lying transverse incision that would lead to a very narrow zone between the new inframammary fold and the mastectomy scar should call into question the appropriateness of this technique.

Preoperative Evaluation and Care

Discussions of alternatives may vary depending on whether the patient is evaluated before or after mastectomy. If it takes place before mastectomy, discussion may often include the question of immediate or delayed breast reconstruction. Immediate reconstruction usually involves consideration of a tissue expander or a permanent implant with total muscle coverage. This is sometimes the definitive reconstruction, but often requires, at an interval, removal of the expander and permanent implant placement. At this second procedure a stable inframammary fold might be formed and implant volume adjustment can be made. Except for the patient with a small, youthful breast, immediate reconstruction may often involve two stages. Lower thoracic advancement inframammary fold formation can be a consideration in the second stage.

In delayed reconstruction, an alternative to a tissue expander is lower thoracic advancement and planned implant expansion (Figs. 32-4 to 32-6). After an appropriate interval following mastectomy, the lower thoracic advancement reconstruction is performed, placing at that time the largest implant that can be accommodated. At an interval of 4 to 6 months, at the time nipple-areola reconstruction is usually undertaken, a small portion of the lateral inframammary incision can be opened and volume supplemented by as much as 50 percent of the original volume. This latter technique of planned implant expansion often saves the frequent office visits required for tissue expander reconstruction, and I find

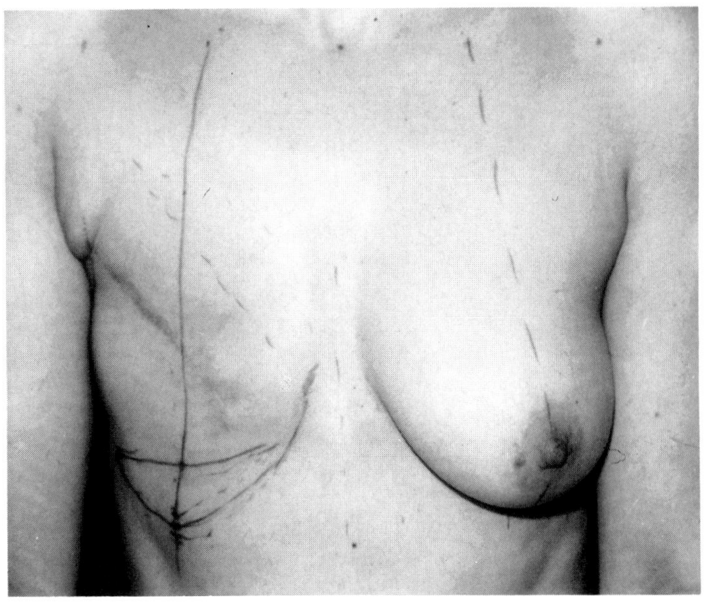

FIGURE 32-4 Seven months after a right modified mastectomy. The chest is marked for first-stage reconstruction with lower thoracic flap advancement and subpectoral implant placement. Note the obliquity of the scar, producing a distinct superomedial zone and inferolateral zone on the thoracic wall. Note also the modest ptosis of the remaining breast, which raises the possibility of left mastopexy or right tissue expansion reconstruction to increase the ptosis. Planned implant expansion was selected in an effort to stretch skin between the edge of the pectoralis major and fixed inframammary fold in order to produce some ptosis and fair symmetry of shape.

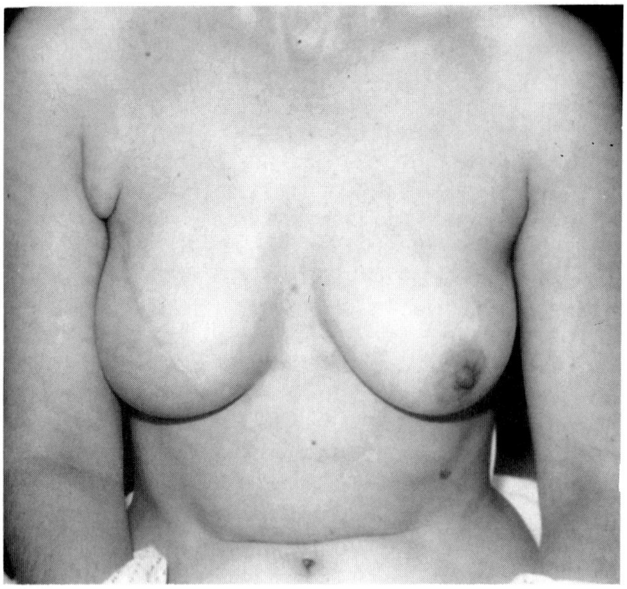

FIGURE 32-5 The same patient 6 months later after first-stage reconstruction and ready for planned implant expansion and nipple-areola reconstruction. The reconstruction has attained a fair element of ptosis, producing quite good symmetry of shape and thus not requiring any alteration of the remaining breast.

it a worthy consideration among the various reconstructive alternatives. The ideal candidate will not need the remaining breast altered and could undergo lower thoracic advancement with permanent implant placement 4 to 6 months following mastectomy or at any time thereafter, with possible planned implant expansion at the time of nipple-areola reconstruction. All patients are admitted the day of surgery and

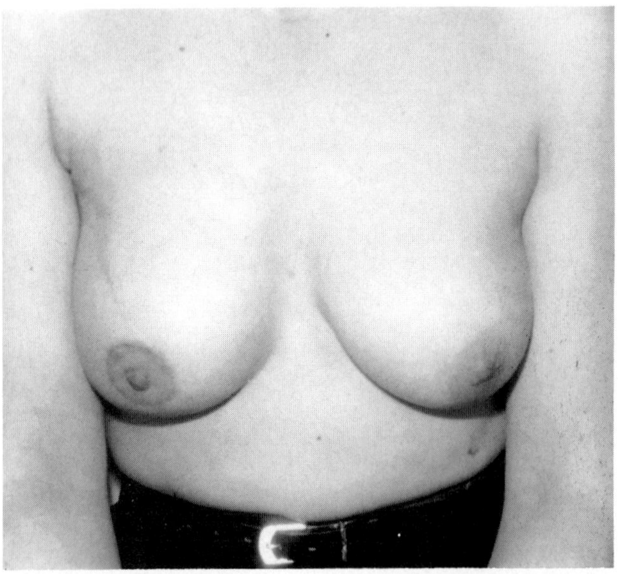

FIGURE 32-6 The same patient 6 months after second-stage reconstruction by planned implant expansion and nipple-areola reconstruction. This has produced symmetry of volume and shape and a modest degree of ptosis to match the remaining breast.

given skin preparation instructions to be used several days preoperatively, as well as sleep medication for one or more nights before admission.

Surgical Technique

The patient is measured and marked in the operating theatre immediately before surgery. She is instructed to wear her brassiere and external prosthesis to the operating room. This is helpful in marking the level at which she comfortably perceives the inframammary fold should be on the mastectomy site (see Fig. 32-4). Likewise, the external prosthesis can be used as a rough index to implant volume by doing a volumetric displacement. The breast meridian is then marked, and between 2 and 4 cm below the inframammary line, in the meridian, the center of the de-epithelialized zone is marked. This zone will be roughly crescent shaped, extending medially on the inframammary fold, to complement the medial extent of the inframammary fold on the opposite breast, and laterally to the anterior axillary line on the inframammary fold (Fig. 32-7). The zone is approximately 1 cm wide in its midportion, tapering toward both ends. The more smooth and uniform the crescent, the easier subsequent tailoring becomes. Thus, in a broader chest the medial and lateral ends are further apart, and a site of 4 cm below the inframammary fold is not nearly so deep in appearance as a very narrow chest with that same central marking. A rough guide to the distance below the inframammary fold is a flap design approximately 1 cm below the inframammary fold in the meridian per 100 ml of planned implant volume. Thus, a 250-ml implant would have a crescent centered some 2.5 cm below the inframammary fold in the meridian. With these markings in place, the patient is carefully positioned supine with arms extended and the table flexed in the midportion. Intraoperatively, the outlined crescent is de-epithelialized. Immediately afterward, the junction of the intact epithelium with the dermis at the superior and inferior edges is back cut for 1 to 2 mm at an angle of about 45 degrees. This allows a better eversion of the epithelium at the time of closure and helps offset the tendency to inversion. A full-thickness incision is then made through the midportion of the de-epithelialized zone from medial to lateral end. Dissection is carried superiorly at the level of the chest wall tissues, in the preserratus fascial plane. This dissection is performed in the anterior axillary line until the edge of the pectoralis major muscle is identified, and then the retropectoral pocket is developed. The lower costal slips of the pectoralis major are taken down under direct visualization with cauterization, great care being taken not to skeletalize the rib, usually the sixth. The parasternal fibers are likewise incised to a site approximately 3 o'clock on the right breast or 9 o'clock on the left, or until a silicone mammary sizer put in

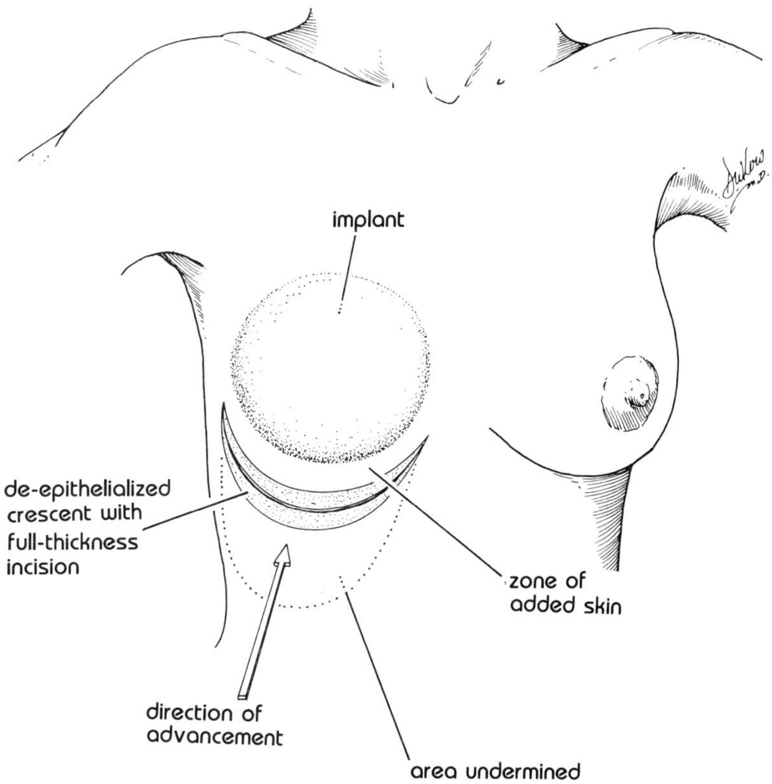

FIGURE 32-7 The markings and planning of the lower thoracic advancement in delayed breast reconstruction. The implant will lie under the outline of the externally worn prosthesis, sitting at the level of the inframammary fold. At an interval of 2 to 4 cm below this in the breast meridian will be the center of the crescent to be de-epithelialized and then incised in its midportion, to allow undermining and flap development. The zone to be undermined inferolaterally to allow advancement in the direction of the meridian will vary, but will approximate at most 1.5 to 2 cm per centimeter of advancement.

place is not restricted at the parasternal zone by remaining muscle slips. If the mastectomy scar and the incision for the lower thoracic advancement cross medially or if there is a very narrow zone between them, care is taken not to extensively undermine the subcutaneous tissue medially, although the underlying muscle slips can be cautiously divided.

Attention is next turned to the inferior dermal edge, which, as the chest wall tissues ascend in the reclining position, will often have elevated on the chest wall very close to the site of the inframammary fold 2 to 2.5 cm simply with reclining and abduction of the shoulder. If it has not ascended to the level of the inframammary fold on the meridian, this usually being right on or above the sixth rib as determined preoperatively in the sitting position, the inferior tissues are elevated off the lower thoracic and upper abdomen tissues to allow a tension-free advancement of the de-epithelialized dermal edge and the subcutaneous tissues. As a rough rule, the most that need be undermined is 1.5 to 2 cm per centimeter of advancement; this much is usually necessary on a fairly tight-skinned individual. The dermal inferior edge is then affixed to the chest wall. The initial suture is a horizontal mattress 2-0 nonabsorbable suture placed in the meridian at the advancing dermal edge. Attention is next turned to the medial and lateral extremes, where a suture halfway between the end of the incision and the meridian suture is placed so as not to leave a contour irregularity or dog-ear at the medial or lateral ends. If there is some gathering of tissues toward the center, this will be more inclined to resolve and smooth out than if it were left at the medial or lateral end.

Likewise, the central half of the advancing dermal flap is affixed to the chest wall tightly with the horizontal mattress sutures, but the lateral and medial portions at their extremes are very loosely attached to the chest wall just as the inframammary fold is better defined and formed centrally than as it extends medially and laterally. A very thick subcutaneous fat layer can make advancement and chest wall suturing difficult. In this situation, I often remove a portion of the subcutaneous fat from beneath the advancing dermal edge to facilitate suturing more free of tension than can occur if this edge is rolled over a very thick subcutaneous fat layer.

The implant sizers are then put in place, and the superior dermal edge can be gently turned over the sizer to gauge the ease of approximation of the superior dermal edge to the inferior dermal edge. This should be free of any excessive tension. If the superior edge needs to be forced under tension for closure, a smaller implant volume will be needed initially. I next irrigate the pocket with a saline solution and corticosteroids and with half-strength povidone-iodine (Betadine) solution. The permanent double-lumen implant is then put in place. The superior dermal edge is brought down and sutured in at least three layers to the inferior dermal edge, again with

2-0 and 3-0 synthetic absorbable sutures. The back cut of the epidermal flap is everted with a continuous 3-0 suture. This gives a modest increase in dermal-to-dermal opposition and facilitates eversion of the closure, which sometimes is further everted with an epidermal suture. The implant is thus covered by the pectoralis major muscle over its superomedial portion but by subcutaneous fat and skin below the edge of the muscle in the inferolateral portion (Fig. 32–8). The wound closure is supported with an inframammary dressing to press the inferior tissues firmly against the chest wall and slightly support the fold. A support brassiere is then put in place. The wound is rarely drained. If the reconstruction is on the patient's dominant hand side, a sling is worn for the first 3 days. The surgery is performed either on an outpatient basis or more commonly with an overnight hospital stay. Postoperative care consists of an office visit in 5 to 7 days for dressing and suture removal, at which time a lighter support brassiere is instituted to be worn for a 2-week period. The patient may begin light activity, e.g., grooming or driving, on the third or fourth postoperative day. However, full range of shoulder motion, particularly heavy lifting, is restricted until the second week and then gradually increased, so that most activities are totally resumed by 4 weeks after surgery.

In 340 delayed breast reconstructions performed with this technique, there have been 14 immediate complications. Six patients had early postoperative hematomas requiring reoperation, and all had immediate replacements of implants and subsequent uneventful healing. Periprosthetic sepsis developed in three patients, two of these being diabetic and two having had drains placed at the time of surgery. These were all treated with implant removal and systemic antibiotics and subsequent successful reconstruction with the same technique. Five patients had wound disruption requiring prosthesis removal and subsequent delayed replacement; two of these were diabetic and four were obese and had elements of subcutaneous fat necrosis. Significantly, the author noted no dermal necrosis at the superior edge of the flap, although colleagues have reported this in patients who were obese or diabetic or in whom the surgery was performed soon after mastectomy. On a delayed basis, 17 patients have required reattachment of the inframammary flap advancement, most of these being only a partial stretching and detachment that was easily redone at the time of nipple-areola reconstruction. In the presence of good pectoralis major function, troublesome periprosthetic capsule formation has been very infrequent.

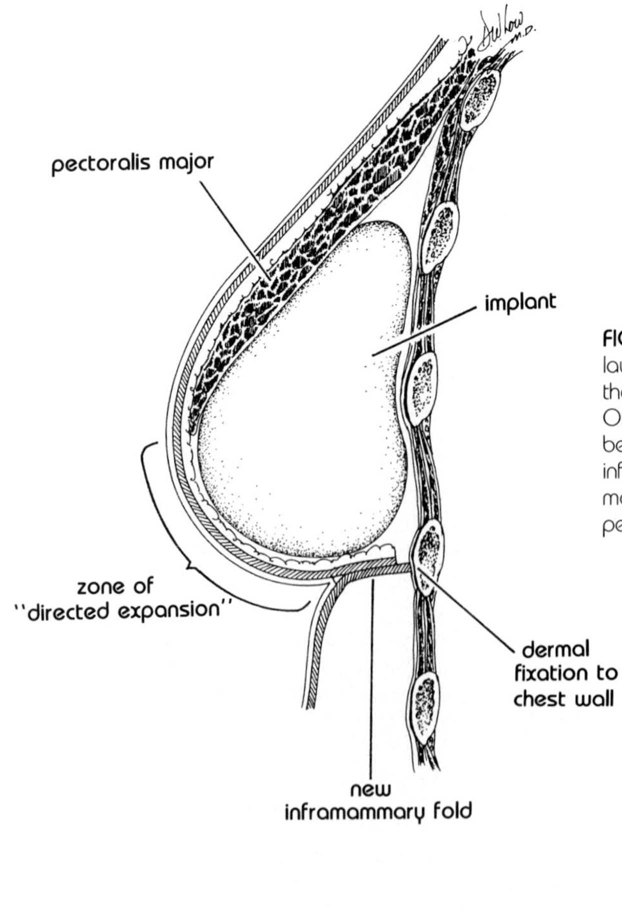

FIGURE 32–8 Cross-sectional presentation of completed delayed breast reconstruction with subpectoral implant and lower thoracic skin supplement with buried dermal inframammary fold. Of particular note is the subsequent occurrence of skin expansion below the inferior edge of the pectoralis major muscle and fixed inframammary fold, which at an interval of approximately 6 months will allow an increase in implant volume of up to 50 percent.

The advantages of the technique are its relative simplicity, reliability, and adaptability. The modest tissue supplement has a good color match, and the formation of a stable and fixed inframammary fold is becoming increasingly appreciated in its contribution to breast shape and patient comfort. The expansion of the skin envelope over the months can be used to great advantage. This expansion occurs between the edge of the pectoralis major and the stable inframammary fold, thus principally in the inferolateral direction where skin deficiency is most notable and is somewhat directed by the forces of muscle contraction, not being a random, undirected expansion. This allows increase of implant volume by about 50 percent at 6 months, and has proved a good alternative to formal use of the tissue expander (Figs. 32-4 to 32-6). However, the technique has definite limitations. It is a delayed reconstruction technique, the skin supplement is modest, and there is a new inframammary scar. Nonetheless, within these restrictions it has proved a helpful alternative in delayed postmastectomy breast reconstruction. The final appearance does take a number of months to evolve and this too must be stressed to the patient. It is not a technique in which what is seen in the operating theatre is in evidence after several months.

References

1. Maxwell GP. Igino Tansini and the origin of the latissimus dorsi musculocutaneous flap. Plast Reconstr Surg 1980; 65:682-692.
2. Tansini I. Nuovo processo, per l'amputazioe della mammaela per cancer. Reforma Med 1846; 12:3.
3. Berson MK. Derma-fat-fascia transplants used in building up breasts. J Surg 1944; 15:451-456.
4. DeCholonolky T. Mastectomies with simultaneous reconstruction of breasts. Surgery 1958; 44:689-697.
5. Letterman G, Schurter M. Total mammary gland excision with immediate breast reconstruction. Am Surg 1955; 21:835-844.
6. Marino H. Glandular mastectomy: Immediate reconstruction. Plast Reconstr Surg 1952; 10:204-208.
7. Cronin T, Gerow F. Augmentation mammoplasty: A new "natural feel" prosthesis. Trans Third Int Congr Plastic Surgeons. New York: Excerpta Medica, 1963; 41-49.
8. Snyderman RK, Guthrie RH. Reconstruction of the female breast following radical mastectomy. Plast Reconstr Surg 1971; 47:565.
9. Lewis JR. Use of a sliding flap from the abdomen to provide cover in breast reconstructions. Plast Reconstr Surg 1979; 64:491-497.
10. Cronin TD, Upton J, McDonough JM. Reconstruction of the breast after mastectomy. Plast Reconstr Surg 1977; 59:114.
11. McCraw JB, Dibbel DG, Carraway JH. Clinical definitions of independent myocutaneous vascular territories. Plast Reconstr Surg 1977; 60:341-352.
12. Bostwick J, Vasconez L, Jurkiewicz M. Breast reconstruction after a radical mastectomy. Plast Reconstr Surg 1978; 61:682-693.
13. Schneider WJ, Hill HL, Brown RG. Latissimus dorsi myocutaneous flap for breast reconstruction. Br J Plast Surg 1977; 30:277-281.
14. Ryan JJ. The planning of breast reconstruction after mastectomy. In: Lewison EF, Montague ACW, eds. Diagnosis and treatment of breast cancer, Baltimore: Williams & Wilkins, 1981:255-287.
15. Ryan JJ. A lower thoracic advancement flap in breast reconstruction after mastectomy. Plast Reconstr Surg 1982; 70:153-158.

CHAPTER 33

Reconstruction with the Latissimus Dorsi Flap

JOHN BOSTWICK III, M.D.

BACKGROUND AND HISTORY

Although Tanzini described a pedicled latissimus dorsi musculocutaneous flap for closure of the radical mastectomy defect as early as the 1890s,[1] this flap did not gain widespread popularity for breast reconstruction until the 1970s. In 1976, the pedicled latissimus dorsi musculocutaneous flap was reintroduced for the management of radiation necrosis of the chest wall,[2] and in 1977 the latissimus dorsi island musculocutaneous flap was introduced for breast reconstruction.[3] At this time, most of the patients who requested breast reconstruction had radical mastectomy deformities with thin, grafted, or irradiated skin. Breast reconstruction with only a silicone breast implant under the available tissue did not provide satisfactory tissue restoration.

It was soon apparent that the latissimus dorsi island musculocutaneous flap offered a viable method for reconstructing the radical mastectomy deformity. It provided autogenous muscle for replacement of the pectoralis major muscle, and an island of skin and subcutaneous fat to replace missing tissue from the excised skin ellipse. Furthermore, the latissimus dorsi insertion could be detached and transposed anteriorly for reconstruction of the anterior axillary fold. With this reconstructive approach, a silicone breast implant was needed for replacement of breast mound volume. Although the latissimus dorsi muscle provided durable cover for a silicone breast implant, it was not a panacea. It unfortunately did not prevent the development of capsular contracture and the subsequent firmness and deformity, a long-term problem associated with this technique.[4]

Today the safety, appearance, and softness of the latissimus dorsi flap breast reconstruction is enhanced by placement of a textured-surface expander at the time of the latissimus dorsi flap procedure. This device is positioned to avoid stress or undue pressure on the newly transferred flap. It is expanded with saline solution in the postoperative period and exhanged for a textured-surface or polyurethane-covered breast implant during a second procedure.[5]

The back donor scar, one of patients' primary objections to this procedure, and the flap design have also been improved. Initially the scar was designed transversely across the back beneath the brassiere. Subsequent designs, laterally for reconstruction of the modified radical mastectomy deformity and now obliquely in the natural skin lines of the back to include the excess "roll" of subcutaneous tissue, create a much more acceptable scar. A combination of these two designs with additional fat harvest now permits the inclusion of enough further autogenous tissue in the flap to permit a totally autogenous latissimus dorsi flap reconstruction that no longer relies on a silicone breast implant for creation of the breast mound.

ESSENTIAL ANATOMY

The latissimus dorsi muscle is analogous to the pectoralis major muscle anteriorly; its triangular shape, thickness, axillary insertion, proximal dominant pedicle, and large surface area contribute to its similarity to and utility for replacing the pectoralis major muscle after a radical mastectomy.

The latissimus dorsi muscle is a superficial muscle of the back originating medially from the lower six thoracic spines, inferiorly from the iliac crest, and inferolaterally with the external oblique muscle where it shares slips of origin. In the lower and middle portion of the back the muscle is relatively thin; its fibers begin to converge at the level of the scapula tip. The proximal muscle thickens as it approaches the axilla. Beginning at the scapula tip, it is lateral to the teres major; however, these muscles are closely associated, and the latissimus dorsi muscle spirals around the teres major muscle as these muscles approach their humeral insertions. These two muscles constitute the primary portion of the posterior axillary fold. The latissimus dorsi muscle inserts at the intertubercular groove of the humerus. This insertion may be detached and the latissimus dorsi tendon reinserted anteriorly to provide a dynamic reconstruction of the anterior axillary fold analogous to that of the pectoralis major muscle.

The blood supply of the latissimus dorsi flap is complex; it derives nourishment from the proximal thoracodorsal pedicle and from additional secondary pedicles related to the teres major, the serratus anterior muscle, and posterolateral intercostal and paraspinal segmental perforators. A profuse and predictable intramuscular blood supply branches from the proximal thoracodorsal pedicle, adding to the reliability and versatility of the flap and permitting the muscle to be split into two or more paddles with skin islands designed over these split muscle portions.

The thoracodorsal pedicle, the primary proximal blood supply of the latissimus dorsi muscle, originates from the axillary vessels. The thoracodorsal artery usually branches from the subscapular artery soon after its origin from the axillary artery. The thoracodorsal vessels are 1.5 to 2.5 mm in diameter, and the thoracodorsal pedicle is usually at least 10 cm in length. This combination of a long pedicle with vessels of sufficient diameter make the latissimus dorsi flap a currently popular choice for free tissue transfer with microsurgical anastomosis.

From the level of the scapula tip toward the axilla, the latissimus dorsi muscle is situated primarily over the serratus anterior muscle. The external fascia of the serratus anterior muscle contains a complex of blood vessels. Branches of these vessels converge toward the axilla and join, by a collateral branch, the thoracodorsal pedicle at its entrance into the latissimus dorsi muscle, about 10 cm below the axillary vessels. The direction of blood flow is normally from the axillary artery via the thoracodorsal artery into the latissimus dorsi muscle, and across the serratus collateral branch to the outer serratus anterior fascia. If the thoracodorsal artery is divided or if its flow is occluded, the flow in the serratus collateral reverses. Blood then flows from the intercostal arteries through the serratus anterior muscle, and via the serratus collateral and into the latissimus dorsi muscle, making it possible for the latissimus dorsi flap to survive on the serratus collateral after thoracodorsal pedicle division. The thoracodorsal pedicle is at risk of injury or may require excision for oncologic reasons during axillary lymph node dissection.[6,7]

The thoracodorsal nerve is contained in the thoracodorsal pedicle and has its origin from roots C6–C8 of the posterior cord of the brachial plexus. Thoracodorsal nerve division results in latissimus dorsi muscle paralysis and denervation atrophy, leading to marked thinning of the muscle and causing it to have an almost transparent appearance. This is most often seen after an axillary lymph node dissection in which the thoracodorsal nerve is excised or divided. Denervation and subsequent paralysis of the latissimus dorsi muscle can be helpful after a latissimus dorsi flap to reduce the uncomfortable pulling or to stop unattractive contractions of the transposed muscle. Complete separation of the latissimus dorsi muscle from the teres major muscle and division of the latissimus dorsi insertion can also reduce the possibility of a tight flap. Because denervation of the latissimus dorsi muscle or anterior transposition of the latissimus dorsi flap causes little noticeable functional loss,[8] the latissimus dorsi flap is also a popular choice for microvascular transfer.

The latissimus dorsi musculocutaneous flap is an excellent example of a musculocutaneous unit.[9] The intramuscular vessels of the latissimus dorsi send perforators upward into the subcutaneous tissue to supply the skin of the back overlying the latissimus dorsi muscle. Based on its proximal thoracodorsal pedicle, the entire latissimus dorsi muscle and its overlying skin and subcutaneous tissue, including the random skin a few centimeters beyond the margins of the latissimus dorsi muscle, can be carried as a musculocutaneous flap. Practically speaking, however, the amount of skin harvested is limited to permit primary closure and the best donor scar. Preoperative tissue expansion can permit a wider skin harvest, usually in the natural skin lines of the back or laterally along the margin of the latissimus dorsi muscle. This area contains the primary intramuscular vessels, and the scar is hidden by the arm and the lateral brassiere.

PATIENT SELECTION

Symmetry is a primary consideration in selecting a breast reconstruction technique. The nonflap techniques of breast reconstruction with available tissue and a breast implant, or a tissue expander followed later with a breast implant, are currently the most frequently used types of breast reconstruction. They provide for the minimal amount of scarring and additional procedures outside the immediate breast region. Additional autogenous tissue is often necessary, however, to provide adequate breast contour. If symmetry is not possible without the addition of autogenous tissue, this requirement must be determined at the initial consultation, and the patient informed of this necessity. The latissimus dorsi flap is an intermediate choice for breast reconstruction. It is selected when the requirements for breast reconstruction indicate the need for some additional tissue, and the pedicled transverse rectus abdominis musculocutaneous (TRAM) flap or a free flap breast reconstruction is not safe, possible, or advisable (Fig. 33-1). The latissimus dorsi flap breast reconstruction technique is also generally considered not to be as major a surgical intervention and not as stressful to the patient as a TRAM flap. In addition, the latissimus dorsi flap has a significant track record of safety and reliability, with generally excellent perfusion of the transposed tissues.

Patients who have undergone suction-assisted lipectomy of the abdominal wall, and those with a previous abdominoplasty or other incisions that preclude safe transfer of the abdominal tissue to the breast region, would not be candidates for a TRAM flap but can be considered for a latissimus dorsi flap. Others appropriate for the latter procedure are those with health habits or conditions that could compromise the safety of the TRAM flap, such as cigarette smoking, obesity, diabetes mellitus, or collagen diseases and other problems affecting the microcirculation (Fig. 33-2). The latissimus dorsi flap is a safer alternative for these patients. Total loss of the latissimus dorsi flap has been seen in less than 1 percent of our patients. The overweight patient who is a high risk for the TRAM flap can still have an autogenous tissue breast reconstruction with the latissimus dorsi flap. The latissimus dorsi flap is hardy and reliable, but patients should refrain from cigarette smoking in the perioperative period to maximize microcirculation and tissue viability.

The latissimus dorsi flap is selected most often for patients who have a tight mastectomy site and a full, ptotic opposite breast with fullness in the lower outer quadrant. With the new fleur-de-lis design and other designs of the latissimus dorsi flap to harvest more autogenous tissue, this flap can often be used without the need for an implant.[10-12] However, patients best suited for a total autogenous latissimus dorsi flap breast reconstruction should either have a minimal tissue requirement for the reconstruction or a significant layer of subcutaneous tissue posteriorly over the latissimus dorsi muscle. An estimate of skin requirements is obtained by measuring the surface dimensions of the opposite breast and comparing them with the measurement at the mastectomy site. When the skin cover discrepancy between the mastectomy site and the opposite breast dimensions is more than 6 to 7 cm and there is little tissue in the upper abdomen or laterally for recruitment with tissue expansion, it is unusual for tissue expansion to

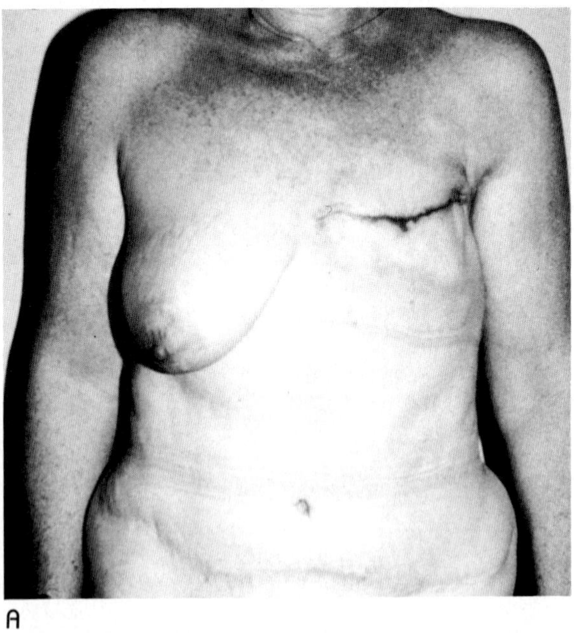

A

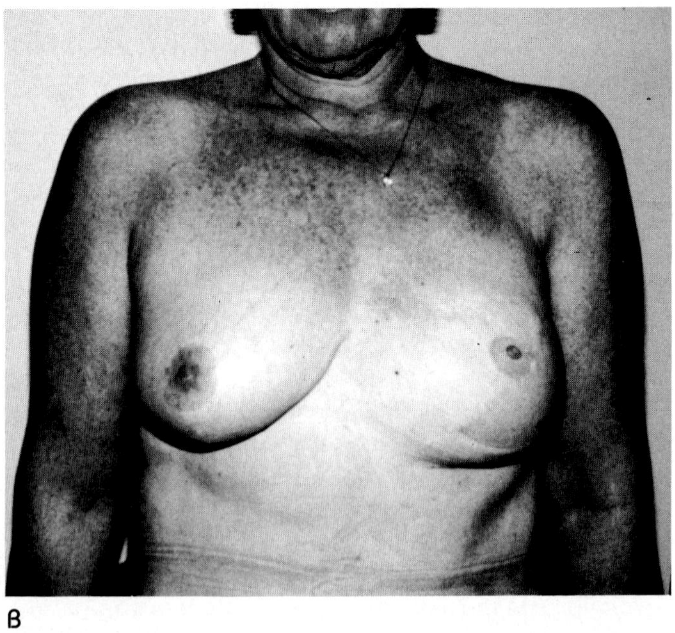

B

FIGURE 33-1 *A*, This 48-year-old woman underwent a left modified radical mastectomy and requested breast reconstruction. She needed autogenous tissue but had received a previous abdominoplasty. A latissimus dorsi flap designed in the natural skin lines of her midback was transposed anteriorly and placed at the level of the opposite inframammary crease after a small reduction mammaplasty. A silicone breast implant was placed at the time of the initial procedure. *B*, Four years after the breast reconstruction with the latissimus dorsi flap and silicone breast implant. Although the symmetry is acceptable, a tissue expander at the time of the breast reconstruction would have given a better opportunity for symmetry. (From Bostwick J. Plastic and reconstructive breast surgery. St Louis: Quality Medical Publishing Co, 1990:675.)

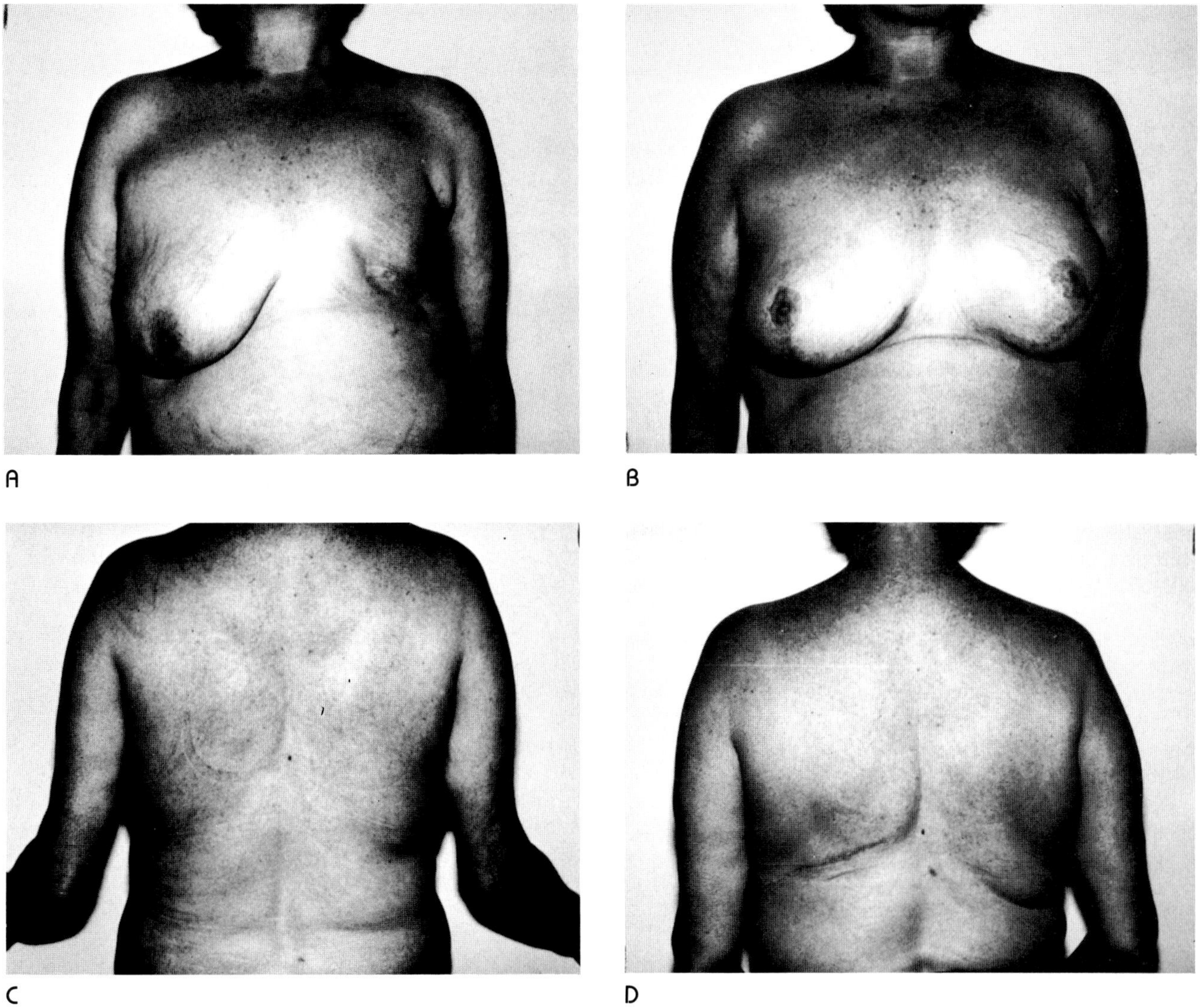

FIGURE 33-2 *A*, This 48-year-old woman underwent a left modified radical mastectomy and requested breast reconstruction. She needed autogenous tissue but was not a good candidate for a transverse rectus abdominis musculocutaneous (TRAM) flap because she was overweight and smoked cigarettes. A latissimus dorsi flap designed in the natural skin lines of her midback was transposed anteriorly and placed at the level of the opposite inframammary crease after a small reduction mammaplasty. A tissue expander was placed at the time of the initial procedure. *B*, Three months later the tissue expander was exchanged for a polyurethane-covered silicone breast implant, and the nipple-areola reconstruction was done. She is shown 2 years later. The breast reconstruction has remained soft and acceptably symmetric. *C*, The patient's back before the procedure. *D*, Her back 2 years later. The scar is thin, but there is some asymmetry of the soft tissues. (From Bostwick J. Plastic and reconstructive breast surgery. St Louis: Quality Medical Publishing Co, 1990:673–674.)

provide enough tissue for an attractive breast reconstruction. Modification of the opposite breast with mastopexy or reduction mammaplasty is an option, but some patients prefer a back scar and symmetry to alteration of an attractive opposite breast.

The latissimus dorsi flap is also considered when the skin flaps of the mastectomy are extremely thin and tissue expansion would contribute further to thinning. The latissimus dorsi muscle provides additional interposed tissue between the implant and the skin, reducing the possibility of extrusion. When a polyurethane-covered implant is used, interposition of latissimus dorsi muscle reduces the ripple effect seen when this device is inserted directly under thin skin. The latissimus dorsi flap is especially considered when the thin flaps are associated with radiation therapy. Radiated tissues expand poorly, and autogenous tissue, either with the TRAM flap, a free flap, or the latissimus dorsi flap, is usually necessary for a breast reconstruction after radiation therapy.

Although the radical mastectomy deformity is

less frequently seen today, some women who underwent the procedure years ago are only now requesting breast reconstruction (Fig. 33-3). Other patients have had pectoralis major muscle excision because of breast cancer recurrence after lumpectomy radiation or for local removal of a deep breast cancer. These patients may not be candidates for the TRAM flap. The latissimus dorsi flap is useful in these situations; the muscle can be transposed to span the anterior axilla and reconstruct the anterior axillary fold, and the skin island can supplement the skin deficit. When a significant subcutaneous tissue deficit remains in the upper chest after a radical mastectomy, the single layer of latissimus dorsi flap needs to be supplemented with a de-epithelialized skin island, a customized polyurethane-covered silicone breast implant, or a free flap or pedicled TRAM flap to provide contour restoration. The latissimus dorsi flap may also be used for optimal anterior axillary fold and upper lateral chest reconstruction in conjunction with a TRAM flap breast reconstruction for patients with a radical mastectomy deformity.

The latissimus dorsi flap is also appropriate for immediate breast reconstruction, which is becoming more accepted and popular. Much the same considerations of patient selection regarding delayed breast reconstruction are applicable to immediate breast reconstruction. When the excision at the site of the mastectomy will leave a tissue deficit that is not amenable to the placement of a breast implant, or when a breast implant or tissue expander will not give an acceptable symmetry, autogenous tissue is considered. The latissimus dorsi flap is a choice for autogenous tissue, but the pedicled TRAM flap is often the first choice when the surgeon is comfortable with the latter, and the patient has sufficient lower abdominal wall tissue, desires an abdominoplasty, and is a safe candidate for a TRAM flap. When the TRAM flap is not considered a safe or viable option, and a free flap is also not appropriate, the latissimus dorsi flap is a good choice for immediate breast reconstruction. The candidate for immediate breast reconstruction with the latissimus dorsi flap should understand that there will be a back incision and scar, and a patch of the flap on the reconstructed breast. However, the latissimus dorsi flap provides a safe predictable source of autogenous tissue for breast reconstruction, and with the techniques of additional autogenous tissue harvest, a breast reconstruction can be performed with the latissimus dorsi flap without the need for a breast implant.

PREOPERATIVE EVALUATION AND CARE

Candidates for a latissimus dorsi flap breast reconstruction should be evaluated for significant psychological, physical, oncologic, aesthetic, and reconstructive factors. They should be psychologically stable and able to undergo the stress of a major surgical procedure, general anesthesia, and a possible prolonged convalescence. They must also be able to cope with postoperative depression and accept a result that may not be ideal. For some patients, the latissimus dorsi flap or other flap procedures, which require additional donor site incisions and scars, may be more involved than they can mentally han-

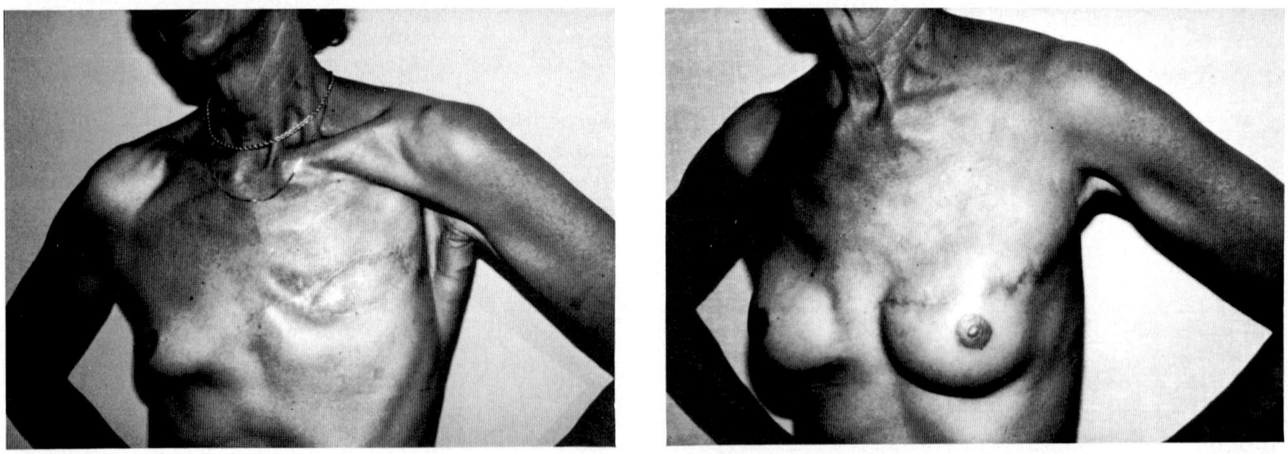

A B

FIGURE 33-3 *A*, This 58-year-old woman underwent a radical mastectomy 8 years before her breast reconstruction. She was thin and her abdomen was not adequate for a TRAM flap. She received a de-epithelialized latissimus dorsi flap and silicone breast implant for the breast reconstruction. At the same procedure an augmentation mammaplasty of the opposite breast was performed. The de-epithelialized flap gave good fill for the infraclavicular region, and the insertion was reattached anteriorly to the divided end of the pectoralis major muscle tendon. *B*, One year after the breast reconstruction with the de-epithelialized latissimus dorsi flap and a silicone breast implant. (From Bostwick J. Plastic and reconstructive breast surgery. St Louis: Quality Medical Publishing Co, 1990:671–672.)

dle, and for these women a simpler method should be chosen.

The latissimus dorsi flap procedure is a major operation. The patient selected for this reconstructive approach must be in good general health. She should not have a life-threatening condition that could be put at risk by general anesthesia and the surgical procedure. Her microcirculatory status also merits consideration. If she is a heavy cigarette smoker and does not stop smoking in the perioperative period, the risks of tissue loss and flap failure are significant, but generally less than those with the pedicled TRAM flap. Other conditions associated with decreased microcirculation, such as diabetes mellitus or collagen vascular diseases, are relative contraindications to the latissimus dorsi flap breast reconstruction. Although a blood transfusion is almost never necessary when a latissimus dorsi flap is ued, one or two units of autogenous blood should be considered.

The patient's oncologic status should also be evaluated. The reconstructive surgeon should consult with the surgical and medical oncologist regarding the stage and status of the tumor, the nature of the treatment, and the patient's current medications. The reconstructive surgeon should carefully assess the local conditions for signs of recurrence, such as nodularity in the mastectomy scar or axillary or supraclavicular adenopathy. Breast cancer patients should also have an updated evaluation by their medical oncologist before breast reconstruction to check for the possibility of detectable systemic disease that could negate the benefits of the reconstructive surgery.

The opposite breast should be examined preoperatively and the patient's risk status carefully considered. Her history, her family history, the pathologic findings concerning the initial breast tumor, and other pathologic changes in the remainder of the breast alert the reconstructive surgeon to the possibility of cancer in the opposite breast and direct the discussion about such a risk to the opposite breast. Preoperative breast imaging is an important component of the oncologic evaluation of the opposite breast before an operative intervention.

Aesthetic considerations during the preoperative planning of breast reconstruction with the latissimus dorsi flap focus on the plan for symmetry. The opposite breast or the modified opposite breast is the model for the breast reconstruction. After careful measurements for skin and volume deficits, a flap is chosen and designed to accurately replace the missing tissues. When sufficient autogenous tissue is not available for latissimus dorsi flap breast reconstruction, the flap is used to replace skin, provide muscle cover, and supply upper breast fill; the breast mound can then be replaced with a silicone breast implant after the tissues have been adequately stretched with a tissue expander.

Specific preoperative evaluation of the chest wall and the anterior axillary fold may indicate that these areas require reconstruction or supplementation, particularly after a radical mastectomy. In these instances, anterior transposition of the latissimus dorsi insertion can be used to reconstruct the anterior axillary fold, and an additional de-epithelialized portion of the skin island will restore upper chest wall and infraclavicular fullness.

The site of the mastectomy scar influences the positioning of the flap. When the scar is low and oblique, the latissimus dorsi flap is placed in the opened scar. When the mastectomy scar is more vertical or higher on the chest wall, the mastectomy scar is not opened, and the latissimus dorsi flap is placed in the lower, outer portion of the reconstructed breast to restore more fullness and breast ptosis; the flap incisions are less noticeable in this position.

The quality and tightness of the skin at the mastectomy site and the presence of skin grafts are assessed. Skin grafts or radiation changes can affect and increase tissue requirements, and usually indicate the need for a flap breast reconstruction. When the skin is very thin and the latissimus dorsi flap is planned, maximal muscle harvest is required to provide complete latissimus dorsi muscle cover protection for the implant or tissue expander. Radiated tissues do not expand normally and may need to be replaced and supplemented with autogenous skin from the back.

The status of the pectoralis major muscle needs to be checked; it can be intact and functioning, or it may be missing, partially excised, or thinned and atrophic. When muscle function is impaired, additional fill is needed in the upper breast region to provide a symmetric upper breast reconstruction.

The innervation, size, contractility, and function of the latissimus dorsi muscle are also evaluated. A functioning latissimus dorsi muscle is a good indication that the thoracodorsal nerve and possibly the thoracodorsal pedicle are intact. Sometimes the surgeon removes the thoracodorsal artery and vein but preserves the thoracodorsal nerve. In this situation the viability of the latissimus dorsi flap depends on an intact serratus collateral vessel nourishing the latissimus dorsi muscle from the intercostal arteries via reversed flow in the serratus collateral. When I am uncertain about the status of the thoracodorsal pedicle after an axillary dissection, I presume that it has been divided and always preserve the serratus collateral vessels. If the latissimus dorsi muscle is nonfunctioning, I assume that the entire thoracodorsal pedicle has been excised. Although a latissimus dorsi flap based on the serratus collateral vessels can survive in this situation, it has limited flap volume and the entire flap may not survive; I therefore prefer to use another flap for the breast reconstruction.

FLAP DESIGN

I use six basic flap designs for tissue harvest, which provide varying amounts of tissue with specific donor scar orientations.

The thinnest, least noticeable donor scars have been in the natural skin lines of the back. Many women, especially those with some excess subcutaneous tissue, have a "roll" of fatty tissue in the direction of this line, which is just below the brassiere line on the middle back (Fig. 33-4). This design creates a relatively wide skin island because of the excess tissue frequently present in the region. A second incision toward the axilla, usually the mastectomy scar or extended mastectomy scar, is needed to complete the upper axillary dissection.

A laterally positioned donor scar avoids a scar across the back, and is concealed beneath the arm and under the lateral portion of the brassiere (Fig. 33-5). This design is used for breast reconstruction after a modified radical mastectomy. The lateral margin of the transposed latissimus dorsi muscle is sutured to the lower outer margin of the pectoralis major muscle to give lower outer quadrant tissue fullness.

For the patient with considerable subcutaneous tissue, the subcutaneous tissue harvest can be extended beyond the margins of the skin island, and because of the nature of this broad musculocutaneous flap, a relatively large volume of subcutaneous fat can be obtained. The harvest is particularly effective in the lumbar region and over the midback expanse. When maximal subcutaneous harvest overlying the latissimus dorsi muscle is combined with the fleur-de-lis skin harvest, it is possible for many patients to have breast reconstruction with autogenous tissue from the back.

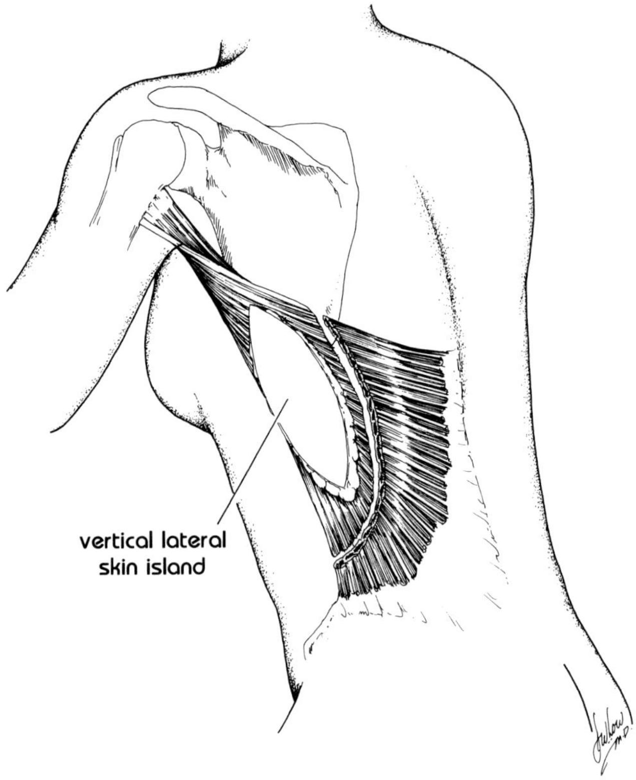

FIGURE 33-5 A laterally positioned skin island avoids a scar across the back and results in a scar concealed beneath the arm and by the lateral portion of the brassiere.

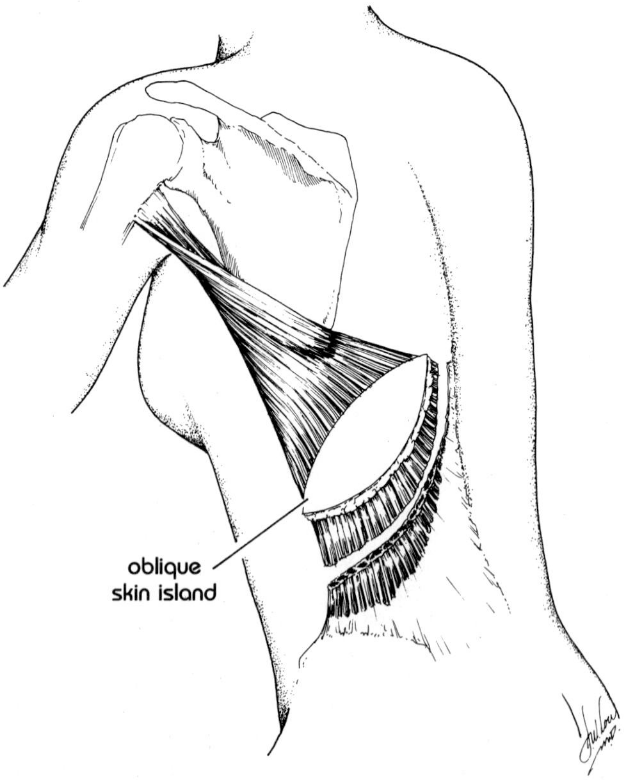

FIGURE 33-4 The natural skin lines of the back course downward from the midline in an oblique direction. An ellipse of skin designed in the direction of these lines results in a wider skin island and usually a less noticeable donor scar.

The maximal latissimus dorsi flap harvest combines these two flap designs and produces an inverted "T" scar. This flap design resembles the fleur-de-lis and is useful for autogenous tissue breast reconstruction.

For reconstruction of the radical mastectomy deformity or to supply tissue for the upper chest wall and anterior axillary fold, an extended lateral flap or a transverse flap across the back, with the donor scar beneath the brassiere, is selected. When the harvest is primarily for muscle, small lateral incisions are made. I use this approach to obtain muscle for breast reconstruction for patients with Poland's syndrome. A transverse axillary incision is necessary to give access to the axillary portion of the dissection.

When more breast mound volume is required than is available from the autogenous tissue of the back, I prefer to place a textured-surface expander at the time of the breast reconstruction. This device is adjusted in the postoperative period to give symmetry with the opposite breast. It is exchanged during the second procedure for a textured-surface or polyurethane-covered implant, and the nipple-areola is reconstructed at this time.

Flap Position

The position of the latissimus dorsi flap anteriorly is determined by the tissue requirements for symmetry and by the need to minimize the visible scars in the breast region. When sufficient breast skin is available or when autogenous tissue breast reconstruction is used after tissue expansion, the latissimus dorsi flap can be de-epithelialized, shaped with sutures, and positioned appropriately subcutaneously to provide an autogenous tissue breast reconstruction without additional scars.

For the modified radical mastectomy deformity, the most natural skin island position is often in the lower outer portion of the reconstructed breast. When the mastectomy scar is high or vertical, it is disregarded and the latissimus dorsi flap skin island is placed in a new incision along the lower outer breast.

For reconstruction of the upper chest wall and anterior axillary fold, the de-epithelialized latissimus dorsi flap and the autogenous tissue are repositioned to provide optimal symmetry. Sometimes I flip the latissimus dorsi flap for upper chest fill and place the de-epithelialized portion deeper against the chest wall, and the deeper, smoother surface of the latissimus dorsi muscle on the outer surface just beneath the skin gives a more natural breast reconstruction.

Markings

The dimensions of the skin island needed for the breast reconstruction anteriorly are determined and marked on the back. The requirements of autogenous tissue are determined and marked relative to the skin ellipse. Usually, an obliquely oriented skin island can be harvested about 8 to 10 cm wide and 25 to 30 cm in length, and the donor site closed primarily. When the latissimus dorsi flap is expanded before harvesting, a larger skin island can be obtained. This permits a primary closure and avoids the necessity for a skin graft at the donor site.

When breast implants are to be used, the dimensions of the opposite breast are taken into account and the dimensions of the breast implant necessary to give symmetry are determined preoperatively. This gives some idea of the limits of the flap elevation of the reconstructed breast, and the tissue and breast implant requirements. During the procedure, breast implant sizers are also helpful to determine the optimal breast implant.

SURGICAL TECHNIQUE

Harvest of Skin Island

The patient is placed in a lateral position for latissimus dorsi flap elevation. The inflatable bean bag helps maintain and stabilize the patient's position during this phase of the procedure. The axilla is prepared in the surgical field, and the arm is placed in a stockinette. An incision is made around the skin island into the subcutaneous tissue. When additional autogenous tissue is to be harvested, the dissection proceeds in the plane just below the subdermal plexus. When only a skin island and the latissimus dorsi muscle are needed, the incision bevels outward to the muscle. The remaining back skin is then elevated from the latissimus dorsi muscle through the extent of the planned flap. Multiple perforators are encountered in this elevation and are controlled with the electrocautery. The flap is then elevated from its deep surface, and the muscle is divided from the adjacent structures, preserving the thoracodorsal pedicle and the serratus collateral vessel.

I divide the latissimus dorsi muscle first in the inferior portion and then in the medial portion. The lateral margin of the latissimus dorsi muscle is identified, and care taken to preserve the external oblique origins, which share some common slips with the latissimus dorsi muscle. The flap is then elevated from inferiorly toward the axilla. Care is taken to identify the serratus anterior muscle and leave it in situ; it should not be elevated with the latissimus dorsi muscle. The serratus anterior muscle is found at the tip of the scapula and extends beneath the latissimus dorsi muscle toward the lateral chest wall. There is a fascial interval and attachment of the serratus anterior muscle to the latissimus dorsi muscle along this inferior margin. This fascia must be divided to permit elevation of the latissimus dorsi muscle while the serratus anterior muscle is left undisturbed.

As the dissection moves toward the axilla, and the latissimus dorsi muscle is elevated from the serratus anterior muscle, the serratus collateral vessels are identified by locating the vessels on the outer surface of the serratus anterior muscle, which converge toward the axilla, and the point of entry of the thoracodorsal pedicle into the latissimus dorsi muscle. These vessels join to form the collateral pedicle, which unites with the thoracodorsal pedicle near its entrance to the latissimus dorsi muscle about 10 cm below the axillary vessels (Fig. 33-6).

The latissimus dorsi muscle must be separated medially from the teres major muscle, which courses with the latissimus dorsi muscle from the scapula tip to their insertions on the humerus. This portion of the dissection is important and must be complete up to the insertions, because it frees the latissimus dorsi flap and permits anterior transposition of the flap without tethering it to the teres major muscle. This

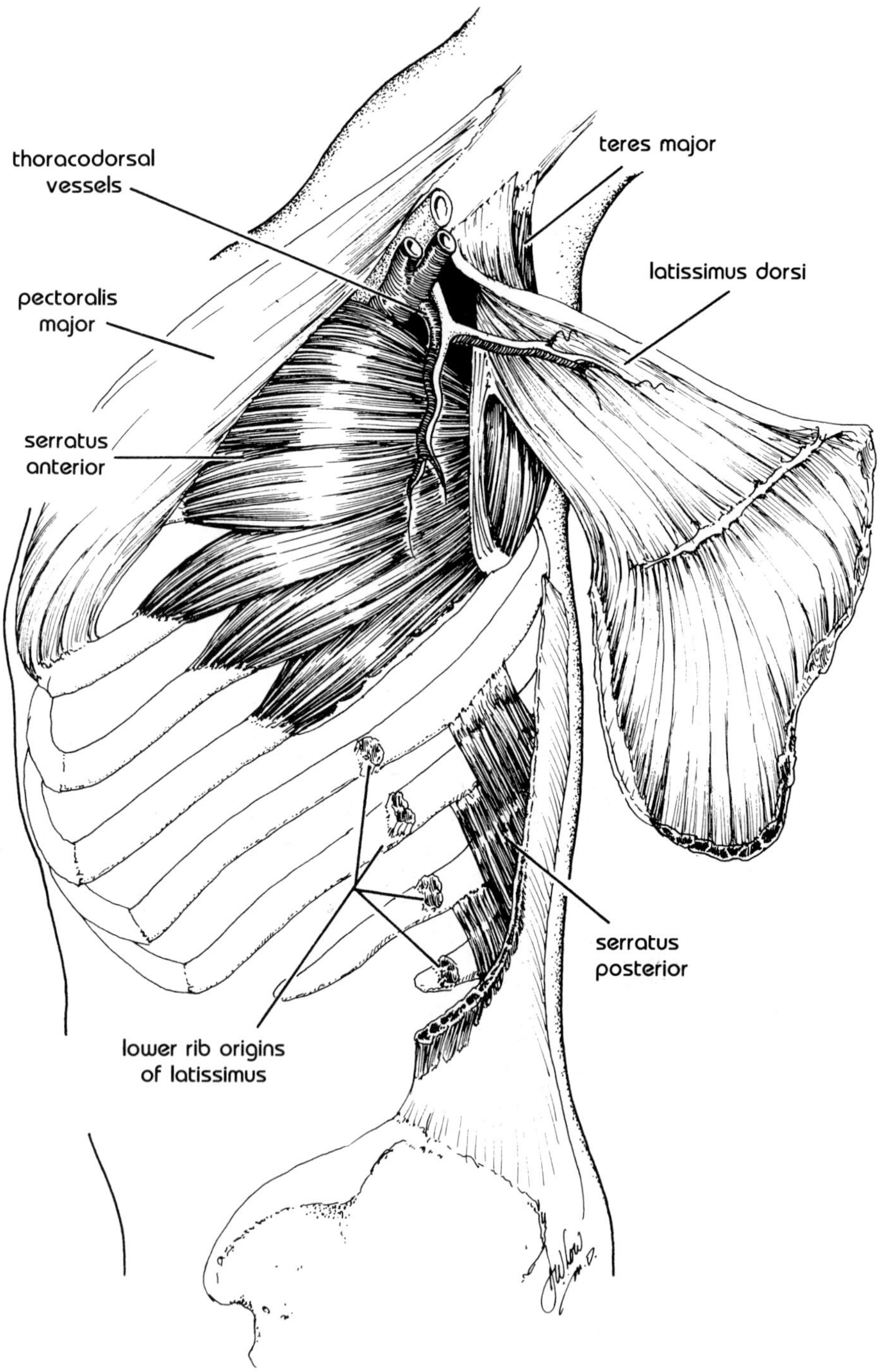

FIGURE 33-6 The serratus collateral vessels are on the surface of the serratus anterior muscle. The collateral pedicle joins near its entrance to the latissimus dorsi muscle, about 10 cm below the axillary vessels.

method of dissection allows safe identification of the thoracodorsal pedicle of the latissimus dorsi muscle.

When anterior transposition of the latissimus dorsi muscle insertion is necessary, it is divided near the intertubercular groove of the humerus after positive identification of the thoracodorsal pedicle. The tendon can then be reinserted anteriorly into position for the insertion of the pectoralis major muscle between the deltoid muscle and the coracobrachialis muscle. It is not usually necessary to divide the insertion of the latissimus dorsi muscle for breast reconstruction after a modified radical mastectomy; however, I do separate it completely from the teres major muscle to avoid tightness and restriction of activity during shoulder motion.

To transpose the latissimus dorsi flap anteriorly and to close the donor site, the anterior chest wall incision is opened and the flaps of the mastectomy are elevated according to the preoperative plan. A subcutaneous tunnel is made high in the axilla, and the flap is brought through this tunnel. It is important to transpose the latissimus dorsi flap through a high tunnel. This orientation permits pedicle positioning to restore axillary fullness; a lower transposition fails to improve the axillary hollowness and creates an unnatural lateral breast fullness.

After hemostasis is attained in the back, a siliconized drain is placed in the dependent portion of the wound, and the back incision is closed in layers, the final one being an intracuticular suture.

LATISSIMUS DORSI FLAP BREAST RECONSTRUCTION WITH IMPLANT OR EXPANDER

After the flap is transposed anteriorly and the back is closed, the patient is placed in the supine position with arms out and secured to the arm boards, so that she can be positioned upright on the operating table. The mastectomy wound is then opened to the limits of the preoperative markings so that the breast reconstruction with the latissimus dorsi flap can be completed.

When the pectoralis major muscle is present and the mastectomy skin flaps are thin, I prefer to position the textured-surface expander in the submuscular position, and therefore elevate the breast flaps with the pectoralis major muscle. When the latissimus dorsi flap is to be positioned in the lower outer quadrant, an incision is made in a predetermined position along the lower and outer margins of the proposed reconstructed breast as well as inferiorly along the inframammary fold. The upper breast flap is elevated with the skin and the pectoralis major muscle. The latissimus dorsi flap is then positioned in the lower outer quadrant of the reconstructed breast. The latissimus dorsi muscle is sutured to the pectoralis major muscle, producing complete muscle cover for the tissue expander or breast implant (Fig. 33-7). When the new incision is made at the inframammary fold, it must be remembered that there is a mastectomy flap below the original mastectomy incision that obtains its vascular supply from the underlying pectoralis major muscle, and these deep attachments must be preserved.

For breast reconstruction after radical mastectomy, the upper portion of the chest wall deformity is an important component of the breast reconstruction. Therefore, dissection of the mastectomy deformity must extend up to the clavicle and out onto the upper arm to the area of the pectoralis major muscle insertion. This point is determined by the position of the insertion of the pectoralis major muscle tendon on the opposite arm. The flap is positioned to give the best anterior axillary fold and upper chest wall

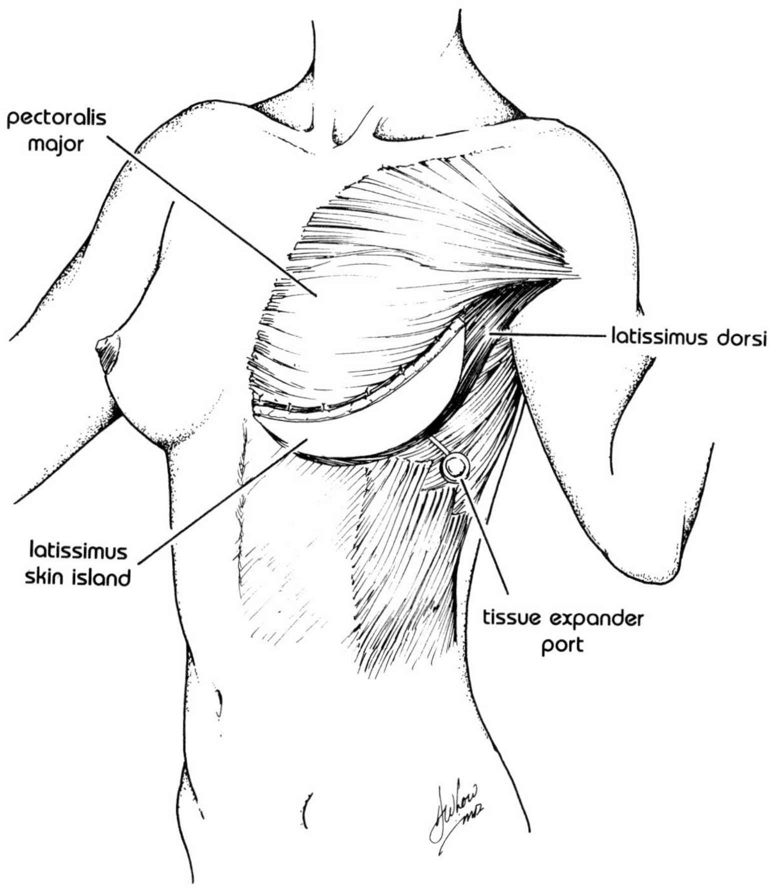

FIGURE 33-7 The skin island is ideally positioned in the lower outer quadrant of the reconstructed breast. The implant or tissue expander is covered by pectoralis major muscle superiorly, and latissimus muscle and skin island inferolaterally.

fill, and usually the latissimus dorsi flap skin island is de-epithelialized to supplement this fullness.

When the latissimus dorsi flap is needed primarily for muscle cover or fullness, it is elevated without a skin island transposed through the axilla and positioned to cover the lower portion of the implant. The upper portion of the implant can usually be covered by the elevated pectoralis major muscle (Fig. 33–8).

Completion of a breast reconstruction with the latissimus dorsi flap often requires placement of a tissue expander or breast implant. The implant size is determined by the dimensions of the defect; implant sizers are helpful for this purpose. If an implant can be selected that provides good symmetry without stressing the flap, I place it at the time of the initial breast reconstruction. If the implant needed for the best symmetry is so large that it will put undue pressure on the latissimus dorsi flap, or if the specific volume for symmetry cannot be determined, I place a textured-surface expander.

The late development of capsular contractures under some latissimus dorsi flap breast reconstructions has led me to use a polyurethane-covered implant under the flap, because it results in a lower incidence of capsular contracture.

NONIMPLANT LATISSIMUS DORSI MUSCLE FLAP RECONSTRUCTION

For breast reconstructions with autogenous tissue only, a similar elevation of the mastectomy flaps is made and the latissimus dorsi flap is de-epithelialized, sutured into the appropriate breast shape, and positioned to give the best symmetry with the opposite breast (Fig. 33–9).

I design an ellipse of skin about 7 to 10 cm wide, depending on the relative tightness of the back tissue. The design of this skin island is in the direction of the natural skin lines and usually incorporates a roll of tissue, which is present if the patient is somewhat overweight. When a maximal amount of autogenous tissue is needed, a vertical ellipse is designed along the lateral margin of the latissimus dorsi muscle. After the skin incision is made, instead of continuing the incision down to the muscle and elevating the skin and subcutaneous tissue off the muscle, the skin is elevated in the superficial area of the superficial fascia to preserve the fat over the muscle. Inferior to the skin island, a similar skin elevation is performed down to the flank region. The incision is then deepened down to the latissimus dorsi muscle, and the latter is elevated from its lower attachments

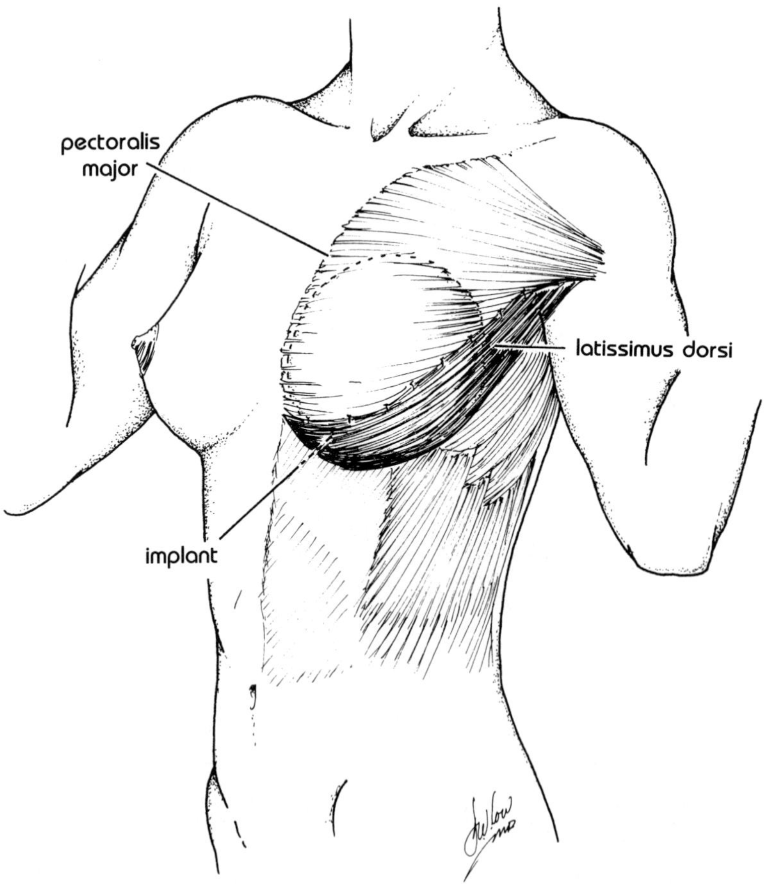

FIGURE 33–8 The latissimus dorsi muscle can be elevated and transposed without a skin island when it is needed primarily for muscle cover. That portion of a silicone implant not covered by pectoralis major muscle can be protected by the latissimus dorsi muscle, which also adds fill to the reconstruction.

from the chest wall. This technique provides a significant amount of subcutaneous tissue to supplement the standard latissimus dorsi flap.

After the latissimus dorsi muscle is transposed anteriorly, the flap is fashioned to provide a breast mound shape symmetric with the opposite breast. When the additional vertical component of the flap is designed, the medial and lateral margins of the lower ellipse are brought up and sutured to this vertical portion, thus giving the flap a fleur-de-lis pattern. This method of suturing gives some coning and projection to the breast shape. The lower fatty tissue and muscle below the transverse skin island is turned underneath and rotated upward to provide additional lower breast projection. If the patient has previously had a tissue expansion or an implant and is not deficient in outer skin cover, the flap is de-epithelialized and buried for the autogenous tissue breast reconstruction.

POSTOPERATIVE CARE

Postoperative care focuses on pain control, management of the back donor site, and management of the breast reconstruction. Postoperatively the patient is placed on a patient-controlled analgesia (PCA) administration device so that she can have timely, appropriate, and responsive pain relief. She is encouraged to get out of bed either the evening of the operation or the next day to reduce the possiblity of deep venous thrombosis. A broad-spectrum antibiotic is prescribed for the first 4 to 5 days postoperatively, particularly if an implant or tissue expander has been placed.

The patient is instructed to avoid excessive shoulder motion to allow the elevated skin of the back to heal to the deeper structures of the back. Significant shoulder motion and activity can shear these new healing attachments and a seroma can develop. Siliconized drains are placed in the back and retained until the drainage is below 20 ml per 12 hours. When a seroma develops, if it is small to moderate in size and not uncomfortable, it usually subsides with time. If it becomes large and uncomfortable, serial aspirations are usually indicated. After several aspirations, if the seroma persists and is uncomfortable, I place a Penrose drain in a dependent region, which usually causes the seroma to subside.

When the anterior axillary fold has been reconstructed and the latissimus dorsi insertion has been transposed anteriorly, I instruct the patient not to abduct her arm for 3 to 4 weeks to permit healing in the region of the axillary reconstruction and avoid stress or detachment of the insertion. After this period has elapsed, the patient is told to perform exercises in front of a mirror to contract the transposed latissimus dorsi muscle and to encourage its contractions. This keeps the bulk and volume of the latissimus dorsi muscle at a maximal level.

When an expander is placed beneath the latissimus dorsi reconstruction, expansion is begun early in the postoperative period when healing seems to be satisfactory. I prefer relatively rapid expansion and often expand or adjust the volume during the hospitalization period to obtain the best symmetry. If flap viability is questionable, however, some of the saline is removed from the tissue expander until flap status is ascertained.

RESULTS

Results of the latissimus dorsi muscle flap reconstruction can be very acceptable but depend on appropriate patient selection, the artistry and experience of the surgeon, the specific technique of breast reconstruction with the latissimus dorsi flap, the amount of autogenous tissue used in the reconstruction, and the behavior of the breast implants and expanders. The best results of breast reconstruction are with maximal use of autogenous tissue. Breast reconstruction with the fleur-de-lis flap technique provides satisfying breast reconstructions whose softness is equal to, and sometimes softer than, that achieved with a TRAM flap reconstruction. The combination of the muscle and fatty tissue appears to be not quite as firm as the lower abdominal fat can be at times. These reconstructions not only are soft and warm, but offer a greater likelihood of sensory reinnervation.

The results of the latissimus dorsi flap procedure with an implant have been improved by use of the textured-surface expander followed by placement of a polyurethane-covered implant to help mitigate the problems of capsular contracture that have characterized long-term results of this technique. The expander permits specific determination of appropriate breast size, symmetric with the opposite breast. The polyurethane-covered implant, with its low incidence of capsular contractures and late deformity, produces softer breasts in the long term.

Management of patients who develop capsular contracture is either with a capsulectomy and replacement with a polyurethane implant, or replacement with autogenous tissue plus a TRAM flap or a free flap. The textured-surface permanent expander implant is also useful in breast reconstruction and particularly so for the very wide breast without significant projection. I presently use a textured-surface expander implant, and when the small valve is used, it can be left in place for a year or more to permit specific adjustments for maximal symmetry.

ADVANTAGES

The latissimus dorsi flap is safe, reliable, and versatile for breast reconstruction. It can be used for

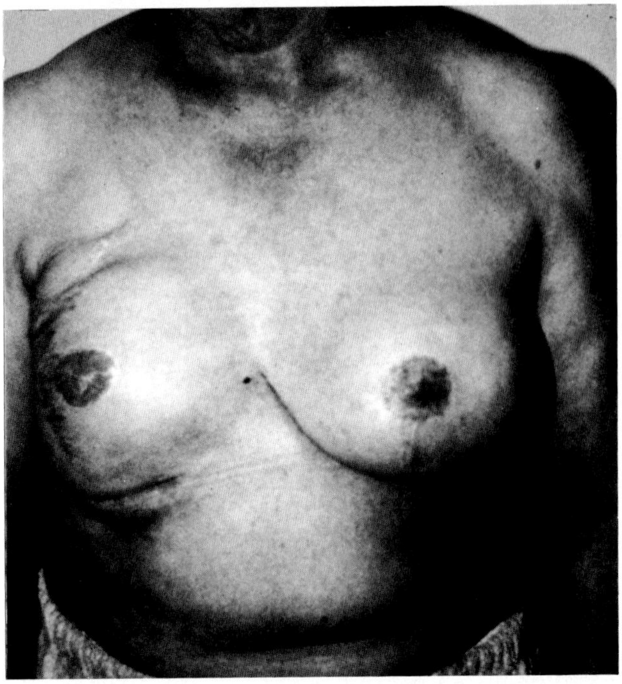

A

FIGURE 33-9 *A*, A 64-year-old woman after a right radical mastectomy, a left modified mastectomy, and bilateral implant reconstruction. After multiple revisions, the right 600-ml implant is firm and contracted laterally, and the inframammary fold is deficient. *B*, A horizontal cutaneous segment is outlined with the patient in the lateral decubitus position. The dotted line depicts the margins of fat to be "carried" on the myoadipocutaneous flap. *Left*, Anterior view. *Right*, Posterior view. *C*, *Left and Right*, Elevation of the back skin from the latissimus dorsi muscle for a distance of 8 to 10 cm above and below the cutaneous segment. *D* (1, 2, 3) *Left*, Preoperative views. *Right*, Postoperative anterior, right oblique and left oblique views. The cutaneous segment of the flap was used to correct the contracture of the lateral breast, and the fat on the surface of the latissimus muscle was used to replace the implant. Note the "upper fill" and the improved breast contour, with better definition of the inframammary fold. (Case report and photographs courtesy of John B. McCraw, M.D.)

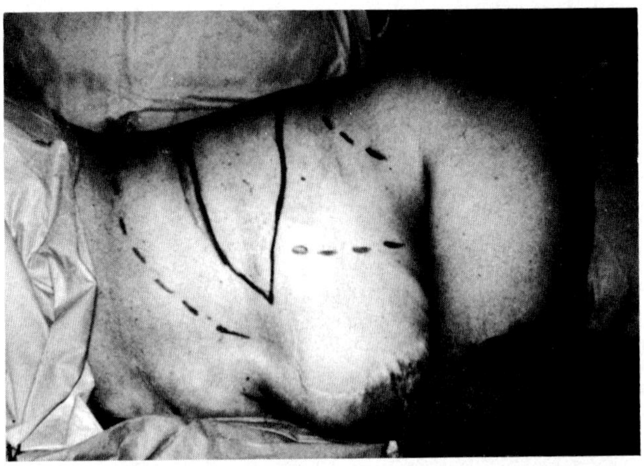

B1

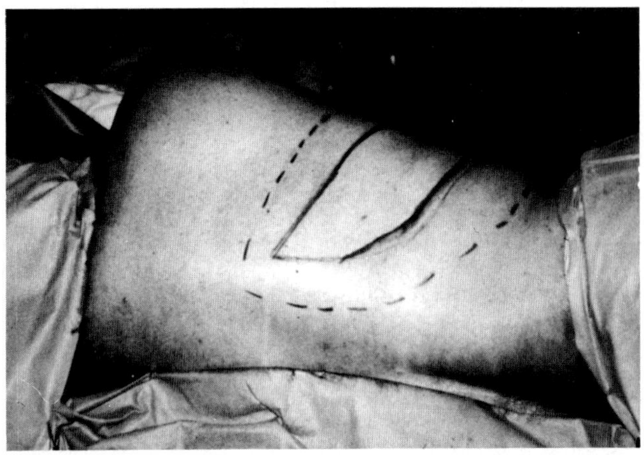

B2

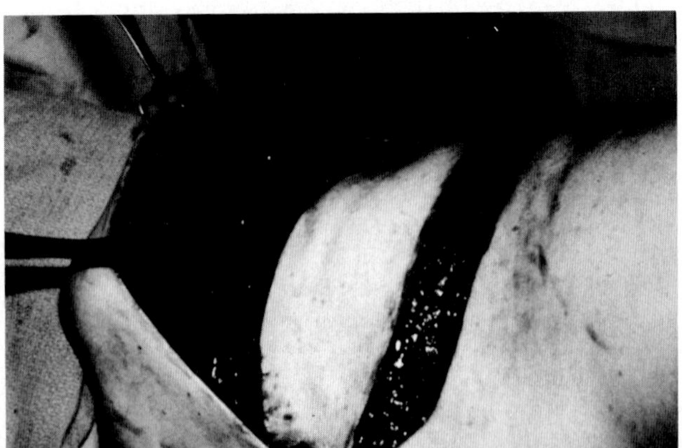

C1

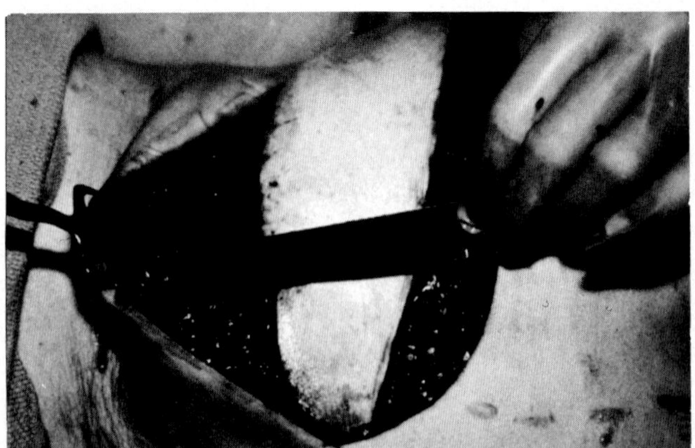

C2

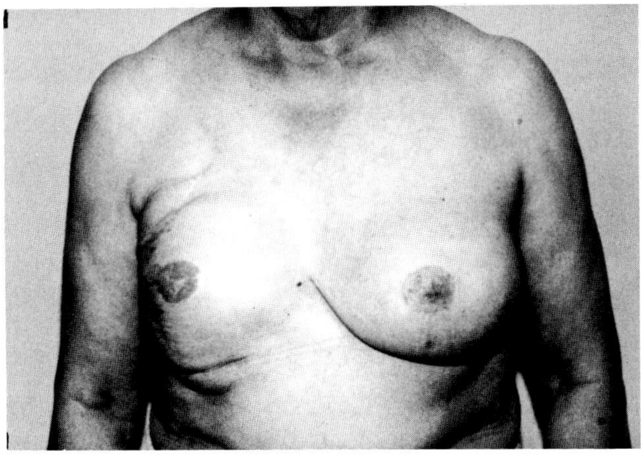
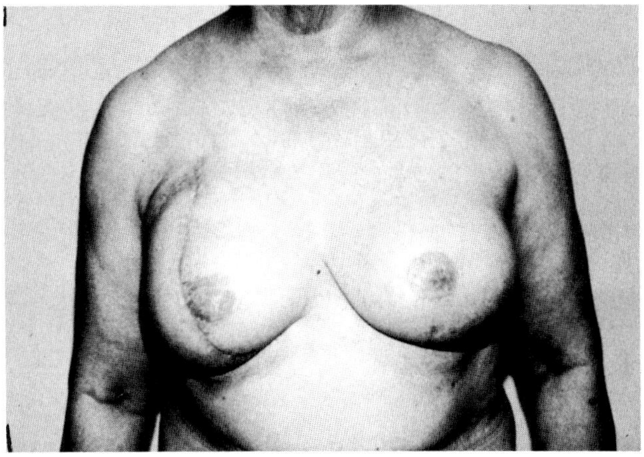

D1 D1

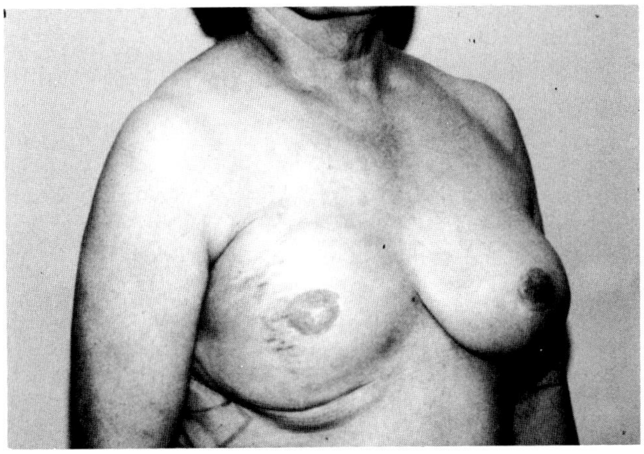
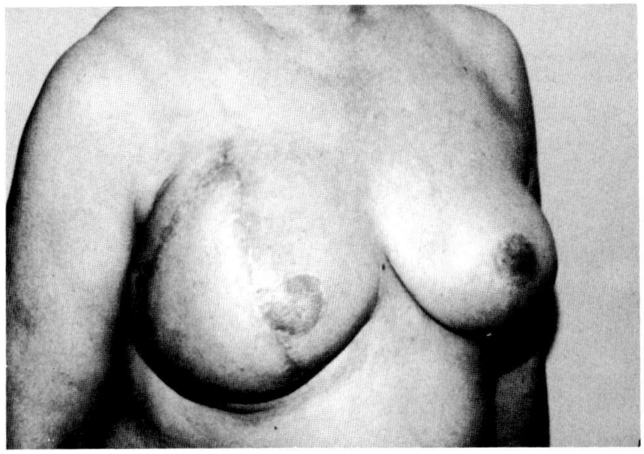

D2 D2

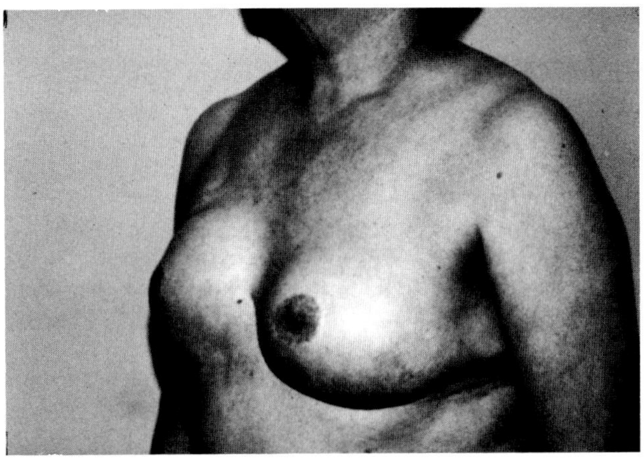
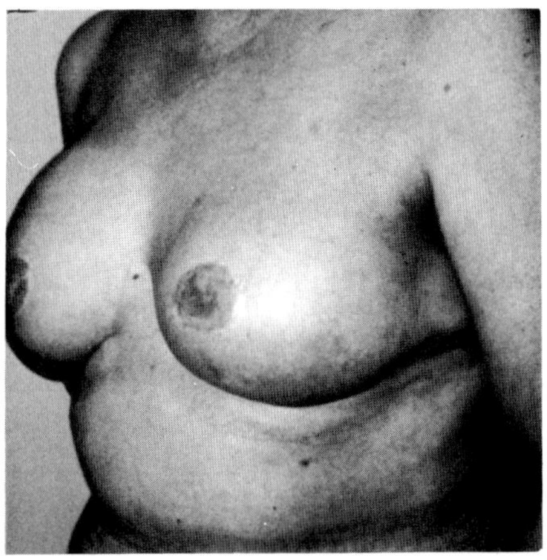

D3 D3

Figure 33-9 *Continued*

the range of primary and secondary mastectomy problems requiring the addition of autogenous tissue, skin, or muscle. The mobility and length of the pedicle permits the latissimus dorsi flap to be placed in virtually any region of the mastectomy deformity; it is even possible to transpose the latissimus dorsi flap to the opposite breast when a chest wall deficit requires closure. Advances in tissue harvesting now permit a totally autogenous tissue latissimus dorsi flap breast reconstruction in many patients.[10-12]

The safety of the latissimus dorsi muscle flap has been documented in the literature. Numerous reports indicate that flap failure caused by poor vascularity is a rarity when the thoracodorsal pedicle remains intact. Even after thoracodorsal pedicle division, the serratus collateral provides reliable flow in over 80 percent of patients. The intramuscular blood supply, multiple perforators, and strong dominant proximal thoracodorsal pedicle ensure flap safety regardless of the skin island design, and permit elevation of subcutaneous tissue over the entire muscle. The flap's versatility stems from its combination of muscle, subcutaneous tissue, and skin.

The newer techniques of autogenous harvesting have broadened the advantages by making total autogenous tissue breast reconstruction possible with the latissimus dorsi flap; this flap can now provide significant autogenous tissue for a nonimplant breast reconstruction. Additional tissue is harvested from the fatty tissue in the central and lower back region overlying the latissimus dorsi muscle, as well as from subcutaneous tissue in the upper back region. An additional skin ellipse along the lateral margin of the latissimus dorsi muscle provides further skin or can be de-epithelialized for additional bulk.

DISADVANTAGES

The back donor site, the complexity of the procedure, the frequent need for silicone breast implants with the associated possibility of capsular contracture, and the necessity to turn the patient during the procedure are all disadvantages of the latissimus dorsi muscle flap. The most acceptable scars have been designed either along the lateral margin of the latissimus dorsi muscle, so that it can be covered by the brassiere and the arm, or in the natural skin line across the midback. The scar from the natural skin line is thin, but it is a permanent scar across the back that can be visible under certain clothing. Scars diagonally placed across the back and against the skin lines can widen and become hypertrophic. The contour of the back is also lost, particularly if a major subcutaneous tissue harvesting is done. Thoracic outlet syndrome has also been caused by a latissimus dorsi flap for breast reconstruction.[13] When significant autogenous tissue is harvested for breast reconstruction, the back donor site can also be somewhat depressed and asymmetric relative to the opposite side, and some patients have requested liposuction of the opposite back to give better symmetry. In the immediate postoperative period, seroma is common and certainly a disadvantage of this procedure.

The complexity of the procedure is another disadvantage, requiring significant planning for positioning the skin island and selecting and positioning an implant or tissue expander. The latissimus dorsi flap also needs to be harvested with the patient in the lateral position, whereas the breast is reconstructed with the patient in the supine position. Therefore the patient must be turned, repositioned, and redraped during the procedure.

In the past, capsular contracture occurred after breast reconstruction with the latissimus dorsi flap at a rate similar to that with breast augmentation. The use of the tissue expander has now permitted improved symmetry, and the polyurethane-covered implant has provided predictably soft breast reconstructions.

AVOIDANCE OF COMPLICATIONS

Primary vascular complications are unusual after the latissimus dorsi flap procedure. The flap's reliability is excellent because of its significant blood flow derived from the thoracodorsal pedicle and from the serratus collaterals. Preoperative determination of the status of the thoracodorsal pedicle helps avoid complications in this region. The latissimus dorsi flap should not be used if the thoracodorsal pedicle and the serratus collateral have been divided.

A seroma in the back is a common occurrence after the latissimus dorsi flap procedure. Its incidence increases with a large flap harvest and when patients have had previous radiation. A siliconized drain and avoidance of shoulder motion appear to decrease the risk of seroma.

Infection after the latissimus dorsi flap procedure is unusual and is rarely seen in the absence of tissue loss. The patient is given broad-spectrum antibiotics before and after surgery to try to minimize this occurrence.

Hematoma after a latissimus dorsi flap procedure may be related to a technical problem in not controlling a specific bleeding vessel, or more commonly may be caused by the patient's taking anticoagulants or medications that affect platelet adhesiveness. Preoperatively counseling the patient to avoid aspirin products, ibuprofen, and other nonsteroidal anti-inflammatory medications can reduce the incidence of hematoma.

Capsular contracture and late breast deformities are also a problem after the latissimus dorsi flap reconstruction. These have been decreased significantly by use of tissue expansion to determine the proper volume for the implant, and to avoid early tightness after placement of a large implant under the latissimus dorsi flap. The tissue expander is later replaced with a polyurethane implant.

Late capsular contracture is treated either by capsulectomy with placement of a polyurethane implant, or placement of autogenous tissue from either a TRAM flap or a free flap.

CONCLUSION

The latissimus dorsi flap is a reliable and versatile source of tissue for breast reconstruction. It provides a valuable source of autogenous tissue, particularly when the abdominal donor site is unavailable or the magnitude of TRAM flap required is considered too great. The modification of the latissimus dorsi flap procedure to provide breast reconstruction with autogenous tissue without an implant has broadened its application and improved long-term results.

References

1. Tanzini I. Sopra il mio nuovo processo di amputatzione della mammella. Gasetta Medica Italiana 1906; 57:141.
2. Olivari N. The latissimus flap. Br J Plast Surg 1976; 29:126.
3. Schneider WJ, Hill HL, Brown RG. Latissimus dorsi myocutaneous flap for breast reconstruction. Br J Plast Surg 1977; 30:277.
4. McCraw JB, Maxwell GP. Early and late capsular "deformation" as a cause of unsatisfactory results in the latissimus dorsi breast reconstruction. Clin Plast Surg 1988; 15:717.
5. Bostwick J III. Plastic and reconstructive breast surgery. St Louis: Quality Medical Publishing Co, 1990.
6. Fisher J, Bostwick J III. Evaluation of the blood supply to the latissimus dorsi muscle after thoracodorsal vessel interruption. Surg Forum 1981; 32:576.
7. Fisher J, Bostwick J III, Powell RW. Latissimus dorsi blood supply after thoracodorsal vessel division: The serratus collateral. Plast Surg 1986; 72:502.
8. Russell RC, Pribaz J, Zook EG, et al. Functional evaluation of latissimus dorsi donor site. Plast Reconstr Surg 1986; 78:336.
9. McCraw J, Dibbell D, Carraway J. Clinical definition of independent myocutaneous vascular territories. Plast Reconstr Surg 1977; 60:341.
10. Hokin JA. Mastectomy reconstruction without a prosthetic implant. Plast Reconstr Surg 1983; 72:810.
11. Hokin JA, Silfverskiold KL. Breast reconstruction without an implant: Results and complications using an extended latissimus dorsi flap. Plast Reconstr Surg 1987; 79:58.
12. McCraw J. The fleur-de-lis latissimus dorsi flap. Presented at the Sixth Annual Southeastern Breast Reconstruction Symposium, Atlanta, GA, January 26–28, 1990.
13. Rubio P-A, Rose F-A. Thoracic outlet syndrome caused by a latissimus dorsi flap for breast reconstruction. Chest 1990; 97:494.

CHAPTER 34

Breast Reconstruction with Rectus Abdominis Flaps

L. FRANKLYN ELLIOTT, M.D.
CARL R. HARTRAMPF, JR., M.D.

The introduction of rectus abdominis flaps for reconstruction of the breast with only autogenous tissue brought a revolutionary change to the entire field of breast reconstruction after mastectomy.[1] The latissimus muscle coverage of implants and the tissue expander were improvements from the previous, generally unacceptable technique of an implant placement beneath the thin skin of the chest wall after mastectomy, but the transverse rectus abdominis myocutaneous (TRAM) flap provided the opportunity to create a new breast after mastectomy with totally autogenous tissue and an acceptable donor site scar. The TRAM flap did more than introduce a standard method for autogenous tissue breast reconstruction that could be repeated by carefully trained surgeons in multiple centers around the world. It stimulated thinking and experimentation with regard to blood flow through musculocutaneous perforators and within subcutaneous fat.[2,3] Development of the TRAM flap has also led to increased understanding of venous outflow in extensive subcutaneous fat flaps.[4] Finally, it has provided greater understanding of blood flow across the midline and between vascular zones.[5] These research efforts have led to the introduction of new, mostly fat flaps — the superficial inferior epigastric artery (SIEA) free flap and the transverse gracilis flap — and has also facilitated the acceptance of other methods of autogenous tissue breast reconstruction, such as the gluteal free flap and the lateral transverse thigh free (LTTF) flap.[6,7] Judged in this light, the TRAM flap has been a significant contribution that may be expected to undergo continued study, improvement, and perfection in the 1990s.

BACKGROUND AND HISTORY

A germinal idea for the eventual development of the TRAM flap was suggested by Brown and colleagues in 1975 with the demonstration of undelayed transverse abdominal flaps based on rectus abdominis perforators.[8] The transverse nature of filling of abdominal fat and overlying skin was therefore demonstrated on the basis of rectus abdominis perforators. Cronin and associates in 1977 used these same transverse abdominal flaps, although based higher on the abdomen, for breast reconstruction with an implant.[9] Again, the transverse concept based on rectus abdominis perforators was used but without extension across the midline or with adequate fat transfer for total autogenous breast reconstruction without an implant. McCraw and colleagues extended these upper rectus abdominis myocutaneous flaps further laterally to create voluminous island tissue transfers for breast reconstruction in 1977.[10] An interesting extension of the transverse concept was introduced on the dorsal surface of the body with the creation of lumbosacral flaps based across the midline on paraspinous perforators, as described by Hill and associates in 1978 (Fig. 34-1).[11] Putting the concept of musculocutaneous perforators to overlying transverse fascia, fat, and skin of the lower abdomen together with blood flow across the midline, Hartrampf and colleagues introduced the transverse abdominal island flap for breast reconstruction in 1982.[1] The vertical rectus abdominis flap for totally autogenous breast reconstruction had previously been introduced but was plagued by the more obvious donor site in the vertical abdominal

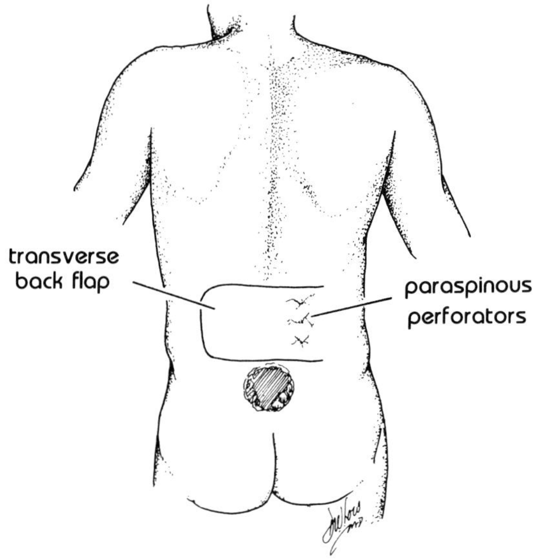

FIGURE 34-1 A concept leading to the development of the TRAM flap was a transverse lumbosacral flap based on paraspinous perforators.

scar.[12] Further refinements of the TRAM flap have been offered in the 1980s and are the subject of this chapter.

ANATOMY

The foundation for the TRAM flap is the rectus abdominis muscle itself, which arises from the fourth or fifth costochondral junction and extends down over the rib margin to insert at the pubic symphysis. Embryologically, the muscle developed in the adult in segments known as somites, which are segments of muscle between the tendinous inscriptions. Each of these segments has its own innervation and secondary blood supply that correspond to the intercostal neurovascular bundles (Fig. 34-2). The main blood supply is the epigastric pedicle, the inferior being a greater contributor than the superior. These two vessels arborize in the mid-rectus abdominis muscle at or near the umbilicus. They also contribute to musculocutaneous perforators, which can be found throughout the anterior surface of the rectus abdominis muscle but have a preponderance in the periumbilical area.[13] The tendinous inscriptions are characterized by a significant thinning of the muscle as well as an attachment to the overlying anterior rectus fascia, but no attachment to the deeper posterior rectus fascia. The attachments to the anterior rectus fascia make dissection of the anterior rectus fascia away from the underlying muscle somewhat more difficult in this location. In addition, the thinness of the muscle at the inscription can lead to injury to the vertical blood supply if extreme care is not used in dissecting the fascia away from the underlying muscle.

A key to the success of a superiorly based TRAM flap is avoidance of injury to the superior epigastric pedicle. Variations have been described,[14] but the location is generally constant, the vessel being just deep to the costal margin in the xiphoid level and continuing in that site until it emanates from under the costal margin and enters the muscle at about the level of the seventh costochondral junction (Fig. 34-2). This anatomic configuration permits further dissection of the superior epigastric pedicle at the costal margin if this is necessary for longer vascular leash in transferring the flap. Either the vessels can be dissected from under the costal margin or costal margins can be resected, to effectively lengthen the vascular leash. With the lower abdominal flap, however, this is not necessary in most cases. Usually, the pedicle exits as a single artery and vein as it enters the superior muscular hilum. At or about that level there is also a large side branch known as the eighth intercostal artery, which should be divided once the pedicle is clearly identified so that the superior portion of the muscle will be deinnervated and the pedicle maximally released from the costal margin.

The deep inferior epigastric pedicle is also relatively constant and enters the inferior muscle at the level of the arcuate line of the posterior sheath, which generally lies midway between the umbilicus and the pubis. The artery measures some 3 to 4 mm and is accompanied by two venae comitantes. The nerves that enter the muscle from the lateral position are accompanied by small vessels, which are insignificant with regard to blood supply to the muscle. The only other vessel of significance frequently found is one that may track from the midportion of the muscle toward the umbilicus. This vessel is usually a single vein and can be sacrificed with impunity. However, its size can often concern the surgeon if this finding is unexpected.

PATIENT SELECTION

The indications for reconstruction with the rectus abdominis flaps must begin with the patient who desires autogenous tissue breast reconstruction rather than implant-expander option. Furthermore, the patient should be willing to accept a transverse scar that extends from beyond the anterior superior iliac spine on each side. The operation is best suited for those who have an excessive amount of lower abdominal fat relative to their body size. However, even patients who are appropriately proportioned in abdominal fat relative to body size and who are within 10 percent of their ideal body weight generally have adequate tissue to reproduce the breast size that is sacrificed at the time of mastectomy. As a

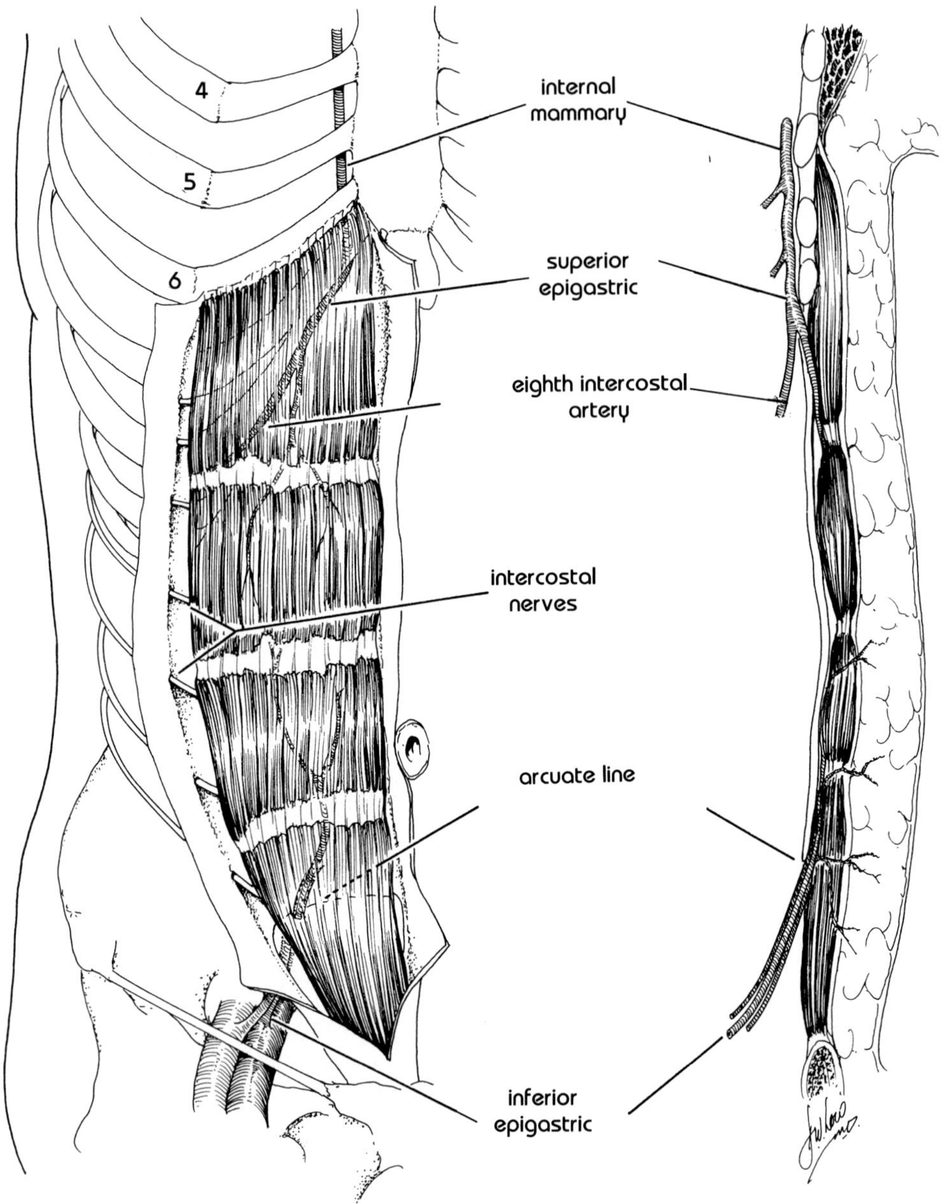

FIGURE 34-2 *Left,* Anterior view of the right rectus abdominis muscle with the anterior fascia reflected. *Right,* Cross section of the vertical midportion of the rectus abdominis muscle. Note the thinness of muscle at the tendinous inscriptions.

general rule, for a unilateral reconstruction, approximately 50 to 60 percent of a total transverse flap is necessary for reconstruction. In a very trim patient, more of the flap may be necessary, in which case methods for augmenting the blood flow to the flap may be chosen. Nonetheless, the TRAM flap is still usually adequate for reconstructing an average-sized breast even for the trim patient.

Our investigations have shown that the flap size can be estimated preoperatively using the following formula: 0.8 (constant) × length × height × thickness = weight in grams.[15] The thickness of the flap is estimated by using soft tissue calipers that can estimate skin fold thickness. This skin fold thickness is divided in half for a single skin thickness measurement. The other measurements are gained by simply measuring the proposed length and height of the flap on the patient. Using this formula, a preoperative estimate of what is available can be made. If more than 60 percent of the flap is necessary for reconstruction, augmentation of the blood supply to the flap is planned. This can be done by using a double pedicle if there is a midline incision or by transferring the TRAM flap as a free flap, which utilizes a larger vascular pedicle.

Patients with larger, more pendulous breasts are generally better candidates for the TRAM flap than for an implant-expander. This is not to say that ptosis and large breasts cannot be reconstructed with the implant-expander, but the TRAM flap is generally more natural and therefore more successful in terms of breast aesthetics. Furthermore, patients with larger breasts have more abdominal adipose tissue for donation and therefore are more prone to accept the TRAM option.

The obese patient is not excluded outright. However, the flap must be handled with care, because shearing or injury to the musculocutaneous perforators can occur owing to the sheer weight of the flap. Preoperative estimates of flap size are again useful in this setting, to help determine how much of the flap is needed to reconstruct the desired breast size. If 50 percent or less of the flap is needed, most of this can be located directly over the muscle pedicle itself without significant extension to the other side (Fig. 34-3). However, if more of the flap is needed in the obese patient, we currently tend to use the free flap technique, again to obtain a better blood supply to a more tenuous flap.

There are no absolute contraindications to the TRAM flap except in the patient who has had a previous TRAM flap, abdominoplasty, or abdominal liposuction. Relative contraindications have been listed in an attempt to rank their order of importance (Table 34-1). However, all these factors are important and the additive effect of multiple factors cannot be denied. There is no question that smoking is the most frequent concern. It is best for any patient who smokes to quit smoking at least 3 months before surgery. Obviously, this is not always possible in the setting of immediate breast reconstruction, but cessation of smoking 2 to 3 weeks before the operation can generally be achieved. In patients with a history of recent smoking, we again tend to choose the type of TRAM flap in which the blood supply is augmented, either the double-pedicle or the free TRAM flap (Fig. 34-4).

Current indications for use of the free TRAM technique are undergoing evolution. Initially, we had specific indications for the free flap technique, i.e., transverse incisions across the upper abdomen, radiation in the sternal or epigastric region, augmentation of an otherwise pedicled flap that appeared compromised in the early postoperative period, or increased tissue needs for the reconstructed breast in patients in whom the double-pedicle technique did not appear superior to the free flap technique. With success in these categories, the indications for the free TRAM flap have expanded to include any patient who is a candidate for a TRAM flap. If the patient needs 60 percent or less of a total TRAM flap based on preoperative measurements and if there are no other risk factors, we continue to choose the superiorly based pedicled TRAM flap. However, in patients with any of the risk factors noted above or in whom more than 60 percent of the flap is needed, the free TRAM technique is considered from the outset and weighed against the single- or double-pedicle TRAM flap. (Fig. 34-5).

PREOPERATIVE EVALUATION AND CARE

After a thorough explanation of all the reconstructive options, an operative plan is chosen in concert with the patient's desires and a consultation with the husband, if the patient wishes. The patient is generally seen in the office 1 or 2 days before surgery for history taking and physical examination. At that time, an operative permit is obtained and the patient is given preoperative instructions. For an uncomplicated case, we do not hesitate to admit the patient the day of surgery even if the operation is to begin at 7:30 A.M. On the other hand, if the patient lives a great distance from the hospital, has some other complicating factor, or is able to secure agreement from the insurance company for admission the day before surgery, she can be admitted the afternoon or evening before surgery. In that event, intravenous fluids are begun that evening and continued at 75 ml an hour. This is intended to fully hydrate the patient, in view of the bowel cleanout that occurs the evening before surgery. We give the patient one bottle of magnesium citrate the evening before surgery and a Fleet enema the morning of surgery. If the patient is to be admitted the morning of surgery, she is told to take the magnesium citrate the night before surgery and is given the Fleet enema on arrival at the hospital. Methylprednisolone, 250 mg, is given at the time of anesthetic induction, at the time of pedicle division, and 6 hours after completion of the operation. The patient is also instructed in the use of the incentive spirometer preoperatively. Finally, she is placed on a liquid diet at 6 P.M. the evening before surgery.

Instructions on smoking will previously have been reviewed extensively with the patient, but if it is desired to document cessation of smoking, a urine nicotine level can be obtained with the preoperative laboratory work.

Our current approach toward blood transfusions is that we generally have not found them to be necessary even after bilateral mastectomies with immediate bilateral TRAM reconstructions. Nonetheless, it is wise to inform the patient of the options for autologous blood or for donor-directed blood from a close friend or family member. If autologous blood is chosen, we would not want a unit to be drawn within 3 weeks of surgery, because the patient does not replete the blood adequately by that time. We also desire a level of 26 to 28 percent hematocrit before consideration of transfusion in the immediate postoperative period. Using these criteria, we have found that only a rare patient needs blood transfusions when undergoing either unilateral or bilateral TRAM flap reconstruction.

SURGICAL TECHNIQUE

The patient is placed on the operating table in the supine position, at which time a Foley catheter is placed and two pillows are positioned under the knees. The umbilicus is cleaned carefully with a cotton-tipped applicator and prep solution, and the superior 1 to 2 inches of pubic hair are shaved. The

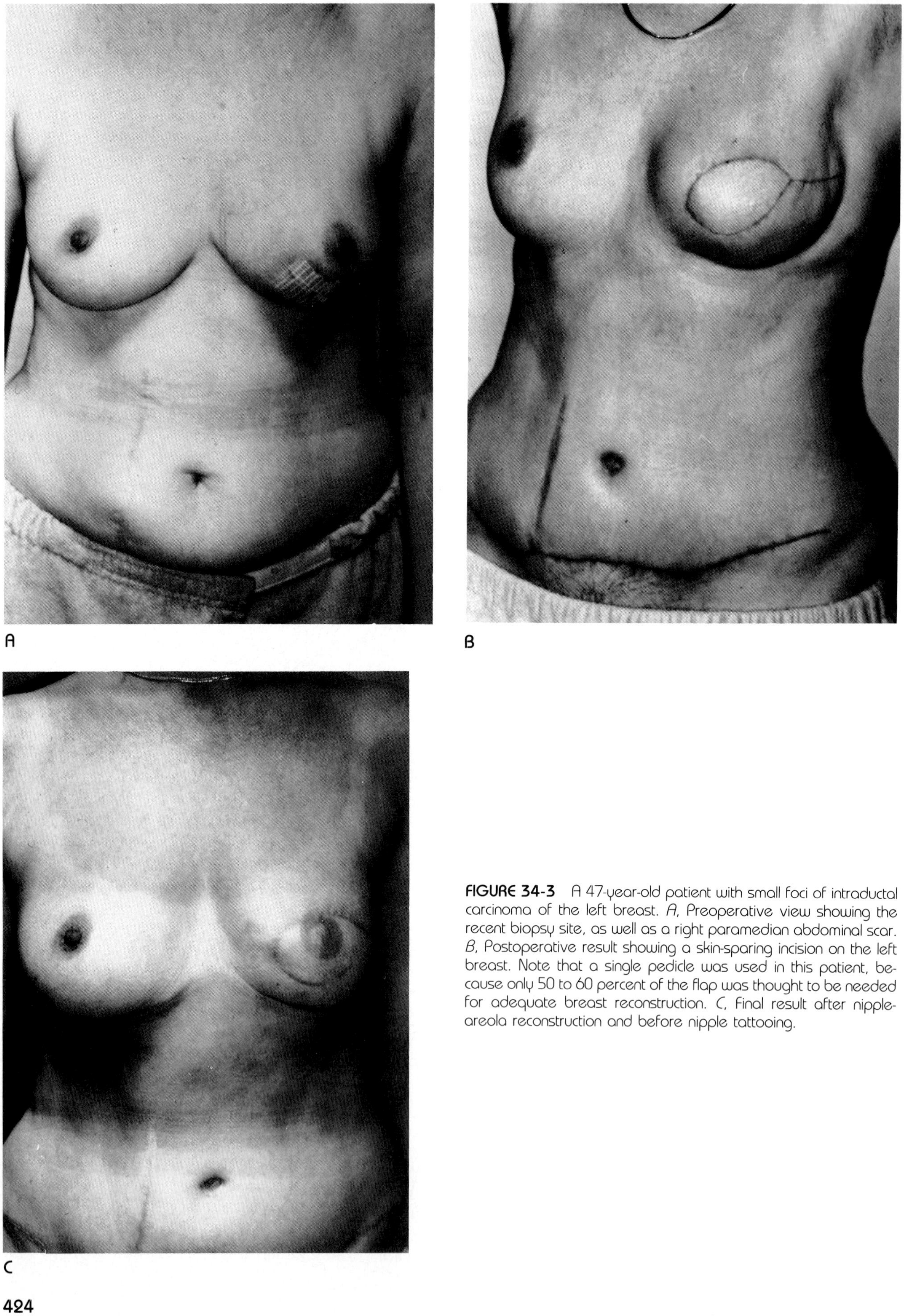

A

B

C

FIGURE 34-3 A 47-year-old patient with small foci of intraductal carcinoma of the left breast. *A*, Preoperative view showing the recent biopsy site, as well as a right paramedian abdominal scar. *B*, Postoperative result showing a skin-sparing incision on the left breast. Note that a single pedicle was used in this patient, because only 50 to 60 percent of the flap was thought to be needed for adequate breast reconstruction. *C*, Final result after nipple-areola reconstruction and before nipple tattooing.

TABLE 34-1 TRAM Operation Risk Factors and Their Severity

Risk Factor	Score (1-10)
OBESITY	
Moderate: <25% above IBW	1
Severe: >25% over IBW	5
SMALL VESSEL DISEASE	
Light to moderate smoking (1+ pack/day for 2-10 years)	1
Chronic heavy smoking (10-20 pack years)	2
Chronic heavy smoking (20-30 pack years)	5
Autoimmune disease (scleroderma, Raynaud's, etc.)	8
Diabetes mellitus—non-insulin dependent	5
Diabetes mellitus—insulin dependent	10
PSYCHOSOCIAL PROBLEMS	
Unstable emotional state (life crisis)	2
Personality disorder	3
Substance abuse	5
ABDOMINAL SCARS	
If "planned out" of flap design	0.5
Disruption of vascular perforators; transection of superior epigastric vessels (Chevron incision, abdominoplasty, etc.)	10
PATIENT'S ATTITUDE	
Patient is unwilling or unable to invest time required for healing, or objects to abdominal scar	10
SURGEON'S INEXPERIENCE	
Less than 10 TRAM flaps	1
A MAJOR SYSTEM DISEASE PROCESS	
Chronic lung disease	10
Severe cardiovascular disease	10

From Hartrampf CR, Bennett GK. Autogenous tissue reconstruction in the mastectomy patient—a critical review of 300 patients. Ann Surg 1987; 205:508.

only markings preoperatively are the inframammary line, the lateral extent of the breast (in the setting of immediate reconstruction), and the midline from the costal margin to the pubis. It is very easy to mislocate the final position of the umbilicus at the end of the operation if the midline is not marked carefully.

Once the patient is anesthetized, prepared, and draped, the abdominal ellipse is marked on the abdomen. This generally extends vertically from one fingerbreadth above the umbilicus to one fingerbreadth above the pubis, extending laterally to approximately 3 to 4 cm beyond the anterior superior iliac spine. All the markings are carefully measured so that the flap is symmetric.

For immediate reconstruction, harvesting of the TRAM flap can begin at the same time that the general surgeon begins the mastectomy. Two sets of instruments are used, and every effort is made to keep the abdominal and chest operative fields separate. This requires cooperation with the oncologic surgeon, who must feel comfortable with this approach. Simultaneous dissection, although not a necessity, is an option that can reduce the overall operative time by 45 to 60 minutes.

The abdominal ellipse is circumscribed and the incisions are beveled away from the flap to the anterior rectus sheath and external oblique. The upper abdominal skin and fat are dissected just superficial to the anterior rectus fascia over the costal margin bilaterally. The umbilicus is then circumscribed, and dissection around the umbilicus is carried down to the anterior rectus sheath, leaving a jacket of fat around the umbilical stalk to help ensure adequate blood supply to the umbilicus.

Single Pedicle

For the single-pedicle technique, the rectus abdominis muscle contralateral to the mastectomy defect is chosen for the flap. The wing of the flap contralateral to the muscle pedicle can then be elevated to the midline just superficial to the anterior rectus fascia. The umbilicus is carefully left in place, and the flap is elevated to a point 1 cm lateral to the medial border of the rectus muscle to be used. The ipsilateral wing of the flap is then elevated 1 cm medial to the lateral border of the rectus muscle to be used. The anterior rectus sheath is incised with the electrocautery unit, beginning at the costal margin, 1 cm medial to its lateral border. This incision continues through the anterior rectus sheath and through the underlying rectus muscle to the posterior rectus sheath, extending inferiorly to a point midway between the umbilicus and the pubis. Here the inferior epigastric pedicle is identified, and with retraction a 2- to 3-cm length of this pedicle is dissected proximally. The pedicle is then ligated and divided. The central segment of the rectus abdominis muscle can be rolled medially and the superior epigastric pedicle either visually or palpably identified. If this identification is not possible at this point, the sterile Doppler is used to locate the pedicle before beginning the medial dissection of the muscle.

Once the pedicle is localized, an incision is made with the electrocautery, 1 cm lateral to the medial border of the rectus muscle, and continued down through the anterior rectus sheath and underlying rectus abdominis muscle to the posterior sheath. This incision is continued from the level of the costal margin to a point midway between the umbilicus and the pubis where it joins the lateral incision. At this point the central segment of the rectus muscle along with the overlying TRAM flap can be elevated out of the bed (Fig. 34-6).

With the superior pedicle in direct view, further dissection continues along the costal margin dividing the eighth intercostal nerve and any other attachments, until the pedicle is dissected within 1 to 2 cm of the xiphoid. This gives adequate range of motion of the flap for practically any kind of positioning on the chest wall. The anterior abdominal wall defect is temporarily closed with skin staples, and an ade-

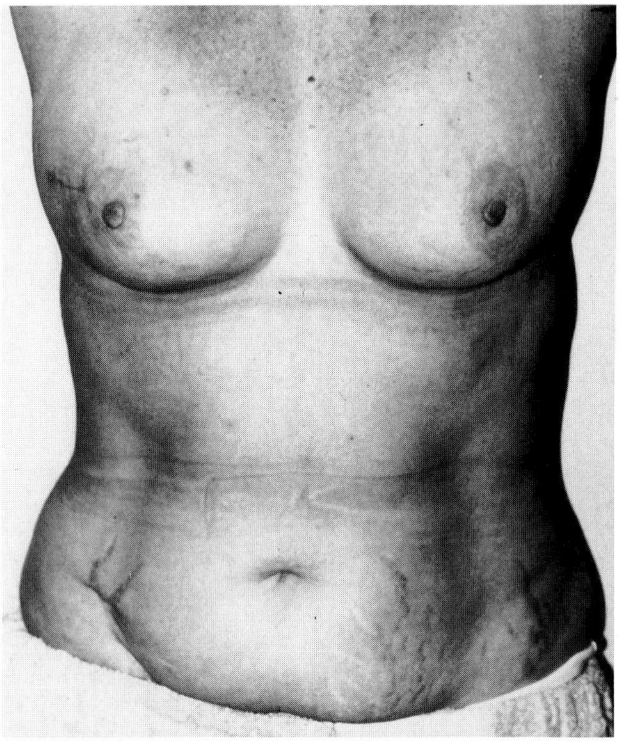

A

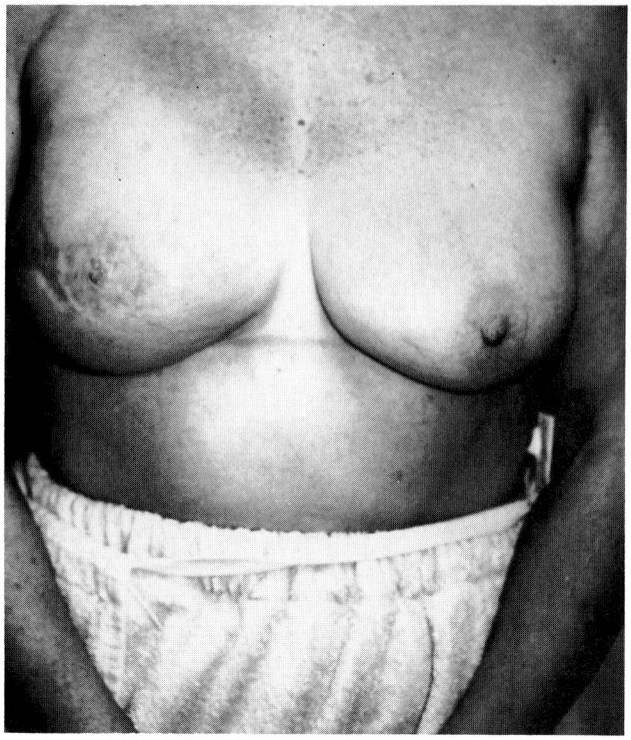

B

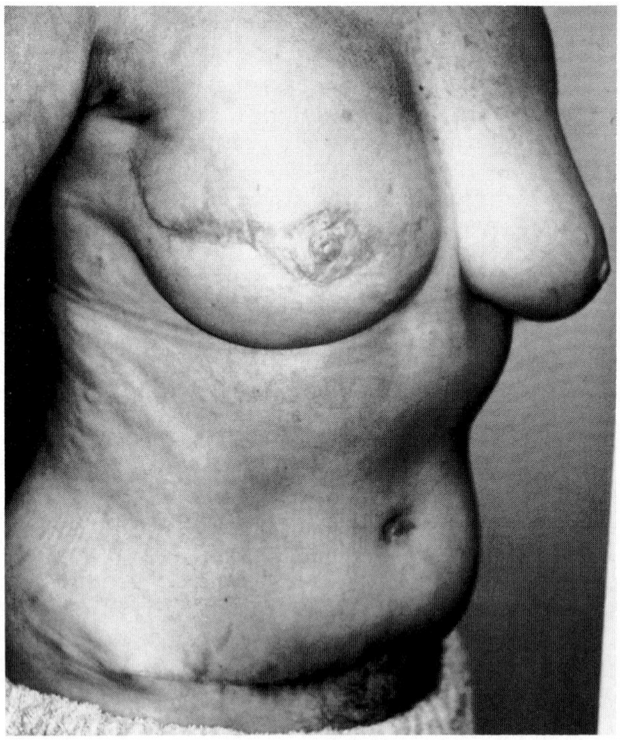

C

FIGURE 34–4 A 54-year-old patient with a recent biopsy of the right lateral breast, confirming the diagnosis of ductal carcinoma. She had a smoking history of two packs per day for 20 years. *A*, Preoperative view showing adequate abdominal donor tissue. *B*, Frontal postoperative result after initial TRAM reconstruction, using the double-pedicle flap. The patient then underwent nipple-areola reconstruction. Note the poor quality of scarring around the nipple-areola reconstruction, characteristic of smokers. It is worthy to note that there was no fat necrosis in the breast, however. *C*, Postoperative oblique view showing the poor scarring result.

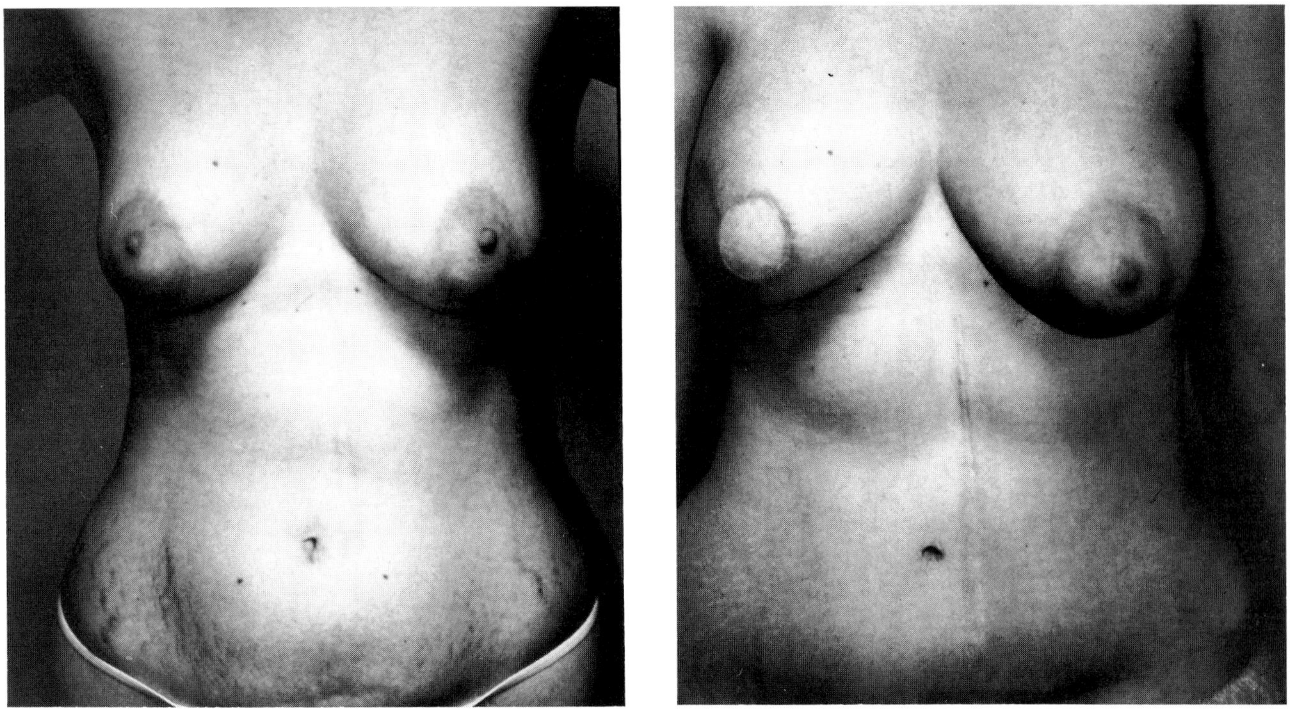

A B

FIGURE 34-5 A 30-year-old patient with biopsy-proved ductal carcinoma of the right breast. She also had a history of Hodgkin's disease 10 years previously, with mantle irradiation, as well as a midline abdominal scar for exploratory laparotomy. Owing to breast size, abdominal scarring, and the irradiation therapy, the free TRAM technique was chosen. *A*, Preoperative view. Note the midline abdominal scar. *B*, Four-month postoperative result before nipple-areola reconstruction.

quate-size tunnel is created through to the chest dissection area. The flap is weighed with a sterile fish scale, and is then passed through the tunnel to the chest area and temporarily stabilized with skin staples.

The abdominal wall defect is closed with a double-stranded 0 monofilament suture from the pubis to the costal margin. The opposite anterior rectus fascia is plicated in a similar manner from the pubis to the costal margin in order to maintain the umbilicus in the midline.

After the appropriate site for the umbilicus is located, drains are placed. The patient is elevated to a near-sitting position and the abdominal wall is closed. A semicircular segment of skin is removed over the umbilical site, and the umbilicus is inset by suturing it to the surrounding skin and to the underlying anterior rectus fascia. Suturing to the underlying fascia ensures that the normal umbilical dimple is more closely simulated.

The shaping of the flap is generally best done by using one of two positions of the flap itself (Fig. 34-7). It is preferable to place the contralateral portion of the flap up toward the axilla, turning the ipsilateral portion of the flap under to give projection to the breast. This ensures adequate filling in the infraclavicular hollow but may not give adequate projection to match the opposite side. The alternative choice is to rotate the flap 180 degrees, placing the former umbilical site at the inferior 6 o'clock position of the breast. The central segment at the umbilical site can be resected in a V-type manner and then closed directly, to give the flap a more conelike shape. In either of these shaping techniques, the lateral wings of the flap are generally sacrificed, because viability in those areas cannot be guaranteed.

The inset of the flap can be previewed using skin staples. Subsequent adjustments, if necessary, can be readily made. Once the shape is acceptable, the flap is de-epithelialized where it is to be buried, and the buried portions are sutured in the pocket superiorly, medially, and laterally. Drains are placed and the skin incisions are closed.

Our dressings include sterile 1-inch paper tape over all incisions and drain sponges around the drains.

Single-Pedicle Free Flap

The positioning of the patient is similar to that described for the superior pedicle technique. It is not necessary to alter the patient's position on the

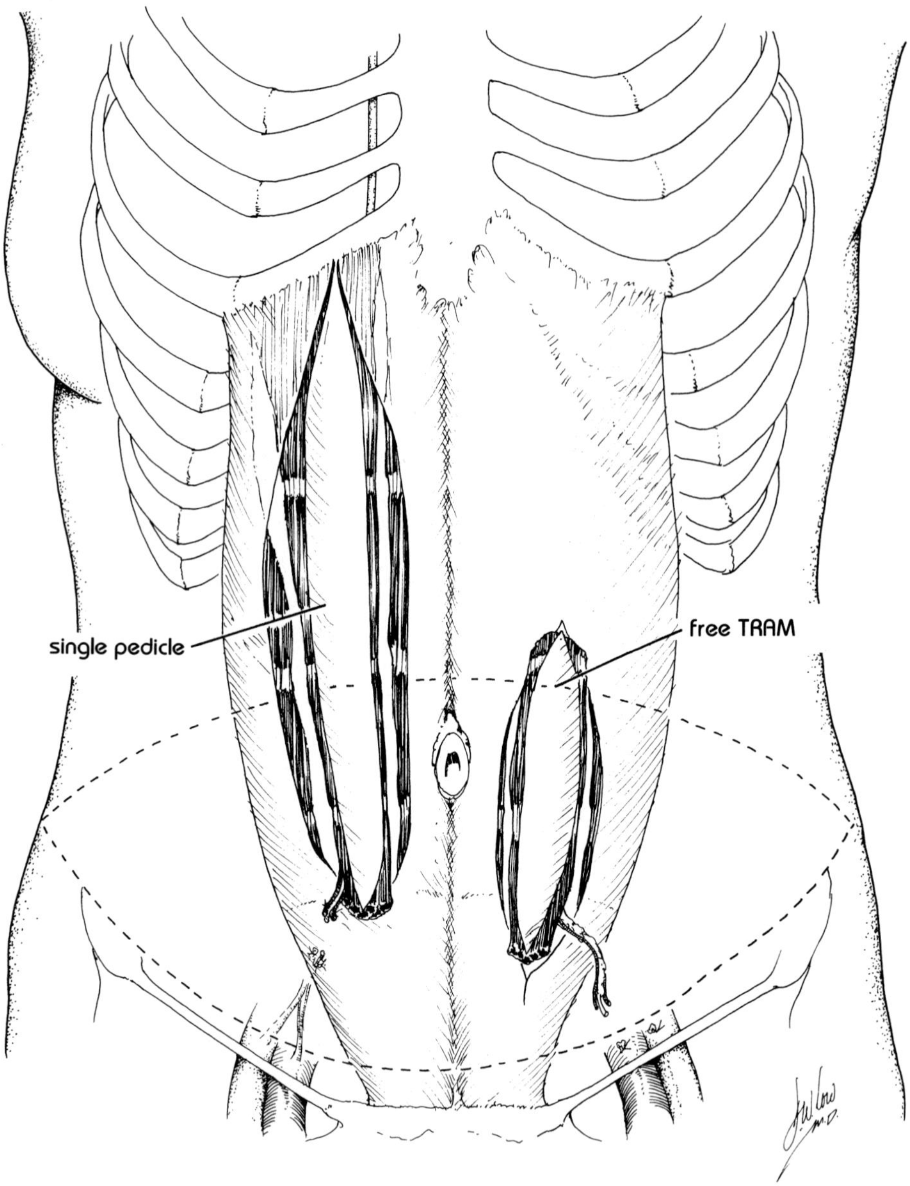

FIGURE 34–6 *Left,* Anterior rectus incisions for a superiorly based flap are illustrated for the right rectus abdominis muscle. Note that the incisions continue well above the costal margin. *Right,* Anterior rectus incisions for a free flap.

table to better visualize the vascular pedicle in the axilla. In fact, this position facilitates the simultaneous dissection by two microsurgeons, one dissecting the pedicle in the axilla and the other preparing the TRAM free flap. However, in the case of immediate reconstruction, the thoracodorsal pedicle is often clearly dissected during the mastectomy, thus limiting the need for further dissection. It is wise to inform the oncologic surgeon of the intention to use the thoracodorsal pedicle so that his dissection can proceed with care in that area.

For the single-pedicle free flap technique, we generally choose the ipsilateral muscle, because this places the vascular pedicle and ipsilateral portion of the flap more superiorly where less volume is needed and allows the contralateral portion of the flap to extend inferiorly to form the mound of the breast. The design of the flap and its elevation are similar except that an incision into the anterior rectus sheath and through the rectus muscle begins approximately midway between the costal margin and the umbilicus (see Fig. 34–6). Thus, approximately half as much rectus muscle is harvested with the inferior technique as with the superior technique. Once the inferior epigastric vessels are identified, we do not hesitate to continue the incision into the midportion of the rectus sheath inferiorly toward the pubis in order to obtain better exposure of the inferior epigastric pedicle. We dissect the pedicle down to the junction of the femoral and iliac vessels and divide it there, giving a pedicle length of some 6 to 8 cm. The pedicle generally is not divided until the vessels are ready in the axilla and the microscope has been moved into the field.

Our first choice for recipient vessels in the axilla is the thoracodorsal pedicle. The crossing vessels to

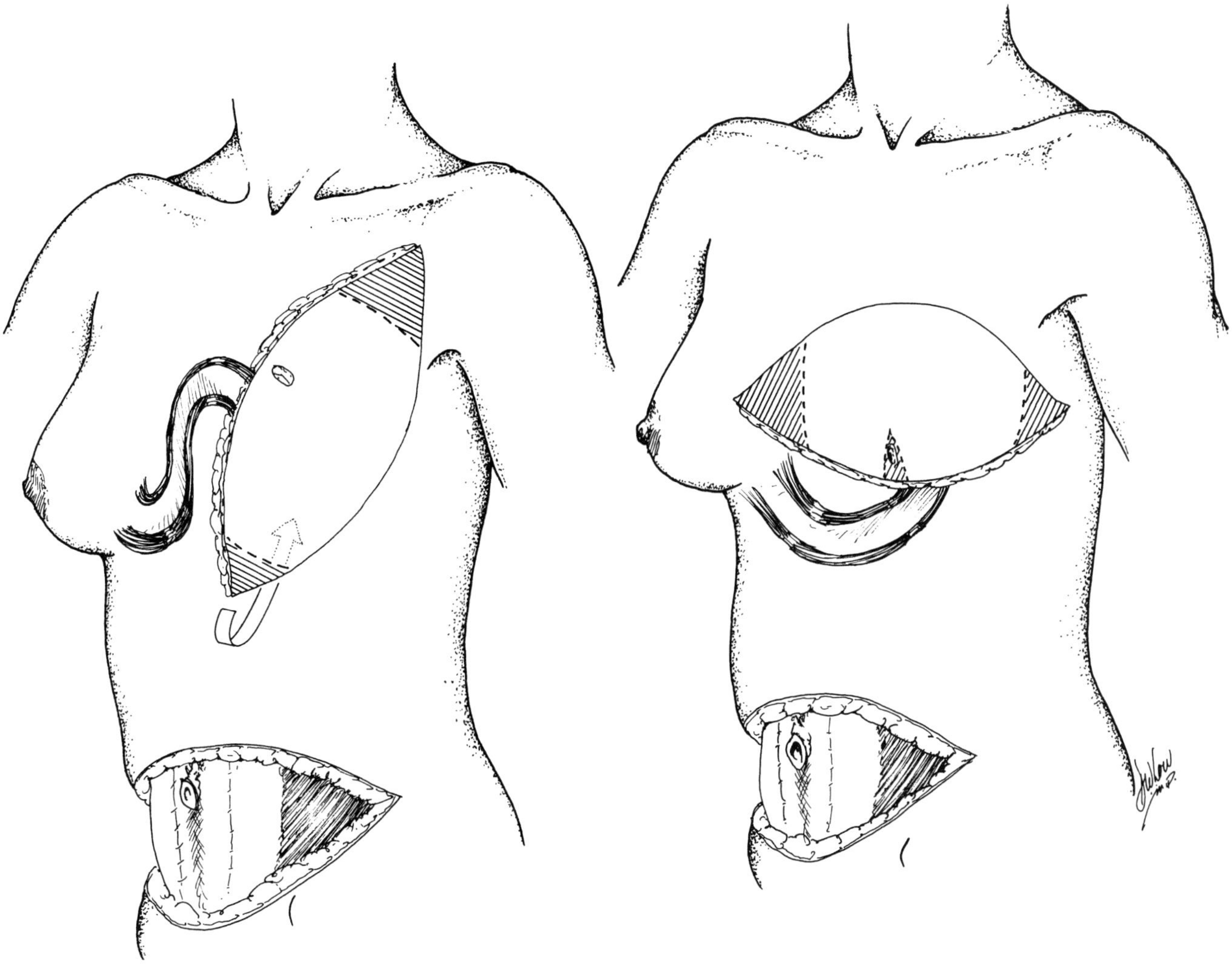

FIGURE 34-7 *Left*, The most common method of flap orientation with the contralateral portion up toward the axilla where usually less filling is needed. *Right*, Rotation of flap 180 degrees. This method may give better projection when the umbilical site is closed.

the serratus are in slightly better proximity to the chest wall than the main trunk of the thoracodorsal vessels, but if the crossing vessels are of inadequate size, we use the main trunk of the thoracodorsal pedicle (Fig. 34-8). If the pedicle is divided in this location, blood supply continues to the latissimus dorsi muscle via the crossing vessels to the serratus anterior.[16] As the microvascular anastomosis is carried out, the vessel lumens are irrigated with heparinized saline. At the conclusion of the anastomoses, the vessels are bathed in a papaverine-lidocaine solution. The microclamps are released and complete filling of the entire flap is observed. The flap is then inset as described above. The abdominal wall is closed as described for the single pedicle.

Double Pedicle

If the double pedicle is deemed necessary for a single-sided reconstruction, one must decide whether the flap will be kept as a single unit or divided into two separate flaps. Unilateral reconstruction is successful with either technique, and this is the surgeon's choice. The split-flap technique may be better when more superior filling is needed or if there is an unusual defect. However, the split-flap technique can be more demanding in that it presents a wider array of variations in shaping the new breast. If the flap is to be harvested as a single flap, the dissection of the first pedicle is carried out as described above, except that the incision in the anterior rectus sheath that is 1 cm lateral from the medial border is made from the posterior surface of the rectus muscle out through the anterior sheath as the flap is rolled from lateral to medial (Fig. 34-9). The inferior pedicle has already been divided through the lateral incision, and this allows rotation of the medial segment of the rectus muscle out of its bed. Dissection of the opposite pedicle proceeds as described for the single-pedicle technique. Dissection of both pedicles must be continued up to within

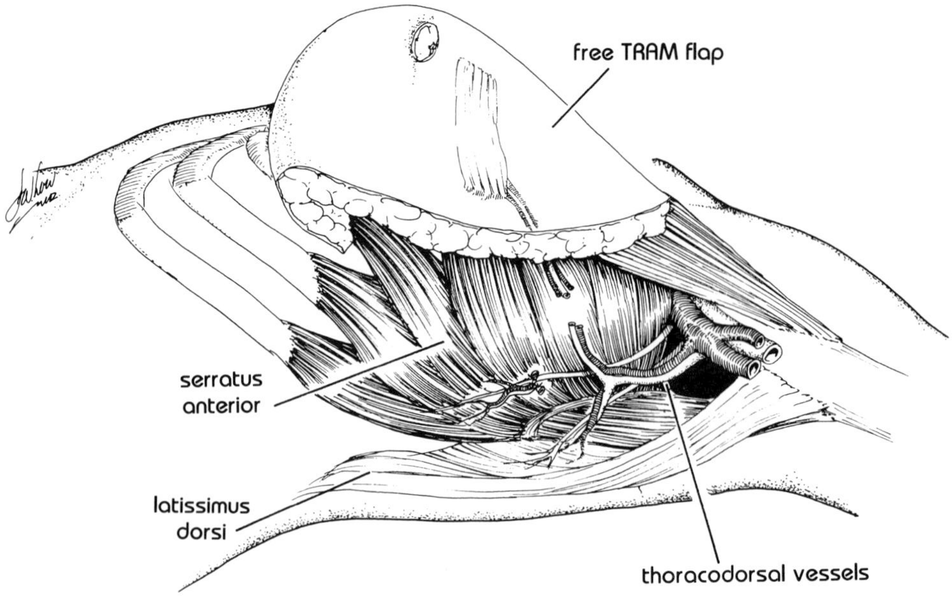

FIGURE 34-8 Left free TRAM flap. Preparations have been made for anastomosis of the inferior epigastric vessels to the crossing vessels to the serratus anterior.

1 cm of the xiphoid so that proper rotations of the pedicles in the tunnel can be achieved. Careful positioning of the pedicles in the tunnel is vitally important to prevent any overlapping of the pedicles or any impingement of the pedicles on each other (Fig. 34-10). If the pedicle lengths are dissected as described, there is as much mobility of the flap for breast shaping as with the single-pedicle technique.

The closure of the abdominal wall defect involves temporary stapling of each anterior rectus sheath defect immediately after it is created. With this temporary closure in place, the permanent closure can be performed, often simultaneously, by again using a double-stranded 0 monofilament suture from the pubis to the costal margin. In 80 to 90 percent of patients, this can be accomplished without the use of synthetic mesh. However, if there is any doubt about the adequacy of the closure, or if the patient has a current smoking history, mesh is added. We also generally add fascial staples to supplement the fascial closure in the case of a bilateral pedicle harvest.

Bilateral Reconstruction

The dissection of the bilateral flaps for bilateral reconstruction proceeds as described for a single-pedicle dissection except that the flap is split in the midline and each flap is dissected separately. There is a slightly different design for the tunnel from the abdominal area to the chest area in that we are bringing the flaps more directly to the chest dissection area and avoiding total undermining of the xiphoid-lower sternum region (Fig. 34-11). Thus, the flap on the right side is brought up at the 5 o'clock position, and the flap on the left side at the 7 o'clock position (Fig. 34-12). Although this does violate the inframammary fold to some degree, creation of a slight amount of ptosis generally obviates this problem in terms of aesthetics. If fullness in that area persists, the pedicle of the flap can be divided at a later date, usually at the time of nipple-areola reconstruction. Abdominal wall closure is similar to that described for the double pedicle.

POSTOPERATIVE CARE

At the end of the operation, the patient is in a flexed position to close the abdominal skin. The patient is transferred from the operating table to the hospital bed in that same position and maintained as such overnight. Low-molecular-weight dextran is infused at a constant rate for 3 to 4 days postoperatively in free flap patients.

On the first postoperative day, the patient is encouraged to be out of bed, the Foley catheter is removed, and the diet is advanced. Usually by the afternoon or evening of that day, the diet has been advanced and the intravenous line removed. Patient-controlled analgesia is utilized while the IV is in place.

Monitoring of the flap, whether pedicled or free, is done during frequent visits by the physicians and nurses. The nurses in our unit have been carefully instructed of the parameters for which to watch, and this has been helpful in noting any early postoperative problems. However, it is best for the physician to visit 4 to 6 hours after surgery to assess the continued good health of the flap.

In patients in whom there is adequate chest wall

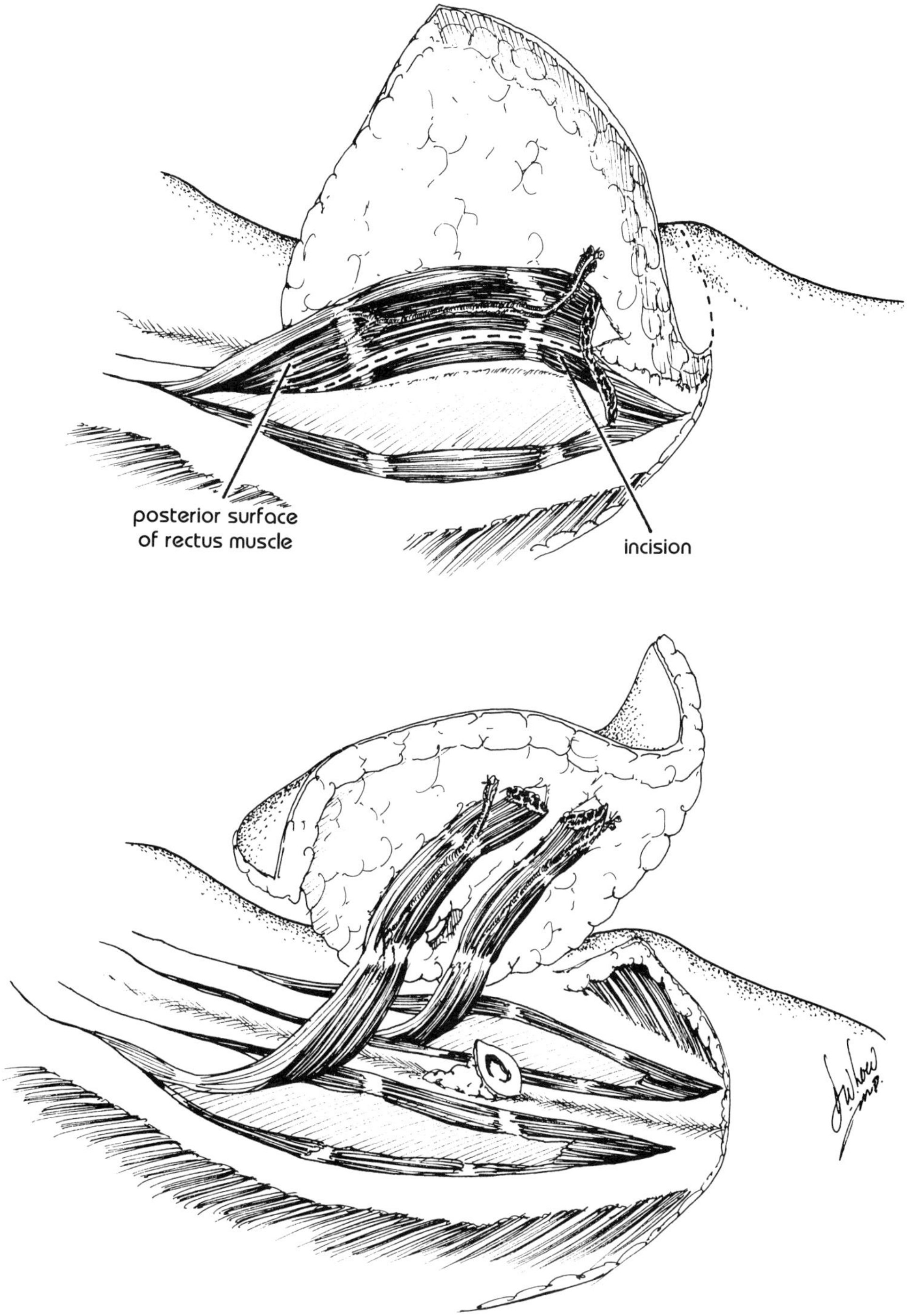

FIGURE 34-9 Dissection of double-pedicle TRAM flap. *Above,* A medial incision in the first muscle pedicle is made from the posterior surface of the muscle. This is extended through the anterior rectus sheath. *Below,* The double-pedicle TRAM flap elevated. Note the 1 cm of anterior rectus fascia and muscle on both sides of the midline.

skin for coverage of the TRAM flap, a small abdominal skin island is left in the incision laterally for monitoring purposes. This can be resected at the time of nipple-areola reconstruction. Another option in patients with minimal breast cancer who have chosen immediate reconstruction is to fill the nipple-areola circle with the TRAM flap skin. This island serves as a monitoring site as well as a subsequent pod for nipple-areola reconstruction.

No attempt is made to advance drain removal rapidly. No drains are removed until the drainage per day is less than 25 ml, so patients are often sent home with drains in position. They are usually discharged on the fourth or fifth postoperative day and are given a sheet of instructions for home activities.

RESULTS

Over the past 10 years, one author (CRH) performed 628 TRAM breast reconstructions in 534 patients.[17] These were both single- and double-pedicle

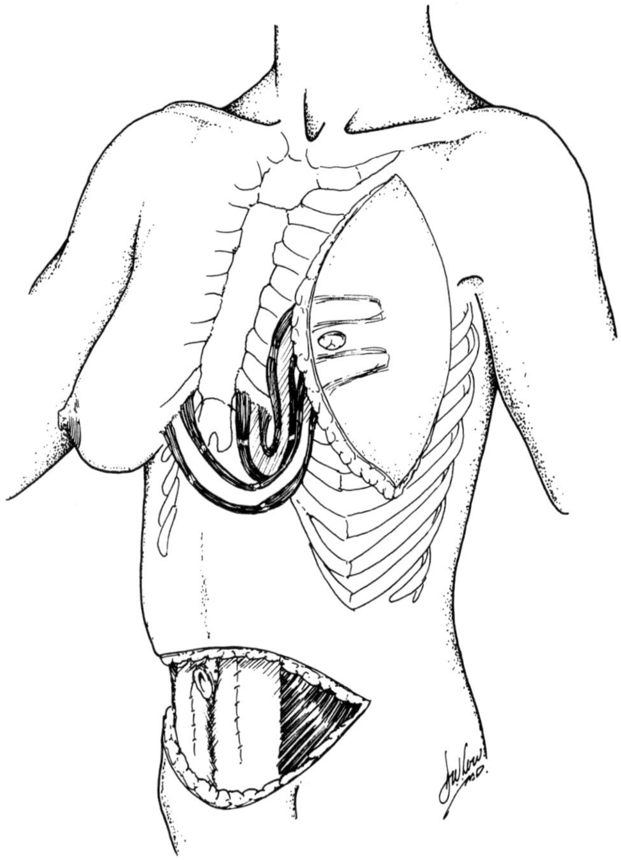

FIGURE 34-10 Double-pedicle TRAM reconstruction. Note the double-sling arrangement of the two muscle pedicles. They should not overlap or cross each other.

TRAM flaps for unilateral breast reconstruction as well as bilateral breast reconstruction using the TRAM flap. None of these operations involved the free TRAM technique. Two patients (0.3 percent) experienced total flap failures in this group and 32 patients (6.7 percent) experienced subtotal flap loss. In the first 119 patients, approximately 15 percent had areas of hardness in the buried portions of the TRAM flap that apparently represented foci of fat necrosis. Abdominal wall hernias developed in six patients (1.3 percent). Almost half of the total group could not perform sit-ups preoperatively, but of those who could, 83 percent with unilateral muscle harvest and 36 percent with bilateral muscle harvest could perform sit-ups postoperatively. Patients' assessment of the operation based on a questionnaire sent to the first 300 patients (with a 97.6 percent response rate) revealed that 98 percent felt that the TRAM flap breast reconstruction was worth the time and effort and would recommend it to other patients.

The free TRAM flap procedure has been performed in ten patients. In two patients, a unilateral free TRAM was performed on one side and a conventional pedicle TRAM on the other side. There has been no flap loss. One patient had a small area of fat necrosis, less than 2 cm. There have been no abdominal wall weaknesses or hernias.

AVOIDANCE OF COMPLICATIONS

Complications may be secondary to poor patient selection, a basic problem that no degree of surgical excellence can overcome. Patients who have several risk factors such as a recent smoking history, obesity, and diabetes mellitus have a higher likelihood of delayed healing, at best, and flap loss, at worst. Despite these admonitions, these patients are often no better candidates for the implant-expander technique either. The most worrisome factor in selection is the patient who is actively smoking. It appears that the free TRAM technique will contribute to reduction of the incidence of fat necrosis in the flap in this clinical setting. However, complications with the skin flaps created by the resecting surgeon on the chest wall or associated with the abdominal closure will not be affected by any alteration of the TRAM technique. Fluoroscein may help in this clinical setting, although we have rarely used it.

The preoperative psychological status of the patient is another area in which patient selection can help avoid postoperative complications. The patient who is unable to grasp or accept the implications of the disease or the postoperative implications of a TRAM flap breast reconstruction is not a suitable candidate for this technique. The complication that will ensue is unhappiness with the postoperative result regardless of its degree of excellence. We do not show pre- and postoperative photographs to all patients, but this may be useful for patients who may not fully understand the operation and its recovery and healing phases. These problems are especially relevant in the patient who anticipates immediate breast reconstruction.

The most common errors in surgical performance that lead to postoperative complications are inadequate dissection of the superior pedicle at the costal margin; twisting, kinking, or overlapping of the pedicle or pedicles in the tunnel; and inadequate closure of the anterior abdominal wall fascia.

It is natural, especially early in one's experience with the TRAM flap, to feel that staying away from the pedicle (not seeing it) will reduce the chance of injuring it. Although avoidance of direct injury to the pedicle is vitally important. It is equally important that an adequate dissection of the superior pedicle be performed to avoid kinking or compromise of the pedicle at the costal margin as the flap is rotated to the chest wall. This most profoundly affects the low-pressure vessel, the vein, and in turn leads to venous hypertension in the flap, cyanosis of the skin island, a large amount of dark venous blood in the drains postoperatively, and eventual fat necrosis or partial

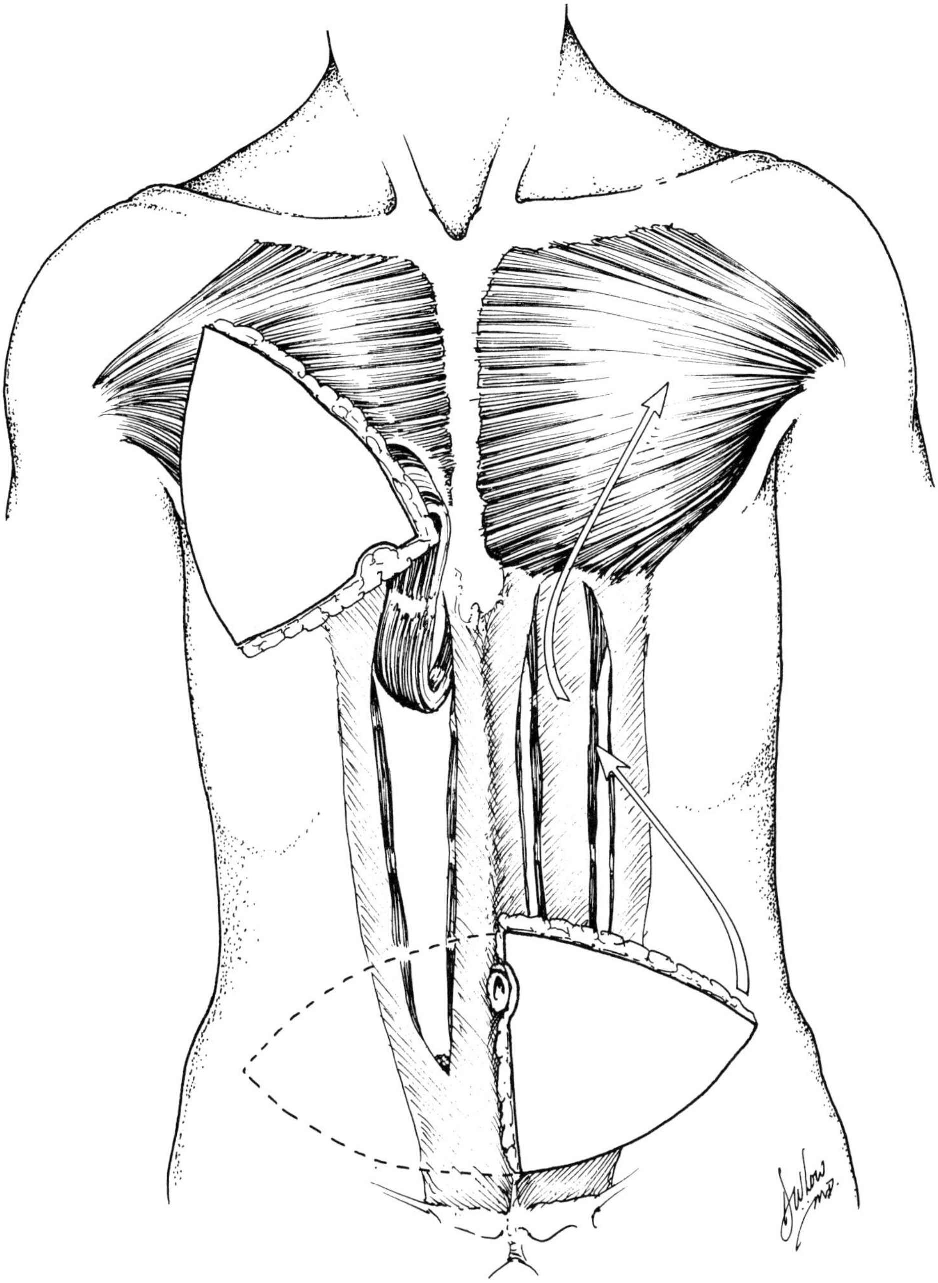

FIGURE 34-11 Bilateral TRAM reconstruction. The arrows demonstrate the tunnel route through which the flap is passed. Undermining of the xiphoid area is avoided.

flap loss. The shift from the preferred inferior epigastric venous drainage to superior epigastric venous drainage when a superior pedicle flap is elevated is accompanied by significant changes in directions of blood flow within the TRAM flap.[18] Any added compromise to the vein will further tip the scales in favor of venous congestion and lead to the spiral that ends in complications. Venous congestion noted during the operation can often be relieved and alleviated by releasing the ligature on the inferior epigastric vein. Periods of release of the vein during the operative procedure can allow an otherwise congested flap to achieve a more normal state before closure of all the incisions. However, if this congestion is not completely relieved, other measures must be taken before skin closure. The first step is to carefully examine the superior epigastric pedicle as it crosses over the costal margin. Often more dissection is needed, not less, to clearly delineate the vascular pedicle and ensure that it is unencumbered by adjacent folded muscle tissue. One should not be reluctant to replace the TRAM flap back in the abdomen to conduct this exploration if venous congestion is not resolved. In the unlikely event that the superior epigastric vein has been injured, a microvascular venous anastomosis can be performed using the

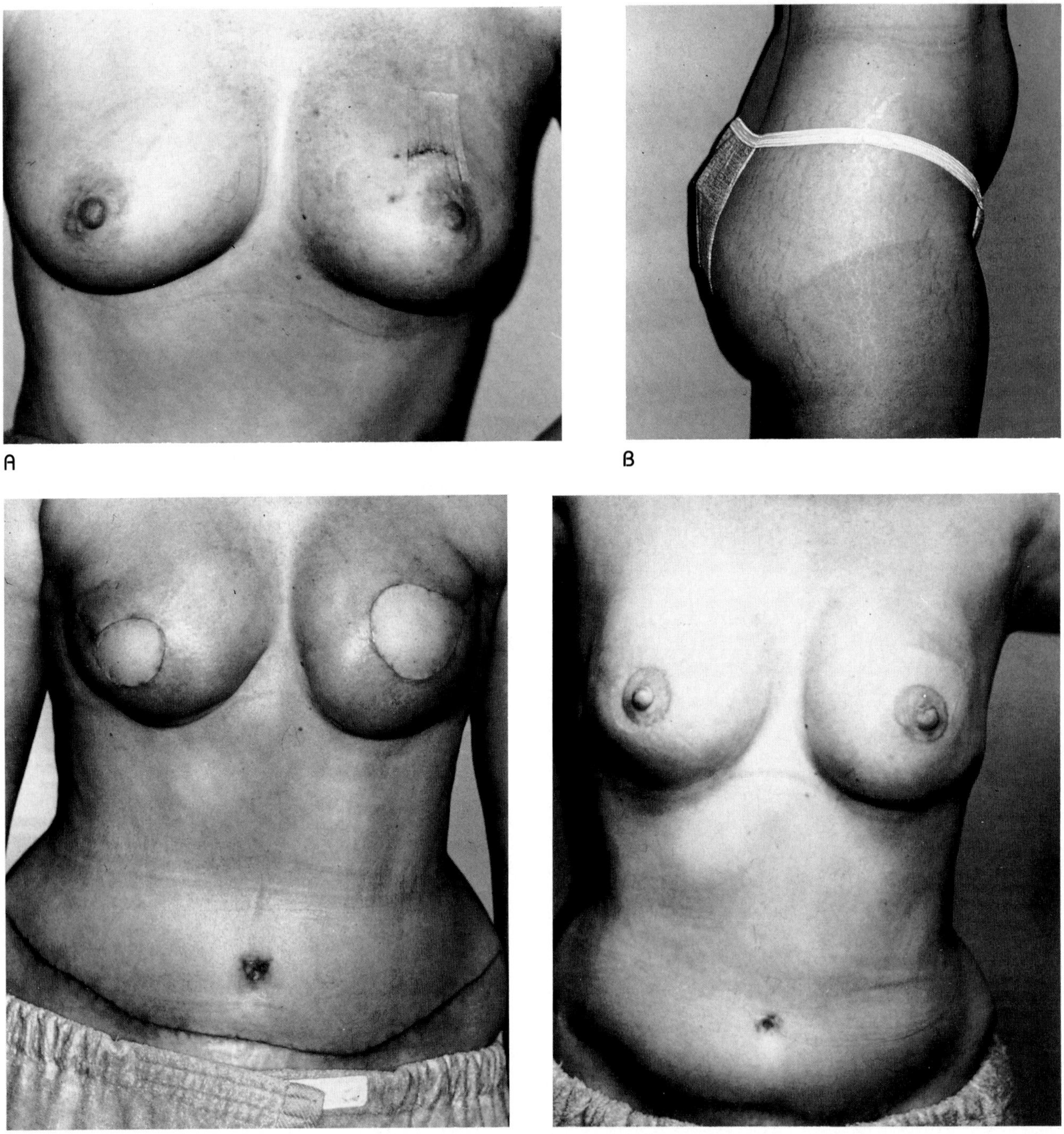

FIGURE 34-12 A 35-year-old patient with biopsy-proved lobular carcinoma of the left breast. She elected to have bilateral mastectomies, with immediate reconstruction. *A*, Preoperative view showing left breast biopsy. *B*, Lateral preoperative view showing the amount of abdominal tissue available for transfer. *C*, Results 2 months after bilateral immediate TRAM breast reconstruction. *D*, One year after bilateral TRAM breast reconstruction and bilateral nipple-areola reconstruction. *E*, Lateral view 1 year after surgery.

inferior epigastric vein, which has been left long at its initial division.

Cyanosis, mottling, or bruising of the flap either intraoperatively or postoperatively all suggest significant compromise, generally in the venous system. Chemotherapeutic agents such as nifedipine (Procardia), dextran, and heparin may all be of some benefit but their use is certainly empirical. Prompt re-exploration is almost always a better answer when a change such as this is observed in a TRAM flap.

Arterial kinking, blockage, or injury can occur in either the dissection or rotation of the pedicle. If the

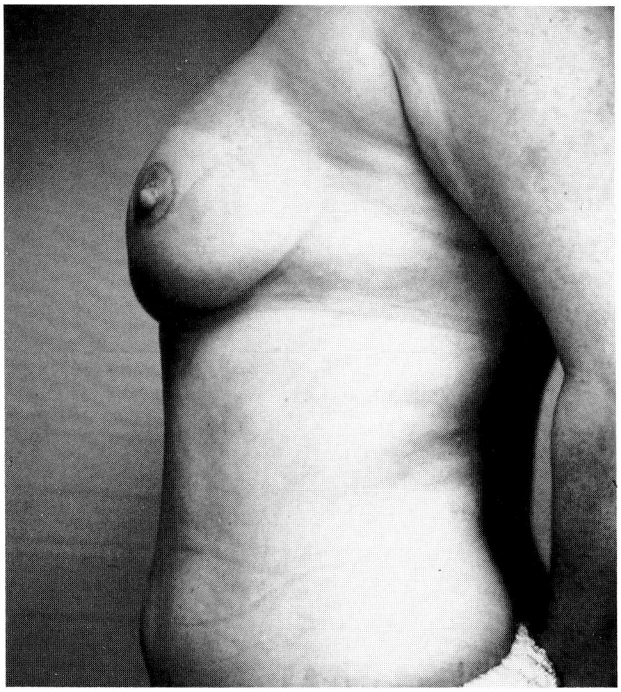

E

Figure 34-12 *Continued*

superior epigastric artery has been directly injured, a microvascular arterial anastomosis can be performed between the inferior epigastric artery and the thoracodorsal pedicle if the diagnosis is made intraoperatively or in the early postoperative period.

Free TRAM flaps go through fewer color changes than the pedicled TRAM flap. Once revascularized, the free TRAM flap should have essentially the same color and temperature as the surrounding skin and should remain that way. Any deviation from this in the setting of a free TRAM flap should dictate immediate exploration. There is generally little problem in performing another microvascular anastomosis and salvaging a flap if the diagnosis is made early and the patient immediately explored. We often use low-dose heparin in this setting, but again its use is empirical and will not overcome a poor microvascular anastomosis. Occasionally, a second venous anastomosis is performed if the first microvascular venous anastomosis is thought to be inadequate. However, in most patients, a single vein is more than adequate to satisfy the flap.

Double-pedicle techniques for single-sided breast reconstruction add the complexity of two muscle pedicles in a single tunnel. Careful dissection to a high level near the xiphoid of both pedicles, along with positioning the pedicles in the tunnel as a "double sling," one beneath the other, generally avoids compromise of either pedicle in the tunnel. However, if problems do arise with vascularity of a double-pedicle flap, this should be the first area to explore.

The importance of a secure abdominal wall closure cannot be overemphasized. Extreme diligence is necessary to ensure that both leaves of the anterior rectus sheath (the components of the internal and external oblique, respectively) are included in the abdominal wall closure (Fig. 34-13). If the inner

FIGURE 34-13 Detail of abdominal wall cross section during the TRAM procedure. *Above*, Incision into the rectus muscle with the overlying attached TRAM flap. Note the medial and lateral segments of muscle that are left. *Below*, Muscle-fascia defect after the TRAM is elevated. The suture is passed through a single leaf medially but two leaves laterally, securing both the internal and external oblique muscle and fascia to the medial rectus abdominis sheath.

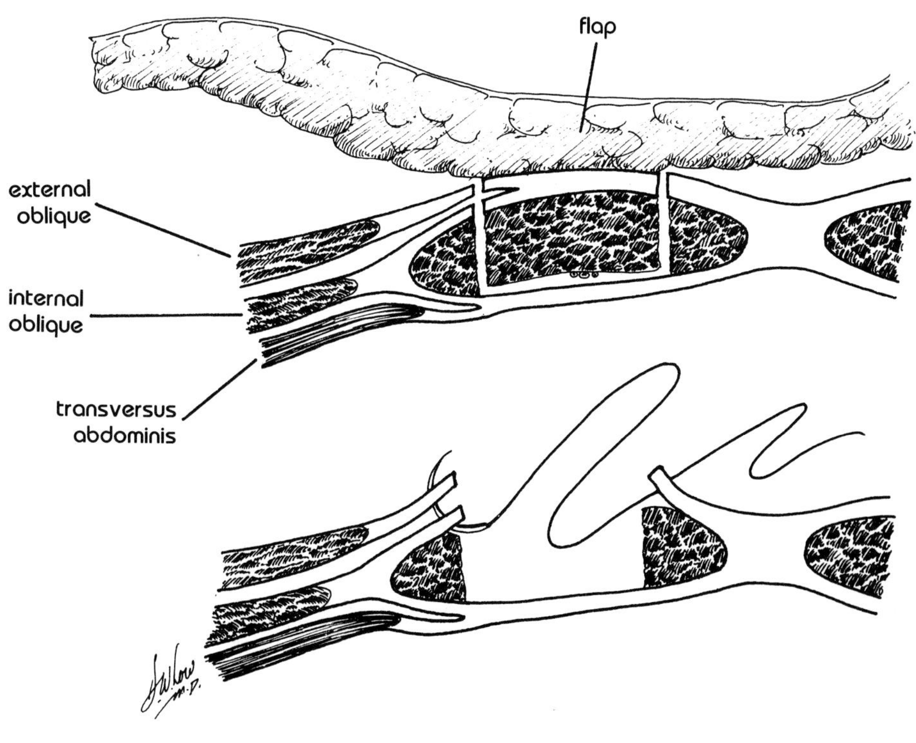

leaf is not included, weaknesses of the abdominal wall will be noted postoperatively. This will not be manifested as a hernia but as a weakness of the abdominal wall that often troubles the patient from an aesthetic standpoint. If the surgeon is concerned with the tightness of the abdominal wall fascial closure, Proline mesh should be overlaid generally from the umbilicus to the pubis. This mesh is sutured with monofilament suture around the periphery. The central portions of the mesh are fused to the underlying abdominal wall tissue with fascial staples. This prevents any herniation beneath the mesh. As mentioned previously, we prefer to use mesh reinforcement in all patients with a significant smoking history.

Cooperation with the oncologic surgeon in the context of immediate breast reconstruction after mastectomy is vitally important to the overall success of the operation. Surgeons' techniques differ in terms of thinness of chest wall flaps, and this must be anticipated. With experience, one can predict those flaps that will be too thin to have consistent primary healing and therefore need to be resected before TRAM breast shaping. It is disheartening to de-epithelialize areas of the TRAM flap that one later finds would have been helpful to fill in areas of overlying skin loss due to chest flaps that do not survive. The reconstructive surgeon must take great care with regard to the chest skin flaps as experience is gained with each oncologic surgeon. There should be no reluctance to resect any questionable areas of skin flaps at the time of reconstruction, because replacement with TRAM flap skin is much easier than trying to cover a denuded area later.

CONCLUSION

Reconstruction of the breast with rectus abdominis flaps has assumed a paramount position among the options for breast reconstruction today. It is the gold standard in terms of a natural result and minimal donor site morbidity. Increased knowledge of all facets of the anatomy and physiology of the TRAM flap over the past decade have led to improvements and refinements in technique. Nonetheless, this technique still involves possible complications that can be disastrous. There is no substitute for training and experience in achieving the highest level of aesthetic result with the lowest incidence of complications. The TRAM flap will continue to have wide application in both the pedicle and microvascular free flap form. The place for the microvascular transfer will eventually be decided by individual surgeons in relation to their ability to perform microsurgery and the specific needs of each patient. In the coming decade, we may perhaps see better control of the microcirculation within a TRAM flap through either mechanical or pharmacologic means. This will probably be most helpful with regard to the venous side, especially in the pedicled TRAM flap. The growth of the TRAM flap's use has been phenomenal, and it will continue to be employed in a significant proportion of patients desiring breast reconstruction.

References

1. Hartrampf CR, Scheflan M, Black PW. Breast reconstruction with a transverse abdominal island flap. Plast Reconstr Surg 1982; 69:216.
2. Boyd JB, Taylor GI, Corlett R. The vascular territories of the superior epigastric and the deep inferior epigastric systems. Plast Reconstr Surg 1984; 73:1.
3. Shaw WW, Fenz L. A comparison of the superior versus the inferior pedicles of the transverse rectus abdominis myocutaneous flap: Implications in breast reconstruction. Plast Reconstr Surg (in press).
4. Taylor GI, Caddy CM, Watterson PA, Crock JG. The venous territories (venosomes) of the human body. Plast Reconstr Surg 1990; 86:185.
5. Taylor GI, Palmer JH. The vascular territories (angiosomes) of the body: Experimental study and clinical applications. Br J Plast Surg 1987; 40:113.
6. Shaw WW. Microvascular free flap breast reconstruction. Clin Plast Surg 1984; 11:333.
7. Elliott LF, Beegle PN, Hartrampf CR. The lateral transverse thigh free flap: An alternative for autogenous tissue breast reconstruction. Plast Reconstr Surg 1990; 85:169.
8. Brown RG, Vasconey LO, Jurkiewicz MJ. Transverse abdominal flaps and the deep epigastric arcade. Plast Reconstr Surg 1975; 55:417.
9. Cronin TD, Upton J, McDonough JM. Reconstruction of the breast after mastectomy. Plast Reconstr Surg 1977; 59:1.
10. McGraw JB, Dibbell DG, Carraway JH. Clinical definition of independent myocutaneous vascular territories. Plast Reconstr Surg 1977; 60:341.
11. Hill HL, Brown RG, Jurkiewicz MJ. The transverse lumbosacral flap. Plast Reconstr Surg 1978; 62:177.
12. Dreaver JM. Total breast reconstruction. Ann Plast Surg 1981; 7:54.
13. Boyd J, Taylor GI, Corlett RJ. The vascular territories of the superior epigastric and deep inferior epigastric systems. Plast Reconstr Surg 1984; 73:1.
14. Miller LB, Bostwick J, Hartrampf CR, et al. The superiorly based rectus abdominis flap: Predicting and enhancing its blood supply based on an anatomic and clinical study. Plast Reconstr Surg 1988; 81:713.
15. Feldman S, Michelow B, Hartrampf CR, et al. Method to preoperatively predict the weight of a TRAM flap. Perspect Plast Surg 1989; 3:91.
16. Stevenson TR, Rohrich RJ, Pollock RA, et al. More experience with the "reverse" latissimus dorsi musculocutaneous flap: Precise location of blood supply. Plast Reconstr Surg 1984; 74:237.
17. Hartrampf CR, Barnthouse JR, Bennett GK. Complications in TRAM flap surgery: Their prevention and management. Instructional Courses Volume IV, Plastic Surgery Educational Foundation, 1991 (in press).

CHAPTER 35

Breast Reconstruction with Free Flaps

WILLIAM W. SHAW, M.D.
CHRISTINA Y. AHN, M.D.

The initial step in breast reconstruction is to evaluate the mastectomy deformity that results from loss of skin surface, breast volume, the nipple-areola complex, symmetry, and contour defects. Currently, two general methods are described to create a suitable breast mound, which is the first step in breast reconstruction:

1. The use of a silicone implant or tissue expander. The latter stretches the skin into the appropriate shape, with the desired volume maintained by permanent implant insertion.
2. The use of autologous tissue to replace the skin and volume.

Although most patients are grateful for the improvement achieved by implants, this method presents several fundamental limitations and problems.[1,2] The implants may become infected, extruded, or ruptured, resulting in the loss of reconstruction and requiring additional surgery. Another inherent and difficult problem is the unavoidable foreign body reaction toward the implants, which results in capsule formations. Hard capsular contractures may result in pain, shifting, and distortion of the reconstructed breast mound even many years after reconstruction. When the overlying skin is thin, patients have complained of "coldness" of the implant and lack of skin sensation.

Autogenous reconstruction methods require the transplantation of suitable skin and bulk from a different part of the body to create the breast mound. Once successfully transplanted, the living tissue can be sculpted to achieve optimal shape and size by filling out specific contour defects and fully restoring symmetry. In time, the warm and soft reconstructed breast becomes easily accepted by the patient. Most patients studied have also described a spontaneous restoration of some sensation in the autogenous transplanted tissue, thereby adding to the sense of wholeness. The main disadvantages of autogenous breast reconstructions are the additional donor site scars and the more complex nature of the surgery.

With the introduction of myocutaneous flaps, small autologous breasts were reconstructed with latissimus dorsi flaps.[3] Since then, variations of the superiorly based rectus abdominis myocutaneous flap have become the main vehicle to transplant excess abdominal tissue to reconstruct the breast mound. Free flaps were initially used only in selected difficult cases. However, they have subsequently been utilized for elective delayed reconstructions as well as immediate reconstructions.

As confidence with free flap surgery is gained, free tissue transfer is likely to become a standard option in autologous breast reconstruction.

INDICATIONS FOR FREE FLAPS

Difficult Surface or Contour Problems

The reconstructive surgeon is still faced with the problems of skin surface and difficult contour resulting from various ablative surgical and adjuvant therapeutic procedures. "Washboard-like" tight-skinned chest from radical mastectomy, skin shortage that results from resection of large fixed tumors, and breast cancer recurrence after radiation are some of the challenging problems in breast reconstruction. Reconstructions using implants or expanders under tight and irradiated skin are prone to implant-related complications. The resultant shapes are disappointing, particularly when pectoralis muscle is absent, contracted, or fibrotic. These deformities require additional autologous tissue for correction. When adjacent local flaps are not available, free flap transfer is the only reconstructive solution.

Unsuitable Regional Flaps

Superiorly based transverse rectus abdominis myocutaneous (TRAM) flaps are unsuitable in patients who have undergone previous abdominoplasty and have upper abdominal surgical and vertical midline lower abdominal surgical scars. Symmetry is also difficult to achieve with a superiorly based TRAM flap in a thin patient with large breasts, because sufficient volume cannot be harvested from the abdomen. Although the loss of the rectus abdominis muscle on one or both sides is well tolerated, this may be a serious concern for athletic patients. In women of childbearing age, the potential risk of pregnancy for the weakened abdominal wall has not yet been fully evaluated.

Failures from Other Reconstructions

Patients in whom implant or tissue expanders have failed often undergo repeated procedures to rectify or salvage disappointing results. When all else fails, autologous tissue reconstruction becomes the only permanent solution, and free flaps offer greater reconstructive versatility for salvage.

Patient Preference

As the general patient population becomes increasingly aware of the various options in breast reconstructive methods, their preference plays an important role in the ultimate selection of procedure. Patients with obese, protuberant, or unsightly lower abdomens may strongly prefer the TRAM flap in order to benefit from the abdominoplasty as well as from their primary breast reconstruction. Others may choose to leave the abdomen alone either for athletic reasons or because of unwillingness to accept the abdominal scar; these may choose gluteal free flap to hide scars in the buttock. Other patients may choose the tensor fascia lata (TFL) free flap to benefit from removal of excess tissue from the lateral thigh area.

Immediate Reconstructions

Because increasing numbers of patients are treated with lumpectomy and radiation, those who develop local recurrences require a wider skin excision than usual when mastectomy is performed. The wound closure at the time of mastectomy may require immediate autologous tissue reconstruction owing to insufficient skin or problems with irradiated skin. Some mastectomy patients choose to have immediate reconstruction with autologous tissue. With a coordinated team approach between general surgeon and reconstructive surgeon, the skin incision and reconstructive needs can be well planned. Because the wound is widely opened by the mastectomy procedure and the recipient vessels are partially exposed, immediate reconstructions can usually be done remarkably expeditiously. The convenience and economic savings, along with minimizing the psychological trauma from the mastectomy deformity, make immediate reconstruction an attractive alternative.

RECIPIENT VESSEL FOR FREE FLAPS

Ideal recipient vessels should have the following characteristics: suitable diameter match, appropriate vascular pedicle length, location outside the zone of injury, and expendability (Fig. 35–1). The axillary vessels and their branches are most commonly used. However, mastectomy or axillary dissection may result in vascular injury and scarring, which makes the axilla an unavailable and undesirable recipient site. For instance, severe scarring of the axilla with denervation of the latissimus muscle would suggest that thoracodorsal vessels are not suitable.

For gluteal free flaps, the internal mammary vessels provide the best insetting. In about 25 percent of patients, however, the internal mammary vein is too small for the gluteal vein, thus making anastomosis very difficult and prone to thrombosis. For these patients, the external jugular or the cephalic vein can be substituted. Finally, vein grafts can be used to lengthen the vascular pedicle in order to reach axillary vessels.

DONOR TISSUES FOR BREAST RECONSTRUCTION

Transverse Rectus Abdominis Myocutaneous (TRAM) Free Flap

The use of the superiorly based pedicled TRAM flap has confirmed the abdomen as a highly desirable source of donor site for breast reconstruction. Currently, TRAM flaps are gradually being used as free flaps rather than as pedicle flaps in both immediate and elective reconstructions.[4–6] This trend is supported by the previous studies that demonstrated the dominance of the inferior epigastric system over the superior epigastric and the excellent results of lower extremity reconstruction with inferiorly based free rectus abdominis flaps.

The free TRAM flap has excellent blood supply within all the regions of harvested flap tissue. The long vascular pedicle allows easy anastomosis with the branches of the axillary artery and provides a much greater freedom and versatility in molding the breast mound (Fig. 35–2). In addition, it is no longer necessary to take the entire muscle; the upper muscle dissection and tunneling can be avoided. There-

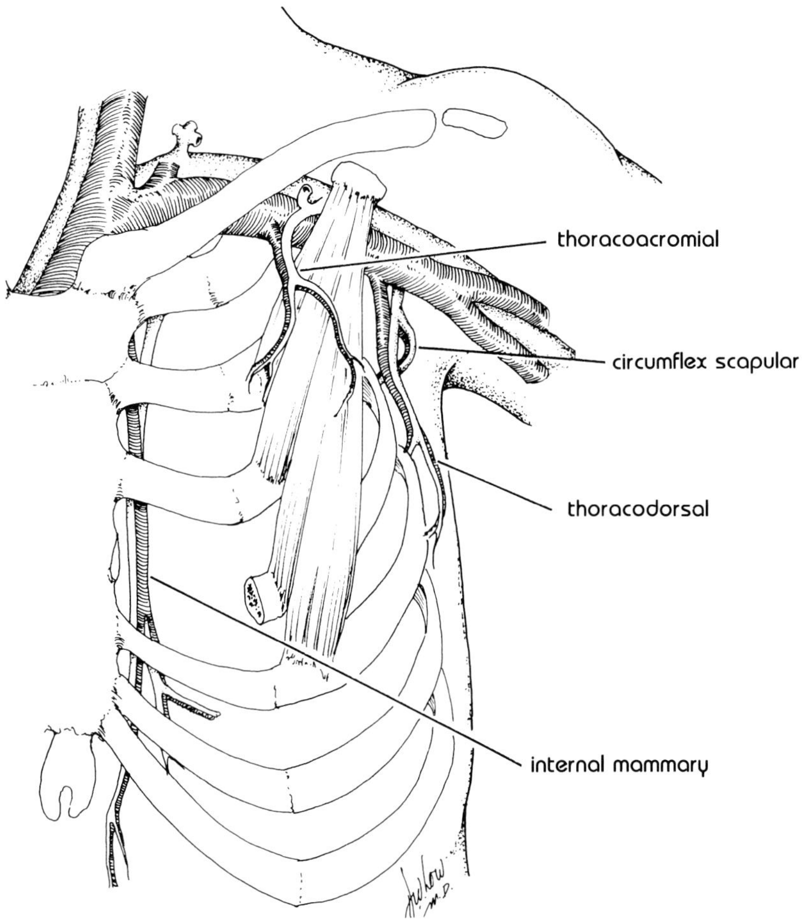

FIGURE 35-1 Recipient vessels for free flap breast reconstruction. The thoracodorsal vessels are the most frequently used for most donor flaps. The internal mammary vessels allow for best insetting of gluteal free flaps.

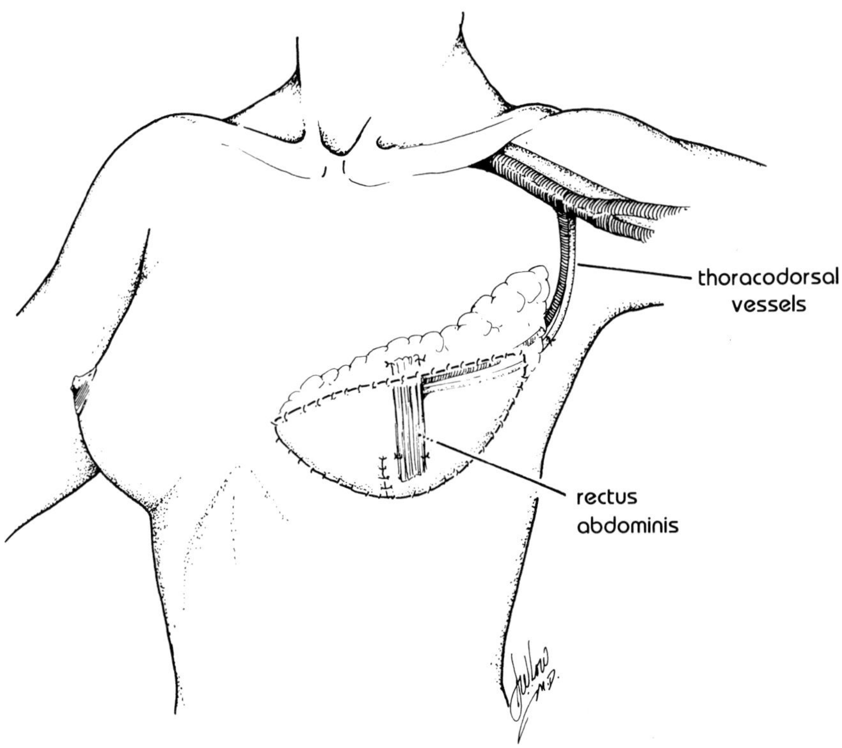

FIGURE 35-2 The long vascular pedicle of the free transverse rectus abdominis myocutaneous (TRAM) flap allows ease of anastomosis with the recipient axillary vessels and versatility in molding the breast mound.

fore, free TRAM flap patients can be ambulating sooner than those who undergo pedicled TRAM flap reconstruction. However, the inferiorly based free TRAM flap may be unsuitable in patients with previous lower abdominal scars because of possible previous injury to the inferior epigastric system.

Attention to technical details is important. Careful flap dissection, preservation of the rectus abdominis muscle and anterior rectus sheath, and meticulous fascial closure generally result in less abdominal discomfort or functional loss. An approximately 5-cm rim of the upper central abdominal fat overlying the anterior rectus sheath should be harvested as the upper part of the free flap; this allows better flap perfusion and a greater volume of flap available. Inferiorly, it is essential to incise superior to the arcuate line to avoid abdominal wall weakness and hernia (Fig. 35-3).

With experience, both the lateral slip of rectus muscle and the majority of the anterior rectus sheath can be preserved. An approximately 4-cm width of anterior rectus sheath needs to be harvested in order to preserve the major perforators to the free flap. The medial fascial incisions can be made approximately 1 cm lateral to the midline (linea alba). It is also beneficial to leave the lateral intercostal nerves undisturbed during the lateral rectus muscle slip dissection. Most important, it is essential to achieve a meticulous anatomic fascial closure of the donor defect to avoid an abdominal hernia and minimize abdominal wall weakness (Fig. 35-4).

Superior Gluteal Free Flap

Fujino and Harashina first performed breast reconstruction using the upper gluteus maximus myocutaneous free flap based on the superior gluteal artery and vein.[7] The vascular pedicle was attached to axillary vessels. Shaw modified the procedure by

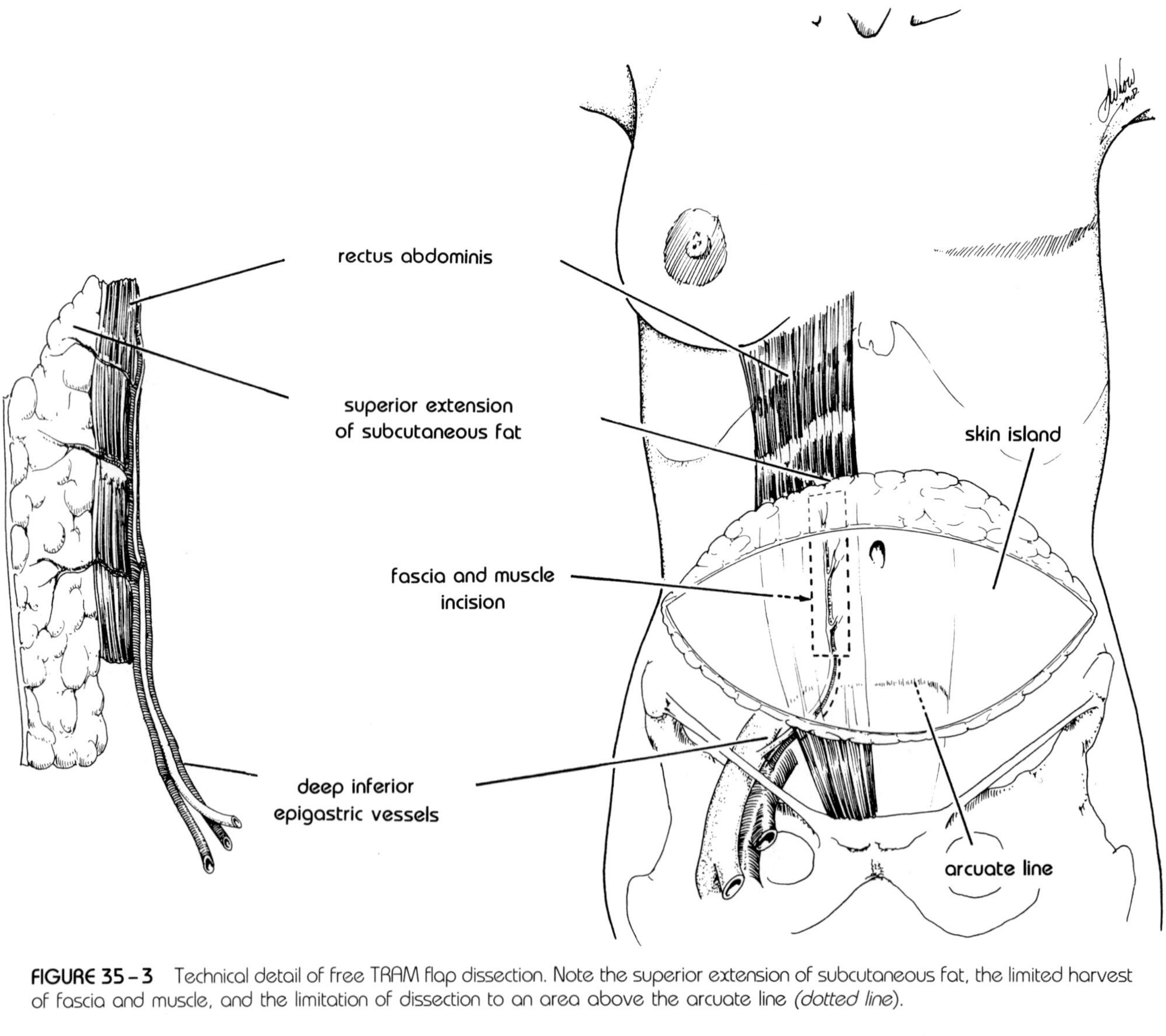

FIGURE 35-3 Technical detail of free TRAM flap dissection. Note the superior extension of subcutaneous fat, the limited harvest of fascia and muscle, and the limitation of dissection to an area above the arcuate line *(dotted line)*.

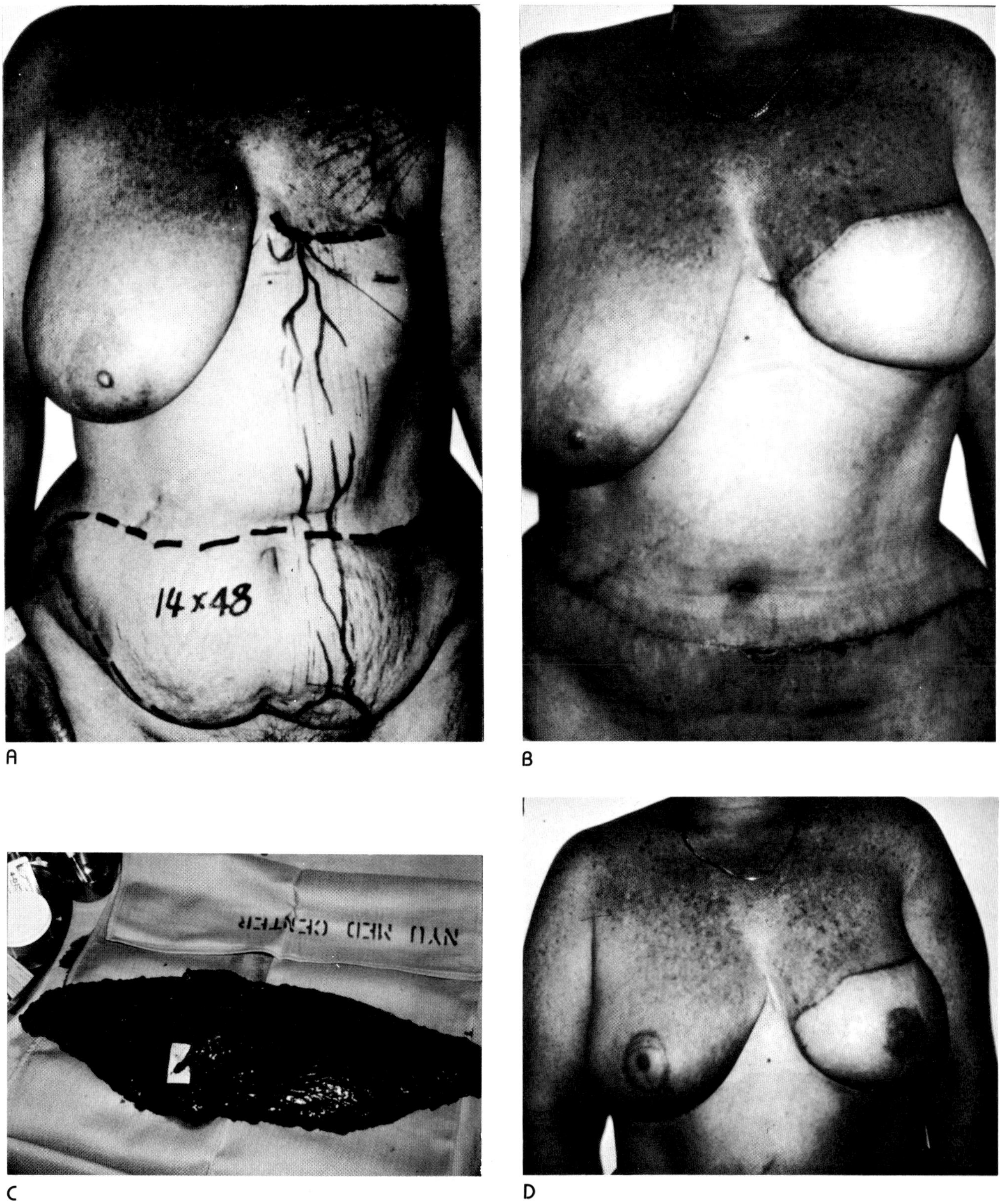

FIGURE 35-4 TRAM free flap reconstruction. *A*, Preoperative markings of the chest and abdominal incisions. *B*, Two weeks after surgery. *C*, Flap harvested with a small amount of rectus abdominis muscle, leaving sufficient muscle and fascia for abdominal wall integrity. *D*, *E*, Anterior and oblique views six weeks after right reduction mammaplasty and left nipple-areola reconstruction.

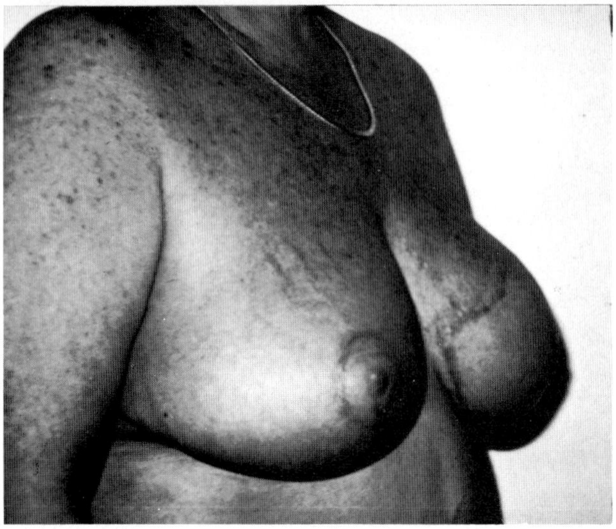

E

Figure 35-4 *Continued*

using the internal mammary vessels to allow proper insetting of the breast mound (Fig. 35-5).[8] Careful patient selection and precise preoperative planning is essential to the achievement of highly gratifying results from this method. The direction and amount of skin and subcutaneous wedge harvest need to be executed in such a way to match the shape and the bulk of the neo-breast mound as closely as possible (Fig. 35-6). It is also important to include approximately 20 percent of the gluteus maximus muscle cuff beneath the subcutaneous fat to ensure viability of the flap and protect the vascular pedicle (Fig. 35-7). Skin widths up to 13 cm have been taken without any difficulty in primary closure or significant contour deformity. Cuff removal of a small amount of gluteus maximus muscle does not result in a noticeable functional loss. Even in thin patients, a generous amount of tissue can be harvested (Fig. 35-8). This is one of the more difficult flaps in terms of flap dissection and vessel anastomosis, thus limiting its use to experienced reconstructive surgeons (Fig. 35-9).

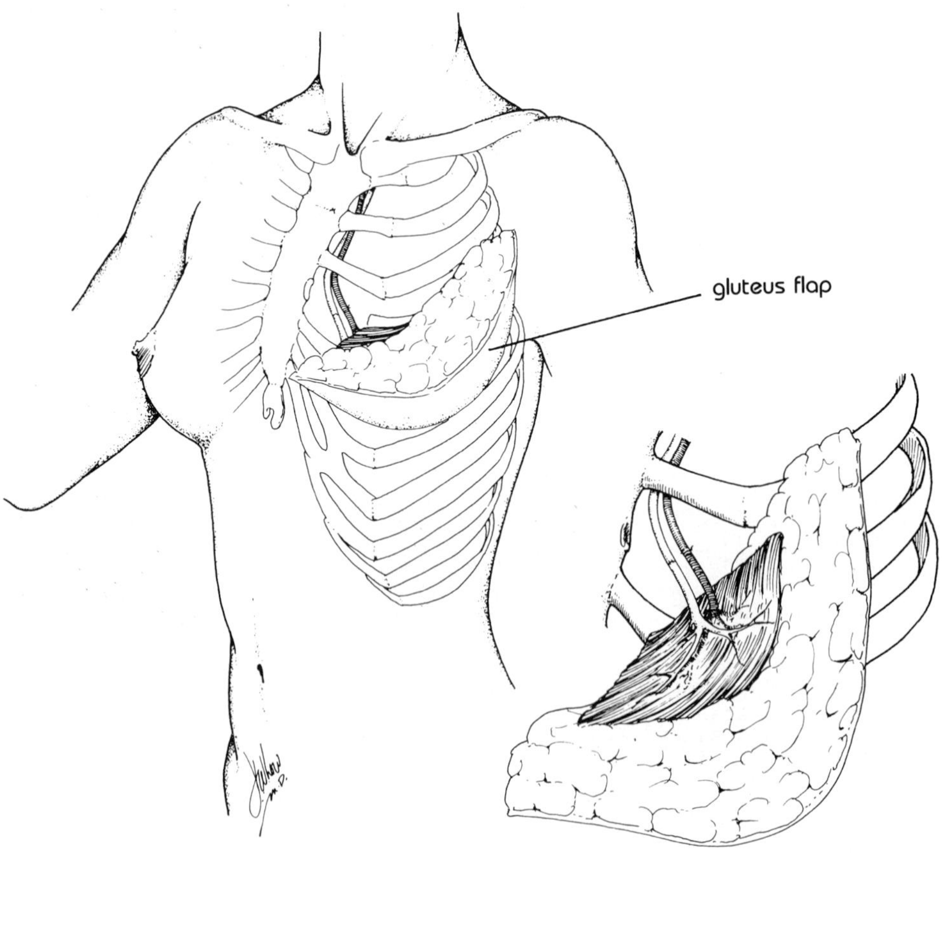

FIGURE 35-5 Insetting of the gluteal free flap is more easily done when the internal mammary vessels are used as recipient vessels.

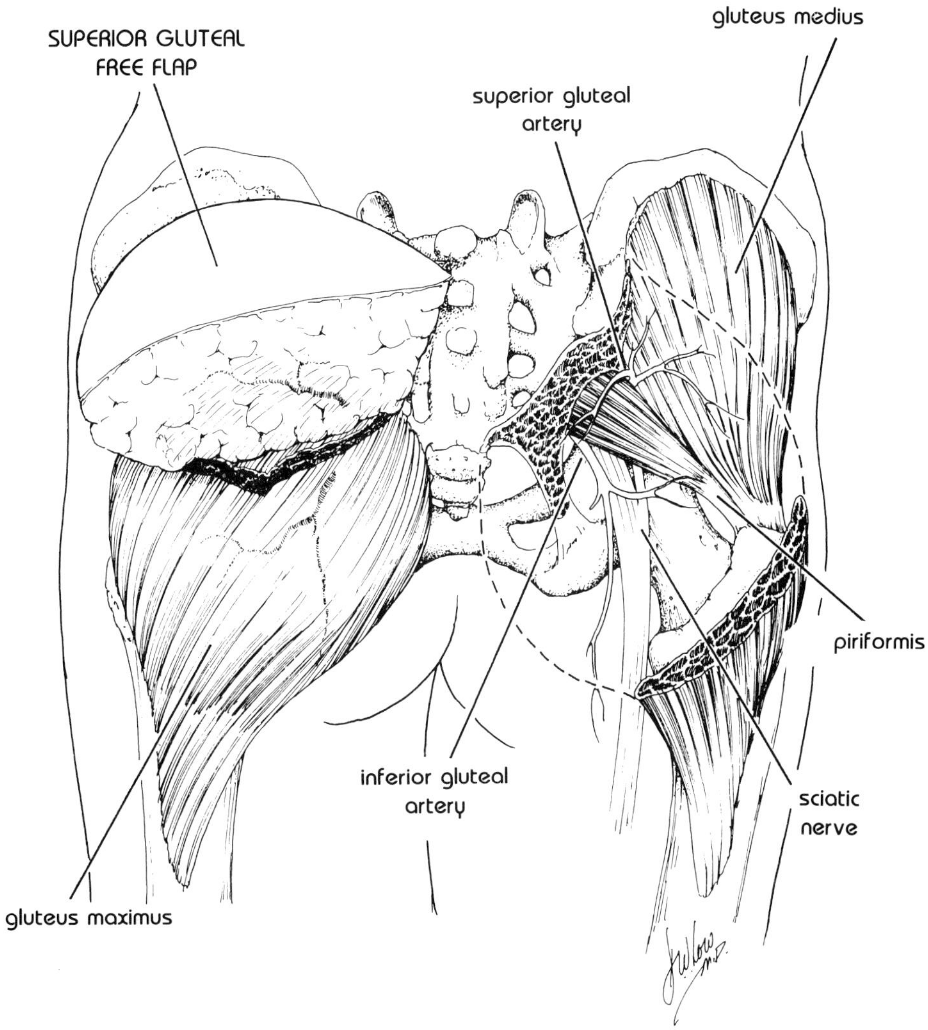

FIGURE 35-6 The superior gluteal free flap is supplied by the superior gluteal vessels and supported by a portion of the superior gluteus muscle. Design of the flap includes a direction of the skin island and wedge of subcutaneous fat sufficient to watch the neo-breast as closely as possible. This careful design minimizes the donor defect.

Inferior Gluteal Free Flap

This flap is based on inferior gluteal vessels that support the lower gluteus maximus muscle, subcutaneous tissue, and skin as a myocutaneous autologous tissue.[8] Although the vascular pedicle is slightly longer than the superior system, it requires careful dissection to preserve the sciatic nerve. The inferior direction, and the location of a donor site scar in an area visible below the underwear or swimsuit line, can be undesirable.

Tensor Fascia Lata (TFL) Flap

Adequate breast volume can be harvested from the lateral thigh in patients with obese, protuberant tissue excess in this region. Patient selection is important and preoperative planning needs to be precise in order to determine the exact volume of the subcutaneous fat to be harvested and to minimize the donor contour defect. It can be harvested using either a transverse or vertical skin paddle. A meticulous closure of the donor site is important to restore lateral thigh contour. Liposuction or a contralateral excisional procedure may be necessary to achieve donor site symmetry. The TFL flap may be considered unsuitable for patients without sufficient excess volume at the donor site or those with a severe skin deficit at the recipient site. The possible donor site contour defect and asymmetry, along with unavoidable, long, visible scars, make this flap a less attractive alternative.[1]

Groin Flap

The free groin flaps were used by Serafin and Georgiade to resurface chest wall skin and to adequately cover implants in radical mastectomy defor-

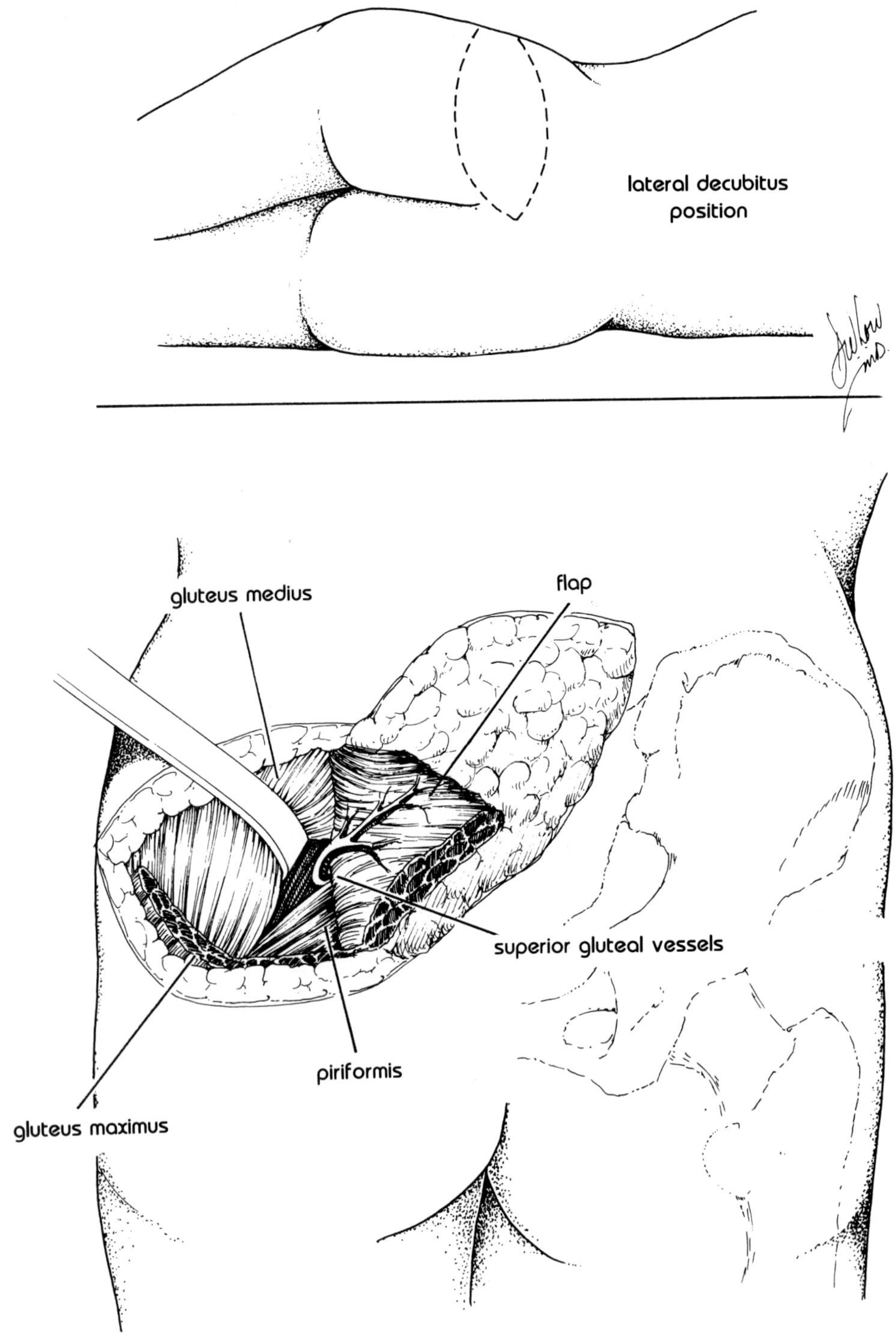

FIGURE 35-7 The lateral decubitus position is best used for harvest of the superior gluteal free flap. After skin and subcutaneous incision, the gluteus maximus muscle is incised to include approximately 20 percent of muscle cuff with the flap. Division of the gluteus from its origin on the sacrum and posterior iliac crest allows visualization of the vascular pedicle arising between the gluteus medius and piriformis muscles. Proximal dissection of the pedicle allows a length of 2 to 3 cm before entry into the muscle.

mities with large areas of skin grafted chest wall.[3] Although this flap has a well-concealed, ideal donor defect, its short and often small-diameter pedicle makes the anastomosis more difficult and often requires vein grafts. It is also difficult to achieve central anterior projection with the groin flap without the use of an implant beneath the flap. This free flap has been made obsolete by the introduction of the TRAM flap.

Contralateral Latissimus Dorsi Flap

This free flap can be used when muscle and skin are needed but the ipsilateral latissimus is either unavailable or insufficient. This may still be a useful flap in selected patients, but the awkward position and the intraoperative redraping make this a less desirable donor site.

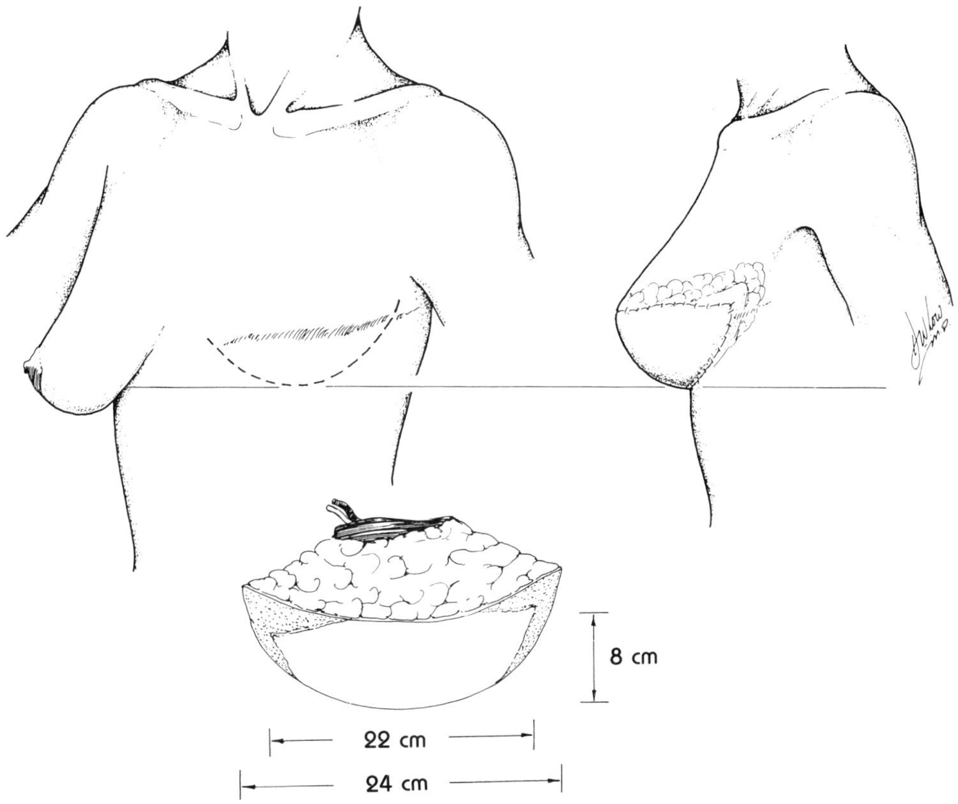

FIGURE 35-8 The gluteal free flap provides good projection of the neo-breast. Skin widths can vary according to the defect and projection of breast tissue desired. An 8-cm distance from the inframammary fold to the central projection of the breast mound is ideal, although widths of the flap up to 13 cm can be taken. The length can also vary, but shape can be developed by placing de-epithelialized portions of the flap past the area designed for the skin island.

Contralateral Breast Wedge

Le-Quang used the lateral half of the contralateral breast based on the lateral thoracic vessels to achieve excellent aesthetic breast reconstruction and also to obtain simultaneous breast reduction.[9] Unfortunately, this is not a well-accepted alternative owing to the increased risk of carcinoma developing in the contralateral breast.

METHOD SELECTION

The patient and the surgeon jointly can establish the most suitable individualized reconstructive plan based on multiple factors. This process begins with the first consultation during which the surgeon discusses with the patient the different methods of breast reconstruction. The relative merits, benefits, risks, and suitability of each method should be discussed. The surgeon then carefully determines the anatomic deformity, specific reconstructive needs, and overall patient risk factors, while inviting the patient to actively voice her preference and participate in the selection of procedure.

Several fundamental anatomic features need to be considered in the planning and selection of the free flap for breast reconstruction. First, the opposite breast must be evaluated to determine its size, shape, and symmetry and the location of the breast mound. The opposite breast may need to be reduced, mastopexed, or augmented to achieve optimal symmetry. A gluteal free flap is most suitable for reconstructing a firm, conical breast, whereas a free TRAM flap is ideal for reconstructing a soft, slightly ptotic breast.

Second, one should carefully review all the technical aspects of the free flap operation with regard to the choice of recipient vessel, skin coverage, insetting, and donor site anatomy.

Finally, the surgeon's experience needs to be taken into account in the selection of the free flap. The TRAM free flap can be safely and relatively easily used by most reconstructive surgeons with moderate microsurgical experience. However, the gluteal free flap requires much more experience and technical expertise to safely harvest and transplant free flaps. It also requires considerable planning to achieve the best results. Thus, use of this flap should not be attempted until the surgeon has gained considerable microsurgical experience and has carefully studied the specific anatomy.

COMMENTS

Free flap transfer offers many inherent advantages in breast reconstruction and remains an important option as an autologous breast reconstructive method in immediate as well as elective cases.

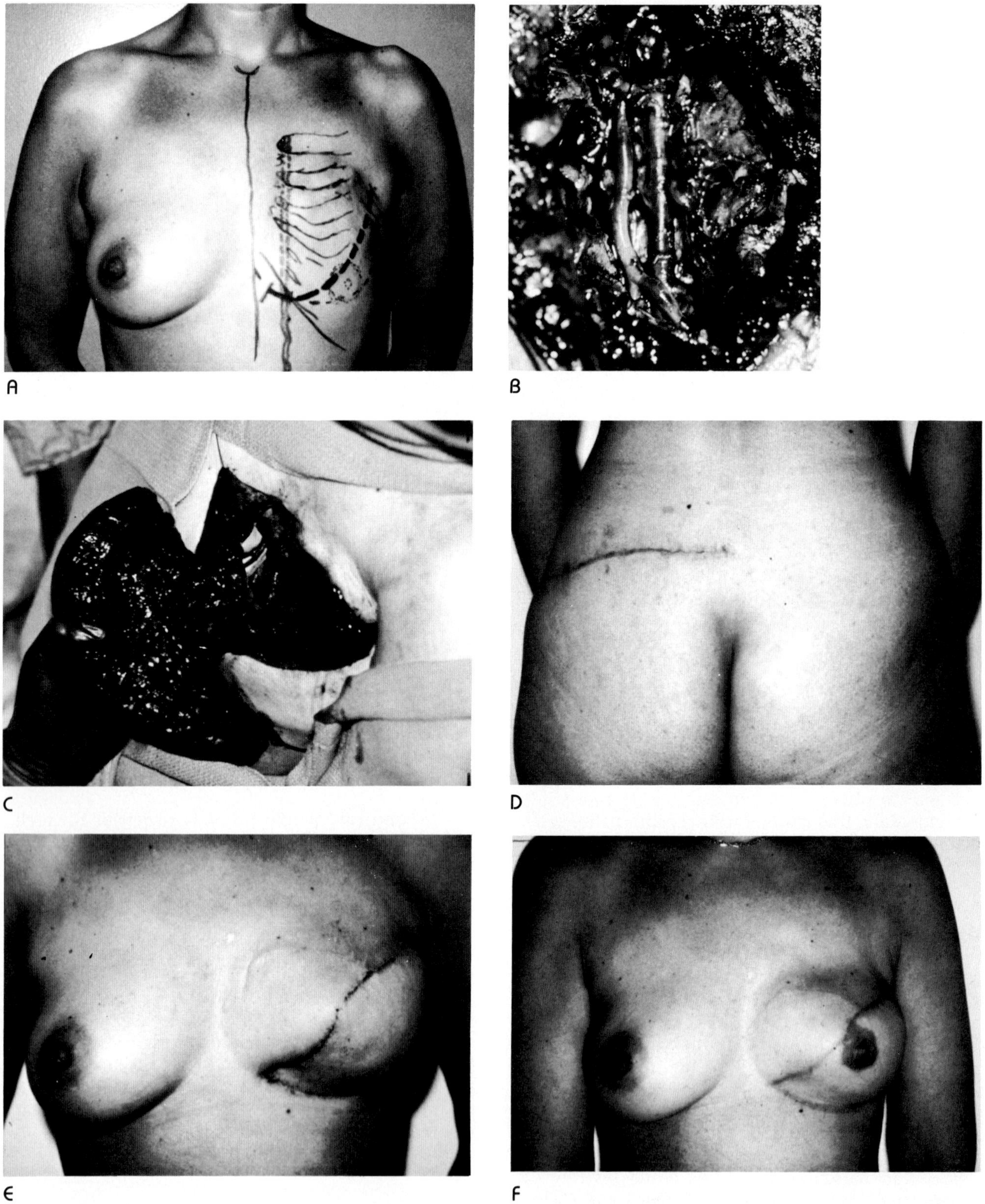

FIGURE 35-9 Autologous breast reconstruction with the superior gluteal free flap. *A*, Skin markings of incision and the location of internal mammary vessels. *B*, These vessels exposed to be used as the recipient vessels. *C*, Superior gluteal flap after anastomosis to the internal mammary vessel. *D*, Donor site, *E*, Two weeks after surgery. *F*, One year following gluteal free flap reconstruction and subsequent nipple-areola reconstruction.

This is due to its excellent blood supply, the versatility in flap design, the great degree of freedom in the shaping of the neo-breast mound, and the minimal donor site morbidity.

Patients who elect to undergo implant reconstruction must be willing to accept the possibility of a 5 to 40 percent late capsule contracture rate and the need for future surgical revisions. Although tissue expanders have provided valuable flexibility in the use of implants, the complication rate is still considerable.

With techniques described in Chapter 34, Hartrampf produced excellent results from the pedicled TRAM flap, with a failure rate of only 2 percent and a low incidence of complications. However, others have experienced considerably more problems with partial flap necrosis or abdominal wall morbidity.

The senior author's experience with more than 140 free flaps for breast reconstruction has shown that the procedure can be performed with a minimal failure rate (1.8 percent). Furthermore, free flaps have produced highly gratifying results, despite a slightly longer initial operating time and the need for microsurgical expertise.

As confidence is gained with more cumulative experience in free flap surgery and a two-team approach in reducing operating time, the free flap is likely to become an excellent option in many breast reconstructions to achieve the most satisfactory results.

References

1. Shaw W. Microvascular free flap breast reconstruction. Clin Plast Surg 1984; 11:333-341.
2. Song RY, Yang PY, Yu HT, Huang HY. Breast reconstruction without a silicone implant. Clin Plast Surg 1982; 9:85-86.
3. Serafin D, Georgiade NG, Ginen KS. Transfer of free flaps to provide well-vascularized thick cover for breast reconstructions after radical mastectomy. Plast Reconstr Surg 1978; 62:527-536.
4. Friedman RJ, Argenta LC, Anderson R. Deep inferior epigastric free flap for breast reconstruction after radical mastectomy. Plast Reconstr Surg 1985; 76:454-458.
5. Pennington DC, Pelly AD. The rectus abdominis myocutaneous free flap. Br J Plast Surg 1980; 33:227-282.
6. Shaw W. Discussion of deep inferior epigastric free flaps for breast reconstruction. Plast Reconstr Surg 1985; 76:459-460.
7. Fujino T, Harashina T, Enomoto K. Primary breast reconstruction after a standard radical mastectomy by a free flap transfer. Plast Reconstr Surg 1976; 58:372-374.
8. Shaw W. Breast reconstruction by superior gluteal microvascular free flaps without silicone implants. Plast Reconstr Surg 1983; 72:490-499.
9. Le-Quang C. Microvascular tissue transfer in plastic surgery. In: Lie TS, ed. Microsurgery: Procedures of the International Congress of the International Microsurgery Society. Amsterdam: Excerpta Medica, 1979:125.

CHAPTER 36

Complications of Breast Reconstruction

J. BRIEN MURPHY, M.D.

PREOPERATIVE ASSESSMENT

Complications can result from any surgical procedure. Many complications can be avoided by careful preoperative planning, selection of the best procedure for the patient, and the ability to know when the operation should not be performed.

Careful preoperative assessment is essential to identify patients with unrealistic expectations. These patients are the most unforgiving if the breast reconstruction falls beneath their expectations. Recognizing the patient with unrealistic expectations may be difficult. The input of the office receptionist or staff nurse is often helpful, as patients frequently reveal their "true colors" well before the interview with the surgeon. Certainly efforts should be made to avoid patients who arrive with a litany of complaints about their previous surgeon or consultant; your name may be added to their list no matter how superbly you judge your operative result.

Interviewing and examining all patients twice prior to surgery is recommended. This may be impossible for those that come a great distance or for those who are planning immediate reconstruction (within the week), but this practice should be encouraged for most patients. The second visit helps to cement the patient-physician relationship, and may also allow the surgeon to recognize social or anatomic nuances that were missed on initial assessment. We encourage patients to bring spouses or family members for either visit as they frequently have their own concerns about additional surgery after living with the emotional trauma of the primary mastectomy and their questions may be more realistic and directed than those of the patient. The patient's idealism will be tempered by this pointed review of all options and complications. A photograph album with average results taken at different postoperative intervals is an additional method used to educate the patient, and helps to illustrate that wound healing in breast reconstruction is not always perfect and predictable. The patient's perspective of her expected result is brought into focus because the photographs illustrate more precisely what to expect. The realistic woman is encouraged by what reconstruction can accomplish, while even good photo results are disappointing to the unrealistic patient.

The surgeon is presented with certain limitations in reviewing reconstructive options with patients undergoing immediate reconstruction because of the short time period between diagnosis and surgery. These patients are scheduled as the last appointment during office hours, which allows an unhurried approach to review surgical options, timing options, and procedural details with the patient who is frequently upset with the recent cancer diagnosis. Working in concert with a well-informed oncologic surgeon is a great help when introducing material to the newly diagnosed patient. The oncologic surgeon presents mastectomy reconstruction as a positive solution to the extirpative surgery and prepares the patient with introductory information prior to our consultation. Previous reconstruction patients who

Editor's Note: This chapter is included to present an overview of the topic of complications following breast reconstruction, and to provide continuity in this section of the textbook. The reader is referred to chapters featuring specific techniques or procedures for detailed discussions of complications and their management. (RBN) have had similar procedures may also be called to assist and give advice to the new patient. Previous patients are often most helpful when new patients are finalizing the decision whether to have reconstruction and to decide between autologous and implant reconstruction. Any patient who is indecisive about options with immediate reconstruction should be seen again even though the time frame is short. If confusion remains, a delayed reconstruction should be considered. Selling an operation to an indecisive patient may only lead to later unhappiness.

In conjunction with the emotional factors involved in selecting a procedure are multiple systemic factors that influence the result and may bias a procedure toward specific complications. Hartrampf and others have attempted to weigh certain factors that may add to morbidity or be an absolute contraindication to autologous reconstruction.[1,2] The latter includes chronic obstructive pulmonary disease, severe cardiovascular disease, uncontrolled hypertension, and insulin-dependent diabetes. Minor contraindications for reconstruction include obesity, patient attitude, and other factors affecting small blood vessels such as autoimmune diseases and smoking. Miller et al took this analysis one step further and retrospectively reviewed all their breast reconstructions both autologous and implant, immediate and delayed, to look at specific influences on complications. Again diabetes was the most significant, while smoking, age greater than 60, obesity and hypertension approached significance for implant loss only in immediate breast reconstruction. This experience should certainly be used to influence choices of patients and procedures and avoid predictable complications in patients with these specific conditions.

All these studies illustrate the importance of careful preoperative screening to avoid postoperative problems. Breast reconstruction, whether delayed or immediate, requires careful preoperative assessment. Attention to detail is essential to determine the specific procedure from which the patient will experience the least morbidity and the greatest benefit.

COMPLICATIONS OF IMPLANT RECONSTRUCTION

Reconstruction using an implant remains the most common procedure for delayed and immediate reconstruction. The variety of implants (saline or gel, permanent or temporary expanders, textured or nontextured) add to the patient confusion when selecting a reconstructive procedure. The surgeon must direct the patient preoperatively through this maze and emphasize the critical deficits of any implant, so that the choice of the specific implant is clear and not clouded by minor product variabilities.

Preoperatively, when discussing the use of an implant, certain questions always surface concerning the safety of the silicone prosthesis. Their long-term influences on local tissue are regarded as potential complications and should be thoroughly reviewed with the patient before surgery both to eliminate any misinformation and to make the patient comfortable with her decision to select implant reconstruction. Patients must be reassured that the presence of an implant will not influence their tumor behavior and not obscure or delay the diagnosis of a local recurrence. Retrospective studies have shown that the long-term prognosis is no different for survival between reconstructed and nonreconstructed patients.[4,5] Recurrences after radical local treatment most often occur in the skin flaps and are frequently accompanied by simultaneous distant disease.[6] Our experience confirms that local recurrences are not masked by the implant. Any postoperative periprosthetic mass is, however, thoroughly investigated by mammography and ultrasound with needle aspiration or open biopsy used for tissue confirmation. This is the only way to guarantee a tissue diagnosis and reassure the patient.

Standard mammographic techniques are not reliable for visualizing the whole breast mound when an implant is in position, because the percentage of glandular tissue obscured by the implant after augmentation mammaplasty varies from 22 to 83 percent. The reconstructed breast should have little, if any, glandular tissue present, but there is a small percent that remains, even after mastectomy performed by the most experienced of surgeons. The current recommendations to maximize tissue visualized are proposed by Eklund et al.[7-9] Five views are routinely used for each breast: the standard mediolateral, oblique, vertical, craniocaudal, and 90 degree mediolateral compression views. This study should be performed yearly after surgery. Silicone gel creates radiodensity. Although other radiolucent fillers such as peanut oil have been proposed, their efficacy and biocompatability have not been proved.[10]

Immediate Complications

Preoperatively, all patients are placed on broad-spectrum antibiotics that are continued 3 days after drain removal. In addition, Phisoderm scrubs of the trunk are initiated twice a day starting 3 days before surgery to minimize potential bacterial surface contamination. Our incidence of infection with implant loss after immediate reconstruction remains constant at 3 percent,[11] and is usually seen in the older, more compromised patient. Persistent pain with low-grade fever and local tissue signs associated with ischemia are the most consistent findings. Removal of the prosthesis with drainage of the pocket is mandated when clinical signs indicate frank infection. Secondary reconstruction using either an implant or autologous tissue transfer is performed when the chest wall scar is mature, usually 6 to 12 months later.

Toxic shock syndrome is a frightening complication now reported with elective breast reconstruction.[12] The clinical course is more fulminating, and potentially lethal, caused by toxins of the staphylococcus organism. The presentation is dramatic with gastrointestinal symptoms followed by high fever, skin rash, and hypotension. Treatment consists of open drainage, copious flushing of the cavity, fluid replacement, antibiotics, and cardiovascular support. Corticosteroid therapy has been recommended because it may inhibit the toxin. Early recognition and aggressive treatment is needed to reverse this potentially fatal course.

Fluid collections, both serous and bloody, at the reconstructed site are seen both early and late during the postoperative period. Early hematomas should be surgically evacuated because they have the potential to serve as a nidus for future capsule formation. Late serous drainage, (more than 50 to 60 cc over a 24-hour interval) is usually seen after a node dissection. Drains are removed after 8 or 9 days despite persistent high drainage and the chest is circumferentially wrapped with a 6-inch Ace bandage. The seroma is allowed to be absorbed but any persistent seroma is aspirated through an intercatheter, displacing the prosthesis anteriorly. These seromas slowly resolve after repeated aspiration although the incidence of significant capsule formation appears higher in this group.

Immediately after surgery there may be displacement of the prosthesis, usually in a cranial or lateral direction. It may be possible to manipulate the prosthesis back to its correct position if the pocket is adequate. Frequently, continued external pressure from an elastic bandage or tape must be used to maintain the prosthesis in this corrected position. If this is not successful, an open capsulotomy and capsulorrhaphy may be required, with placement of a textured prosthesis to maintain symmetric positioning.

Marginal necrosis along the wound edge was the most common problem encountered before expandable implants were available. This was usually observed in patients who smoked tobacco, and so had thin flaps when a large prosthesis was placed to create better symmetry with the opposite side. The expander has allowed a smaller volume to be placed initially while awaiting total flap healing before expanding the reconstructed breast to symmetry.

Wound edge ischemia is best treated conservatively, with antibacterial ointment and dry dressings. The eschar is allowed to separate spontaneously to allow for secondary healing. Cellulitis and other systemic signs of deeper involvement are reviewed with the patient during this stage to avoid prosthetic involvement and exposure. Oral antibiotics are not given routinely unless the wound appears moist or erythema is increasing. Spontaneous separation of the eschar with epithelialization will occur over 2 to 3 weeks. Eschar removal must not be expedited by debridement. These attempts may expose the prosthesis, which may have been stable beneath the eschar preventing uneventful healing. Marginal wound necrosis should not delay chemotherapy, although the latter may slow wound healing.

Localized inflammation is seen both early and late postoperatively, and may be due to traumatic introduction of bacteria along a slow healing wound edge or seeding from a distant site. Oral or parenteral antibiotics are indicated depending on patient symptoms and breast appearance, to prevent bacterial threat to the prosthesis. All patients are cautioned about any infection in the involved limb and hand, and even small lacerations are treated with topical ointment or oral antibiotics.

Late Complications

The most common drawback to implant reconstructions remains capsular contracture, which is seen at some level in most patients. A small capsule can be appreciated even in the softest of reconstructed breasts, usually lateral or inferior where the muscle brassiere may be incomplete and the prosthesis is potentially subcutaneous. This capsule is usually asymptomatic and appreciated more by the examining physician than the patient. The patient with the painful capsule or prosthesis distorted by the thick capsule remains an enigma regarding both the capsule's etiology and a successful permanent solution. The former is well debated and remains unsolved with a plethora of potential causes.[13] Surgery is less than an ideal answer but the only option for the distorted and symptomatic capsule seen in 10 to 15 percent of all implant reconstructed patients. The surgery for capsule contracture includes (1) circumferential capsulotomy for the periphery of the capsule base with radial incision of the anterior roof, or (2) capsulectomy. The latter is helpful for the recurrent thick or calcified capsule. Resection involves only the anterior capsule, and leaves the floor intact unless there is evidence for prosthetic fracture and silicone bleed in this posterior capsule wall. Intra- and postoperative bleeding is more significant with capsulectomy and drainage is almost always required. Any capsule resected must be submitted for pathologic exam to rule out microscopic recurrence. The latter may be confused with calcification within the capsule. In addition, with capsular distortion of the prosthesis, external positioning alone with tape and dressings to maintain prosthetic position cannot be relied on. Internal capsulectomy in conjunction with replacement with a textured or polyurethane covered prosthesis with simultaneous external dressings has proved the best combination to correct the high positioned prosthesis.[14,15] The introduction of the textured and coated prosthesis will hopefully reduce the overall incidence of capsular complications. The long-term tissue effect of the polyurethane is another parameter that needs to be followed closely over the long term before any stamp of approval is unanimously accepted.

Breast pain at the reconstructed site 2 to 3 months after surgery is unusual and is usually associated with capsular contracture. Specific-point tenderness, however, has been associated with a neuritis or neuroma of the chest wall. These may respond to anti-inflammatory medication or local inflammation control with corticosteroid injection if the specific area can be localized. Pain refractory to conservative treatment will require open exploration and capsulectomy with implant replacement. Jabaley and Das reported two patients with polyurethane implants with similar findings;[15] both had contracture of the capsule between the outer polyurethane covering and inner silicone shell. Capsulectomy and replacement with a standard implant improved the symptoms. Lateral breast mound pain with depression superomedially and bulging laterally may be due to detachment of the serratus anterior muscle from the rib cage along the posterior axillary line as reported by Huang.[16] Repair of the defect or implant removal is the treatment. In all cases of persistent pain, work-up must rule out cancer recurrence; a negative work-up indicates exploration with repair of the defect or capsulectomy and implant change.

The association of silicone implants with "human adjuvant disease" has been suggested.[17,18] Scleroderma is the most common diagnosis with pulmonary and arthritic symptoms seen both early and up to 21 years after implantation. Symptoms may abate with implant removal, but frequently the disease process is ongoing and is treated in standard fashion. Any patient with a history of connective tissue disease or unusual symptoms prior to reconstruction should be considered for autologous reconstruction alone until a better understanding between silicone and human adjuvant disease is established.

Implant reconstruction remains the most common method for breast reconstruction. There have been significant technologic improvements in the prosthetic product, but much more is unknown about prosthetic-tissue relationships. Continued investigation with honest reporting of our results and complications will allow us to develop the best prosthetic reconstruction with the least morbidity.

COMPLICATIONS OF AUTOGENOUS RECONSTRUCTION

The transverse rectus abdominis myocutaneous flap (TRAM) remains the standard against which all other autogenous tissue transfers are measured for breast reconstruction. The flap can be raised and transferred with its superior epigastric vascular pedicle intact or transferred as a free flap based on the inferior epigastric artery. The flap has excellent predictable results with a complication rate inversely related to the experience of the surgeon.[19–21]

Certain preoperative precautions should be taken to minimize morbidity. We have previously reviewed Hartrampf's contraindications to surgery and the importance of these cannot be overemphasized.[1] The obese patient in particular has been singled out as a high-risk patient, with complications approaching 40 percent in this group.[23] It must be emphasized, however, that these are complications and not failures, and this may be the only realistic procedure for selected obese patients. Postoperative subcutaneous heparin, and antiembolism hose, both active and passive, as well as early postoperative ambulation are recommended to minimize deep vein thrombosis. The operating room environment as well as all patient fluids and gases should be warmed to minimize vasoconstriction and flap compromise during the procedure. The double pedicled flap or supercharged unilateral flap should be considered for the indicated patient with a smoking history.

Total flap loss is a technical misadventure and not even reported in the large series.[1,19,20,23,24] Immediate re-exploration is indicated to correct the vascular compromise that is usually venous and related to the positioning of the flap beneath the tunnel. Perioperative steroids may decrease edema and improve the patient's overall well being, but should not be used in place of sound surgical judgement with a compromised flap.

Partial flap loss is reported in 2 to 6 percent of all patients, and almost uniformly involves the more random area of the flap.[23] This may present initially as firmness or drainage at the suture line, but with time full thickness loss or fat necrosis is apparent. Aggressive surgical debridement in an office facility, simple wound care, and packing is frequently all that is required to allow secondary healing. Subsequent revision with wound maturation may be required and can be timed with the nipple/areolar reconstruction.

More extensive fat necrosis is a problem that may require outpatient surgical debridement to prevent prolonged packing and emotional wear on the patient. Late fat necrosis in the healed incision is sometimes difficult to delineate from local cancer recurrence. Mammography is not helpful and biopsy with resection is essential to establish the diagnosis; exploration should not be delayed, even if fat necrosis is suspected. At surgery, all involved fat should be resected.

Postoperative seromas are unusual if large drains are used and sequentially removed. Slavin reported pseudocyst formation as a late sequel of unrecognized seromas occurring 3 to 6 months after surgery.[25] These may present as a mass of the epigastrium or chest wall and are clinically distinct from a hernia. CAT scan or ultrasound is helpful for diagnosis, but biopsy with resection of the anterior cyst wall is essential to rule out breast cancer recurrence or possible hernia.

Revision of the flap is necessary in approximately 20 percent of patients and can be timed with the nipple/areolar reconstruction. Contour defects of the abdomen and axilla or suture line revisions secondary to tissue loss are the most common indications. The suction cannula has proved invaluable for removing small irregularities due to flap or chest wall soft tissue redundancies. The midline bulge created by the turnover of the rectus muscle is more apparent in the thin patient and can be resected directly if it is still present 4 months after surgery. Slavin reported that 3 percent of patients required a small implant (100 to 125 cc) placed beneath the flap to improve superior projection when hollowing is apparent.[23] The infraclavicular add-on polyurethane prosthesis may also be helpful to correct this deformity when autologous tissue cannot be advanced for correction.

True hernia or bulging secondary to weakness of the abdominal wall remains a distressing complication reported as high as 43 percent in some series.[24] Minimizing fascial resection, especially beneath the arcuate line with careful reapproximation of the fascial line at the time of the primary surgery, is the best safeguard to ensure abdominal wall integrity. Relaxing incisions and mobilization of the external oblique fascia to reinforce the midline fascial wall are all helpful to minimize tension and to prevent hernia. Local tissue, or Marlex and Gortex mesh should be used primarily to reinforce the fascia if there is any question about the security of the primary fascial repair. This selection demonstrates good surgical judgement and not an admission of lesser surgical skills. Postoperatively, all the activity restrictions are enforced for 4 to 6 weeks to maintain the repair. If a hernia should occur, early exploration and repair by the surgical oncologist ensures minimal patient discomfort or progression of the defect.

Distortion of the umbilicus and lateral fullness of the superior apron flap of the abdominoplasty are the most significant aesthetic deformities of the abdomen. The umbilicus is best managed at the initial reconstruction by taking excess length with the umbilic stalk and by imbricating the periumbilical fascia opposite the donor rectus with permanent sutures when closing the abdomen. This pulls the umbilicus back toward the midline to partially correct the distortion created by the paramedian fascial closure. The extra length of the umbilicus allows it to be approximated toward the midline without tension. The contour defects are best treated by suction lipectomy at a second procedure.

The long-term effect of the loss of the rectus abdominis muscle has not been well-investigated clinically. The chief function of the rectus abdominis is flexion of the trunk against resistance and, in the supine position, lifting of the chest, and indirectly of the head.[24] The rectus muscle may also assist in breathing. Hartrampf has shown that 20 percent of the unilateral and 65 percent of the bilateral reconstructions lost their ability to perform sit-ups post surgery.[1] Normal activities and posturing, however, were unaffected and the latter with back pain may have actually improved. Preservation of the lateral rectus muscle does not preserve the muscle function because of denervation of this segment with removal of the medial half.[25] Prospective clinical investigation will be helpful in assessing the long-term effect of muscle loss as well as the minimum amount of muscle needed to maintain flap vascularity yet preserve some function.

The TRAM flap limitations appear to be directly related to patient choice as well as the experience of the surgeon. The free inferior TRAM flap may be used more frequently because of the minimal violation of the muscle and sheath as well as the absence of upper abdominal contour deformities.

COMPLICATIONS OF LATISSIMUS DORSI RECONSTRUCTION

The success of the transverse rectus abdominis musculocutaneous (TRAM) flap has placed the latissimus dorsi flap (LDF) in the role of the "forgotten sister." However, for those patients needing autogenous tissue who are not TRAM candidates, and for those who have had TRAM reconstruction in the past and face the increasing incidence of secondary primary carcinomas in the opposite breast, the LDF has again taken an active role in breast reconstruction. The LDF can be used with an implant or as a pure autologous flap and each has common and unique complications.[26]

The blood supply to the LDF is vigorous and loss of the flap due to vascular compromise is usually a result of technical difficulties. Minor tissue loss is seen in less than 5 percent and most complications with this flap are related to donor site difficulties and capsule problems when a prosthesis is used.

The most common problem with the LDF donor site is seroma formation. At least two large No. 10 French drains are used for immediate drainage of all donor sites, and they are removed sequentially only after a maximum 30 to 35 cc of fluid is collected for the 24-hour interval. A 6-inch Ace dressing is placed circumferentially after drain removal for compression of the donor site until it is certain that no fluid is collecting or, if fluid is present, that it is being passively absorbed. Seromas will still develop despite these precautions and should be drained as often as necessary to prevent wound compromise or expansion of the seroma into the mastectomy site. An angiocatheter can be placed in a sterile and atraumatic fashion at the most dependent point of the donor site, with the patient moving from a sitting to lateral decubitus position to milk all fluid from the area. A binder or Ace bandage is then used for compression. We have not had to open any donor site to resect the bursa using this simple and conservative method.

The donor site scar is a significant trade-off for this procedure but is frequently related to the initial width of the LDF skin flap. The latter should be smaller than 8 cm or a spreading scar or hypertrophy is ensured. Tissue expansion of the skin and muscle can be used preoperatively to expand the proposed island if the procedure is a delayed reconstruction and an adequate time interval is left for expansion.[27,28] This may prove to be especially helpful in the fleur-de-lis flap where a second vertical scar is added to the standard transverse incision. However, the potential for seroma would appear to be higher because of the pseudobursa created by the expander and the latter may need to be removed at the time of flap elevation.

Contour defects are common when a significant amount of soft tissue is removed with the flap. This can vary from flatness of the donor site with muscle loss in the thin individual to true cavitation in the obese patient where the flap was used with extended subcutaneous tissue for autologous breast reconstruction. This donor site can be improved by secondary suctioning of the high points and irregularities 6 to 8 months after surgery. A small Mercedes cannula introduced through the scar can be directed toward the defect edges to soften the contour.

Large skin islands greater than 10 to 12 cm will require skin grafting and potential donor site deformity. Maruyama and Iwahira have used a reversed ipsilateral LDF from the residual inferior muscle.[27] To minimize the contour defect, this flap is based on the 9th through the 11th intercostal perforating vessels, which are spared with removal of the superior flap. This provides an aesthetic solution to the large defect, seen especially with the fleur-de-lis flap.

The functional loss of the muscle is largely overlooked when results are reported for the LDF. Russell et al reported mild to moderate shoulder weakness involving all muscles when compared to the unoperated side.[30] In addition, shoulder motion was decreased. This was thought to be due to both scarring in the axillary dissection site and stiffness because of pain from limited motion. Recruitment of synergistic muscles improves these limitations but physical therapy directed at strengthening these muscles should be an ongoing part of recovery to minimize permanent loss or persistent weakness.

A distressing late complication reported by McCraw and Maxwell is capsular contracture around the implant placed with this breast flap, usually seen longer than 5 years after reconstruction.[31] The capsule incidence is higher in the radical mastectomy group (75 percent versus 39 percent in the modified group) in whom the muscle brassiere is incomplete and the implant is not fully covered by muscle. Secondary attempts at total muscle coverage, however, did not guarantee resolution of the capsule and the authors have postulated that in certain patients the capsule will always be unremitting. In these patients, autologous tissue transfer, the use of polyurethane implants, or controlling the capsule using an expansile pocket with a permanent expander for volume addition appear to be plausible solutions.

The LDF has had highs and lows in its use over the past 15 years. The recent introduction of the fleur-de-lis flap coupled with a better understanding and control of the complications related to this flap, will certainly elevate the LDF nearer center stage. The LDF will again prove to be valuable as secondary and tertiary breast reconstruction begins to evolve.

FREE-FLAP AUTOLOGOUS RECONSTRUCTION

The superior gluteal and inferior rectus microvascular free flaps are the most widely used free tissue for breast reconstruction. Both are used in unique circumstances and require a competent team of microvascular reconstructive surgeons to initiate and complete the tissue transfer, aiming to achieve flap loss rates less than 5 percent.

Shaw has written widely on the use of the superior gluteal flap and has shown excellent long-term donor and recipient results.[32,33] The superior gluteal artery was chosen for its accessibility and ease of dissection and has been the vessel for the gluteus flap of choice. Paletta et al have proposed the use of the inferior gluteal artery based flap.[34] The vascular pedicle is longer and the autologous tissue transferred is more abundant and may give better projection to the new breast because of its fat distribution above the superior muscle. Both flaps leave a potentially disfiguring donor site scar and contour defect. The superior flap incision is directly across the buttock, while the inferior flap donor site is closer to the buttock crease. Patient preference and physician experience may dictate which of the above gluteal flaps and incisions to use. The donor contour defect can be improved by secondary surgery with selective suctioning, done in combination with nipple-areolar reconstruction.

The superior and inferior gluteal flaps both create a potential functional deficit that is not well described when results with these flaps are reviewed. The superior half of the muscle is a key factor in hip abduction and the inferior muscle assists in hip extension and external rotation. There will be definite permanent weakness of these functions and the patient should be aware of this deficit when options are presented. Physical therapy directed at improving these deficits is essential to the postoperative recovery.

Grotting has shown excellent results with minimal complications in over 70 patients with free transfer of the transverse rectus abdominis myocutaneous free flap based on the inferior epigastric vasculature.[35] Two patients required immediate reoperation because of venous problems, but no flap was lost totally and only two showed partial loss. There were no donor site abdominal wall deficits because of the small amount of rectus fascia and muscle removed with the inferior epigastric artery. Grotting emphasized a two-surgeon approach for this procedure to maintain an operative time of under 4 hours and to minimize subsequent morbidity. The inferior TRAM eliminates the functional and donor site problems of the gluteal flap and appears to be the free flap of choice for the future in free tissue breast reconstruction.

CONCLUSION

Most complications can be avoided with careful patient selection and planning of the correct procedure for each individual patient. Honest evaluation of results and acceptance of complications will assist the surgeon in avoiding future misadventures. No surgeon is immune from complications.

References

1. Hartrampf CR, Jr. The transverse abdominal island flap for breast reconstruction: A 7-year experience. Clin Plast Surg 1988; 15(4):703-716.
2. Kroll SS, Netscher DT. Complications of TRAM flap breast reconstruction in obese patients. Plast Reconstr Surg 1989; 84:886.
3. Miller AP, Falcone E. Breast reconstruction: Systemic factors influencing local complications. Presented ASPRS/PSEF/ASMS Annual Convention, San Francisco, CA 1989.
4. Georgiade GS, Riefkohl R, Cox E, et al. Long-term clinical outcome of immediate reconstruction after mastectomy. Plast Reconstr Surg 1985; 76:415.
5. Webster DJ, Mansel RE, Hughes LE. Immediate reconstruction of the breast after mastectomy. Is it safe? Cancer 1984; 53:1416-1419.
6. Bruce J, Vandergrift MS, Diner WC. Mammography and breast implants. Plast Reconstr Surg 1988; 82:1-6.
7. Eklund GW, Busby RC, Miller SH, et al. Improved imaging of the augmented breast. Am J Roentgenol 1989; 151:469-473.
8. Miller S, Ecklund GW. Mammography of the augmented breast. (Letter) Plast Reconstr Surg 1988; 82:922.
9. Silverstein MJ, Gierson ED, Gamagami P, et al. Breast cancer diagnosis and prognosis in women augmented with silicone gel-filled implants. Cancer 1990; 66:97-101.
10. Gumucio CA, Pin P, Young VL, et al. The effect of breast implants on the radiographic detection of microcalcification and soft-tissue masses. Plast Reconstr Surg 1989; 84:772-782.
11. Noone RB, Murphy JB, Spear SL, Little JW III. A six-year experience with immediate reconstruction after mastectomy for cancer. Plast Surg 1985; 76:258-269.
12. Tobin G, Shaw RC, Goodpasture HC. Toxic shock syndrome following breast and nasal surgery. Plast Reconstr Surg 1987; 80:111-114.
13. Baker J, Donis R. Genesis and management of the hard augmented breast. Adv Plast Reconstr Surg 1990; 6:249-270.
14. Hester TR, Nahai F, Bostick J, Cukic J. A 5-year experience with polyurethane-covered mammary prostheses for treatment of capsular contracture, primary augmentation mammoplasty, and breast reconstruction. Clin Plast Surg 1988; 15:569-585.
15. Jabaley M, Das S. Late breast pain following reconstruction with polyurethane-covered implants. Plast Reconstr Surg 1986; 78:390-395.
16. Huang TT. Breast and subcapsular pain following submuscular placement of breast prostheses. Plast Reconstr Surg 1990; 86:275-280.
17. Spiera H. Scleroderma after silicone augmentation mammaplasty. JAMA 1988; 260:236.
18. Weisman M, Vecchione T, Albert D, et al. Connective tissue disease following breast augmentation: A preliminary test of the human adjuvant disease hypothesis. Plast Reconstr Surg 1988; 82:626-630.
19. Scheflan M. Building a breast without a prosthesis: The transverse abdominal island flap. Clin Plast Surg 1984; 11:303.
20. Scheflan M. The transverse abdominal island flap: Part I. Indications, contraindications, results, and complications. Ann Plast Surg 1983; 10:25-35.
21. Hartrampf CR Jr, Bennett GK. Autogenous tissue reconstruction in the mastectomy patient. A clinical review of 300 patients. Ann Surg 1987; 205:508.
22. Kroll SS, Netscher DT. Complications of TRAM flap breast reconstruction in obese patients. Plast Reconstr Surg 1989; 84:886-892.
23. Slavin SA, Goldwyn RM. The mid-abdominal rectus abdominis myocutaneous flap: Review of 236 flaps. Plast Reconstr Surg 1988; 81:189-199.
24. Slavin SA, Howrigan PJ, Goldwyn RM. Pseudocyst formation after rectus flap breast reconstruction: Diagnosis and treatment. Plast Reconstr Surg 1989; 83:670-675.
25. Duchateau J, Declety A, Lejour M. Innervation of the rectus abdominis muscle: Implications for rectus flaps. Plast Reconstr Surg 1988; 82:223-228.
26. Hokin J, Silfverskiold K. Breast reconstruction without an implant: Results and complications using an extended latissimus dorsi flap. Plast Reconstr Surg 1986; 79:58-67.
27. Maruyama Y, Iwahira Y. Latissimus dorsi musculocutaneous flap: Correction of donor-site defect with reverse latissimus flap. Plast Reconstr Surg 1987; 80:858-861.
28. Radovan, C. Tissue expansion in soft-tissue reconstruction. Plast Reconstr Surg 1984; 74:482.
29. Argenta LC. Controlled tissue expansion in reconstructive surgery. Br J Plast Surg 1984; 37:520.
30. Russell RC, Pribaz J, Zook EG, et al. Functional evaluation of latissimus dorsi donor site. Plast Reconstr Surg 1986; 78:336-344.
31. McCraw JB, Maxwell GP. Early and late capsular "deformation" as a cause of unsatisfactory results in the latissimus dorsi breast reconstruction. Clin Plast Surg 1988; 15:717-726.
32. Shaw WW. Microvascular free flap breast reconstruction. Clin Plast Surg 1984; 2(2):333-341.
33. Shaw WW. Breast reconstruction by superior gluteal microvascular free flaps without silicone implants, Plast Reconstr Surg 1983; 72:490-499.
34. Paletta CE, Bostwick J, Nahai F. The inferior gluteal free flap in breast reconstruction. Plast Reconstr Surg 1989; 84:875-883.
35. Grotting JC. Personal Communication, 1990.

CHAPTER 37

Deformities After Conservative Breast Cancer Treatment

JEAN-YVES PETIT, M.D.
MARIO RIETJENS, M.D.

Treatment of breast cancer has changed remarkably in the last few decades, evolving from classical radical mastectomy to modified radical mastectomy, and now tumorectomy and axillary dissection with postoperative radiotherapy. The latter is used for all tumors of less than 30 mm at the Gustave-Roussy Institute and for those of up to 4 or 5 cm in other institutions.

Because the overall and disease-free survival rates from conservative treatment for small tumors were no different from those from modified radical mastectomy, as reported by three randomized controlled trials in Italy, France, and the United States,[1-3] conservative treatment is becoming more popular as the therapy of choice.

The cosmetic result is an important factor in conservative treatment. Good to excellent results have been reported.[4,5] However, breast deformity does occur and can be perceived.[6] These deformities are due not only to the size and shape of the breast,[5,7,8] the location of the tumor, and radiation and chemotherapy,[7,9-11] but also to the surgical techniques.[5,12-14]

In our Institute, we have used conservative treatment since 1970. Our goal is both to remove the tumor and to achieve the best cosmetic result possible.

COSMETIC EVALUATION OF PATIENTS WHO RECEIVED CONSERVATIVE TREATMENT

From 1967 to 1989, conservative treatment was given to approximately 3,000 patients at our Institute. Most were classified as T1 or T2, N0 or N1 and M0 (UICC TNM classification) with a tumor measuring 30 mm or less with no other criteria of exclusion such as age, breast size, histologic findings, or hormonal status.

In an attempt to reach better objectivity, the cosmetic evaluation of such treatment was made on the basis of the results of three different studies.

The first study was performed in 1983 in 89 patients whose cosmetic evaluation was made at least 5 years after their treatment. Most were treated at the start of our breast-saving protocol.

The second study, the results of which were published,[15] was undertaken under the responsibility of the radiotherapists of our Institute. The study deals with the cosmetic evaluation entered in the chart of 592 patients by the radiotherapists themselves at each follow-up visit. One of the interests of such a study is to provide an opportunity to observe the evolution of the cosmetic results with time.

The third study reported the cosmetic results of 140 patients several days after the surgical stage, in order to evaluate the surgical sequelae before the first radiation or chemotherapy.

These three studies provide evaluation of patients treated with the same radiosurgical protocol, including a wide tumorectomy, axillary dissection and radiotherapy for the breast (45 Gy on the whole gland with an additional 15 Gy on the tumor bed). However, these treatments were performed at different times. For instance, the tumorectomy performed in the 1970s was often a quadrantectomy, whereas the same category of patients underwent a wide tumorectomy in the late 1980s. Therefore, any comparison between results must take into account these technical variations. They will therefore be discussed independently.

First Cosmetic Evaluation

Material

Of 100 patients called to our clinics, 89 responded and were included in the study. The 100 were chosen randomly among the total series performed at the Institute between 1972 and 1978. All the cases were classified Stage I or small Stage II with a tumor size less than 2.5 cm. All the women who came to the outpatient clinics were examined by a surgical team that was not responsible for their treatment.

The surgical treatment consisted of a quadrantectomy in nearly 40 percent of patients and a wide tumorectomy in 60 percent. A lymph node dissection was performed at the same time.

Radiotherapy was given during the 5 to 6 week interval after the surgery at a dose of 45 Gy on the breast by external beam (Co-60) with an additional 15 Gy on the tumor bed. Moreover, almost all the patients with positive nodes received 15 Gy on the internal mammary chain, and 70 percent of this group were given 45 Gy to the axillary and supraclavicular areas.

Assessment of Cosmesis

A standard protocol, including six different views, was carried out for each patient by professional photographers. Different criteria were rated from 0 to 3 points according to their degree:

1. Radiodystrophy, telangiectasia.
2. Radiosclerosis around the scar.
3. Scar contraction.
4. Glandular defect.
5. Areolar deformity.
6. Global contraction of the breast.

The harmonious shape of the treated breast was rated as "yes," "no," or "more or less." The degree of symmetry was given 0 to 3 points.

The location of the scar, the number of scars (unique or separated), and the location of the final deformity were also noted. Finally, a global evaluation of the cosmetic results was rated 0 to 5. An estimation was given retrospectively of the opportunity of a surgical repair and which type of surgery could have been proposed.

This information provides different approaches to evaluate the sequelae and cosmetic result for each patient.

Results

The percentage rates of the different sequelae are shown in Table 37-1. It is difficult to differentiate precisely the various sequelae because of the different types of treatment. However, the percentage of sequelae most likely caused by surgery, such as scar contraction or glandular defect, is higher than the percentage of sequelae related to the radiotherapy: 50 and 41 percent versus 22 and 38 percent.

TABLE 37-1 Percentage of Sequelae (89 Patients)

	Nil or Moderate (0 or 1 point)	Medium or Important (2 or 3 points)
Scar contraction	50% (45)	50% (44)
Glandular defect	59% (52)	41% (37)
Areolar deformity	75% (67)	25% (22)
Radiodystrophy	78% (70)	22% (19)
Radiosclerosis	62% (55)	38% (34)
Global contraction of breast	70% (62)	30% (27)

Although the percentage rates of sequelae are high, the shape of the treated breast has been rated as harmonious independently of the contralateral breast in 65 percent, "more or less" in 20 percent, and disharmonious in 15 percent of the cases. Symmetry was good to excellent (2 to 3 points) in 79 percent and poor (0 to 1 point in 21 percent of cases. The global cosmetic evaluation rated from 0 to 5 points was found to be good to excellent (4 to 5 points) in 52 percent, fair (2 to 3 points) in 28 percent, and poor (0 to 1 point) in 20 percent (Fig. 37-1).

In order to reach a better objectivity, we compared the global cosmetic evaluation rated from 0 to 5 divided into three groups with the results obtained by addition of the points resulting from the sequelae also divided into three groups: excellent (up to 5 points), fair (6 to 10 points), and poor (more than 10 points).

Evaluation by addition of sequelae gives a lower percentage of excellent results and increases the percentage of fair results, whereas the poor results are not consistently different, as shown in Table 37-2. Moreover, the cosmetic results are related to the location of the tumor in the breast. The percentage of fair and poor results is significantly higher when the tumor is in the lower quadrants of the breast: 86 percent (12/14) versus 33 percent (18/54) (Fig. 37-2).

The interest of such a study is to provide a more objective evaluation of the poor cosmetic results after conservative treatment in a population treated more than 5 years previously. Whatever the type of approach, either global or by rating of the sequelae or the symmetry, the percentage of poor results varies from 15 to 20 percent. In addition, the surgical technique appears to be responsible for at least 50 to 60 percent of the disabling results, indicating that

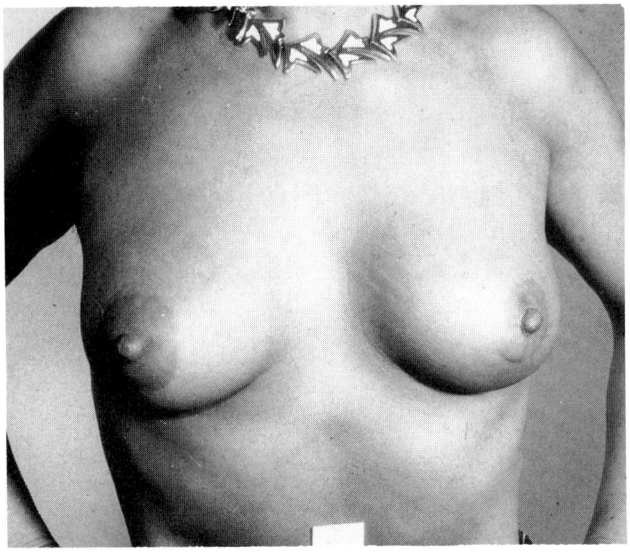

A

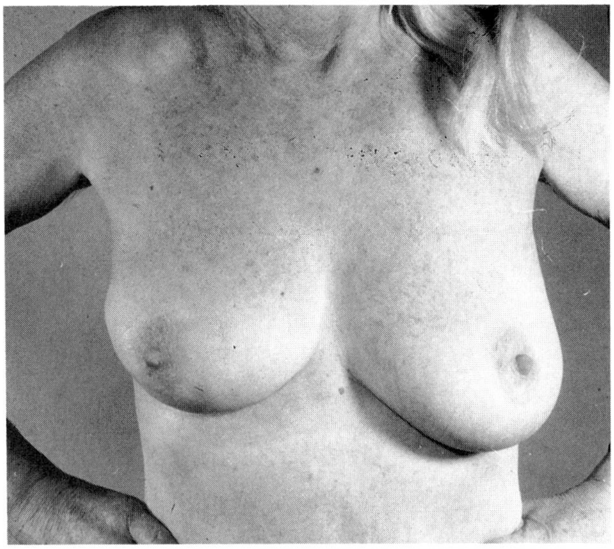

B

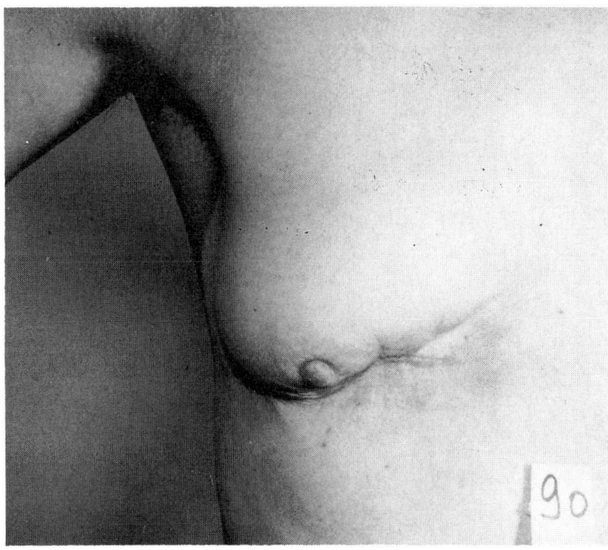

C

FIGURE 37–1 Cosmetic evaluation of results after tumorectomy and radiation therapy were rated good (*A*), fair (*B*), and poor (*C*).

improvement of the surgical procedure might produce better overall cosmetic results.

Considering the type of sequelae observed in the photographs, the reviewers discussed the theoretical opportunity of a plastic surgical repair. According to them, 36 percent of the patients could have been candidates for an improvement of the cosmetic result by means of plastic surgery. The type proposed is shown in Table 37-3.

TABLE 37-2 Comparison Between Global Cosmetic Evaluation and Rating of Sequelae

	Global Evaluation	Addition of Sequelae
Excellent	52% (46)	46% (41)
Fair	28% (25)	36% (32)
Poor	20% (18)	18% (16)

Second Cosmetic Evaluation

Between 1970 and 1982, 592 women with T1, small T2, N0 N1 M0 breast cancer and managed by lumpectomy, axillary dissection, and radiotherapy were followed and cosmetically evaluated by the radiotherapists of the Institute. The overall cosmetic result and degree of asymmetry, fibrosis and telangiectasia of the treated breasts were assessed by the radiation oncologist at each follow-up visit. The changes in these cosmetic parameters with time are shown in the study. The cosmetic results were graded as excellent, good, or fair/poor. These were defined as:

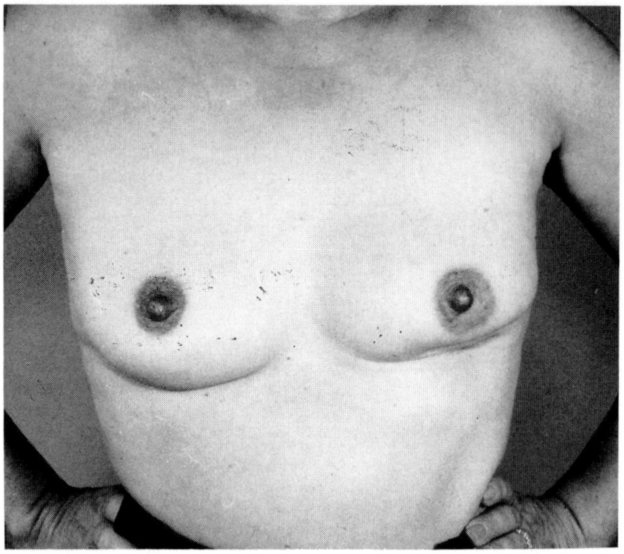

FIGURE 37-2 Cosmetic results are related to the location of the tumor in the breast. Treatment of lower quadrant lesions carries a higher percentage of poor results.

TABLE 37-3 Surgical Repair of Sequelae

Method	Number of Cases
Glandular mammaplasty	5
Mastopexy, ipsilateral or contralateral	12
Lastissimus dorsi flap	7
TRAM flap	4
Prosthesis	1
Z-plasty	3

Excellent: No defect or only a barely perceptible defect. It is difficult to detect the treated breast on a front view.

Good: Moderate deformity or asymmetry visible on a front view but not requiring surgical repair.

Fair/Poor: Gross deformity or asymmetry for which it is mandatory to propose a surgical improvement.

At 5 years the overall cosmetic result was excellent in 58 percent, good in 38 percent, and fair/poor in 8 percent. At 10 years this had fallen to 34, 54, and 22 percent respectively (Fig. 37-3). The most significant factors were tumor size, the presence of defect after surgery, and the daily applied dose per fraction to the breast. Surgical and radiotherapy technique (especially alternate-day fractionation) can significantly affect the cosmetic result obtained.

A multivariate analysis was performed of the factors associated with a cosmetic defect. The overall cosmetic results reported in this series are comparable with other reports.[16-18] However, it should be noted that the results tended to deteriorate with time, thus confirming the importance of reporting results actuarially.

Not surprisingly, a postsurgical defect had a significantly adverse effect on both the overall cosmetic result and the degree of asymmetry (Fig. 37-4). On multivariate analysis this was independent of tumor size, suggesting that surgical technique was itself important.

The technique of breast irradiation did not change during the period considered and the radiotherapy protocol was adhered to. Thus, no effect of dose or fractionation was apparent. Similarly, all patients received a boost to the tumor bed with little variation in technique.

Daily applied dose per fraction did, however, have a consistently significant effect. Our data clearly illustrate the increase in late radiation effects seen in normal tissue with the large daily dose frac-

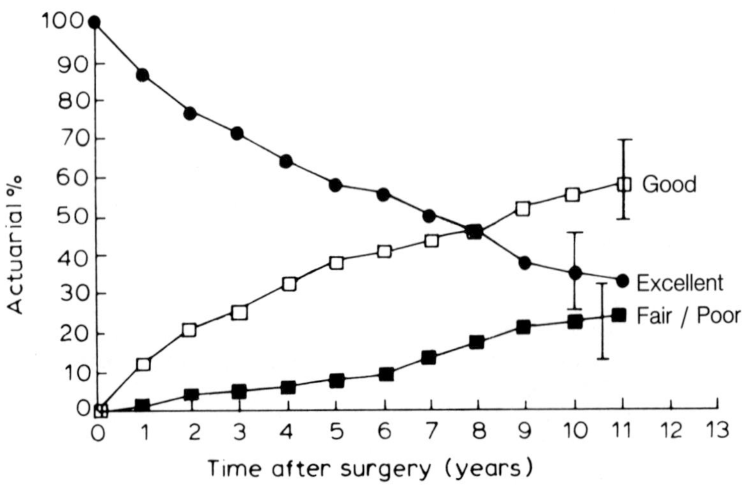

FIGURE 37-3 Changes in the overall cosmetic result with time are plotted actuarially.

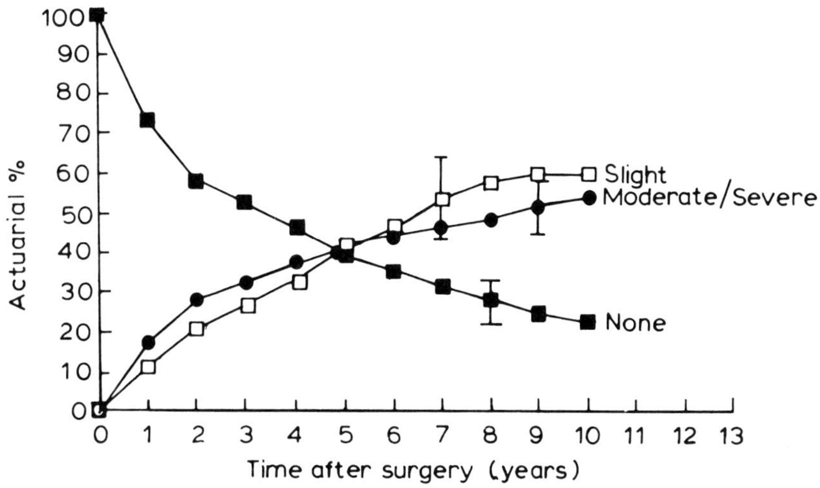

FIGURE 37-4 Postsurgical deformities were graded as none, slight, and moderate/severe. Over time the surgical defect had a significantly adverse effect on breast symmetry, plotted actuarially.

tions used in alternate-day treatment schedules. Accordingly, we recommend that alternate-day fractionation should be avoided.

This study underlines the deterioration of cosmetic results with time especially in regard to the radiologic sequelae. This may explain the apparently better results reported by others, with less than 5 percent of poor results.[1,5,13,15,16] A longer observation of the documented cases could have erased such differences.

Third Cosmetic Evaluation

We randomly chose 140 patients operated on since 1984 who had tumorectomy with at least 1 to 2 cm of clear margins and axillary dissection, in order to evaluate the surgical sequelae in their breasts before their first radiation and/or chemotherapy.

The evaluators looked for skin retraction, breast retraction, glandular defects, and the absence of deformity in three different views (front view of both breasts, lateral views of each breast) taken just before postoperative treatment was begun, approximately 2 to 3 weeks after surgery. The findings are listed in Table 37-4. Most notable were skin retraction (16 percent) and glandular defects (20 percent). In 3 percent of patients the breast appeared globally smaller than the opposite breast without any localized defect. The evaluators could find no deformity in 73 percent.

TABLE 37-4 Surgical Complications in 140 Patients Treated by Tumorectomy and Axillary Dissection

Deformity	N	%
Skin retraction	23	16
Breast retraction	4	3
Glandular defects	29	20
No deformity	102	73

Sum of percentage is greater than 100 percent because several deformities may be found in the same breast.

Further reviews of patients with skin retractions and glandular defects revealed that the operators did not adhere to surgical guidelines for tumorectomy and axillary dissection at our Institute. These patients had no complete elevation of the glandular tissue from the pectoral fascia to allow for glandular reconstruction, one long straight continuous incision for both tumorectomy and axillary dissection, and periareolar incision for tumors in the lower part of the inferior half of the breast.

Breast retractions were found mainly in patients with small breasts. The tumorectomy with a good 1 to 2 cm of clear margins in these patients amounts to more or less a quadrantectomy.

Comparing these results with those of the first study, the percentage of surgical disorders such as glandular defect or skin retraction is significantly lower in the patients included in the last study: 16 and 20 percent versus 50 and 41 percent. This may indicate an improvement due to the technique itself, because the selection of patients remained the same during the two periods.*

PREVENTION OF MORPHOLOGIC DAMAGE AFTER CONSERVATIVE TREATMENT

On the basis of our extensive experience in conservative treatment, we have implemented surgical guidelines for tumorectomy and axillary dissection in our department. These were designed to obtain as pleasant a cosmetic result as possible, as one of the main purposes of conservative treatment is to avoid a mutilated breast.

***Editors note** Comparison of the two groups of patients is difficult, because radiation therapy was used in the first group. Some of the post-treatment deformities thought to be caused by surgery alone may have been a result of combination therapy.

For lesions situated in the upper breast, we use an arciform incision; lesions in the lower breast are removed via a radial incision. A submammary or paramammary incision in the anterior axillary line is used for lesions deep in the breast at the level of the chest wall, or for exploration of a diffuse lumpy breast (Fig. 37–5*A*). After the incision is made, the entire breast is dissected off the pectoral fascia. This is usually easy. A "bimanual" examination of the breast can then be made, and any prominent cyst or tumor that was not palpable preoperatively can then be found readily. By way of this incision, the entire posterior surface of the breast can be everted toward the operative field and examined, and any lesion situated anywhere in the breast can be resected.

Some surgeons recommend excision of the skin overlying the tumor.[1] In our experience histologic studies of the specimen showed that this is not needed unless on physical examination the tumor is found to be very superficial or adherent to the overlying skin.

Many surgeons today do not recommend a quadrantectomy if a complete excision with clear margins of the primary tumor can be made.[16] This tumorectomy alone, instead of a quadrantectomy, if it can be done, not only is sufficient to remove the tumor but also permits a better cosmetic result. The quadrantectomy is actually a partial mutilation of the breast that leaves a more severe postoperative deformity, and repairing it is often difficult, especially in small breasts.

In performing the tumorectomy after the skin incision has been made, we grasp the tumor with the fingertips, then sharply transect the glandular tissue, at least 1 cm around the tumor, down to the pectoral fascia. This entire piece of breast tissue is next dissected from the pectoralis major muscle and sent to the pathology department. The transection down to the pectoralis then permits us to elevate the whole breast off the pectoral fascia (Fig. 37–5*B*). Bimanual examination of the breast can then be made and the edges of the gland approximated to cover the defect.

Certain authors have stated that the tumorectomy defect is rapidly filled by serum and blood so that the cosmetic result is constantly good even for a large tumor. We disagree, because the serum and blood are reabsorbed in a few months and the patient usually returns with at best a skin retraction over the defect, or at worst a severe alteration in the form of the breast. This loss of breast tissue with subsequent skin retraction is found in 41 percent of patients in the first study and 16 percent in the third. This difference is probably related to the improvement in technique between both studies. We believe

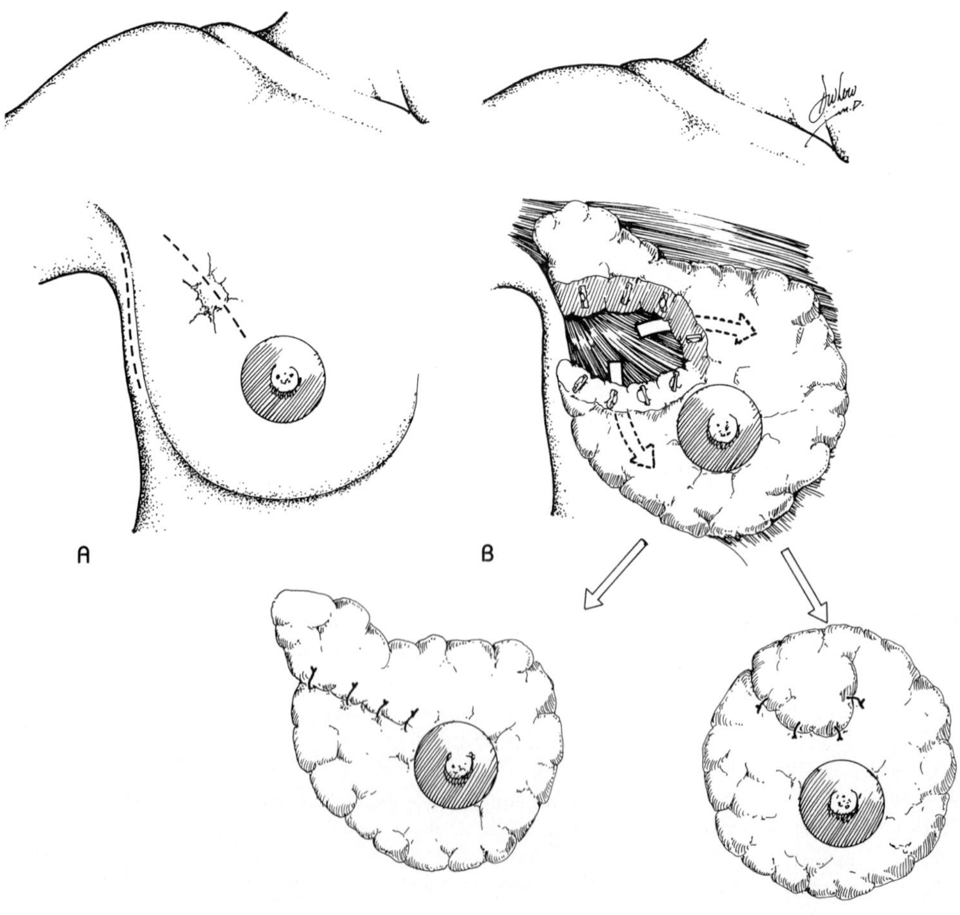

FIGURE 37–5 *A (upper left),* A radial or arciform incision may be made over the tumor without skin excision, unless the tumor is superficial in the breast tissue or adherent to the skin. A submammary or paramammary incision is used for deep lesions at the chest wall level or for exploration of a diffusely lumpy breast. *B (right),* The glandular tissue is resected to the pectoral fascia, with at least a 1-cm margin around the tumor. The edges of remaining breast parenchyma are marked with metallic clips. Undermining of the entire breast parenchyma from the pectoral fascia then permits closure of the remaining breast tissue *(lower left).* A flap of glandular tissue may be needed to close the defect *(lower right).*

that a few simple sutures to approximate the edges of the defect after elevation of the breast from the chest wall can readily prevent this loss.

After a large tumorectomy in a small or medium-sized breast, a glandular flap may be needed to repair the defect. This flap can be advanced or rotated into the defect after being released from the pectoralis major and the subcutaneous tissue (Fig. 37-5*B*). Before this, the tumor bed is marked with metallic clips for postoperative radiotherapy or simple follow-up on mammography.

If in situ radiation is planned, a radiotherapist will place catheters before closure for later insertion of internal needles.

The wound is closed in two layers after a suction drain or a small Penrose drain is placed. A running absorbable suture is used for the subcutaneous layer and a 4-0 nylon used for the skin.

At this stage, we also evaluate the symmetry of the breasts by placing the patient in a sitting position. The opposite breast is always draped in the operative field. Sometimes, especially after wide tumorectomy that has required a large glandular flap to remodel the gland, the operated breast appears too small and too high compared with the untreated breast. Such uncommon asymmetry can be improved by a mastopexy or mammaplasty in the untreated breast. This contralateral breast surgery is rarely performed and only if there is marked disproportion.

Taking advantage of the surgical techniques in plastic surgery, we sometimes propose to remove the tumor through a reduction mammaplasty approach. If the tumor is in the lower quadrants, the superior pedicle technique is used (Fig. 37-6). If it is in the upper quadrants, the inferior pedicle technique is preferred (Fig. 37-7).

Although these techniques provide an excellent approach for wide tumorectomies, they also require in most patients contralateral surgery to obtain final good symmetry.

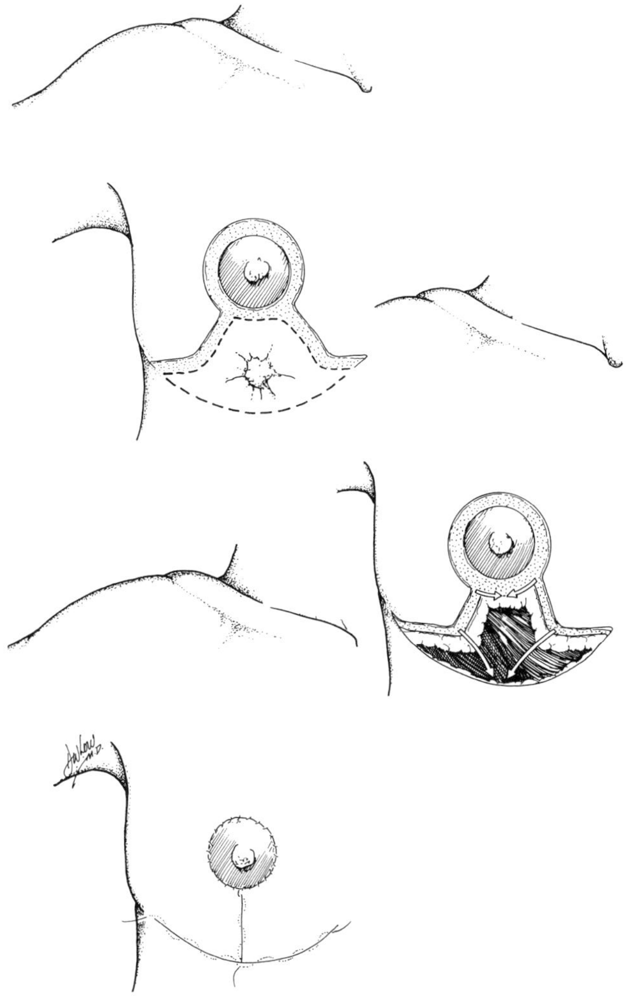

FIGURE 37-6 Tumorectomy for lesions in the inferior breast may be performed with the technique of superior pedicle mammaplasty. A surgical margin of at least 1 cm is needed. The nipple pedicle is de-epithelialized (*above*). Breast parenchyma is approximated (*center*). Skin closure is similar to that for reduction mammaplasty (*below*).

SURGICAL TREATMENT OF MORPHOLOGIC DAMAGE AFTER CONSERVATIVE TREATMENT

Global Asymmetry

The most common deformity observed after conservative treatment is an asymmetry between the two breasts, the treated one remaining too firm and partially upwardly retracted while the non-treated breast looks soft and more pendular.

Improvement of the cosmetic aspect in most cases can be provided by a mastopexy of the non-treated breast. A good result is easily obtained provided that the opposite treated breast is globally retracted with no local glandular defect. In our experience, the contralateral mastopexy has been the operation most frequently used for improvement of poor aesthetic results after CT (45 %) Fig. 37-8 *A*, *B*.

Glandular Defects

The second most common deformity leading patients to seek surgical improvement is the glandular defect. Such defects are more visible in the lower part of the breast. They are often hard to repair because of healing difficulties in radiated tissues. Local glandular flaps, which can be a good solution to prevent the defect at the time of the tumorectomy, are usually no longer available for secondary reconstruction (Fig. 37-9).

Local skin flaps are not bulky enough to achieve a partial reconstruction, but they can be associated

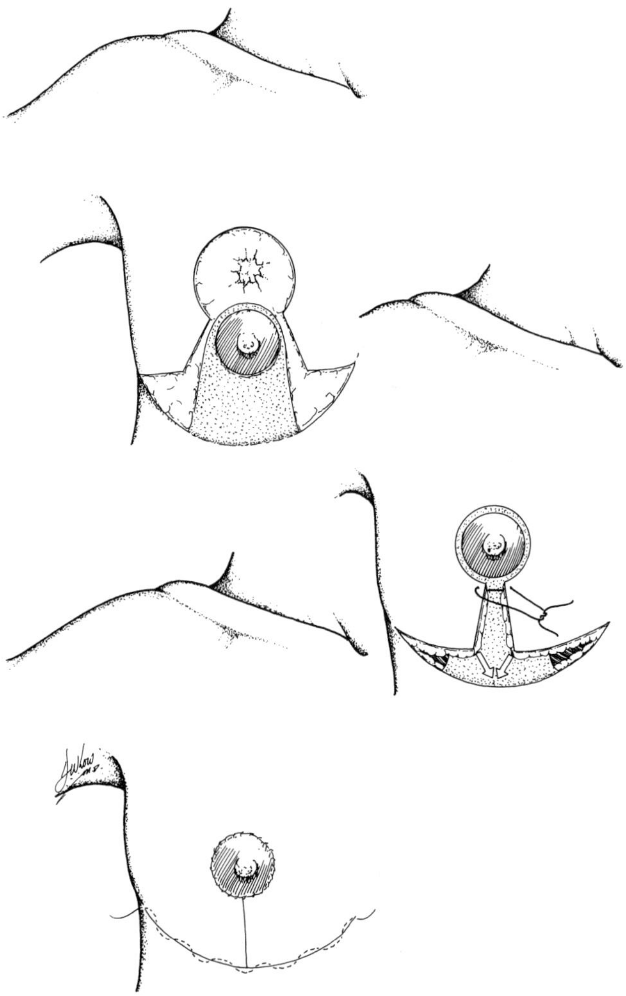

FIGURE 37–7 If the tumor is in the superior position in the breast, resection is done after incisions for inferior pedicle mammaplasty (*above*). Skin flaps are elevated and closed over the de-epithelialized inferior pedicle (*center*), and conventional skin closure completes the procedure (*below*).

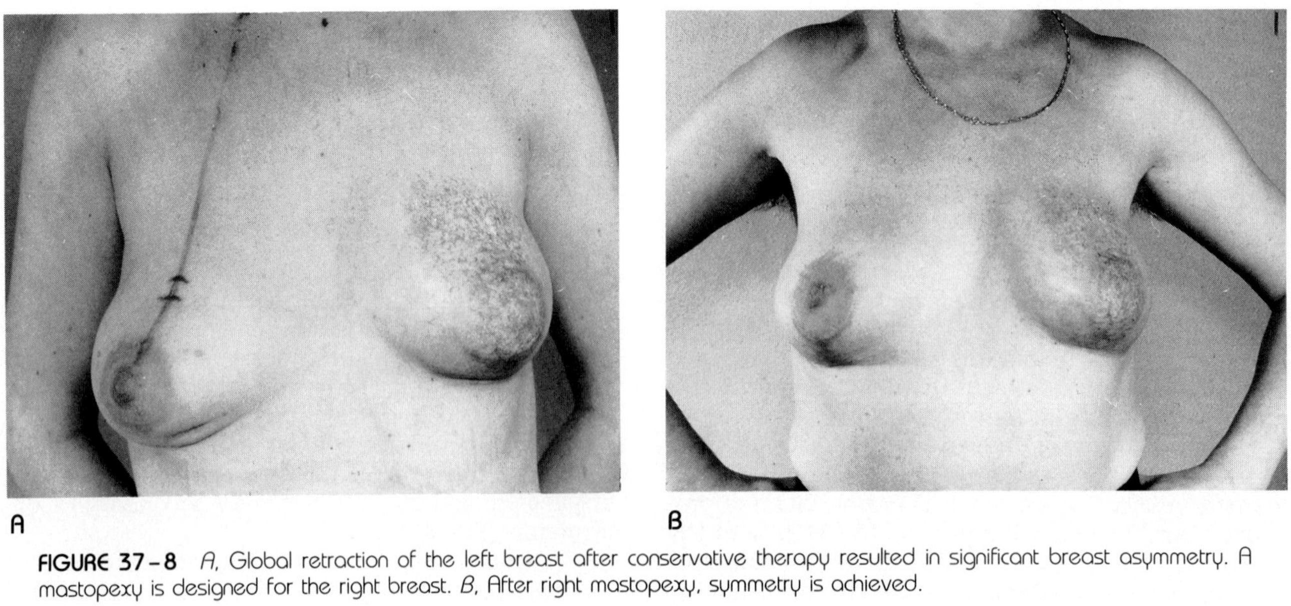

A

B

FIGURE 37–8 *A*, Global retraction of the left breast after conservative therapy resulted in significant breast asymmetry. A mastopexy is designed for the right breast. *B*, After right mastopexy, symmetry is achieved.

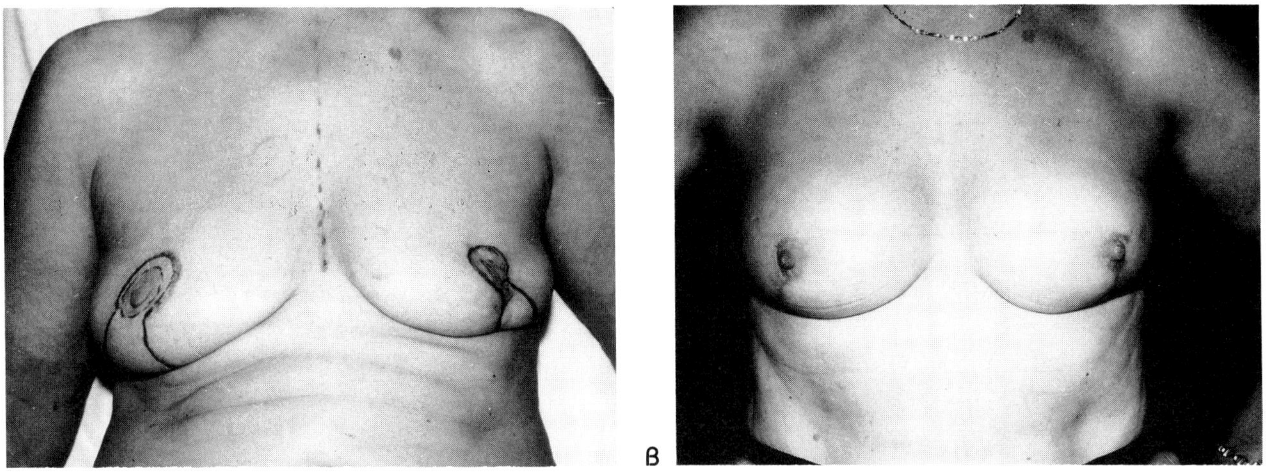

FIGURE 37-9 *A*, A glandular flap is planned to correct the left breast deformity after conservative therapy. Right mastopexy is planned. *B*, The satisfactory result obtained is not common in radiated tissues.

with either an implant or an autotissue transfer such as an omentoplasty or a de-epithelialized musculocutaneous flap.

The great omentum provides a well-vascularized and well-adapted tissue according to the texture. The omental mesh can be prepared through a short subcostal incision and brought up to the mammary site to fill the glandular defect. Such repair has had a satisfactory final result in our experience (Fig. 37-10).

Another way to fill the defect by providing adequate volume is to use a musculocutaneous flap. The latissimus dorsi flap is better used for defects of the upper quadrants of the breast (Fig. 37-11); the transverus rectus abdominis musculocutaneous (TRAM) flap is more adequate for defects of the lower or inner quadrants (Fig. 37-12). These flaps can be partially de-epithelialized to fill the defect under the gland. A double de-epithelialized TRAM flap was used with success in place of prosthetic implants in a woman with a Baker Grade IV capsular contracture after subcutaneous mastectomy.

If the defect is associated with skin radiodystrophy or necrosis, the best solution is provided by an appropriate musculocutaneous flap. However, the final cosmetic result is often impaired by the color and texture of the flap, which appears as a patch on the remaining breast. The upper rectus abdominis flap can be considered for repair of the lower inner quadrants. However, it usually provides too much bulk in the inner part of the inframammary fold. The lower rectus flap, with its long muscular pedicle, is more versatile and provides better material to model the contour of the breast.

Local glandular defects may sometimes be repaired with local glandular flaps without distant tissue transpositions. For example, for defects in the upper quadrants, cosmetic improvement can be obtained by a mastopexy procedure. It is advisable to perform the same mastopexy on the contralateral side to reach a better symmetry.

Defects in the lower part of the breast can also occasionally be repaired by the techniques of reduction mammaplasty or mastopexy, using the upper pedicle technique for lower defects and the lower pedicle for upper defects. However, these procedures are available only for broad-breasted women.

Scar Contraction

Another deformity results in a skin contraction along the scar, especially after a long incision in the upper outer quadrant for removal of the tumor together with lymph node dissection. This deformity is best prevented by making a double separate incision at the time of the CT main conservative procedure, or at least by breaking the incision line in the middle to avoid the usual contraction of long scars. Otherwise, it is necessary to repair the retracted scar by a Z-plasty in order to provide additional length to the skin.

Areolar Deformity

More often, these scar contractions lead to areolar deformities or displacements, especially when there is a glandular defect in addition to the scar contraction. The best procedure to repair such "hooklike" deformities of the areola complex is to use some additional skin, fat, and muscle with a latissimus dorsi flap to reconstruct the upper outer quadrant. In some cases the distortion of the areola is so significant that it requires a total transposition of the nipple-areola as a free graft (see Fig. 37-10). Another solution to improve the location of the nipple-areola is to transpose it as a free graft after de-

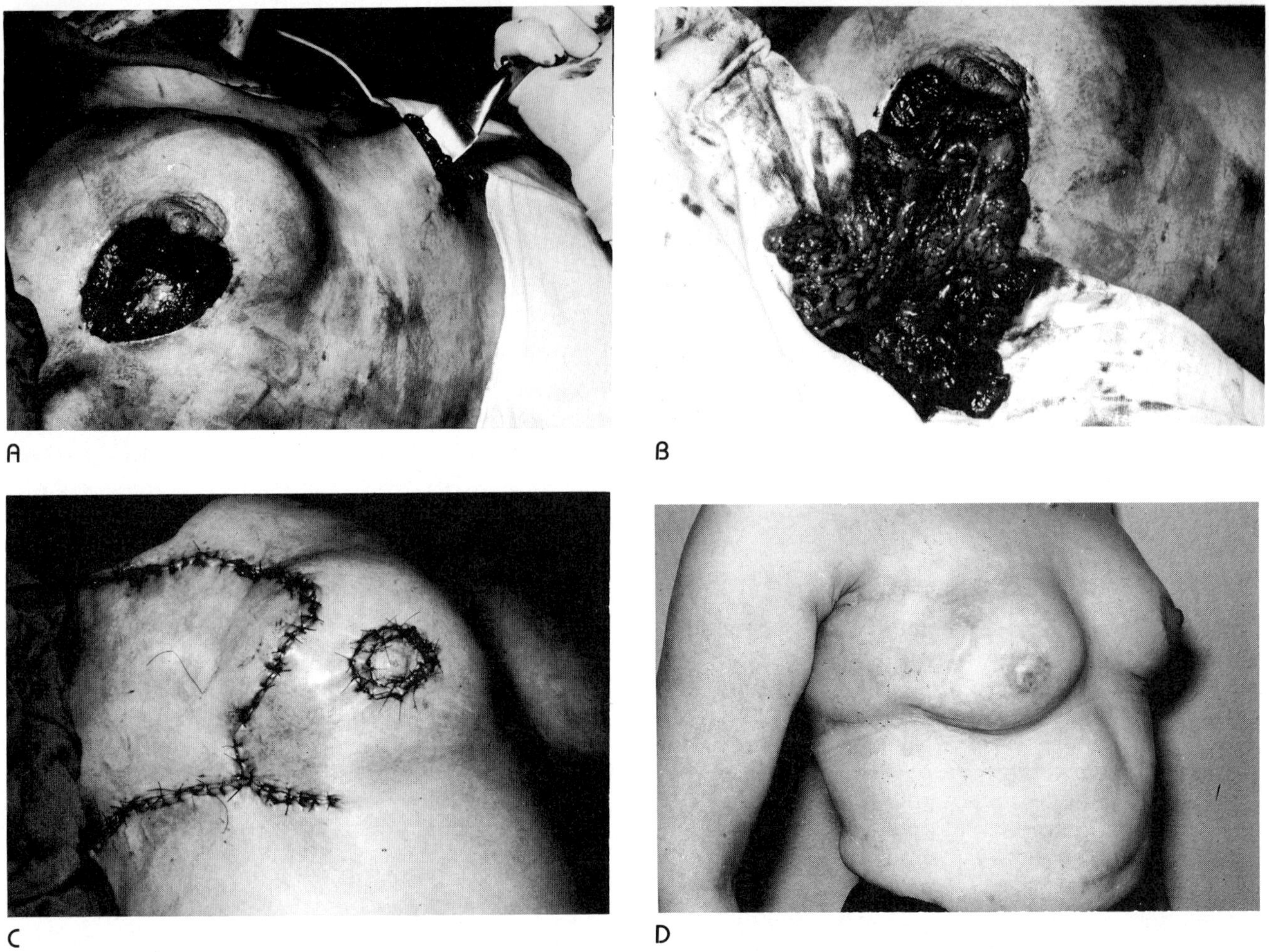

FIGURE 37–10 *A*, Surgical defect after resection of retracted skin and breast fibrosis. A subcostal incision is made to deliver the great omentum to the chest defect. *B*, The omentum is well vascularized and provides plentiful tissue to fill the surgical defect. *C*, A rotation skin flap covers the omental flap. *D*, One year after surgery a good cosmetic result is maintained.

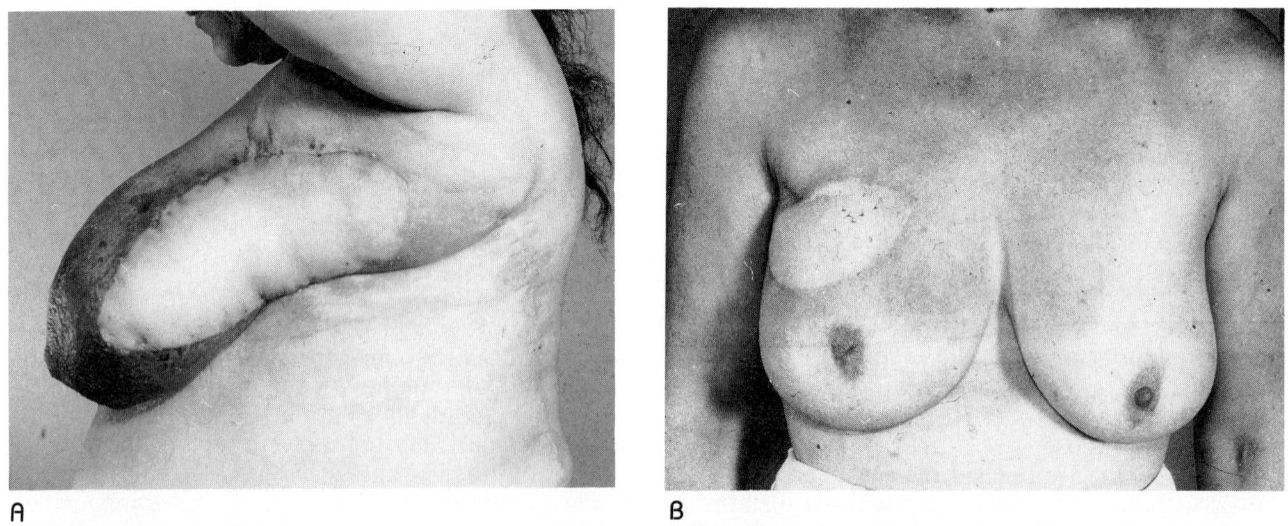

FIGURE 37–11 *A*, Postoperative result of reconstruction of a superolateral deformity after conservative therapy. A latissimus dorsi flap filled the surgical defect after resection of a contracted, fibrotic breast. *B*, The latissimus dorsi flap is the treatment of choice for deformities in the superior breast.

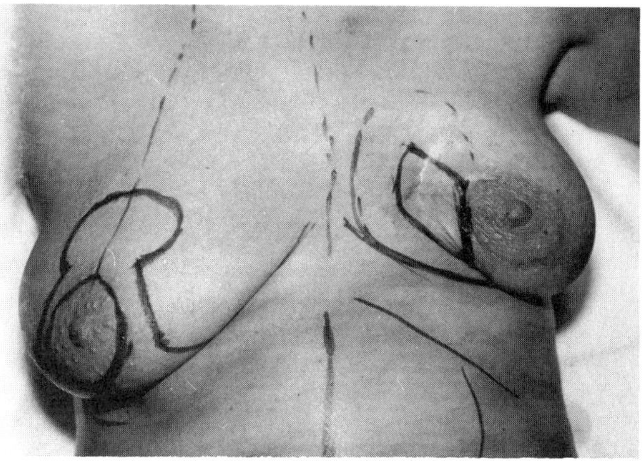
A

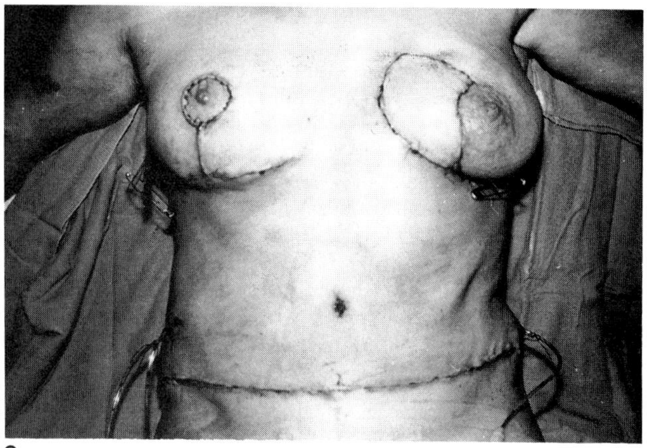
B

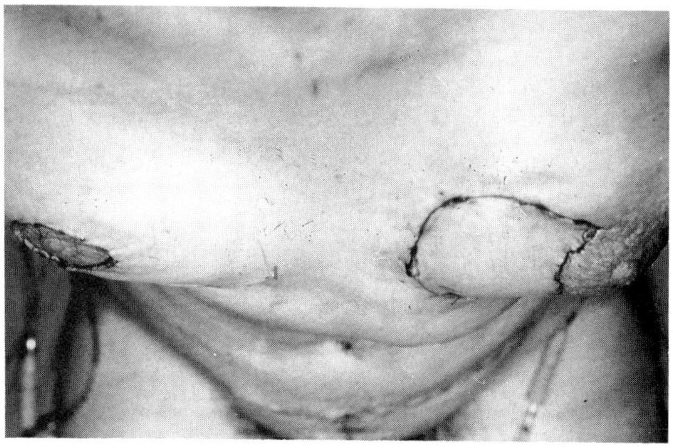
C

FIGURE 37 – 12 *A*, For conservative treatment deformities in the inner or lower quadrants, TRAM flap reconstruction is indicated. The plan of resection is outlined on the left breast. A simultaneous reduction mammaplasty is planned for the right breast. *B*, *C*, Immediate improvement in symmetry is demonstrated at completion of surgery.

epithelialization of a crescent of skin on one side. This crescent is switched on the opposite side of the areola to cover the lack of skin left by the nipple transposition. However, this maneuver usually leads to poor cosmetic results.

Crippled Breast After Conservative Treatment

Resulting from intensive radiotherapy for an inflammatory cancer or from radiotherapy performed by earlier methods of treatment, crippled breasts presenting with extensive radiodystrophy or radionecrosis cannot be repaired with partial reconstructions. Moreover, the clinical and radiologic follow-up of such patients is not reliable. Sometimes, radiated breasts are painful. It therefore may be mandatory in certain cases, after giving detailed information to the patient, to propose a mastectomy with immediate breast reconstruction. Such reconstruction almost always requires a musculocutaneous flap; the lower rectus flap appears to be the most appropriate. A complete histologic examination of the breast removed is essential.

References

1. Veronesi U, Saccozi R, Del Vecchio M, et al. Comparing radical mastectomy with quadrantectomy, axillary dissection and radiotherapy in patients with small cancers of the breast. N Engl J Med 1981; 305:6.
2. Sarrazin D, Le M, Rouesse J, et al. Conservative treatment versus mastectomy in breast cancer tumors with macroscopic diameter of 20 mm or less. Cancer 1984; 53:1209.
3. Fisher B, Bauer M, Margolese R, et al. Five year results of randomized clinical trial comparing total mastectomy and segmental mastectomy with or without radiation in the treatment of breast cancer. N Engl J Med 1985; 312:665.
4. Danoff BF, Pajak TF, Solin LJ, Goodman RL. Excisional biopsy, axillary node dissection and definitive radiotherapy for stages I and II breast cancer. Int J Radiat Oncol Biol Phys 1985; 11:479.
5. Ray GR, Fish VJ. Biopsy and definitive radiation therapy in stage I and II adenocarcinoma of the female breast: Analysis of cosmesis and the role of electron beam supplementation. Int J Radiat Oncol Biol Phys 1983; 9:813.
6. Pearl RM, Wisnicki J. Breast reconstruction following

lumpectomy and irradiation. Plast Reconstr Surg 1985; 76:83.

7. Clarke D, Martinez A, Goffinet DR. Analysis of treatment results and complications in the radiotherapeutic management of early stage breast cancer. Int J Radiat Oncol Biol Phys 1981; 7:1219.
8. Westdahl PR. Selection, work-up and surgical technique of conservation surgery and axillary dissection. Front Radiat Ther Oncol 1983; 17:48.
9. Browde S, Nissenbaum MM. Primary radiotherapy after tumor excision as an alternative to mastectomy for early breast cancer. Rationale and preliminary results of a prospective study. S Afr Med J 1983; 64:531.
10. Levitt SH. Primary treatment of early breast cancer with conservation surgery and radiation therapy. The effect of adjuvant chemotherapy. Cancer 1985; 55:2140.
11. Danoff BF, Goodman RL, Glick JH, et al. The effect of chemotherapy on cosmesis and complications in patients with breast cancer treated by definitive irradiation. Int J Radiat Oncol Biol Phys 1983; 9:1625.
12. Clarke D, Martinez A, Cox RS. Analysis of cosmetic results and complications in patients with stage I and II breast cancer treated by biopsy and irradiation. Int J Radiat Oncol Biol Phys 1983; 9:1807.
13. Bedwinek J. Treatment of stage I and II adenocarcinoma by tumor excision and irradiation. Int J Radiat Oncol Biol Phys 1981; 7:1553.
14. Harris JR, Martin B, Levene MD, et al. Analysis of cosmetic results following primary radiation therapy for stage I and II carcinoma of the breast. Int J Radiat Oncol Biol Phys 1979; 5:257–261.
15. Dewar JA, Ben Hamou S, Ben Hamou E, et al. Cosmetic results following lumpectomy axillary dissection and radiotherapy for small breast cancers. Radiother Oncol 1988; 12:273.
16. Beadle GF, Silver B, Botnick L, et al. Cosmetic results following primary radiation therapy for early breast cancer. Cancer 1984; 54:2911–2918.
17. Calle R, Vilcoq JR, Pilleron JP, et al. Conservative treatment of operable breast carcinoma by irradiation with or without limited surgery. Ten year results. In: Harris JR, Hellman S, Silen W, eds. Conservative management of breast cancer. Philadelphia: JB Lippincott, 1983:3.

CHAPTER 38

Nipple-Areola Reconstruction and Correction of Inverted Nipple

JOHN WILLIAM LITTLE, M.D.

The breast has been emblematic of woman and her nurturing role in civilized society. This symbolism continues today, evoking powerful emotions on both societal and personal levels. The visual concentration of such symbolism occurs at the functional outlet of the breast, the nipple-areola. Through its color contrast and its responsive three-dimensional qualities, the nipple-areola focuses the aesthetic, erotic, and sexual appeal of the breast. When the nipple-areola is absent from the breast for any reason, the visual and symbolic impact of that breast is profoundly weakened. A major benefit of breast reconstruction is reversal of the mastectomy defect and its negative implications concerning health, survival, and femininity. This appreciation occurs on multiple levels, but the most important remains the visual aspect. Thus, the quick glance in the dressing-room mirror becomes an unconscious reassurance to the survivor of breast cancer who perceives her balanced bosom with its symmetric pair of pigmented nipples-areolae. It is this casual glance that reminds her that all is well and that her life crisis is behind her.

The absent nipple-areola has many etiologies. Just as there may be polythelia, supernumerary nipples, along the milk line, so there may be athelia, congenital absence of the nipple-areola, or a rudimentary presentation in an otherwise perfectly formed breast. A more common congenital deficiency presents as a component of the broader deformity of Poland's syndrome, in which aspects of the breast mound, shoulder girdle, and forearm and hand may also be deficient. Traumatic absence may follow any local integumentary loss, most commonly burn. Iatrogenic trauma and loss remains fortunately rare, but may follow ischemic complications of reduction mammaplasty or injudicial biopsy of the prepubescent breast bud. Most cases of nipple-areolar loss occur through the treatment of neoplasms of the breast, not from direct tumor involvement of that structure but as a component of established surgical therapy for breast malignancy. The overwhelming example remains mastectomy for carcinoma, although localized treatment of Paget's disease or tumorectomy with radiation for central carcinomas of the breast are further examples. Finally, a limited deformity of the nipple-areola complex involves the inverted nipple, which most often is congenital, but occasionally follows episodes of infection or trauma and, of particular significance, subjacent neoplasm.

In the past, there was a lack of enthusiasm on the part of some plastic surgeons and not a few of their patients for nipple-areolar reconstruction, which was regarded as an unnecessary further burden on the breast reconstruction patient. Since the acceptance of medical tattoo for nipple-areolar coloration, however, any aspects of the surgery that may have been considered burdensome have been eliminated. Certainly, there remains no significant morbidity from the surgery itself or from scars at specialized tissue sites that were previously necessary for the purpose of producing pigmented grafts. Nipple-areolar reconstruction, as well as correction of the inverted nipple, is a procedure easily performed in the most rudimentary of surgical offices without the need for premedication or adjuvant pharmacology, and either can be accomplished without the production of new scars remote from the nipple site. Common wisdom once held that nipple-areolar reconstruction cannot salvage the aesthetic success of an inartistic breast reconstruction, but that a poor nipple-areola reconstruction can detract from one otherwise satisfactory. Today, however, I believe that the results of nipple-areola reconstruction are so predictably realistic that an artistic reconstruction on an otherwise indifferent breast mound may considerably aid the patient's overall acceptance of the reconstructive result (Fig. 38–1). This view is supported by our retrospective psychological survey of patients which compared those who had opted for nipple-areola reconstruction with those who had not. There was a highly significant correlation between overall patient satisfaction with the breast reconstruction and the presence of the nipple-areola.

There are a number of goals in nipple-areolar reconstruction, some important and achievable, others not. The most important, and frequently difficult, goal is that of proper positioning. This may be straightforward when the resultant breast mound reconstruction is excellent and nearly symmetric with the opposite breast, as typically occurs after reconstruction by autogenous tissue techniques. It is equally straightforward in cases of bilateral reconstruction when the reconstructive techniques have been the same for both breasts and there is again a high degree of symmetry. However, when there remain significant differences between the two breasts, as with an alloplastic reconstruction of one breast and significant ptosis in the remaining natural breast, proper positioning may be difficult to achieve. In this common situation the requirements for such positioning remain complex. Symmetry, of course, must be pursued for the two nipple-areola complexes, but a key question is whether the symmetry should be in the undressed state or in the typical supported state, whereby the brassiere lifts the natural ptotic breast a significant degree and the reconstructed breast little, if at all. These considerations are important because a good nipple reconstruction will be subtly evident through many forms of clothing. Despite the need for symmetric positioning with the opposite nipple-areola, each complex must remain centric in its relationship with its own breast. Clearly, then, the final position in such situations must represent a compromise among these various goals. Because the difficulty of such positioning increases with the degree of asymmetry between the breast mounds, a prudent rule suggests that nipple-areola reconstruction be delayed until a state of reasonable symmetry has been previously accomplished between the two breasts. Generally, it is recommended that nipple-areola reconstruction be postponed to the second stage of nearly all breast reconstructions and not uncommonly to a third or later stage. It must be remembered that any significant nipple-areola malposition will detract significantly from the final result of breast reconstruction and will present a difficult challenge for secondary correction.

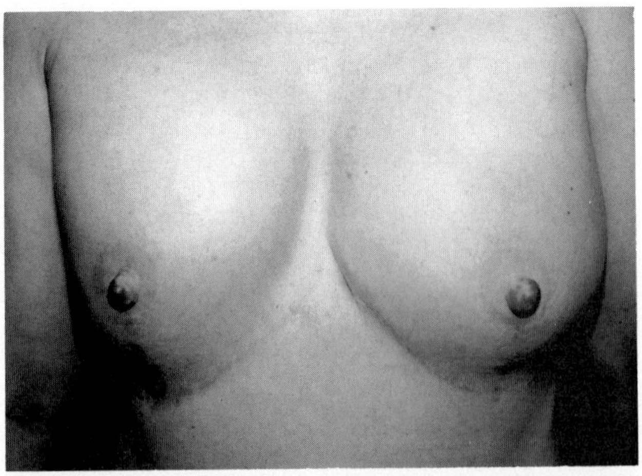

FIGURE 38–1 Strong nipple-areola reconstructions by skate technique on top of flat grafted remnants can enhance patient acceptance of otherwise poor breast mound reconstructions.

After proper positioning, the next important goal is that of symmetric shape and size of the areolae. This has become a straightforward goal to accomplish through the use of delayed tattoo for coloration. At a final office visit the surgeon merely transposes the mirror image of the opposite areola, whatever its shape and size, to the new breast by intradermal tattoo. Another important goal is that of symmetric size and shape of the nipples themselves. Until recently, consistent and lasting nipple projection remained elusive. This is no longer the case, as a number of techniques produce reliable and lasting projection today. A final desired goal remains symmetry of color and tone for both nipples and areolae, which is more attainable today through the use of tattoo than with previous techniques, but which even so remains too often unfulfilled. Efforts at color match continue to improve, however, with the increasing array of professional tattoo pigments available and the growing experience of the individual tattoo artist-surgeon. The least important of attainable goals remains symmetry of texture and surface quality, because these details are not easily discernible at common viewing distances, such as the combined distances to and from the typical bedroom mirror. Finally, at least two goals are still out of reach. The reconstructed nipple must remain an inert structure of fixed proportions and cannot yet be reconstructed as a dynamic unit capable of erectile response to various stimuli. Erotic sensibility also remains essentially unobtainable, although more than a few patients have described the return of such sensation to the area of the reconstructed nipple-areola complex. This must be accepted as evidence of the great potential of the human forebrain rather than any particular surgical accomplishment in the chest wall.

AREOLA RECONSTRUCTION

Reconstruction of the two-dimensional areola has traditionally been straightforward. Options have included banking, sharing,[2-6] free tissue grafting,[7-9] and tattoo.[10-14] Of these I consider that tattoo offers the greatest advantage today. The practice of banking the nipple-areola from a cancerous breast in the groin for later retransfer has the proved potential for transplantation of malignant cells, even when the primary tumor is remote from the nipple-areola, and subjacent pathologic sections of the specimen appear tumor free.[15-21] Equally to the point, however, such twice-transferred structures invariably lose color and projection and compare unfavorably with those reconstructed de novo. The sharing of full-thickness areolar tissue from the periphery of an opposite and enlarged areola that is undergoing reduction through mastopexy or reduction mammaplasty remains a natural choice, involving, as it does, reconstruction in kind. Any other form of areolar sharing, such as split grafting from the surface, imposes unacceptable alterations to the donor structure. Free tissue grafting for areolar simulation has required the use of specialized donor sites to produce heightened pigmentation in the matured grafts. Most of these have been genital or paragenital sites associated with significant surgical and psychological morbidity. Furthermore, areolae reconstructed from the once popular site of the upper inner thigh have routinely lost pigmentation over time, so that long-term results typically are indistinguishable from surrounding breast skin. Finally, the use of such grafts as circular structures of a given diameter has produced areolar shapes and sizes asymmetric with the opposite areola. The shape of many areolae remains discoid and noncircular with an axis of obliquity that changes with differing positions of the breast, as when standing or reclining. Rigid, round skin grafts naturally do not possess this fluid aspect of shape. In addition, many such grafted structures have contracted in unpredictable ways, producing yet further asymmetry. Intradermal tattoo, on the other hand, fulfills most of the requirements for reconstruction in two dimensions. Color match may be inexact and may also fade with time, but color control is far greater with the use of selected earth pigments than with the spontaneous darkening that follows the transfer of specialized grafts, and the addition of further color requires only an office visit of trivial inconvenience. Release from the requirement of specialized donor sites for pigmented grafts essentially eliminates any significant morbidity from nipple-areolar reconstruction and makes the procedure appropriate for the most squeamish of patients. Furthermore, the final act of tattoo, performed some 4 months after nipple-areolar reconstruction, allows mirror-image simulation of the opposite areola with a fluid patch of color. If the nipple reconstruction itself has been misplaced from the symmetric ideal, the areolar tattoo can be placed in the symmetric position, allowing the nipple a somewhat eccentric position within the color pattern. Thus, the overall impression of symmetry is enhanced. Typically, the only skin graft used at the areolar site is the small graft taken to close the donor site of nipple reconstruction. This is taken as a small full-thickness strip of skin along a portion of the mastectomy scar, a flap donor site scar, or any pre-existing surgical scar; closure produces concomitant scar revision. When desired, the need for such a graft can often be eliminated altogether by advancing the undermined margins of the small defect to the reconstructed nipple base. The only governing principle here is that the final pattern and size of any graft placed as a component of nipple reconstruction fall within the anticipated pattern of final tattoo. The tattoo is later added without regard for the graft pattern.

NIPPLE RECONSTRUCTION

Reconstruction of the three-dimensional nipple was traditionally unreliable until recent years, but today a number of techniques offer predictable results with lasting projection. Options again have historically included banking, sharing, and free grafting,[4,8,9,22-27] as well as local flaps.[28-47] Among these, the local flap is still the only option that produces a final result with maximal projection of both the reconstructed and the remaining nipple. If the naturalness of the final result in breast reconstruction is enhanced through artistic nipple-areola addition, then the more projectile and three-dimensional the nipple, the greater is this enhancement. As mentioned, banking of any portion of the nipple-areola complex from a cancerous breast is unjustified and inappropriate. The practice of sharing the remaining nipple by removing a free composite graft of approximately half the bulk of that structure is time-honored and continues in use today. Certainly the most expedient form of nipple-areola reconstruction is the transfer of such a nipple graft to a tattooed areolar bed. Although this may be appropriate for the patient with a truly outsized nipple, it is not the most advantageous option for other women. Perhaps most important, it represents an assault against the one remaining area of erotic breast sensibility in the mastectomy patient. Furthermore, the potential projection of the nipple reconstruction is reduced by half for both nipples. Therefore, the finished pair of nipples-areolae, however symmetrically and artistically rendered, are less projectile and less three-dimensional than otherwise possible. It is exactly this three-dimensional quality that brings heightened realism, not only to the nipple-areola, but to the overall result of the reconstructed breast. Furthermore, this realism can be appreciated both in and out of clothing. Therefore, it is preferable to respect the remaining nipple-areola and its full degree of projection and to match it de novo. Free grafts other than the shared composite nipple graft remain dismally ineffective in producing any degree of acceptable projection and are therefore inappropriate.

Local flap techniques have finally fulfilled the promise of reliable and lasting projection so that virtually any opposite nipple can be matched today. Local flap reconstruction of the nipple has followed two basic designs: an island flap based on a central subcutaneous pedicle or stalk, and a conventional flap elevation based on a subdermal blood supply. The former has proved insufficiently consistent in producing lasting projection and, except as a secondary technique, can be forgotten. A number of techniques of the latter design, on the other hand, can be relied on to produce consistent results with nipples of any desired projection. Among these, the skate technique is especially appealing in the aesthetic appearance of the final nipple contour; the reliability, simplicity, and rapidity of the technique; the ease of postoperative care; the minimal donor site distortion; and the lasting, long-term projection (Fig. 38–2). During my initial experience with this technique, before confidence had been gained in long-term results, early nipples, raised to the full potential of the design, were of such Brobdingnagian proportions that all required secondary reduction by amputation.

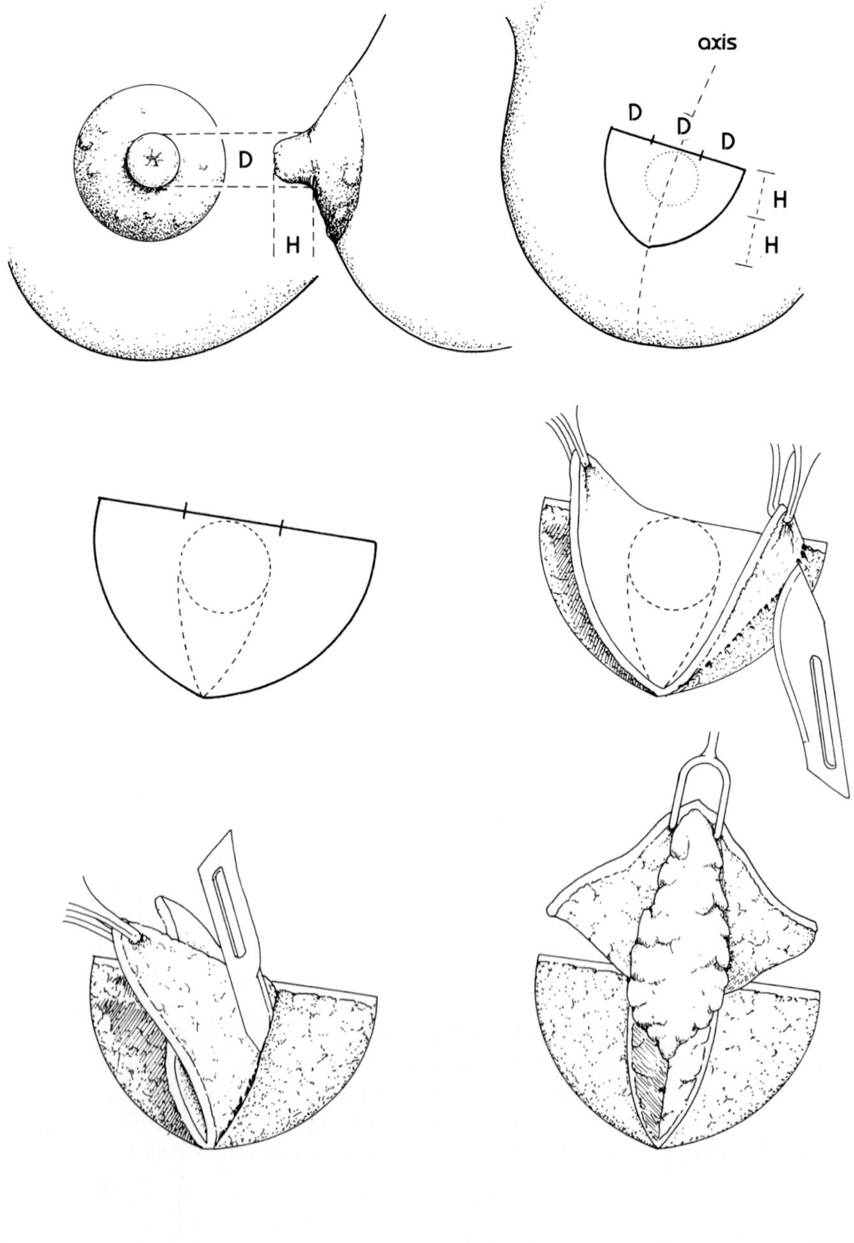

FIGURE 38–2 Artist's rendering of the skate technique. The projection of the contralateral nipple (H) provides a guide for design of the height of the skate (2H). The contralateral nipple diameter (D) is tripled to result in the width of the skate "wings." Partial-thickness elevation of the wings is converted to full-thickness incision into subcutaneous tissue to form the nipple core. The wings are closed around the core when the subcutaneous trough is closed. After the flap donor site is narrowed, the defect remaining is resurfaced with a full-thickness skin graft. Addition of areola is by intradermal tattoo at a later procedure.

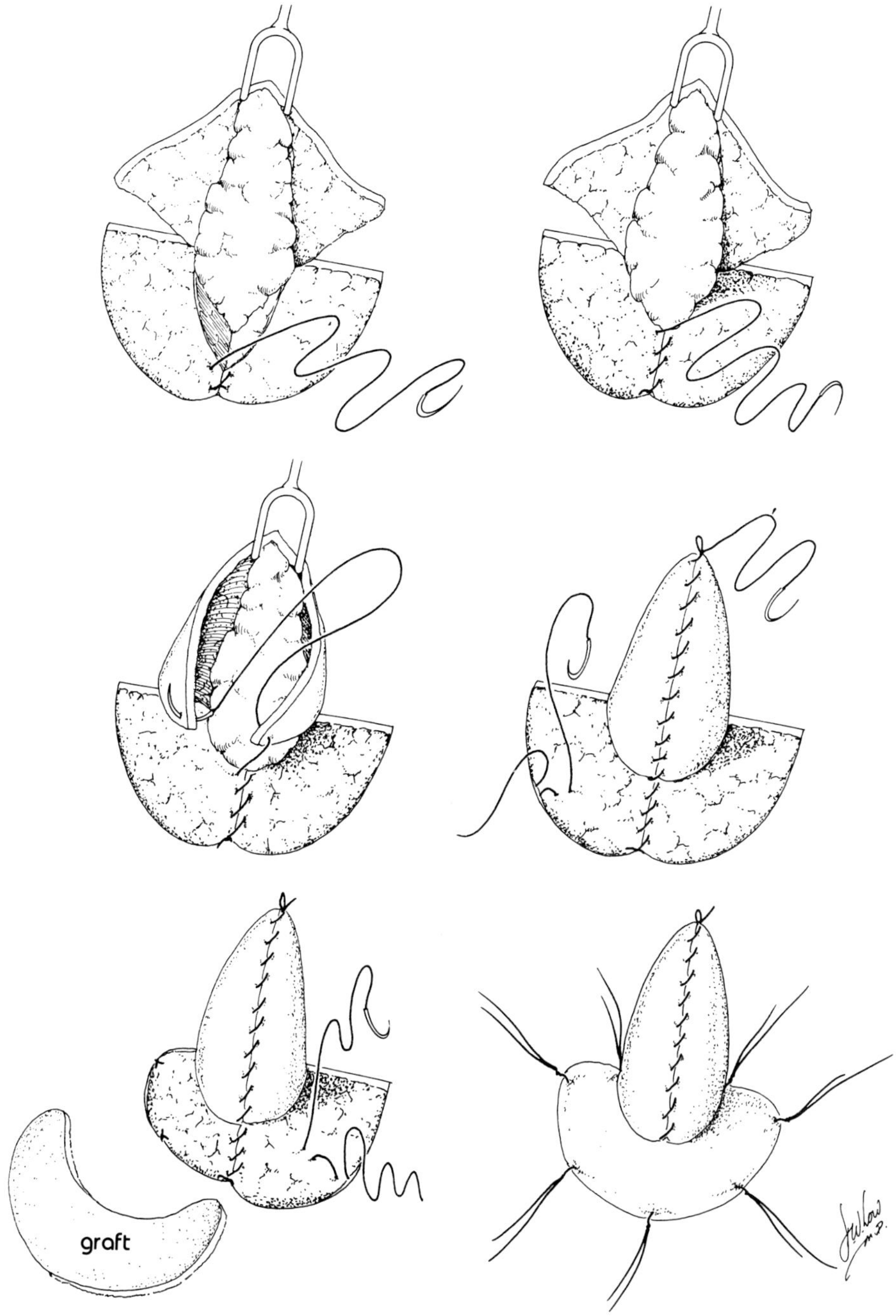

Figure 38-2 *Continued*

Nipple-Areolar Reconstruction With Tattoo: The Author's Technique

Skate Nipple Reconstruction

Nipple-areola reconstruction is usually performed on an outpatient basis with the premedicated patient under local anesthesia as part of the planned second stage of breast reconstruction. It may, however, be performed at a third or later stage, as a component of further alteration of the breast mound, or as an isolated procedure in the office. The patient is placed in a sitting position on the operating table to determine the optimal position for the nipple-areola. Sternal notch-to-nipple, midsternal line-to-nipple, and midclavicular line-to-nipple distances are transposed from the normal to the reconstructed side. The nipple position is indicated and a faint areolar circle roughly drawn about this point so that the gestalt of symmetry can be appreciated as the surgeon moves back a distance (Fig. 38-3*A*). Further adjustments are then made from the aesthetic point of view. Once the final position is determined, the patient is placed supine on the table with arms akimbo, hands behind the buttocks, and elbows abducted away from the axillae. This position gives full

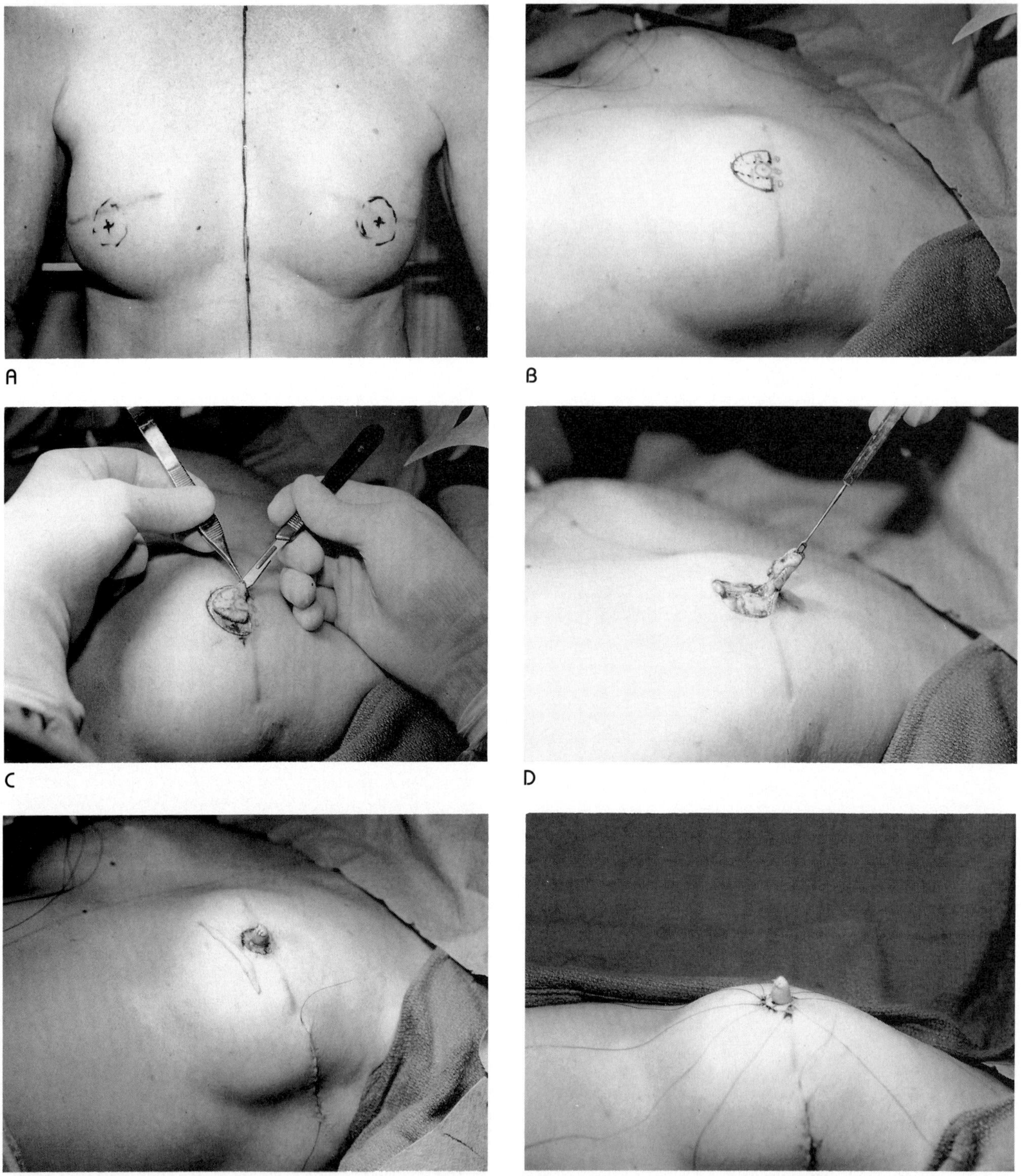

FIGURE 38–3 Skate technique. *A*, Preoperative positioning. *B*, Preoperative design. *C*, Wings elevated to split thickness. *D*, Composite body cut free and elevated to vertical. *E*, Donor bed diminished, awaiting a graft from the lateral scar. *F*, Finished skate nipple awaiting a tieover dressing. *G*, *H*, Postoperative appearance 4 days after removal of tieover dressings. (Photography by Maryallys Finical.)

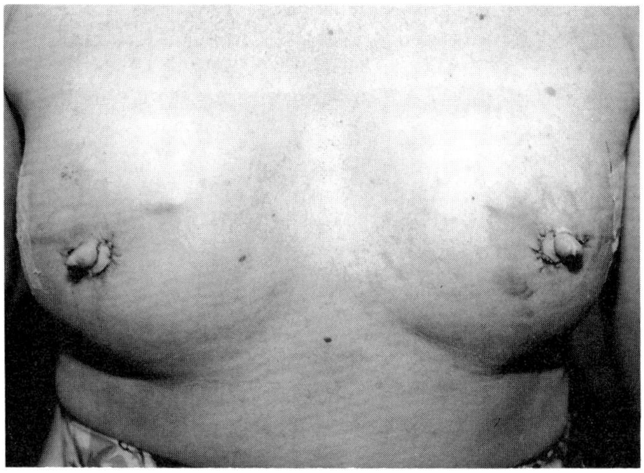

G

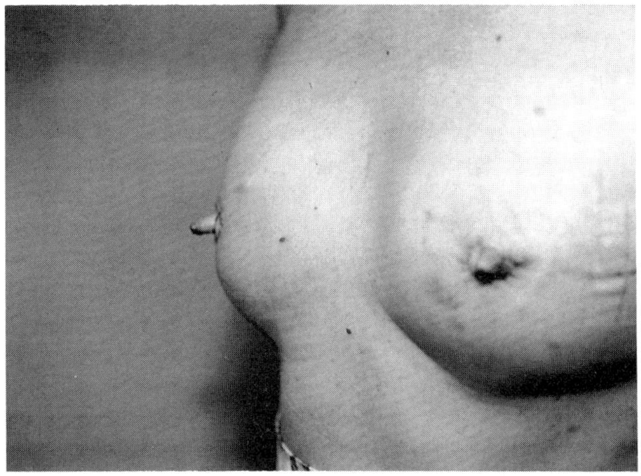

H

Figure 38-3 *Continued*

access to the lateral thorax and axilla for anesthesia and surgery. A circle the exact diameter of the opposite nipple is drawn about the nipple point. A decision is made about the direction of axis for the skate flap. Two considerations are necessary here: (1) if the mastectomy scar crosses near the nipple point, it will be necessary to rotate the axis of the skate design so that the wings and body of the skate are not violated by the scar; (2) if there are no such considerations, the surgeon assesses the radius of maximal laxity about the nipple point and orients the flap in this direction so that the minor dermal defect that lies in the wake of flap elevation closes with greatest ease. If neither factor appears important, the flap is designed with its axis at the 6 o'clock position so that the resulting nipple seam will fall on the undersurface of the new nipple. Once the axis of the flap is determined, a base tangent is placed perpendicular to the axis. This line will determine the squared-off posterior margin of the wings of the flap. The length of this segment, or wing width, will be one additional nipple diameter to each side, so that the total length of the base line will be three such diameters. Next the desired height of the nipple is determined; my rule of thumb suggests twice the height of the opposite stimulated and erect nipple. The distance of two such opposite nipple heights is then marked out along the axis from the tangent base, with a small additional distance included at the apex for infolding as the flap is cinched closed.

A curvilinear, ellipsoid line is drawn to connect the three points, determining the margins of the flap wings. This arc begins at the point of the lateral extremity of one wing base, curves through the apex point on the flap axis, and returns to the lateral point of the opposite wing base. Dotted lines are then used to denote the width of the composite body of the flap, the central third of the tangent base, and are extended as parallel lines that later taper to meet at the design apex. These dotted lines are necessary to remind the surgeon not to undermine excessively during development of the wings, so that the composite body is cut full width, or one nipple diameter wide (Fig. 38-3*B*). A small amount of local anesthetic with vasoconstrictor is added in the subdermal plane. Surgery is begun by incising the ellipsoid wing margins and the two wing bases. The central portion of the baseline corresponding to the original nipple width is not incised. The partial-thickness wings are then dissected up to the dotted lines (Fig. 38-3*C*). This dissection is performed at the deepest possible split-thickness level, leaving behind a minimal reticular pattern of deep dermis covering the subcutaneous tissues. The surgeon should resist the temptation to elevate the wings at the full-thickness level, because this is unnecessary for their survival. Moreover, the suture-holding ability of the small amount of retained dermis is important in closing the areolar defect and avoiding contour depression. Such dermis also presents a stable base on which to advance the areolar defect margins. Finally, if a small skin graft is required to close the wound, its take is predictably better on the dermal bed. As the partial-thickness dissection of the wings is completed at the level of the dotted lines, the dissection turns abruptly from horizontal to vertical. The wings are lifted and the remaining dermis is incised perpendicularly through the subjacent subcutaneous tissue. This maneuver is performed on either side, creating a thick composite flap body. As the body is cut free at the apex and dissected centrally toward the nipple, care must be taken to include a significant subcutaneous tongue along the entire length of the flap. When the subcutaneous elements are scant, as may occur in the breast reconstructed by a submuscular tissue expander, underlying muscle is included to enhance both the bulk and the heartiness of the flap. The most likely errors in execution of the skate technique are the cutting free of too little fat or muscle to nurture the flap and give it adequate bulk, or rough handling of the elevated flap that detaches the delicate subcutaneous tissues from the dermal undersurface.

It is important that a significant three-dimensional trough remain in the wake of flap elevation. As the dissection proceeds centrally, the undercutting of the fatty element of the flap is halted when the nipple disc itself is reached, so that there remains an intact subjacent vertical blood supply through the fat into the new nipple. The dermal elements on either side of the nipple disc, however, are divided back to the tangent line, care again being taken not to undercut the central subcutaneous stalk. Thus, the final flap is provided with a double blood supply: that of a subjacent subcutaneous stalk as well as a conventional subdermal blood supply coming into the nipple at the flap base. At this point the composite flap can be lifted freely into a vertical orientation without resistance by dermal elements (Fig. 38–3*D*).

Closure of the areolar defect is begun with a running absorbable suture (5-0 Vicryl). The dermal margins of the areolar trough or defect are approximated about half the distance to the nipple, and a third point of dermis is included in the suture at the periphery of the skin defect at 6 o'clock. When the suture is tied, the margin of the ellipsoid defect is pulled in toward the nipple column. The suture is then rapidly continued in running fashion up the areolar defect, taking small bites of dermis, until the appropriate position at the near margin of the new nipple base is reached. At this point the suture is locked and the pointed extremities of the two wings are brought together around the exposed composite belly or undersurface of the flap. The continuing suture is then run up the nipple, approximating the margins of the two flap wings, closing the flap cylinder. The cylinder apex is closed in running "pursestring" fashion after any pointed aspect has been blunted with a scissors. Additional sutures of the same material are added at the sides to stabilize the new nipple column to the dermal base at 3 and 9 o'clock. The resulting flap, impressively tall, stands perpendicular to the plane of the breast. Again, the same suture material is used to advance the remaining margins of the periphery of the defect in toward the nipple itself. Five or six such interrupted sutures are usually required to minimize the remaining dermal defect, so that the smallest of grafts will suffice for wound closure. It is frequently possible to advance the skin margins up to the nipple itself so that no skin graft is necessary. This presents little advantage, however, over the harvesting of a minor graft along one of the scars and using this to wrap around the small remaining margin of exposed dermis. Such marginal advancement toward the nipple should be limited if contour flattening is produced at the breast apex. The desire to avoid a skin graft is insufficient justification for the production of any shape distortion; more important, it must not be allowed to limit the initial design and proportions of the nipple flap to less than those necessary to create an ultimate match. A further small skin graft around a part of the base of the nipple is a trivial addition and its avoidance represents a minuscule victory, one that must not detract in any way from the ultimate goal of a projectile, symmetric nipple.

If a skin graft is necessary to close the donor site wound, it need never exceed 1 centimeter in width and is often narrower. Such a narrow graft is typically removed from alongside a portion of the mastectomy scar for a distance of 3 cm, so that a scar revision is accomplished with closure of the defect. The graft is then defatted and thinned of excess dermis and applied to the U-shaped defect about the nipple base (Fig. 38–3*E*, *F*). It is rapidly sewn in place with fine silk sutures left long for tieover. An additional 6-0 nylon suture is run locking-style to close any gaps that remain. The small graft and the nipple are covered with a greasy gauze dressing, on top of which a wet cotton bolus around a rigid sleeve is added and tied in place. The rigid portion of the dressing is made by removing 1 centimeter from the base of a plastic syringe barrel, utilizing a disposable ophthalmic cautery. Through such a tieover dressing, pressure is provided to the small skin graft, while the nipple flap remains protected within the rigid sleeve. Finally, the tieover dressing is covered with an additional gauze square taped in place to stabilize the apparatus. This dressing is removed at precisely 4 days along with the tieover sutures, so that no stitch marks remain (Fig. 38–3*G*, *H*). The 6-0 nylon suture is left for later removal and the nipple and graft are recovered with a simple, greasy gauze dressing. No special aftercare is required and at the subsequent office visit, 1 week after surgery, the fine nylon suture is removed. Full activity is permitted, including bathing and showering. Occasionally a partial-thickness desquamation may occur along the seam of the new nipple, representing the most distal portions of the partial-thickness wing flaps. This is treated by daily application of a greasy dressing or ointment. Any minor eschar that develops is allowed to separate and heal without special attention. Any greater degree of necrosis is almost always indicative of improper technique and insufficient attention to the inclusion of composite subcutaneous or muscular elements. If the final nipple projection proves inadequate, the error almost invariably lies in the initial design, most often an insufficient primary height of the pattern. All surgeons lend their own stamp to the execution of this or any design. The two-to-one formula works for me in estimating final height, but a different ratio may be appropriate to the style of the individual surgeon; experience will determine this. For the beginning surgeon, the best advice is to err on the side of too much projection initially. The surgeon must also resist the temptation to amputate an exuberant result prematurely, at 3 months for example, because the nipple may end up wanting after 1 year. Some have agitated for immediate tattoo and coloration of the nipple at the time of its creation, but such impatience defeats the considerable advantage of tattoo as an ultimate fine-tuning tool that does more than simply color the local flap. If one is concerned about textural adjuncts, as when the opposite areola presents especially prominent Montgomery glands, the best approach is that of Becker and Prysi,[48] who embed small portions of the mastectomy scar into areolar stab wounds. This can be done at the time of nipple creation, except in that portion of the future areola that is covered with the small skin graft. Alternatively, if a larger areolar graft has been required, this can be added at some office visit before the tattoo procedure. In practice, I almost never add this embellishment to the finished nipple-areola, although I am happy to do so for any perfectionistic patient.

Tattoo

The intradermal tattoo is postponed 4 or more months after nipple-areola reconstruction, for multiple reasons. Assuming that a second-step alteration of the reconstructed breast mound was included during the previous procedure, a certain time is required to determine the final result. One of the advantages of late areolar tattoo is that small discrepancies in nipple position can be ameliorated with this technique, and such subtle decisions cannot be made until the two breast mounds are in a stable state, with the postsurgical phase essentially resolved. Furthermore, it is important that the color of any grafted tissues required to close the donor wound has returned toward its normal state, so that decisions regarding color are not complicated by temporary graft pigments. Also, just as the final and exact areolar size and shape are determined at tattoo, so this minor procedure provides the opportunity for final adjustment and tailoring of the nipple itself. Although such tailoring is only occasionally performed, it may be appropriate to narrow a nipple column that is broad and splayed compared with its mate, and this is done by de-epithelialization and closure of a portion of its circumference. One must resist the temptation, however, to amputate a nipple that is only moderately more projectile than the ideal, especially if the timing is as early as 3 or 4 months after nipple reconstruction.

To those who might decry yet a third stage in the routine design for breast reconstruction, it must be pointed out that the tattoo procedure involves no more than a routine office visit in terms of inconvenience to either patient or surgeon. The patient is placed in the sitting position and the size, shape, and orientation of the normal areola is transferred in mirror-image fashion onto the opposite breast with a marking pen. If the exact nipple position has been somewhat off the symmetric ideal, this fact is ignored and the areola is drawn as symmetrically to the other side as possible. An eccentric position of the nipple within the areolar field is more acceptable than asymmetry of the highly visible areolar position. Thus, it is possible to truly fine-tune the final position of most nipple-areolar placements. Many areolae take on an ellipsoid shape in the sitting position, and this variation is carefully recorded in mirror-image fashion during the marking. Any pattern of small graft necessary to close the nipple donor site is ignored, because it falls well within the areolar pigment design.

The patient is now placed supine and the area of the breast apex prepared with an alcohol swab. A local anesthetic with a vasoconstrictor is used to infiltrate beneath the base of the design, as much to diminish the blood flow that may complicate the coloration process as to provide anesthesia. If the nipple is to be tailored, this is now performed with closure by fine chromic catgut sutures. Next, the tattoo is undertaken. Multiple pigments are currently available from most tattoo supply houses, both surgical and lay, including a range of pigments appropriate to areolar tones. It is often possible to select one that closely simulates the color of the opposite areola. In earlier years, I mixed all my areolar colors from a basic supply of white, brown, and red pigments, so that custom mixing remains an option, but it can be troublesome and is largely unnecessary today. Fortunately, the severe tissue reactions against certain tattoo pigments, most notably reds and yellows, are no longer a danger. The mercury and cadmium oxides once necessary to produce these bright colors are discontinued by most tattoo supply houses. I have seen no such reaction in my 8 years of tattooing.

The selected or mixed pigment is painted alongside the opposite areola with a cotton swab to judge the general color; as mentioned earlier, exact final color match is difficult and requires artistic experience. Some changes occur from the appearance of the appliqué to that of the finished tattoo 3 or more months later. In the first place, the appliqué color immediately appears different as it is embedded. As one begins the tattoo process, the color may appear lighter than the appliqué suggested. As the tattoo progresses in time, however, and especially as more and more red cells with their hemosiderin pigment are embedded, the tattoo becomes progressively, even shockingly, darker. The surgeon must not be dissuaded by this, because the appearance at tattoo must be significantly darker if the final match is to be close. Exaggerated darkening clears rapidly within the first 3 weeks as blood and hemosiderin products are removed from the tattoo site. Beyond that, there will be a definite progressive loss of pigment over time, and this should be taken into account. If the tattoo equipment is sufficiently powerful, the needles are appropriately sharp, and the surgeon is experienced, the pigment will be embedded in the deep dermis and hence resistant to early fading. If, on the other hand, the embedding process has been superficial, much of the early pigment will be lost. Even a good tattoo, however, fades subtly but inexorably over time. All patients should understand this, and an individual patient may wish to return for additional color in the future. In fact, few avail themselves of this opportunity. However, secondary tattoo is an especially rapid procedure, no time being lost in determining shapes and patterns; it can be as quick as any office visit during a busy day. There are a range of options in tattoo equipment, of both medical and lay design. A number are offered by surgical supply houses and are designed specifically for medical tattoo. These tend to present a more attractive apparatus and are more delicate to use, but are significantly more expensive than those available from lay tattoo houses. On the other hand, they tend to produce less torque and power for imbedding pigments. Easily the most important consideration in the purchase of tattoo equipment should be the adequacy of torque to power the needle deeply into the dermis. Systems designed for embedding pigments in the fine skin of the eyelid cannot be expected to perform well in the thick dermis of a latissimus dorsi flap. For this reason, I prefer the powerful and inexpensive, if somewhat more cumbersome, equipment of the lay tattoo artist. Not only is the initial investment less, but the cost of tattoo needles is trivial and therefore allows disposal after one-time use; thus, needles are always sharp and sterile. Needles are available in a variety of arrangements, from single needles to clusters of eight or more. I prefer a single row of four or five, likening this to a paintbrush.

The basic technique of tattoo is not difficult to learn and can be practiced on pigs' feet purchased at the local supermarket. One dips the needle into the pigment mixture and begins painting the area marked for the areola much as one might paint or fill in a coloring book. The tattoo device is held at approximately 45 degrees to the plane of the working surface with the painting motion toward the operator, so that the needles do not jam or stick into the skin. The action should be patient and repetitive, developing the whole surface before going back to apply yet more pigment. It is essentially a pointillist technique, and as the individual dots become more dense, the appearance of color becomes deeper and darker. If one works too rapidly or overworks a given area, significant trauma may occur to the surface epithelium. This then develops a fine eschar that later sloughs with much of the pigment, leaving a faint area with little color. When the areolar pattern has been covered by pigment, the excess surface pigment and blood is removed with alcohol swabs to ascertain the amount of color that remains intradermal. Another treatment is performed over the entire area with the same cleaning process to check the appearance. This sequence is continued until the proper depth of color is achieved. The nipple, because of its mobility and contour, is a more difficult structure to tattoo than the areola. If it is especially mobile, it may be necessary to fix it in place with a toothed forceps during the tattoo process. Another option is a multiple jab technique rather than a painting one to color its limited irregular surface. In addition, many nipples have a color tone different from that of the surrounding areolae, the red color associated with vascular erectile tissue often presenting in a subtle or not so subtle fashion. Thus, red pigments can be added to the pigment mix or embedded as pure red tones to enhance the match and realism of the final result. After completion of the tattoo, the treated area is painted with a final surface appliqué of pigment and covered in turn with a greasy dressing, which is left in place for 5 days. After its removal, no special care is required (Fig. 38-4). Occasionally, a patient presents with a subtle, lightly colored opposite areola and it may not be possible to match such faint coloration. A practical solution may be to tattoo both structures with the same pigment, presenting a darker but symmetric final appearance to both. Again, a realistic, eye-catching nipple-areolar reconstruction does much to visually authenticate the overall result of breast reconstruction. Just as a protuberant, projectile nipple aids in this effect, so, within limits, does a darker, more visible areolar coloration.

Secondary Reconstruction

In the past, when nipple reconstruction was wanting in terms of projection, I advocated a nipple pullout technique with a wraparound graft as an expedient to further boost projection.[43] In truth, the small graft required for this technique is not significantly smaller than that required for the full skate elevation. I therefore now prefer to perform the skate technique on top of the failed remnants. It is equally effective atop the remnants of inadequate previous nipple reconstruction by other techniques, flattened remnants after free grafting of the nipple-areola during reduction mammaplasty or subcutaneous mastectomy (Fig. 38-1), and those remaining after nipple-areolar necrosis and loss from any cause (Fig. 38-5). Any surviving areolar elements are included within the design of the skate wings and become components of the final nipple. If there has been intact subjacent nerve supply, the resulting nipple may in fact have erectile properties. The resultant nipple column is frequently misshapen because of the inclusion of existing remnants, but any such untidiness is easily corrected by straightforward tailoring when the tattoo is added.

INVERTED NIPPLE

The volume of literature on the subject of the inverted nipple[49-64] suggests a complexity in its correction that some have not found.[65-67] There are

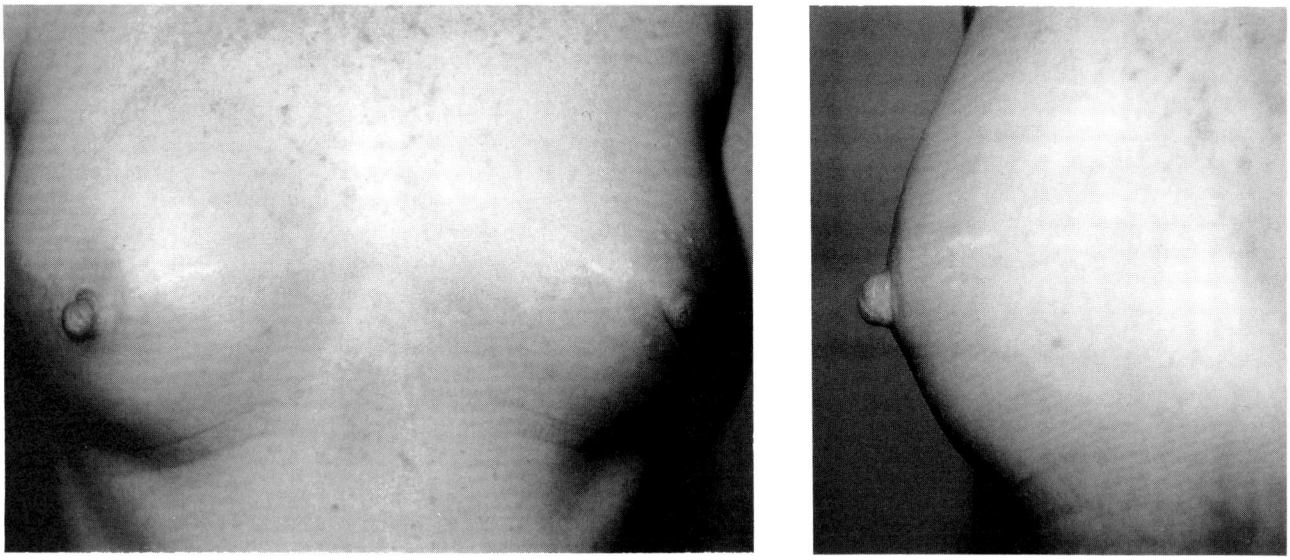

A B

FIGURE 38-4 *A, B,* Late result after right modified radical mastectomy with immediate reconstruction by submuscular prosthesis and subsequent right nipple-areolar reconstruction performed 1 year earlier by the skate technique.

many classifications of the deformity, some indicating whether the nipple inversion is intermittent or constant, others whether the nipple can or cannot be withdrawn into an everted position. The salient aspect of the deformity pertinent to its correction, however, is the integumentary adequacy of the height (or depth, while inverted) of the nipple column. If such height is adequate, the constancy or rigidity of the inversion makes no difference. If, on the other hand, the nipple column is inadequate and poorly formed, its correction to an everted state will reproduce little that is nipple like. In this situation, the best solution remains nipple reconstruction by skate flap atop the inadequate structures. When nipple column height is adequate but inverted, a simple eversion technique suffices.

Correction of Inverted Nipple: The Author's Technique

With the patient supine on the office operating table, the inverted nipple and its areola complex is treated with a local anesthetic and a vasconstrictor, including a portion of the subjacent breast. The nipple is everted to the greatest degree possible and held in this position by a stout, transfixing needle. A lower, hemicircumferential incision is placed at the base of the nipple, cutting full thickness through the areolar skin into subjacent breast. It is necessary to divide nipple ducts with any accompanying congenital or acquired bands in order to achieve satisfactory and lasting eversion. Although this precludes later lactation function, it must be remembered that the uncorrected, inverted nipple is itself an established preventive to breast feeding, so that no existing function is lost. The correction must be seen as essentially aesthetic, because it cannot restore an outlet for lactation. The governing principle in the successful execution of this surgery is that the everted nipple column must possess a volume of retained ductal tissue and breast parenchyma adequate to fill, and preferably exceed, its volumetric capacity after its release from deeper breast elements. The historical error in this technique has been the division of such elements at or near the dermis of the inverted nipple. The resultant empty nipple column has a decided propensity to contract into a flattened or depressed posture, despite efforts to block such recurrence with local tissue transplantations or mechanical sutures. Thus, as the central subjacent core of ductal tissue is divided, it is done so well down into the breast at some distance below the lowest reaches of the inverted nipple cap. This maneuver is performed sharply with the scalpel so that the nipple everts without resistance and remains so after the needle is withdrawn. Because it is unnecessary to divide tissue peripherally near the dermis, the nerve supply and sensation to the nipple remain intact. As the nipple rises with its all-important subjacent plug of breast elements, both are captured in this position with a fine, nonabsorbable, internal "pursestring" suture delicately placed about the periphery of the nipple base, but avoiding direct suturing into the dermis. This single suture is tied loosely with only enough cinch effect to prevent the descent of the

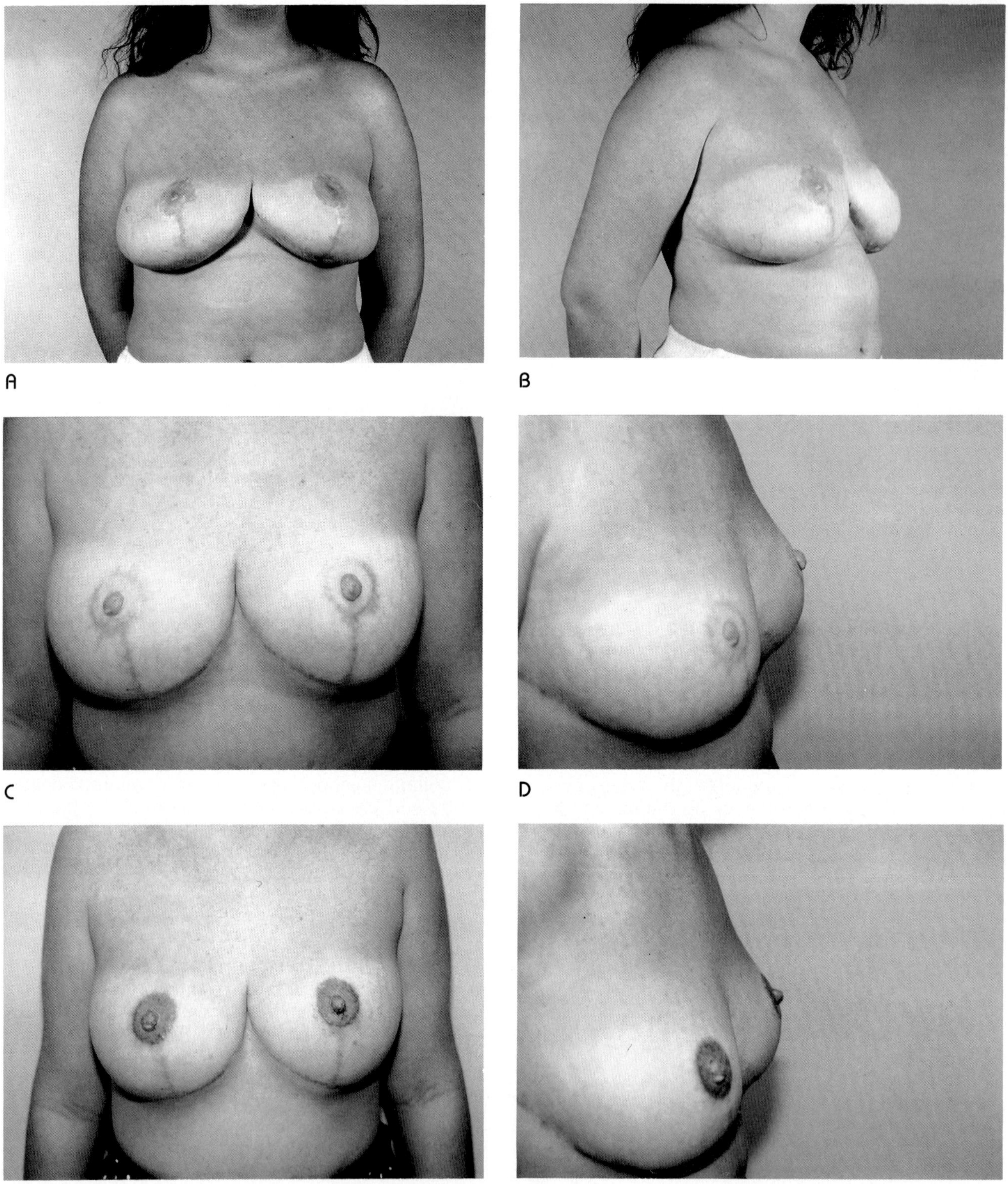

A B C D E F

FIGURE 38–5 Result of inexpert reduction mammaplasty. *A, B,* Flat, splayed breasts with wide scars and overelevated areolae with loss of nipple projection. *C, D,* Six-month results after revision mammaplasties and with skate nipple reconstructions performed over previous remnants. *E, F,* Result immediately after nipple tailoring and tattoo; the nipples are erectile and responsive to stimuli.

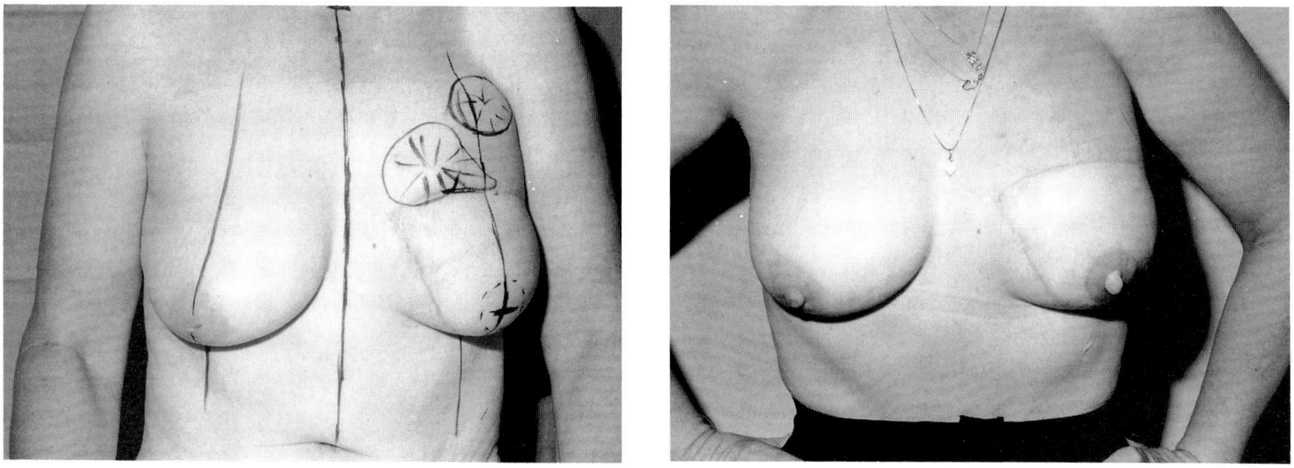

A B

FIGURE 38-6 Inverted nipple, left breast. *A*, Inversion to be corrected during contralateral nipple-areolar reconstruction. *B*, Result after 4 months; skate nipple awaits tailoring and tattoo.

ductal bolus back to its contracted origins. The skin incision is closed with fine interrupted chromic catgut sutures (Fig. 38-6). Hematoma and recurrence of inversion are potential complications, but I have no personal experience with either after this simple maneuver.

CONCLUSION

Nipple-areola reconstruction enhances the realism of breast reconstruction and increases patient satisfaction with the final results. The addition of this symbolic appurtenance is an excellent example of a low-investment, high-yield return in plastic surgery. Since the advent of tattoo coloration over the transplantation of specialized tissues, results have been enhanced and morbidity has essentially been eliminated. Nipple reconstruction by the skate technique provides artistic results that can reliably match any opposite nipple, removing the temptation to alter the remaining structure. Finally, aesthetic correction of the inverted nipple is straightforward.

References

1. Wellisch DK, Schain W, Noone RB, Little JW. The psychological contribution of nipple addition in breast reconstruction. Plast Reconstr Surg 1987; 80:699.
2. Cronin TD, Upton J, McDonough JM. Reconstruction of the breast after mastectomy. Plast Reconstr Surg 1977; 59:1.
3. Klein D. Correction of loss of the areola mammae. Plast Reconstr Surg 1952; 10:469.
4. Millard DR. Nipple and areolar reconstruction by split graft from the normal side. Plast Reconstr Surg 1986; 77:676.
5. Schwartz AW. Reconstruction of the nipple and areola. Br J Plast Surg 1976; 29:230.
6. Wexler MR, O'Neal RN. Areola sharing to reconstruct the absent nipple. Plast Reconstr Surg 1973; 51:176.
7. Broadbent RR, Woolf RH, Metz PS. Restoring the mammary areola by a skin graft from the upper inner thigh. Br J Plast Surg 1977; 30:220.
8. Gruber RP. Method to produce better areolae and nipples on reconstructed breasts. Plast Reconstr Surg 1977; 60:505.
9. Gruber RP. Nipple-areola reconstruction: A review of techniques. Clin Plast Surg 1979; 6:71.
10. Becker H. The use of intradermal tattoo to enhance the final result of nipple-areola reconstruction. Plast Reconstr Surg 1986; 77:673.
11. Conway H, Hugo NW, Tulenko JF, eds. Surgery of tumors of the skin, 2nd ed. Springfield, IL: Charles C Thomas, 1966.
12. Little JW. Discussion of Becker H. The use of intradermal tattoo to enhance the final result of nipple-areola reconstruction. Plast Reconstr Surg 1986; 77:676.
13. Rubin JR. The burned breast. NY State J Med 1975; 75:865.
14. Spear SL, Convit R, Little JW. Intradermal tattoo as an adjunct to nipple-areolar reconstruction. Plast Reconstr Surg 1989; 83:907.
15. Allison AB, Howorth MG Jr. Carcinoma in a nipple preserved for heterotropic auto-implantation. N Engl J Med 1978; 298:1132.
16. Andersen JA, Pallesen RM. Spread to the nipple and areola in carcinoma of the breast. Ann Surg 1979; 189:367.
17. Andersen JA, Gram JB, Pallesen RM. Involvement of the nipple and areola in breast cancer; value of clinical findings. Scand J Plast Reconstr Surg 1981; 15:39.
18. Bouvier B. Problems in breast reconstruction. Med J Aust 1977; 1:937.
19. Lagios MD, Alpert B. Frequency and type of nipple involvement in mammary cancer as a function of tumor location and size. Am J Clin Pathol 1979; 72:648.
20. Quinn RH, Barlow JF. Involvement of the nipple and

areola by carcinoma of the breast. Arch Surg 1981; 116:1139.
21. Rose EH. Carcinoma in a transplanted nipple. Arch Surg 1980; 116:1131.
22. Adams WM. Labial transplant for correction of loss of the nipple. Plast Reconstr Surg 1949; 4:295.
23. Brent B, Bostwick J III. Nipple-areola reconstruction with auricular tissues. Plast Reconstr Surg 1977; 60:353.
24. Cocke WM Jr. Breast reconstruction following mastectomy for carcinoma. Boston: Litle, Brown, 1977.
25. Kiskadden WS. Case report on split grafting of the nipple. Plast Reconstr Surg 1950; 5:184.
26. Klatsky SA, Manson PN. Toe pulp free grafts in nipple reconstruction. Plast Reconstr Surg 1981; 68:245.
27. Rose EH. Nipple reconstruction with four-lobe composite auricular graft. Ann Plast Surg 1985; 15:78.
28. Berson MI. Construction of the pseudoareola. Surgery 1946; 20:808.
29. Basch G, Ramirez M. Reconstruction of the nipple: A new technique. Plast Reconstr Surg 1984; 73:977.
30. Chang WHJ. Nipple reconstruction with a T flap. Plast Reconstr Surg 1984; 73:140.
31. Cohen IK, Ward J. Pinwheel nipple-areolar reconstruction. Plast Reconstr Surg 1986; 77:995.
32. DiPirro EJ. Reconstruction of the nipple and areola after a burn. Plast Reconstr Surg 1970; 46:299.
33. Dubin DB. A new simplified method for nipple reconstruction. Presented at the Annual Meeting of the American Society of Plastic and Reconstructive Surgeons, New Orleans, 1980.
34. Hartrampf C, Culbertson J. A dermal-fat flap for nipple reconstruction. Plast Reconstr Surg 1984; 73:982.
35. Kon M. Two- and three-flap nipple reconstruction. Plast Reconstr Surg 1985; 75:284.
36. Kroll SS, Hamilton S. Nipple reconstruction with the double-opposing-tab flap. Plast Reconstr Surg 1989; 84:520.
37. Little JW, Munasifi T, McCulloch DT. One-stage reconstruction of a projecting nipple: The quadrapod flap. Plast Reconstr Surg 1983; 72:422.
38. Little JW. Nipple reconstruction by quadrapod flaps (letter). Plast Reconstr Surg 1983; 72:422.
39. Little JW. Nipple-areola reconstruction. Clin Plast Surg 1984; 11:351.
40. Little JW. Nipple-areola reconstruction. Adv Plast Surg 1987; 3:43.
41. Little JW, Spear SL. The finishing touches in nipple-areolar reconstruction. Perspect Plast Surg 1988; 2:1.
42. Little JW. Nipple-areolar reconstruction. In: Marsh JL, ed. Current therapy in plastic surgery. Philadelphia: BC Decker, 1989:55.
43. Little JW, Spear SL. Nipple-areolar reconstruction and tattoo. In: Russell RC, ed. Instructional Courses, Vol 2. St Louis: CV Mosby, 1989:199.
44. Muruci D, Jose J, Nogueira LR. Reconstruction of the nipple-areola complex. Plast Reconstr Surg 1978; 61:558.
45. Serafin D, Georgiade M. Nipple-areola reconstruction after mastectomy. Ann Plast Surg 1982; 8:29.
46. Silversmith PE. Nipple reconstruction by quadrapod flaps (letter). Plast Reconstr Surg 1983; 72:422.
47. Snyder CC, Pickens JE, Slater TB. Surgery of the areola-nipple complex. In: Masters FW, Lewis JR, eds. Symposium on aesthetic surgery of the face, eyelid and breast. St Louis: CV Mosby, 1972:192.
48. Becker H, Prysi MF. A new technique for reconstructing Montgomery's tubercles. Plast Reconstr Surg 1990; 86:147.
49. Broadbent TR, Woolf RM. Benign inverted nipple, trans-nipple-areolar correction. Plast Reconstr Surg 1976; 58:1.
50. D'Assumpcao EA, Rosa EM. Correcting the inverted nipple. Br J Plast Surg 1977; 30:249.
51. Elsahy NJ. An alternative operation for inverted nipples. Plast Reconstr Surg 1976; 57:436.
52. Elsahy NJ. Correction of deformed areola and nipple. Acta Chir Plast (Praha) 1977; 19:224.
53. Gangal JT, Gangal MH. Suction method for correcting flat nipples or inverted nipples. Plast Reconstr Surg 1978; 61:294.
54. Goodman RM, Bonne-Tamir B, Ashbel S, et al. Genetic studies in a family with inverted nipples (mamillae invertitia). Clin Genet 1979; 15:346.
55. Herman GE. Kehrer's operation for depressed nipple. Lancet 1889; 2:12.
56. LaMont E. Congenital inversion of the nipple in identical twins. Br J Plast Surg 1973; 26:178.
57. Letterman G, Schurter M. The surgical correction of inverted nipples. South Med J 1967; 60:724.
58. Otte MJ. Correcting inverted nipples—an aid to breast feeding. Am J Nursing 1975; 75:454.
59. Schwager RG, Smith JW, Gray GF, et al. Inversion of the human female nipple, with a simple method of treatment. Plast Reconstr Surg 1974; 54:564.
60. Skoog T. An operation for inverted nipples. Br J Plast Surg 1953; 5:65.
61. Skoog T. Surgical correction of inverted nipples. J Am Med Wom Assoc 1965; 20:931.
62. Spina V. Inverted nipple. Plast Reconstr Surg 1957; 19:63.
63. Teimourian B, Adham MH. Simple technique for correction of inverted nipple. Plast Reconstr Surg 1980; 65:504.
64. Wolfort FG, Marshal KA, Cochran TC. Correction of the inverted nipple. Ann Plast Surg 1978; 1:294.
65. Bostwick J. Plastic and reconstructive breast surgery. St Louis: Quality Medical Publishing, 1990:487.
66. Hamilton JM. Inverted nipples. Plast Reconstr Surg 1980; 65:507.
67. Hartrampf CR, Schneider WJ. A simple direct method for correction of inversion of the nipple. Plast Reconstr Surg 1976; 58:678.

CHAPTER 39

Salvage Mastectomy and Reconstruction

SUMNER A. SLAVIN, M.D.

Conservative surgery and radiotherapy have gained widespread recognition as effective treatment for early-stage breast cancer. Both retrospective[1-7] and prospective[8-10] studies have demonstrated that this combination of conservative therapies is an acceptable alternative to mastectomy, in terms of both the equivalent survival rates provided and the local tumor control achieved.[11-14] It is likely that breast-conserving surgery and radiotherapy will be used with increasing frequency as patients seek to avoid the mutilation of mastectomy and gain an optimal cosmetic result. The growing popularity of this approach poses certain unique reconstructive challenges for plastic surgeons. Two important clinical entities have emerged from breast-sparing regimens: (1) the patient with a breast that has been reduced and altered by one or more local excisions and (2) the patient with cancer recurrence in a previously irradiated breast. Plastic surgeons need to study these vastly different situations in order to develop the most appropriate reconstructive solutions for each.

COSMETIC RESULTS AFTER CONSERVATIVE SURGERY AND RADIOTHERAPY

In general, the long-term cosmetic results after conservative surgery and radiation therapy have been extremely satisfying.[15-17] Earlier reports that evaluated patients 3 years after treatment noted that 86 percent had a good to excellent scored cosmetic result. More recently the long-term results at 7 and 10 years after initial treatment have become available,[18] indicating that 90 to 95 percent of patients have either acceptable or very good cosmetic results at 10 years. Previous fears regarding the long-term stability of an early favorable cosmetic appearance have not proved justified. Researchers have noted, however, that a constellation of physical findings consisting primarily of breast edema, retraction, and telangiectasia formation can adversely affect the cosmetic outcome. The chronology of change is different for each component: breast edema usually occurs within the first year of treatment and improves with further evolution of healing, usually over a period of 4 to 8 years; in contrast, retraction and telangiectasia formation occur later but remain unchanged after 3 and 7 years.

More than any other single factor, tumor size influences the final cosmetic outcome. Significant degrees of breast deformity result when progressively larger resections of breast tissue are necessitated. Clearly, at some as yet undetermined point, extensive local resection exceeds the aesthetic boundaries that are the cornerstone of breast conservation. Reconstruction of these partial mastectomy defects, discussed later in this chapter, is a complex problem.

LOCAL RECURRENCE

Because neither mastectomy nor conservative surgery coupled with radiation therapy can exert any therapeutic influence on existing distant metastases, local tumor control has received considerable attention as the singular measure of treatment success. The concept of local recurrence is defined in terms of cancer reappearance on or about the involved breast. From a prognostic point of view, local recurrence after conservative surgery and radiation is associated with a more substantially improved outlook than is recurrence after mastectomy.[19] The principal factors influencing the development of a recurrence have been identified as (1) the extent of the original breast surgery, especially whether the gross excision of the tumor was complete or incomplete; (2) the histologic features of the tumor; and (3) the dose of radiation therapy. For patients with early stage breast cancer (clinical Stages I and II), local recurrence rates after lumpectomy or wider excision have been 5 to 10 percent in most series at 5 years.[12, 20–23] However, recurrences develop as late as 15 years after this combined therapy.

Diagnosis of Recurrence

When local relapse does occur, it is characteristically within the breast and has been identifiable by either physical examination or mammography in most cases.[24] In approximately 25 percent of patients, mammography may be the only means of detecting these relapses. Clinical examination and mammography tend to detect different manifestations of recurrence; invasive carcinomas were more likely to be found on physical examination, whereas intraductal carcinoma relapses or tumors with minimal or no invasive features were detected principally by mammography.

Detection of a relapse requires careful inspection of sites other than within the breast parenchyma. The most common extraparenchymal sites have included the cutaneous surface of the breast, associated axillary lymph nodes, and contiguous areas of chest wall. Fibrotic changes on the surface of the breast, induced by either radiation therapy or surgery, can potentially obscure the visible and palpable evidence of breast cancer recurrence (Fig. 39-1). Most of these relapses are attributed to a failure of control of the original tumor. Recurring lesions are generally considered to represent de novo tumor growth when they are discovered in quadrants different from the original.

Biopsy is mandated in all situations, not only to establish the specific histologic characteristics of the recurrence, but also to assist in identification of the rare radiation-induced sarcoma that can appear in this scenario.

Prognosis After Recurrence

Unlike local recurrence after mastectomy, which may be associated with distant metastases in 25 to 50 percent of patients at the time of diagnosis, failure after conservative surgery and radiotherapy carries a much better prognosis. For patients in whom the recurrence consists primarily of noninvasive disease, the prognosis is particularly excellent. Several series have demonstrated that 45 to 70 percent of all patients with evidence of relapse were alive at 5 years, and half were free of distant disease.[26–30] These favorable statistics are substantiated by a fail-

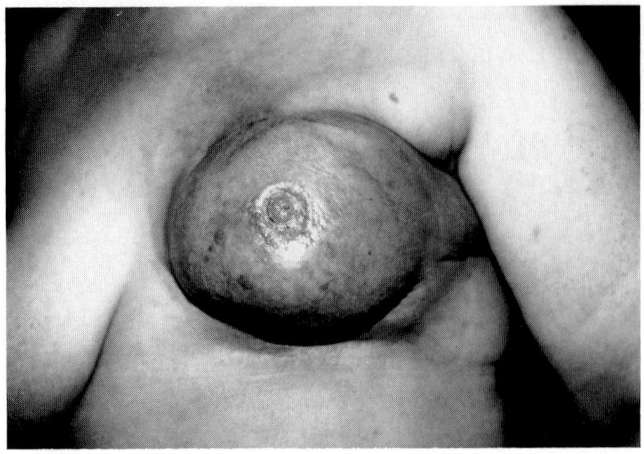

FIGURE 39-1 This 56-year-old woman had undergone lumpectomy and radiation therapy for infiltrating ductal carcinoma. She developed postradiation changes consisting of edema, retraction, and skin ulceration, which initially obscured recurrent breast cancer. A biopsy of the ulcerated periareolar area demonstrated tumor cells.

ure to identify any distant metastases later than 6 years after the initial recurrence. The yearly risk of a recurrence (approximately 1 percent per year) tends to be an isolated event in all but a small fraction of patients.

Most inoperable failures of treatment occur early. Other factors associated with a grim prognosis include a relapse occurring in the context of extensive locoregional disease, or manifesting an aggressive tumor biology. Also, patients who on initial presentation had pathologically positive lymph nodes have a worsened prognosis. However, if axillary lymph nodes are involved at the time of recurrence, the effect on survival appears to be negligible. Similarly, the size of the recurrent tumor is not known to be a predictive factor. With these circumstances as exceptions, most patients with relapse, as many as 75 to 88 percent in some series, will be either cured or palliated by repeat wide excision or salvage mastectomy. Some authors have suggested that the survival of patients with isolated local recurrences lacking histologic evidence of invasion (or having only minimal invasion) who are treated with a secondary surgical procedure is essentially equivalent to the survival of patients who have never relapsed.

Treatment After Recurrence: Role of Salvage Mastectomy

In view of these optimistic survival statistics, most patients with recurrence should be considered favorable candidates for salvage mastectomy and plastic surgical reconstruction.[31] After salvage mastectomy for breast relapse, up to 80 percent of patients appear disease free for follow-up periods extending to 67 months. Certainly, these statistics are superior to those achieved for patients with local (chest wall) recurrence after mastectomy, in whom a disease-free survival exceeding 5 years is uncommon. In other series, the 5-year recurrence rate was 37 percent for 65 patients undergoing salvage mastectomy and has been reported to be as low as 12 percent. Evaluation of these results reveals that the single most important factor determining the success of salvage mastectomy was the histologic features of the recurrent tumor: patients with predominantly noninvasive lesions or minimal focal invasion had no further recurrences. Unfortunately, patients with infiltrating tumors suffered from a 38 percent incidence of locoregional recurrence or distant disease.

Postoperative complications after salvage mastectomy appear to be unusual, judging by the paucity of such reports.[32] Delayed wound healing has been described, but the frequency of this complication is less than might be expected in this group of patients with significant antecedent radiation to the breast. The few reports of delayed wound healing described trauma to the chest wall with the subsequent formation of nonhealing ulcers. Similarly, the complication rate following wide local excision has been extremely low.[33] The application of myocutaneous flaps for the reconstruction of both partial and complete mastectomy defects is discussed later in this chapter.

Salvage Mastectomy Versus Wide Excision

It is not yet clear whether salvage mastectomy or wide surgical excision is the superior treatment in terms of subsequent locoregional control or survival. Insofar as breast cosmesis may have been a critical influencing factor in the initial treatment selection, it is not surprising that patients seeking a salvage procedure might prefer wide excision over mastectomy. In some series, patients either have refused mastectomy or were assessed as medically inoperable.[24] Of 55 patients treated with wide (wedge) excision at the Marseilles Cancer Institute, the survival rate was 79 percent at 5 years and 66 percent at 8 years. Although eight patients developed further recurrences, five were able to undergo successful local control by repeat excision. Other authors have confirmed the ability of repeated wedge excision to control local disease and compare favorably with survival achieved by salvage mastectomy.[34] These investigators noted that the risk of a future recurrence in the breast after reexcision approximates that of segmental mastectomy (36 percent at 5 years). Given the low probability of subsequent chest wall recurrence after either salvage mastectomy or salvage wide excision—12 percent at 5 years—patients with a particular concern for breast preservation may choose the lesser procedure. For small, well-localized recurrences, wide excision has gained increased popularity.

Wide local excision may be less advantageous for patients with multicentric disease at the time of relapse. It has been theorized, but not substantiated, that wide excision could prove to be inadequate treatment for this particular group of patients. The incidence of histologic multicentricity in mastectomy specimens obtained at salvage mastectomy has ranged from 14 to 22 percent.[35] On the basis of this information, it might be possible to determine the feasibility of wide local excision in terms of the presence or absence of multicentric breast disease. In uncertain situations when the clinical or radiologic evidence is inconclusive, salvage mastectomy should be the treatment of choice. Although the histologic presence of predominantly invasive disease in the relapsed area has been demonstrated to affect survival, it is not known whether tumor histology is a determinant for the selection of a specific salvage procedure. Therefore, the ultimate treatment choice for salvage remains controversial. At the Joint Center for Radiation Therapy in Boston, mastectomy has been preferred for operable candidates in whom conservative surgery and radiation have failed.[19]

Other centers have reported similar experiences with and preference for salvage mastectomy rather than repeated wedge resection.[31] Of 27 patients successfully treated for recurrence, 25 underwent salvage mastectomy and two had wide excision. There were only two subsequent local failures in this group. The small numbers of patients in each category (salvage mastectomy and wide excision) precluded a definitive opinion regarding the efficacy of the respective techniques. The authors concluded that both techniques provided a high salvage rate for patients experiencing failure after initial conservative excision and radiotherapy.

Role of Adjuvant Therapy for Recurrence

In addition to salvage mastectomy and repeat wide excision, consideration has been given to the potential role of chemotherapy after local recurrence. There is little, if any, information regarding the use of chemotherapy, either in conjunction with a salvage procedure or in substitution for it. No discernible differences in outcome with or without chemotherapy have been observed.[19] However, metastatic carcinoma has been found in four of 11 patients in whom ipsilateral axillary sampling was performed at the time of the recurrence.[27] Perhaps patients with a high risk of metastatic disease might benefit from systemic therapy. Possible candidates for such treatment could include those with positive axillary nodes at the time of breast failure; evidence of muscle, blood vessel, or lymphatic invasion; or skin involvement. In addition, any patient with an aggressive tumor biology might be a reasonable candidate for chemotherapy.

It is difficult to find data regarding further treatment of local recurrence with radiation therapy. Certainly, such treatment could be expected to affect breast cosmesis adversely. Other complications such as ulceration, skin necrosis, or osteonecrosis are feared possibilities. The concomitant use of a myocutaneous flap at the time of salvage mastectomy would, theoretically, present an opportunity for further radiation therapy. A few patients have undergone additional courses of radiation to the myocutaneous flap breast reconstruction site.[37] Although none have developed ulcerations or osteonecrosis, the skin and soft tissues of the flap react in a manner similar to a radiated breast; most of the changes observed have consisted of cutaneous thickening, hyperpigmentation, subcutaneous fibrosis, and capsular fibrosis in patients with myocutaneous flaps covering an accompanying breast implant. No breakdown of previously healed areas has occurred, nor has there been extrusion of implants situated beneath a radiated flap. Whether additional radiation therapy after salvage mastectomy will prove to be effective remains to be determined; its feasibility, in the context of salvage mastectomy and myocutaneous flap reconstruction, is suggested by the few cases studied.

SELECTION OF PATIENTS AND INDICATIONS FOR SURGERY

Much concern has been expressed over which patients are appropriate candidates for salvage mastectomy and reconstruction. Clearly, evidence described earlier in this chapter suggests that most patients in whom conservative surgery and radiation have failed will be alive 5 years after salvage surgery, and half will be free of disease. The data following salvage mastectomy indicate that this palliative and sometimes life-saving procedure should be offered to all Stage I and II patients. Stage III patients can also be treated with a salvage operation, which if necessary can be performed in conjunction with additional chemotherapy or radiation therapy.[37] Therefore, it appears that patients whose anatomy permits myocutaneous flap reconstruction and whose constitution will tolerate it are all potential candidates for this technique. There is scant evidence to exclude from eligibility either diabetic patients or those who smoke.[38, 39]

The presence of ulceration or osteoradionecrosis in association with local recurrence has not precluded salvage mastectomy and reconstruction with myocutaneous flaps. Even extensive radiation-induced fibrosis and thickening of the cutaneous surface of an entire hemithorax (and beyond) have proved amenable to this approach. More than any other factor, the advent of the myocutaneous flap era has provided an opportunity for the safe performance of salvage mastectomy and concomitant reconstruction.

Preoperative Evaluation

Most patients requiring salvage mastectomy for local recurrence need either a latissimus dorsi or a rectus abdominis myocutaneous flap to reconstruct the resulting postmastectomy defect. These patients should be evaluated for the feasibility of either type of procedure. The involved breast should be carefully examined to determine the extent of radiation injury to both ipsilateral and contralateral cutaneous surfaces. Measurements of the anticipated defect aid in selecting the proper single flap or determining the possible need for multiple flaps.

The tumor recurrence site is an important determinant of the ultimate aesthetic result. Tumors located in either a periareolar position or anywhere along the lower pole of the breast can be included in a standard mastectomy incision that allows preservation of infraclavicular and supra-areolar native skin of the chest wall. Recurrences in superior, superomedial, or superolateral locations mandate sacrifice of skin in those areas in order to ensure complete inclusion of the lesion. Under these circumstances, the entire reconstruction is unavoidably shifted to a medial, superior, or lateral location that compromises the aesthetic result. In general, salvage mastectomy tends to encompass generous skin borders for two reasons: first, there is a need to extend the excision beyond the zone of radiated skin to new, healthier, margins; second, the procedure seeks to eradicate the local recurrence and eliminate any further tumor reappearance in the wound.

The chest wall should be inspected for evidence of injury to either the pectoralis major or the ipsilateral and contralateral latissimus muscles. These latter structures can be tested for denervation or diminished contractility. Pectoralis major muscle atrophy implies that the flap selected must serve the dual purposes of chest wall and breast reconstruction. Evidence of osteoradionecrosis, noted not only on physical examination but also on chest x-ray and chest computed tomography (CT), may require reconstruction with prosthetic material for enhanced chest wall integrity. It is unusual to resort to angiographic evaluation of the thorocodorsal or deep superior epigastric arterial pedicle in the absence of a previous procedure that could have caused interruption; conservative surgery and radiation therapy do not usually cause major pedicle compromise.

Similarly, physical examination should rule out the myriad potential contraindications to rectus abdominis flap surgery, including subcostal and midline incisions, lower abdominal (cesarean and hysterectomy) scars, hernias, or areas of weakness. Subcostal incisions in particular may transgress the midline at a subcutaneous level, thus compromising the respective vascular pedicles of both rectus muscles. In view of the extreme importance of flap viability in a radiated setting, any suspected unilateral injury to the deep epigastric arterial system makes it wise to base the flap on the other, healthy side. When this choice does not exist, a preoperative presumption of either vascular unity or disruption may require confirmation by angiography.

CHOICE OF SURGICAL TECHNIQUE

Latissimus Dorsi Myocutaneous Flap

For over a decade, this workhorse of myocutaneous flaps has proved a reliable source of well-vascularized skin, soft tissue, and muscle.[40-43] It is usually available for salvage mastectomy reconstruction except in situations, such as radical mastectomy, that can endanger its vascular supply. Various authors have documented the area of transposition of this flap,[44] extending beyond the ipsilateral chest wall to neck, sternum, and contralateral hemithorax. More recently, the contralateral latissimus flap was shown to reach the opposite chest wall, a feat of transposition not originally thought possible.[45] Use of the latissimus dorsi myocutaneous flap as a free flap unit[46] or in combination as an extended myocutaneous flap/free flap complex[47] has been applied to the radiated defect intrinsic to salvage mastectomy.

In terms of advantages, this flap uniquely provides a large surface area of muscle for coverage of the chest wall. As an adjunct to other flaps, such as the rectus, it can supplement difficult closure problems adjacent to clavicle or axilla. The extraordinary vascularity and resilience of the muscular component allows the inclusion of an implant in wounds characterized by severe postradiation changes (Fig. 39-2).

The skin island is, however, more restrictive. It has the disadvantage of not permitting bilateral flap elevation because of the lateral decubitus positioning requirement. Even in the more common situation of unilateral salvage mastectomy and breast reconstruction, the use of a latissimus flap usually requires repositioning of the patient from a supine position for mastectomy to a lateral decubitus position for flap elevation. Occasionally, both the mastectomy and the latissimus flap elevation can be performed with the patient in a lateral decubitus position, necessitating only one intraoperative repositioning for insetting and contouring of the flap on the chest wall after flap transposition and closure of the donor site has been performed.

In my experience,[37] flap necrosis or even partial necrosis is unusual. Seroma predominates as the most commonly encountered complication, occurring in 10 to 20 percent of patients and almost always confined to the back donor site. Back donor site dehiscence, a complication that causes significant morbidity because of the resultant prolonged delay in wound healing, has also been an extremely infrequent problem, noted in only one patient. Implant migration and extrusion have been rare, despite the unfavorable conditions attendant on these radiated wounds. Similarly, there has been virtually no need for blood transfusion; the salvage mastectomy tends to be a bloodless procedure performed in a vascularly depleted, radiation-fibrosed field.

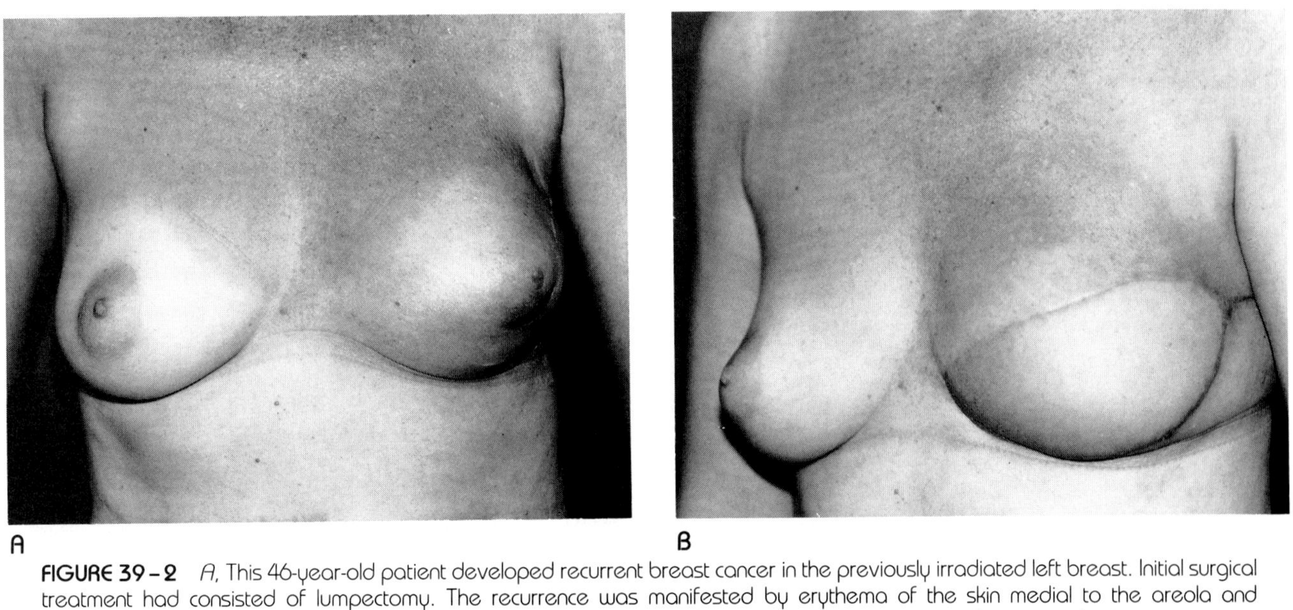

A B

FIGURE 39-2 *A,* This 46-year-old patient developed recurrent breast cancer in the previously irradiated left breast. Initial surgical treatment had consisted of lumpectomy. The recurrence was manifested by erythema of the skin medial to the areola and palpable subcutaneous thickening. *B,* After salvage mastectomy for the recurrent breast cancer, a latissimus dorsi myocutaneous flap, including an implant placed beneath it, were used to reconstruct the defect. Uncomplicated healing ensued, unaffected by placement of a foreign body (implant). The excellent vascularity of the expansive latissimus dorsi muscle is a reliable choice in such situations.

Rectus Abdominis Myocutaneous Flap

The rectus abdominis myocutaneous flap, pioneered and developed by a number of contributors,[48–54] has been recognized as a safe and reliable source of well-vascularized autogenous tissues. Unlike the more restrictive donor area of the latissimus dorsi myocutaneous flap, the rectus flap can incorporate an extensive cutaneous surface area from the middle and lower abdomen. Previous authors[55,56] have conceived a myriad of flap designs, extending from the epigastric skin to the most inferior portions of the abdomen. Because of the abundance of periumbilical perforating vessels from the deep epigastric arterial system located there, the midabdominal cutaneous island, with or without an extension of lower abdominal skin, has become popular.[57]

The rectus abdominis myocutaneous flap is particularly well suited for salvage mastectomy and breast reconstruction. Its attributes include not only a large cutaneous surface area, but also a superbly vascularized muscle whose transposition arc extends equally well to ipsilateral or contralateral hemithorax. This outstanding vascularity permits application of the flap to patients with a history of radiation therapy. More complex reconstruction problems, including osteoradionecrosis of rib and sternum, often in association with recurrent tumor and infection, are appropriate for this technique. Although a single pedicled transverse rectus flap possesses an excellent blood supply, some have augmented its vascularity by inclusion of the other muscle.[58] This double-pedicled rectus flap (Fig. 39–3) can resurface most of the hemithorax and beyond. For many plastic surgeons, either the single- or the double-pedicled transverse rectus flap is the one of choice when breast cancer recurs after conservative surgery and radiation therapy.

The use of a rectus abdominis microvascular free flap has been proposed for immediate breast reconstruction patients.[59,60] Data about large series of previously radiated patients undergoing salvage mastectomy and reconstruction is lacking, but there are individual reports of success under these circumstances. The free transverse rectus flap allows preservation of innervated rectus muscle both medially and laterally. Its blood supply from the deep inferior epigastric arterial system surpasses that of the superiorly based pedicled rectus flap. Other advantages include enhanced abdominal wall integrity and strength, decreased abdominal native flap undermining, and improved aesthetic contouring. Previous radiation therapy has not precluded anastomosis of the flap vessels to either thorocodorsal or internal mammary recipients.

Complications[61–63] among patients undergoing rectus flap breast reconstruction after salvage mastectomy have included flap loss, partial necrosis, delayed healing, infection, bleeding, hernia, seroma, umbilical necrosis, fat necrosis, pseudocyst formation,[64] and a need for blood transfusion. There has also been concern that a rectus flap procedure might adversely affect labor or vaginal delivery in patients of childbearing age and capability. A recent report of a normal delivery in a patient who had a rectus flap breast reconstruction at least partially allays these fears.[59]

Finally, it is important to note that the rectus flap salvage patients, like those with latissimus flap

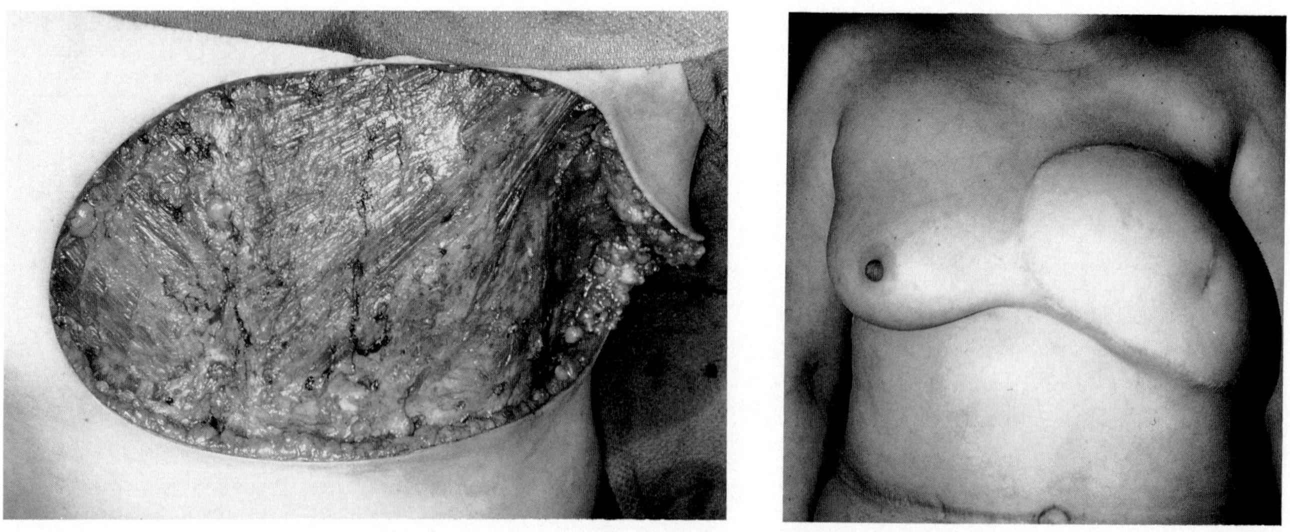

A B

FIGURE 39–3 *A*, A 32-year-old woman with inflammatory breast cancer required salvage mastectomy after failed chemotherapy and radiation therapy. The mastectomy defect was extensive, necessitated by diffuse tumor growth. *B*, A large, double-pedicled midabdominal rectus abdominis myocutaneous flap, measuring 16 by 42 cm, provided the necessary cutaneous and muscular tissues for resurfacing most of the left hemithorax, including the presternal area.

salvage, can potentially be given further radiation treatment to the reconstructed breast and chest wall area. Unfortunately, there are neither controlled studies nor reports of long-term follow-up in these isolated cases.

Chemotherapy can also be administered to patients after salvage mastectomy and rectus flap reconstruction, but again data are lacking regarding the efficacy of such treatment.

Salvage Mastectomy and Free Flap Reconstruction

Sometimes neither the latissimus dorsi nor the rectus abdominis myocutaneous flap is available for reconstruction after salvage mastectomy. This situation most commonly occurs when the muscle and its associated blood supply have been divided by previous operations or injured by radiation therapy. The use of microvascular free flaps, harvested from the gluteus maximus muscle and based on the superior gluteal artery, has been proposed for this situation.[65-67] Among the advantages of this donor site are its general availability and the provision of substantial soft tissues that resemble the fatty composition of normal breast tissue. Proponents claim that a flap of excellent vascularity and aesthetic quality is created by this technique. Unfortunately, thrombosis of the venous anastomosis has been a significant problem, culminating in flap loss. Most of these flaps have not been used in a previously irradiated wound, nor has use of the flap for salvage mastectomy been well established.

In addition to the free gluteus maximus flap, the groin, contralateral latissimus, and tensor fascia lata free flaps have been described.[68] Flap loss has also occurred in these patients, especially when previously radiated axillary vessels were chosen for the microvascular anastomoses. Patients with stigmata of radiation injury, including cutaneous fibrosis, brachial plexus neuropathy, and clavicular or sternal osteoradionecrosis, should alert the plastic surgeon to the increased risk of microvascular thrombosis. Most authors have recommended strict avoidance of vessels lying within the radiation zone of injury; selection of healthy vessels outside the radiated zone becomes essential under these conditions. Alternative suitable vessels may be found in the neck or even the face, where branches of the external carotid artery and facial vein offer a better chance of success.

Despite the impressive advances of microsurgery over the past decade, the feasibility of free flap breast reconstruction after salvage mastectomy has not been proved in any large series. The prolonged operating room time needed for this type of reconstruction constitutes a potential disadvantage, as does the 3 to 5 percent incidence of flap loss. With further experience, however, this technique could graduate from a choice of last resort to a reliable optional source of healthy autogenous tissue.

DETECTION OF BREAST CANCER RECURRENCE AFTER SALVAGE MASTECTOMY

The issue of breast cancer surveillance and detection after salvage mastectomy for failed conservative surgery and radiation is an important one for plastic surgeons. Most studies[69-71] have focused on the subject of immediate reconstruction, usually with submuscular implants or inflatable expanders, and generally performed on patients who have not received antecedent radiation therapy. These reports have shown that neither survival nor cancer recurrence rates are affected by immediate reconstruction in this group of primarily clinical Stage I and II patients. In addition, the performance of immediate reconstruction did not impede treatment of primary or secondary disease. Concerns that immediate reconstruction might delay diagnosis or compromise the treatment of locoregional recurrence were not realized. Overall, these authors concluded that immediate reconstruction with implants and expanders is a safe option that is compatible with optimal cancer management.

However reassuring this may be, little information is available on the fate of patients undergoing salvage mastectomy and reconstruction with myocutaneous flaps. Does the presence of a myocutaneous flap conceal a recurrence or delay its recognition? This question, partially answered by anecdotal reports or limited series,[12,19] is currently under investigation.[37] Patterns of locoregional recurrence were reviewed in patients who underwent salvage mastectomy and immediate myocutaneous flap breast reconstruction for invasive breast carcinoma. Preliminary findings showed that recurrences develop in axillary and supraclavicular nodes, and most commonly in the native skin flaps of the chest wall that border the flap reconstruction. All such recurrences were clinically detectable. To date, not a single recurrence appears to have been hidden by the flap. On the basis of this evidence, it appears that salvage mastectomy and reconstruction for invasive breast cancer using either rectus or latissimus flaps (with and without implants) not only provides the requisite well-vascularized soft tissues for previously radiated breast and chest wall areas, but also does not compromise the diagnosis and treatment of further recurrence.

Finally, the psychological benefits that patients derive from immediate reconstruction, in the context of either primary breast cancer therapy or salvage mastectomy, deserve mention.[72,73] There is ample documentation of the improved adaptation and enhanced satisfaction with body image that follow breast reconstruction. Certainly, the salvage mastectomy patient, whose initial attempt to preserve her breast has been unsuccessful, is in great need of the psychological advantages provided by immediate breast reconstruction.

POSTQUADRANTECTOMY BREAST DEFORMITY

Although the most commonly encountered reconstructive problem among breast cancer patients after failed conservative surgery and radiation is the postsalvage mastectomy defect, there is an increasing number of patients with a variant of this condition that has become known as the postquadrantectomy deformity.[74] Quadrantectomy represents an extension of the concept of wide excision for recurrence. Essentially synonymous with other resection terms such as partial mastectomy, segmentectomy, and extended tylectomy, this procedure usually denotes excision of an entire quadrant of the breast along with the skin overlying it and the associated deep border of pectoralis muscle fascia. This technique, which has gained popularity in Europe,[75] has supplanted lumpectomy and radiation therapy in some centers. Because it involves removal of portions of skin and glandular tissues in excess of most wide excisions, the defect can be a formidable one. In addition, the presence of the residual breast components, altered in varying degrees by radiation therapy and subsequent fibrosis, creates a reconstructive challenge often more complex than a postmastectomy defect.

The range and variety of reconstructive problems have been classified under four categories: Type I, distortion and dislocation of the nipple-areola complex; Type II, deformity characterized by localized skin and subcutaneous and glandular tissue deficiency; Type III, breast retraction; and Type IV, the severely radiated breast associated with marked radiation-induced changes of skin, subcutaneous tissue, and breast parenchyma. For each group, a specific reconstructive procedure has been recommended. Type I patients respond to placement of subpectoral implants and revision of long linear scars with Z-plasties or the addition of local flaps. Type II patients are treated with the addition of a myocutaneous flap, most commonly a latissimus, to correct the cutaneous and glandular abnormalities. For Type III problems, the author has recommended submuscular augmentation. For Type IV deformities (the most severe), flap reconstruction with either a latissimus or rectus flap is effective. Unfortunately, the authors did not provide information regarding results and complications of these various reconstructive solutions. Of 54 patients, many (81 percent) were assessed as needing some reconstructive procedure. In this scenario of significant tissue loss and heavy irradiation (6,000 rads), it would seem risky to attempt local flap transpositions or major scar revisions in previously radiated areas. Myocutaneous flap reconstruction, preferably with the adjacent latissimus dorsi muscle, is the logical procedure for well-vascularized donor tissues. In view of the myriad appearances of postquadrantectomy deformities, latissimus dorsi myocutaneous flaps incorporating varying amounts of skin and muscle can provide successful customized solutions.

From a technical point of view, it is important initially to resect scar and fibrotic breast tissues in order to establish the entirety of the defect. Skin islands should always be designed in excess of the defect (at least twice the size) so that some portions can be de-epithelialized and buried if necessary. Some areas of skin may have altered integrity as the procedure progresses; it may become necessary to debride marginal skin edges and supply greater surfaces of skin than were originally measured. The latissimus muscle can be taken in its entirety, or portions left with an intact hemineurovasculature. Folding and sculpting of the muscle is ideal for these partial defects.

It is difficult to find any reports documenting impeded detection of future recurrence in this population of patients after myocutaneous flap breast reconstruction. However, regular physical examination and mammography are absolutely essential. In the author's experience, the detection of local recurrence has not been a problem.

References

1. Amalric R, Santamaria F, Robert F, et al. Radiation therapy with or without primary limited surgery for operable breast cancer. A 20-year experience at the Marseilles Cancer Institute. Cancer 1982; 49:30–34.
2. Bedwinek J, Perez C, Kramer S, et al. Irradiation as the primary management of stage I and II adenocarcinoma of the breast: Analysis of the RTOG breast surgery. Cancer Clin Trials 1980; 3:11–18.
3. Calle R, Vilcoqu JR, Pilleron JP, et al. Conservative management of operable breast carcinoma by irradiation with or without limited surgery—ten-year results. In: Harris JR, Hellman S, Silen W, eds. Conservative management of breast cancer. Philadelphia: JB Lippincott, 1983:3–9.
4. Chu A, Cope O, Russo R, et al. Treatment of early stage breast cancer by limited surgery and radical irradiation. Int J Radiat Oncol Biol Phys 1980; 6:25–30.
5. Clark RM, Wilkinson RH, Mahoney LJ, et al. Breast cancer. A 21-year experience with conservative surgery and radiation. Int J Radiat Oncol Biol Phys 1982; 8:967–975.
6. Harris JR, Botnick LE, Bloomer WD, et al. Primary radiation therapy for early breast cancer. The experience at the Joint Center for Radiation Therapy. Int J Radiat Oncol Biol Phys 1981; 7:1549–1559.
7. Montague ED, Ames FC, Schell SR, et al. Conservative

surgery and irradiation as an alternative to mastectomy in the treatment of clinically favorable breast cancer. Cancer 1984; 54:2668-2672.
8. Osborne MP, Ormiston N, Harmer CL, et al. Breast conservation in the treatment of early breast cancer. A 20-year follow-up. Cancer 1984; 53:349-355.
9. Pierquin B, Owen R, Mayiin C, et al. Radical radiation therapy of breast cancer. Int J Radiat Oncol Biol Phys 1980; 6:17-24.
10. Prosnitz LR, Goldenberg JS, Packard RA, et al. Radiation therapy as initial treatment for early stage cancer of the breast without mastectomy. Cancer 1977; 39:917-923.
11. Romsdahl MM, Montague ED, Ames FC, et al. Conservation surgery and irradiation as treatment for early breast cancer. Arch Surg 1983; 118:521-528.
12. Recht A, Silver B, Schnitt S, et al. Breast relapse following primary radiation therapy for early breast cancer: I. Classification, frequency, and salvage. Int J Radiat Oncol Biol Phys 1985; 11:1271-1276.
13. Sarrazin D, Le M, Rouesse J, et al. Conservative treatment versus mastectomy in breast cancer with macroscopic diameter of 20 millimeters or less. The experience of the Institut Gustave-Roussy. Cancer 1984; 53:1209-1213.
14. Veronesi U, DelVecchio M, Greco M, et al. Results of quadrantectomy, axillary dissection, and radiotherapy (QUART) in T_1N_0 patients. In: Harris JR, Hellman S, Silen W, eds. Conservative management of breast cancer. Philadelphia: JB Lippincott, 1983:91-99.
15. Beadle GF, Silver B, Botnick L, et al. Cosmetic results following primary radiation therapy for early breast cancer. Cancer 1984; 54:2911-2918.
16. Ray GR, Fish VJ. Biopsy and definitive radiation therapy in stage I and II adenocarcinoma of the female breast: Analysis of cosmesis and the role of electron beam supplementation. Int J Radiat Oncol Biol Phys 1983; 9:813-818.
17. Clarke D, Martinez A, Cox RS. Analysis of cosmetic results and complications in patients with stage I and II breast cancer treated by biopsy and irradiation. Int J Radiat Oncol Biol Phys 1983; 9:1807-1813.
18. Rose MA, Olivotto R, Cady B, et al. Conservative surgery and radiation therapy for early breast cancer. Long-term cosmetic results. Arch Surg 1989; 124:153-157.
19. Recht A, Hayes DF. Specific sites and emergencies: Local recurrence. In: Harris JR, Hellman S, Henderson IC, Kinne DW, eds. Breast diseases. Philadelphia: JB Lippincott; 1987:508-524.
20. Clark RM. Alternatives to mastectomy—the Princess Margaret Hospital experience. In: Harris JR, Hellman S, Silen W, eds. Conservative management of breast cancer. Philadelphia: JB Lippincott, 1983: 35-46.
21. Fisher B, Bauer M, Margolese R, et al. Five-year results of 3 randomized clinical trials comparing total mastectomy and segmental mastectomy with or without radiation in the treatment of early breast cancer. N Engl J Med 1985; 312:665-673.
22. Danoff BE, Pajak TE, Solin LL, et al. Excisional biopsy axillary node dissection and definitive radiotherapy for stages I and II breast cancer. Int J Radiat Oncol Biol Phys 1985; 11:479-483.
23. Montague ED. Conservation surgery and radiation therapy in the treatment of operable breast cancer. Cancer 1984; 53:700-704.
24. Kurtz JM, Amalric R, Brandone H, et al. Local recurrence after breast-conserving surgery and radiotherapy. Frequency, time course, and prognosis. Cancer 1989; 63:1912-1917.
25. Kurtz JM, Spitalier JM, Amalric R. Late breast recurrence after lumpectomy and irradiation. Int J Radiat Oncol Biol Phys 1983; 9:1191-1194.
26. Kurtz JM, Amalric R, Delouche G, et al. The second ten years: Long-term risks of breast conservation (abstr). Int J Radiat Oncol Biol Phys (Suppl 1) 1985; 11:184-185.
27. Schnitt SJ, Connolly JL, Recht A, et al. Breast relapse following primary radiation therapy for early breast cancer. II. Detection, pathologic features, and prognostic significance. Int J Radiat Oncol Biol Phys 1984; 11:1277-1284.
28. Recht A, Schnitt SJ, Connolly JL, et al. Prognosis following local or regional recurrence after conservative surgery and radiotherapy for early stage breast carcinoma. Int J Radiat Oncol Biol Phys 1989; 16:3-9.
29. Harris JR, Recht A, Amalric R, et al. Time course and prognosis of local recurrence following primary radiation therapy for early breast cancer. J Clin Oncol 1984; 2:37-41.
30. Kurtz JM, Spitalier JM, Amalric R. Late breast recurrence after lumpectomy and irradiation. Int J Radiat Oncol Biol Phys 1983; 9:1191-1194.
31. Hafty B, Goldberg N, Rose M, et al. Conservative surgery with radiation therapy in clinical stage I and II breast cancer. Arch Surg 1989; 124:1266-1270.
32. Leung S, Otmezguine Y, Calitchi E, et al. Locoregional recurrences following radical external beam irradiation and interstitial implantation for operable breast cancer—a twenty-three year experience. Radiother Oncol 1986; 5:1-10.
33. Kurtz JM, Amalric R, Brandone H, et al. A second chance to preserve the breast: Results of wide excision after lumpectomy and irradiation (abstr). Int J Radiat Oncol Biol Phys (Suppl 1) 1985; 11:103.
34. Kurtz JM, Spitalier JM, Amalric R, et al. Results of wide excision for local recurrence after breast-conserving therapy. Cancer 1988; 61:1969-1972.
35. Fisher ER, Sass R, Fisher B, et al. Pathologic findings from the National Surgical Adjuvant Breast Project (Protocol 6). II. Relation of local breast recurrence to multicentricity. Cancer 1986; 57:1717-1724.
36. Spitalier JM, Gumbarelli J, Brandone H, et al. Breast-conserving surgery with radiation therapy for operable mammary carcinoma: a 25 year experience. World J Surg 1986; 10:1014-1020.
37. Slavin SA, Love SM, Goldwyn RM. Breast cancer recurrence and detection in patients undergoing immediate reconstruction and salvage mastectomy with myocutaneous flaps. Presented at the 59th Annual Scientific meeting of the American Society of Plastic and Reconstructive Surgeons, Plastic Surgery Educational Foundation, American Society of Maxillofacial Surgeons, Boston, MA, October 23, 1990.
38. Rees TD, Liverett DM, Guy CL. The effect of cigarette smoking on skin flap survival in the facelift patient. Plast Reconstr Surg 1984; 73:911-915.
39. Nolan J, Jenkins RA, Kurihara K, et al. The acute effects of cigarette smoke exposure on experimental skin flaps. Plast Reconstr Surg 1985; 74:544-549.
40. McCraw JB, Penix JO, Baker JW. Repair of major defects of the chest wall and spine with the latissimus

dorsi myocutaneous flap. Plast Reconstr Surg 1978; 62:197-206.

41. Bostwick J III, Nahai F, Wallace JG, et al. Sixty latissimus dorsi flaps. Plast Reconstr Surg 1979; 63:31-41.
42. Bostwick J III, Scheffan M. The latissimus dorsi musculocutaneous flap: One stage breast reconstruction. Clin Plast Surg 1980; 7:71-78.
43. Larson DL, McMurtrey MJ. Musculocutaneous flap reconstruction of chest-wall defects: An experience with 50 patients. Plast Reconstr Surg 1984; 73:734-740.
44. Dinner MI, Peter CR. The arc of the latissimus dorsi myocutaneous flap. Ann Plast Surg 1979; 3:425-429.
45. Matsuo K, Hirose T, Hayashi R, et al. Chest wall reconstruction by contralateral latissimus dorsi musculocutaneous flap. Plast Reconstr Surg 1988; 82:994-999.
46. Harashina T, Takayama S, Ikuta Y, et al. Reconstruction of chest-wall radiation ulcer with free latissimus dorsi muscle flap and meshed skin graft. Plast Reconstr Surg 1983; 71:805-808.
47. Harii K, Iwaya T, Kawaguchi N. Combination myocutaneous flap and microvascular free flap. Plast Reconstr Surg 1981; 68:700-710.
48. Drever JM. The epigastric island flap. Plast Reconstr Surg 1977; 59:343-346.
49. Robbins TH. Rectus abdominis myocutaneous flap for breast reconstruction. Aust NZJ Surg 1979; 49:527-530.
50. Hartrampf CR, Scheflan M, Black PW. Breast reconstruction with a transverse abdominal island flap. Plast Reconstr Surg 1982; 69:216-224.
51. Dinner MI, Labandter HP, Dowden RV. The role of the rectus abdominis myocutaneous flap in breast reconstruction. Plast Reconstr Surg 1982; 69:209-214.
52. Bunkis J, Walton RL, Mathes SJ, et al. Experience with the transverse lower rectus flap abdominis operation for breast reconstruction. Plast Reconstr Surg 1983; 72:819-827.
53. Scheflan MD, Dinner MI. The transverse abdominal island flap: Part I. Indications, contraindications, results and complications. Ann Plast Surg 1983; 10:24-35.
54. Scheflan MD, Dinner MI. The transverse abdominal island flap: Part II. Surgical technique. Ann Plast Surg 1983; 10:120-129.
55. Scheflan M. Building a breast without a prosthesis. The transverse abdominal island flap. Clin Plast Surg 1984; 11:303-315.
56. Slavin SA. Rectus abdominis myocutaneous flaps (letter to the editor). Plast Reconstr Surg 1983; 72:738.
57. Slavin SA, Goldwyn RM. The midabdominal rectus abdominis myocutaneous flaps: Review of 236 flaps. Plast Reconstr Surg 1988; 81:189-197.
58. Ishii CH, Bostwick J III, Raine TJ, et al. Double-pedicle transverse rectus abdominis myocutaneous flap for unilateral breast and chest wall reconstruction. Plast Reconstr Surg 1985; 76:901-907.
59. Grotting JC, Urist MM, Maddox WA, et al. Conventional TRAM flap versus free microsurgical TRAM flap for immediate breast reconstruction. Plast Reconstr Surg 1989; 83:828-841.
60. Friedman RJ, Argenta LC, Anderson R. Deep inferior epigastric free flap for breast reconstruction after radical mastectomy. Plast Reconstr Surg 1985; 76:455-458.
61. Georgiade GS, Voci VE, Riefkohl R, Scheflan M. Potential problems with the transverse rectus abdominis myocutaneous flap in breast reconstruction and how to avoid them. Br J Plast Surg 1984; 37:121-125.
62. Scheflan M, Kalisman M. Complications of breast reconstruction. Clin Plast Surg 1984; 11:343-350.
63. Slavin SA, Howrigan P, Goldwyn RM, LoVerme W. Abdominal wall function after rectus flap breast reconstruction. Presented at the 55th Annual Scientific Meeting of the American Society of Plastic and Reconstructive Surgeons, Plastic Surgery Educational Foundation, American Society of Maxillary and Facial Surgeons, Los Angeles, CA, October 27, 1986.
64. Slavin SA, Howrigan P, Goldwyn RM. Pseudocyst formation following rectus flap breast reconstruction: Diagnosis and treatment. Plast Reconstr Surg 1989; 83:670-675.
65. Fujino T, Harashina T, Enomoto K. Primary breast reconstruction after a standard radical mastectomy by a free flap transfer. Plast Reconstr Surg 1976; 58:372-374.
66. Shaw WW. Breast reconstruction by superior gluteal microvascular free flaps without silicone implants. Plast Reconstr Surg 1983; 72:490-499.
67. Shaw WW. Microvascular free flap breast reconstruction. Clin Plast Surg 1984; 11:333-341.
68. Serafin D, Voci VE, Georgiade NG. Microsurgical composite tissue transplantation: Indications and technical considerations in breast reconstruction following mastectomy. Plast Reconstr Surg 1982; 70:24-34.
69. Noone RB, Murphy JB, Spear SL, et al. A 6 year experience with immediate reconstruction after mastectomy for cancer. Plast Reconstr Surg 1985; 76:258-269.
70. Georgiade GS, Riefkohl R, Cox E, et al. Long-term clinical outcome of immediate reconstruction after mastectomy. Plast Reconstr Surg 1985; 76:415-420.
71. Dowden RV, Blanchard JM, Greenstreet RL. Breast reconstruction: Selection, timing, and local recurrence. Ann Plast Surg 1983; 10:265-269.
72. Schain WS, Jacobs E, Wellisch DK. Psychosocial issues in breast reconstruction. Clin Plast Surg 1984; 11:237-251.
73. Stevens LA, McGrath MH, Druss RG, et al. The psychological impact of immediate breast reconstruction for women with early breast cancer. Plast Reconstr Surg 1984; 73:619-626.
74. Berrino P, Campora E, Santi P. Postquadrantectomy breast deformities: Classification and techniques of surgical correction. Plast Reconstr Surg 1987; 79:567-572.
75. Veronesi V, Saccozzi R, Deluecchio M, et al. Comparing radical mastectomy with quadrantectomy, axillary dissection, and radiotherapy in patients with small cancers of breast. N Engl J Med 1981; 305:6-11.

CHAPTER 40

Breast and Chest Wall Reconstruction After Radiation Therapy

N. BRADLY MELAND, M.D.
PHILLIP G. ARNOLD, M.D.

The primary or adjunctive treatment of radiation therapy for breast cancer has undoubtedly saved many lives and prolonged others. Nonetheless, the benefits received from radiation therapy can cause significant physiologic changes to the tissues of the chest wall. The smallest amount of trauma may frequently result in an open wound that gradually increases in size until it becomes a threat to life. The ever-present risks of recurrent or persistent malignancy and late, radiation-induced sarcomas are a major consideration for the surgeon who undertakes the treatment of these disorders.

The current management of breast cancer is perhaps more complex and confusing to the patient than that of any other disease. The current enigma about who should have minimal surgery, with or without radiation, is not yet fully solved, although the reports of local recurrence rates from segmental or partial mastectomies alone range from 18 to 37 percent.[1,2]

Because local recurrence with "minimal surgery" or with large breast cancers is possible, radiation therapy as an adjunctive treatment is now relatively commonplace. The radiotherapy sequence is time consuming, delivering approximately 5,000 rads over a 5-week period. Interstitial implants placed around the site of the tumor may also be used to deliver a boost of an additional 1,000 to 1,500 rads. Currently, doses of over 6,000 rads are infrequently used because of the high incidence of local complications.[3-6] The present trend in the management of this disease is toward more liberal use of forms of radiation therapy.[6] Continued advances in isotopes, linear accelerators, and interstitial implants have led to less catastrophic injury and complications.[6] The plastic and reconstructive surgeon will continue to be faced with problems of reconstruction around the breast and chest wall, and we will discuss and review these. The current common indications for postoperative radiation therapy for breast cancer are listed in Table 40–1.[7]

RADIATION THERAPY

Historical Aspects

Light waves, heat waves, radiowaves, ultraviolet waves, x-rays, and gamma waves are all forms of electromagnetic radiation. They are made up of small bundles of energy called photons that travel in waves with a velocity ranging from 3×10^8 m per sec or 186,000 miles per sec in a vacuum. The various forms of electromagnetic radiation all have different wavelengths. The electromagnetic waves of interest in radiation oncology are very short with a very high frequency (Table 40–2).[6] Therefore, the energy associated with one photon is greater, giving more tissue penetration. With the discovery of x-rays by Roentgen in 1925, its effects on cells, and indeed on cancer, were rapidly discovered, and shortly thereafter radiation was used to treat breast cancer.[6] However, the equipment available at that time to deliver the x-ray dose was poor, and high doses were re-

TABLE 40-1 Relative Indications for Postoperative Radiotherapy After Radical Mastectomy

Centrally located tumor
Inner quadrant tumor
Positive lymph nodes
Primary greater than 5 cm in size
Skin or chest wall involvement
High-grade tumor or close surgical margins

From Fletcher GH, Montague ED, Taple N, Barker JL. Breast. In: Fletcher GH, ed. Textbook of radiotherapy, 3rd ed. Philadelphia: Lea & Febiger, 1980:527-583.

quired to achieve appropriate tissue depths, causing serious skin injury. Local tumor control was difficult to achieve and normal tissue was damaged consistently. With the discovery of radium by the Curies, a radioactive source that emitted a highly penetrating photon wave provided an alternative technique to the treatment of breast cancer. Interstitial implants were then found to be effective. The first clinical study of such interstitial implant techniques was made by Keynes.[8,9]

In the 1940s, high-energy orthovoltage x-ray machines providing more tissue penetration and less surface injury became available. McWhirter first advocated limited surgery with radiation in 1948.[10,11] Baclesse encountered problems with skin intolerance associated with his orthovoltage equipment.[12] He developed techniques of prolonged radiation and concluded that external beam radiation alone would cure breast cancer in some patients. Cosmetic deformity frequently resulted.

In the 1950s, supervoltage radiation such as cobalt 60 and linear accelerators was developed, permitting the delivery of homogenous irradiation doses to the breast and lymphatic drainage areas with better epidermal sparing. Present-day treatment includes the external supervoltage delivery sources as well as refined radiation implants for interstitial delivery systems.[6]

TABLE 40-2 Electromagnetic Spectrum

Wave Length in Cm		Type of Radiation
0.0001	(10^{-4})	Visible light
0.00001	(10^{-5})	
0.000001	(10^{-6})	Ultraviolet
0.0000001	(10^{-7})	
0.00000001	(10^{-8})	X-rays
0.000000001	(10^{-9})	
0.0000000001	(10^{-10})	Gamma rays
0.00000000001	(10^{-11})	
0.000000000001	(10^{-12})	Cosmic rays

Definition

Ionizing radiation is defined as the absorption of energy by some matter from a radiation beam resulting in "excitation" or "ionization" in the atoms of the irradiated material. This results in raising the electrons of the atoms in that radiation material to a higher energy level, the process called "excitation." "Exposure" is the quantity that describes the output of an x-ray or gamma ray generator. It is the charge that results when a unit mass of air is exposed to ionizing radiation. The Fifth International Congress of Radiology in 1937 accepted the "roentgen" as the international dosage unit for x-ray or gamma ray exposure. "The roentgen is equivalent to one electrostatic unit of electricity liberated from 1 cc of air at standard temperature and pressure (0°C, 760 mm of mercury) upon exposure to ionizing radiation."

The Seventh International Congress of Radiology adopted the "rad" as the "unit of absorbed dose of any ionizing radiation equal to 100 ergs per gram by any absorber." It has been recommended, however, that a special unit called the "gray" (Gy) should now replace the rad as the common unit of absorbed dose measured. "One gray is equivalent to 1 jewel per kilogram." Currently, however, most radiation oncologists continue to use the rad as the unit for absorbed dose of radiation.[13]

Effect of Radiation on Tissue

The histologic changes seen after radiation injury are not specific. Similar patterns are seen in other forms of tissue injury, including burns, frostbite, infection, and ischemia. Radiation-injured cells demonstrate changes in both the nucleus and the cytoplasm. The nuclei become swollen and pyknotic, with clumping of chromatin. Cytoplasmic changes include vacuole formation, endoplasmic reticulum disintegration, and rupture of plasma membranes. Tissues having the most radiosensitivity are those with the greatest mitotic activity, least differentiation, and rapid cell turnover.[14]

The effects of ionizing radiation can be categorized as somatic or genetic, and acute or chronic. Acute effects are observed within minutes or as long as 30 to 60 days. Chronic effects develop over months to many years. The discussion in this chapter is limited to changes affecting the epidermis and tissues that are encountered in breast and chest wall wounds.

The effects of radiation on the epidermis are many. The epidermal cells are extremely sensitive to radiation injury because of their active proliferation and mitotic activity in replacing desquamating epidermal cells. Postirradiation erythema usually presents at 48 hours and reaches a peak 2 to 3 weeks after the injury. The skin is frequently tender to palpation and feels thick and firm owing to interstitial and intercellular edema. Within a few weeks, the skin usually appears to be recovered. The deeper epidermal and dermal changes continue to progress and are dose dependent. Basement membranes become thickened and reduplicated. Stellate and spindle-shaped radiated fibroblasts are often found scattered throughout the cellular matrix. Also found in the dermis are small ectatic vessels with endothelial atypia. Muscles show striking fiber atrophy, multinucleate atypia, and interstitial fibrosis.[15,16] Late skin changes include thinned epithelial layer, usually without rete pegs. Parakeratosis and hyperkeratosis of the nuclei of the epithelial cells is usually extensive. Loss of sebaceous glands and hair follicles is seen, but the very resistant sweat glands are usually present in fewer numbers. Elastic fibers in the dermis are destroyed, with considerable hyalinization of the dermal collagen. Fibroblasts in the dermis and subcutaneous tissue usually enlarge and become neoplastic. Lymphatics and small capillaries are noted to be suspiciously absent or are enveloped in thick, fibrous tissue. [17,18] Late changes in the muscle include vacuolated cells that are also replaced in scar tissue with few blood vessels. Bone is frequently devitalized, with obliteration of the vessels in the periosteal layer, and to a lesser extent in the endosteum.[19]

The physician should be aware of the clinical signs and pathognomonic changes of chronic radiation dermatitis: (1) slick, shiny, patchy, parchment-like appearance of the skin secondary to scarring and atrophy, with loss of elastic fibers; (2) dryness, cracking, and depilation due to loss of sebaceous glands, hair follicles, and a decreased amount of sweat glands; (3) light or brown patches due to pigmentation and/or depigmentation from melanocytic and malanosomal injury; (4) telangiectasias thought to be secondary to thrombosis of the superficial venules and small arteries; (5) raised, rough nodules from hyperkeratosis and papillomatosis of the epidermis; and (6) encrusted dark spots, small punched-out ulcers, ulcers with raised margins around skin defects with dirty, yellow-gray bases (again secondary to endarteritis and arterial thrombosis), and firm, reddish-brown, diffuse areas of plaques, connotating subcutaneous fibrosis.[15]

RADIATION THERAPY FOR BREAST CANCER

The classic indications for radiation therapy for breast cancer have broadened in the modern era. Many authors have recommended it as a primary treatment for breast carcinoma without excisional surgery.[20,21] Although this form of therapy is common in Europe, it still has not achieved complete acceptance in the United States, for many reasons.[16] At the present time, there is little dispute that postoperative radiation therapy is effective at reducing local and regional recurrence.[6] However, the risks of radiation therapy for breast cancer must also be realized by clinicians. It has been known for many years that radiation injury can induce breast cancer, including adenocarcinomas of the adnexal structures, as well as sarcomatous change in the fibrous structures.[22-26] The astute clinician must keep these problems clearly in mind when evaluating patients with radiation-induced changes to the chest wall and breast, because recurrent or radiation-induced sarcomas and carcinomas of soft tissue and bone must be ruled out.

The effects of breast implants on irradiation in one postmastectomy patient have been studied in three research-oriented papers. All of these showed that breast implants neither hinder nor interfere in any way with radiation therapy.[27-29]

Complications After Radiation Therapy

The reconstructive surgeon must be familiar with breast changes through the entire spectrum of the biologic response to radiation, from the acute epidermal changes previously discussed to the late radiation injury changes of fibrosis and ulceration. Conservative breast surgery followed by radiation therapy is now a common primary treatment for breast cancer. Radiation therapy is also an integral part of the treatment of chest wall mediastinal and supraclavicular areas in most patients with Stage 2 disease. Reconstructive surgeons should be concerned with patients in whom radiation problems are encountered after surgery. In order to further differentiate this and sequential treatment, Bostwick and colleagues devised a classification system for the sequelae of breast irradiation (Table 40-3), based on the treatment of 54 patients with radiation complications after breast cancer treatment.[30] The authors concluded that this system has facilitated their understanding of the process of injury and simplified their treatment strategies. Recommended reconstructive programs include a rectus abdominis myocutaneous flap for primary reconstruction in patients

TABLE 40-3 Classification of Radiation Sequelae of Breast Irradiation

Breast necrosis
After lumpectomy and primary radiation therapy
After treatment of advanced local breast cancer
Radionecrosis and chest wall ulceration
After adjunctive radiation therapy
After radiation therapy for recurrent breast cancer
Accelerated coronary atherosclerosis with median sternotomy wound failure after coronary revascularization
Brachial plexus pain and paresis
Lymphedema and axillary cicatrix
Radiation-induced neoplasia

From Bostwick J, Stevenson TR, Nahai F, et al. Radiation to the breast—complications amenable to surgical treatment. Ann Surg 1984; 200:543.

in Categories 1, 2, and 6; latissimus dorsi flaps for Categories 2, 3, and 5; and an omentum flap for Category 4. A transposed omental flap is highly reliable for patients in Categories 2, 3, 4, and 6. Reconstruction of the deformed radiated breast by partial breast excision and reconstruction with latissimus dorsi flaps have also been reported.[31, 32] We advocate completion mastectomy and autologous tissue reconstruction in most of these patients.

BREAST RECONSTRUCTION IN THE IRRADIATED PATIENT

Breast reconstruction is now commonplace in the repertoire of the reconstructive surgeon. The options for treatment of patients requesting breast reconstruction after radiation therapy are similar to those for patients seeking breast reconstruction without radiotherapy. They include (1) not accepting the patient for reconstruction, (2) simple submuscular silicone implant placement, (3) expander implant placement as a two-stage procedure, (4) permanent expander implant placement, (5) implant placement covered with a local cutaneous or myocutaneous flap, (6) autologous reconstruction using a regional myocutaneous flap, and (7) autologous reconstruction with a free tissue transfer.

The decision can also be complicated by the question of timing of the reconstruction. It must be individualized to the patient, depending on her expectations, the condition and availability of tissue, and the surgeon's experience and expertise.

Historically, early breast reconstruction was done with the use of local flap and/or breast-sharing procedures, using tubed pedicles from the opposite breast or from other areas of the body. This had the drawbacks of a random blood supply and multiple procedures over a prolonged period with variable cosmetic results (Figs. 40-1, 40-2).[33-38]

Local cutaneous flaps from the lateral chest or advancement sliding flaps of the abdominal wall have also been advocated and used to cover breast implants. However, their use is not recommended in patients with a history of radiation scarring, contracture, necrosis, and ulceration. Implant exposure can be expected when such local cutaneous tissues are used in these marginal situations.[39-41]

With the advent of Silastic implants for breast reconstruction (Cronin and Gerow, 1963), the reconstructive surgeon received an overwhelming array of prosthetic materials with which to reconstruct the breast.[42] The ingenious development of the tissue expander by Radovan in the 1970s was also a major advance.[43] In our practice we have been extremely conservative in breast reconstruction of the radiated chest wall with prosthetic material, but Stabile and associates reported successful silicone breast implant reconstruction after radiation therapy in eight patients.[44] All eight were alive and well 8 months to 6½ years after irradiation and 3 months to 3 years after breast reconstruction; the results were gratifying.

In our current practice, we are not recommending silicone breast implant placement in the irradiated chest wall. We believe, like others, that place-

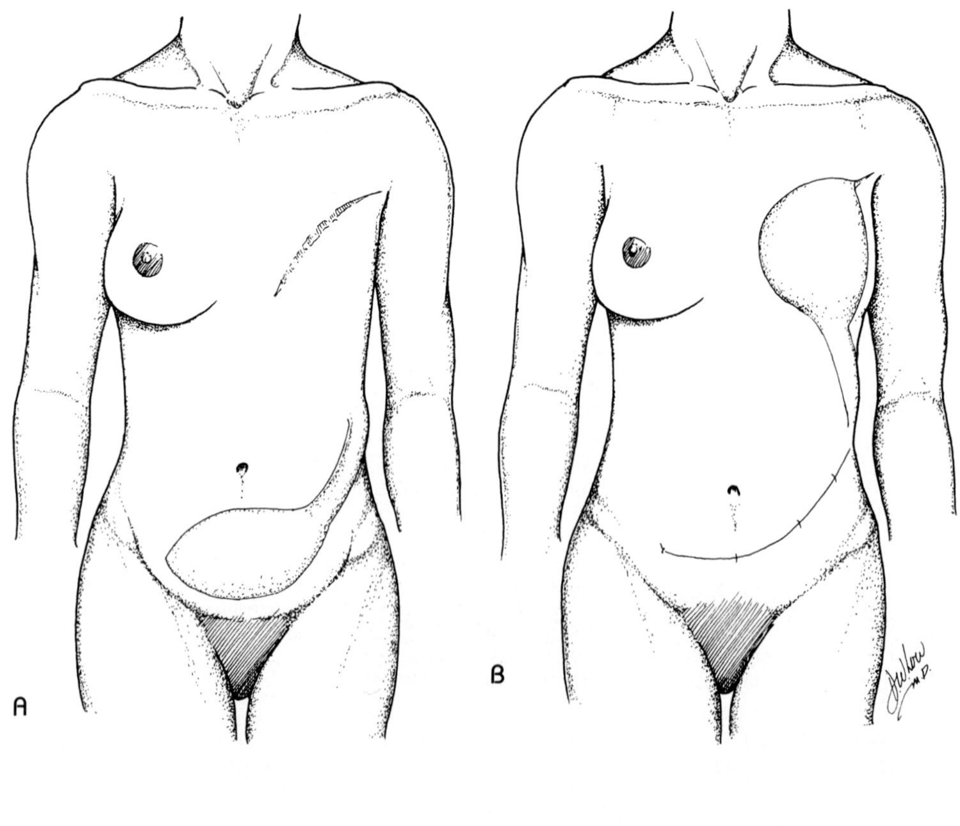

FIGURE 40-1 *A and B, Technique of breast reconstruction with the tubed abdominal flap, initially credited to Gillies.*

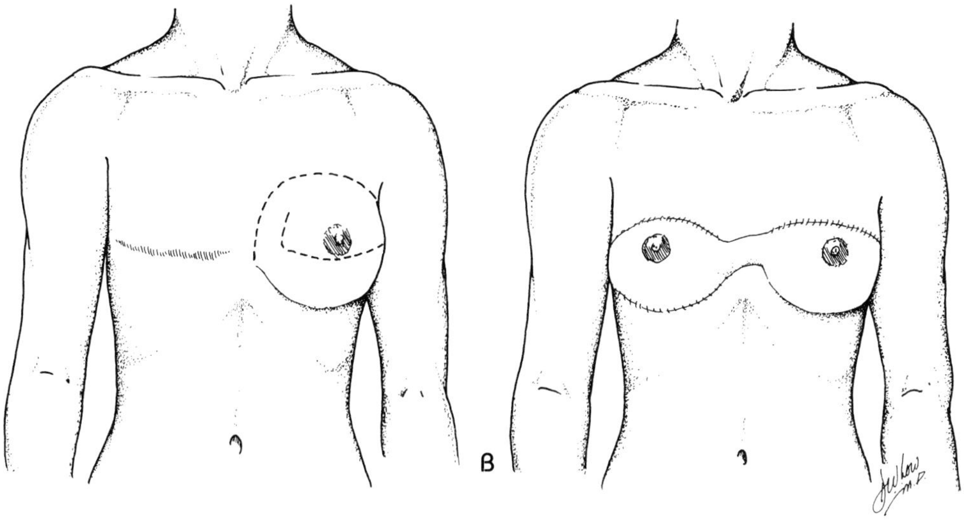

A B

FIGURE 40-2 *A* and *B*, One of the many techniques of shared breast reconstruction with a tubed pedicled flap of breast tissue, refined by Millard.

ment of silicone prostheses or tissue expanders in a previously irradiated chest wall is fraught with a high frequency of exposure, infection, or wound complications. The final reconstructive effort is often less than that desired owing to the inability of the skin to stretch, redrape, and form a proper breast mound. It is advisable to use musculocutaneous flap transposition or free flaps, with or without silicone implants, as the procedure of choice for patients seeking breast reconstruction after failed conservative therapy with radiation. Those desiring reconstruction after postoperative chest wall radiation can be treated with a latissimus dorsi flap with or without implant, a rectus abdominis myocutaneous flap, or a free tissue transfer to achieve the most pleasing aesthetic result with the fewest complications.[45-48] These techniques are discussed more fully in other chapters.

We have had acceptable results in immediate breast reconstruction with the permanent expander prosthesis placed immediately after mastectomy and sequentially expanded to the appropriate size to match the opposite breast. We have performed immediate breast reconstruction with the permanent soft tissue expander, followed by chemotherapy and radiation therapy, on several occasions, with often satisfactory results, albeit limited follow-up (Figs. 40-3*A* and *B*).

CHEST WALL RECONSTRUCTION

Historical Aspects

Ambroise Paré in his ten books of surgery published in 1564, stated: "gangrene and other mortifications can occur as complications of some forms of

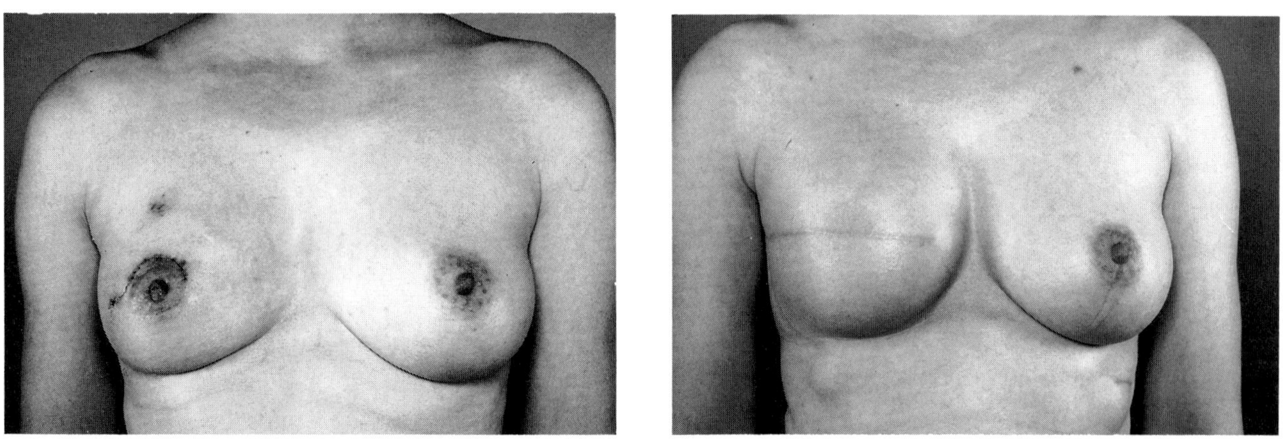

A B

FIGURE 40-3 *A*, Preoperative mastectomy for immediate reconstruction. *B*, One year after immediate breast reconstruction with Becker permanent implant. Chemotherapy and local radiation therapy to the chest wall were given after the immediate reconstruction procedure.

treatment. These complications gave more evil to the surgeons and the patients than the maladies in which they occur."[49] The reconstructive surgeon today can certainly identify with Paré's concepts when confronted with the patient with massive radiation necrosis of the chest wall. Early in our surgical heritage, Brown and colleagues showed us convincingly that the surgeon must use nonradiated, well-vascularized tissue where previous radiation has occurred in order to achieve, or to hope to achieve, a healed wound.[50] The common simple procedures of primary or delayed primary wound closure and split-thickness skin grafts rarely, if ever, produced satisfactory complete and long-term wound closure in obvious irradiated tissue.[14]

Kiricuta championed the use of the greater omentum. His original work in 1956 demonstrated its successful use in the treatment of vesicovaginal fistulas. In 1963 he extended the omentum's usefulness in the repair of chest wall defects.[51,52] During the 1980s muscle and musculocutaneous flaps became common in the armamentarium of plastic surgeons and are reliable means of managing chest wall defects.[53–59]

Fortunately, the chest wall is an accessible area for several large, well-vascularized musculocutaneous units. Free tissue transfers for coverage are not commonly required, but should be considered for difficult cases in which local muscle flaps are not available. They also serve as reliable back-up procedures for any reconstructive effort. In some situations, free flap transfer may be the first choice.

General Considerations in Irradiated Chest Wall Defects

The reconstructive surgeon presented with an irradiated chest wall wound should initially consider several general questions:

1. Is recurrent or persistent malignancy still present in the wound?
2. Will the lesion presented require a full-thickness or partial-thickness chest wall resection? If full-thickness, what is the status of the underlying lung parenchyma and pulmonary reserve?
3. Is it resectable?
4. If the lesion or tumor is not resectable, is a subtotal resection and reliable coverage a reasonable therapeutic alternative? The surgeon must remember: "first do no harm." When the question of resectability and malignancy is answered, the best procedure must then be selected to reconstruct that particular chest wall defect.
5. If the procedure fails, what are the reliable back-up procedures?
6. Can I, as a reconstructive surgeon, do an adequate job in this patient on my own or should I have assistance from another subspecialized surgeon?

If we in reconstructive surgery can remember these six simple points, patients presenting to us with these difficult wounds will be managed appropriately and, it is hoped, with acceptable results.

Preoperative Evaluation

Most patients are referred from oncologists and the presence or absence of malignant or metastatic disease has already been determined. In the presence of a chest wall radiation ulcer, resection and reconstruction should be *considered* even in the face of metastatic disease. In many of these very difficult situations, the quality of life can be vastly improved, pain can be diminished, and the patients can live out their remaining months or years in relative comfort.[41]

After clinical examination, the true extent of the disease process must be understood. Computed tomography (CT) or magnetic resonance imaging (MRI) have proved very helpful in our practices in addition to other more standard radiographic tools. Either of these two modalities frequently delineate conditions of the underlying lung parenchyma and the mediastinal structures. The presence of mediastinal abscess, pulmonary parenchymal abscess, or empyema is critical to the operative planning and types of resection required. If there is a history of herald bleeding or persistent bleeding with these ulcers in the anterior chest wall, preoperative angiography must be considered; unexpected involvement of the great vessels or even the heart itself has been encountered by the unwary surgeon. Ulcerations of recent onset, commonly seen along the parasternal area, deserve very careful observation, because erosion of the internal mammary vessel with life-threatening hemorrhage is possible. At the completion of a complete history taking, physical examination, laboratory studies, and specialized interventional tests, the surgeon should be ready to proceed with resection.

Resection of the Irradiated Chest Wall

Frozen section availability is extremely important at the time of the chest wall resection. The pathologist should be informed preoperatively about the problem, and multiple cuts and frozen section biopsies of all suspicious areas and surgical margins should be examined in the resected specimen. In resecting a lesion that shows radiation damage without any recurrent or radiation-induced malignancy, a more conservative resection is appropriate. The goal is to remove all obvious nonvital tissue. This most frequently involves large areas of skin and any bone and particularly cartilage that are obviously affected (i.e., not bleeding or sequestered). This resection often leaves a thickened, scarred pleura or lung parenchyma itself. If the pleura is also excised, pneumothorax is rare because of the extensive scarring from the previous radiation injury, although one should be prepared for it. The lung parenchyma is usually adherent to the internal thoracic wall. If lung parenchyma is obviously nonvital, it also must be resected until bleeding tissue is identified. Cartilage and bone that are nonviable or sequestered and left behind will eventually result in continued drainage, no matter how well vascularized the coverage used. Above all, we have found that removal of exposed cartilage and obvious necrotic bone is perhaps the most important way to prevent future infection and drainage. If there is any question about the adequacy of resection, it can be done in stages. The wound must be kept moist between dressing changes, and the patient can be returned to the operating room at a later date. The disadvantage of this is that the wound can desiccate very rapidly, and radiated tissue that is allowed to desiccate may become nonviable in the interim, thus setting up a nonending cycle. When the wound has been completely debrided and all obvious nonviable tissue removed, reconstruction should be carried out rapidly.

Reconstruction

Choice of reconstructive material for the partially excised or partial-thickness chest wall debridement is, of course, dependent on the location of the problem. Several muscle flaps have proved very helpful for this reconstruction, including the external oblique myocutaneous, latissimus dorsi, and rectus abdominis flaps. However, we have been pleased with omental transposition for partial-thickness defects. This has provided good coverage with very low morbidity.

The omentum has no structural strength and seems to work much better when placed on a stable surface, such as with partial-thickness excisions. It is not as useful for full-thickness chest wall defects that require a stable anterior chest wall. These flap options are discussed in more detail later in the chapter.

Radiation Damage with Recurrent Cancer

In patients with persistent or recurrent cancer, the resection almost always involves full-thickness skin, subcutaneous tissue, thoracic skeleton, and pleura. The physiologic and surgical defect associated with this type of resection is much more severe. The surgeon must achieve air-tight closure with healthy tissue and as much chest wall stability as possible to allow for independent ventilation by the patient. These defects are more appropriately treated with a muscle or musculocutaneous flap than with omentum.[54,60-62]

In patients with radiation ulcers and open wounds, we do not use alloplastic materials to reconstruct the chest wall. In these patients, coverage of the full-thickness debrided chest wall with a large myocutaneous flap has resulted in adequate coverage and sufficient stability for the patient to maintain ventilation independently. Most of these wounds are contaminated; and thus placement of an alloplastic mesh in the wound for reconstruction is not appropriate. Infection may result in entire wound breakdown with eventual removal of the mesh and failure of the initial intended reconstructive procedure.[55,63]

Technical Aspects and Indications for Flap Coverage

Omentum

The greater omentum as a transposition flap is invaluable to cover partial-thickness chest wall defects (Figs. 40-4*A* and *B*). The omentum is based on the gastroepiploic artery and veins, originating from the gastroduodenal artery on the right, and a branch of the splenic artery on the left. It is harvested via a laparotomy incision and then tunneled to the chest wall through a subcutaneous tunnel over the rib margin. It can be based on either the right or left gastroepiploic vessel, depending on the anatomic location of the chest wall defect. Care should be taken to avoid kinking of the gastric outlet, and we have found it helpful to tack the omentum intra-abdominally to the falciform ligament or the peritoneal surface in order to reduce the incidence of internal herniation. The techniques of omental elongation and harvesting have been well described by several authors (Fig. 40-5).[52,64-66]

Pectoralis Major Muscle

The pectoralis major muscle is our first choice to close any superior midline chest wall defect, although this is rarely indicated in the irradiated breast wound. The muscle may be damaged by previous mastectomy and radiation injury, so its use in the context of these patients is limited. The muscle is based on the thoracoacromial artery and vein and can be lifted as a muscular or musculocutaneous flap. It originates from the sternum, the medial portion of the clavicle, and the first five ribs. It inserts into the intratrabecular groove of the humerus, and this insertion can be taken down to increase the extent of muscle coverage for medial defects. Its thoracoacromial artery is a short branch of the second portion of the axillary artery. It passes on the medial border of the pectoralis minor muscles and pierces the clavipectoral fascia to divide into four branches: pectoral,

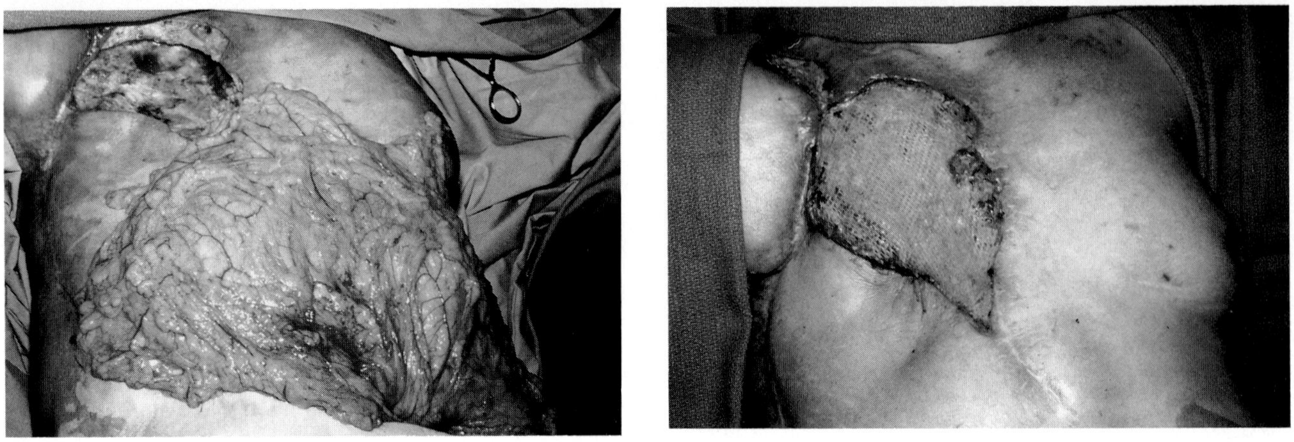

A B

FIGURE 40-4 *A*, A debrided radiation ulcer 18 years after mastectomy. The omentum has been elevated and draped over the abdominal wall. *B*, Postoperative course showing skin graft coverage of the omentum.

acromial, clavicular, and deltoid. The pectoral branch is the largest and serves as the primary blood supply to the pectoralis major and minor muscles. This is found at the level of the midclavicle. The muscle can also be used to cover radiation defects of the axilla and anterior shoulder (Figs. 40-6*A* and *B*).[63]

Latissimus Dorsi Muscle

The latissimus dorsi is a large muscle with its lateral border forming the posterior axillary fold. It originates from the lumbodorsal fascia and from the iliac crest posteriorly, and inserts into the lesser tubercle and intratrabecular groove of the humerus

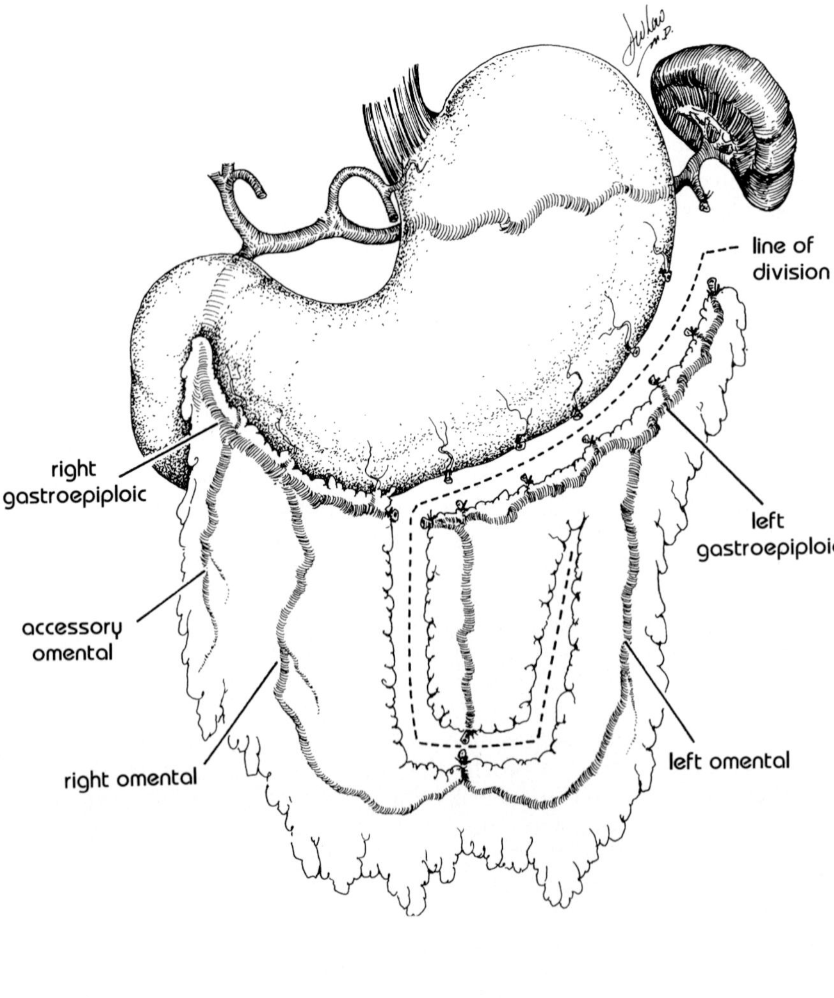

FIGURE 40-5 The surgical anatomy of the omentum and the lines of incision between the omental vessels for pedicle elongation.

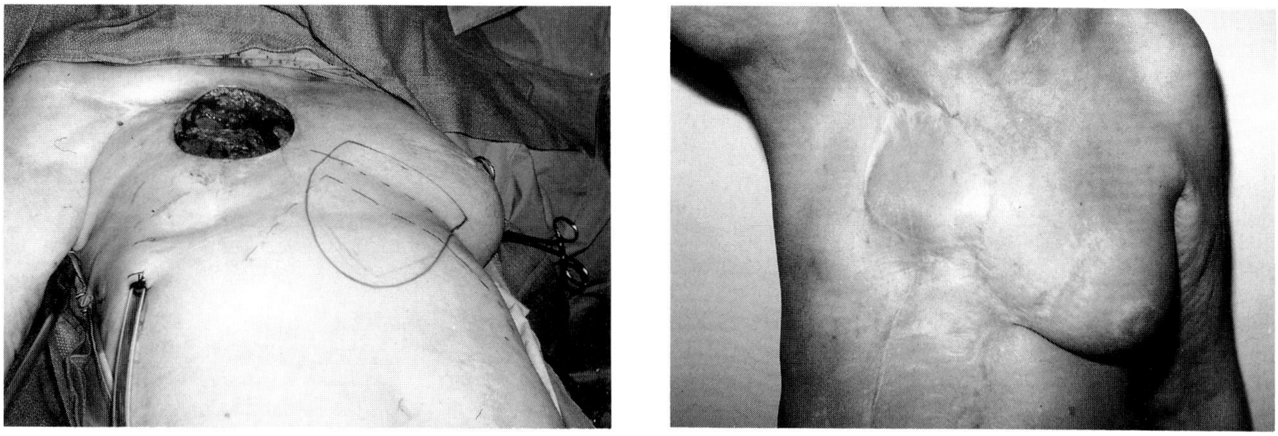

A B

FIGURE 40-6 *A*, The pectoralis major myocutaneous flap paddle is marked. *B*, Healed wound with flap elevated into place and minimal distortion of the left breast.

just posterior to the teres major muscle. The muscle is supplied primarily by the thoracodorsal artery and vein, which are primary branches of the subscapular artery and vein. If this vessel has been sacrificed by radiation injury or during the mastectomy, it will survive on its serratus or circumflex scapular branches.[67,68] The latissimus dorsi muscle has proved very useful for anterior chest wall defects, axillary and shoulder defects, and high clavicular defects after radiation necrosis or recurrent tumor excision of the chest wall. The donor defect, if a large myocutaneous flap is raised, can be skin grafted. However, skin breakdown and hyperkeratosis is common if skin grafting is done over exposed scapula.

External Oblique Muscle

The external oblique is the largest, strongest, and most superficial of the flat abdominal wall muscles. It originates from the posterior aspect of the sixth to the 12th ribs, and interdigitates with the latissimus dorsi and serratus anterior muscles. The fibers insert onto the anterior half of the iliac crest, and the superior fibers form the external oblique aponeurosis, which eventually contributes to the anterior rectus sheath. Its blood supply is from deep perforators that arise from the sixth to the 12th intercostal vessels and enter the undersurface of the muscle at or near the posterior axillary line. This raised muscle forms a large musculocutaneous or muscular flap. It has also proved useful in covering wounds of the lower anterior chest wall after radiation necrosis or for recurrent breast cancer after mastectomy. The flap is easy to raise, has excellent vascularity, and can be transposed up to the level of the inframammary fold. Often its donor defect must be skin grafted, but this has been well tolerated in our experience (Figs. 40-7*A* and *B*).[69,70]

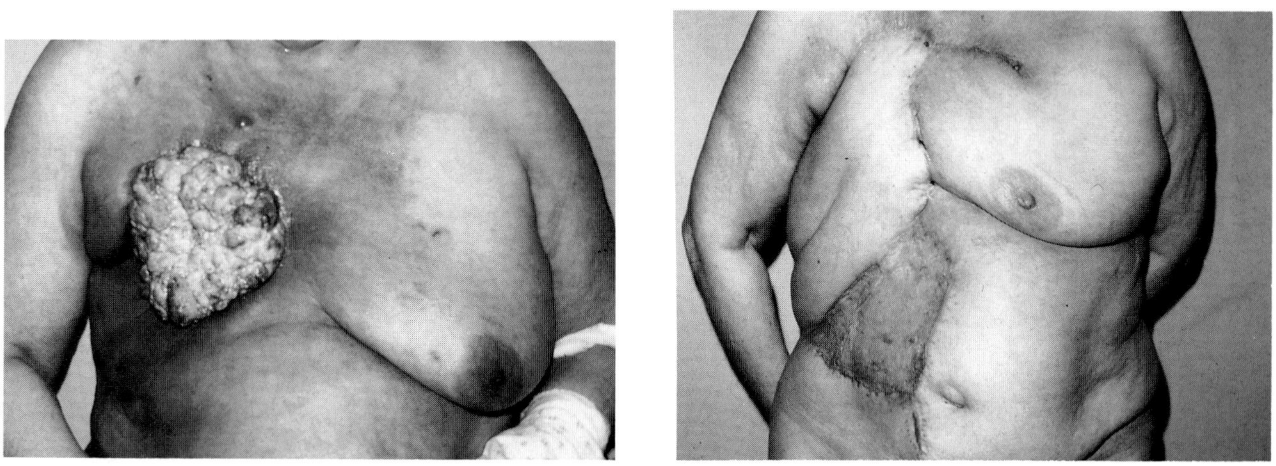

A B

FIGURE 40-7 *A*, Recurrent adenocarcinoma 6 years after mastectomy and radiation therapy. The tumor was widely excised, including full-thickness chest wall. *B*, Reconstruction was carried out with an external oblique transposition flap. (Courtesy of John E. Woods, M.D.)

Rectus Abdominis Muscle

The rectus abdominis is a paired muscle running on either side of the abdominal midline. It originates from the lower three costochondral junctions and sternum and inserts into the anterior pubic crest. Its blood supply is dual: a continuation of the internal mammary artery as the superficial epigastric vessel, and primarily from the external iliac artery and vein, the deep inferior epigastric vessels. The flap can be raised as a large myocutaneous unit and transposed to cover large irradiated or necrotic lesions of the anterior chest wall based on the superficial epigastric artery and vein. In our practice, because of the threat of internal mammary artery radiation injury, we have not considered the rectus abdominis as a frontline muscle to be used in radiation-damaged tissues of the chest wall. However, it should not be forgotten and it has been used in a salvage procedure in several of our patients (Figs. 40-8*A* to *C*).[63,71-73]

Trapezius Muscle

The trapezius can be used for high clavicular anterior chest wall lesions, but because of dual positioning and the closer locale of other musculocutaneous flaps, it has not been used for anterior chest wall defects in our practice. Its blood supply is based on the descending branch of the transverse cervical artery and vein, from the common carotid thyrocervical trunk. The donor site can be closed primarily.[65]

CONCLUSION

The single most important consideration for the reconstructive surgeon facing a radiation wound is adequate debridement. Inadequate debridement is the cause of many failures, both early and late, and is a natural consequence when the surgeon is trying not to hurt or to be kind to an already devastated patient. This "kindness" may result in inadequate removal of necrotic tissue and can require a second, more complex surgical procedure in an effort to reclaim a losing situation. One of the most perplexing situations that the reconstructive surgeon can encounter is to have removed radiation-damaged tissue and transposed a musculocutaneous flap, only to watch the radiated tissues around the periphery

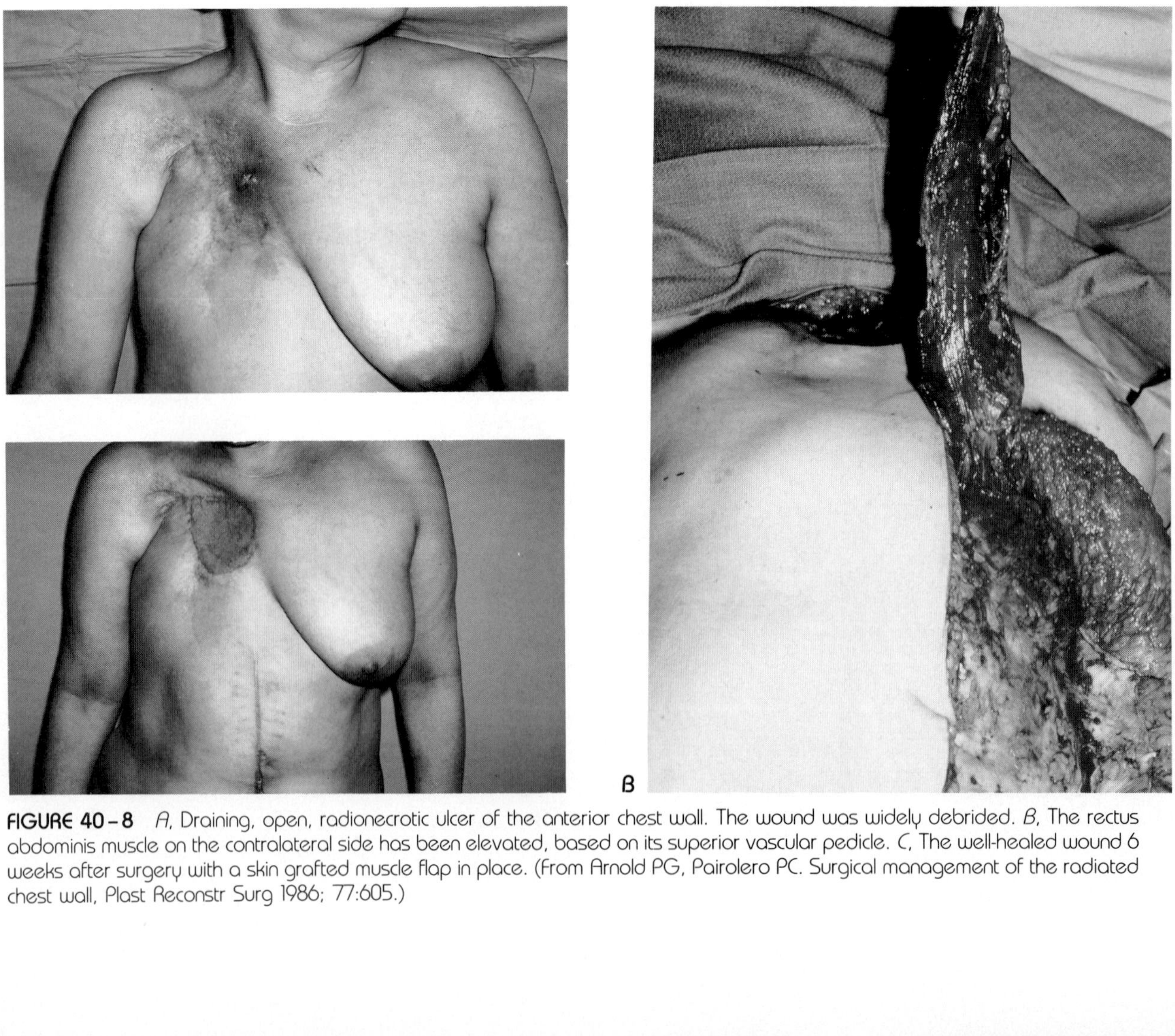

FIGURE 40-8 *A*, Draining, open, radionecrotic ulcer of the anterior chest wall. The wound was widely debrided. *B*, The rectus abdominis muscle on the contralateral side has been elevated, based on its superior vascular pedicle. *C*, The well-healed wound 6 weeks after surgery with a skin grafted muscle flap in place. (From Arnold PG, Pairolero PC. Surgical management of the radiated chest wall, Plast Reconstr Surg 1986; 77:605.)

slowly die, resulting in a viable musculocutaneous flap in a sea of necrotic radiated tissue. We have found the greater omentum a very dependable alternative and, in fact, a first-line reconstructive option in many of these patients.

Although the complications that follow radiation-related wounds of the chest wall are impressive in appearance and truly life-threatening, many patients can be helped by careful preoperative assessment, thoughtful resections, and planned reconstructions. One must consider the magnitude of risk that may be involved in any attempt to close these wounds. In some patients, routine conservative management may be the wisest choice. If pain is not a dominant feature and if the patient's life style is not severely affected, moist dressings may be the only treatment required. Topical antibiotics may also be helpful.

There is no doubt that the reconstructive surgeon will continue to manage these radiation-induced wounds. Four points introduced by Jack C. Fisher provide advice for all surgeons attempting to prevent these catastrophic events.

1. "We should discourage the use of ionizing radiation for benign disease."
2. "More radiation wounds should be anticipated early in the course of treatment. If the skin is thin or prior surgery has interrupted blood supply to an area, it would be helpful for the plastic and reconstructive surgeon to intercept the problem early and offer reconstructive skills before the patient becomes miserably acute with a serious, life-threatening problem."
3. "Continued participation on tumor boards offers reconstructive surgeons the best opportunity to stimulate consideration of long-term as well as short-term sequelae in the treatment choices for malignancy, i.e., surgical, radiologic, and chemotherapeutic. Our input is important."
4. "We as physicians should all demand from our clinical investigators and journal editors that reports of the outcome after cancer treatment include valid expressions of all late after effects. It is not appropriate to simply report traditional declarations of survival time. Life quality should also be mentioned."[74]

References

1. Crile GC. The incidence of local recurrences of carcinoma of the breast. Surg Gynecol Obstet 1983; 156:497.
2. Fisher B, Bauer M, Margolese R, et al. Five-year results of a randomized clinical trial comparing total mastectomy and segmental mastectomy, with and without radiation, in the treatment of breast cancer. N Engl J Med 1985; 312:665.
3. Veronesi U, Saccozzi R, Del Vecchio M, et al. Comparing radical mastectomy with quadrantectomy, axillary dissection, and radiotherapy in patients with small cancers of the breast. N Engl J Med 1981; 305:6.
4. Fletcher GH, Montague E, Nelson AJ. Combination of conservative surgery and irradiation for cancer of the breast. Am J Roentgenol Rad Ther Nucl Med 1976; 126:216.
5. Alpert S, Ghossein NA, Stacey P, et al. Primary management of operable breast cancer by minimal surgery and radiotherapy. Cancer 1978; 42:2054.
6. Harris JR, Beadle JF, Hellman S. Clinical studies on the use of radiation therapy as primary treatment of early breast cancer. Cancer 1984; 53:705.
7. Fletcher GH, Montague ED, Taple N, Barker JL. Breast. In: Fletcher GH, ed. Textbook of radiotherapy, 3rd ed. Philadelphia: Lea & Febiger, 1980:527–583.
8. Keynes G. The treatment of primary carcinoma of the breast with radium. Acta Radiol 1929; 10:393.
9. Keynes G. Conservative treatment of cancer of the breast. Br Med J 1937; 2:643.
10. McWhirter RV. The value of simple mastectomy and radiotherapy in the treatment of cancer of the breast. Br J Radiol 1948; 21:599.
11. McWhirter RV. Simple mastectomy and radiotherapy in the treatment of breast cancer. Br J Radiol 1955; 28:128.
12. Baclesse F. Roentgen therapy as the sole method of treatment of cancer of the breast. Am J Roentgenol 1949; 62:311.
13. Johns HE, Cunningham JR. Basic concepts. In: The physics of radiology, 4th ed. Springfield, IL: Charles C Thomas, 1983:3–36.
14. Rubin P, Casarett GW. Radiation histopathology. In: Clinical radiation pathology. Philadelphia: WB Saunders, 1968:38–61.
15. Robinson DW. Surgical problems in the excision and repair of radiated tissue. Plast Reconstr Surg 1975; 55:1, 41.
16. Friedman N. The effects of irradiation on breast cancer. The Breast. CA 1988; 38:368.
17. Teloh HA, Mason ML, Wheelock MD. Histopathologic study of radiation injuries of the skin. Surg Gynecol Obstet 1949; 88:609.
18. Wells FR. The lymphatic vessels in radiodermatitis—a clinical and experimental study. Br J Plast Surg 1969; 16:243.
19. Marchetta FC, Sako K, Holyoke ED. Treatment of osteoradionecrosis by intraoral excision of the mandible. Surg Gynecol Obstet 1967; 125:1003.
20. Spitalier J. Brandone H, Ayme Y, et al. Cesium therapy of breast cancer—a five year report on 400 patients. Int J Radiat Oncol Biol Phys 1977; 2:231.
21. Prosnitz LR, Goldenberg IF. Radiation therapy as a primary treatment for early stage carcinoma of the breast. Cancer 1975; 35:1587.
22. Wanebo CK, Johnson KG, Sato K. Breast cancer after exposure to atomic bombings of Hiroshima and Nagasaki. N Engl J Med 1968; 279:667.
23. Land CE. Low dose radiation—a cause of breast cancer? Cancer 1980; 46:868.
24. Lamobec J, Sus-Krasovec M. Malignant phyllodes tumor following radiation of the breast. J Pathol Res Pract 1985; 180:727.
25. Cipher AE. Radiation-induced injuries of the chest wall. Surg Gynecol Obstet 1988; 167:129.
26. Squire R, Bianchi A, Jakate SM. Radiation-induced sar-

coma of the breast in a female adolescent. Cancer 1988; 60:2444.
27. Shedbalker AR, Devata A, Padanilam T. A study of effects of radiation on silicone prostheses. Plast Reconstr Surg 1980; 65:805.
28. McGinley PH, Powell WR, Bostwick J. Dosimetry of silicone breast prostheses. Radiology 1980; 135:223.
29. Krishnan L, St. George FJ, Mansfield CM, Krishnan EC. Effects of silicone gel breast prostheses on electron and photon dose distributions. Med Phys 1983; 10:96.
30. Bostwick J, Stevenson TR, Nahai F, et al. Radiation to the breast—complications amenable to surgical treatment. Ann Surg 1984; 200:543.
31. Nash AG, Taylor PR. Breast reconstruction after failed conservation. Ann R Coll Surg Engl 1985; 67:303.
32. Bostwick J, Paletta C, Hartrampf CR. Conservative treatment for breast cancer—complications requiring reconstructive surgery. Ann Surg 1986; 203:481.
33. Holdsworth WG. A method of reconstructing the breast. Br J Plast Surg 1956; 9:161.
34. DelaPlaza R. Post-mastectomy reconstruction by a contralateral abdominal mammary flap. Ann Plast Surg 1981; 6:2.
35. Harris HI. Automammoplasty. J Int Coll Surg 1949; 12:827.
36. Millard DR. Breast reconstruction after radical mastectomy. Plast Reconstr Surg 1976; 58:283.
37. Marshall DR, Danstee EJ, Marshall DR, et al. Post-mastectomy breast reconstruction using a breast-sharing technique. Br J Plast Surg 1981; 34:426.
38. Millard DR. Reconstructive mammoplasty using an economical flap from the opposite breast. Ann Plast Surg 1981; 6:374.
39. Snyderman RK, Guthrie RA. Reconstruction of the female breast following radical mastectomy. Plast Reconstr Surg 1971; 47:565.
40. Lewis JR. Use of a sliding flap from the abdomen to provide cover in breast reconstruction. Plast Reconstr Surg 1979; 64:491.
41. Woods JE, Arnold PG, Masson JK, et al. Management of radiation necrosis and advanced cancer of the chest wall in patients with breast malignancy. Plast Reconstr Surg 1979; 63:235.
42. Cronin TD, Gerow FJ. Augmentation mammoplasty: A new natural feel prosthesis. Transactions of Third International Congress of Plastic & Reconstructive Surgery. Amsterdam: Excerpta Medica, 1963.
43. Radovan C. Breast reconstruction after mastectomy using a temporary expander. Plast Reconstr Surg 1982; 69:195.
44. Stabile RJ, Santoro E, Dispaltro F, Sanfilippo LJ. Reconstructive breast surgery following mastectomy and adjunctive radiation therapy. Cancer 1980; 45:2738.
45. Hartrampf CR, Scheflan MS, Black PW. Breast reconstruction with a transverse abdominal island flap. Plast Reconstr Surg 1982; 69:216.
46. Scheflan M, Dinner MI. The transverse abdominal island flap: Part I. Indications, contraindications, results, and complications. Ann Plast Surg 1983; 10:24.
47. Millard DR. Variations in the design of the latissimus dorsi flap in breast reconstruction. Ann Plast Surg 1981; 7:269.
48. Ruetschi MS, LeWinn LR, Chaglassian TA. Variation of latissimus dorsi skin island design for post-mastectomy reconstruction. Ann Plast Surg 1981; 6:171.
49. Paré A. Ten books of surgery. Translated by Linkler RW, Womack N. Atlanta: University of Georgia Press, 1969.
50. Brown JB, Fryer MP, McDowell F. Application of permanent pedicle blood carrying flaps. Plast Reconstr Surg 1951; 8:335.
51. Kiricuta I. L'Emploi du grand epiploon dans la chirurgie du sein cancereux. Presse Med 1963; 71:15.
52. Kiricuta I. The use of omentum in plastic surgery. Elmsford, NY: Pergamon Press, 1980.
53. Arnold PG, Pairolero PC. Chest wall reconstruction: Experience with 100 consecutive patients. Ann Surg 1984; 199:725.
54. Larson DL, McMurtrey MJ, Howe HJ, et al. Major chest wall reconstruction after chest wall irradiation. Cancer 1982; 49:1286.
55. Larson DL, McMurtrey MJ. Musculocutaneous flap reconstruction in chest wall defects and experience with 50 patients. Plast Reconstr Surg 1984; 73:734.
56. Latham WD. Operative treatment for post-radiation defects of the chest wall. Report of six cases. Am Surg 1966; 32:700.
57. Pairolero PC, Arnold PG. Thoracic wall defects: Surgical management of 205 consecutive patients. Mayo Clin Proc 1986; 61:557.
58. Seyfer AE. Radiation associated lesions of the chest wall. Surg Gynecol Obstet 1988; 167:129.
59. Woods JE, Irons GB, Masson JK. Use of muscular, musculocutaneous and omental flaps to reconstruct difficult defects. Plast Reconstr Surg 1977; 59:191.
60. McCraw JB, Penix JO, Baker JW. Repair of major defects of the chest wall and spine with a latissimus dorsi myocutaneous flap. Plast Reconstr Surg 1978; 62:197.
61. Heinz GL, Lee G. Osteoradionecrosis of the chest wall. Management of post-resection defects using Marlex mesh in rotated latissimus dorsi myocutaneous flaps. Am Surg 1983; 49:608.
62. Arnold PG, Pairolero PC. Surgical management of the radiated chest wall. Plast Reconstr Surg 1986; 77:605.
63. McCraw JB, Arnold PG. McCraw & Arnold's atlas of muscle and musculocutaneous flaps. Norfolk, VA: Hampton Press, 1986.
64. Arnold PG, Witzke DJ, Irons GB, Woods JE. Use of omental transposition flaps in soft tissue reconstruction. Ann Plast Surg 1983; 11:508.
65. Arnold PG, Irons GB. The greater omentum: Extensions in transposition and free tissue transfer. Plast Reconstr Surg 1981; 67:169.
66. Alday ES, Goldsmith HS. Surgical technique for omental lengthening based on arterial anatomy. Surg Gynecol Obstet 1972; 135:103.
67. Maxwell JP, McGibbon BM, Hoopes JE. Vascular considerations in the use of latissimus dorsi myocutaneous flap after mastectomy with axillary dissection. Plast Reconstr Surg 1979; 64:771.
68. Fisher J, Bostwick J, Powell RW. Latissimus dorsi blood supply after thoracodorsal vessel division: The serratus collateral. Plast Reconstr Surg 1983; 72:502.
69. Meland NB, Ivy EJ, Woods JE. Coverage of chest wall and pelvic defects with the external oblique musculofasciocutaneous flap. Ann Plast Surg 1988; 21:297.
70. Hodgkinson DJ, Arnold PG. Chest wall reconstruction using the external oblique muscle. Br J Plast Surg 1980; 33:216.
71. Meland NB, Fisher J, Irons GB, et al. Experience with

80 rectus abdominis free tissue transfers. Plast Reconstr Surg 1989; 83:481.
72. Maruyama Y, Onishi K, Iwahira Y. Reconstructing chest walls with vertical abdominal fasciocutaneous flaps. Scand J Plast Reconstr Surg 1986; 20:79.
73. Reed WP, Spence RJ. Vertical rectus abdominis musculocutaneous flap for breast reconstruction after radiation. South Med J 1987; 80:287.
74. Fisher JC. Complications in radiation therapy. In: Georgiade NG, Georgiade GS, Riefkohl R, Barwick WJ, eds. Essentials of plastic maxillofacial and reconstructive surgery. Baltimore: Williams & Wilkins, 1987.

CHAPTER 41

Burns and Trauma of the Breast

R. MICHAEL McCLELLAN, M.D.
FRANCIS X. DELONE, JR., M.D.

Probably one of the earliest depictions of the human figure in art form was during the Paleolithic period. The *Nude Woman* from the La Magdeleine Cave is a rock carving of Penne (Torn), France, c. 15,000 to 10,000 B.C. The *Venus of Willendorf* in Austria, c. 15,000 to 10,000 B.C., is a 4¾-inch stone female figurine with a round belly and large pendulous breasts signifying sexuality, fertility, and fecundity. *Mycerinus and His Queen* from the third pyramid at Giza, c. 2500 B.C., provides Egyptian emphasis on female beauty in the soft, swelling form of the queen through a thin and close-fitting gown. This true beauty in form is universally acknowledged and any alteration or disfigurement is tragic.

> *As objectively as we can imagine, breasts are the most visible sign, the most universal symbol, and one of the most important embodiments of being a woman—a member of that half of humanity with the capacity to feed a baby directly and completely from her own body.*
>
> *Today we are coming to see that our own conventional separation of the human organism into mind and body, though analytically convenient, is inevitably artificial and ultimately limiting in concept. We can now better accept and appreciate the natural presumption each of us has about themselves. That is, the maintenance of our bodies as close to their natural state as possible for our mental and spiritual, as well as physical health.*
>
> *The healthy human being is indeed a thing of beauty. To borrow from Plato, beauty is the combination of three essential elements: wholeness, unity and radiance. A thing of beauty has a wholeness—uniqueness, boundaries, and an identity of its own that separates it from its background. It has a unity—internal consistency, harmony, and integrity that make us feel it belongs together as it is. And it has radiance—a quality of inspiration, life, light, and emission of energy that creates pleasure in the mind and emotions.*
>
> *A woman's breasts are a part of her natural beauty—her naturally integrated, radiant individuality. If her body's integrity has been compromised, by disease, accident or other cause, she has the right to seek whatever remedy she chooses to restore to her her sense of wholeness, unity and radiance—her sense of beauty—without anyone questioning her motives or mentality.*[2]

The breast may be injured in many ways, but ranks low in organs injured in terms of overall incidence.[3] Burns, then, become one of the most common traumas of the breast, excluding surgical procedures. Approximately 61,000 burn injuries require hospital admission yearly.[4] The commonly considered high-risk groups remain the same for breast burns as for other anatomic areas, and these often include the young, elderly, and handicapped. Males are at higher risk than females for breast and chest burns due to occupational hazards and certain types of work, but they infrequently require later reconstruction. The upper anterior chest is an area at relatively high risk, just as are the face and hands, for thermal injury of many causes. In children suffering from hot liquid spills, clothing ignition burns, or caustic injuries, the anterior chest is often involved to some degree.

A burn deep into the parenchymal substance is uncommon, but a circumferential burn of the breast may result in a cicatrix that prevents normal growth and breast projection.

Any meaningful discussion of breast reconstruction must begin with a firm grasp of the female development and the anatomic changes that go along with that growth. This is especially appropriate for breast trauma and burns because the decision-making process changes, depending on the age and relative state of development of the injured patient.

At the sixth week of intrauterine life, the primordium of the mammary gland is first seen as the mammary (milk) line or ridge. This thickening of ectoderm extends from the axilla to the groin. Only a portion of this line is identifiable at the eighth week. At the site of future mammary gland development, the epithelial cells grow down, penetrate, and later proliferate in the subcutaneous mesenchyme. By the end of prenatal life, the epithelial sprouts are cannulized, forming lactiferous ducts. At the approach of puberty, the gland changes in females. The breast enlarges owing to an increase in glandular tissue, particularly the ducts, and to a deposit of adipose tissue.[5,6]

The extent to which the glands proliferate and the amount of fat deposition determine ultimate breast size, which is generally complete at age 16 years. It would be considered normal, however, to complete breast development as early as age 14 or as late as age 18 years.[7] It should be remembered that a patient requires frequent assessment over the years of thelarche.

RECONSTRUCTION

In a discussion of injury to the breast and consequent reconstruction, it seems appropriate to divide individuals into three distinct groups: prepubescent, pubescent (adolescent), and adult. The first groups can be further subdivided, depending on the presence or absence of the nipple-areola complex.[8–10]

Prepubescent

Although most surgical breast trauma is a result of neoplasm ablation, some instances of breast trauma can occur in children as a result of lesions occurring early in life. Thus, trauma other than that from burns may lend itself to similar reconstructive methods. Young children before the onset of pubertal development may present with unilateral or bilateral breast tissue. When this enlargement occurs in the subareolar area with no other signs of sexual precocity, the entity is termed "juvenile breast hypertrophy." The areola and nipple are not pigmented at this phase of development. An injudicious biopsy of this condition, which tends to happen more often unilaterally, may severely damage the breast and result in partial or complete failure of its development. There may also be some degree of scar tethering of one of the breast quadrants.

Abscess formation is unusual in a child but most frequently occurs in the first 2 months of life, probably because the infant breast secretes transiently. Untreated abscesses or overzealous incision and drainage can traumatize the breast at this tender age, and may affect breast size and shape as a result of permanent parenchymal tissue loss or scar formation.

Thermal injury affects this age group much more commonly. Significant thermal injury to the anterior chest wall involving the nipple-areola complex in prepubescent females causes much anxiety for parents and surgeon.[8] It is important to remember that in the acute phase of burn treatment involving the prepubescent breast, an extremely conservative approach is necessary.[9] As stated earlier, the breast bud is deep in the subcutaneous tissue, and it requires a very deep burn to injure this tissue. Loss of the nipple-areola complex often does *not* mean loss of underlying breast bud. Even in third-degree burns, the nipple is often regenerated from the proliferating epithelium of the milk ducts. Therefore, late, rather than early, tangential excision is essential to protect and preserve the breast tissue.

Nipple-Areola Complex Absent

In the prepubescent acute burn, early aggressive debridement in the area of the nipple-areola complex must be avoided; this is particularly true when the complex is not apparent. It is best to allow the eschar to demarcate over the breast bud area in females. Treatment by blunt eschar separation and split-thickness skin grafting is then mandatory.[9] The technique of early aggressive tangential excision can lead to difficulties in this anatomic area. Tangential or sequential excision down to a viable bed and split-thickness skin grafting, if done, should be performed late in the course of therapy for an acute burn rather than early. The local anatomy of the nipple-areola complex area should be avoided at all costs if late tangential excision is chosen during the grafting phase.

Some authors advocate nonoperative treatment of prepubescent burns as long as there is not a large defect.[10] They note that the most common injury is a scald burn caused by a child pulling hot water from the stove onto her head and chest, which usually produces superficial and deep partial-thickness injuries. These authors are content to allow healing by wound edge contracture supported by relatively high elasticity of the soft tissue. Only functionally necessary scar releases are performed until puberty and the eventual start of breast development. At that time, total excision of the tethering scars and grafts is performed. However, as previously stated,[9] if conservative separation or excision of eschar and grafting is performed late in the acute burn, subsequent scar excision can be avoided. This may be more aesthetically pleasing early in the child's development.

If larger burn wounds are allowed to heal on their own, later complete excision of the mature scar at puberty is the treatment of choice, because single releases and split-thickness skin grafting do not release the entire breast mound adequately.[9] Complete excision of hypertrophic scars as a release should also be performed at puberty, as it may provide a more symmetric breast release and a better cosmetic result.

Nipple-Areola Complex Present

If the complex is present (Fig. 41-1), early conservative release of contractures can be performed for better breast contour. This should be considered only when the complex is dramatically distorted. Care should be taken not to injure the breast bud beneath the complex. Conservative scar release or excision should be followed by split-thickness skin grafting. Again, this approach is not often indicated. Most scar releases in this age group are reserved for the axilla and other functional areas.[10] This is particularly true in patients who underwent grafting in the acute phase, because the nipple-areola complex will not be significantly distorted.

Pubescent

In this group the breast is starting to develop. For the sake of discussion, the adolescent or pubescent group will be defined as individuals aged 9 to 18 years.[11] Thelarche is defined as the onset and progress of breast development. The average age of onset of thelarche is 11 years, and the average duration approximately 4 years. It is important to correct contour deformities before reconstructing the nipple-areola complex.[9] This is accomplished by release and thick split-thickness skin grafts, local flaps, or myocutaneous flaps.[10,12-14] Correction of contour deformities assists breast development in the pubescent patient with intact breast buds. The breast skin expands and bulges in nonscarred areas if early release is not achieved (Fig. 41-2). The developing breast mound is entrapped in a scar envelope, release of which is indicated when the breast develops (Fig. 41-3).

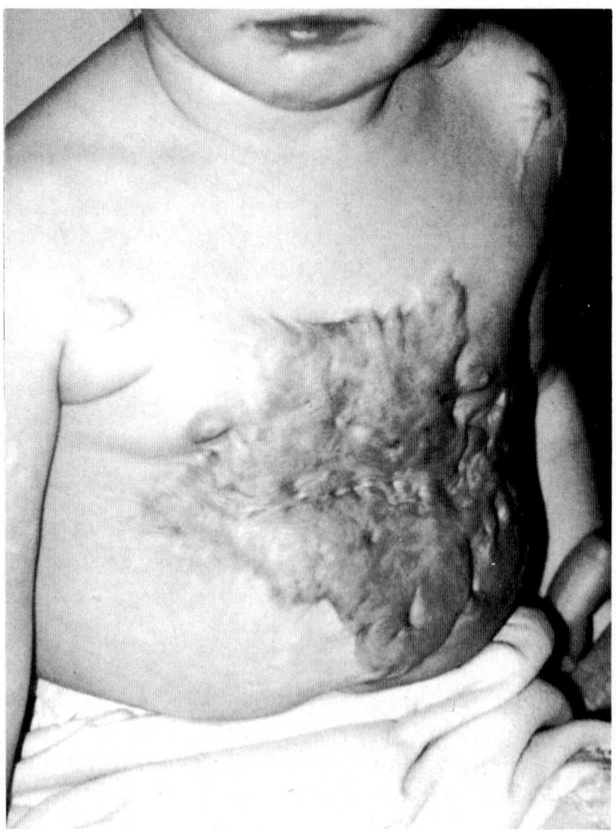

FIGURE 41-1 A prepubescent child with chest scarring secondary to burn. The nipple-areola complex is present.

Nipple-Areola Complex Absent

When the complex is destroyed in prepubescent patients, it is usually advisable to await puberty and the onset of breast development before attempting reconstruction. Otherwise, release of contractures may be at the wrong level, i.e., possibly through the breast bud. In this case, the inframammary fold matches the opposite nonburned breast, or is created at the inferior edge of the developing breast. Similarly, lateral contracture release can be accomplished if breast development is present. Release is performed at the edge of the bulging tissue, usually at the anterior edge of the latissimus dorsi muscle.

Nipple-Areola Complex Present

When the nipple-areola complex is present and is distorted, earlier release is possible because the normal landmarks are present. With the patient standing, the normal distance from the inferior edge of the areola to the inframammary fold is approximately 5 to 6 cm.[12] Surgical technique begins by measuring down this distance, or if possible equaling the opposite nonburned distance. The release may be made to gain maximal symmetry. In addition, if the complex is distorted, circumferential release of the areola can be performed at the same time. The goal is an adequate "one-time" release.[9] Inframam-

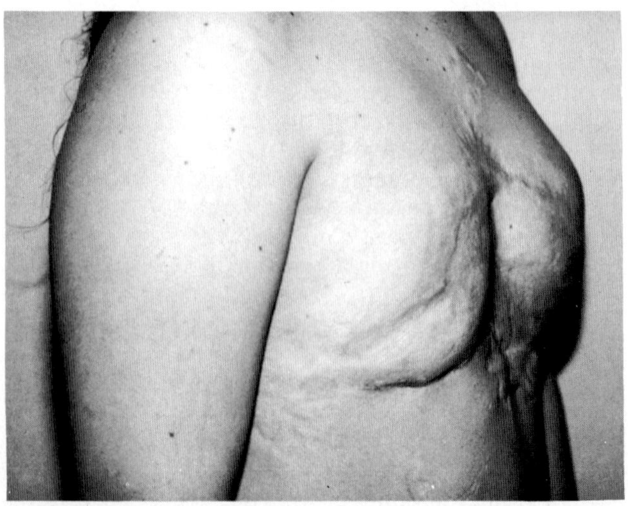

FIGURE 41-2 An adolescent in early thelarche demonstrating bulging of breast tissue above the inferior burn scar.

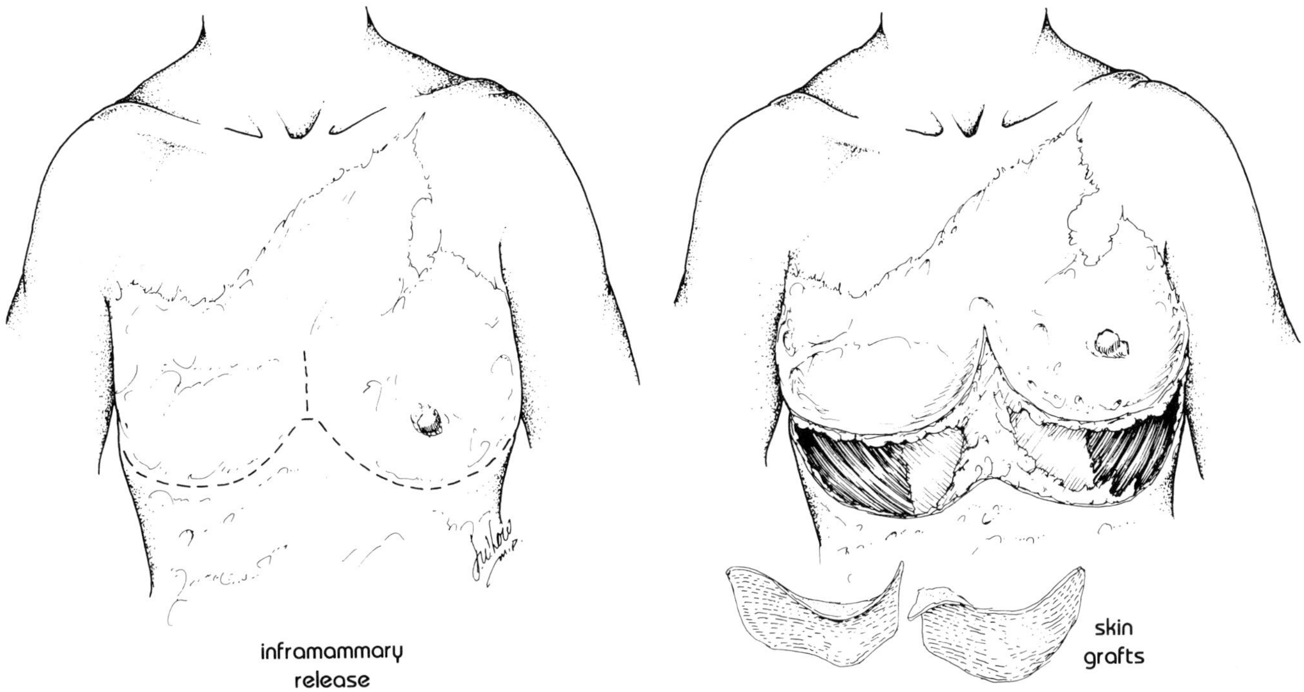

FIGURE 41–3 Release of the burn scar envelope is indicated when breast development begins. Incisions in the inframammary fold should extend to unscarred chest muscle. Thick split-thickness skin grafts are placed in the defect.

mary release is made down to the muscle fascia, with as little undermining of breast tissue as possible performed. However, the scar must be fully released to allow upward rotation or repositioning of the skin. The gap is then filled with a split-thickness skin graft (Fig. 41–4), local flaps, or a myocutaneous flap, depending on the amount of local tissue damage or adjacent burned skin. In cases of larger surface area burns with most of the breast previously grafted, graft releases may blend in with the surrounding tissue better than flaps. This is because the "normal" skin in the flap may provide a significant contrast, appearing as an island or normal skin surrounded by graft and scar tissue.

In some patients the release of medial or lateral contracture bands can be accomplished with local skin flaps (i.e., Z-plasties) rather than by release and skin grafting (Figs. 41–5, 41–6).[10] Incisions over the sternum should be avoided because hypertrophic scarring is common in this area. Planning should keep scars limited to the inframammary fold when possible. In preoperative marking and throughout surgery the arm is fully abducted to ensure adequate upward positioning of the breast. Postoperative shoulder abduction may be maintained with a shoulder spica or airplane splints as required.

When there is distraction of the breast laterally, an incision is made over the anterior edge of the latissimus dorsi muscle down to the fascia.[15] Dissection is then carried to the pectoralis major muscle (Fig. 41–7). Again, if the nipple-areola complex is present, this surgery can be performed early in puberty because the landmarks are intact. If the complex is not present, one should await breast development to know exactly where the release is to be made. Once the breast has developed, release is made at the edge of the bulging tissue (Fig. 41–8).

Postoperatively, after complete "take" of the grafts, patients are required to wear Uvex or silicone

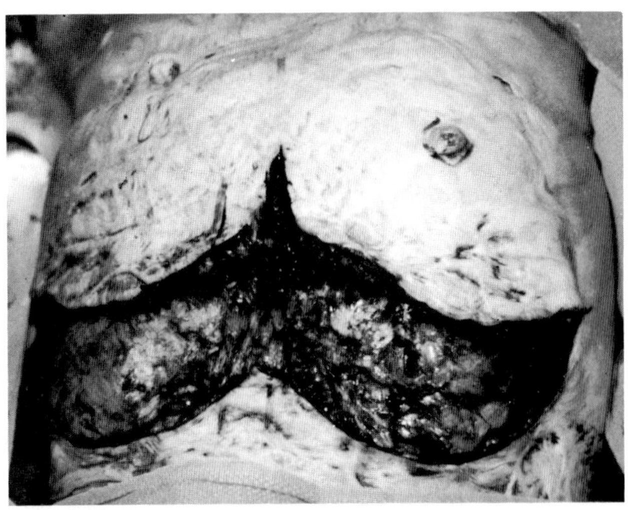

FIGURE 41–4 When the scar is released fully, upward rotation of the skin creates a large defect in the inframammary area. This is covered with a skin graft.

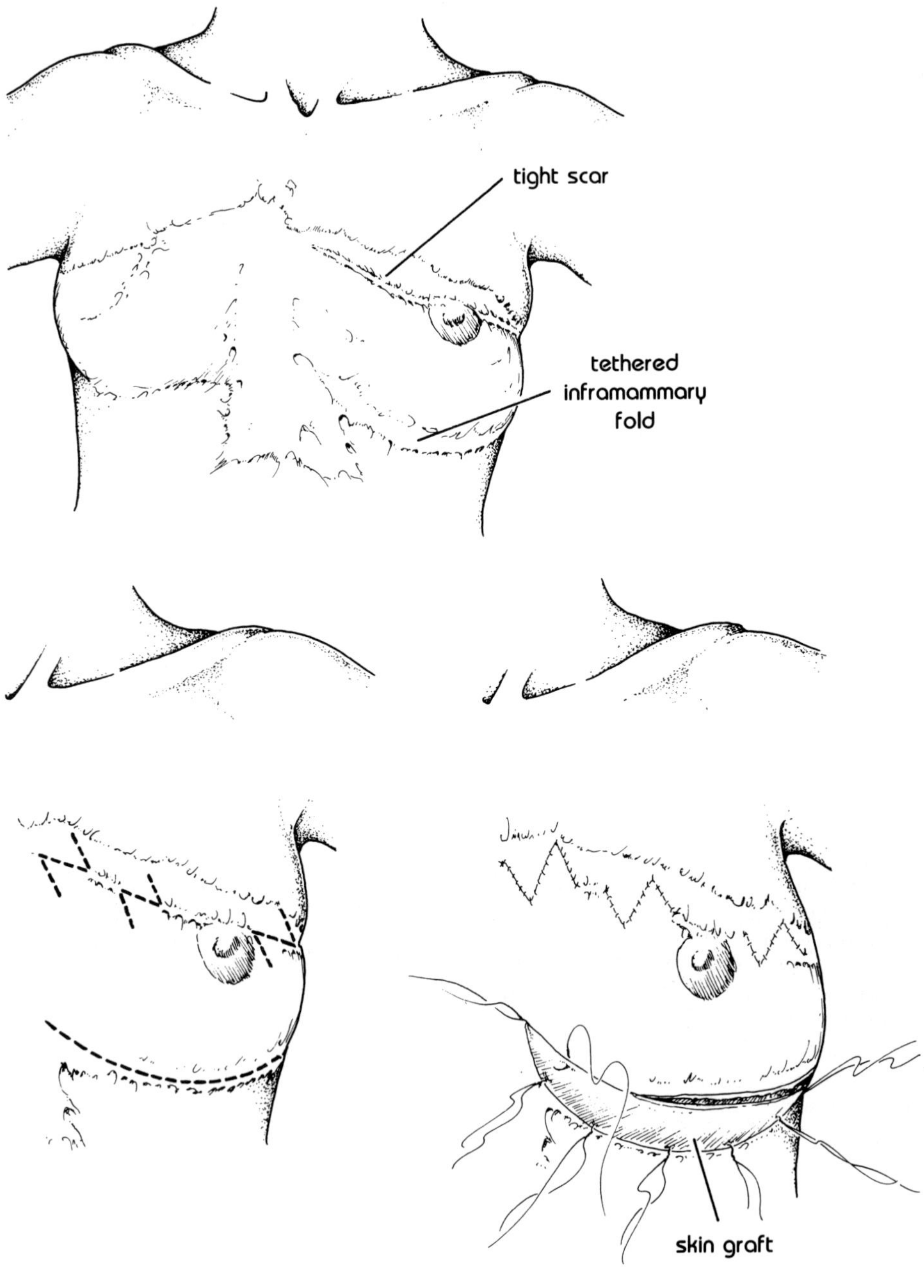

FIGURE 41-5 Medial or lateral contracture bands can be released with Z-plasties, planned to avoid incisions over the sternum. Local flap procedures in one area of the breast can be combined with inframammary release and skin graft.

conformers. Usually by 2 weeks after surgery the grafts can withstand standard pressure garments, and these should be continued until the scar is thought to have fully matured.[14,16] This often takes as long as 1 year or slightly longer. If flaps are used for the release, this is not necessary in many cases. The availability of unburned skin for latissimus dorsi, TRAM, or other free flap donor sites is often limited in these patients. The degree of bilateral involvement also dictates the choice of reconstructive procedure: for example, the unilateral breast burn lends itself uniquely to a TRAM flap.

Adults

If the breast bud is injured (e.g., in a fourth-degree burn) or excised as a result of early aggressive treatment in a prepubescent patient, the breast fails to develop. Several modes of reconstruction are available. If hypertrophic scarring is present, the scars may be excised and the area skin grafted. This is followed in several months to a year with the insertion of a tissue expander under the pectoralis major muscle (see Fig. 41-6).[17,18] The incision for the insertion is made at the intended inframammary

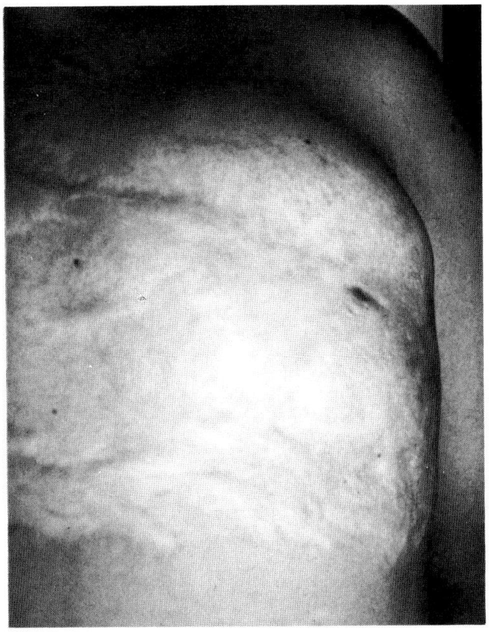

A

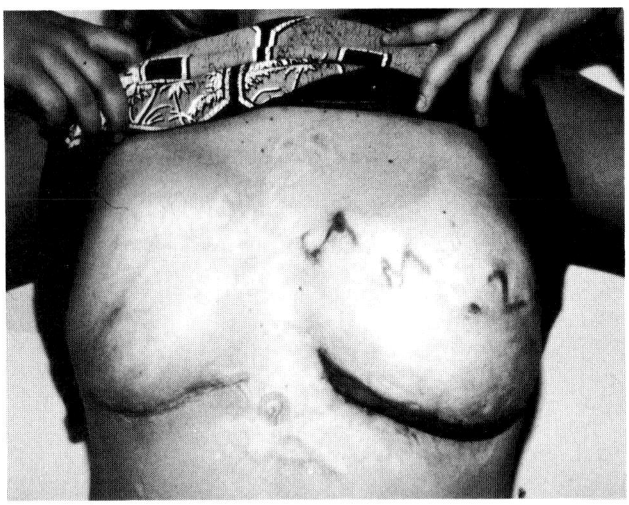

B

FIGURE 41-6 *A*, A burn during breast development produced a tethering effect of the scar across the upper one third of the breast. *B*, Six weeks after contracture release with multiple Z-plasties and inframammary release with skin graft. Tissue expander inserted in left breast via inframammary incision.

fold; this essentially creates the fold. If the patient is burned on only one side and is not fully developed on the normal side, the expansion may then keep pace with the opposite breast development (see Fig. 41-7).[19] When the breast is fully developed, the expander is removed and replaced with a permanent implant. Alternatively, a Becker expander-prosthesis may be used so that after full inflation only the injector port needs to be removed.[20]

The opposite nonburned breast may need to be reduced to match a reconstructed smaller breast. The patient with a ptotic or excessively large, nonburned opposite breast, and who prefers not to have surgery for that breast, will require a flap for sufficient soft tissue. This is also true for patients with extremely deep burns involving muscle.[21] The latissimus dorsi flap (especially the extended or fleur-de-lis pattern), with or without an implant, and particularly the TRAM flap can provide sufficient soft tissue to produce ptosis to match the opposite nonburned breast.[22-25] In cases of excessive size differences, a tissue expander may be placed under the muscle to stretch the flap for later implantation with a permanent larger prosthesis.[26] A gluteal free flap may also be of benefit in these patients.[27]

In the adult breast with normal development but caudal (downward) displacement, release is accomplished as described for the pubescent patient, depending again on the presence or absence of the nipple-areola complex. Release is made at the inframammary fold down to the fascia. Thick split-thickness skin grafts or local flap coverage are best.

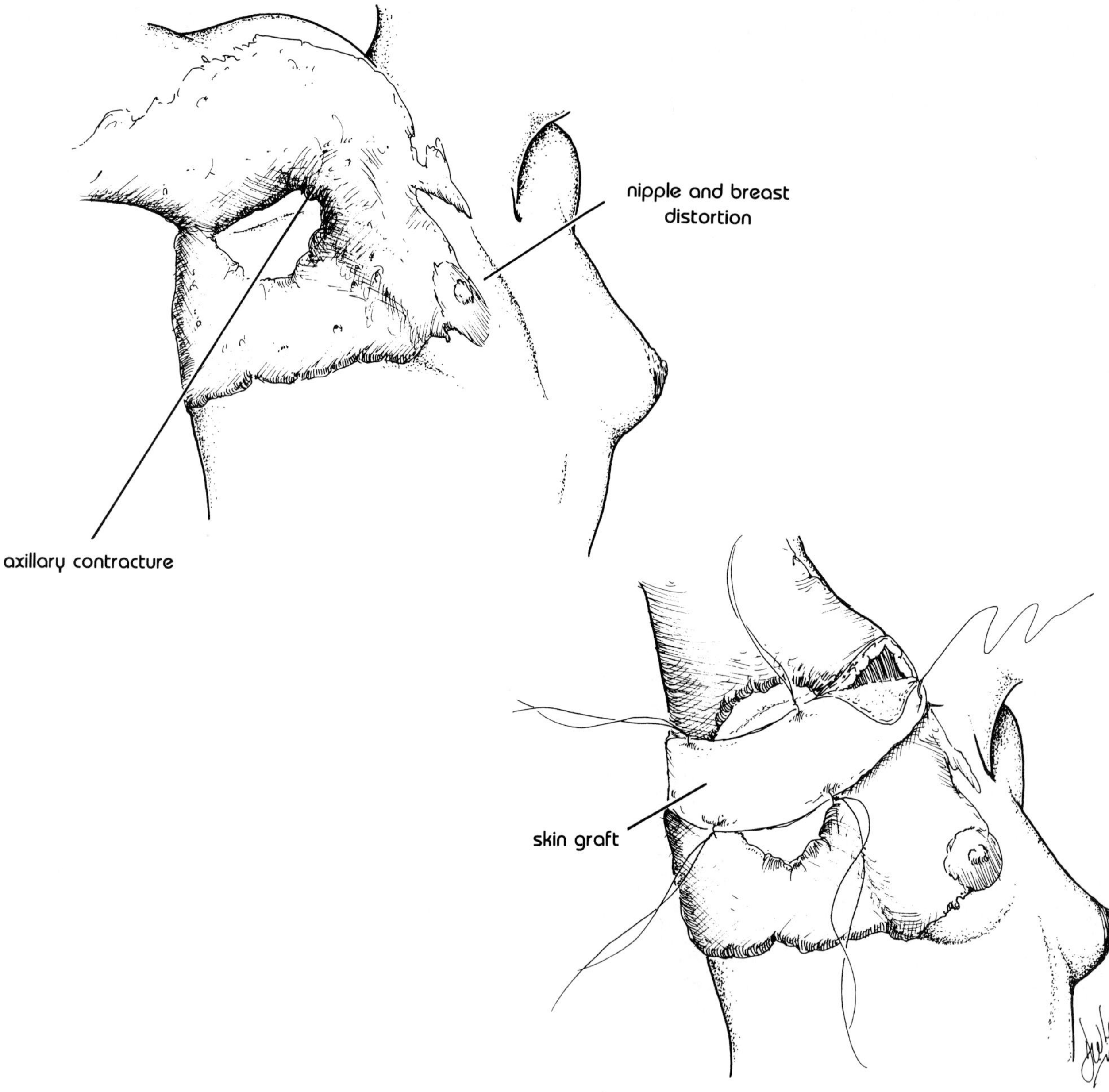

FIGURE 41-7 Axillary burn scar contracture can distort the breast laterally and toward the axilla. Release of the contracture extends to the latissimus dorsi and pectoralis major muscles. A thick split-thickness skin graft fills the defect.

Again, if scars are hypertrophic, scar excision is performed as a part of the release and skin grafting is then utilized. If band contractures are present, Z-plasty flaps are used. If split-thickness skin grafts are used, silicone or Uvex molds are employed, with appropriate accompanying pressure garments.[14,16]

For the extremely scarred, caudally displaced breast, at least one author has advocated excision of all inferior scar tissue and release of the nipple-areola complex circumferentially.[28] Using a superior pedicle advancement with a Wise pattern and grafting inferiorly, this completes reconstruction of the breast. This, of course, requires essentially normal skin superiorly, and also reduces the size of the reconstructed burned breast. Nonburned skin superiorly is a unique situation.

COMPLICATIONS

Complications after burn reconstruction of the breast are for the most part the same as those encountered in any breast reconstruction. These include infections (with or without prosthesis loss), skin graft loss, partial or complete flap loss, delayed wound healing, asymmetry, hypertrophic scars, and residual breast deformity. Uniquely in burn patients, another more subtle area of deformity may become

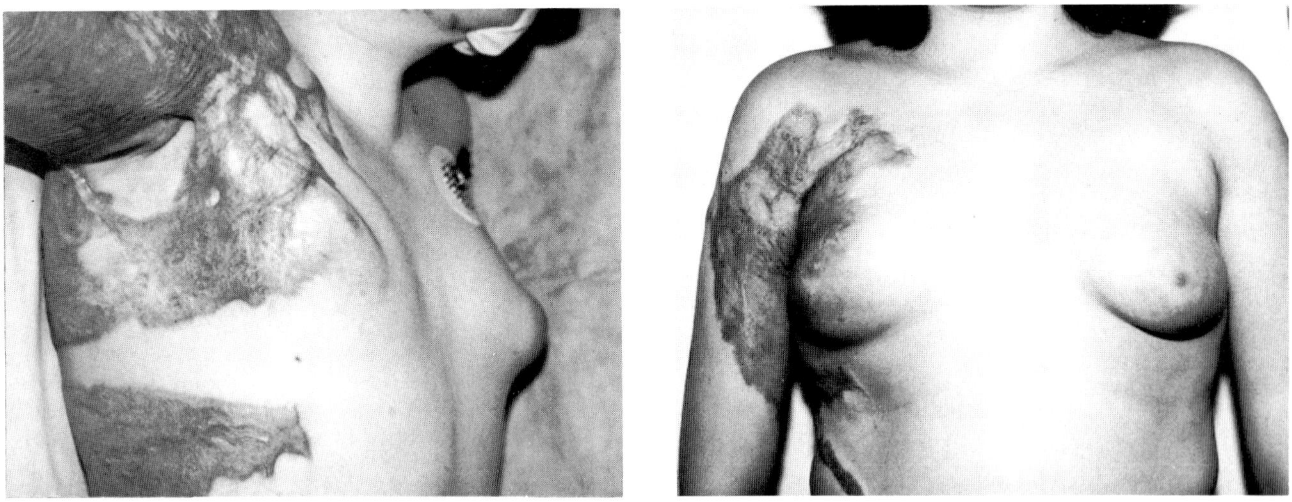

A B

FIGURE 41-8 *A*, Nipple and breast tissue distortion is seen from a burn scar contracture of the superior and lateral breast and axilla. *B*, After axillary release with skin graft, an improvement in symmetry of the nipple-areola complex is seen.

apparent when releasing a particular area of scar contracture.

TISSUE EXPANSION

Grafts or hypertrophic scars of moderate size can be obliterated by the use of tissue expanders placed in subcutaneous pockets under normal skin adjacent to the scar or graft. The normal skin is then expanded to adequate dimensions by weekly injections. A mandatory waiting period of 1 month without injections should then elapse before scar or graft excision is undertaken, to allow maximal skin growth and laxity. If surgery is attempted before this time, the skin may retract to its original size when the expanders are removed and tension is relaxed or released. After excision and tissue expander removal, the defect is closed with the newly stretched and expanded skin.

Complications of tissue expanders must be considered and may be slightly higher in this population owing to the placement through grafted skin. This may result in delayed primary healing. The authors' experience suggests another reason may be the direct compression that the nonyielding scar envelope exerts on the expander, which may result in an increase in port leakage with subsequent deflation or may prevent the completion of the expander inflation. The technique of gradual inflation of the tissue expander during thelarche progression may lead to clinically significant capsule formation, because of the protracted time that the expander needs to stay in place. This can be handled with closed or open capsulotomy, as indicated, allowing further expansion to ensue. This is a consideration in counseling a family about their child's breast reconstruction. In the future this may be less of a problem as textured expanders undergo more intensive clinical scrutiny.

NIPPLE-AREOLA RECONSTRUCTION

Nipple-areola reconstruction is best left until the breast is fully developed and all the reconstructions have matured.[9] Careful search must be made for the existing nipple; the patient may help in this endeavor. If the nipple is present, it should be used. This may require periareolar nipple release. A full-thickness skin graft for the areola to allow the nipple to protrude is a useful technique. If the nipple is small but the surrounding skin is intact, local dermal skin flaps such as the "S,"[29,30] "tab,"[31] "pinwheel,"[33] quadrapod,[34] or skate flaps[35] can be used because the blood supply is adequate. Local dermal flaps should be avoided when the nipple is absent or if split-thickness skin grafts have been used, because the blood supply will not be adequate to sustain such flaps. Consideration may be given to delaying the local flaps in some instances.

If the opposite breast is normal, nipple sharing can be employed, especially if the opposite nipple is protuberant. Other choices include ear lobes or toe pulp; toe pulp harvesting, however, may be painful.[36-38] The problems with nipple reconstruction include long-term settling of the nipple height, with ultimate flattening and loss of projection. It is better to overestimate the size of the nipple if local flaps are used.

Areola reconstruction is best achieved with areola sharing from the opposite nonburned breast or with full-thickness inner thigh grafts that are later tattooed.[39-43] Earlier use of labia minora skin grafts has resulted in hyperpigmented grafts;[44] the inner thigh skin grafts may become hypopigmented. Because it has full-thickness dermis, the full-thickness thigh graft will retain a tattoo pigment. It has been suggested that full-thickness skin graft may be tattooed on the undersurface before grafting, obviating the second-stage tattooing procedure.[45]

Failures or complications of this reconstructed phase parallel some of those previously mentioned. These include partial or complete loss of flaps or grafts, asymmetry, loss of nipple projection, and pigmentation variations.

CONCLUSIONS

In summary, several points must be emphasized. In early childhood a conservative approach to skin grafting and wound healing must be taken to preserve the breast bud. Any releases before puberty are for functional reasons only. At puberty, scar contractures of the breast may be released when the breast tissue starts to bulge. Nipple-areola reconstruction is best left until the breast is fully developed and all the reconstructions have matured.

> *For all our knowledge, we have not unraveled the mysteries of a woman's breast. We might just as well stop trying. If we did so, men might feel unburdened and grateful, and women might feel relieved and at last truly appreciated.*
>
> *In the final analysis, all we can really say in the case of any particular woman is that it is more than likely that her breasts are tightly bound to her most intimate sense of self, her womanhood and her personhood. Without prying further, it is our duty and pleasure to respect that bond and to assume the responsibility to help her maintain it as best we can.*[2]

Acknowledgement

The authors gratefully acknowledge the contribution to the introduction and summary by Randy C. Rolfe.

References

1. Hummer TR. Bluegrass wasteland. In: The 18,000-ton Olympic dream. New York: Quill/Morrow, 1990:62.
2. Rolfe RC. Personal correspondence.
3. Accident facts. Chicago: National Safety Council, 1989.
4. Frank HA, Berry C, Wachtel TL, et al. The impact of thermal injury. J Burn Care Rehabil 1987; 8:260.
5. Moore KL. The developing human—clinically oriented embryology. 4th ed. Philadelphia: WB Saunders, 1988:427.
6. Gray's Anatomy. 13th ed. Clemente CD ed. Philadelphia: Lea & Febiger, 1985:1582.
7. Marshall WA, Tanner JM. Variation in pattern of pubertal changes in girls. Arch Dis Child 1969; 44:291.
8. McCauley RL, Beraja V, Rutan L, et al. Longitudinal assessment of breast development in adolescent female patients with burns involving the nipple-areola complex. Plast Reconstr Surg 1989; 83:676.
9. Neale HW, Smith GL, Gregory RO, MacMillan BG. Breast reconstruction in the burned adolescent female (an 11-year 1157 patient experience). Plast Reconstr Surg 1982; 70:718.
10. Kunert P, Schneider W, Flory J. Principles and procedures in female breast reconstruction in the young child's burn injury. Aesthetic Plast Surg 1988; 12:101.
11. Souler M. Adolescent amenorrhea. Pediatr Clin North Am 1987; 34:4.
12. Bishop JP, Fisher J, Bostwick J. The burned female breast. Ann Plast Surg 1980; 41:25.
13. Inanove NP, Bolkovtinova LA. Surgical repair of mammary gland scar deformities caused by burn injuries. Acta Chir Plast 1988; 19:25.
14. Sunhuey CP. Correction of postburn contractures of the breast. Br J Plast Surg 1982; 70:718.
15. Salisbury RE, Brown AG. Atlas of reconstructive burn surgery. Philadelphia: WB Saunders, 1981:196.
16. Parks DH, Baur PS, Larson DL. Late problems in burns. Clin Plast Surg 1977; 4:547.
17. Argenta LC, Marks MW, Grabb WC. Selective use of serial expansion in breast reconstruction. Ann Plast Surg 1988; 11:185.
18. Argenta LC, Marks MW, Pasyk KA. Advances in tissue expansion. Clin Plast Surg 1988; 12:159.
19. Marks MW, Argenta LC, Thornton JW. Burn management: The role of tissue expansion. Clin Plast Surg 1987; 14:543.
20. Becker H. Breast reconstruction using an inflatable breast implant with detachable reservoir. Plast Reconstr Surg 1984; 73:678.
21. Hokin JA, Silfverskiold KL. Breast reconstruction without an implant: Results and complications using an extended latissimus dorsi flap. Plast Reconstr Surg 1987; 79:58.
22. Santi P, Berrino P, Calli A, et al. Anterior transposition of the latissimus dorsi muscle through minimal incisions. Scand J Plast Reconstr Surg 1986; 20:89.
23. McShane R, Omotunde O, Weatherly-White RCA. Individualized muscle coverage implants in breast reconstruction. Plast Reconstr Surg 1981; 67:318.
24. Millard DR. Breast aesthetics when reconstructing with the latissimus dorsi musculocutaneous flap. Plast Reconstr Surg 1982; 70:161.
25. Hartrampf CR, Scheflan M, Black PW. Breast reconstruction with a transverse abdominal island flap. Plast Reconstr Surg 1982; 69:216.
26. Thornton JW, Marks MW, Izenburg PH, Argenta LC. Expanded myocutaneous flaps: Their clinical use. Clin Plast Surg 1987; 14:529.
27. Shaw W. Breast reconstruction by superior gluteal microvascular free flaps without silicone implants. Plast Reconstr Surg 1983; 72:490.
28. Guan W-X, Jin Y-T, Cao H-P. Reconstruction of postburn female breast deformity. Ann Plast Surg 1988; 21:65.

29. Couin ED, Ureys DH, Ruis-Raguea A. Nipple reconstruction—the S flap. Plast Reconstr Surg 1988; 81:783.
30. Weiss J, Hern O, Rosenberg L, Shafir R. The S nipple-areolar reconstruction. Plast Reconstr Surg 1989; 83:904.
31. Kroll SS, Hamilton S. Nipple reconstruction with the double-opposing tab flap. Plast Reconstr Surg 1989; 84:520.
32. Little JW. Nipple-areolar reconstruction. Adv Plast Reconstr Surg 1987; 3:43.
33. Coler IK, Ward SA, Chandrasekhar B. The pinwheel flap nipple barrier areolar graft reconstruction. Plast Reconstr Surg 1986; 77:995.
34. Little JW III, Manasif T, McCulloch DT. One-stage reconstruction of a projecting nipple: The quadrapod flap. Plast Reconstr Surg 1983; 71:126.
35. Little JW, Spear S. Skate flap—nipple-areolar reconstruction. Perspect Plast Surg 1988; 2:1.
36. Dipirro E. Reconstruction of the nipple and areola after a burn. Plast Reconstr Surg 1970; 46:299.
37. Klatsky SA, Manson PN. Toe pulp free grafts in nipple reconstruction. Plast Reconstr Surg 1981; 68:245.
38. Wexler RM, O'Neal RM. Areola sharing to reconstruct the absent nipple. Plast Reconstr Surg 1973; 51:176.
39. Rees TD. Reconstruction of the breast areola by intradermal tattooing and transfer. Plast Reconstr Surg 1975; 55:620.
40. Becker H. The use of intradermal tattoo to enhance the final result of nipple-areolar reconstruction. Plast Reconstr Surg 1986; 77:673.
41. Spear SL, Convit R, Little JW III. Intradermal tattoo as an adjunct to nipple-areolar reconstruction. Plast Reconstr Surg 1988; 83:907.
42. Masser M, DiMeo L, Hobby JAE. Tattooing in reconstruction of the nipple and areola: A new method. Plast Reconstr Surg 1989; 84:677.
43. Becker H. Nipple-areolar reconstruction using intradermal tattoo. Plast Reconstr Surg 1988; 81:450.
44. Adams WM. Labia transplant for correction of loss of the nipple. Plast Reconstr Surg 1949; 4:295.
45. Areuer J. Tattooing the reconstructed areola without a tattoo machine (letters). Plast Reconstr Surg 1988; 81:995.

INDEX

Index

An "*f*" following a page number indicates a figure
A "*t*" following a page number indicates a table